ROUTLEDGE INTERNATIO
HANDBOOK OF WOMEN'S SEXUAL
AND REPRODUCTIVE HEALTH

The *Routledge International Handbook of Women's Sexual and Reproductive Health* is the authoritative reference work on important, leading-edge developments in the domains of women's sexual and reproductive health.

The handbook adopts a life-cycle approach to examine key milestones and events in women's sexual and reproductive health. Contributors drawn from a range of disciplines, including psychology, medicine, nursing and midwifery, sociology, public health, women's studies, and indigenous studies, explore issues through three main lenses:

- the biopsychosocial model
- feminist perspectives
- international, multidisciplinary perspectives that acknowledge the intersection of identities in women's lives.

The handbook presents an authoritative review of the field, with a focus on state-of-the-art work, encouraging future research and policy development in women's sexual and reproductive health. Finally, the handbook will inform health care providers about the latest research and clinical developments, including women's experiences of both normal and abnormal sexual and reproductive functions.

Drawing upon international expertise from leading academics and clinicians in the field, this is essential reading for scholars and students interested in women's reproductive health.

Jane M. Ussher is Professor of Women's Health Psychology at Western Sydney University, Australia. She is the author of 11 books, including *The Madness of Women: Myth and Experience* and *Managing the Monstrous Feminine: Regulating the Reproductive Body*. Jane is also editor of the Routledge *Women and Psychology* book series.

Joan C. Chrisler, PhD, is The Class of '43 Professor Emerita of Psychology at Connecticut College, USA. She is the founding editor of the journal *Women's Reproductive Health*, co-author of *Woman's Embodied Self: Feminist Perspectives on Identity and Image* and author of dozens of articles and chapters on women's embodiment and health.

Janette Perz is Professor of Health Psychology and Director of the Translational Health Research Institute (THRI) at Western Sydney University, Australia. She has undertaken a significant research program in sexual and reproductive health, including premenstrual syndrome, menopause, and concerns about fertility and sexuality after cancer.

The Routledge International Handbook Series

For more information about this series, please visit: www.routledge.com/Routledge-International-Handbooks-of-Education/book-series/HBKSOFED.

ROUTLEDGE INTERNATIONAL HANDBOOK OF WOMEN'S SEXUAL AND REPRODUCTIVE HEALTH

Edited by Jane M. Ussher, Joan C. Chrisler and Janette Perz

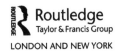

Routledge
Taylor & Francis Group

LONDON AND NEW YORK

First published 2020
by Routledge
4 Park Square, Milton Park, Abingdon, Oxon OX14 4RN

and by Routledge
605 Third Avenue, New York, NY 10017

First issued in paperback 2022

Routledge is an imprint of the Taylor & Francis Group, an informa business

Publisher's Note
The publisher has gone to great lengths to ensure the quality of this reprint but points out that some imperfections in the original copies may be apparent.

British Library Cataloguing-in-Publication Data
A catalogue record for this book is available from the British Library

Library of Congress Cataloging-in-Publication Data
A catalog record has been requested for this book

ISBN 13: 978-1-03-247524-0 (pbk)
ISBN 13: 978-1-138-49026-0 (hbk)
ISBN 13: 978-1-351-03562-0 (ebk)

DOI: 10.4324/9781351035620

Typeset in Bembo
by Swales & Willis, Exeter, Devon, UK

https://www.routledgehandbooks.com/

CONTENTS

Contents

AUTHOR BIOGRAPHIES

Verónica Alcalá-Herrera PhD is Professor of Psychology at the Universidad Nacional Autónoma de México, Mexico City, Mexico.

Jessica L. Barnack-Tavlaris PhD is an Associate Professor of Psychology at The College of New Jersey, Ewing, New Jersey, USA.

Deborah Bateson MBBS is Medical Director of Family Planning NSW, Clinical Associate Professor in the Discipline of Obstetrics, Gynaecology and Neonatology at the University of Sydney, and Adjunct Professor at the Centre for Social Research in Health at UNSW Sydney, Australia.

Linda Bauld PhD is Bruce and John Usher Professor of Public Health at The University of Edinburgh, UK.

Jessica R. Botfield MIPH is a Senior Research Officer at Family Planning NSW, Australia, and a casual Research Associate at the Centre for Social Research in Health, University of New South Wales, Sydney, Australia.

Kirsten I. Black PhD is Associate Professor in the Discipline of Obstetrics, Gynaecology and Neonatology at the University of Sydney, Australia.

Jan Burns PhD is a Professor of Clinical Psychology in the Salomons Institute of Applied Psychology, Canterbury Christ Church University, UK.

Hilary Burrage is Adjunct Professor, Northwestern University, Chicago, Illinois, USA, and a member of the Advisory Board of the Global Media Campaign to End FGM. She lives in London, UK.

Abigail Bray PhD is an independent social scientist and consultant based in London, UK.

Joanne Cacciatore PhD is an Associate Professor at Arizona State University, Tempe, Arizona, USA, and the founder of the MISS Foundation, an international NGO that aids grieving parents. Her daughter, Cheyenne, died during birth at term in 1994.

Maxime Charest is an MA candidate in Clinical and Counselling Psychology at the University of Toronto, Canada.

Joan C. Chrisler PhD is The Class of '43 Professor Emerita of Psychology at Connecticut College, New London, Connecticut, USA.

Courtney Cronley PhD, MSSW, is an Associate Professor in the College of Social Work at the University of Tennessee, Knoxville, Tennessee, USA.

Hannah H. Dahlen PhD is the Professor of Midwifery and Higher Degree Research Director at the School of Nursing and Midwifery, Western Sydney University, Australia.

Cristyn Davies is a senior research associate in the Discipline of Child and Adolescent Health, Faculty of Medicine and Health at the University of Sydney, and the Children's Hospital Westmead, Sydney, Australia.

Heather Dillaway PhD is Professor of Sociology, Director of the Bachelor of Science in Public Health Program, and Associate Dean of the College of Liberal Arts and Sciences, at Wayne State University in Detroit, Michigan, USA.

Elaine Denny PhD is Professor Emerita of Health Sociology at Birmingham City University, Birmingham, UK.

Pat Dudgeon PhD is from the Bardi people of the Kimberley in Western Australia, and is a Professor in the School of Indigenous Studies, University of Western Australia.

Tracey Feltham-King PhD is Senior Lecturer in Critical Studies in Sexualities and Reproduction and in the Psychology Department of Rhodes University, South Africa.

Jane R. W. Fisher PhD is Professor of Global and Women's Health in Public Health and Preventive Medicine at Monash University, Melbourne, Australia.

Heather Fritz PhD is an Assistant Professor at the Institute of Gerontology and in the Occupational Therapy Program in the Department of Healthcare Sciences, at Wayne State University in Detroit, Michigan, USA.

Jenifer A. Gorman MA is Senior Lecturer in Psychology at Connecticut College, New London, Connecticut, USA.

Karin Hammarberg PhD is Senior Research Fellow in Public Health and Preventive Medicine at Monash University, Melbourne, Australia.

Alexandra J. Hawkey PhD is Associate Research Fellow at the Translational Health Research Institute at Western Sydney University, Sydney, Australia.

Annemarie Hennessy is Distinguished Professor and Dean of the School of Medicine at Western Sydney University, Sydney, Australia.

Myra S. Hunter PhD is Professor Emerita of Clinical Health Psychology at the Institute of Psychiatry, Psychology, and Neuroscience at King's College London, UK.

Camille J. Interligi PsyD is a staff clinician at the University of Pittsburgh Counseling Center, Pittsburgh, Pennsylvania, USA.

Yasmin Jayasinghe PhD is a Gynaecologist and co-chair of the Fertility Preservation Taskforce at the Royal Children's Hospital Melbourne, and a Senior Lecturer in the Department of Obstetrics and Gynaecology, University of Melbourne, Australia.

Nancy J. Kenney PhD is Associate Professor of Psychology and Gender, Women's, and Sexuality Studies at the University of Washington, Seattle, Washington, USA.

Peggy J. Kleinplatz PhD is Professor in the Faculty of Medicine and Director of Sex and Couples Therapy Training at the University of Ottawa, Ontario, Canada.

Jill Wieber Lens JD is an Associate Professor of Law at the University of Arkansas, Fayetteville, Arkansas, USA. She is also the mother of a stillborn child, Caleb Marcus Lens.

Larissa Lewis BA is a Qualitative Researcher and Project Coordinator at The Kirby Institute, UNSW Sydney, Australia.

Catherine Lysack PhD is Professor of Occupational Therapy and Interim Dean of the Eugene Applebaum College of Pharmacy and Health Sciences, at Wayne State University, Detroit, Michigan, USA.

Catriona Ida Macleod PhD is SARChI Chair of Critical Studies in Sexualities and Reproduction and Distinguished Professor of Psychology at Rhodes University, South Africa.

Jeanne Marecek PhD is Senior Research Professor and William Kenan Professor of Psychology Emerita at Swarthmore College, Swarthmore, Pennsylvania, USA.

Jennifer Marino PhD is an epidemiologist and research fellow in the Department of Obstetrics and Gynaecology, Faculty of Medicine, Dentistry and Health Sciences at the University of Melbourne, Australia.

Maria Luisa Marván PhD is a Researcher at the Institute of Psychological Research at the Universidad Veracruzana, Xalapa, Mexico.

Brianna Marzolf is a medical student in the College of Osteopathic Medicine at Michigan State University in East Lansing, Michigan, USA.

Maureen C. McHugh PhD is a Distinguished University Professor in Psychology at Indiana University of Pennsylvania (IUP), Indiana, Pennsylvania, USA.

Ruth P. McNair PhD is a practicing general practitioner and Honorary Associate Professor at the Department of General Practice, University of Melbourne, Australia.

Sonia Milani BA is a Research Coordinator at the University of British Columbia Sexual Health Laboratory, Vancouver, Canada.

Shamsun Nahar MSW is a doctoral candidate in the School of Social Work at the University of Texas at Arlington, Texas, USA.

Felix Naughton PhD is Senior Lecturer in Health Psychology at the University of East Anglia, UK.

Paula Nicolson PhD is Emeritus Professor of Health and Social Care at Royal Holloway, University of London, and a Fellow of the British Psychological Society.

Kyja Noack-Lundberg PhD is a Researcher in the Translational Health Research Institute at Western Sydney University, Australia.

Caitlin Notley PhD is Senior Lecturer in Mental Health at the University of East Anglia, UK.

Miriam O'Connor MBBS MPH is an Australian Obstetrician and Gynaecologist working mainly in global reproductive health in low and middle income countries.

Chloe Parton PhD is an Adjunct Fellow at the Translational Health Research Institute at Western Sydney University, Sydney, Australia.

Michelle Peate PhD is the Program Leader of the Psychosocial Health and Wellbeing Research (emPoWeR) Unit, Department of Obstetrics and Gynaecology, University of Melbourne, Australia.

Janette Perz PhD is Director of the Translational Health Research Institute (THRI) and Professor of Psychology in the School of Medicine, Western Sydney University, Australia.

Niva Piran PhD is a clinical psychologist and Professor Emerita in Applied Psychology at the Ontario Institute for Studies in Education of the University of Toronto, Canada.

Jennifer Power PhD is a Senior Research Fellow at the Australian Research Centre in Sex, Health and Society, La Trobe University, Melbourne, Australia.

Jerilynn C. Prior MD is Professor of Endocrinology and Metabolism and Scientific Director of the Centre for Menstrual Cycle and Ovulation Research at the University of British Columbia, Vancouver, Canada.

Heather Rowe PhD is Senior Research Fellow at the School of Public Health and Preventive Medicine, Monash University, Melbourne, Australia.

Lianne A. Rosen PhD is a clinical and health psychologist in Ottawa, Ontario, Canada.

Virginia Schmied is Professor in the School of Nursing and Midwifery at Western Sydney University, Australia.

S. Rachel Skinner PhD is Professor in the Child and Adolescent Health Faculty of Medicine and Health, Sydney University, and a consulting Adolescent Physician at the Children's Hospital Westmead, Australia.

Sahar Sobhgol is a Registered Midwife at Westmead Hospital and PhD candidate at Western Sydney University, Australia.

Alyson K. Spurgas PhD is Assistant Professor of Sociology and Women's, Gender, & Sexuality Studies at Trinity College, Hartford, Connecticut, USA.

Lesley Stafford PhD is Head of Clinical Psychology in the Centre for Women's Mental Health, Royal Women's Hospital, and Associate Professor of Psychology at the University of Melbourne, Australia.

Margaret L. Stubbs PhD is Professor Emerita of Psychology at Chatham University, Pittsburgh, Pennsylvania, USA.

Wassim Tarraf PhD is an Assistant Professor at the Institute of Gerontology and in the Occupational Therapy Program in the Department of Healthcare Sciences, at Wayne State University in Detroit, Michigan, USA.

Cheryl B. Travis PhD is Professor Emerita of Psychology at the University of Tennessee, Knoxville, Tennessee, USA.

Jane M. Ussher PhD is Professor of Women's Health Psychology in the Translational Health Research Institute (THRI) and School of Medicine, Western Sydney University, Australia.

Michael Ussher PhD is Professor of Behavioural Medicine at St George's, University of London, UK, and at The University of Stirling, UK.

Olga B. A. van den Akker PhD is Professor of Health Psychology at Middlesex University, London, UK.

Julia Velten PhD is a Licenced Psychotherapist and a Research Associate at the Mental Health Research and Treatment Center, Ruhr University Bochum, Germany.

Sam Warner PhD is a consultant clinical psychologist and Honorary Lecturer, Salford University, UK.

Annalise Weckesser PhD is a Senior Research Fellow at the Centre for Social Care and Health-Related Research, Birmingham City University, Birmingham, UK.

Nancy Fugate Woods PhD, RN, FAAN, FGSA is Professor Emerita of Biobehavioral Nursing and Health Informatics and Dean Emerita of the School of Nursing at the University of Washington, Seattle, Washington, USA.

INTRODUCTION

Joan C. Chrisler, Jane M. Ussher and Janette Perz

Improved sexual and reproductive health is a key pillar of the overall health, empowerment, and human rights of individuals and of the sustainable and equitable development of societies. Ill-health from causes related to sexual and reproductive health, including too many, too early and too frequent pregnancies, remains a major cause of death and disability among women and girls, particularly among the most vulnerable, marginalized and underserved. Poor sexual and reproductive health contributes significantly to poverty, thereby limiting socio-economic development. Conversely, achieving sexual and reproductive health empowers individuals and communities to participate in economic development

World Health Organization, United Nations Fiftieth Commission on Population and Development, New York, USA, 3–7 April 2017

The United Nations (UN) and its partner agencies, including the World Health Organization (WHO), have long recognized the importance of health and health care to human rights and quality of life. Particular attention has often been paid to women's sexual and reproductive health, neglect of which has resulted in high rates of morbidity and mortality for women and girls around the world. For example, the UN Declaration of Human Rights (UN General Assembly, 1948) includes the right to a *standard of living adequate for health and well-being (with special assistance and care for mothers and children)*. The UN Convention on the Elimination of All Forms of Discrimination Against Women (CEDAW; UN, 1979) includes an explicit statement that reproductive rights are essential to gender equality and women's ability to participate fully in political, civil, economic, cultural, and social life. At the UN-sponsored International Conference on Population and Development in Cairo in 1994, representatives from almost 200 countries agreed that reproductive rights are human rights and that the governments of their countries would protect women's ability to make reproductive decisions and to control their fertility (Center for Reproductive Rights, 2009). The UN's Millennium Development Goals (MDGs), which were designed to eliminate poverty, disease, illiteracy, and environmental degradation by the year 2000, included specific goals to reduce maternal mortality and end discrimination against women (UN, 2015). The MDGs were replaced by the Sustainability Development Goals (SDGs), designed to promote economic, social, and environmental development, and focused primarily on eradicating poverty and recognizing women's health as essential to that goal (UN, 2015). The WHO statement above concisely illustrates the central importance of women's sexual and reproductive health for women and their families, as well as for policy makers, health providers, and researchers (WHO, 2017).

The United Nations International Conference on Population and Development Programme of Action states that "reproductive health … implies that people are able to have a satisfying and safe sex life and that they have the capability to reproduce and the freedom to decide if, when and how often to do so" (UNPF, 2019). Implicit in this condition are women's right to say no to sex, and to be informed about and to have access to safe, effective, affordable, and acceptable methods of family planning, as well as other methods of their choice for regulation of fertility that are not against the law, and the right of access to appropriate health care services that will enable women to go safely through pregnancy and childbirth and provide them with the best chance of having a healthy infant.

According to the World Health Organization, health, including sexual and reproductive health, is not simply the absence of disease. It is "a complete state of physical, mental, and social well-being" (WHO, 1948). Reproductive health includes the reproductive system and its processes and functions at all stages of life; it is a crucial part of general health and human development. It is key during adolescence and early adulthood, sets the stage for women's health beyond the reproductive years, and affects the health of the next generation, as the health of infants is largely a function of their mothers' health and access to reproductive health care. Sexual health includes the enhancement of quality of life and intimate relationships; it is not merely access to counselling and treatment of sexually transmitted infections or dysfunctions.

Sexuality and reproduction cannot be understood solely as biological phenomena; they are social, cultural, and political practices, with socially and culturally prescribed meanings and experiences (Braun, Gavey, & McPhillips, 2003; Ussher, 2006). A complex array of socioeconomic, cultural, political, personal, and interpersonal factors is implicated in women's sexual and reproductive health. Principal among these is the place of women in society. Women's rights and gender equality are particularly important for their ability to exercise control over their own bodies in terms of reproductive choices and lifestyles (e.g., to choose their own sexual partners, to obtain education, to work outside their homes, to have access to fertility control). But other issues also contribute to how women experience their reproductive and sexual health. These include systemic and structural issues, such as access to quality health services (WHO, 2014), privacy and confidentiality, and representations of girls and women in the media (American Psychological Association Task Force on the Sexualization of Girls, 2007). These issues also include risk factors, such as violence, abuse of drugs or alcohol, and powerlessness to control sexual and reproductive behaviour and decision making. Finally, women's health is influenced by psychosocial factors, such as beliefs and expectations associated with sexual and reproductive health, women's experiences of their bodies, and their self-confidence and self-esteem. The discursive meanings ascribed to sex and reproduction, which vary across history and culture, also influence women's experience and ability to have agency and control (Ussher, 2006).

Sexual and reproductive health issues overlap with many other research and programmatic areas, including education, health promotion, violence prevention, socialization of gender roles and sexuality, and mental health concerns. Thus, women's sexual and reproductive health and rights cannot be achieved without promotion of gender equality and equality of marginalized groups, such as culturally and linguistically diverse women, disabled women, and those who are lesbian, bisexual, queer, transgender, or intersex. Some groups of women have not benefited from the overall improvements in the area of sexual and reproductive health experienced by many socially advantaged women in higher-income countries. Social disadvantage greatly affects access to health services and sexual and reproductive health information and resources. For example, migrant and refugee women are less likely to access sexual and reproductive healthcare services (Botfield, Newman, & Zwi, 2016) and, consequently, are less likely to utilise reliable methods of contraception (Omland, Ruths, & Diaz, 2014), or participate in cervical cancer screening (Beckett, 2016). Despite UN resolutions and WHO policies and projects, there remains a significant need for targeted sexual and reproductive health education, health promotion, and prevention strategies, particularly for "at risk" or marginalized population groups.

Framework

The authors of this handbook have examined women's sexual and reproductive health across the lifespan through three main lenses: (1) feminist perspectives; (2) the biopsychosocial model; and (3) international, multicultural perspectives that acknowledge the intersection of identities in women's lives. These three lenses provide an essential framework for any consideration of women's sexual and reproductive health because, as discussed above, these matters rely so much on women's cultural, social, political, and environmental context.

Feminist perspectives

This book was conceived, and the authors instructed to write, from a feminist perspective. There are many forms of feminism, including mid-20th-century Western philosophical approaches (e.g., radical, liberal, Marxist) and more recent, more diverse approaches (e.g., intersectional, transnational, standpoint, womanist, indigenous) (see Nelson, 2015; Rutherford, 2011). Our authors were not restricted in the perspectives they could choose. The most important point, which is reflected in most chapters, is a wholistic and intersectional focus on women in the context of their lives. Our authors place women in the centre, rather than on the margins, of the discussion. A focus on how women experience their sexual and reproduction health or illness, how and why they make the decisions they do, what they need (as opposed to what physicians or public health officials think is best), constitutes a feminist approach (Spain & Spain, 2016). As the UN and WHO documents have noted for decades, gender equality and empowerment of women are essential to women's health and well-being and that of their families. In cultures where women's oppression is greater, and sexual and reproductive rights are minimal, women's health is worse. In low-income countries and families, where resources are scarce and what is available is directed mainly to men and boys, women's and girls' health suffers.

Consciousness-raising was a main focus of the second wave of feminism, also known as the Women's Liberation Movement. Women gathered in small groups to speak truths to each other about their lives (Engdahl, 2012). In doing so, they realized the ways in which their experiences were similar, which gave rise to the slogan "the personal is political." For example, they learned that violence against women is so common that individual women could no longer be blamed for their victimization (Gavey, 2005). In many chapters in this book, the political and sociocultural context of women's lives is illuminated to show its effects on the "personal" matter of women's sexual and reproductive health. If women are unable to make their own decisions about whether and when to become pregnant or which contraceptives to utilize to avoid pregnancy, their health may suffer as they give birth to children too closely spaced (Hawkey, Ussher, & Perz, 2018). If women are sexually assaulted, they are unable to protect themselves from sexually transmitted infections or unwanted conception (Gavey, 2005). If physicians and clinics have reputations as transphobic or unwelcoming of lesbian, bisexual, or queer women and girls, then people who need their services will delay seeking treatment or avoid it altogether, with potentially serious consequences to their physical and mental health (McNair, Szalacha, & Hughes, 2011).

Sometimes simply moving women's experiences from the margin to the center, or "flipping the script," can raise consciousness in ways that promote health and well-being. Gloria Steinem's (1978) classic essay "If Men Could Menstruate" is an example. As Steinem pondered the stigma attached to menstruation, it occurred to her that the stigma would disappear if men were the ones who menstruated. She imagined, for example, that menstrual management supplies would be funded by governments and free to all who need them. Furthermore, a heavy flow would be seen as a badge of honour and coping with cramps a sign of courage. In a similar, but more serious vein, some of our authors ask readers to re-consider "common knowledge" about women's sexual and reproductive health. Is menopause a "condition" that requires medical monitoring, or is it a normal developmental transition (like puberty)? Is adolescent pregnancy a public health emergency, or is it easier on women's bodies to give birth at younger ages? Is premenstrual distress a sign of hormonal dysfunction, or is it an understandable response to the conditions of women's lives? Reading this book with an open mind may suggest many more such questions.

The biopsychosocial model

A feminist perspective does not negate biology, or, indeed, biomedical aspects of women's sexual and reproductive health (Dan, 1993). However, the biopsychosocial model (Engel, 1977, 1980) is an increasingly accepted advance over the biomedical model which held sway in Western medicine for the previous 300 years. Unlike the single-factor, reductionistic biomedical model, which assumes mind–body dualism, the biopsychosocial model is multifactorial, wholistic, assumes that the state of the mind and body (with both conceptualized in a social context) influence each other, and focuses on health as well as illness. It is a good fit with WHO's (1948) definition of health as encompassing "physical, mental, and social well-being."

In order to assess a person's health, and to prevent illness, health care providers must consider biological factors (e.g., tumors, infections, injuries), psychological factors (e.g., stress, anxiety, depression), and social factors (e.g., social support, oppression, empowerment). Spirituality (e.g., religious faith, access to the arts, access to nature) is often considered among the psychological factors, as its presence can promote resilience and good coping and its absence can promote alienation and depression. Culture is often considered among the social factors, as traditions and beliefs can promote positive or negative health behaviours, including whether and when to seek health care. Cultural traditions and beliefs about which social roles are open to women and which are not influence the degree of gender equality and the extent of women's empowerment to make decisions about their health and health care. Cultural beliefs about "normal" sexuality and reproduction influence women's experiences of their bodies and their ability to exercise choice and control. The state of the environment in which people live is also an important determinant of people's health, and may be considered a social (and economic) factor. For example, is the air and water clean, or is it polluted? Are there dangers in the workplace or local environment (e.g., sexual harassment, toxic waste from industry, gang violence)? Are there physicians, midwives, or other health care providers available nearby? How far away is the closest clinic or hospital? Do women have access to sex education and information about fertility control?

The menstrual cycle is a good example of a biopsychosocial phenomenon. It is a physiological process that involves gradual changes in the release and circulation of several hormones that cause the development and release of an ovum, which might be fertilized and result in pregnancy if the woman is heterosexually active and contraceptives are not used. Although people generally think of the physiology of menstruation as the same for every woman, it is not. The length of women's cycles varies, the amount and length of menstrual flow varies, and women who use oral contraceptives do not actually have menstrual cycles, although they may have light break-through bleeding every fourth week. Some other women do not have menstrual cycles, such as those who are too thin (e.g., ballet dancers, long-distance runners, women with anorexia nervosa), or who have had chemotherapy treatments for cancer that resulted in early menopause, or those who use continuous oral contraceptives or Depo-provera (known as menstrual suppression medications). Furthermore, some transgender men and non-binary individuals do menstruate. The hormones associated with the menstrual cycle have various effects on the body as they circulate, such as causing water retention or uterine cramps. How annoying or painful these experiences are depends on psychosocial factors, such as tradition (e.g., stigma, belief that menstruation is punishment from God), attitudes and beliefs (e.g., menstruation is debilitating or shameful, emotions and behaviours cannot be controlled during certain times of the cycle), personal (e.g., resilience, control, stress) and interpersonal (e.g., social support or lack of it), and economic or environmental factors (e.g., affordability of menstrual management supplies; availability of diuretics, pain relief, and other medicines; ability to take time to rest). A similar description could be written about most of the topics covered in this handbook, and readers will see this model reflected in many of the chapters.

International, multicultural perspectives

The biopsychosocial model and various feminist perspectives (perhaps especially intersectional, transnational, indigenous, standpoint, and Marxist approaches) remind us to consider women's context whenever we think about their health and well-being. We asked our authors to take an international, multicultural approach to their topics and consider women in countries with various levels of economic development and different cultural and spiritual beliefs and traditions. This proved to be a challenge for many authors, as the majority of research on women's sexual and reproductive health has been conducted in Western developed nations, especially Australia and countries in Western Europe and North America. In cases where little research and few statistics were available beyond these countries, our authors have pointed to what type of research needs to be done and which populations have been neglected.

Macro-level factors (e.g., the quality and extent of health care systems, cultural traditions) are as important as micro-level factors (e.g., women's ability to pay for medications and services, genetics) in determining women's sexual and reproductive health and well-being. Cultural traditions, for example, play a role in whether women are willing and able to use contraceptives, which type of birth attendant they prefer (e.g., grandmother, midwife, physician), and where they would like to give birth to their children (e.g., at home, in a clinic or hospital, in a specific special location such as their own country or town of birth).

Indigenous Australian women often resist urgings to give birth in city hospitals as they believe childbirth should take place in locations with spiritual importance that promote maternal and child well-being (see Dudgeon & Bray, Chapter 36, this volume). Recent studies in Nigeria (Moore, Alex-Hart, & George, 2011), Uganda (Sagna & Sparks, 2016), and Saudi Arabia (Dhaler, 2017) show low use of reproductive health services in rural areas where clinic visits can require a long journey from home. Transportation costs are a barrier to sexual and reproductive health care even in developed countries for low-income women and in cities and towns where hospitals have ceased to offer obstetric services (Miles-Cohen, 2018; Ramaswamy, Unruh, & Comfort, 2018). For example, in the U.S., political divisions have led to the closing of abortion clinics such that more than one half of American women have no abortion services in their county of residence (Jones & Jerman, 2017), and attempts are regularly made to defund clinics that offer low-cost contraception, routine gynecological care, and STI testing (Sagrestano & Finerman, 2018). American politics have an impact on women's health around the world, as presidential administrations alternately (depending upon which political party is in power) fund and defund sexual and reproductive services for women in low-income countries. And, of course, poverty, homelessness, and social exclusion have a profound impact on health and well-being everywhere they exist.

Cultural traditions, laws, religion, and societal hierarchies influence every aspect of women's lives, including their sexual and reproductive health. Our authors consider women's health in terms of their cultural and social contexts, as well as in the context of their everyday lives, family organizations, and intimate relationships. We acknowledge that culture is dynamic and relational, rather than static and fixed, and often changes rapidly (Hall & Graham, 2012). We also acknowledge the intersection of identity positions and its impact on women's sexual and reproductive health and well-being, with particular attention to gender, race/ethnicity, culture, social class, sexuality, age, ability status, and relationship context (Davis, 2008).

Organization of the handbook

The handbook is organized thematically into six sections: Menarche, menstruation, and menopause; reproductive and gynaecological disorders; contraception and infertility; pregnancy and childbirth; sexuality and sexual health; and marginalized women's health, all of which encompass a range of disciplinary standpoints, including psychology, medicine, nursing, midwifery, sociology, gender studies, public health, and indigenous studies.

In the first section (menarche, menstruation, and menopause), our authors cover menarche in the context of pubertal development (Stubbs), psychosocial and cultural aspects of the experience of menarche (Marván & Alcalá-Herrera), the normal menstrual cycle (Prior), attitudes toward menstruation and behavioural concomitants of the cycle (Chrisler & Gorman), premenstrual mood and distress (Ussher & Perz), and menopause and midlife from a psychosocial perspective (Hunter).

The second section (reproductive and gynecological disorders) covers polycystic ovary syndrome, dysmenorrhea, and menstrual migraine (Woods & Kenney), endometriosis (Denny & Weckesser), breast and reproductive cancers (Travis), and psychosocial aspects of cancer and its treatment (Parton).

In the third section (contraception and infertility), our authors cover contraception (Bateson), abortion (Marecek), women's experiences of infertility (Barnack-Tavlaris), cancer and fertility (Peate, Stafford, & Jayasinghe), and assisted conception techniques and surrogate motherhood (van den Akker).

The fourth section (pregnancy and childbirth) covers adolescent pregnancy (Macleod & Feltham-King), smoking during pregnancy (Ussher, Naughton, Notley, & Bauld), medical aspects of pregnancy (Hennessy), miscarriage (Rowe & Hawkey), stillbirth (Cacciatore & Lens), psychological aspects of pregnancy (Fisher & Hammarberg), childbirth and sexuality (Dahlen & Sobhgol), postpartum adjustment (Nicolson), and perinatal mental health (Schmied).

In the fifth section (sexuality and sexual health), our authors cover sexual health and embodiment (Piran), adolescents' sexual health (Skinner, Davies, Marino, Botfield, & Lewis), older women's sexual health (Interligi & McHugh), sexual dysfunctions and interventions (Veltten & Milani), critical analyses of sexual dysfunctions (Kleinplatz, Rosen, Charest, & Spurgas), HIV and STIs (Power), sexual violence (Noack-Lundberg), child sexual abuse (Warner), genital mutilation and genital surgeries (Burrage).

The sixth section (marginalized women's health) provides a deeper focus on the sexual and reproductive health of migrant and refugee women (Hawkey), homeless women (Cronley & Nahar), Indigenous women and girls (Dudgeon & Bray), women in low- and middle-income countries (Black & O'Connor), women with physical (Dillaway, Marzolf, Fritz, Tarraf, & Lysack) and intellectual (Burns) disabilities, and lesbian, bisexual, queer, and transgender women (McNair).

Goals of the handbook

Our first goal for this handbook was to provide an authoritative reference work for researchers, health care providers, and students who wish to obtain a balanced overview of important, leading-edge developments in particular domains of women's sexual and reproductive health. We aimed to strike a balance between an authoritative review of the field and a focus on state-of-the-art work, and we attempted to produce an excellent and engaging source of contemporary scholarship that will be of interest to a multidisciplinary group of readers.

A second goal was to encourage research and policy development in areas of women's sexual and reproductive health where more work (in some cases, *much more* work) is needed. We hope that our readers will be inspired to think about projects they might undertake that could shed light on these important topics, especially as they pertain to understudied, marginalized women. Many of our authors point out inconsistences in research findings, methodological errors, gaps in the literature, and understudied topics and populations, which should assist researchers and students in finding ways to contribute. Public policy that empowers women, and promotes gender equality, leads to welcoming and sensitive health care for all women, and provides comprehensive health and sex education that will lead to improvements in women's sexual and reproductive health and well-being.

A third goal, but certainly not the least of the three, is to educate health care providers about the latest research and, especially, about women's experiences of both normal (e.g., menstruation, pregnancy, childbirth) and abnormal (e.g., STIs, sexual pain, dysmenorrhea, infertility, cancer) sexual and reproductive functions, in the context of social and environmental factors that influence women's health (e.g., sexual violence, smoking, cultural marginalization, social and gendered inequalities). We hope that a better, more comprehensive, understanding of women's health and health care experiences and a biopsychosocial approach to assessment and treatment will lead to provision of more sensitive care. Greater sensitivity might mean listening closely to women and asking them questions about what they need and want, offering treatment and interventions that take women's relational, cultural, and spiritual context into account, and taking the time to educate women about their bodies, their health, and their options.

Conclusion

The field of women's sexual and reproductive health is at the forefront of discussion for researchers, policy makers, and health care providers. In particular, researchers and policy makers are moving away from the conceptualization of sexual and reproductive health as purely a biomedical experience toward a biopsychosocial perspective that acknowledges the importance of a woman's environment and the way in which embodied experiences are influenced by cultural discourse and practice. As such, important interdisciplinary research is currently being conducted on women's sexual and reproductive health across the lifespan.

Such research is giving rise to findings that challenge established conceptual frameworks and leading to new theories as well as important refinements to existing conceptual models. The growth that is currently taking place in women's sexual and reproductive health research and theory makes it especially timely to survey the field so as to take stock of emerging trends and debates. This book presents such a survey, and we hope that it will be helpful to our readers in their work – wherever in the world they live and in whatever way they work to promote women's sexual and reproductive health and well-being.

References

American Psychological Association Task Force on the Sexualization of Girls (2007). Report of the APA Task Force on the Sexualization of Girls. Retrieved from www.apa.org/pi/women/programs/girls/report.

Beckett, M. (2016). The borders that remain: Prevention of cervical cancer in refugee and immigrant women in Canada. *University of Ottawa Journal of Medicine, 6*(2), 61.

Botfield, J. R., Newman, C. E., & Zwi, A. B. (2016). Young people from culturally diverse backgrounds and their use of services for sexual and reproductive health needs: A structured scoping review. *Sexual Health, 13*(1), 1–9.

Braun, V., Gavey, N., & McPhillips, K. (2003). The `fair deal'? Unpacking accounts of reciprocity in heterosex. *Sexualities, 6*(2), 237–261.

Center for Reproductive Rights (2009, January 20). *Repro rights are human rights*. Retrieved from www.reproductiverights.org/feature/repro-rights-are-human-rights.

Dan, A. J. (1993). Integrating biomedical and feminist perspectives on women's health. *Women's Health Issues, 3*, 101–103.

Davis, K. (2008). Intersectionality as buzzword: A sociology of science perspective on what makes a feminist theory successful. *Feminist Theory, 9*(1), 67–85.

Dhaler, E. A. (2017). Access to reproductive health care services for women in the southern region of Saudi Arabia. *Women's Reproductive Health, 4*, 126–140.

Engdahl, S. (2012). *The women's liberation movement* (1st ed.). Detroit, MI: Greenhaven Press.

Engel, G. L. (1977). The need for a new medical model: A challenge for biomedicine. *Science, 196*, 129–136.

Engel, G. L. (1980). The clinical application of the biopsychosical model. *American Journal of Psychiatry, 137*, 535–544.

Gavey, N. (2005). *Just sex? The cultural scaffolding of rape*. London, UK: Routledge.

Hall, K. S. & Graham, C. A. (2012). *The cultural context of sexual pleasure and problems: Psychotherapy with diverse clients*. New York, NY: Routledge.

Hawkey, A., Ussher, J. M., & Perz, J. (2018). "If you don't have a baby, you can't be in our culture": Migrant and refugee women's experiences and constructions of fertility and fertility control. *Women's Reproductive Health, 5*, 75–98.

Jones, R. K. & Jerman, J. (2017). Abortion incidence and service availability in the United States, 2014. *Perspectives on Sexual and Reproductive Health, 49*, 3–14.

McNair, R., Szalacha, L. A., & Hughes, T. L. (2011). Health status, health service use, and satisfaction according to sexual identity of young Australian women. *Women's Health Issues*, *21*(1), 40–47.

Miles-Cohen, S. (2018). Gardening and women's maternal care in the U.S. capital: The unacceptable chasm. *Women's Reproductive Health*, *5*, 20–24.

Moore, B., Alex-Hart, B., & George, I. (2011). Utilization of health care services by pregnant mothers during delivery: A community based study in Nigeria. *Journal of Medicine and Medical Science*, *2*, 864–867.

Nelson, J. (2015). *More than medicine: A history of the feminist women's health movement.* New York, NY: New York University Press.

Omland, G., Ruths, S., & Diaz, E. (2014). Use of hormonal contraceptives among immigrant and native women in Norway: Data from the Norwegian prescription database. *BJOG: An International Journal of Obstetrics and Gynaecology*, *121*(10), 1221–1228.

Ramaswamy, M., Unruh, E., & Comfort, M. (2018). Navigating social networks, resources, and neighborhoods: Facilitators of sexual and reproductive health care use among women released from jail. *Women's Reproductive Health*, *5*, 44–58.

Rutherford, A. (2011). From the ground up: Feminist approaches, methods, and critiques. *Psychology of Women Quarterly*, *35*, 175–179.

Sagna, M. L. & Sparks, P. J. (2016). Institutional birth in Uganda: The interplay of individual characteristics, physical accessibility, and social context. *Women's Reproductive Health*, *3*, 30–44.

Sagrestano, L. M. & Finerman, R. (2018). Does the government own my body? The reproductive health of women. In J. Nadler & M. Lowery (Eds), *War on women in the United States? Battlefields, battles, and skirmishes* (pp. 157–182). Santa Barbara, CA: Praeger.

Spain, D. & Spain, D. (2016). *Constructive feminism: Women's spaces and women's rights in the American city.* Ithaca, NY: Cornell University Press.

Steinem, G. (1978, October). If men could menstruate. *Ms.*, p. 110.

United Nations (UN) (1979). Convention on the elimination of all forms of discrimination against women. *GA Res. 34/180. UN GAOR, 34th Sess. Supp. No. 46 at 193 UN Doc. A/34–46 adopted 3 September 1981.*

United Nations (UN) (2015). *The millennium development goals report 2015.* New York, NY: United Nations. Retrieved from www.un.org/millenniumgoals/2015_MDG_Report/pdf/MDG%202015%20rev%20July%201).pdf.

United Nations General Assembly (1948). *Universal declaration of human rights.* New York, NY: United Nations. Retrieved from www.un.org/en/universal-declaration-human-rights.

United Nations Population Fund (UNPF) (2019). *Sexual and reproductive health.* New York, NY: United Nations. Retrieved from www.unfpa.org/sexual-reproductive-health.

Ussher, J. M. (2006). *Managing the monstrous feminine: Regulating the reproductive body.* London, UK: Routledge.

World Health Organization (WHO) (1948). *Constitution of the World Health Organization.* Geneva, Switzerland: World Health Organization. Retrieved from www.who.int/governance/eb/who_constitution_en.pdf.

World Health Organisation (WHO) (2014). *Ensuring human rights in the provision of contraceptive information and services: Guidance and recommendations.* Geneva, Switzerland: World Health Organization. Retrieved from http://apps.who.int/iris/bitstream/10665/102539/1/9789241506748_eng.pdf.

World Health Organization (WHO) (2017). *Statement delivered on behalf of the World Health Organization.* Geneva, Switzerland : World Health Organization. Retrieved from www.who.int/reproductivehealth/CPD-statement.pdf.

PART I

Menarche, menstruation and menopause

1

PUBERTAL DEVELOPMENT AND MENARCHE

Physiological and developmental aspects

Margaret L. Stubbs

Development in puberty includes complex biological processes that result in the physical maturation of the reproductive system and related physical growth. Some of these begin during childhood, but reproductive or sexual maturity (i.e., the biological capacity to reproduce) culminates in adolescence. Adolescence is more broadly recognized as a transitional period of development between childhood and adulthood, which includes not only pubertal changes but also changes in cognitive abilities, self-perception, and social relations with family members and peers. For girls, menarche is a major pubertal event, but it is only one such event, and a late occurring one at that. Menarche is sometimes noted as a marker for, a signal of, or synonymous with puberty, but these notions obscure the complexity of pubertal growth that develops over time within childhood and adolescence. This chapter addresses how menarche is situated within puberty as girls become reproductively and psychosocially mature. The information to follow related to the physiological aspects of pubertal development comes from studies conducted in the United States or other developed countries unless specially stated.

Physiological aspects of puberty

This physiology is multifaceted and not completely understood. One pubertal process is clinically known as gonadarche, involving the reactivation of the hypothalamus-pituitary-gonadal (HPG) axis. This axis is active in fetal development but becomes inactive until puberty when the hypothalamus secretes gonadotropin-releasing hormone (GnRH), which stimulates the anterior pituitary to release luteinizing hormone (LH) and follicle stimulating hormone (FSH) to the gonads, in girls, the ovaries. In turn, LH and FSH stimulate the ovaries to produce estradiol. The increase in estradiol is first externally noticeable with breast bud development, known as thelarche (Dorn & Rotenstein, 2004). Along with an increase in other hormones throughout early puberty, menarche eventually occurs in mid to late puberty; menstruation becomes cyclical and ovulatory later, about one year after menarche, for most girls (Hillard, 2014).

Research into what influences the reactivation of the HPG axis at puberty indicates that nutritional support is needed to begin and maintain pubertal development. Leptin, a hormone produced by fat cells, plays a key role. Leptin levels signal the hypothalamus when there is enough nutritional support for pubertal development to begin and proceed (Dorn & Biro, 2011). Researchers have identified additional neurotransmitters, neuropeptides, notably Kisspeptin and its receptor, growth factors, and metabolic signals that contribute to the onset of puberty (Manfredi-Lozano et al., 2016). How these factors interact to stimulate the reactivation of GnRH by the hypothalamus has yet to be fully revealed (Biro, Greenspan, & Galvez, 2012).

Another pubertal process is the activation of the hypothalamic-pituitary-adrenal (HPA) axis. This process, known as adrenarche, involves the maturation of the adrenal glands and their production of certain androgens (Dorn & Biro, 2011). Adrenarche begins in children aged 6–8, although no outward signs of the process appear until later in puberty when increased androgen levels result in observable pubic hair growth (i.e., pubarche), other ancillary body hair, body odor, and perhaps acne (Abrue & Kaiser, 2016; Dorn & Biro, 2011). Typically, pubarche occurs before thelarche, and menarche occurs last. However, variations in this sequence also occur, such as thelarche before pubarche, or pubarche and thelarche appearing together (Biro, Huang, Daniels, & Lucky, 2008). In studying peripubertal girls, Biro et al. (2014) found that hormonal changes related to adrenarche occurred before those associated with gonadarche, suggesting that two pathways may represent the onset of puberty.

While adrenarche and gonadarche are thought to be distinct processes, research continues to explore their timing as sequential, oppositional, or coactivated (Shirtcliff et al., 2015). Some have noted that, in addition to its function in advancing pubertal changes, the HPA axis also regulates the stress response. To maximize the body's capacity to perceive and defend against a threat, the stress response has been found to suppress other physiological systems, including reproductive function (Chrousos & Gold, 1992). Although this oppositional relationship between the stress response and reproductive function has been demonstrated in adults, Ruttle, Shirtcliff, Armstrong, Klein, and Essex (2013) suggested that it may not occur in adolescence. They argue that it makes more sense that coactivation, or positive coupling, would advance the development of both axes during adolescence, as opposed to the suppression of one by the other. As Shirtcliff et al. (2015) pointed out, "Stress and puberty can, and frequently do, co-occur" (p. 646), certainly an understatement.

An evolutionary/life history theory of development supports the notion of coactivation (Belsky, Steinberg, & Draper, 1991). This perspective differentiates between various kinds of stress and evolutionary strategies employed to manage them within specific contexts. Within this explanation, early puberty given significant childhood adversity may be adaptive in an evolutionary sense to maximize reproductive success, though not without associated costs (e.g., early sexual activity). Several studies have demonstrated a relationship between early menarche and stressful aspects of family adversity, including early maternal harshness (Belsky, Steinberg, Houts, & Halpern-Felsher, 2010), father absence (Tither & Ellis, 2008), maternal depression, and stepfather presence (Ellis & Garber, 2000). Researchers continue to explore relationships between HPA hormones and specific kinds of early life adversity in girls (and boys), though no consistent results have yet emerged (Negriff, Saxbe, & Trickett, 2015).

Related research regarding increases in children's and adolescents' body weight (Jasik & Lustig, 2008) has prompted investigations of "excessive" weight as a contributor to early puberty onset. Heavy weight children typically experience puberty earlier than their average or underweight peers, both in the U.S. (Kaplowitz & Bloch, 2016) and many other countries, e.g., India (Banik, Mendez, & Dickinson, 2015), Korea (Lee, Kim, Oh, Lee, & Park, 2016), and Turkey (Tekgül, Saltik, & Vatansever, 2014).

These data are in line with the theory that reproductive function requires enough nutritional support to occur, but when does "enough" lead to "excessive"? Castilho and Nucci (2015) noted that, with the improvement in economic conditions in Brazil, many fewer people experience food shortage and, instead of eating the healthier food provided in the public schools, children often prefer to consume junk food. Though lack of access to a healthy diet persists in many locations, where it does exist, healthy eating is not necessarily ensured.

Further, food intake is entwined with socioeconomic status. Researchers have documented earlier menarche in girls in the lowest levels of income in U.S., despite the general downward trend in menarcheal age in that country (Kreiger et al., 2015). Similar results come from research conducted elsewhere, e.g., Ghana (Ameade & Garti, 2016) and China (Meng, Li, Duan, Sun, & Jia, 2017). How might lower socioeconomic status, and poverty in particular, impact menarche? More often poverty is associated with lack of access to improved/healthier food and later menarche in many secular trend studies. However, living in poverty is a significant stressor (Kreiger et al., 2015). Thus, along with adverse family interactions, poverty could be considered to contribute to earlier pubertal development. This is especially relevant considering the functional relationships between the HPA and HPG axes during puberty that are currently being explored.

Finally, naturally occurring and manufactured endocrine-disrupting chemicals (EDCs) have been noted throughout the world as impacting pubertal physiology. In the U.S., the Endocrine Society (Gore et al., 2015) has documented the relationship between early breast development and exposure to EDCs, as does the International Federation of Obstetrics and Gynecology (Di Renzo et al., 2015). Some data indicate a relationship between EDCs and early menarche in the U.S. (Boswell, 2014). However, in a review of studies from the U.S., Europe, and Asia, Mouritsen et al. (2010) concluded that the link between exposure to EDCs and early thelarche is stronger than that between EDC exposure and early menarche. At the same time, studies show that specific compounds (e.g., lead) have been found to be related to late or delayed aspects of pubertal development in girls (Schoeters, Hond, Dhoog, van Larebeke, & Leijs, 2008). These researchers stressed that the relationships that may occur between the myriad of EDCs and disruptions of the endocrine process throughout the lifespan have yet to be fully understood, and called for more studies of EDC exposure related to human health. Importantly, Shakeel, George, Jose, Jose, and Mathew (2010) noted the disproportionate exposure to EDCs worldwide and associated negative health consequences among low-income people. They called specifically for more studies in developing countries, emphasizing that results from developed countries cannot be generalized to low-income or resource-poor countries.

A trend in earlier pubertal onset?

Determination by the timing of breast bud development

A key study by Herman-Giddens et al. (1997) raised clinical concern about earlier pubertal onset. Previous data had indicated that the average age of thelarche was 11.5 years (Marshall & Tanner, 1969), but Herman-Giddens et al. (1997) reported that the average age was 9.96 years for European American girls and 8.87 years for African American girls. Their study was criticized for its lack of a representative sample and for the use of inspection rather than palpation to evaluate breast bud development. However, subsequent studies with methodological corrections have shown similar results (Jasik & Lustig, 2008).

One outcome of these studies was renewed concern about precocious puberty. Kaplowitz and Bloch (2016) recommended that girls who experience breast bud development assessed by palpation before the age of 8 be referred for an evaluation of precocious puberty. Observable signs of adrenarche before age 8, especially the appearance of pubic hair, should also be referred to investigate a diagnosis of premature adrenarche (Kaplowitz & Bloch, 2016). Premature adrenarche has been studied in relation to the development of polycystic ovarian syndrome (PCOS) and other related health issues that might ensue (Dorn & Biro, 2011). Despite these concerns, Kaplowitz and Bloch (2016) defined central precocious puberty in girls as the full activation of the HPG axis, and further, that true precocious puberty entails increased development and growth of breasts, though pubic hair may not exist. Diagnosis usually includes bone age determination and hormonal assays. Studies of the incidence of precocious puberty have also occurred in other parts of the world, e.g., in Korea (Kim, Huh, Won, Lee, & Park, 2015), and Pakistan (Atta et al., 2014), albeit with various diagnostic indicators. It is important to note that precocious puberty is distinct from early puberty.

Determination by the timing of menarche

Interest in documenting girls' pubertal onset is often framed as concern about potential consequences for health and well-being, not the least of which is early sexual activity and pregnancy (see Marvàn & Alcalá-Herrera, Chapter 2, this volume). Accordingly, many studies world-wide have investigated location-specific population norms, or a secular trend, in the decline in age of pubertal onset. Deriving these norms is complicated, as it can take 1–7 years to complete pubertal growth (Mendel, 2014). Many of these studies focus on girls' pubertal timing, whereas research on boys' pubertal timing is not as plentiful but has been increasing (Hermann-Giddens et al., 2012; Mendel & Ferrero, 2012). The age of menarche is very often used as a marker of pubertal onset, even though it is a late occurring pubertal event. Although breast bud development is currently the best indicator of the reactivation of the HPG axis, Wacharasindhu (2009) explained that it is rarely used by researchers, partly because participants can more easily recall the age of menarche than the age of thelarche. He also noted that, in some locations, physical examination of the breast is not considered polite or an accepted procedure.

Further, many factors, some mentioned previously, are investigated as contributors to menarcheal timing in these studies. For example, ethnicity, location, and religious differences have been explored. In the U.S., Black and Hispanic girls have been found to experience earlier menarche than non-Hispanic White and Asian girls (Hillard, 2014). In China, the downward trend in the age of menarche was documented for girls from rural but not urban areas (Meng et al., 2017). In India, Christian and Muslim women reported earlier menarche than women who practice Hindu, Sikh, and other religions Pathak, Tripathi, and Subramanian (2014).

Unlike early thelarche, a trend in earlier menarche has not been found in the U.S. over the past 50 years (Cabrera, Bright, Frane, Blethen, & Lee, 2014). The average age of menarche prior to 1950 in the developed world fell from 16–17 to about 13 years of age and then leveled off. Papadimitriou (2016) reported that the average age of menarche in the U.S. is 12.3 years, based on data from girls born in 1993, which is similar to that of girls born in 1980. Similarly, Juul, Change, Brar, and Parekh (2017) documented a declining menarcheal age in many developed countries throughout the world. A simple Google Scholar search of "secular trends in age at menarche" resulted in a plethora of studies conducted in low-, middle-income, and resource-poor countries. This general decline throughout the world over time has been attributed to improved economic conditions and better nutrition (Papa-dimitriou, 2016), as well as political transformation in countries such as Poland (Gomula & Koziel, 2017) and South Africa (Said-Mohamed et al., 2018).

It is also worth noting that results from studies of secular trends pertain not only to specific countries but also to specific populations studied within those countries. However, location-specific findings preclude generalization. Yet these studies can yield additional information of use in designing effective interventions to improve the health and well-being of vulnerable subgroups of girls who experience early thelarche or menarche.

Taken together, the data reviewed thus far come from a vast literature on physiological pubertal processes and reveal their complicated interconnections. Relationships between the HPA and HPG functioning during pubertal development have yet to be fully delineated and will continue to be studied, including exploration of factors that contribute to variations in pubertal onset and development.

Psychological experiences of pubertal development and menarche

Methodological considerations

It is difficult to isolate or generalize about girls' reactions to pubertal events. Because many studies of secular trends in pubertal development focus on menarche to the exclusion of other pubertal events, reported reactions to puberty are conflated with reported reactions to menarcheal experience and subsequent early menstrual experience. Summers-Effler (2004) has warned that generalizing about developing girls without closer investigation of their psychosocial reactions to their experiences does them a disservice. She noted that girls' experiences of the more visible aspects of early development, such as breast development, which itself can vary in terms of whether growth is large or small, likely result in very different approaches used to navigate early development. Both Summers-Effler (2004) and Mendel (2014) have suggested that more attention be paid to the tempo of how fast or slow pubertal events occur.

Mendel (2014) also suggested more detailed study of pubertal synchrony. Most of these investigations have focused on synchrony related to the typical sequence of physiological changes, but Mendel suggested that differences in timing and tempo can impact girls' reactions to them related to their co-occurrence with other events in adolescence (e.g., trying out for sports teams or school plays). Summers-Effler (2004) noted that girls regard breast development as a positive or negative event depending on the social context in which it occurs and the responses of others in those contexts. For some U.S. girls in her study, early and large breast development led to exclusion as "different" from their peer group and resulted in unwanted sexual attention from boys and men. For one girl, this led to body shame, hiding breast development with baggy clothes and adopting a negative attitude towards men. Some girls who reported feeling isolated from their undeveloped peers were supported by parents with practical interventions, such as bringing home all kinds of bras until together they found one that enabled the girls to continue the sports they loved without embarrassment. Other girls, who had felt excluded from their peers in early grades, found that their breast development became an asset in later grades and brought them popularity based on attention from, and early sexual activity with, boys.

Girls' subjective timing (i.e., whether they think of themselves as early, average, or late maturers) has also been a focus in studies of pubertal events. Although results from a physical examination may be more accurate, subjective timing has been found to be more important than actual timing related to menarcheal experience (Rierdan, Koff, & Stubbs, 1989). Mendel (2014) argued that, beyond simple self-categorization, girls' subjective perceptions might be the most telling, especially if they reveal more of what girls think about their own experiences of various aspects of pubertal change, whether considered independently or as they relate to one another in specific contexts.

Developmental considerations

Girls' experiences of puberty are biopsychosocial in nature. Physical development occurs not just in terms of reproductive capacity, but together with other changes such as height, muscle growth, and brain development. How girls react to pubertal change is related to their cognitive development, which varies with age. Because children in middle childhood (6–11 years) and in adolescence (the teen years) can experience puberty, it is important to recognize that biological, cognitive, and social aspects of development vary significantly during these two periods. Following are highlights of development during these two periods, drawn primarily from Berger (2017), with the acknowledgment that these generalizations may not fully describe girls in non-western locations.

Middle childhood is generally a healthy time when children have become more independent physically. They also become more aware of themselves in relation to others and engage in social comparison. Peers become very important in terms of making friends and determining values. In terms of cognitive development, children in middle childhood are concrete thinkers and are best at solving problems when engaged in hands-on learning opportunities using concrete props. They are avid collectors of information. Because of their concrete thinking, they can be very rigid when using rules to classify and categorize people and behavior (e.g., appropriate behavior for girls and for boys). At the same time, special needs in terms of physical and cognitive development, as well as experiences of childhood adversity, can occur and may become important concrete attributes used in judging themselves as alike, or different from, peers.

Brain development in adolescence results in more advanced cognitive ability in problem solving. Adolescents can think abstractly so that they can rely less on concrete props to solve problems. They can entertain a variety of possibilities in doing so, thus demonstrating creativity, though not always reflecting reality. At the same time, they are learning to use deductive reasoning (i.e., starting from a general premise to arrive at probable specific examples). However, they also often use inductive thinking (i.e., beginning with a specific example and using that, perhaps as the sole evidence, to derive a general principle). It takes time to develop the ability to use a systematic process to solve problems, including social problems, as opposed to relying on a hunch, or personal experience.

Adolescents, of course, do not always use more advanced thinking just because they can. Concerns about personal identity and socializing may take precedence, related in part to the development of feelings of sexual desire, explorations of sexual activity, and, for some, sexual orientation or gender identity. One's peer group is very important in adolescence, as they may feel a need to conform to peer group values and behaviors and to minimize appearances of being different. Self-consciousness as a means of appraising one's relationship to one's peers is also characteristic of adolescents. Cognitive limitations, such as egocentrism, may also influence peer relationship appraisals and play a part in relationships with their parents and other adults. For example, adolescents may think that they are the center of attention of an imaginary audience, such that everyone else can see what they perceive as their flaws. Or they may present two kinds of personal fable: on the one hand, they may believe that they are unique and no one understands them, or, on the other hand, that they are invincible and nothing dangerous will happen to them.

In addition, adolescents can be very impulsive, influenced more at times by an immediate reward than longer-term consideration of the results of an action (Steinberg & Scott, 2003). During puberty the limbic system, which includes the amygdala, contributes to the experience of intense emotions, including both fear and pleasure. It develops sooner than the prefrontal cortex, which contributes to reflection and analysis and is not thought to develop fully until the mid-20s. As a result, and especially during early puberty, emotions can and often do drive adolescents' actions and reactions. Steinberg, Cauffman, Woolard, Graham, and Banich (2009) reported that psychosocial maturity is distinct from general cognitive maturity and develops later in adolescence. They suggested that cognitive problem solving as unhurried logical reflection develops by about age 16. Problem solving that requires the coordination of both affect and more advanced executive functioning, especially in emotional situations or when decisions must be made more quickly, develops later. Their work implies that adolescents younger than 16 may indeed be able to apply deductive reasoning in many situations, but we should not expect them to be able do so in socioemotional situations until later in development. Finally, it should also be recognized that early adolescents, like children in middle childhood, are more likely to rely on concrete, as opposed to abstract, deductive thinking.

Developmental considerations and girls' experiences of pubertal events

Girls who experience puberty and menarche before the teen years have access to fewer developmental resources, including cognitive ability, to process their physical changes. With respect to the anticipation of menarche, the youngest girls will be wondering about related concrete details, and sometimes the information offered is not concrete enough to be readily understood. For instance, girls talking with this author have asked whether "menstrual flow" is like a waterfall or water rushing from a faucet and whether "having an accident" while menstruating is like falling off a bicycle. These kinds of questions reveal how young girls typically apply concrete thinking in learning about something new.

Similarly, the notion that beginning to menstruate signifies that a girl is now a woman and can have children is perhaps too remote from girls' experiences of childhood to be very meaningful in a practical sense. Some early work does indicate a shift in girls' self-perception from more childlike to more grown up related to the event of menarche, but also noted that girls' endorsement of feeling more grown up was perhaps related to the repetition of "now you are a woman" in educational materials and menstrual management product advertisements then aimed at U.S. girls (Koff, 1983). In subsequent work, Koff and Rierdan (1995) highlighted the notion that "now you are a woman" was too abstract a concept to be very meaningful for young, less cognitively mature girls. In more recent research in which adult refugee and immigrant women who had relocated to Canada or Australia were asked to recall their memories of menarche (Hawkey, Ussher, Perz, & Metusela, 2017), one Somali woman aptly explained the discrepancy between being told "you are a woman" and the reality of being a child:

> When you get your period … [You're] not running around anymore, just being like a woman, act[ing] like a woman. Actually, you are not … because, when you

are 11 like my age when I got period, 11 is not a woman it's just a young girl, but you act as you are a woman.

(p. 1477)

Findings from multicountry studies indicate that, in many locations, when girls develop breasts, begin menstruation, and thus transition to "being a woman," gender norms impose very concrete restrictions on their everyday activities. These include how to dress, which household tasks they undertake, increased time indoors, avoidance of men and boys, and, paradoxically, also being regarded as available for sexual activity, ready to marry, and start a family (Coast, Presler-Marshall, & Lattof, 2017; UNESCO, 2014). Hawkey et al. (2017) noted that, in the absence of concrete details about how menstruation relates to pregnancy or sex, some women thought, as young postmenarcheal girls, that if they touched a boy or man, they might get pregnant. Further, expectations for marriage can result in girls dropping out of school altogether, not only to turn their attention to preparing for family life, but also to avoid sexual harassment related to others knowing that they are postmenarchal (Coast et al., 2017; UNESCO, 2014).

Girls in the developed world also experience concrete behavioral restrictions during the pubertal transition. Based on over 25 years of research on the body experiences of Canadian girls and women, Piran (2017) documented how body constraints imposed during childhood can lead to an erosion of the comfort girls may have felt with respect to their bodies. Some of these constraints are as simple as pressure to wear more feminine and/or revealing clothing, even when participating in sports, or to engage in more feminine, and fewer physical, activities. Piran noted that these constraints intensify as girls become aware of both the need to adhere to contemporary beauty standards that emphasize a sexy appearance and the prejudicial and objectifying treatment that girls and women often experience. Brown and Gilligan (1992) found that girls become keenly aware of these cultural values during the transition from childhood to adolescence. Examples of the struggle to make sense of these messages came from their interviews with U.S. girls over time. They noted that, as girls got older, their self-references shifted from expressions of the strong "I" of childhood (I like …, I feel …) to those that reflected the "eye of culture" (I should …, I don't know …) in adolescence (p. 167). Brown and Gilligan stressed that an important developmental task during this transitional time is how girls come to know and maintain their own feelings and perceptions in the face of contradictory cultural representations of how they *should* feel.

The typical description of a menstrual period in many menstrual education materials provides generalized details about how long a period lasts, how much blood is lost, and what negative aspects of menstruation (e.g., cramps, moodiness) can be expected. Younger girls who are concrete, rule-bound thinkers try to see if their menstrual experiences fit this description of what is normal; they may feel abnormal if they do not have cramps or mood swings or if their period is "too long" or "too short" or they lose "too much" or "too little" menstrual fluid (Stubbs, 2013). Practical support, along with accurate factual information, is necessary to help younger, especially early developing, girls to evaluate and integrate both personal and external information about growing up.

Egocentrism may reinforce older girls' self-consciousness about pubertal changes, especially if their development is different from that of their peer group. Referring to an imaginary audience, girls may worry that everyone can tell when they have their periods. For girls in developing countries, who lack privacy and effective materials to manage their periods, or who avoid school during menstruation, it may be true that people can identify them as menstruators. Menstrual stigma thus presents a developmental dilemma for girls in terms of having to integrate the notion that menstruation is a normal bodily process but is culturally regarded as a predominantly negative experience. Menstrual stigma persists both in developed (Chrisler & Johnston-Robledo, 2018) and developing (Dutta, Badloe, Lee, & House, 2016; Sommer et al., 2016) countries, despite efforts to reduce it and activism to raise public awareness of related issues.

The development of sexual feelings and explorations of sexual activity in adolescence can also complicate adjustment to menstrual life, particularly as girls self-objectify to present themselves as sexually attractive and available. Roberts and Waters (2004) noted that girls and women engage in many self-objectifying practices to achieve the beauty ideal, including self-monitoring, dieting, and concealing menstrual status. These practices distract girls (and women) from noticing important internal cues about their own bodily functioning, including menstruation. Roberts (2004) demonstrated that women who self-objectify also hold negative attitudes toward menstruation. The current representation of menstruation as unnecessary may encourage women to reduce the number of menstrual periods they experience or to eliminate them all together. This representation, along with an emphasis on menstruation as inconvenient, has been reinforced since the advent of cycle-reducing or stopping contraception in the mid-2000s (Stubbs, 2008; Woods, 2013). Adolescent girls are not immune from this representation, as they are avid readers of material for adult women and accomplished seekers of information about sexuality and reproduction via the internet and social media (Hall, Sales, Komro, & Santelli, 2016). In the U.S., health care practitioners also promote these notions to girls, as both the American Academy of Pediatrics (2014) and the American College of Obstetrics and Gynecology (2017, 2018) have endorsed the use of long-acting, reversible contraception as a first line of defense in curtailing unwanted pregnancy among adolescents.

Data on the experiences of late maturing girls are not as prevalent in the literature. It should be noted, however, that late maturing girls (and boys) do receive clinical attention and treatment (Dunkle & Quinton, 2014). Late maturing girls also experience some of the same negative psychosocial outcomes as early maturing girls, such as body image issues, depression, and lower self-esteem and self-confidence (e.g., Benoit, Lacourse, & Claes, 2013). Research based on U.S. samples suggests that late maturing girls who see themselves as off-time may worry about whether they are "normal" until their menstruation begins (Rierdan & Koff, 1985).

Although not directly queried about timing, and the adult refugee and immigrant women interviewed by Hawkey et al. (2017) generally described menstruation as a welcome sign of fertility, one Somali woman said:

> When I started bleeding, I kind of felt happy … I was really waiting because it kind of lessened my anxiety because I was asking myself, oh my goodness, I'm not going to be have children … it was kind of a relief.
>
> *(p. 1477)*

In related research, Hawkey, Ussher, and Perz (2018) reported that motherhood is so central to identity in some locations that women unable to bear children soon after marriage are denigrated, stigmatized, and distressed. Although motherhood is also a cultural value in the West, they pointed out that other avenues for self-development are available there to women who do not want or cannot have children.

Menstrual knowledge

Girls' experiences of and related responses to puberty, menarche, and menstruation are connected to what they know (e.g., are formally or informally taught, absorbed from cultural representations) about these processes. A review of studies primarily conducted in the U.S. and Europe indicates that, in general, girls' knowledge about menarche and menstruation is inadequate (Stubbs, 2008). One recent study of a small group of preadolescent girls and boys aged 7–12 in the U.S. indicated that they know very little about human reproduction and anatomy on which instruction about pubertal development could build (Hurwitz et al., 2017). The authors noted a dearth of studies about the menstrual knowledge and experiences of U.S. ethnic minority girls, as older studies of girls' menstrual knowledge and experience primarily included girls from middle- and upper-class White families. However, based on their review of studies that do exist, they concluded that minority girls are also uninformed. Future studies of the current menstrual knowledge and experiences among girls from developed countries are needed to update older findings.

In contrast, an abundance of data regarding girls' knowledge of pubertal changes, including menstruation, comes from developing countries. Two reviews of this literature document these girls' inadequate knowledge about pubertal change and negative pubertal experiences (e.g., Coast et al., 2017; UNESCO, 2014). Both sources indicate that many girls begin menstruation without knowing what is happening to them and that what they do know is often related to what they have learned from tradition (e.g., cultural representations of menstruation as dirty and menstruating women as impure). These variables are related to anxiety, fear, and self-doubt as girls' emotional reactions to menarche and menstruation.

These sources further emphasize that (especially younger) girls who are out-of-school or have disabilities are not receiving the menstrual education or menstrual hygiene management efforts that do exist. Because talking about pubertal issues is considered private and hard to do in public, in-school programs are often compromised. Both sources note the lack of pubertal education to address girls' sexual desires as they develop during this time. Even talking with parents can be difficult because of social norms that discourage discussions of sexuality.

An important focus within much of the literature on girls' menarcheal and menstrual experience in developing and resource-poor countries highlights issues related to menstrual hygiene (Coast et al., 2017; UNESCO, 2014). Chandra-Mouli and Patel (2017) discussed in detail that, in addition to a general lack of information about menstruation, information about how and where to manage menstruation is also inadequate, including limited access to menstrual managements products. Lack of privacy in public places (especially in schools) and deficient latrines, water supply, and disposal facilities are also noted as problematic. Rheinländer, Gyapong, Akpakli, and Konradsen (2019) pointed out that girls are often shamed for the ways they try to cope with these practical problems (e.g., urinating behind a bush while menstruating for lack of a sanitary, private place to do so), which is likely to undermine a positive response to menstrual life. Inadequacies related to hygiene are recognized in this literature as impeding girls' adjustment to menstrual life, threatening their physical and psychological health, and curtailing their education, which together contribute to diminishing girls' capacity to achieve economic and social equality.

Improving menstrual education

Providing girls with adequate information about pubertal development and menstruation remains a challenge in developed as well as developing countries. As her review of books on puberty and menstruation available to girls in the U.S. revealed, Stubbs (2013) found many problematic aspects. In most, puberty was described as problematic: a period of instability, upheaval, and being out of control or being under the control of one's hormones. When menstruation was discussed, it was only one of many pubertal topics covered; other topics competed for the readers' interest, such as beginning to date or dealing with acne, body hair, or body odor. Content generally emphasized the biological aspects of the menstrual cycle, with less attention paid to sociocultural aspects. The relationship between menstruation and sex was often only vaguely mentioned or woefully understated. Negative aspects of menstrual experience (e.g., cramps) were mentioned as typical, and these were described as "symptoms." Describing menstrual changes as symptoms connotes disease (Chrisler, 1996), which may be confusing if girls have been told that menstruation is "normal." In the books reviewed, these changes were often identified as premenstrual syndrome (PMS), which was also described as normative. Cramps and cycle irregularity were often described as both symptoms and as normative. Both can indicate underlying conditions worthy of further medical evaluation, but are often overlooked by health care professionals because they too see these as normative in girls (Hillard, 2014).

Positive premenstrual changes *do* exist (King & Ussher, 2012), but none were mentioned in the books reviewed by Stubbs (2013), nor was any information given about menstruation as a vital sign, which has been promoted by both the American Academy of Pediatrics (2016) and the American College of Gynecology and Obstetrics (2015). This omission in menstrual education material prevents girls from learning about menstrual health and its connection to overall well-being. Given these predominately negative representations of puberty and menstruation, preadolescent girls might very well be apprehensive or less than enthusiastic about upcoming developmental changes.

Clinical state-of-the-art information about "what's normal and what's not" regarding the biological aspects of menstrual experience in early adolescence *does* exist (Hillard, 2008, 2014). Yet there is no evidence-based curriculum based on results of that research or from findings exploring the psychosocial aspects of menstruating. Instead, in many U.S. schools, menstrual education is often offered by menstrual product manufacturers with no program known to evaluate its effectiveness (Sterling, 2018). These materials have long been critiqued as presenting mostly negative representations of menstruation (Chrisler & Johnston-Robledo, 2018), promoting a neat, clean body that does not leak (Erchull, Chrisler, Gorman, & Johnston-Robledo, 2001), and providing mixed messages to girls, for example, that menstruation is important, but girls should act like they would on any other day (Charlesworth, 2001). Furthermore, the menstrual cycle is not featured in core areas and outreach within U.S. public health initiatives (Sterling, Karczmarczyk, & Ivabze, 2017). In sum, advocates of girls' reproductive health in both the developed and developing world can agree on the paucity and quality of menstrual education to date.

It should go without saying that updated, evidenced-based, and culturally sensitive information regarding menarche and early menstrual experience should be foundational to all menstrual education. In addition, menstrual educators should describe various trajectories within pubertal development and consider developmental differences in girls' cognitive abilities when presenting information. We know that preparing girls with quality menstrual education before menarche can result in positive attitudes toward menstruation and that these are related to more positive menarcheal and later menstrual experiences, body positivity, and even later sexual agency (see Marvàn & Alcalá-Herrera, Chapter 2, this volume).

Conclusion

As this chapter has only briefly detailed, the biological changes related to puberty and menarche are complex, as are the cultural contexts in which girls experience them. But so too are other complex topics that have been successfully introduced to children at very young ages by teachers and others who design curricula based on information gleaned from human development research (Stubbs, 2016). We can and must take the same approach to education about the development of reproductive capacity, including the very central role of menstruation's broader connection to girls' and women's well-being.

References

Abrue, A. P. & Kaiser, U. B. (2016). Pubertal development and regulation. *Lancet Diabetes and Endocrinology, 4*, 254–264.

Ameade, E. P. K. & Garti, H. A. (2016). Age at menarche and factors that influence it: A study among female university students in Tamale, Northern Ghana. *PLoS ONE, 11*, e0155310.

American Academy of Pediatrics. (2016). Menstruation in girls and adolescents: Using menstruation as a vital sign. *Pediatrics, 137*(3), e20154480.

American Academy of Pediatrics, and Committee on Adolescence (2014). Contraception for adolescents. *Pediatrics, 134*, e1224.

American College of Obstetrics and Gynecology, Committee on Adolescent Health Care (2015). Menstruation in girls and adolescents: Using the menstrual cycle as a vital sign. [ACOG Committee Opinion No 651]. *Obstetrics & Gynecology, 126*, e143–146.

American College of Obstetrics and Gynecology, Committee on Adolescent Health Care (2017). Adolescent pregnancy, contraception, and sexual activity. *Obstetrics and Gynecology, 129*, e142–149. Retrieved from www.acog.org/-/media/Committee-Opinions/Committee-on-Adolescent-Health Care/co699.pdf?dmc=1&ts=20181126T1849100104.

American College of Obstetrics and Gynecology, Committee on Adolescent Health Care Long-Acting Reversible Contraception Work Group (2018). Adolescents and long-acting reversible contraception: Implants and intrauterine devices. *Obstetrics and Gynecology, 131*, e130–139. Retrieved from www.acog.org/Clinical-Guidance-and-Publications/Committee-Opinions/Committee-on-Adolescent-Health-Care/Adolescents-and-Long-Acting-Reversible-Contraception?IsMobileSet=false.

Atta, I., Laghari, T. M., Khan, Y. N., Lone, S. W., Ibrahim, M., & Raza, J. (2014). Precocious puberty in children. *Journal of the College of Physicians and Plastic Surgeons Pakistan, 25*, 124–128. Retrieved from https://jcpsp.pk/query-result.php.

Banik, S. D., Mendez, N., & Dickinson, F. (2015). Height growth and percentage of body fat in relation to early menarche in girls from Merida, Yucatan, Mexico. *Ecology of Food and Nutrition, 54*, 644–662.

Belsky, J., Steinberg, L., & Draper, P. (1991). Childhood experience, interpersonal development, and reproductive strategy: An evolutionary theory of socialization. *Child Development, 62*, 647–670.

Belsky, J., Steinberg, L., Houts, R. M., & Halpern-Felsher, B. L. (2010). The development of reproductive strategy in females: Early maternal harshness –> earlier menarche –> increased sexual risk taking. *Developmental Psychology, 46*, 120–128.

Benoit, A., Lacourse, E., & Claes, M. (2013). Pubertal timing and depressive symptoms in late adolescence: The moderating role of individual, peer, and parental factors. *Development and Psychopathology, 25*, 455–471.

Berger, K. (2017). *The developing person though the lifespan* (10th ed.). New York, NY: Worth.

Biro, F. M., Greenspan, L. C., & Galvez, M. P. (2012). Puberty in girls of the 21st century. *Journal of Pediatric and Adolescent Gynecology, 25*, 289–294.

Biro, F. M., Huang, B., Daniels, S. R., & Lucky, A. W. (2008). Pubarche as well as thelarche may be a marker for the onset of puberty. *Journal of Pediatric and Adolescent Gynecology, 28*, 323–328.

Biro, F. M., Pinney, S. M., Huang, B., Baker, E. R., Chandler, D. W., & Dorn, L. D. (2014). Hormone changes in peripubertal girls. *Journal of Clinical Endocrinology & Metabolism, 99*, 3829–3835.

Boswell, H. B. (2014). Normal pubertal physiology in females. In J. E. Dietrich (Ed.), *Female puberty: A comprehensive guide for clinicians* (pp. 7–30). New York, NY: Springer.

Brown, L. M. & Gilligan, C. (1992). *Meeting at the crossroads: Women's and girls' development*. Cambridge, MA: Harvard University Press.

Cabrera, S. M., Bright, G. M., Frane, J. W., Blethen, S. L., & Lee, P. A. (2014). Age of thelarche and menarche in contemporary US females: A cross-sectional analysis. *Journal of Pediatric Endocrinology and Metabolism, 27*, 47–51.

Castilho, S. M. & Nucci, L. B. (2015). Age at menarche in schoolgirls with and without excess weight. *Jornal de Pediatria, 91,* 75–80.

Chandra-Mouli, V. & Patel, S. V. (2017). Mapping the knowledge and understanding of menarche, menstrual hygiene, and menstrual health among adolescent girls in low- and middle-income countries. *Reproductive Health, 14,* 1–14.

Charlesworth, D. (2001). Paradoxical constructions of self: Educating women about menstruation. *Women & Language, 24,* 13–20.

Chrisler, J. C. (1996). PMS as a culture-bound syndrome. In J. C. Chrisler, C. Golden, & P. D. Rozee (Eds), *Lectures on the psychology of women* (1st ed., pp. 107–121). New York, NY: McGraw Hill.

Chrisler, J. & Johnston-Robledo, I. (2018). *Women's embodied self: Feminist perspectives on identity and body image.* Washington, DC: American Psychological Association.

Chrousos, G. P. & Gold, W. P. (1992). The concepts of stress and stress system disorders. *Journal of the American Medical Association, 267,* 1224–1252.

Coast, E., Presler-Marshall, E., & Lattof, S. R. (2017). *An agenda for policy and action to support girls through puberty and menarche.* London, UK: Gender and Adolescence Global Evidence. Retrieved from www.gage.odi.org/sites/default/files/201707/P%20and%20M%20Digest%20%20FINALpdf.

Di Renzo, G. C., Conry, J. A., Blake, J., DeFrancesco, M. S., DeNicola, N., Martin, J. N., McCue, K. A., Richmond, D., Shah, A., Sutton, P., Woodruff, T. J., van der Poel, S. Z., & Giudice, L. C. (2015). International Federation of Gynecology and Obstetrics opinion on reproductive health impacts of exposure to toxic environmental chemicals. *International Journal of Gynecology and Obstetrics, 131,* 219–225.

Dorn, L. D. & Biro, F. M. (2011). Puberty and its measurement: A decade in review. *Journal of Research on Adolescence, 21,* 180–195.

Dorn, L. D. & Rotenstein, D. (2004). Early puberty in girls: The case of premature adrenarche. *Women's Health Issues, 14*(6), 177–183.

Dunkle, L. & Quinton, R. (2014). Transition in endocrinology: Induction of puberty. *European Journal of Endocrinology, 170,* R229–239.

Dutta, D., Badloe, C., Lee, H., & House, S. (2016). *Supporting the rights of girls and women through Menstrual Hygiene Management (MHM) in the East Asia and Pacific Region: Realities, progress, and opportunities.* Bangkok: UNICEF East Asia and Pacific Regional Office (EAPRO). Retrieved from http://www.cswashfund.org/sites/default/files/MHM_Realities_Progress_and_Opportunities Supporting_opti.pdf.

Ellis, B. J. & Garber, J. (2000). Psychosocial antecedents of variation in girls' pubertal timing: Maternal depression, stepfather presence, and marital and family stress. *Child Development, 71,* 485–501.

Erchull, M. J., Chrisler, J. C., Gorman, J. A., & Johnston-Robledo, I. (2001). Fact or fiction? A content analysis of education materials about menstruation. *Journal of Early Adolescence, 22,* 1304–1317.

Gomula, A. & Koziel, S. (2017). Secular trend and social variation in age at menarche among Polish school girls before and after the political transformation. *American Journal of Human Biology, 30,* e23048.

Gore, A. C., Chappell, V. A., Fenton, S. E., Flaws, J. A., Nadal, A., Prins, G. S., Toppari, J., & Zoeller, R. T. (2015). Executive summary to EDC-2: The Endocrine Society's second scientific statement on endocrine-disrupting chemicals. *Endocrine Reviews, 36,* 593–602.

Hall, K. S., Sales, J. M., Komro, K. A., & Santelli, J. (2016). The state of sex education in the United States. *Journal of Adolescent Health, 58,* 595–597.

Hawkey, A. J., Ussher, J. M., Perz, J., & Metusela, C. (2017). Experiences and constructions of menarche and menstruation among migrant and refugee women. *Qualitative Health Research, 27,* 1473–1490.

Hawkey, A. J., Ussher, J. M., & Perz, J. (2018). "If you don't have a baby, you can't be in our culture": Migrant and refugee women's experiences and constructions of fertility and fertility control. *Women's Reproductive Health, 5,* 75–98.

Hermann-Giddens, M. E., Slora, E. J., Wasserman, R. C., Bourdony, C. J., Bhapkar, M. V., Koch, G. G., & Hasemeier, C. M. (1997). Secondary sexual characteristics and menses in young girls seen in office practice: A study from the pediatric research in office setting network. *Pediatrics, 99,* 505–512.

Hermann-Giddens, M. E., Steffes, J., Harris, D., Slora, E., Hussey, M., Dowshen, S. A., & Reiter, E. O. (2012). Secondary sexual characteristics in boys: Data from the pediatric research in office settings network. *Pediatrics, 130*(5), e1058–e1068.

Hillard, P. J. (2008). Menstruation in adolescence: What's normal, what's not. *Annals of the New York Academy of Sciences, 1135,* 29–35.

Hillard, P. J. (2014). Menstruation in adolescents: What do we know? And what do we do with the information? *Journal of Pediatric & Adolescent Gynecology, 27*, 309–319.

Hurwitz, L. B., Lauricella, A. R., Hightower, B., Sroka, I., Woodrullf, T. K., & Wartella, E. (2017). "When you're a baby you don't have puberty": Understanding of puberty and human reproduction in late childhood and early adolescence. *Journal of Early Adolescence, 37*, 925–947.

Jasik, C. B. & Lustig, R. H. (2008). Adolescent obesity and puberty: The "perfect storm". *Annals of the New York Academy of Science, 1135*, 265–279.

Juul, F., Chang, V. W., Brar, P., & Parekh, N. (2017). Birth weight, early life weight gain and age at menarche: A systematic review of longitudinal studies. *Obesity Reviews, 18*, 1272–1288.

Kaplowitz, P. & Bloch, C. (2016). Evaluation and referral of children with signs of early puberty. *Pediatrics, 37*(1), e20153732.

Kim, S. H., Huh, K., Won, S., Lee, K.-W., & Park, M.-J. (2015). A significant increase in the incidence of central precocious puberty among Korean girls from 2004 to 2010. *PLoS ONE, 10*, e0141844.

King, M. & Ussher, J. M. (2012). It's not all bad: Women's construction and lived experience of positive premenstrual change. *Feminism & Psychology, 23*, 399–417.

Koff, E. (1983). Through the looking glass of menarche: What the adolescent girl sees. In S. Golub (Ed.), *Menarche* (pp 77–86). Lexington, MA: D. C. Heath Publishers.

Koff, E. & Rierdan, J. (1995). Preparing girls for menstruation: Recommendations from adolescent girls. *Adolescence, 30*, 795–811.

Kreiger, N., Kiang, M. V., Kosheleva, A., Waterman, P. D., Chen, J. T., & Beckfield, J. (2015). Age at menarche: 50-year socioeconomic trends among US-born Black and White women. *American Journal of Public Health, 105*, 388–397.

Lee, M.-H., Kim, S. H., Oh, M., Lee, K.-W., & Park, M.-J. (2016). Age at menarche in Korean adolescents: Trends and influencing factors. *Reproductive Health, 13*, 1–7.

Manfredi-Lozano, M., Roa, J., Ruiz-Pino, F., Piet, R., Garcia-Galiano, D., Pineda, R., & Tena-Semoere, M. (2016). Defining a novel leptin—melancocortin—kisspeptin pathway involved in the metabolic control of puberty. *Molecular Metabolism, 5*, 844–857.

Marshall, W. A. & Tanner, J. M. (1969). Variations in pattern of pubertal changes in girls. *Archives of Disease in Childhood, 44*, 291–303.

Marvàn, M. L. & Alcalá-Herrera, V. (2020). Menarche: Psychosocial and cultural aspects. In J. Ussher, J. Chrisler, & J. Perz, (Eds), *Routledge international handbook of women's sexual and reproductive health*, (pp. xx–xx). Abingdon, UK: Routledge.

Mendel, J. (2014). Beyond pubertal timing: New directions for studying individual differences in development. *Current Directions in Psychological Science, 23*, 215–219.

Mendel, J. & Ferrero, J. (2012). Detrimental psychological outcomes associated with pubertal timing in adolescent boys. *Developmental Review, 32*, 49–66.

Meng, X., Li, S., Duan, W., Sun, Y., & Jia, C. (2017). Secular trend of age at menarche in Chinese adolescents born from 1973 to 2004. *Pediatrics, 140*, e20170085.

Mouritsen, A., Aksglaede, L., Sørensen, K., Morganson, S., Leffers, H., Main, K. M., & Juul, A. (2010). Hypothesis: Exposure to endocrine-disrupting chemicals may interfere with the timing of puberty. *International Journal of Andrology, 33*, 346–359.

Negriff, S., Saxbe, D. E., & Trickett, P. K. (2015). Childhood maltreatment, pubertal development, HPA axis functioning, and psychosocial outcomes: An integrative biopsychosocial model. *Developmental Psychobiology, 57*, 984–993.

Papadimitriou, A. (2016). The evolution of the age at menarche from prehistorical to modern times. *Journal of Pediatric & Adolescent Gynecology, 29*, 527–630.

Pathak, P. K., Tripathi, N., & Subramanian, S. V. (2014). Secular trends in menarcheal age in India: Evidence from the Indian Human Development Survey. *PLoS One, 9*, e111027.

Piran, N. (2017). *Journeys of embodiment at the intersection of body and culture: The developmental theory of embodiment.* Cambridge, MA: Academic Press.

Rheinländer, T., Gyapong, M., Akpakli, D. E., & Konradsen, F. (2019). Secrets, shame and discipline: School girls' experiences of sanitation and menstrual hygiene management in a peri-urban community in Ghana. *Health Care for Women International, 40*, 13–32.

Rierdan, J. & Koff, E. (1985). Timing of menarche and initial menstrual experience. *Journal of Youth and Adolescence, 14*, 237–244.

Rierdan, J., Koff, E., & Stubbs, M. L. (1989). Timing of menarche and initial menstrual experience: Replication and further analysis in a prospective study. *Journal of Youth and Adolescence, 18*, 413–426.

Roberts, T.-A. (2004). Female trouble: The menstrual self-evaluation scale and women's self- objectification. *Psychology of Women Quarterly*, *28*, 22–26.

Roberts, T.-A. & Waters, P. L. (2004). Self-objectification and that "not so fresh feeling": Feminist therapeutic interventions for healthy female embodiment. *Women & Therapy*, *27*(3–4), 5–21.

Ruttle, P. L., Shirtcliff, E. A., Armstrong, J. M., Klein, M., & Essex, M. J. (2013). Neuroendocrine coupling across adolescence and the longitudinal influence of early life stress. *Developmental Psychobiology*, *57*, 688–704.

Said-Mohamed, R., Prioreschi, A., Nyati, L., van Heerden, A., Munthali, R. J., Kahn, K., Tollman, S. M., Gómez-Olivé, F. X., Houle, B., Dunger, D. B., & Norris, S. A. (2018). Rural-urban variation in age at menarche, adult height, leg-length and abdominal adiposity in Black South African women in transitioning South Africa. *Annals of Human Biology*, *5*, 123–132.

Schoeters, G., Hond, E. D., Dhooge, W., van Larebeke, N., & Leijs, M. (2008). Endocrine disruptors and abnormalities of pubertal development. *Basic & Clinical Pharmacology and Toxicology*, *102*, 168–175.

Shakeel, M. K., George, P. S., Jose, J., Jose, J., & Mathew, A. (2010). Pesticides and breast cancer risk: A comparison between developed and developing countries. *Asian Pacific Journal of Cancer Prevention*, *10*, 173–180.

Shirtcliff, E. A., Dismukes, A. R., Marceau, K., Ruttle, P. L., Simmons, J. G., & Han, G. (2015). A dual-axis approach to understanding neuroendocrine development. *Developmental Psychobiology*, *57*, 643–653.

Sommer, M., Caruso, B. A., Sahin, M., Calderon, T., Cavill, S., Mahon, T., & Phillips-Howard, P. A. (2016). A time for global action: Addressing girls' menstrual hygiene management needs in schools. *PLOS Medicine*, *13*(2), e1001962.

Steinberg, L., Cauffman, E., Woolard, J., Graham, S., & Banich, M. (2009). Are adolescents less mature than adults? Minors' access to abortion, the juvenile death penalty, and the alleged APA "flip-flop". *American Psychologist*, *61*, 583–594.

Steinberg, L. & Scott, E. S. (2003). Less guilty by reason of adolescence: Developmental immaturity, diminished responsibility, and the juvenile death penalty. *American Psychologist*, *58*, 1009–1018.

Sterling, E. W. (2018, November). *Menstrual health education in the United States: Opportunities for improvement and barriers to change.* San Diego, CA: American Public Health Association.

Sterling, E. W., Karczmarczyk, D., & Ivabze, I. (2017, November). *Menstrual health is public health: The importance of menstrual cycle education.* Paper presented at the meeting of the American Public Health Association, Atlanta, GA.

Stubbs, M. L. (2008). Cultural perceptions and practices around menarche and adolescent menstruation in the United States. *Annals of the New York Academy of Sciences*, *1135*, 55–66.

Stubbs, M. L. (2013, June). *Current menstrual education resources: Still room for improvement.* Paper presented at the 20th biennial conference of the Society for Menstrual Cycle Research, New York, NY.

Stubbs, M. L. (2016). A developmental perspective on adolescents' reproductive self-care. *Women's Reproductive Health*, *3*, 100–105.

Summers-Effler, E. (2004). Little girls in women's bodies: Social interaction and the stigmatizing of early breast development. *Sex Roles*, *52*, 29–24.

Tekgül, N., Saltik, D., & Vatansever, K. (2014). Secular trend of menarche in an immigrant urban city in Turkey: İzmir. *Turkish Journal of Pediatrics*, *56*, 138–143.

Tither, J. M. & Ellis, B. J. (2008). Impact of fathers on daughters' age at menarche: A genetically and environmentally controlled sibling study. *Developmental Psychology*, *44*, 1409–1420.

United Nations Educational, Scientific and Cultural Organization (UNESCO) (2014). *Good policy and practice in health education: Puberty education and menstrual hygiene management.* Paris, France: UNESCO.

Wacharasindhu, S. (2009). A trend of normal puberty around the world. *Siriraj Medical Journal*, *61*, 1–2.

Woods, C. S. (2013). Repunctuated feminism: Marketing menstrual suppression through the rhetoric of choice. *Women's Studies in Communication*, *36*, 267–281.

2

MENARCHE

Psychosocial and cultural aspects

Maria Luisa Marván and Verónica Alcalá-Herrera

Menarche is probably the most important change of puberty for girls because it is a landmark of physical maturity and it occurs suddenly and without warning unlike other gradual physical changes. Menarche not only involves a biological transformation in girls' bodies, but also demands emotional and social adjustments to them. Moreover, the way in which menarche is experienced may exert a later impact on women's reproductive health, sexuality, and lifestyle behaviors (Estanislau, Hardy, & Hebling, 2011).

Although the particular meaning of menarche varies considerably in different cultures, it is always a significant event with a profound impact on girls' lives. In fact, memories of menarche are retained over a long time with surprising clarity. Kauder (2009), then an undergraduate student, edited an anthology of accounts about menarche from women and girls around the world, who shared their thoughts and feelings. The accounts range from the first half of the last century to the first decade of this century, and were written by women who differed in age, race, religion, and sociocultural background. All of the women remembered their first periods with many details: where and when it happened, who was with them, whom they told about it, how they reacted, etc. It is worth noting that, although every woman has vivid memories of her menarche, almost none talk openly about it, probably because of feelings of embarrassment, shame, or disgust. However, the perception of menarche and the menstrual body by younger generations is changing, at least in some societies (Lee, 2009; Polak, 2006); some women even use the taboo of menstruation to their own advantage (Sharifi, 2018). In this chapter we discuss the main factors that influence how a girl experiences menarche, such as the sociocultural context in which she lives, the preparation she had received, and the age at which her menarche occurs.

Cultural meanings of menarche

The specific meaning of menarche varies widely across cultures. Although celebrations of menarche are rare, it is commemorated in some societies as a rite of passage that acknowledges that a girl is moving into womanhood. For example, in Zambia, girls stay at home until their first period finishes; they do not do any work and are treated like "queens." In some places in India, a large party is organized for the menarcheal girl, and she receives gifts of jewelry. However, not all the rituals involve gifts or celebrations; for instance, in another region of India menarche is associated with an internal wound that needs healing, and dietary changes are thought to be necessary to strengthen the reproductive system. In rural Turkey, a menarcheal girl gets a slap from her mother or another woman who is present at the time she gets her first period, as a symbolic act to remind the girl that she has reached a new stage in her development and thus has to be careful and prudent (Hawkey, Ussher, Perz, & Metusela, 2017; Soumya & Sequira, 2016; Uskul, 2004). In a cross-cultural study, college students from Lithuania, the US, Malaysia, and Sudan were asked to write an account of their first menstruation. Although no woman mentioned any public celebration, some of them mentioned that an adult relative (mainly mothers) had congratulated them or given them a gift (Chrisler & Zittel, 1998).

In most Western societies menarche is usually a private event that is treated as a hygiene crisis. That is, the first menstrual period has been reduced from a sign of womanhood to a problem that needs to be managed in a confidential and hygienic way using the "right" products; this approach de-emphasizes the emotional and other developmental aspects of puberty. Moreover, girls are taught that menstruation is a normal, natural event, but told it should be hidden (Stubbs, 2008), a paradoxical message that implies that menstruation is both healthy and stigmatized. Although there have been attempts to promote the celebration of menarche and menstruation, positive messages could be minimized by the stigmatizing messages; girls may become confused about how to celebrate something that is supposed to be hidden (Johnston-Robledo & Chrisler, 2013). The first author's research team asked a group of postmenarcheal girls and their mothers to list words that define the concept "menstruation." There were some similarities between how a mother defined menstruation and how her daughter did. Both mothers and daughters used more words with negative connotations than with positive connotations, and they defined menstruation as something natural but annoying. Mothers also defined menstruation as "dirty" (Marván, Cortés-Iniestra, & González-Aguilera, 2014). If adults believe that menstruation is annoying and dirty, they will transmit this view to their young daughters before the girls experience their menarche.

The taboo of menstruation is broadly seen worldwide, and euphemisms have been invented in many languages to avoid saying the words "menstruation" or "menses," both in daily informal talks and in the popular press. Some examples are "my moon," "the curse," "Aunt Flo," "big red," "my friend's visit," "those days," "monthly bill," "my communist friend," "red aunt," "red king," "cardinals," "bloated," "the illness," "bad time," and "bingo" (Delaney, Lupton, & Toth, 1988; Kauder, 2009; Sveen, 2016). Most girls try to keep their menses secret, especially from boys, who generally use what they know of the menses to taunt girls (Marván & Bejarano, 2005). According to some authors, knowing about menstruation provides boys with the opportunity to practice male power by ridiculing and oppressing girls (Diorio & Munro, 2000). Others have claimed that both the stigma and taboo of menstruation contribute to women's lower social status (Johnston-Robledo & Chrisler, 2013).

Advertisements for menstrual products have strengthened the taboo of menstruation by highlighting secrecy attitudes, which have also been reinforced by popular culture. In some content analyses of menstrual product advertisements from magazines directed to young adolescents, it has been shown that the ads portray menstruation as an annoying and secretive event with which girls have to struggle (Marván & Cortés-Iniestra, 2008). Premenarcheal girls are influenced by these messages, which affect their views about menarche and menstruation. For example, in a study conducted with premenarcheal Mexican girls, their most prevailing attitudes towards menstruation were secretive; the girls believed that it would be too embarrassing if menstrual blood or hygiene products became visible (Marván, Espinosa-Hernàndez, & Vacío, 2002). These beliefs, together with negative messages from mothers, as well as advertisements and other media messages, might lead premenarcheal girls to form negative attitudes toward menstruation, which in turn influence how they experience their menarche and their subsequent menses. If menstruation were discussed more openly, it would be easier for girls to acknowledge the positive aspects of it, and their experience of menarche might also be more positive. There is some evidence to suggest that discussions about menstruation among American girls are changing in tone; an analysis of forums in which young adolescents share information, such as message boards, chat rooms, and online social networking sites, indicate that girls talk openly about menstrual experiences and even encourage each other to talk about menstruation with their boyfriends (Polak, 2006). It is important for researchers to conduct similar analyses in other countries where there are more secretive attitudes toward menarche and menstruation.

In the cross-cultural study by Chrisler and Zittel (1998), some Malaysian and Sudanese women mentioned that their behavior became restricted when they reached menarche and that the freedom of childhood was over. One Malaysian woman wrote that she had told the boys that she could not play with them anymore because she had "asthma." This narrative is similar to others found in a recent study carried out with Jordanian adolescent girls (Al Omari, Abdel Razeq, & Fooladi, 2016). By the time of menarche, girls had realized how to distinguish between appropriate and inappropriate behaviors during menstruation (Sharifi, 2018), and they began to change their daily activities. The fact that premenarcheal girls were taught about activities that they should and should not do while menstruating predicts that years later they will still believe that menstruation implies limitations in daily activities (Lee & Sasser-Coen, 1996; Marván & Trujillo, 2010). This is an example of how cultural constructions of menstruation put women in a restrictive and disadvantaged position with respect to men from the time they reach menarche. Although girls around the world are taught to restrict their behavior during menstruation, there are specific behavioral prescriptions and proscriptions that prevail in some cultures more than in others.

Emotional reactions to menarche

The experience of menarche is influenced by several factors, such as the kind of preparation a girl has received, her knowledge, her expectations, her age, the emotional support from her family, and her own personality traits. In several studies conducted in the US and Canada during last century, menarche was associated with a series of contradictory beliefs and feelings, and girls reported having experienced a mixture of positive and negative feelings at the same time, such as happiness and fear; enthusiasm and anger; excitement and nervousness; anxiety and pleasure; acceptance and rejection; support and loneliness; self-control and loss of control (Andrews, 1985; Golub & Catalano, 1983; Morse & Doan, 1987; Petersen, 1983). Unlike those findings, in a more recent study conducted with undergraduate students in the US, women remembered menarche as "no big deal" (p. 625) and reported more positive experiences of menarche and less shame and humiliation than in the past, even though secrecy surrounding menstruation was still present (Lee, 2009). However, after a review of the literature from 2000 to 2014 on the puberty experiences of low-income girls in the US, the authors concluded that most girls report having had negative experiences of menarche, such as embarrassment, fear, confusion, and annoyance (Herbert et al., 2016).

Other studies conducted during the current century in developing countries, such as Pakistan (Ali & Rizvi, 2009), India (Kumar & Srivastava, 2011), Iran (Hagikhani-Golchin, Hamzehgardeshi, Fakhri, & Hamzehgardeshi, 2012), and Brazil (da Silva, Tadini, Dias de

Freitas, & Goellner, 2012), also show that many adolescents report fear and worry at menarche. Hawkey et al. (2017) recently conducted a study with migrant and refugee women resettled in Australia and Canada who were from Afghanistan, Iraq, Somalia, South Sudan, Sudan, Sri Lanka, and various South American countries. Although the women had different cultural and religious backgrounds, they expressed similar negative constructions of menarche and menstruation. The researchers concluded that, as a result of menstrual shame and stigma, many women experience menarche with a complete absence of knowledge about their bodies. In a study carried out with a large sample of more than 1,500 Chinese postmenarcheal girls, almost 85% of them reported having felt annoyed and embarrassed at menarche; however, despite these negative feelings, many girls also reported having felt as if they were becoming more feminine (Tang, Yeung, & Lee, 2003). Other studies have also shown that girls still experience menarche in an ambivalent way (Fernández, 2012). Although menstruation is more openly discussed today, becoming a menstruating woman may still create confusion in girls because they receive mixed messages (Marván, Morales, & Cortés-Iniestra, 2006): menarche is upsetting and traumatic, but girls must behave normally; menarche is a symbol of sexual maturity, but it is also a secretive and mysterious event (Brooks-Gunn & Ruble, 1980; Kissling, 1996).

Emotional responses to menarche are largely influenced by attitudes toward menstruation, which are shaped by the immediate environment and the culture in which a girl grows up. Prior to menarche, girls internalize many of the prevailing cultural views of menstruation; unfortunately, these views are mainly negative. Attitudes toward menstruation as a healthy sign of womanhood predict the most positive menarcheal experiences (Rierdan & Koff, 1990). Positive emotional reactions to menarche are also associated with perceptions of menstruation as a natural event and rejection of negative attitudes toward menstruation; on the contrary, negative emotional responses to menarche are related to perceptions of menstruation as a negative event (Tang et al., 2003).

At the same time, early menstrual experiences are related to menstrual attitudes later in life. Adult women who had had extremely negative menarcheal experiences report more current negative menstrual attitudes than do women who had had more positive menarcheal experiences (McPherson & Korfine, 2004). In a recent study in which undergraduate women were asked to complete the phrase "my first menstruation was …" with single words, it was shown that positive emotional reactions to menarche predict later pleasant attitudes toward menstruation, whereas negative reactions predict secretive attitudes (Marván & Chrisler, 2018).

Reaching menarche earlier or later than peers may play an important role in how menarche is experienced. Both early and late maturers are viewed as "out of step" with their peers, which could be either an advantage or disadvantage, depending on the values of the peer group (Greif & Ulman, 1982). In general, early maturers show higher anxiety and a greater degree of worry about menstruation than their peers do (Natsuaki, Leve, & Mendle, 2011; Stubbs, Rierdan, & Koff, 1989), are more likely to have felt scared and sad at menarche, and tend to endorse secretive attitudes (Marván & Alcalá-Herrera, 2014).

Preparing girls for menarche

Preparation for menarche has been associated with menarcheal experience, as well as with later attitudes toward menstruation. Women who considered themselves more prepared, as compared with those who think they were unprepared, had a more positive experience of menarche and hold more positive attitudes toward menstruation (Marván & Molina, 2012;

Rierdan & Koff, 1990; Tang et al., 2003). However, the information given to girls is not always timely nor is it necessarily adequate. After a review of the literature published between the years 2000 and 2015 regarding the experience of girls from 25 different low- and middle-income countries, Chandra-Mouli and Patel (2017) concluded that many girls are uninformed and unprepared for menarche. Moreover, in some places girls are frequently not informed about menstruation until after menarche; for example, in a recent study conducted in rural Varanasi (India), only one-third of the girls surveyed were aware of menstruation before menarche (Kansal, Singh, & Kumar, 2016).

For many decades, both researchers and practitioners of health education have been concerned about the poor preparation that premenarcheal girls generally receive, probably due to the silence surrounding menstruation, because much of the information is impersonal and difficult for girls to assimilate and because girls frequently have difficulty expressing their feelings about pubertal issues. But there are also other problems inherent to preparation for menarche; for example, girls who live with their father as the primary caretaker find it embarrassing to discuss menstruation with him even if they have a close relationship. They believe that their father lacks credibility concerning menstrual issues, and therefore behave in a distancing way and do not feel comfortable asking their fathers anything about the issue (Kalman, 2003). Moreover, at the first indication of pubertal development, there are some girls who, because they do not want their bodies to change, "decide" they will not grow up and will not have menses, regardless of the information received. They may excuse themselves from learning about something that they believe could not happen to them because they will never menstruate (Gillooly, 2004). It is important that girls learn to conceptualize abstract concepts such as menstruation and that adults prepare them to handle the onset of physical maturity and reproductive life. After pubertal changes, the body could be positioned as a site of shame or as healthy and normal.

Prior to menarche, girls in most countries are exposed to various formal and informal sources of information about menstruation and menarche, such as from mothers, other adult family members, siblings, friends, teachers, books, booklets, websites, medical personnel, magazines, and films. Despite this variety of sources, mothers typically remain the primary source. How a mother discusses issues related to menarche and menstruation with her premenarcheal daughter influences the girl's experience of menarche. If mothers transmit a positive view of menarche, then their daughters, for the most part, develop more positive, or, at least, less negative, attitudes. On the contrary, if mothers transmit a negative view, the daughters are more likely to develop more negative attitudes.

Mothers are not necessarily comfortable or competent when they discuss menstruation with their premenarcheal daughters, due to embarrassment, lack of knowledge, lack of experience in how to handle the discussion, a poor mother–daughter relationship, or because they are uncomfortable with the idea that their daughters will soon be capable of sexuality and reproduction (Bhartiya, 2013; Cooper & Knoch, 2007; Costos, Ackerman, & Paradis, 2002; Herbert et al., 2016). Unfortunately, many mothers regard the task of preparing their daughters for menarche as something necessary but difficult to initiate (Gillooly, 2004). Sometimes, even though mothers explicitly depict menstruation as a natural event in a woman's life, the way in which they express this may inadvertently suggest the opposite to their daughters (Kissling, 1996). As mothers have a fundamental role in preparing their daughters for menarche, they should try to develop positive attitudes, be well informed on the topic, and be emotionally supportive. Although maternal emotional support at the time of menarche has been associated with positive experiences of menarche, some women who had maternal emotional support still recall negative memories of menarche (Lee, 2008).

Teaching about menstruation is not restricted to mothers; schools also play an important role in menstrual education. Therefore, the first author's research team explored how Mexican premenarcheal girls and their teachers view the preparation for menstruation received at school (Marván & Bejarano, 2005). Both teachers and students agreed that the most discussed topics in class were hygiene and body function, but there were some important discrepancies between what girls and teachers said. For example, although most teachers claimed they had discussed the emotional aspects of menses, few girls said the same. Another worrisome inconsistency was that teachers believed that their students were better prepared for menarche than the students considered themselves to be. When education focuses only on hygiene and biological aspects of menstruation, it can cause a disconnection between knowledge and a girl's own bodily experience that makes it difficult for girls to relate the received information to themselves and their bodies. Practical and biological information need to be combined with discussion of the emotional aspects of the menses (Koff & Rierdan, 1995).

Since the early 1980s, women have stressed that information about menstruation as a biological event is insufficient preparation for menarche; they need to be more informed about the concrete experience of menstruating (Rierdan, Koff, & Flaherty, 1983). However, it seems that not much has changed since then in most countries. Girls would be better prepared than they currently are if they were told about the emotional aspects of menarche and menstruation. In fact, girls who had discussed the emotional and experiential aspects prior to menarche are more likely than their peers to report that they had felt prepared to start menstruating when they got their first period and more likely to show positive attitudes toward menstruation when they become postmenarcheal (Marván & Molina, 2012).

Is age at menarche important?

Age at menarche varies among women across cultures; in developed countries where individuals have the longest life expectancies, menarche is earlier, which has been associated with better nutritional conditions. Moreover, age at menarche also differs between women in well-off and underprivileged conditions within the same country (Thomas, Renaud, Benefice, de Meeus, & Guegan, 2001; Yermachenko & Dvornyk, 2014).

There was a trend toward a lower age at menarche during the 20th century, which was more evident in the industrialized countries, probably because of the improvement in socioeconomic conditions (Papadimitriou, 2016). Whether this trend is continuing or not in the current century is a matter of debate. According to some authors, this trend has tended to slow down or stabilize in the most developed nations (Karapanou & Papadimitriou, 2010; Papadimitriou, 2016), whereas age at menarche has continued to lower in some developing countries (Marván, Castillo, Alcalá-Herrera, & del Callejo, 2016).

The trend towards earlier ages at menarche may have multiple health implications that are important to take into consideration even though the mechanisms of them are not clear (Jae-Hoo, 2016). It is also important to take into account that this trend has coincided with later ages of psychosocial maturity and, therefore, physical maturity is outpacing cognitive and emotional development. This gap between physical and psychosocial maturity could cause girls to engage in risky behaviors such as substance abuse, antisocial behavior, or deliberate self-harm (Mendle, 2014; Moffitt, 1993; Patton & Viner, 2007).

Although body mass index and genetic heritage play an important role in determining age at menarche, psychosocial factors have also been associated with menarcheal timing. For example, menarche occurs at an earlier age among girls raised in stressful family circumstances, such as divorce, increased family conflict, or longer durations of father absence (Jean et al., 2011; Mendle et al., 2006). Sexual abuse and subjective perception of environmental danger are other stressful life experiences that have been associated with early menarche (Amir, Jordan, & Bribiescas, 2016; Gamble, 2017; Mendle, Leve, Ryzir, Natsuaki, & Ge, 2011).

Reaching menarche earlier than one's peers could have important consequences for girls because they do not have enough time to acquire, integrate, and strengthen adaptive and coping skills to guarantee an effective transition from childhood to adolescence, which leads to an asynchrony between physical and cognitive and social maturity (Allison & Hyde, 2013). For example, due to their early physical development, older people may perceive these girls as having greater maturity and therefore force them to face certain challenges before they are emotionally or cognitively prepared to do so (Mendle, Turkheimer, & Emergy, 2007). In this sense, early maturing girls are more vulnerable to older peer pressures, and are more likely than later maturing girls to have older peers who engage in deviant behaviors (Ge et al., 1996), such as alcohol and drug use or engagement in petty crimes. Early menarche is also a risk factor for sexual harassment because the development of visible secondary sexual characteristics could attract the attention and interest of older boys and men (Allison & Hyde, 2013). Another consequence is social victimization; if a boy supposes that a girl has had her first period when she is too young, he may tease or bully her (Allison & Hyde, 2013).

Researchers have found that early menarche may predispose girls to other emotional problems, such as depressive symptoms, anxiety, eating disorders, social isolation, antisocial behavior, self-harming behaviors, substance abuse, or suicidal ideation (Alcalá-Herrera & Marván, 2014; Copeland et al., 2010; Deng et al., 2011; Gaudineau et al., 2010; Meghan & Oinonen, 2011; Mendle, Ryan, & McKone, 2018; Platt, Colich, McLaughlin, Gary, & Keyes, 2017). Some of these emotional problems may continue into adulthood (Mendle et al., 2018). Early menarche has also been associated with early sexual initiation, early pregnancy and childbirth, and sexually transmitted infections (Ibitoye, Choi, Tai, Lee, & Sommer, 2017). As we pointed out above, some researchers who focus on menarcheal timing and girls' experiences of menstruation have concluded that menarche is more difficult for early maturers.

In recent years it has been demonstrated that sex hormones are not only related to reproductive maturity, but also to brain maturity. There is an accelerated growth of neural connections in adolescents' brains; of particular importance are the limbic-cortical circuits that participate in the analysis of risk situations, decision making, planning, self-regulation of behaviors, and impulse control (Sawyer, Azzopardi, Wickremarathne, & Patton, 2018; Vigil et al., 2011). Frontal cortical areas reach their full maturity in early adulthood to consolidate intellectual capacity and emotional regulation, and strengthen social relationships (Sawyer et al., 2018). In girls with early menarche the activation of these systems is accelerated (Jetha & Segalowitz, 2012; Van Wingen, Ossewaarde, Bäckström, & Hermans, 2011); thus, earlier age at menarche has been associated with higher performance IQ (Noipayak, Rawdaree, Supawattanabodee, & Manusirivitthaya, 2016), although not all the researchers have found the same result. Moreover, some years later, adolescents who experienced early menarche use fewer non-productive coping strategies than their peers do. Due to the vulnerability caused by reaching their menarche so early, they could have been confronted with more difficult situations to manage, and, consequently, they have learned not to use non-productive coping strategies (Alcalá-Herrera & Marván, 2014). Despite these abilities, early maturers need special support to diminish the gap between their physical and psychosocial maturity.

On the other hand, by the time that most girls have reached menarche, the few girls who have not yet experienced it may feel uncomfortable with their maturational status and look forward to experiencing, as their peers do, the visible manifestations of puberty that come along with menarche. Therefore, compared with their peers, they are more likely to have more positive reactions to menarche as well as more positive attitudes toward menstruation (Marván & Alcalá-Herrera, 2014).

Conclusion

As menarche is a biological event permeated with cultural, social, and personal significance, it is important for girls to be well prepared to experience it. However, girls are more often advised about how to cope with practical aspects of menstruation than about how to deal with their feelings. Becoming a menstruating woman usually creates confusion in girls because they so often receive mixed messages; they are taught that menarche is a proud marker of womanhood but, ironically, that it is important to hide any of trace of it. During the current century there has been greater openness about menstruation in some countries, but, despite this increased openness, preparing girls for menarche remains problematic.

The findings described in this chapter stress the necessity of intensifying our efforts to provide a more complete menstrual education in which more emphasis should be put on discussion of the emotional aspects of menarche. Parents, teachers, and health educators should be aware of the emotional and cognitive development of girls that allows them to conceptualize abstract concepts such as menstruation and prepares them for coping with the beginning of physical maturity. Educators should be able to relate to girls, maintain open communication with them, and willingly discuss girls' concerns.

References

Al Omari, O., Abdel Razeq, N. M., & Fooladi, M. M. (2016). Experience of menarche among Jordanian adolescent girls: An interpretive phenomenological analysis. *Journal of Pediatric and Adolescent Gynecology*, *29*, 246–251.

Alcalá-Herrera, V. & Marván, M. L. (2014). Early menarche, depressive symptoms, and coping strategies. *Journal of Adolescence*, *37*, 905–913.

Ali, T. S. & Rizvi, S. N. (2009). Menstrual knowledge and practices of female adolescents in urban Karachi, Pakistan. *Journal of Adolescence Health*, *33*, 531–541.

Allison, C. & Hyde, J. S. (2013). Early menarche: Confluence of biological and contextual factors. *Sex Roles*, *68*, 55–64.

Amir, D., Jordan, M. R., & Bribiescas, R. G. (2016). A longitudinal assessment of associations between adolescent environment, adversity perception, and economic status on fertility and age of menarche. *PLoS ONE*, *11*(6), 1–16.

Andrews, S. (1985). The experience of menarche: An exploratory study. *Journal of Nurse-Midwifery*, *30*(1), 9–14.

Bhartiya, A. (2013). Menstruation, religion, and society. *International Journal of Social Science and Humanity*, *3*, 523–527.

Brooks-Gunn, J. & Ruble, D. (1980). Menarche: The interaction of physiological, cultural, and social factors. In A. J. Dan, E. A. Graham, & C. P. Beecher (Eds), *The menstrual cycle* (pp. 141–159). New York: Springer.

Chandra-Mouli, V. & Patel, S. (2017). Mapping the knowledge and understanding of menarche, menstrual hygiene, and menstrual health among adolescent girls in low- and middle-income countries. *Reproductive Health, 14*(1), 30–47.

Chrisler, J. C. & Zittel, C. B. (1998). Menarche stories: Reminiscences of college students from Lithuania, Malaysia, Sudan, and the United States. *Health Care for Women International, 19*, 303–312.

Cooper, S. C. & Knoch, B. P. (2007). "Nobody told me nothing": Communication about menstruation among low-income African-American women. *Women's Health, 46*(1), 57–78.

Copeland, W., Shanahan, L., Miller, S., Costello, J., Angold, A., & Maughan, B. (2010). Outcomes of early pubertal timing in young women: A prospective population-based study. *The American Journal of Psychiatry, 167*, 1218–1225.

Costos, D., Ackerman, R., & Paradis, L. (2002). Recollections of menarche: Communication between mothers and daughters regarding menstruation. *Sex Roles, 46*, 49–59.

da Silva, B. J., Tadini, A. C., Dias de Freitas, M. J., & Goellner, M. B. (2012). Meaning of menarche according to adolescents. *Acta Paulista de Enfermagem, 25*, 249–255.

Delaney, J., Lupton, M. J., & Toth, E. (1988). *The curse: A cultural history of menstruation.* Urbana: University of Illinois Press.

Deng, F., Tao, F., Wan, Y., Hao, J., Su, P., & Cao, Y. X. (2011). Early menarche and psychopathological symptoms in young Chinese women. *Journal of Women's Health, 20*, 207–213.

Diorio, J. & Munro, J. (2000). Doing harm in the name of protection: Menstruation as a topic for sex education. *Gender and Education, 12*, 347–366.

Estanislau, M., Hardy, E., & Hebling, E. (2011). Menarche among Brazilian women: Memories of experiences. *Midwifery, 27*, 203–208.

Fernández, O. D. (2012). Los tabúes de la menarquia: Un acercamiento a la vivencia de jóvenes escolares chilenas [The taboos of menarche: An approach to the experiences of Chilean schoolgirls]. *Revista de Psicología, 21*(1), 7–29.

Gamble, J. (2017). Puberty: Early starters. Girls are entering puberty at ever younger ages. What are the causes, and should we be worried? *Nature International Journal of Science, 550*, 10–11.

Gaudineau, A., Ehlinger, V., Vayssiere, C., Jouret, B., Arnaud, B., & Godeau, E. (2010). Factors associated with early menarche: Results from the French health behaviour in school-aged children (HBSC) study. *BioMed Central Public Health, 38*, 385–387.

Ge, X., Conger, R. D., & Eldar, Jr., G. H. (1996). Coming of age too early: Pubertal influences on girls' vulnerability to psychological distress. *Child Development, 67*, 3386–3400.

Gillooly, J. B. (2004). Making menarche positive and powerful for both mother and daughter. In J. C. Chrisler (Ed.), *From menarche to menopause* (pp. 23–35). New York: Haworth Press.

Golub, S. & Catalano, J. (1983). Recollections of menarche and women's subsequent experiences with menstruation. *Women & Health, 8*(1), 49–61.

Greif, E. B. & Ulman, K. J. (1982). The psychological impact of menarche on early adolescent females: A review of the literature. *Child Development, 53*, 1413–1430.

Hagikhani-Golchin, N. A., Hamzehgardeshi, Z., Fakhri, M., & Hamzehgardeshi, L. (2012). The experience of puberty in Iranian adolescent girls: A qualitative content analysis. *BioMed Central Public Health, 12*(698), 1–8.

Hawkey, A. J., Ussher, J. M., Perz, J., & Metusela, C. (2017). Experiences and constructions of menarche and menstruation among migrant and refugee women. *Qualitative Health Research, 27*, 1473–1490.

Herbert, A. C., Ramirez, A. M., Grace, L., North, J. S., Askari, S. M., West, L. R., & Sommer, M. (2016). Puberty experiences of low-income girls in the United States: A systematic review of qualitative literature from 2000 to 2014. *Journal of Adolescent Health, 60*, 363–379.

Ibitoye, M., Choi, C., Tai, H., Lee, G., & Sommer, M. (2017). Early menarche: A systematic review of its effect on sexual and reproductive health in low- and middle-income countries. *PLoS One, 12*(6), e0178884.

Jae-Hoo, Y. (2016). Effects of early menarche on physical and psychosocial health problems in adolescent girls and adult women. *Korean Journal of Pediatrics, 59*, 355–361.

Jean, R. T., Wilkinson, A., Spitz, M., Prokhorov, A., Bondy, M., & Forman, M. (2011). Psychosocial risk and correlates of early menarche in Mexican-American girls. *American Journal of Epidemiology, 173*, 1023–1210.

Jetha, K. M. & Segalowitz, J. S. (2012). *Adolescent brain development: Implications for behavior.* Atlanta: Elsevier.

Johnston-Robledo, I. & Chrisler, J. C. (2013). The menstrual mark: Menstruation as social stigma. *Sex Roles, 68,* 9–18.

Kalman, M. B. (2003). Adolescent girls, single-parent fathers, and menarche. *Holistic Nursing Practice, 17*(1), 36–40.

Kansal, S., Singh, S., & Kumar, A. (2016). Menstrual hygiene practices in context of schooling: A community study among rural adolescent girls in Varanasi. *Indian Journal of Community Medicine, 41*(1), 39–44.

Karapanou, O. & Papadimitriou, A. (2010). Determinants of menarche. *Reproductive Biology and Endocrinology, 8*(1), 115.

Kauder, N. R. (2009). *My little red book.* New York: Twelve.

Kissling, E. A. (1996). Bleeding out loud: Communication about menstruation. *Feminism & Psychology, 6,* 481–504.

Koff, E. & Rierdan, J. (1995). Preparing girls for menstruation: Recommendations from adolescent girls. *Adolescence, 30,* 795–811.

Kumar, A. & Srivastava, K. (2011). Cultural and social practices regarding menstruation among adolescent girls. *Social Work in Public Health, 26,* 594–604.

Lee, J. (2008). "A Kotex and a smile": Mothers and daughters at menarche. *Journal of Family Issues, 29,* 1325–1347.

Lee, J. (2009). Bodies at menarche: Stories of shame, concealment, and sexual maturation. *Sex Roles, 60,* 615–627.

Lee, J. & Sasser-Coen, J. (1996). *Blood stories. Menarche and the politics of the female body in contemporary U.S. society.* New York: Routledge.

Marván, M. L. & Alcalá-Herrera, V. (2014). Age at menarche, reactions to menarche, and attitudes towards menstruation among Mexican adolescent girls. *Journal of Pediatric and Adolescent Gynecology, 27,* 61–66.

Marván, M. L. & Bejarano, J. (2005). Premenarcheal Mexican girls' and their teachers' perceptions of the preparation that students receive about menstruation at school. *Journal of School Health, 75*(3), 86–89.

Marván, M. L., Castillo, R. L., Alcalá-Herrera, V., & del Callejo, D. (2016). The decreasing age at menarche in Mexico. *Journal of Pediatric and Adolescent Gynecology, 29,* 454–457.

Marván, M. L. & Chrisler, J. C. (2018). Menarcheal timing, memories of menarche, and later attitudes toward menstruation. *Cogent Psychology, 5,* 1525840.

Marván, M. L. & Cortés-Iniestra, S. (2008). *Menstruación: Qué es y qué no es.* [Menstruation: What it is and what it is not]. Mexico City, Mexico: Pax.

Marván, M. L., Cortés-Iniestra, S., & González-Aguilera, R. (2014). Significado psicológico de la menstruación en madres e hijas [Psychological meaning of menstruation in mothers and daughters]. *Psicología Y Salud, 24*(1), 89–96.

Marván, M. L., Espinosa-Hernàndez, G., & Vacío, A. (2002). Premenarcheal Mexican girls' expectations concerning perimenstrual changes and menstrual attitudes. *Journal of Psychosomatic Obstetrics & Gynecology, 23,* 89–96.

Marván, M. L. & Molina, A. M. (2012). Mexican adolescents' experience of menarche and attitudes toward menstruation: Role of communication between mothers and daughters. *Journal of Pediatric and Adolescent Gynecology, 25,* 358–363.

Marván, M. L., Morales, C., & Cortés-Iniestra, S. (2006). Emotional reactions to menarche among Mexican women of different generations. *Sex Roles, 54,* 323–330.

Marván, M. L. & Trujillo, P. (2010). Menstrual socialization, beliefs, and attitudes concerning menstruation in rural and urban Mexican women. *Health Care for Women International, 31,* 53–67.

McPherson, M. E. & Korfine, L. (2004). Menstruation across time: Menarche, menstrual attitudes, experiences, and behaviors. *Women's Health Issues, 14,* 193–200.

Meghan, A. R. & Oinonen, K. A. (2011). Age at menarche is associated with divergent alcohol use patterns in early adolescence and early adulthood. *Journal of Adolescence, 34,* 1065–1076.

Mendle, J. (2014). Beyond pubertal timing: New directions for studying individual differences in development. *Current Directions in Psychological Science, 23,* 215–219.

Mendle, J., Leve, L., Ryzir, M., Natsuaki, M., & Ge, X. (2011). Associations between early life stress, child maltreatment, and pubertal development among girls in foster care. *Journal of Reasearch on Adolescence, 21,* 817–880.

Mendle, J., Ryan, R. M., & McKone, M. P. (2018). Age at menarche, depression, and antisocial behavior in adulthood. *Pediatrics, 141*(1), 1–10.

Mendle, J., Turkheimer, E., D'Onofrio, B. M., Lynch, S. K., Emery, R. E., Slutske, W. S., & Martin, N. G. (2006). Family structure and age at menarche: A children-of-twins approach. *Developmental Psychology, 42,* 533–542.

Mendle, J., Turkheimer, E., & Emergy, R. E. (2007). Detrimental psychological outcomes associated with early pubertal timing in adolescent girls. *Developmental Review, 27,* 151–171.

Moffitt, T. E. (1993). Adolescent-limited and life-course persistent antisocial behavior: A developmental taxonomy. *Psychological Review, 100,* 674–701.

Morse, J. M. & Doan, H. M. (1987). Adolescents' response to menarche. *Journal of School Health, 57,* 385–389.

Natsuaki, M. N., Leve, L. D., & Mendle, J. (2011). Going through the rites of passage: Timing and transition of menarche, childhood sexual abuse, and anxiety symptoms in girls. *Journal of Youth and Adolescence, 40,* 1357–1370.

Noipaya, P., Rawdaree, P., Supawattanabodee, B., & Manusirivitthaya, S. (2016). Age at menarche and performance intelligence quotients of adolescents in Bangkok, Thailand: A cross-sectional study. *BioMed Central Pediatric, 16,* 87–92.

Papadimitriou, A. (2016). The evolution of the age at menarche from prehistorical to modern times. *Journal of Pediatric and Adolescent Gynecology, 29,* 527–530.

Patton, G. C. & Viner, R. (2007). Pubertal transitions in health. *Lancet, 369,* 1130–1139.

Petersen, A. C. (1983). Menarche: Meaning of measures and measuring meaning. In S. Golub (Ed.), *Menarche* (pp. 63–76). Lexington: Lexington Books.

Platt, J. M., Colich, N. L., McLaughlin, K. A., Gary, D., & Keyes, K. M. (2017). Transdiagnostic psychiatric disorder risk associated with early age of menarche: A latent modeling approach. *Comprehensive Psychiatry, 79,* 70–79.

Polak, M. (2006). From the curse to the rag: Online URLs rewrite the menstruation narrative. In Y. Jiwani, C. Steenbergen, & C. Mitchell (Eds), *Girlhood: Redefining the limits* (pp. 191–207). New York: Black Rose Books.

Rierdan, J. & Koff, E. (1990). Premenarcheal predictors of the experience of menarche: A prospective study. *Journal of Adolescent Health Care, 11,* 404–407.

Rierdan, J., Koff, E., & Flaherty, J. (1983). Guidelines for preparing girls for menstruation. *Journal of the Academy of Child Psychiatry, 22,* 480–486.

Sawyer, M. S., Azzopardi, S. P., Wickremarathne, D., & Patton, C. G. (2018). The age of adolescence. *Lancet Child & Adolescent Health, 2,* 223–228.

Sharifi, N. (2018). *Female bodies and sexuality in Iran and the search for defiance.* London: Palgrave Macmillan.

Soumya, L. & Sequira, L. (2016). A descriptive study on cultural practices about menarche and menstruation. *Journal of Health Science, 6,* 10–13.

Stubbs, M., Rierdan, J., & Koff, E. (1989). Developmental differences in menstrual attitudes. *Journal of Early Adolescence, 9,* 480–498.

Stubbs, M. L. (2008). Cultural perceptions and practices around menarche and adolescent menstruation in the United States. *Annals of the New York Academy of Sciences, 1135,* 58–66.

Sveen, H. (2016). Lava or code red: A linguistic study of menstrual expressions in English and Swedish. *Women's Reproductive Health, 3,* 145–159.

Tang, C. S., Yeung, D. Y., & Lee, A. M. (2003). Psychosocial correlates of emotional responses to menarche among Chinese adolescent girls. *Journal of Adolescent Health, 33,* 193–201.

Thomas, F., Renaud, F., Benefice, E., de Meeus, T., & Guegan, J. F. (2001). International variability of ages at menarche and menopause: Patterns and main determinants. *Human Biology, 73,* 271–290.

Uskul, A. K. (2004). Women's menarche: Stories from a multicultural sample. *Social Science & Medicine, 59,* 667–679.

Van Wingen, G., Ossewaarde, L., Bäckström, T., & Hermans, E. F. (2011). Gonadal hormone regulation of the emotion circuitry in humans. *Neuroscience, 191,* 38–45.

Vigil, P., Orellana, R., Cortés, M., Molina, C., Switzer, B., & Klaus, H. (2011). Endocrine modulation of the adolescent brain: A review. *Journal of Pediatric and Adolescent Gynecology, 24,* 330–337.

Yermachenko, A. & Dvornyk, V. (2014). Nongenetic determinants of age at menarche: A systematic review. *BioMed Research International, 2014,* 1–14.

3

THE MENSTRUAL CYCLE

Its biology in the context of silent ovulatory disturbances

Jerilynn C. Prior

The menstrual cycle is a unique expression of an individual woman's integrated genetic, metabolic, physiological, and sociocultural life history (Mishra, Cooper, Tom, & Kuh, 2009). Further, an individual woman's experience of her menstrual cycles shapes her perceptions and ways of being in the world while also profoundly, often imperceptibly, altering her biology/physiology. Normal menstrual cycles are essential for women's holistic health as defined by the World Health Organization (2006) charter: "a state of complete physical, mental and social well-being and not merely the absence of disease or infirmity." In this chapter I provide an integrated physiological framework for the biology of the menstrual cycle and discuss its importance to women's sexual and reproductive health.

Biological understanding of menstrual cycles has undergone a revolution in the last 25 years (Prior, Vigna, Schechter, & Burgess, 1990). We now know that predictable, average-length menstrual cycles (defined as 21–35 days long; Abraham, 1978) may or may not involve release of an egg (the latter is known as *anovulation*). Or a cycle may be regular and ovulatory, but with a time of progesterone production from ovulation until the next flow that is too short for normal physiology and fertility (*short luteal phase*). The cycles that are clinically normal but with either anovulation or short luteal phases are described as *subclinical ovulatory disturbances*. This means that, rather than having a normal balance of progesterone and estrogen, the cycle is wholly or partially dominated by estrogen (actually *estradiol*) levels.

Estrogen and progesterone together make up a woman's hormonal reproductive *system* and are key partners. In every cell and tissue of women's bodies, estrogen acts as a powerful and continuous stimulant of cell growth (Clarke & Sutherland, 1990). Progesterone, by contrast, is briefly growth-stimulating in all the same tissues as estrogen, and then develops its major action to promote cellular maturation and continuously inhibit estrogen-stimulated cellular "overgrowth" (Clarke & Sutherland, 1990).

The presence or absence of ovulation and the duration/amount of progesterone production are highly variable within and between women; progesterone levels are higher, even in conception cycles, in women from economically well-off than women from lower-income countries (Vitzthum, Spielvogel, & Thornburg, 2004). Progesterone production is normally and universally lower (in amount and duration) in the several years following menarche and prior to the final menstrual flow. That this variability of ovulation and progesterone production is subclinical and silent (not perceptible to women or to health care providers) within "normal" cycles makes its self-knowledge and scientific documentation difficult. Furthermore the concept of subclinical ovulatory disturbances within regular cycles is highly contested by gynecologists (Malcolm & Cumming, 2003). The concept of *silent ovulatory disturbances* is revolutionary because it both changes and explains previously inexplicable data; it also integrates mind and body in ways that could lead to effective prevention of many diseases as well as to improved treatment of women's reproductive disturbances.

Ill health (in its broadest sense) predicts ovulatory disturbances, and ovulatory disturbances, in turn, are an important but clinically silent, risk factor for ill health. The good news is that these disturbances are usually totally reversible (Prior, Yeun, Clement, Bowie, & Thomas, 1982), but only if all dimensions of ill-health are healed (Michopoulos, Mancini, Loucks, & Berga, 2013; Prior, Vigna, Barr, Rexworthy, & Lentle, 1994). Furthermore, women with reversible cycle disturbances must *not* be inappropriately "treated" with the hypothalamus-suppressing high-dose estrogen in combined hormonal contraceptives (CHC) (Falsetti, Gambera, Barbetti, & Specchia, 2002; Prior, 2016). In avoiding and treating ovulatory disturbances, we could prevent the majority of pre-menopausal bone loss that leads to osteoporotic fractures (Prior, 2018), women's earlier (ages 40–60) heart attacks (Prior, 2014), most breast (Fournier, Berrino, & Clavel-Chapelon, 2008), and almost all endometrial cancers.

For the majority of women, periodic bleeding (menstruation) is normally present for 30–45 years, or for almost half of their lifespans. Because much of what we know about menstrual cycles is biased because it was derived from women seeking medical treatment (Kaufert & Syrotvik, 1981), the focus of this chapter is on population-based data. Therefore, I share how neuroendocrine variables are assessed, and interpret the social, physical, and internal nutritional environments that cause adaptations of reproduction that may lead to ovulatory disturbances. These ovulatory changes are the least disruptive of any potential reproductive adaptations for an individual woman's long-term, healthy survival and may help preserve her potential for later fertility.

Most women do not know (other than the "typical" 28 days) how long a menstrual cycle *should* last (from Day 1—the start of flow—to the day before the next flow), or how many days of menstrual bleeding are too many. Nor do they realize that women's normal menstrual cycle subtly influences how much they eat (Barr, Janelle, & Prior, 1995), the function of the heart's electrical system (Tisdale et al., 2016), the supply of oxygen to exercising muscles (Lebrun, McKenzie, Prior, & Taunton, 1995), and whether they are losing or gaining bone (Kalyan & Prior, 2010). Such ignorance is not bliss. It results in a fundamental "mind–body" disassociation that is ultimately damaging to women's health locus of control (Wallston, Wallston, & DeVellis, 1978) and makes them vulnerable to cultural bias (Kissling, 2006) and medical misogyny (e.g., Wilson, 1966).

That normally ovulatory cycles foretell later life bone health, fewer early-in-menopause heart attacks, and likely the prevention of many breast and most endometrial cancers is actively being censored by Medicine. This includes granting agencies, editors of major medical journals, peer reviewers of unknown gender and academic status, and in multiple other ways (Inhorn & Whittle, 2001). We need to acknowledge that silent ovulatory disturbances could be prevented by a more egalitarian society, by sex and gender equality, and by universal access to basic health care services (including counselling and social support).

Menstrual cycle organization and control

Menstruation's complex neuroendocrinology means that there is still much to be understood. Although summarized elsewhere (Navarro & Kaiser, 2013; Prior, 1987; Vitzthum, 2009), it is worth re-looking at the hormonal changes across the ideal menstrual cycle (Figure 3.1).

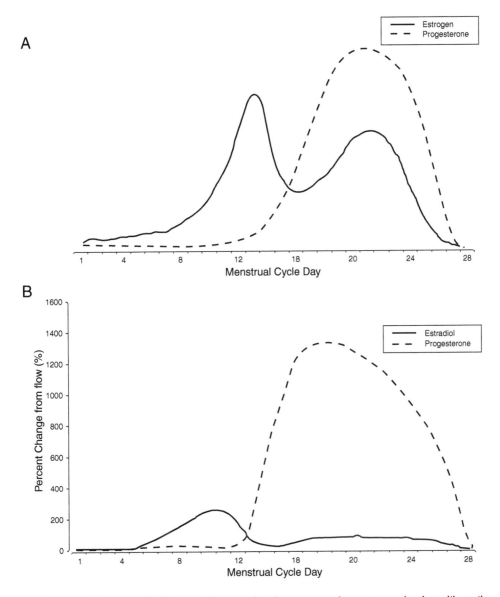

Figure 3.1 A: A typical unit-less diagram of menstrual cycle estrogen and progesterone levels readily available on the Internet. B: The percentage changes of menstrual cycle estradiol and progesterone levels related to their respective low levels during flow/early follicular phase in normal, ovulatory menstrual cycles. Redrawn from data in (Nielsen, Brixen, Bouillon, & Mosekilde, 1990).

Estradiol is produced in pmol/L amounts and is in moderate–high levels for the majority of menstrual cycle days. Progesterone, however, is secreted in nmol/L quantities (nmols are a thousand-fold larger unit than pmols) but is only at above-baseline levels for less than half of the normal cycle (Nielsen et al., 1990). Thus, although progesterone is elevated for fewer days than estradiol, in a healthy cycle the total progesterone production is greater than estradiol production. This fact is obscured by typical "Google images" (Figure 3.1) of cycle

41

hormones without any units that show estradiol's peak as higher than, similar to, or only slightly less than progesterone's peak. The cultural tendency to focus only on estradiol is illustrated by a recent *Nature* publication by world-recognized experts that included a menstrual cycle diagram that omitted progesterone entirely (Davis et al., 2015).

The control of this adaptive system occurs in and is integrated with nutritional, emotional/behavioral, temperature, and other neuroendocrine signals in the hypothalamus, where nerve impulses are transformed into pulsatile hormonal signals (Figure 3.2).

Gonadotrophin-releasing hormone (GnRH) pulsatile secretion can be documented in peripheral blood as rhythmic peaks of the pituitary's luteinizing hormone (LH). This integration involves insulin receptors (for adequacy of nutrition related to balance of caloric intake/expenditure), emotional signals (from the limbic system), hypothalamic temperature assessments (related to exercise, illness, and progesterone's actions to raise core body temperature), assessment of sleep, as well as feedback from levels of the ovarian hormones (estrogen and progesterone).

There is a continuum of women's potential reproductive responses to physiological and psychosocial experiences (Table 3.1). The so-called "functional" hypothalamic amenorrhea (no menstrual flow for 3–6 months) and oligomenorrhea (cycles longer than 35 days but less than 3 months) are rare in the spectrum of adaptive reproductive suppression. The most common are regular menstrual cycles with anovulation or with short luteal phases. Across a year, short luteal phases (≥2 per year) occur for 42% of women initially documented in two cycles to be normally ovulatory (Prior et al., 1990a). Anovulation is less common, and occurs for 20% of initially ovulatory women (Prior et al., 1990a). This continuum has not yet been recognized by most women's health experts (Gordon et al., 2017), who continue to discuss only low estrogen/estradiol and ignore low or absent progesterone levels.

Menstrual cycles and ovulation across the life cycle

Adolescence: maturation of menstruation and ovulation

In childhood, usually between ages 6 and 9, the neuroendocrine and hormonal changes that eventually lead to menarche and menstrual cycling are initiated. The pulses of LH that have been low and almost imperceptible become increased in size, slower, and more adult-like but only during sleep. By menarche the larger LH peaks of adulthood are also present during the day.

The age at menarche varies in different populations but it is accepted to be ages 11–13 for the majority in the advantaged world and somewhat later in other countries. First cycles are usually unpredictable, occasionally too close together, and often too far apart (longer than 45 days) with a mean of 33 days (American College of Obstetricians and Gynecologists, 2015; van Hooff et al., 1998) (Figure 3.3).

In addition, adolescents' first cycles are usually anovulatory, but by the end of the first year may develop ovulation with short luteal phases; within 5 years cycles will be intermittently normally ovulatory (Apter, Viinikka, & Vihko, 1978) (Figure 3.3). In prospective data, Vollman (1977) used a quantitative mean temperature method to document ovulation/luteal phase length (later validated by Prior, Vigna, Schulzer, Hall, & Bonen, 1990), and discovered that it took about 12 years following menarche before the most consistent, normal ovulation occurred.

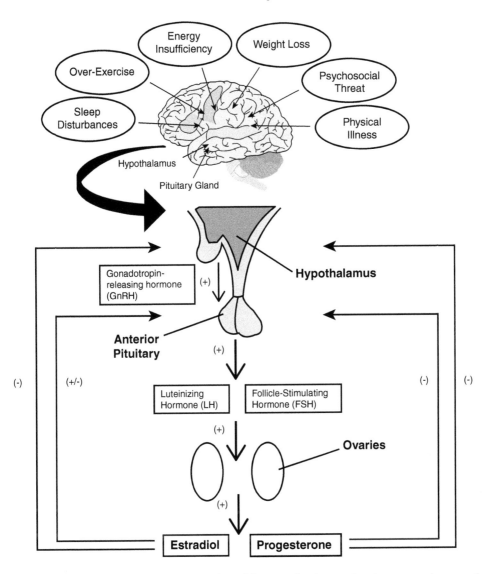

Figure 3.2 Diagram showing the inter-relationships of the internal and external environments as interpreted in the brain, pituitary, ovary and feedback of hormones and environmental variables that create an adaptable ovulatory menstrual cycle. Drawn by D. Kalidasan from a concept by Prior.

Age at menarche is associated with various health and disease characteristics. Early menarche (ages 11 or earlier, where the mean was 12.9 years), in a Canada-wide adolescent-to-adult population study with measured anthropomorphic data, was related to a significantly higher adult body mass index (BMI) with obesity in those with the earliest menarche ages (Harris, Prior, & Koehoorn, 2008). Other populations have shown the same pattern (Ahn et al., 2013), including that there is a 9% decreased risk for type 2 diabetes mellitus per year later age at menarche (Lakshman et al., 2008). Early menarche (in Great Britain characterized as <12 years, mean 13) was associated with a 20% increased risk for cardiovascular diseases and cancers plus overall mortality (Lakshman

Table 3.1 Hypothalamic Menstrual Cycle Adaptations—the spectrum of possibilities from amenorrhea to normal length, regular/predictable cycles; from regular anovulatory cycles to ovulatory but short luteal phase cycles—in addition, this outlines their hormonal changes and potential treatments.

Issue	Manifestation	Hormonal situation	Explanation and/or treatment
Hypothalamic Amenorrhea	No flow for 6 months (mo) (now often considered amenorrhea if flow is absent for 3 mo)	Very low estrogen and often progesterone. Moderately low estrogen and absent progesterone.	More common in the first 10 years after menarche. No flow after 14 days of cycle ★progesterone Flow after 14 days of ★progesterone.
Hypothalamic Oligomenorrhea	"Long cycles" >35 to <180 days or now 90 days	Moderately low estrogen; progesterone production usually but not always absent.	Treat with cyclic ★progesterone—14 days on and14 days off.
Subclinical Hypothalamic Ovulatory Disturbances—*Anovulatory Cycles*	Clinically normal cycling	Estrogen cyclic without any luteal phase progesterone levels.	Treat with cyclic ★progesterone—cycle days 14–27.
Subclinical Hypothalamic Ovulatory Disturbance—*Short Luteal Phase Cycles*	Clinically normal cycling	Estrogen cyclic; but progesterone high for fewer than 10 days.	Treat with cyclic ★progesterone—cycle days.

Note: ★Progesterone's physiological "luteal phase replacement" dose (given that it can be taken only at bedtime) is 300 mg per day.

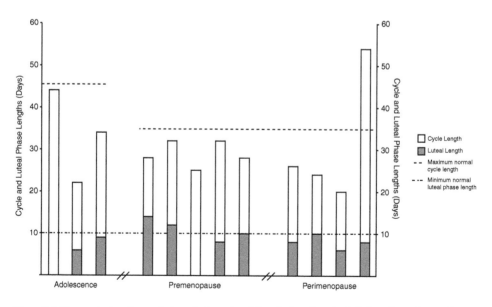

Figure 3.3 Bar graph showing cycle lengths (open) and luteal phase lengths (solid) with ovulatory changes that are typical across the menstruating lifecycle. Drawn by D. Kalidasan from a sketch by Prior.

et al., 2009); a 10% increased all-cause mortality with early menarche (ages 10–11, where the mean was 14) was confirmed by a 37-year longitudinal, whole-population Norwegian study (Jacobsen, Heuch, & Kvale, 2007). A later age at menarche (older than 15) was associated with decreased all-cause mortality in a European population-based study (Merritt et al., 2015).

The largest gain in height occurs around the time of menarche, and hip bone mineral density reaches its peak during ages 16–19 based on prospective, population data (Berger et al., 2010). There is evidence that progesterone (and thus the development of ovulation), as well as estrogen, is responsible for breast growth and transformation (Prior, Vigna, & Watson, 1989).

Premenopause: the peak of menstruating life and fertility

The normal *premenopausal* menstrual cycle length of 21–35 days (Abraham, 1978) has a population average of 27–29 days. Flow normally lasts 2–6 days. Normal ovulation is present in about two thirds of all normal-length menstrual cycles in women ages 20–49, mean age 42 (Prior, Naess, Langhammer, & Forsmo, 2015).

Normal cycle lengths between 21 and 35 days are usual from the early 20s until the mid-30s or whenever perimenopause begins (Figure 3.3). Flow of 2–6 days is associated with 30–60 milliliters (ml) of blood loss, which requires 6–12 soaked normal-sized menstrual management products (each holding ~5 ml or a teaspoon) (Hallberg, Hogdahl, Nillson, & Rybo, 1966). However, menorrhagia, which almost always causes iron deficiency anemia, is associated with blood loss of >80 ml/period (>16 soaked products; Hallberg et al., 1966). Heavy flow is characterized by needing to change (often large or "maxi" sized) sanitary products every 1–2 hours (or empty a 30 ml menstrual cup every 8–12 hours), clotting, and often increased cramping. Although premenstrual symptoms may occur during the premenopausal years and be managed by increasing exercise (Prior, Vigna, & Alojado, 1986), intense symptoms (ascertained in a population-based cohort with its purpose masked) are quite rare (Ramcharan, Love, Frick, & Goldfien, 1992).

Women's usual way of assessing whether they ovulate is to rely on "regular cycles"; some may also describe noticing "fertile mucus" at mid-cycle (i.e., several days of clear, egg-white type, stretchy secretion with a maximal thread-stretch of over 3 centimeters). This mucus is specific for cervical gland secretion in response to high mid-cycle estradiol levels (Figure 3.1). However, a mid-cycle estrogen peak (noted by the stretchy mucus) or an LH peak (documented with a urine stick) does not mean that those normal pre-ovulatory signals have actually triggered egg release and progesterone (Brown, 2011). Nor does it mean that, if ovulation occurs, the luteal phase length is long enough for implantation and thus fertility. Quantitative basal temperature [QBT] data require 10-day luteal phases (Vollman, 1977) or 11–12 days by urine LH data (Cole, Ladner, & Byrn, 2009) to define a fertile cycle.

Can women perceive an ovulatory cycle because they *feel different* in the luteal phase? Some believe that non-troublesome premenstrual experiences (called "molimina") accurately indicate ovulation (Magyar, Boyers, Marshall, & Abraham, 1979). However, attempts to validate this have so far failed (Goshtasebi et al., 2017). As progesterone raises the core temperature by ~0.2 degrees Celsius (Landau, Bergenstal, Lugibihl, & Kascht, 1955) and this is reliably measured first thing in the morning, temperature testing seems ideal. However, basal temperature data have been shown to be inaccurate (Bauman, 1981). Quantitative basal temperature (QBT) uses a 3-day running average and assesses means during the follicular and luteal phases. The temperature shift day correlates highly with (r = ~0.9) but lags 1–3 days behind the serum LH peak (Prior et al., 1990b). The mean temperature QBT (all of cycles' temperatures added together and divided by the number of days of data) is simpler. The luteal phase begins when the actual temperature rises above and stays above the mean temperature and lasts until the start of the next flow (CEMCOR, 2019; Prior et al., 1990b).

There is a growing appreciation that the (estrogen-only) follicular and the (progesterone-estrogen) luteal phases of the menstrual cycle differ in physiological and metabolic character-istics. Healthy, weight-stable younger women eat about 300 kilo-calories more during the luteal phase (Barr et al., 1995), likely because of energy requirements of ovulation-related elevated temperatures. Insulin resistance is increased during the late follicular phase, and estrogen's influence is stronger than progesterone's and insulin resistance is highest in anovulatory cycles (Yeung et al., 2010). In a study of 60 healthy, normal-weight, non-smoking women, daily self-report of feelings of frustration, depression, and anxiety were not higher during the luteal than the follicular phase nor related to hormone levels (Harvey, Hitchcock, & Prior, 2009). Sixty-six initially ovulatory women recorded QBT, exercise, and menstrual cycles and reported fluid retention as greatest on the first day of flow (White, Hitchcock, Vigna, & Prior, 2011). Oxidative stress marker levels have been shown to be higher during follicular than luteal phases and most strongly related to higher estrogen (Schisterman et al., 2010).

Perimenopause: the unpredictable and chaotic end of menstrual cycles

An estrogen/progesterone imbalance with estrogen dominance characterizes perimenopause (Santoro, Rosenberg, Adel, & Skurnick, 1996) with loss of the usual feedback suppression of estrogen by higher endogenous/exogenous estrogen levels (Weiss, Skurnick, Goldsmith, Santoro, & Park, 2004). Beyond the mid-30s and usually in the mid-40s cycles stay "regu-lar" but gradually become shorter until they often average ≤25 days in very early perimeno-pause (Prior, Seifert-Klauss, & Hale, 2012) (Figure 3.3). Cycles then become slightly or definitely irregular and unpredictable (early menopause transition) before the first skipped menstruation that signals the late menopause transition. Perimenopause is the normal mid-life transition from premenopausal menstrual cycles to menopause; it may be perceived only for a short time if mild, but women who are highly symptomatic often experience peri-menopausal changes/symptoms for over 10 years (Freeman, Sammel, Lin, Liu, & Gracia, 2011; Prior et al., 2012). A comprehensive older survey of the experiences of women in different reproductive life phases showed that adolescent and perimenopausal women shared many physiological and psychosocial experiences (Neugarten & Kraines, 1965), perhaps because both were experiencing major social status as well as physiological transitions.

The usual age at onset of unpredictable or irregular cycles (early menopause transition) (Harlow et al., 2012) (Figure 3.4) is 46–48 years in population data from the USA (McKinlay, Brambilla, & Posner, 1992).

Defining the onset of perimenopause by menstrual cycle changes, however, does women a disservice because the hormonal changes of perimenopause (higher estradiol and lower progesterone levels) have *already begun despite maintaining regular menstruation* (Moen, Kahn, Bjerve, & Halvorsen, 2004; Prior, 1998, 2006; Santoro et al., 1996).

Normal perimenopause may begin as early as age 35 and still end with a normal meno-pause (defined as 1 year beyond the last flow) at 40–45 years. Although about 80% of women have few symptoms in perimenopause, approximately one third of women seeking

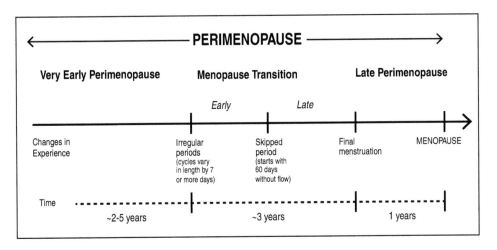

Figure 3.4 The four phases of perimenopause including very early perimenopause when women's experiences and hormones have changed but before the consensus (Harlow et al., 2012) says that the "menopause transition" has begun. Reprinted with permission from Prior et al., 2012.

medical help report very heavy flow (Kaufert, 1986). Other women become troubled by mid-sleep awakening and night sweats that tend to occur cyclically around flow (Hale, Hitchcock, Williams, Vigna, & Prior, 2003). As midlife women are often most symptomatic before their menstrual periods become irregular, it is useful to recognize those with night sweats, sleep disturbances, and shorter cycles as entering perimenopause (Prior, 2005). Other experience changes that may also indicate perimenopause onset while flow is regular are worsening cramps, heavy flow, new/worsening migraines, breast tenderness/lumpiness, premenstrual symptoms, and weight gain despite little change in diet/exercise (Prior, 2005). Any three of the nine above-listed experience changes can be used to make a diagnosis of very early perimenopause (Figure 3.4) (Prior, 2005).

Following a time of irregular cycles (during which heavy flow may still occur and daytime hot flushes may begin) (Figure 3.4) women will then experience a skipped period (or cycle length >60 days) that marks the beginning of the late menopause transition (Harlow et al., 2012). This may be followed within 1–2 years by the final menstruation. The last phase of perimenopause is very late perimenopause, which characterizes the final year of menstrual life. During this year, breast tenderness and cramps have usually gone (unless they are predicting flow) and often vasomotor symptoms (VMS) reach their peak lifetime intensity (Dennerstein, Dudley, Hopper, Guthrie, & Burger, 2000).

An individual woman's path through perimenopause is marked by considerable variation rather than a predictable progression (Kaufert, Gilbert, & Tate, 1987; Mansfield, Carey, Anderson, Barsom, & Koch, 2004). The further women move from the onset of perimenopause, according to Australian population-based data, the less symptomatic they become except that some experience lower libido, more VMS (both day and night), and more frequent headaches (Dennerstein et al., 2000). Perimenopause may, and often does, last 5–10 years.

Symptomatic perimenopause is currently commonly treated with combined hormonal contraceptives (CHC) or menopausal-like ovarian hormone therapy (OHT). However, if estrogen levels are high and poorly suppressible (Prior, 1998), more estrogen is unlikely to help. One study (Casper, Dodin, Reid, & Study Investigators, 1997) showed no significant changes from placebo or CHC related to quality of life, heavy flow, or hot flushes.

Perimenopausal heavy flow, in my clinical experience, improves with ibuprofen (200–400 mg with each meal on every day of flooding menstruation) plus oral micronized progesterone in a physiological luteal phase dose of 300 mg at bedtime daily (Simon et al., 1993). In perimenopausal heavy flow, progesterone needs to be given for 3 months continuously to overcome the cumulative effects of higher estrogen levels, rather than cyclically as in premenopausal women (Prior, 1997). Another effective non-surgical option is the levonorgestrel-releasing IUD (Lethaby, Hussain, Rishworth, & Rees, 2015). Only if there is documented endometrial cancer should hysterectomy be used to "treat" perimenopausal menorrhagia. The natural history of mid-life heavy flow is that it improves the longer a woman is in perimenopause.

Cramps also tend to increase in perimenopause. Ibuprofen, or another non-steroidal anti-inflammatory agent, initially and then "on demand" also works in this situation. A recent randomized controlled trial (RCT) of oral micronized progesterone for perimenopausal VMS showed a daily diary trend to overall improvement, but women perceived significantly improved night sweats in both early and later perimenopause (Prior et al., 2018). It is well documented in RCTs that 300 mg of micronized progesterone at bedtime improves sleep (Caufriez, Leproult, L'hermite-Baleriaux, Kerkhofs, & Copinschi, 2011; Hitchcock & Prior, 2012; Schussler et al., 2008) and that this is progesterone's major "side effect."

Menopause: a new flow-less life phase

Menopause refers to the life phase that begins for a woman who has been 12 months without flow. (The term "postmenopause" should no longer be used because it refers to the now-obsolete definition of "menopause" as the literal last menstrual flow.) The normal age at menopause is officially 40–58 years, with an average age of 49–52, depending on the country. Those few who become menopausal at age 45 or younger may be at higher risk for cardiovascular diseases as well as osteoporosis. The perimenopausal woman who had a difficult time will, in general, be less symptomatic in menopause (although she may have VMS for several more years depending on how early in perimenopause they began) (Freeman et al., 2011).

The 12-month landmark is a statistical "fact": 90% of women aged 45 years or older at menopause onset will not experience a further flow (Wallace, Sherman, Bean, Treloar, & Schlabaugh, 1979). That means that 10% of women will bleed again, and as many as 20% of women younger than 45 at menopause may have flow after 12 months of amenorrhea. Asymptomatic menopausal bleeding (in women not taking OHT) is strongly associated with endometrial cancer (Kaaks, Lukanova, & Kurzer, 2002). Women experiencing flow after amenorrhea for 12 months will usually be scheduled for endometrial biopsies to exclude cancer. If women describe cramp-like pelvic pain, sore breasts, nausea, or bloating before flow, they are experiencing a *normal* flow, as all of those are signs of the higher estrogen levels that triggered the extra menstrual period. Unfortunately for them, the "12-month clock" then starts all over again. Only if they have further flow, within 3 years of the last flow, with no preceding symptoms, should they be investigated for endometrial cancer.

New understanding of symptomatic menstrual cycles

When a cycle includes only estrogen and not progesterone, there is a fundamental hormonal imbalance. Our built environment that causes stress, produces light and noise pollution, interferes with sleep, tempts with fast foods and sweet drinks related to population obesity, includes environmental contaminants that act like estrogen, and promotes decreased physical activity also promotes excess estrogen exposure. The common menstrual cycle problems women face originate with estrogen overbalancing progesterone. I will briefly describe the most frequent disturbances. For further information see www.cemcor.ca.

Menstrual cramps help shed the uterine lining during flow. They are a common experience; for 10–20%, cramps cause severe pain (dysmenorrhea) associated with missing school or work. Menstrual cramps are caused by endometrial and uterine muscle production of prostaglandins (a long fatty acid-type hormone) that increase uterine spasms. Higher prostaglandins are produced if the cervix is tight (as in a woman who has not borne a child, has had an IUD inserted, or has experienced a miscarriage/abortion). In studies with monkeys, estrogen increases and progesterone decreases uterine prostaglandin production (Eldering, Nay, Hoberg, Longcope, & McCracken, 1990). These data suggest that cramps may be worse in shorter cycles with higher estrogen levels (Landgren, Unden, & Diczfalusy, 1980) and in normal-length but *anovulatory* cycles.

Treatment of menstrual cramps involves understanding what causes them, exercise and gradual weight loss (if needed, which decreases high estrogen production), and use of one of the over-the-counter, inexpensive medications (e.g., ibuprofen) in the non-steroidal anti-inflammatory drug (NSAID) family (Marjoribanks, Ayeleke, Farquhar, & Proctor, 2015). However, most NSAIDs' and ibuprofen's inhibition of prostaglandin production appears short-lived, therefore, to control cramps effectively, a woman must take two standard-sized tablets (200 mg X 2) at the first hint and then take a further 200 mg tablet as soon as the cramps *start to come back*, even if that is only 1–2 hours after the last dose. Taking ibuprofen every 6 hours means that 46% of women may not have adequate control of their cramps (Marjoribanks et al., 2015). Combined hormonal contraceptives decrease cramps in premenopausal women, but scientific testing and evidence is lacking about whether they are effective in adolescents and perimenopausal women (Marjoribanks et al., 2015).

Menorrhagia (heavy flow) is associated with an over-thickened endometrium related to higher estrogen and lower progesterone levels. Heavy flow is associated with an imbalance of endometrial prostaglandins, and it decreases by 20–50% with NSAIDs (Lethaby, Augood, & Duckitt, 2002). One 200 mg ibuprofen tablet with each of three meals on every heavy flow day is sufficient.

Heavy flow is more common in adolescent and perimenopausal women because both have higher estrogen levels and lower progesterone levels. Although CHC are commonly recommended, cyclic oral micronized progesterone (300 mg at bedtime for 14 days on and 14 days off) provides a more physiological and usually effective heavy flow therapy for adolescent and premenopausal women (Prior, 1997). Heavy flow is associated with anemia, therefore a blood count and bone marrow iron level (ferritin) need to be assessed and low dose iron therapy taken for a full year if anemia is present. Heavy flow in perimenopause is discussed above.

Endometriosis is caused by cells of the normal uterine lining that have flowed backwards up the fallopian tubes and spilled into the abdominal cavity (most commonly in the pelvis, but they can travel anywhere, including in the lung and eye). Although no clear population data on the question are available, it is likely that endometriosis arises in a setting of chronic, silent anovulation also associated with immune changes that are poorly characterized. It is likely that cyclic progesterone would prevent endometriosis if given prophylactically to young women with a family history of endometriosis.

Fibroids are benign growths within the muscular uterine wall that estrogen stimulates and progesterone inhibits. They increase with age, the majority of women have them, and they usually cause no clinical symptoms. Fibroids are often blamed for perimenopausal heavy flow. However, both fibroids and heavy flow are related to the higher estrogen/lower progesterone levels of perimenopause. Less than 10% of the time fibroids push into the endometrium (sub-mucus) and thus *could* cause heavy flow. In a study of women with heavy flow who had had hysterectomies (once standard heavy flow treatment), only 6 of 99 had sub-mucus fibroids at examination of pathology tissue (Seltzer, Benjamin, & Deutsch, 1990).

Infertility that is related to silent ovulatory disturbances is highly treatable, but this is usually not considered. Cyclic progesterone for ovulatory infertility needs to start after the midcycle LH peak or mucus has disappeared, to avoid interfering with egg release, and then continued for 14 days.

Polycystic ovary syndrome (PCOS) would be better called *anovulatory androgen excess* (AAE) (Prior, Kalyan, & Seifert-Klauss, 2014) because ovarian cysts *simply mean cycles without ovulation*. Besides cycle and ovulatory disturbances in PCOS/AAE, exposure to high levels of ovarian testosterone is essential. Given that rapid LH pulses may cause PCOS/AAE (Blank, McCartney, & Marshall, 2006) and progesterone normally slows LH pulsatility, cyclic progesterone therapy may be a therapeutic option (Prior, 1997).

Conclusion

Women's menstruation is resilient, new life-promoting, and health-producing, yet still is often viewed with negativity, squeamishness, or disgust. This chapter presents a life-affirming view of the menstrual cycle with the goal of better acquainting those who menstruate with the amazing vitality of this reproductive system. In the context of centuries-old social stigma and misogyny it is no wonder that we have not learned until recently that regular cycles may lack ovulation or have short luteal phases and thus produce infertility. Even more important is that increasing obesity in the population and the "estrogen dominance" of anovulatory cycles mean that menstrual cycle-related disturbances increase, women become symptomatic, and then begin to view their reproduction cycle as a problem. In this chapter my goal was to re-acquaint women both with the dynamic and protective responsiveness that lead to silent ovulatory disturbances and the woman-empowering ways to promote ovulatory cycle recovery and later life health.

References

Abraham, G. E. (1978). The normal menstrual cycle. In J. R. Givens (Ed.), *Endocrine causes of menstrual disorders* (1st ed., pp. 15–44). Chicago: Year Book Medical Publishers.

Ahn, J. H., Lim, S. W., Song, B. S., Seo, J., Lee, J. A., Kim, D. H., & Lim, J. S. (2013). Age at menarche in the Korean female: Secular trends and relationship to adulthood body mass index. *Annals of Pediatric Endocrinology & Metabolism, 18,* 60–64.

American College of Obstetricians and Gynecologists (2015). Menstruation in girls and adolescents: Using the menstrual cycle as a vital sign. *Obstetrics & Gynecology, 126,* e143–e146.

Apter, D., Viinikka, L., & Vihko, R. K. (1978). Hormonal pattern of adolescent menstrual cycles. *Journal of Clinical Endocrinology and Metabolism, 47,* 944–954.

Barr, S. I., Janelle, K. C., & Prior, J. C. (1995). Energy intakes are higher during the luteal-phase of ovulatory menstrual cycles. *American Journal of Clinical Nutrition, 61,* 39–43.

Bauman, J. (1981). Basal body temperature: Unreliable method of ovulation detection. *Fertility and Sterility, 36,* 729–733.

Berger, C., Goltzman, D., Langsetmo, L., Joseph, L., Jackson, S., Kreiger, N., Tenenhouse, A., Davison, K. S., Josse, R. G., Prior, J. C., Hanley, D. A., & the CaMos Research Group (2010). Peak bone mass from longitudinal data: Implications for the prevalence, pathophysiology, and diagnosis of osteoporosis. *Journal of Bone and Mineral Research, 25,* 1948–1957.

Blank, S. K., McCartney, C. R., & Marshall, J. C. (2006). The origins and sequelae of abnormal neuro-endocrine function in polycystic ovary syndrome. *Human Reproduction Update, 12,* 351–361.

Brown, J. B. (2011). Types of ovarian activity in women and their significance: The continuum (a reinter-pretation of early findings). *Human Reproduction Update, 17,* 141–158.

Casper, R. F., Dodin, S., Reid, R. L., & Study Investigators (1997). The effect of 20 ug ethinyl estradiol/1 mg norethindrone acetate (Minestrin^TM), a low-dose oral contraceptive, on vaginal bleeding patterns, hot flashes, and quality of life in symptomatic perimenopausal women. *Menopause, 4,* 139–147.

Caufriez, A., Leproult, R., L'hermite-Baleriaux, M., Kerkhofs, M., & Copinschi, G. (2011). Progester-one prevents sleep disturbances and modulates GH, TSH, and melatonin secretion in postmenopausal women. *Journal of Clinical Endocrinology & Metabolism, 96,* E614–E623.

Centre for Menstrual Cycle and Ovulation Research (CeMCOR) (2019). Documenting Ovulation with Quantitative Basal Temperature (QBT). Vancouver: Author. Retrieved from www.cemcor.ca/resources/qualitative-basal-temperature-qbt-method-ovulation-detection.

Clarke, C. L. & Sutherland, R. L. (1990). Progestin regulation of cellular proliferation. *Endocrine Reviews, 11,* 266–301.

Cole, L. A., Ladner, D. G., & Byrn, F. W. (2009). The normal variabilities of the menstrual cycle. *Fertil-ity and Sterility, 91,* 522–527.

Davis, S. R., Lambrinoudaki, I., Lumsden, M., Mishra, G. D., Pal, L., Rees, M., Santoro, N., & Simoncini, T. (2015). Menopause. *Nature Reviews Disease Primers,* 15004.

Dennerstein, L., Dudley, E. C., Hopper, J. L., Guthrie, J. R., & Burger, H. G. (2000). A prospective population-based study of menopausal symptoms. *Obstetrics & Gynecology, 96,* 351–358.

Eldering, J., Nay, M., Hoberg, L., Longcope, C., & McCracken, J. (1990). Hormonal regulation of pros-taglandin production by rhesus monkey endometrium. *Journal of Clinical Endocrinology & Metabolism, 71,* 596–604.

Falsetti, L., Gambera, A., Barbetti, L., & Specchia, C. (2002). Long-term follow-up of functional hypo-thalamic amenorrhea and prognostic factors. *Journal of Clinical Endocrinology & Metabolism, 87,* 500–505.

Fournier, A., Berrino, F., & Clavel-Chapelon, F. (2008). Unequal risks for breast cancer associated with different hormone replacement therapies: Results from the E3N cohort study. *Breast Cancer Research & Treatment, 107,* 103–111.

Freeman, E. W., Sammel, M. D., Lin, H., Liu, Z., & Gracia, C. R. (2011). Duration of menopausal hot flushes and associated risk factors. *Obstetrics & Gynecology, 117,* 1095–1104.

Gordon, C. M., Ackerman, K. E., Berga, S. L., Kaplan, J. R., Mastorakos, G., Misra, M., Murad, M. H., Santoro, N. F., & Warren, M. P. (2017). Functional hypothalamic amenorrhea: An Endocrine Society clinical practice guideline. *Journal of Clinical Endocrinology & Metabolism, 102,* 1413–1439.

Goshtasebi, A., Brajic, T. S., Scholes, D., Lederer Goldberg, B. L., Berenson, A., & Prior, J. C. (2017). Adolescent use of combined hormonal contraceptives and peak areal bone mineral density accrual in prospective studies: A meta-analysis. *Journal of Bone and Mineral Research, 3,* S308.

Hale, G. E., Hitchcock, C. L., Williams, L. A., Vigna, Y. M., & Prior, J. C. (2003). Cyclicity of breast tenderness and night-time vasomotor symptoms in mid-life women: Information collected using the daily perimenopause diary. *Climacteric, 6,* 128–139.

Hallberg, L., Hogdahl, A. M., Nillson, L., & Rybo, G. (1966). Menstrual blood loss: Variation at differ-ent ages and attempts to define normality. *Acta Obstetrics and Gynecology Scandinavia, 45,* 320–351.

Harlow, S. D., Gass, M., Hall, J. E., Lobo, R., Maki, P., Rebar, R. W., Sherman, S., Sluss, P. M., & de Villiers, T. J. (2012). Executive summary of the stages of reproductive aging workshop +10: Address-ing the unfinished agenda of staging reproductive aging. *Journal of Clinical Endocrinology & Metabolism, 97,* 1159–1168.

Harris, M. A., Prior, J. C., & Koehoorn, M. (2008). Age at menarche in the Canadian population: Secu-lar trends and relationship to adulthood BMI. *Journal of Adolescent Health, 43,* 548–554.

Harvey, A., Hitchcock, C. L., & Prior, J. C. (2009). Ovulation disturbances and mood across the men-strual cycles of healthy women. *Journal of Psychosomatic Obstetrics & Gynaecology, 30,* 207–214.

Hitchcock, C. L. & Prior, J. C. (2012). Oral micronized progesterone for vasomotor symptoms in healthy postmenopausal women: A placebo-controlled randomized trial. *Menopause, 19,* 886–893.

Inhorn, M. C. & Whittle, K. L. (2001). Feminism meets the "new" epidemiologies: Toward an appraisal of antifeminist biases in epidemiological research on women's health. *Social Science and Medicine, 53,* 553–567.

Jacobsen, B. K., Heuch, I., & Kvale, G. (2007). Association of low age at menarche with increased all-cause mortality: A 37-year follow-up of 61,319 Norwegian women. *American Journal of Epidemiology, 166*, 1431–1437.

Kaaks, R., Lukanova, A., & Kurzer, M. S. (2002). Obesity, endogenous hormones, and endometrial cancer risk: A synthetic review. *Cancer Epidemiology, Biomarkers, & Prevention, 11*, 1531–1543.

Kalyan, S. & Prior, J. C. (2010). Bone changes and fracture related to menstrual cycles and ovulation. *Critical Reviews in Eukaryotic Gene Expression, 20*, 213–233.

Kaufert, P. A. (1986). Menstruation and menstrual change: Women in midlife. *Health Care for Women International, 7*, 63–76.

Kaufert, P. A., Gilbert, P., & Tate, R. (1987). Defining menopausal status: The impact of longitudinal data. *Maturitas, 9*, 217–226.

Kaufert, P. A. & Syrotvik, J. (1981). Symptom reporting at menopause. *Social Science and Medicine, 15E*, 185–193.

Kissling, E. A. (2006). *Capitalizing on the curse: The business of menstruation.* Boulder, CO: Lynne Rienner.

Lakshman, R., Forouhi, N., Luben, R., Bingham, S., Khaw, K., Wareham, N., & Ong, K. K. (2008). Association between age at menarche and risk of diabetes in adults: Results from the EPIC-Norfolk cohort study. *Diabetologia, 51*, 781–786.

Lakshman, R., Forouhi, N. G., Sharp, S. J., Luben, R., Bingham, S. A., Khaw, K. T., Wareham, N. J., & Ong, K. K. (2009). Early age at menarche associated with cardiovascular disease and mortality. *Journal of Clinical Endocrinology & Metabolism, 94*, 4953–4960.

Landau, R. L., Bergenstal, D. M., Lugibihl, K., & Kascht, M. E. (1955). The metabolic effects of progesterone in man. *Journal of Clinical Endocrinology & Metabolism, 15*, 1194–1215.

Landgren, B. H., Unden, A. L., & Diczfalusy, E. (1980). Hormonal profile of the cycle in 68 normally menstruating women. *Acta Endocrinoligica Copenhagen, 94*, 89–98.

Lebrun, C. M., McKenzie, D. C., Prior, J. C., & Taunton, J. E. (1995). Effects of menstrual cycle phase on athletic performance. *Medicine and Science in Sports and Exercise, 27*, 437–444.

Lethaby, A., Augood, C., & Duckitt, K. (2002). Nonsteroidal anti-inflammatory drugs for heavy menstrual bleeding. *Cochrane Database of Systematic Reviews*, CD000400.

Lethaby, A., Hussain, M., Rishworth, J. R., & Rees, M. C. (2015). Progesterone or progestogen-releasing intrauterine systems for heavy menstrual bleeding. *Cochrane Database of Systematic Reviews*, CD002126.

Magyar, D. M., Boyers, S. P., Marshall, J. R., & Abraham, G. E. (1979). Regular menstrual cycles and premenstrual molimina as indicators of ovulation. *Obstetrics & Gynecology, 53*, 441–444.

Malcolm, C. E. & Cumming, D. C. (2003). Does anovulation exist in eumenorrheic women?. *Obstetrics & Gynecology, 102*, 317–318.

Mansfield, P. K., Carey, M., Anderson, A., Barsom, S. H., & Koch, P. B. (2004). Staging the menopausal transition: Data from the TREMIN Research Program on Women's Health. *Women's Health Issues, 14*, 220–226.

Marjoribanks, J., Ayeleke, R. O., Farquhar, C., & Proctor, M. (2015). Nonsteroidal anti-inflammatory drugs for dysmenorrhoea. *Cochrane Database of Systematic Reviews*, CD001751.

McKinlay, S. M., Brambilla, D. J., & Posner, J. G. (1992). The normal menopause transition. *Maturitas, 14*, 103–115.

Merritt, M. A., Riboli, E., Murphy, N., Kadi, M., Tjonneland, A., Olsen, A., Overvad, K., Dossus, L., Dartois, L., Clavel-Chapelon, F., Fortner, R. T., Katzke, V. A., Boeing, H., Trichopoulu, A., Laglou, P., Trichopoulos, D., Palti, D., Sieri, S., Tumino, R., Sacerdote, C., Panico, S., Bueno-de-Mesquita, H. B., Peeters, P. H., Lund, E., Nakamura, A., Welderpass, E., Quiros, J. R., Agudo, A., Molina-Montes, E., Larranaga, N., Dorronsoro, M., Cirera, L., Barricarte, A., Olsson, A., Butt, S., Idahl, A., Lundin, E., Wareham, N. J., Key, T. J., Nrennan, P. Ferrari, P., Wark, P. A., Norat, T., Cross, A. J., & Gunter, M. J. (2015). Reproductive factors and risk of mortality in the European prospective investigation into cancer and nutrition: A cohort study. *BMC Medicine, 13*, 252.

Michopoulos, V., Mancini, F., Loucks, T. L., & Berga, S. L. (2013). Neuroendocrine recovery initiated by cognitive behavioral therapy in women with functional hypothalamic amenorrhea: A randomized, controlled trial. *Fertility and Sterility, 99*, 2084–2091.

Mishra, G. D., Cooper, R., Tom, S. E., & Kuh, D. (2009). Early life circumstances and their impact on menarche and menopause. *Women's Health, 5*, 175–190.

Moen, M. H., Kahn, H., Bjerve, K. S., & Halvorsen, T. B. (2004). Menometrorrhagia in the perimenopause is associated with increased serum estradiol. *Maturitas, 47*, 151–155.

Navarro, V. M. & Kaiser, U. B. (2013). Metabolic influences on neuroendocrine regulation of reproduction. *Current Opinion in Endocrinology, Diabetes, and Obesity, 20*, 335–341.

Neugarten, B. L. & Kraines, R. J. (1965). Menopausal symptoms in women of various ages. *Psychomatic Medicine, 27*, 266–273.

Nielsen, H. K., Brixen, K., Bouillon, R., & Mosekilde, L. (1990). Changes in biochemical markers of osteoblastic activity during the menstrual cycle. *Journal of Clinical Endocrinology & Metabolism, 70*, 1431–1437.

Prior, J. C. (1987). Physical exercise and the neuroendocrine control of reproduction. *Baillieres Clinical Endocrinology and Metabolism, 1*, 299–317.

Prior, J. C. (1997, February). Ovulatory disturbances: They do matter. *Canadian Journal of Diagnosis, 14*, 64–80.

Prior, J. C. (1998). Perimenopause: The complex endocrinology of the menopausal transition. *Endocrine Reviews, 19*, 397–428.

Prior, J. C. (2005). Clearing confusion about perimenopause. *British Columbia Medical Journal, 47*, 534–538.

Prior, J. C. (2006). Perimenopause lost: Reframing the end of menstruation. *Journal of Reproductive and Infant Psychology, 24*, 323–335.

Prior, J. C. (2014). Progesterone within ovulatory menstrual cycles needed for cardiovascular protection: An evidence-based hypothesis. *Journal of Restorative Medicine, 3*, 85–103.

Prior, J. C. (2016). Adolescents' use of combined hormonal contraceptives for menstrual cycle-related problem treatment and contraception: Evidence of potential lifelong negative reproductive and bone effects. *Women's Reproductive Health, 3*, 73–92.

Prior, J. C. (2018). Progesterone for the prevention and treatment of osteoporosis in women. *Climacteric, 21*, 366–374.

Prior, J. C., Cameron, A., Hitchcock, C. L., Fung, M., Janssen, P., Brief, E., Lee, T., Sirrs, S. M., Kalyan, S., & Singer, J. (2018). Oral micronized progesterone beneficial for perimenopausal hot flushes/flashes and night sweats. *Endocrine Reviews, 39*(2).

Prior, J. C., Ho Yeun, B., Clement, P., Bowie, L., & Thomas, J. (1982). Reversible luteal phase changes and infertility associated with marathon training. *Lancet, 1*, 269–270.

Prior, J. C., Kalyan, S., & Seifert-Klauss, V. (2013). Re-naming PCOS: Suggest anovulatory androgen excess [Letter to the editor]. *Journal of Clinical Endocrinology & Metabolism, 98*, 4325–4328.

Prior, J. C., Naess, M., Langhammer, A., & Forsmo, S. (2015). Ovulation prevalence in women with spontaneous normal-length menstrual cycles: A population-based cohort from HUNT3, Norway. *PLOS One, 10*, e0134473.

Prior, J. C., Seifert-Klauss, V. R., & Hale, G. (2012). The endocrinology of perimenopause: New definitions and understandings of hormonal and bone changes. In V. Dvoryk (Ed.), *Current topics in menopause* (pp. 54–83). Sharjah, UAE: Bentham Science Publishers.

Prior, J. C., Vigna, Y. M., & Alojado, N. (1986). Conditioning exercise decreases premenstrual symptoms: A prospective controlled three month trial. *European Journal of Applied Physiology, 55*, 349–355.

Prior, J. C., Vigna, Y. M., Barr, S. I., Rexworthy, C., & Lentle, B. C. (1994). Cyclic medroxyprogesterone treatment increases bone density: A controlled trial in active women with menstrual cycle disturbances. *American Journal Medicine, 96*, 521–530.

Prior, J. C., Vigna, Y. M., Schechter, M. T., & Burgess, A. E. (1990a). Spinal bone loss and ovulatory disturbances. *New England Journal of Medicine, 323*, 1221–1227.

Prior, J. C., Vigna, Y. M., Schulzer, M., Hall, J. E., & Bonen, A. (1990b). Determination of luteal phase length by quantitative basal temperature methods: Validation against the midcycle LH peak. *Clinical & Investigative Medicine, 13*, 123–131.

Prior, J. C., Vigna, Y. M., & Watson, D. (1989). Spironolactone with physiological female gonadal steroids in the presurgical therapy of male to female transexuals: A new observation. *Archives of Sexual Behavior, 18*, 49–57.

Ramcharan, S., Love, E. J., Frick, G. H., & Goldfien, A. (1992). The epidemiology of premenstrual symptoms in a population-based sample of 2,650 urban women: Attributable risk and risk factors. *Journal of Clinical Epidemiology, 45*, 377–392.

Santoro, N., Rosenberg, J., Adel, T., & Skurnick, J. H. (1996). Characterization of reproductive hormonal dynamics in the perimenopause. *Journal of Clinical Endocrinology and Metabolism, 81*(4), 1495–1501.

Schisterman, E. F., Gaskins, A. J., Mumford, S. L., Browne, R. W., Yeung, E., Trevisan, M., Hediger, M., Zhang, C., Perkins, N. J., Hovey, K., & Wactawski-Wende, J. (2010). Influence of endogenous reproductive hormones on F2-isoprostane levels in premenopausal women: The BioCycle Study. *American Journal of Epidemiology, 172*, 430–439.

Schussler, P., Kluge, M., Yassouridis, A., Dresler, M., Held, K., Zihl, J., & Steiger, A. (2008). Progesterone reduces wakefulness in sleep EEG and has no effect on cognition in healthy postmenopausal women. *Psychoneuroendocrinology, 33*, 1124–1131.

Seltzer, V. I., Benjamin, F., & Deutsch, S. (1990). Perimenopausal bleeding patterns and pathological findings. *Journal of the American Medical Women's Association, 45*, 132–134.

Simon, J. A., Robinson, D. E., Andrews, M. C., Hildebrand, III, J. R., Rocci, Jr., M. L., Blake, R. E., & Hodgen, G. D. (1993). The absorption of oral micronized progesterone: The effect of food, dose proportionality, and comparison with intramuscular progesterone. *Fertility and Sterility, 60*, 26–33.

Tisdale, J. E., Jaynes, H. A., Overholser, B. R., Sowinski, K. M., Flockhart, D. A., & Kovacs, R. J. (2016). Influence of oral progesterone administration on drug-induced QT interval lengthening: A randomized, double-blind, placebo-controlled crossover study. *JACC: Clinical Electrophysiology, 2*, 765–774.

van Hooff, M. H., Voorhorst, F. J., Kaptein, M. B., Hirasing, R. A., Koppenaal, C., & Schoemaker, J. (1998). Relationship of the menstrual cycle pattern in 14–17 year old adolescents with gynaecological age, body mass index and historical parameters. *Human Reproduction, 13*, 2252–2260.

Vitzthum, V. J. (2009). The ecology and evolutionary endocrinology of reproduction in the human female. *American Journal of Physical Anthropology, 140*(Suppl 49), 95–136.

Vitzthum, V. J., Spielvogel, H., & Thornburg, J. (2004). Interpopulational differences in progesterone levels during conception and implantation in humans. *Proceeding of the National Academy of Sciences, 101*, 1443–1448.

Vollman, R. F. (1977). The menstrual cycle. In E. A. Friedman (Ed.), *Major problems in obstetrics and gynecology* (Vol. 7, 1st ed., pp. 11–193). Toronto: W. B. Saunders.

Wallace, R. B., Sherman, B. M., Bean, J. A., Treloar, A. E., & Schlabaugh, L. (1979). Probability of menopause with increasing duration of amenorrhea in middle-aged women. *American Journal of Obstetrics and Gynecology, 135*, 1021–1024.

Wallston, K. A., Wallston, B. S., & DeVellis, R. (1978). Development of the Multidimensional Health Locus of Control (MHLC) scales. *Health Education Monographs, 6*, 160–170.

Weiss, G., Skurnick, J. H., Goldsmith, L. T., Santoro, N. F., & Park, S. J. (2004). Menopause and hypothalamic-pituitary sensitivity to estrogen. *Journal of the American Medical Association, 292*, 2991–2996.

White, C. P., Hitchcock, C. L., Vigna, Y. M., & Prior, J. C. (2011). Fluid retention over the menstrual cycle: 1-Year data from the prospective ovulation cohort. *Obstetrics & Gynecology International, 2011*, 138451.

Wilson, R. A. (1966). *Feminine forever*. New York: M. Evans & Co.

World Health Assemblies (2006). *Constitution of the World Health Organization* (Rep. No. 54 edition, Supplement).

Yeung, E. H., Zhang, C., Mumford, S. L., Ye, A., Trevisan, M., Chen, L., Browne, R. W., Wactawski-Wende, J., & Schisterman, E. F. (2010). Longitudinal study of insulin resistance and sex hormones over the menstrual cycle: The BioCycle Study. *Journal of Clinical Endocrinology & Metabolism, 95*, 5435–5442.

4

THE MENSTRUAL CYCLE
Attitudes and behavioral concomitants

Joan C. Chrisler and Jenifer A. Gorman

Menstruation is a stigmatized status (Johnston-Robledo & Chrisler, 2013), and aspects of it are taboo in many cultures. Common taboos in both developed and developing countries include communication (i.e., one should not talk openly about menstruation) and sex (i.e., vaginal sexual activities are avoided during menstruation). Taboos that are less common than they once were, but still occur in some societies, include bans on cooking, entering places of worship, working in the fields (or caring for houseplants), engaging in other strenuous activities, swimming/bathing, and touching members of the other sex (Fahs, 2011, 2014; Golub, 1992; Kissling, 1996). In some places taboos are strongly enforced and have negative effects on the lives of women and girls. For example, to enforce the taboo against touching or otherwise contaminating others, some cultures have secluded menstruators in huts away from the family home. Although this practice was outlawed in Nepal in 2005, it is still practiced in rural areas, where two girls died in 2017 due to accidents while alone in a hut (BBC, 2017). In other places (e.g., Mexico), girls are advised to avoid various activities, such as swimming, carrying heavy objects, eating certain foods, or drinking cold beverages (Marván, Ramírez-Esparza, Cortés-Iniestra, & Chrisler, 2006). They are not punished for going against such advice, but accepting it interferes with daily life, including school, work, and family roles. These traditions both influence people's attitudes toward menstruation and are influenced by cultural beliefs and attitudes.

In this chapter we discuss the sources of attitudes toward and beliefs about the menstrual cycle and their possible effects on girls and women, review studies of attitudes toward menstruation in different cultures and countries, and consider the possible effects a woman's attitude can have on her psychological and physical health and well-being. We then review research on psychological and behavioral concomitants of the menstrual cycle, show how the results do and do not support stereotypes about women, and consider why this topic has been (and remains) of such popular scientific interest.

Attitudes toward menstruation

Sources of attitudes and beliefs

Taboos associated with menstruation have ancient roots. They arose when people did not understand how women could bleed without a wound or why the blood loss did not do damage to their health (Frazer, 1951). Some cultures developed beliefs that menstrual blood is poisonous and, consequently, that menstruating women are dangerous. For example, beliefs that men will sicken or die if touched by a menstruating woman, that a drop of menstrual blood in a field will cause crops to wither, and that certain foods and beverages (e.g., beer, wine, milk, jam) go bad if a menstruating woman touches them (Frazer, 1951) have been reported in many countries. In Nepal, people in rural areas still believe that a menstruating woman in the house is bad luck: the house could catch fire, the family could become ill, or a tiger could attack (Gettleman, 2018). As late as the 1930s scientists were trying to isolate menotoxins (i.e., poisonous elements) in menstrual fluid (Delaney, Lupton, & Toth, 1987), and the belief that the menstrual cycle makes women dangerous lives on today in stereotypes of premenstrual women as angry, impulsive, and aggressive. Other cultures developed beliefs that menstruation is magical or spiritual. For example, the Yurok people of the American Northwest believed that menstruation is the time when women are at the height of their spiritual powers, thus they should be freed from mundane tasks so that they can concentrate on meditation and other spiritual pursuits (Buckley, 1982). Traditional beliefs like these could influence attitudes toward menstruation in a positive or negative direction. Given that most cultures are patriarchal, attitudes toward menstruation are largely negative.

Religion has been a major source of menstrual taboos. Hinduism "places a special emphasis on purity and pollution" (Gettleman, 2018, p. A6), and women's bodies are seen as polluted during menstruation and for a while after childbirth. In Judaism and Islam, ritual bathing is required after menstruation (Cicurel, 2000; Goldenberg & Roberts, 2004) to restore purity. Although pollution is probably not on the minds of contemporary, educated people, it may be the source of the stigma attached to menstrual blood in both developed and developing countries. In Zambia, where menstrual hygiene supplies are often inaccessible and public restrooms often lack privacy and running water, girls and women may have to miss school or work during menstruation because any sign of blood on their skirts would result in bullying, harassment, and consequent stress and shame (e.g., Lahme & Stern, 2017). In psychology experiments in the US, even the sight of a clean, unused tampon led to expressions of disgust (Rozin, Haidt, McCauley, Dunlop, & Ashmore, 1999) and dislike of and distancing from a woman who dropped a tampon (Roberts, Goldenberg, Power, & Pyszczynski, 2002).

The stigma of menstruation and the communication taboo often extend to language, as people do not like to talk about menstruation. For example, in Ethiopia, the slang word *adef*, which means dirty or unclean, is frequently used to refer to menstruation (Smiles, Short, & Sommer, 2017). English and Swedish speakers often use euphemisms (e.g., period, Aunt Flo, that time of the month, red flower) and dysphemisms (e.g., shark week, closed for repairs, lava, code red) instead of biological terms (i.e., menstruation, the menses) (Ernster, 1975; Sveen, 2016). Euphemisms suggest that menstruation should be secret and unmentionable; dysphemisms render it dangerous, reinforce the sex taboo, or insult and stereotype women under the guise of humor. Themes of danger and negativity can also be found in definitions related to the menstrual cycle in *Urban Dictionary*, a crowd-sourced Internet site. For example, the most "popular" definition of PMS in 2016 was "A powerful spell that women are put under about once every month, which gives them the strength of an ox, the stability of a Window's OX, and the scream of a banshee. Basically, man's worst nightmare" (Gorman et al., 2017). Note the allusion to magic ("spell") and monsters ("banshee").

Perhaps the most common beliefs about the menstrual cycle today in Western societies are the debilitation hypothesis (i.e., the belief that women's abilities are diminished during menstruation) and the "hormonal" hypothesis (i.e., the belief that women are moody, tense, and angry during the premenstrual phase of the cycle). These beliefs are on ample display in popular culture, which contains many stigmatizing messages about menstrual and premenstrual women. These messages have been found in films, television programs, advertisements, magazines, books, social media, and Internet sites (e.g., Chrisler & Levy, 1990; Johnston-Robledo & Chrisler, 2013; King, Ussher, & Perz, 2014; Kissling, 2002; Rosewarne, 2011; Thornton, 2013), and they contribute to gender role stereotypes of women as moodier and less competent than men (Chrisler, 2002). A quick Google search of "period brain" turned up a number of articles and blog posts that assert that women are often confused, mentally "foggy," and unable to think clearly during the menses.

Studies of attitudes and stereotypic beliefs

Women's negative attitudes toward menstruation, based on stigma, shame, inaccurate beliefs, and painful cramps, have been documented in many countries, including Ethiopia, Iceland, India, Mexico, Nepal, South Africa, Turkey, and the US (e.g., Çevirme, Çevirme, Karaoglu, Ugurlu, & Korkmaz, 2010; Crawford, Menger, & Kaufman, 2014; Hoerster, Chrisler, & Rose, 2003; Marván & Trujillo, 2010; Padmanabhanunni & Fennie, 2017; Rose, Chrisler, & Couture, 2008; Smiles et al., 2017; Sveinsdóttir, 2018). Negative attitudes typically reflect concerns about pain and debilitation, the need to keep menstruation secret, the bother of having to manage menstrual hygiene, worries about shame and stigma if menstrual status is discovered, and the need to engage in or avoid certain activities. Some studies indicate that rural, less educated, and older women have more strongly held negative attitudes than urban, more educated, and younger women.

Men and boys have also reported negative attitudes toward menstruation in recent studies conducted in Australia, Taiwan, and the US (Allen, Kaestle, & Goldberg, 2011; Chang, Hayter, & Lin, 2011; Peranovic & Bentley, 2017). Men have reported that they learned misinformation about menstruation, which usually does not get corrected until they have a mature relationship with a woman, as either a romantic partner or close friend, who explains reality to them. They recognize stigma attached to menstruation and often endorse the communication and sex taboos. In one study (Erchull & Richmond, 2015), fathers reported that they would be more likely to discuss negative (e.g., "mood swings") aspects of the menstrual cycle with sons than with daughters, thus enforcing men's negative views. High scores on a measure of hostile sexism have also been shown to predict negative attitudes toward menstruation and toward menstrual and premenstrual women in both Mexico and the US (Chrisler, Gorman, Marván, & Johnston-Robledo, 2014; Marván, Vázquez-Toboada, & Chrisler, 2014).

It is common for women and girls to report ambivalent attitudes toward menstruation, as they typically recognize that it has both positive and negative aspects. For example, they might consider menstruation to be both natural and bothersome, or they might report pride in their womanhood and the need to keep menstruation a secret, or they might consider menstruation a pleasant sign that they could become pregnant and describe it as painful and debilitating. Few studies have focused on positive attitudes toward menstruation, but some researchers have shown that positive priming yields more positive attitudes toward menstruation and reports of more positive (e.g., affectionate, orderliness, feelings of well-being, bursts of energy) and fewer negative (e.g., headaches, water retention, crying) cycle-related changes (e.g., Aubeeluck & Maguire, 2002; Chrisler, Johnston, Champagne, & Preston, 1994; Rose et al., 2008). Higher scores on a measure of body appreciation also predict more positive attitudes toward menstruation in a US sample (Chrisler, Marván, Gorman, & Rossini, 2015). These studies suggest that, if girls and women were exposed to more positive messages about menstruation (e.g., in health education classes or popular culture), their attitudes would become more positive. Indeed, a study of midwifery students in Slovenia showed that attitudes toward menstruation became more positive over the course of the program as students gained knowledge of female physiology and respect for the power of the reproductive body (Dosler & Mivsek, 2015).

Attitudes toward menstruation can affect women's health and well-being. Women whose attitudes are particularly negative report greater self-objectification (Johnston-Robledo, Sheffield, Voigt, & Wilcox-Constantine, 2007; Roberts, 2004; Sveinsdóttir, 2018), the tendency to internalize a critical gaze. Self-objectification has been shown in other studies to be related to depression, eating disorders, sexual dysfunction (Moradi & Huang, 2008), and negative attitudes toward breastfeeding (Johnston-Robledo, Wares, Fricker, & Pasek, 2007), pregnancy (Morris, Goldenberg, & Heflick, 2014), and menopause (Rubinstein & Foster, 2013). Negative attitudes toward menstruation are also associated with interest in or use of Depo-Provera and other cycle-suppressing contraceptives (Johnston-Robledo et al., 2007; Morrison, Larkspur, Calibuso, & Brown, 2010; Rose et al., 2008) and reluctance to use alternative menstrual products (e.g., cups, reusable pads), which are more eco-friendly than traditional products (Grose & Grabe, 2014).

Negative attitudes, especially beliefs that menstruating and premenstrual women are vulnerable, moody, and debilitated contribute to the idea that women are unsuited to roles in the public sphere where effects of their hormonal changes could endanger the smooth functioning of society. This idea is strongly held across many cultures and has inspired hundreds of studies, most of which have been conducted in Western countries.

Menstrual cycle concomitants

In line with the debilitation hypothesis (i.e., pain and changes associated with the menstrual cycle), the hormonal hypothesis (i.e., hormones associated with the menstrual cycle cause women to lose control of their emotions), and, more recently, evolutionary psychology theory, a multitude of studies of psychosocial changes (e.g., behavioral, cognitive, emotional) that were believed to be associated with the menstrual cycle have proliferated. Evolutionary psychologists have been interested in whether menstrual cycle phase affects women's sexual behavior or their attractiveness. Below we review some of this research and consider its value.

Women's performance and cognitive abilities across the menstrual cycle

It has long been assumed that women's performance and abilities are at the mercy of their "raging hormones" (Sommer, 1983). When women entered the workforce in large numbers during World War II, there was a sudden spike in research that tested women's performance across the menstrual cycle. Seward (1944) reviewed some of these earlier studies and found no evidence of performance decline during menstruation. Harlow (1986) reviewed research conducted from the 1920s to the 1980s and reported that most show no changes in performance efficiency and no significant absenteeism due to menstrual pain. Yet, Dalton (1983) claimed that the decline in women's work as a result of cycle-related issues "cost

British industry 3% of its total wage bill … and 8% in America" (p. 100). This misguided concern for the economy has contributed to workplace discrimination against women for decades.

Research on women's work performance across the menstrual cycle has been criticized as having poor ecological validity because many of the studies were conducted with undergraduates in laboratories (Black & Koulis-Chitwood, 1990). The studies that have been conducted in the workplace have shown little to no variation in work performance across the menstrual cycle (Black & Koulis-Chitwood, 1990; Harlow, 1986). Sommer (1983) summarized the results of 29 published and unpublished studies about women's cognitive, perceptual, and motor abilities across the menstrual cycle, abilities that are relevant to work and school performance. Eleven of the studies showed cycle effects, including some negative phase effects (e.g., poorer backward subtraction performance in the pre-ovulatory phase; verbal dysfluencies during menstruation and post-ovulation) and some positive phase effects (e.g., optimum speed of arithmetic premenstrually; better human figure drawing in the post-ovulatory phase; a menstruating group performed better on verbal tasks than a non-menstruating group). Eighteen studies demonstrated no phase differences in performance on cognitive tasks, such as reasoning, perceptual speed, verbal fluency, and arithmetic.

There have been many methodological improvements in performance studies over the years. The most recent research about the menstrual cycle and cognitive functioning has been conducted by neuroscientists who use advanced methods for steroid hormone analyses across the cycle. Sundstrom-Poromaa and Gingnell (2014, p. 1) conducted a review of "methodologically sound menstrual cycle studies" of cognitive functioning and emotion processing in healthy women. They reported mixed results in studies of mental rotation, visuospatial tasks, verbal skills, memory, and emotion processing, and concluded that differences across the menstrual cycle in mental rotation, verbal fluency, memory, and visuospatial ability are "small and difficult to replicate" (p. 12). Thus, there is no conclusive evidence that the work and cognitive performance of healthy women (without any cycle-related medical conditions) is significantly or detrimentally impaired during any phase of the cycle.

Does the menstrual cycle affect women's athletic performance? Paula Ratcliffe, who broke the world record in 2002 when she ran the Chicago Marathon on the first day of her menses (Lewis, 2015), would probably say no. Despite widespread acceptance of the belief that performance is affected by the menstrual cycle, studies have failed to corroborate this claim. For women who do not suffer from severe cycle-related conditions, there do not seem to be conclusive and reliable variations in performance across the menstrual cycle. Eston (1984) reviewed more than 90 studies that used survey research, physical and psychological assessments, and physiological measurements across the menstrual cycle. He found that, in many of the categories in which differences in performance were found, there were either conflicting results about in which phase changes occurred or no differences were detected. For example, there were no changes across the menstrual cycle in simple reaction times, maximum oxygen uptake, and cardiac output during exercise or rest. Eston concluded that the wide variability in the literature is probably a result of many individual variables (e.g., type of sport, nature of the exercise, menstrual symptoms/experiences, nutrition, overall health).

The majority of the early research on athletic performance and the menstrual cycle was based on retrospective studies, such as survey results of women's perceptions of their own performance. When performance was measured in real-time, cycle phase was often calculated based on the calendar method (i.e., counting the number of days since the last menses), yet the most accurate way to determine cycle phases is by hormone assay (Shimoda, Campbell, & Barton,

2018). In a study where cycle phase was confirmed by assay (Lebrun, McKenzie, Prior, & Taunton, 1995), the researchers concluded that athletic performance was not affected by cycle phase for the majority of their tests (e.g., anaerobic capacity, isokinetic strength, endurance), but noted that there may be a slight decrease in aerobic capacity (VO_{2max}) during the luteal phase, although others (Nicklas, Hackney, & Sharp, 1989) have found slight increases in endurance during the luteal phase.

In their review of studies of athletic performance, Rechichi, Dawson, and Goodman (2009) suggested that inconsistencies in the results of research are due to small numbers of participants, invalid verification of menstrual cycle phases, variability in menstrual experiences, and high variability in estrogen and progesterone concentrations both between and within subjects (note that these methodological issues occur in studies of all sorts of possible cycle-related concomitants). The relationship between ovarian hormones and athletic performance is complex. Thus, even when menstrual phase has been adequately verified among a group of women, it is difficult to collapse them into phase groups and make meaningful comparisons.

Sensation and perception across the menstrual cycle

Researchers with an evolutionary perspective have theorized that women have some sensory advantages during high fertility times of the month and during pregnancy (see review by Doty & Cameron, 2009). For example, it has been hypothesized that women have better olfactory acuity during ovulation so that they can smell their potential sexual partners' pheromones, and sensitivity to odors may be higher during pregnancy so that women can beware of dangers (e.g., noxious gasses, rancid food). Some have suggested that olfactory abilities also routinely differ between women and men as a result of reproductive hormones (Evans, Cui, & Starr, 1995; Russell, Switz, & Thompson, 1980). In one of the first studies (Le Magnen, 1952) that systematically tested olfactory sensitivity during different phases of the menstrual cycle, women's sensitivity to crystalline exaltolide (a musky odor) increased after menstruation; however, the number of days after menstruation varied, and some increases occurred in a bimodal pattern (after menstruation and again during the late luteal phase). Thus, concrete conclusions and generalizations could not be made.

Other researchers have also found that women's olfactory sensitivity to exaltolide and other odorants peaks at different times of the menstrual cycle; however, there are conflicting results about at what point in the cycle olfactory sensitivity increases or decreases and to what odorants (e.g., Doty, Hall, Flickinger, & Sondheimer, 1982; Good, Geary, & Engen, 1976). For example, it has been found that olfactory sensitivity increases (e.g., Mair, Bouffard, Engen, & Morton, 1978) *and* decreases around ovulation (e.g., Navarrette-Palacios, Hudson, Reyes-Guerrero, & Guevara-Guzman, 2003) and that there are no differences in olfactory sensitivity across the menstrual cycle (e.g., Hummel, Kobal, Gudziol, & Mackay-Sim, 2007).

In a study of women who were and were not taking oral contraceptives (OCs), researchers found that olfactory sensitivity peaked during the mid-luteal phase, during the second half of the menses, and also mid-cycle for all women, regardless of whether they were taking OCs (Doty, Snyder, Huggins, & Lowry, 1981). However, others (e.g., Landis, Konnerth, & Hummel, 2004) have found that women who are taking OCs have higher olfactory sensitivity and better odor identification than women who are not, and that the longer a woman takes OCs, the better her olfactory acuity (Derntl, Schopf, Kollndorfer, & Lanzenberger, 2013). The conflicting findings might be explained by the types of odorants that were used as stimuli. Taken together, these studies show that women's naturally-occurring hormones seem to affect olfaction, but the mechanisms by which they influence olfaction and the exact patterns of olfactory sensitivity across the cycle are not predictable.

Parlee (1981) and Sommer (1983) conducted extensive reviews of the research on changes in sensory functioning across the menstrual cycle. Their reviews showed no consistent cycle-related changes in temperature sensitivity, two-touch (haptic) thresholds, or taste. There was a trend toward lower pain sensitivity during the premenstrual and menstrual phases, higher olfactory and visual sensitivity around the time of ovulation, and higher auditory acuity at ovulation and at the onset of menstruation. However, the sample sizes were often small (e.g., 4–12 participants), and the experimental procedures, type and frequency of measurements, and ways in which the cycle phases were operationalized varied greatly, which makes it difficult to draw conclusions (Parlee, 1981; Sommer, 1983).

In more recent research wherein hormone levels were assessed, correlations have been found between hormones and enhanced visual processing of emotional stimuli. Wassell, Rogers, Felmingam, Pearson, and Bryant (2015) examined 20 women during their follicular phase (low progesterone), 20 women during their mid-luteal phase (high progesterone), and 24 men. A recall test 2 days later revealed that women with higher progesterone had stronger mental imageries for the negative images than did men and low-progesterone women. However, a stronger test of the hypothesis would require within-subject measurements.

Van Wingen et al. (2008) demonstrated via fMRI imaging that amygdala reactivity increased when women's progesterone levels increased, which suggests a role for progesterone in processing emotional images. Andreano and Cahill (2010) examined the effects of high progesterone and estrogen levels (during the luteal phase) on women's responses to negative emotional images. They found that progesterone, but not estrogen, levels correlated with brain activity in the amygdala. However, when Mareckova et al. (2014) examined the effects of progesterone and estrogen on blood oxygen level-dependent (BOLD) responses to faces, they found BOLD responses increased as a function of estrogen, not progesterone, when women viewed angry and ambiguous faces. Pearson and Lewis (2005) found differences in women's facial recognition of fear between high- and low-estrogen phases of the cycle; participants more accurately recognized fear when estrogen levels were high (late pre-ovulatory phase) than during menstruation when estrogen levels were low. Derntl et al. (2008, p. 1032) suggested that "raised progesterone levels bias behavioral tendencies toward threatening stimuli with the possible aim of protection from any source of threat or danger which might be especially relevant during a possible pregnancy." However, the discrepancies in the literature make it unclear as to whether progesterone or estrogen, or a combination of both, affects emotional processing.

Women tend to be better than men at recognizing the gender of faces and identifying the emotional expression in faces, particularly negative emotions (Schroeder, 2010). To determine whether the menstrual cycle is related to this skill, Derntl et al. (2008) asked women in either their follicular or luteal phases to identify the emotional expression in pictures of faces, including anger, disgust, fear, sadness, happiness, and neutral as their brains were scanned for amygdala activation. Behavioral results showed no differences across cycle phase in accuracy of emotion recognition. There was, however, a negative correlation between amygdala activation and progesterone levels for fearful, neutral, and sad faces. Thus, progesterone levels might mediate a fear-reducing effect, which could improve mood and help with social interactions.

Women's attraction, attractiveness, and sexual behavior across the menstrual cycle

Evolutionary psychology theory purports that heterosexual women are more attracted to high-fitness gene qualities (e.g., physical attractiveness, facial symmetry, muscularity) in men when they are ovulating than during other phases of the cycle (Gangestad, Simpson, Cousins, Garver-Apgar, & Christensen, 2004). But, do women's preferences for men change across the menstrual cycle? Gildersleeve, Haselton, and Fales (2014) conducted a meta-analysis of the existing research about the "ovulatory shift" hypothesis (i.e., women are more sexually attracted to men with "good genes" on high- than on low-fertility days). They examined 50 studies that yielded 134 effects, 96 of which supported the ovulatory shift hypothesis. However, Wood, Kressel, Joshi, and Louie (2014) published a similar meta-analysis of 58 studies, and they concluded that fertile women did *not* prefer to have short-term sexual experiences with men who had high-fitness genetic qualities. In fact, they reported that 30 of the 91 effects were in the opposite direction.

What could cause such a large discrepancy in the results of these studies? Wood and Carden (2014) suggested that there are two main issues with these studies and the meta-analyses of them. First, authors of both meta-analytic studies decided which studies to include and whether to consider both published and unpublished reports. Many of the unpublished reports showed null effects; thus, there is likely a publication bias in that the studies that did not show phase effects of attractiveness were not published. Second, the methods that were used in the studies to estimate women's cycle phases are inconsistent and probably often inaccurate (e.g., hormone levels were often not tested). In a study of women's sexual attraction to men across the menstrual cycle, Shimoda et al. (2018) collected hormone samples to track the menstrual cycle and found that 45% of ovulations were incorrectly labeled when the women used the calendar method to estimate their cycle phases. This is a common limitation in menstrual cycle research. When hormones are assayed, phase effects seem to diminish. For example, Jones et al. (2018) conducted one of the largest longitudinal studies of women's preferences for masculine characteristics in men's faces across the menstrual cycle. They used salivary steroid hormone levels to track cycle phase and found no evidence that women's preference for masculinity increases when women are most fertile. There were no differences between fertile and non-fertile phases, which disconfirms the evolutionary theory.

From an evolutionary perspective, "shifts across the menstrual cycle in sexual desire and arousal may have evolved to promote sexual behavior and saliency of sexual stimuli when probability of conception is heightened during the mid-follicular and ovulatory phases" (Shirazi, Bossio, Puts, & Chivers, 2018, p. 45). Although heterosexual women's attraction to specific characteristics of men during different phases of the menstrual cycle is questionable, there is some evidence to suggest that young women are more sexual, in general, during different times of the cycle (see the review by Motta-Mena & Puts, 2017). For example, some research has shown that women have higher sexual desire and engage more often in sexual activities on the day before and the day of ovulation (Gangestad & Thornhill, 2008). However, Brewis and Meyer (2005) found no differences in women's sexual behavior across the menstrual cycle. Brown, Calibuso, and Roedl (2011) suggested that the conflicting findings about women's sexuality across the cycle may be a result of behavioral factors, such as how attracted the women were to their partners, whether the women had consistent sexual partners, and whether the women were sexually active with women or men.

Other sexually attractive behaviors that have been tested across the menstrual cycle include flirtatiousness (Miller, Tybur, & Jordan, 2007; Puts et al., 2013), women's gait and speed of walking in front of men (Gueguen, 2012), and women's clothing choices (Durante & Haselton, 2008; Eisenbruch, Simmons, & Roney, 2015; Haselton, Mortezaie, Pillsworth, Bleske-Rechek, & Frederick, 2007). These studies have mixed results and serious methodological limitations. The most that can be concluded is that *some* "women show greater interest for social contact with men in the fertile phase of their menstrual cycle," and they try "to appear more attractive in order to attract more men" (Gueguen, 2012, p. 621).

Evolutionary theory also predicts that women will be most sexually active around the time of ovulation, and some researchers have found peak sexual interest and activity at mid-cycle in women who were not using oral contraceptives (e.g., Morris & Urdry, 1982). However, sexuality is complex, and researchers do not agree on what should be measured (e.g., desire, arousal, fantasies, "interest," masturbation, orgasm, self-initiated activity, responsiveness to partner), thus, as in other areas reviewed above, results of studies are mixed. In one interesting study (Wallis & Englander-Golden, 1985, as cited by Golub, 1992), women who were unaware of the purpose of the diary study reported three peaks in sexual arousal: at mid-cycle, during the premenstrual phase, and on Day 4 (toward the end of menses). The mid-cycle peak can be explained by evolutionary theory, but the others cannot. They can, however, be explained by adherence to the sex taboo.

Moods and the menstrual cycle

The hormonal hypothesis, which is widely accepted in the US and other Western countries, suggests that changes in hormone patterns across the menstrual cycle affect women's moods. People used to expect the most negative moods to appear during the menses, but, since 1980, when premenstrual syndrome (PMS) became well known, people expect the most negative moods to occur before the menses begin. (For more about the history of PMS and the medicalization of women's moods, see Chrisler & Caplan, 2002, or Chrisler & Gorman, 2015.) In keeping with the debilitation hypothesis, researchers have focused their attention on negative moods; positive effects of the cycle on moods have rarely been studied (Chrisler et al., 1994; Parlee, 1980).

The results of research on mood, like that of the other cycle concomitants discussed above, are mixed. A review of 47 studies conducted in Western countries shows that 18 reported no association of mood with the menstrual cycle, 18 reported an association between mood and both the premenstrual phase and another phase, and 7 reported mood associated only with the premenstrual phase (Romans, Clarkson, Einstein, Petrovic, & Stewart, 2012). Thus, mood changes are not reliably demonstrable, and, when they do appear, they are weaker than expected. For example, Golub (1976) tracked participants' scores on measures of anxiety and depression across several cycles. She found significant increases in both measures during the premenstrual phase. However, the average premenstrual anxiety scores were lower than average scores others had reported during orientation for new college students and lower than students' scores during exam week. In other words, although the premenstrual scores were statistically significant, they were not clinically significant. Other researchers have found that stress (Wilcoxon, Schrader, & Sherif, 1976) and day of the week (Englander-Golden, Sonleitner, Whitmore, & Corbley, 1986; Ripper, 1991) have a greater effect on women's mood than does the menstrual cycle and that mood fluctuates as much in men as it does in women over the course of 28 days (Parlee, 1980; Rogers & Harding, 1981).

In a recent, well-designed study that used hormone assays to determine cycle phase, Lorenz, Gesselman, and Vitzthum (2017) collected daily reports of depression, anxiety, irritability, and fatigue from 27 women across two to six consecutive menstrual cycles. The majority of the variance in mood (79–98%) was due to daily, not cycle-related, fluctuations. That study, and the others cited above, were conducted prospectively. Retrospective studies, in which women are asked to think back on the last month or two and indicate when they experienced mood changes, often show that participants report negative moods during the premenstrual phase. It may be that women are so familiar with the stereotype of premenstrual women as anxious, tense, and depressed that they incorrectly "remember" any negative moods as having occurred at that point in their cycle rather than more randomly through the cycle. Their reports may be an illusory correlation; because we expect certain patterns, we notice instances when those patterns happen, but we do not remember instances when the pattern does not hold. The expected pattern (learned through cultural stereotypes) leads people to attribute changes in mood to changes in hormones associated with the menstrual cycle (Koeske & Koeske, 1975). Furthermore, research has shown that when participants are aware that a study concerns the menstrual cycle, they report more mood variability than when they do when they are unaware of the study's purpose (AuBuchon & Calhoun, 1985; Englander-Golden et al., 1986). These results could be due to social expectancies or to demand characteristics (i.e., attempts to please the researchers by focusing attention on what participants believe researchers want) (AuBuchon & Calhoun, 1985).

Taken together, these studies show that cycle-related mood changes are not typical of healthy, regularly cycling women. They do *not* show that *no* women experience cycle-related mood changes. For example, some researchers (Halbreich & Endicott, 1987; Mitchell, Woods, & Lentz, 1994) have observed that women who have been diagnosed with depression report that their depression is worse when they are premenstrual, a phenomenon that Nancy Fugate Woods and her team called PMM – premenstrual magnification of existing symptoms. PMM has also been observed in patients with other disorders (e.g., multiple sclerosis, migraine) (Taylor, 2002). There is a difference between being premenstrual and having premenstrual syndrome, a distinction that is lost in popular culture.

Conclusion

The menstrual cycle is a biopsychosocial phenomenon. The biological changes that occur across the cycle can, of course, affect women's behavior, but they are also affected by women's behavior and interpreted in light of women's beliefs about and attitudes toward the menstrual cycle. Attitudes, beliefs, and behaviors are shaped by the sociocultural context in which they were formed. Women differ biologically (e.g., genetics, cycle length, age), psychologically (e.g., positive, negative, or ambivalent attitudes), culturally (e.g., beliefs, habits), and in terms of their physical and mental health. Thus, women's experience of the menstrual cycle and its concomitants is highly variable.

Negative attitudes toward and beliefs about menstruation and menstruating women (e.g., moodiness, unpredictability), and taboos against sex and engagement in strenuous activities during menstruation, have undoubtedly influenced scientists' interest in documenting behavioral, cognitive, sexual, and emotional changes across the menstrual cycle. Even when results of studies do not support cycle effects, researchers continue to look for them because cultural beliefs are so strong, social expectancies are so high, and, of course, evidence of cycle-related debilitation would support the notion that women are the weaker sex and thus uphold the gender status quo and enhance men's political power.

The debilitation hypothesis, the hormonal hypothesis, and evolutionary psychology theory do not hold up in carefully designed empirical investigations. That means that most women's work and athletic performance, sensation and perception, sexual behavior, and mood are not significantly affected by their menstrual cycle. That does not mean, however, that no women experience any mood or sexuality changes or behavioral or cognitive deficits or enhancements at various points in the cycle. Information about cycle-related disorders (e.g., dysmenorrhea, premenstrual syndrome) that could cause such effects can be found in other chapters in this *Handbook*.

References

Allen, K. R., Kaestle, C. E., & Goldberg, A. E. (2011). More than just a punctuation mark: How boys and young men learn about menstruation. *Journal of Family Issues, 32,* 129–156.

Andreano, J. M. & Cahill, L. (2010). Menstrual cycle modulation of medial temporal activity evoked by negative emotion. *NeuroImage, 53,* 1286–1293.

Aubeeluck, A. & Maguire, M. (2002). The menstrual joy questionnaire items alone can positively prime reporting of menstrual symptoms and attitudes. *Psychology of Women Quarterly, 26,* 160–162.

AuBuchon, P. G. & Calhoun, K. S. (1985). Menstrual cycle symptomatology: The role of social expectancy and experimental demand characteristics. *Psychosomatic Medicine, 47,* 35–45.

Black, S. L. & Koulis-Chitwood, A. (1990). The menstrual cycle and typing skill: An ecologically-valid test of the "raging hormones" hypothesis. *Canadian Journal of Behavioral Science, 22,* 445–455.

Brewis, A. & Meyer, M. (2005). Demographic evidence that human ovulation is undetectable (at least in pair bonds). *Current Anthropology, 46,* 465–471.

British Broadcasting Corporation (BBC) (2017, August 10). Nepal criminalises banishing menstruating women to huts. Retrieved January 29, 2018 from www.bbc.com/news/world-asia-40885748.

Brown, S. G., Calibuso, M. J., & Roedl, A. L. (2011). Women's sexuality, well-being, and the menstrual cycle: Methodological issues and their interrelationships. *Archives of Sexual Behavior, 40,* 755–765.

Buckley, T. (1982). Menstruation and the power of Yurok women: Methods in cultural reconstruction. *American Ethnologist, 9,* 47–60.

Çevirme, A. S., Çevirme, H., Karaoglu, L., Ugurlu, N., & Korkmaz, Y. (2010). The perception of menarche and menstruation among Turkish married women: Attitudes, experiences, and behaviors. *Social Behavior and Personality, 38,* 381–394.

Chang, Y.-T., Hayter, M., & Lin, M.-L. (2011). Pubescent male students' attitudes toward menstruation in Taiwan: Implications for reproductive health education and school nursing practice. *Journal of Clinical Nursing, 21,* 513–521.

Chrisler, J. C. (2002). Hormone hostages: The cultural legacy of PMS as a legal defense. In L. H. Collins, M. R. Dunlap, & J. C. Chrisler (Eds), *Charting a new course for feminist psychology* (pp. 238–252). Westport, CT: Praeger.

Chrisler, J. C. & Caplan, P. (2002). The strange case of Dr. Jekyll and Ms. Hyde: How PMS became a cultural phenomenon and a psychiatric disorder. *Annual Review of Sex Research, 13,* 274–306.

Chrisler, J. C. & Gorman, J. A. (2015). The medicalization of women's moods: Premenstrual syndrome and premenstrual dysphoric disorder. In M. C. McHugh & J. C. Chrisler (Eds), *The wrong prescription for women: How medicine and media create a "need" for treatments, drugs, and surgery* (pp. 77–98). Santa Barbara, CA: Praeger.

Chrisler, J. C., Gorman, J. A., Marván, M. L., & Johnston-Robledo, I. (2014). Ambivalent sexism and attitudes toward women in different stages of their reproductive lives: A semantic, cross-cultural approach. *Health Care for Women International, 35,* 634–657.

Chrisler, J. C., Johnston, I. K., Champagne, N. M., & Preston, K. E. (1994). Menstrual joy: The construct and its consequences. *Psychology of Women Quarterly, 18,* 375–387.

Chrisler, J. C. & Levy, K. B. (1990). The media construct a menstrual monster: A content analysis of PMS articles in the popular press. *Women & Health, 16*(2), 89–104.

Chrisler, J. C., Marván, M. L., Gorman, J. A., & Rossini, M. (2015). Body appreciation and attitudes toward menstruation. *Body Image, 12,* 78–81.

Cicurel, I. E. (2000). The Rabbinate versus Israeli (Jewish) women: The Mikvah as a contested domain. *Nashim, 3,* 164–190.

Crawford, M., Menger, L. M., & Kaufman, M. R. (2014). "This is a natural process": Managing menstrual stigma in Nepal. *Culture, Health, & Sexuality, 16*, 426–439.

Dalton, K. (1983). *Once a month* (rev. ed.). Claremont, CA: Hunter House.

Delaney, J., Lupton, M. J., & Toth, E. (1987). *The curse: A cultural history of menstruation* (rev. ed.). Chicago, IL: University of Illinois Press.

Derntl, B., Schopf, V., Kollndorfer, K., & Lanzenberger, R. (2013). Menstrual cycle phase and duration of oral contraception intake affect olfactory perception. *Chemical Senses, 38*(1), 67–75.

Derntl, B., Windischberger, C., Robinson, S., Lamplmayr, E., Kryspin-Exner, I., Gur, R. C., Moser, E., & Habel, U. (2008). Facial emotion recognition and amygdala activation are associated with menstrual cycle phase. *Psychoneuroendocrinology, 33*, 1031–1040.

Dosler, A. J. & Mivsek, A. P. (2015). Does midwifery philosophy affect perceptions of students regarding female reproduction?. *Health Sociology Review, 24*, 175–185.

Doty, R. L. & Cameron, E. L. (2009). Sex differences and reproductive hormone influences on human odor perception. *Physiology and Behavior, 97*, 213–228.

Doty, R. L., Hall, J. W., Flickinger, G. L., & Sondheimer, S. J. (1982). Cyclical changes in olfactory and auditory sensitivity during the menstrual cycle: No attenuation by oral contraceptive medication. In W. Breipohl (Ed.), *Olfaction and endocrine regulation* (pp. 35–42). London, UK: IRL Press.

Doty, R. L., Snyder, P. J., Huggins, G. R., & Lowry, L. D. (1981). Endocrine, cardiovascular, and psychological correlates of olfactory sensitivity changes during the human menstrual cycle. *Journal of Comparative Physiology and Psychology, 95*, 45–60.

Durante, K. M. & Haselton, M. G. (2008). Changes in women's choice of dress across the ovulatory cycle: Naturalistic and laboratory task-based evidence. *Personality and Social Psychology Bulletin, 34*, 1451–1460.

Eisenbruch, A. B., Simmons, Z. L., & Roney, J. R. (2015). Lady in red: Hormonal predictors of women's clothing choices. *Psychological Science, 26*(8), 1332–1338.

Englander-Golden, P., Sonleitner, F. J., Whitmore, M., & Corbley, G. (1986). Social and menstrual cycles: Methodological and substantive findings. In V. L. Olesen & N. F. Woods (Eds), *Culture, society, and menstruation* (pp. 77–96). Washington, DC: Hemisphere.

Erchull, M. J. & Richmond, K. (2015). "It's normal ... Mom will be home in an hour": The role of fathers in menstrual education. *Women's Reproductive Health, 2*, 93–110.

Ernster, V. L. (1975). American menstrual expressions. *Sex Roles, 1*, 3–13.

Eston, R. (1984). The regular menstrual cycle and athletic performance. *Sports Medicine, 1*, 431–445.

Evans, W. J., Cui, L., & Starr, A. (1995). Olfactory event-related potentials in normal human subjects: Effects of age and gender. *Electroencephalography and Clinical Neurophysiology, 95*, 293–301.

Fahs, B. (2011). Sex during menstruation: Race, sexual identity, and women's accounts of pleasure and disgust. *Feminism & Psychology, 21*, 155–178.

Fahs, B. (2014). Genital panics: Constructing the vagina in women's qualitative narratives about pubic hair, menstrual sex, and vaginal self-image. *Body Image, 11*, 210–218.

Frazer, J. G. (1951). *The golden bough.* New York: Macmillan.

Gangestad, S. W., Simpson, J. A., Cousins, A. J., Garver-Apgar, C. E., & Christensen, P. N. (2004). Women's preferences for male behavioral displays across the menstrual cycle. *Psychological Science, 15*, 203–207.

Gangestad, S. W. & Thornhill, R. (2008). Human oestrus. *Proceedings of the Royal Society London B, 275*, 991–1000.

Gettleman, J. (2018, June 20). Nepal's grim superstition, known to lead to a death by shame. *New York Times*, pp. A1, A6.

Gildersleeve, K., Haselton, M. G., & Fales, M. R. (2014). Do women's mate preferences change across the ovulatory cycle? A meta-analytic review. *Psychological Bulletin, 140*, 1205–1259.

Goldenberg, J. L. & Roberts, T.-A. (2004). The beast within the beauty: An existential perspective on the objectification and condemnation of women. In J. Greenberg, S. L. Koole, & T. Pyszczynski (Eds), *Handbook of experimental existential psychology* (pp. 71–85). New York: Guilford.

Golub, S. (1976). The effect of premenstrual anxiety and depression on cognitive function. *Journal of Personality and Social Psychology, 34*, 99–104.

Golub, S. (1992). *Periods: From menarche to menopause.* Newbury Park, CA: Sage.

Good, P. R., Geary, N., & Engen, T. (1976). The effect of estrogen on odor detection. *Chemical Senses and Flavour, 2*, 45–50.

Gorman, J. A., Barney, A., Chrisler, J., Krasner, B., Pavitt, L., Pepin, H., Rosadini, S., Tutino, R., & Wang, Y. (2017, June). *What is PMS? A content analysis of "definitions" from Urban Dictionary*. Poster presented at the meeting of the Society for Menstrual Cycle Research, Kennesaw, GA.

Grose, R. G. & Grabe, S. (2014). Sociocultural attitudes surrounding menstruation and alternative menstrual products: The explanatory role of self-objectification. *Health Care for Women International, 35*, 677–694.

Gueguen, N. (2012). Gait and menstrual cycle: Ovulating women use sexier gaits and walk slowly ahead of men. *Gait and Posture, 35*, 621–624.

Halbreich, U. & Endicott, J. (1987). Dysphoric premenstrual changes: Are they related to affective disorders? In B. E. Ginsburg & B. F. Carter (Eds), *Premenstrual syndrome: Ethical and legal implications in a biomedical perspective* (pp. 351–367). New York: Plenum Press.

Harlow, S. D. (1986). Function and dysfunction: A historical critique of the literature on menstruation and work. In V. L. Olesen & N. F. Woods (Eds), *Culture, society, and menstruation* (pp. 39–50). Washington, DC: Hemisphere.

Haselton, M. G., Mortezaie, M., Pillsworth, E. G., Bleske-Rechek, A., & Frederick, D. A. (2007). Ovulatory shifts in human female ornamentation: Near ovulation, women dress to impress. *Hormones and Behavior, 51*, 40–45.

Hoerster, K. D., Chrisler, J. C., & Rose, J. G. (2003). Attitudes toward and experiences with menstruation in the US and India. *Women & Health, 38*(3), 77–95.

Hummel, T., Kobal, G., Gudziol, H., & Mackay-Sim, A. (2007). Normative data for the "sniffin' sticks" including tests of odor identification, odor discrimination, and olfactory thresholds: An upgrade based on a group of more than 3,000 subjects. *European Archives of Oto-Rhino-Laryngology, 264*, 237–243.

Johnston-Robledo, I. & Chrisler, J. C. (2013). The menstrual mark: Menstruation as social stigma. *Sex Roles, 68*, 9–18.

Johnston-Robledo, I., Sheffield, K., Voigt, J., & Wilcox-Constantine, J. (2007). Reproductive shame: Self-objectification and young women's attitudes toward their reproductive functioning. *Women & Health, 46*(1), 25–39.

Johnston-Robledo, I., Wares, S., Fricker, J., & Pasek, L. (2007). Indecent exposure: Self-objectification and young women's attitudes toward breastfeeding. *Sex Roles, 56*, 429–437.

Jones, B. C., Hahn, A. C., Fisher, C. I., Wang, H., Kandrik, M., Han, C., Fasolt, V., Morrison, D., Lee, A. J., Holzleitner, I. J., O'Shea, K. J., Roberts, S. C., Little, A. C., & DeBruine, L. M. (2018). No compelling evidence that preferences for facial masculinity track changes in women's hormonal status. *Psychological Science, 29*, 1–10.

King, M., Ussher, J. M., & Perz, J. (2014). Representations of PMS and premenstrual women in men's accounts: An analysis of online posts from PMSBuddy.com. *Women's Reproductive Health, 1*, 3–20.

Kissling, E. A. (1996). Bleeding out loud: Communication about menstruation. *Feminism & Psychology, 6*, 481–504.

Kissling, E. A. (2002). On the rag on screen: Menarche in film and television. *Sex Roles, 46*, 5–12.

Koeske, R. K. & Koeske, G. F. (1975). An attributional approach to moods and the menstrual cycle. *Personality and Social Psychology, 31*, 473–481.

Lahme, A. M. & Stern, R. (2017). Factors that affect menstrual hygiene among adolescent schoolgirls: A case study from Mongu District, Zambia. *Women's Reproductive Health, 4*, 198–211.

Landis, B. N., Konnerth, C. G., & Hummel, T. (2004). A study on the frequency of olfactory dysfunction. *Laryngosope, 114*, 1764–1769.

Lebrun, C. M., McKenzie, D. C., Prior, J. C., & Taunton, J. E. (1995). Effects of menstrual cycle phase on athletic performance. *Medicine and Science in Sports and Exercise, 27*, 437–444.

Le Magnen, J. (1952). Olfactory-sexual phenomena in man. *Physiological Sciences Archive, 6*, 125–160.

Lewis, A. (2015, January 22). *Curse or myth: Do periods affect performance?* Retrieved from www.bbc.com/sport/tennis/30926244.

Lorenz, T. K., Gesselman, A. N., & Vizthum, V. J. (2017). Variance in mood symptoms across menstrual cycles: Implications for premenstrual dysphoric disorder. *Women's Reproductive Health, 4*, 77–88.

Mair, R. G., Bouffard, J. A., Engen, T., & Morton, T. H. (1978). Olfactory sensitivity during the menstrual cycle. *Sensory Processes, 2*, 90–98.

Mareckova, K., Perrin, J. S., Khan, I. N., Lawrence, C., Dickie, E., McQuiggan, D. A., Paus, T., & the IMAEN Consortium (2014). Hormonal contraceptives, menstrual cycle, and brain response to faces. *Social, Cognitive, and Affective Neuroscience, 9*, 191–200.

Marván, M. L., Ramírez-Esparza, D., Cortés-Iniestra, S., & Chrisler, J. C. (2006). Development and validation of a new scale to measure Beliefs about and Attitudes toward Menstruation (BATM): Data from Mexico and the United States. *Health Care for Women International, 27*, 453–473.

Marván, M. L. & Trujillo, P. (2010). Menstrual socialization, beliefs, and attitudes concerning menstruation in rural and urban Mexican women. *Health Care for Women International, 31*, 53–67.

Marván, M. L., Vázquez-Toboada, R., & Chrisler, J. C. (2014). Ambivalent sexism, attitudes toward menstruation, and menstrual cycle-related symptoms. *International Journal of Psychology, 49*, 280–287.

Miller, G., Tybur, J. M., & Jordan, B. D. (2007). Ovulatory cycle effects on tip earnings by lap dancers: Economic evidence for human estrus? *Evolution and Human Behavior, 28*, 375–381.

Mitchell, E. S., Woods, N. F., & Lentz, M. J. (1994). Differentiation of women with three perimenstrual symptom patterns. *Nursing Research, 43*, 25–30.

Moradi, B. & Huang, Y.-P. (2008). Objectification theory and psychology of women: A decade of advances and future directions. *Psychology of Women Quarterly, 32*, 377–398.

Morris, K. L., Goldenberg, J. L., & Heflick, N. A. (2014). Trio of terror (pregnancy, menstruation, and breastfeeding): An existential function of literal self-objectification among women. *Journal of Personality and Social Psychology, 107*, 181–198.

Morris, N. M. & Urdry, J. R. (1982). Epidemiological patterns of sexual behavior in the menstrual cycle. In R. C. Friedman (Ed.), *Behavior and the menstrual cycle* (pp. 129–154). New York: Marcel Dekker.

Morrison, L. A., Larkspur, L., Calibuso, M. J., & Brown, S. (2010). Women's attitudes about menstruation and associated health and behavioral characteristics. *American Journal of Health Behavior, 34*, 90–100.

Motta-Mena, N. V. & Puts, D. A. (2017). Endocrinology of human female sexuality, mating, and reproductive behavior. *Hormones and Behavior, 91*, 19–35.

Navarrette-Palacios, E., Hudson, R., Reyes-Guerrero, M. S., & Guevara-Guzman, R. (2003). Correlation between cytology of the nasal epithelium and the menstrual cycle. *Archives of Otolaryngology-Head and Neck Surgery, 129*, 460–463.

Nicklas, B. J., Hackney, A. C., & Sharp, R. L. (1989). The menstrual cycle and exercise: Performance, muscle glycogen, and substrate responses. *International Journal of Sports Medicine, 10*, 264–269.

Padmanabhanunni, A. & Fennie, T. (2017). The menstruation experience: Attitude dimensions among South African students. *Journal of Psychology in Africa, 27*(1), 54–60.

Parlee, M. B. (1980). Positive changes in mood and activation levels during the menstrual cycle in experimentally naïve subjects. In A. J. Dan, E. A. Graham, & C. P. Beecher (Eds), *The menstrual cycle: A synthesis of interdisciplinary research* (pp. 247–263). New York: Springer.

Parlee, M. B. (1981). Menstrual rhythm in sensory processes: A review of fluctuations in vision, olfaction, audition, taste, and touch. *Psychological Bulletin, 93*, 539–548.

Pearson, R. & Lewis, M. B. (2005). Fear recognition across the menstrual cycle. *Hormones and Behavior, 47*, 267–271.

Peranovic, T. & Bentley, B. (2017). Men and menstruation: A qualitative exploration of beliefs, attitudes, and experiences. *Sex Roles, 77*, 113–124.

Puts, D. A., Bailey, D. H., Cardenas, R. A., Burriss, R. P., Welling, L. M., Wheatley, J. R., & Dawood, K. (2013). Women's attractiveness changes with estradiol and progesterone across the ovulatory cycle. *Hormones and Behavior, 63*, 13–19.

Rechichi, C., Dawson, B., & Goodman, C. (2009). Athletic performance and the oral contraceptive. *International Journal of Sports Physiology and Performance, 4*, 151–162.

Ripper, M. (1991). Comparison of the effect of the menstrual cycle and the social week on mood, sexual interest, and self-assessed performance. In D. L. Taylor & N. F. Woods (Eds), *Menstruation, health, and illness* (pp. 19–32). Washington, DC: Hemisphere.

Roberts, T.-A. (2004). Female trouble: The menstrual self-evaluation scale and women's self-objectification. *Psychology of Women Quarterly, 28*, 22–16.

Roberts, T.-A., Goldenberg, J. L., Power, C., & Pyszczynski, T. (2002). "Feminine protection": The effects of menstruation on attitudes toward women. *Psychology of Women Quarterly, 26*, 131–139.

Rogers, M. L. & Harding, S. S. (1981). Retrospective and daily menstrual distress measures using Moos' instruments (Forms A and T) and modified versions of Moos' instruments. In P. Komnenich, M. McSweeney, J. A. Noack, & N. Elder (Eds), *The menstrual cycle: Research and implications for women's health* (pp. 71–81). New York: Springer.

Romans, S., Clarkson, R., Einstein, G., Petrovic, M., & Stewart, D. (2012). Mood and the menstrual cycle: A review of prospective data studies. *Gender Medicine, 9*, 361–384.

Rose, J. G., Chrisler, J. C., & Couture, S. (2008). Young women's attitudes toward continuous use of oral contraceptives: The effect of priming positive attitudes toward menstruation on women's willingness to suppress menstruation. *Health Care for Women International, 29*, 688–701.

Rosewarne, L. (2011). *Periods in pop culture: Menstruation in film and television.* Lanham, MD: Lexington Books.

Rozin, P., Haidt, J., McCauley, C., Dunlop, L., & Ashmore, M. (1999). Individual differences in disgust sensitivity: Evaluations of paper-and-pencil versus behavioral measures. *Journal of Personality, 33*, 330–351.

Rubinstein, H. R. & Foster, J. H. (2013). "I don't know whether it is to do with age or to do with hormones and whether it is to do with a stage in your life": Making sense of menopause and the body. *Journal of Health Psychology, 18*, 292–307.

Russell, M. J., Switz, G. M., & Thompson, K. (1980). Olfactory influences on the human menstrual cycle. *Pharmacology, Biochemistry, and Behavior, 13*, 737–738.

Schroeder, J. A. (2010). Sex and gender in sensation and perception. In J. C. Chrisler & D. R. McCreary (Eds), *Handbook of gender research in psychology* (Vol. 1, pp. 235–257). New York: Springer.

Seward, G. H. (1944). Psychological effects of the menstrual cycle in women workers. *Psychological Bulletin, 41*, 90–102.

Shimoda, R., Campbell, A., & Barton, R. A. (2018). Women's emotional and sexual attraction to men across the menstrual cycle. *Behavioral Ecology, 29*, 51–59.

Shirazi, T. N., Bossio, J. A., Puts, D. A., & Chivers, M. L. (2018). Menstrual cycle phase predicts women's hormonal responses to sexual stimuli. *Hormones and Behavior, 103*, 45–53.

Smiles, D., Short, S. E., & Sommer, M. (2017). "I didn't tell anyone because I was very afraid": Girls' experiences of menstruation in contemporary Ethiopia. *Women's Reproductive Health, 4*, 185–197.

Sommer, B. (1983). How does menstruation affect cognitive competence and psychophysiological response? *Women & Health, 8*(2/3), 53–90.

Sundstrom-Poromaa, I. S. & Gingnell, M. G. (2014). Menstrual cycle influence on cognitive function and emotion processing – From a reproductive perspective. *Frontiers in Neuroscience, 8*, 1–16.

Sveen, H. (2016). Lava or code red: A linguistic study of menstrual expressions in English and Swedish. *Women's Reproductive Health, 3*, 145–159.

Sveinsdóttir, H. (2018). Menstruation, objectification, and health-related quality of life: A questionnaire study. *Journal of Clinical Nursing, 27*, e503–e513.

Taylor, D. (2002). *Taking back the month.* New York: Penguin.

Thornton, L.-J. (2013). "Time of the month" on Twitter: Taboo, stereotype, and bonding in a no-holds barred public arena. *Sex Roles, 68*, 41–54.

Van Wingen, G. A., van Broekhoven, F., Verkes, R. J., Petersson, K. M., Backstrom, T., & Buitelaar, J. K. (2008). Progesterone selectivity increases amygdala reactivity in women. *Molecular Psychiatry, 13*, 325–333.

Wassell, J., Rogers, S., Felmingam, K. L., Pearson, J., & Bryant, R. A. (2015). Progesterone and mental imagery interactively predict emotional memories. *Psychoneuroendocrinology, 51*, 1–10.

Wilcoxon, L. A., Schrader, S. L., & Sherif, C. W. (1976). Daily reports of activities, life events, mood, and somatic changes during the menstrual cycle. *Psychosomatic Medicine, 38*, 399–417.

Wood, W. & Carden, L. (2014). Elusiveness of menstrual cycle effects on mate preferences: Comment on Gildersleeve, Haselton, and Fales (2014). *Psychological Bulletin, 140*, 1265–1271.

Wood, W., Kressel, L., Joshi, P. D., & Louie, B. (2014). Meta-analysis of menstrual cycle effects on women's mate preferences. *Emotion Review, 6*, 229–249.

5

PREMENSTRUAL MOOD DISORDERS

A feminist psychosocial perspective

Jane M. Ussher and Janette Perz

Premenstrual change in mood and embodied sensation first appeared in the biomedical literature in the 1930s, described as "premenstrual tension" (PMT) (Frank, 1931). Premenstrual "disorders" were renamed "premenstrual syndrome" in the 1950s, to incorporate a broader range of symptoms (Dalton, 1959), Late Luteal Phase Dysphoric Disorder (LLPPD) in the 1980s, and now sit in the *Diagnostic and Statistical Manual of Mental Disorders* (*DSM-5*) as Premenstrual Dysphoric Disorder (PMDD), an official psychiatric diagnosis (American Psychiatric Association, 2013). It is estimated that 2–5% of women in North America, Western Europe, and Australia meet a PMDD diagnosis; around 40% meet the lesser diagnosis of PMS – the same basic conglomeration of symptoms, just experienced to a lesser degree (Hartlage, Freels, Gotman, & Yonkers, 2012). Recognition of the continuum of premenstrual distress, and overlap between the diagnostic categories PMS and PMDD, has led to the adoption of the term "Premenstrual Disorders" (PMDs) by an expert advisory panel (Nevatte et al., 2013).

Premenstrual disorders include emotional and behavioural symptoms that can have a significant impact on a woman's quality of life during the premenstrual phase of the menstrual cycle, but the symptoms are absent after menstruation and before ovulation. The symptoms most commonly reported include irritability, anger, depression, mood swings, anxiety, concentration difficulties, feelings of loss of control, and tiredness, often combined with physical symptoms such as bloating, breast tenderness, headache, and general body aches (Rapkin & Lewis, 2013). Within the annals of biomedicine, PMDs are positioned as a biological phenomenon, "an extreme variant of a physiological influence of sex steroids on the brain and other organs" (Nevatte et al., 2013, p. 304). Associated with rises in serum progesterone and estradiol, or variations in monoamine serotonin, biomedical interventions include anxiolytics and hormone treatments to suppress ovulation; oophorectomy; and serotonin reuptake inhibitor (SSRI) anti-depressants (Nevatte et al., 2013; Rapkin & Lewis, 2013).

However, the very notion of premenstrual change as deserving of "diagnosis" has been questioned by many feminist critics (Chrisler, 2004; Ussher, 1989), and the inclusion of PMDD in the appendix of *DSM-IIIR* and *IV* strongly opposed, on the grounds of lack of validity as a distinct "mental illness" (Cosgrove & Caplan, 2004). Biomedical theories and interventions have also been criticised for not taking account of the complex mechanisms underlying premenstrual distress, which are not adequately accounted for by physiology alone (Ussher & Perz, 2017). Such theories also cannot explain why a significant proportion of women do not experience premenstrual distress (Lorenz, Gesselman, & Vitzthum, 2017), or indeed experience heightened distress at any phase of the menstrual cycle (see Romans, Clarkson, Einstein, Petrovic, & Stewart, 2012). In this chapter, we adopt a feminist psycho-social perspective, and draw on a series of research studies we have conducted in the UK and Australia, to examine women's experience of premenstrual distress and strategies of coping (Ussher, 2006). Our focus on psychosocial aspects of premenstrual experience does not negate the role of biology, which is covered in detail in other chapters in this volume. We adopt a material-discursive-intrapsychic (MDI) model (Ussher, 1999; Ussher, Hunter, & Browne, 2000), which provides a multidimensional analysis of the interconnections between the embodied and psychological experience of premenstrual change; the material and rela-tional context of women's lives that may precipitate distress; socially constructed representa-tions of PMDs and the premenstrual woman; and the psychological negotiation in which women engage to make sense of their experience. In the analysis below we use the term "PMS" to refer to women's accounts of moderate-to-severe premenstrual distress, as this is the term used by the majority of women.

PMS as a culture-bound syndrome

Premenstrual distress across cultural contexts

The bodily functions we understand as a sign of "illness" vary across culture and across time. Women's interpretation of psychological and bodily changes as "symptoms" of PMDs cannot be understood outside of the social and historical context in which they live, as interpretation is influenced by the *meaning* ascribed to these changes in a particular cultural context (Ussher, 2006). In this vein, feminist critics have argued that premenstrual changes are a normal part of women's experience, which is only positioned as PMDs because of Western cultural constructions of the premenstrual phase of the cycle as a time of psycho-logical disturbance and debilitation (e.g., Chrisler & Levy, 1990; Rittenhouse, 1991; Rodin, 1992). In cultures such as Hong Kong (Chang, Holroyd, & Chau, 1995), China (Yu, Zhu, Li, Oakley, & Reame, 1996), or India (Chaturvedi & Chandra, 1991; Hoerster, Chrisler, & Gorman Rose, 2003), where menstruation is more likely to be conceptualised as a natural event, women report premenstrual water retention, pain, fatigue, and increased sensitivity to cold, but rarely report negative premenstrual moods or other forms of premenstrual distress. Other studies have shown that people in some non-Western cultures are less likely to see premenstrual change as a serious problem that warrants medical attention (Chandraratne & Gunawardena, 2011; Wong & Khoo, 2011). In research we conducted with recent migrant and refugee women living in Australia, we found absence of a construct of PMS (Ussher et al., 2017), indeed, there was laughter at the very notion that the concept could exist (Ussher et al., 2012). Such research findings support the conclusion that culture shapes the physical and psychological changes that are deemed to be "symptoms" and that PMS is a culture bound syndrome (Chrisler & Caplan, 2002).

Rates of premenstrual distress vary significantly across Western cultures, which suggests that cultural factors also influence awareness of symptoms or perceptions of symptom severity (Den-nerstein, Lehert, Bäckström, & Heinemann, 2009). Equally, within Western cultures PMS is not universal. For example, a study that compared immigrant and U.S.-born women who iden-tified as Asian, Black, or Latina found that the likelihood of reporting premenstrual distress increased with length of duration of U.S. residence, which suggests that exposure to mainstream U.S. culture is associated with diagnosis of PMDs (Pilver, Kasl, Desai, & Levy, 2011).

Idealised femininity and self-identification as a PMS sufferer

Biomedical discourse provides the framework wherein premenstrual change is understood and experienced as an illness within Western cultures, resulting in women's self-positioning as "PMS sufferers" (Ussher, 2003b). The Western conceptualisation of emotion as stable, consistent, and under control is also central to the conceptualisation of premenstrual change as pathology. Chrisler (2008) has described PMS as an archetypal example of a disorder where absence of self-regulation, particularly in relation to the expression of anger, is positioned as pathology. The fear of being overwhelmed by the "menstrual monster" is thus a "recipe for psychological disaster," as women are socialised to believe that they "need to work at self-control in every waking hour" (Chrisler, 2008, p.2). Women monitor premenstrual moods and behaviour in relation to often unrealistic feminine ideals of calmness, consistency, and capability (Brooks, Ruble, & Clarke, 1977; Ussher, 2004), and blame themselves, or their bodies, for perceived transgressions, which facilitates identifying as "PMS sufferers" (Chrisler & Johnston-Robledo, 2002).

This was evident in our research with UK and Australian women who described a range of "unfeminine" emotions as characterising "PMS," including feeling "irritable," "cranky," "short-tempered," "snappy," "confrontational," "bitey," "impatient," "grumpy," "stroppy," "frustrated," "stressed," "annoyed," and "teary" (Ussher & Perz, 2013a). Such emotions were considered problematic because women felt "out of control": "I physically feel like I can't stop it. It's just this physical feeling of I don't know, anger inside"; "I don't have control over how I feel at all" (Ussher, 2003b; Ussher & Perz, 2013b). These accounts show that women accept the premise at the core of biomedical conceptualisations of PMDs: that "normal" emotions are constant, and therefore fluctuations in mood, sensation, or reaction to others are a personal failing or pathology (Chrisler, 2008; Ussher, 2003b).

Premenstrual embodiment: self-objectification and dehumanisation

Cultural constructions of idealised femininity are also implicated in Western women's experiences of premenstrual embodiment. It has been reported that body image "distortion" and body dissatisfaction is higher during the premenstrual phase of the cycle for "normal" Western women who do not self-position as "PMS sufferers" (Kaczmarek & Trambacz-Oleszak, 2016; Teixeira, Dias, Damasceno, Lamounier, & Gardner, 2013). In those women who do present with PMDs, levels of premenstrual symptom severity have been reported to be associated with body image disturbance (Muljat, Lustyk, & Miller, 2007) and with body dissatisfaction (Kleinstäuber et al., 2016). In this vein, the majority of women we interviewed reported negative feelings towards their bodies, and by implication their very selves, when they were premenstrual; they described themselves as "fat," "ugly," "a blimp," "gross," "frumpy," "sluggish," "disgusting," "lumpy," "sludgy," and "unattractive." In these accounts, negative feelings were attributed to perceptions of embodied change premenstrually, such as "bloating," "tenderness in the breasts," and "breasts that feel bigger." Women explicitly described these changes as acting to annihilate their "self-confidence," "sense of being attractive," and "self-esteem" – their very sense of self as a woman. As one woman told us: "Yes I hate myself, I don't have any self-confidence and don't even want to look in any mirror" (Ussher & Perz, 2019).

These accounts suggest a form of self-objectification (Fredrickson & Roberts, 1997), wherein women have internalised a critical gaze that finds them wanting, because the "bloated," "fat" premenstrual body does not conform to the slim, contained, feminine ideal. Similar accounts of surveillance and internalised judgement have been found in interviews with women who position themselves as "overweight" or "obese" (Tischner, 2013). Women's body fat is discursively positioned as ugly and stigmatising within Western cultures and often associated with loathing, disgust, and revulsion (Lupton, 2013). Women expected to discipline and regulate the body, and thus the self, to maintain a slim, contained form (Bordo, 1993; Chrisler, 2011). Body fat is positioned as both a threat to health and morality (Lupton, 2013), with "excess" fat a sign of women "letting themselves go" at both levels (Chrisler, 2011, p. 205). Hatred of the body, and by implication the self, was evident in accounts of many women we interviewed, and animalistic metaphors were often used. For example, "I feel like an elephant, very unattractive"; "I look at myself and I go 'You big fat pig', I hate it"; "I feel like a whale and hate my body during this time" (Ussher & Perz, 2017). Women who are animalised are dehumanised; positioned as creatures of emotion, nature, and desire; and deemed inferior to men (Tipler & Ruscher, 2017); the pig and whale metaphors, in particular, signify depravity (Haslam, Loughnan, & Sun, 2011). Such dehumanisation is also associated with the objectification of the female body (Morris, Goldenberg, & Boyd, 2018), and thus self-positioning as animalistic serves both to denigrate the reproductive body and to reinforce women's self-objectification during the premenstrual phase of the cycle.

The relational context of PMDs

Understanding PMD as a culture bound syndrome does not mean that the reality of premenstrual distress is denied. There is convincing evidence that some women do experience embodied and psychological change during the premenstrual phase of the cycle, which is frequently accompanied by increased sensitivity to emotions or to external stressors (Sabin Farrell & Slade, 1999; Ussher & Wilding, 1992). Anger, sadness, and irritability – as well as joy, creativity, and sexual desire – can also feel more powerful than usual premenstrually (Chrisler, Johnston, Champagne, & Preston, 1994; King & Ussher, 2013), and the multitasking that is a normal part of many women's lives can be more difficult to manage premenstrually (Slade & Jenner, 1980). Such experiences often lead to distress when the responsibilities of home and work cannot be accommodated at the same time to the woman's usual standards (Hardy & Hardie, 2017; Ussher & Perz, 2010). In order to understand this process, we need to examine the psychosocial context of women's lives.

A growing body of research shows an association between relationship strain and premenstrual symptomatology, which suggests that problems in relationships may be associated with women's premenstrual distress (Coughlin, 1990; Kuczmierczyk, Labrum, & Johnson, 1992; Ussher & Perz, 2013a) and that relationship satisfaction can deteriorate premenstrually (Clayton, Clavet, McGarvey, Warnock, & Weiss, 1999; Frank, Dixon, & Grosz, 1993; Ryser & Feinauer, 1992). Direct expression of emotion has been found to be lower in relationships where women report PMS (Kuczmierczyk et al., 1992), which increases the likelihood of premenstrual change being experienced or viewed as problematic. Conversely, effective communication between couples has been associated with lower levels of premenstrual distress (Mooney-Somers, Perz, & Ussher, 2008; Schwartz, 2001). Many women also report that "PMS" has an impact on their partners and their children (Halbreich, Borenstein,

Pearlstein, & Kahn, 2003; Robinson & Swindle, 2000) and that the responsibilities of child-rearing and domestic responsibilities are associated with PMDs (Coughlin, 1990; Ussher, 2003a, 2004; Ussher & Perz, 2010). Indeed, partnered women report greater disruption of daily living as a result of premenstrual symptoms than single women do (Dennerstein, Lehert, Keung, Pal, & Choi, 2010). In combination, this suggests that the most commonly reported psychological "symptoms" of PMDs – anger and irritation – could be conceptualised as a legitimate response to the material circumstances of women's lives, including over-responsibility, lack of support, or relationship tension (Figert, 2005; Ussher, 2004). As one woman told us, "everything comes up at that time, yeah. Everything that might just be a slight pinch normally comes up at the PMT time and it's intensified" (Ussher & Perz, 2013a, p. 135). Another woman said:

> my true feelings come out at a time like that; I get angry that I am the only one who cares about the housework. I get angry on behalf of all women everywhere who have to pick up after everyone else.

These accounts could be characterised as a rupture in self-silencing, where the feminine ideal of controlled and caring compliance that women enact for three weeks of the month is replaced by anger and assertiveness (Perz & Ussher, 2006; Ussher, 2004; Ussher & Perz, 2010). However, expression of anger or discontent is pathologised because women are deemed "out of control," which results in legitimate emotion being dismissed as "just PMS" (Ussher & Perz, 2010, 2013a). Self-positioning as a PMS sufferer acts to maintain and reproduce the boundaries of femininity, as some premenstrual women judge themselves as bad, mad, or insane in relation to the ideal (Chrisler, 2011; Ussher, 2006, 2011). This is evident in accounts of women who position themselves as suffering from PMS, who say that they have failed, or are not good enough, as women (Cosgrove & Riddle, 2003; Ussher & Perz, 2008).

PMS has been described as a gendered phenomenon (Figert, 1995; Markens, 1996), as it is often frustration or anger associated with the self-renunciating role of wife and mother that is expressed premenstrually and then dismissed as PMS (Rodin, 1992; Ussher & Perz, 2010). However, self-renunciation and self-silencing are not simply an enactment of a feminine gendered role, they are also an enactment of hetero-femininity, where women are expected to put the needs of their male partner and children first, or risk relationship loss (Jack, 1991). The majority of research conducted to date on PMDs has focussed on heterosexual women, either by explicit intention, or by omission, as women who take part in research on PMS are generally not asked about their sexual orientation, but our research suggests that gender and sexual identity intersect in relation to Western women's experience of premenstrual change (Ussher & Perz, 2008, 2013a).

Negotiating premenstrual distress in heterosexual and lesbian relationships

The use of belittling or demeaning constructions of PMS on the part of men has been reported to be common in North America, Western Europe, and Australia (King, Ussher, & Perz, 2014; Koch, 2006; Laws, 1983; Sveinsdottir, Lundman, & Norberg, 2002), and it reinforces a gendered power imbalance where menstruating women are positioned as dangerous or dysfunctional (Ussher, 2006). In these cultural contexts, the responses of male partners to premenstrual change have been found to be particularly influential; for example, partner support is associated with lower levels, and lack of support with higher levels, of distress in premenstrual women (Cortese & Brown, 1989;

Ussher, 2003a; Ussher, Perz, & Mooney-Somers, 2007). Indeed, in couples where men demonstrated empathy, understanding, and awareness, marital satisfaction is higher and women's coping with premenstrual distress is more effective (Frank et al., 1993), thus partners appear to act as "moderators" of distress (Jones, Theodos, Canar, Sher, & Young, 2000; McDaniel, 1988). In a study where we compared the experiences of heterosexual and lesbian women, negative constructions of PMS on the part of a woman's partner and absence of partner support were common in heterosexual relationships, which exacerbated distress and resulted in women being pathologised premenstrually (Ussher & Perz, 2013a; Ussher et al., 2007). For example, one woman told us that her male partner saying "I don't know who I'm talking to" when she was premenstrual made her feel like a "paranoid schizophrenic." Another woman said that her male partner had got to the stage where "he really wanted me to go live in another house for two weeks of the month, which is a bit detrimental to a marriage"; she said that she felt so bad about this that it was "slit your wrists time" (Ussher & Perz, 2013a). This confirms a U.S. report that avoidance or rejection on the part of male partners exacerbates women's premenstrual distress (Cortese & Brown, 1989).

Conversely, support and normalisation of premenstrual change were found in all of the lesbian relationships, which allows women to engage in effective coping strategies (e.g., taking time out to be alone or engage self-care) and thus to avoid premenstrual self-pathologisation as mad or bad. Understanding and acceptance of premenstrual change is a key feature of this support; as one lesbian woman commented: "In terms of the response ... it's just really understanding and I guess supportive ... Like, it's not that big an issue that it becomes an issue ... it's just like, 'This is how I'm feeling. That's okay'" (Ussher & Perz, 2013a). Another woman said that her female partner would "go off and make me a tea, or remember little things that are going to comfort me, practical things" (p. 142). A number of male partners did adopt a non-judgemental position in relation to premenstrual change and offered support. For example, one woman said that when she cried premenstrually her husband "usually comes and gives me a cuddle, and says 'oh, don't worry about it, it's that time of the month'" (p. 142). However, such accounts were in the minority in heterosexual relationships.

These accounts suggest that women's experiences of premenstrual change and distress are influenced by both gendered roles and the constructions of femininity adhered to by women and their partners, as well as differences in communication, conflict resolution, and support within heterosexual and lesbian relationships. Previous U.S. research has shown that premenstrual distress is associated with femininity, as more feminine women report higher levels of distress (Cosgrove & Riddle, 2003). Lesbians have been reported to be less likely to conform to the traditional feminine gender role (see Smith & Stillman, 2002) and to experience greater egalitarianism in relationships, manifested as "highly flexible decision making and household arrangements" (Green, Bettinger, & Zacks, 1996, p. 197). Gendered non-adherence has also been linked to the greater instrumentality, combined with expressiveness, that has been found in U.S. research on lesbian, in comparison with heterosexual, relationships (Kurdek, 1987); for example, lesbian couples are reported to demonstrate a greater capacity for mutual empathy, empowerment, and relational authenticity (Mencher, 1990). Premenstrual distress needs to be understood in the context of these reported differences in lesbian and heterosexual relationships, as discourses of hetero-normativity may influence women's experience of premenstrual change, self-pathologisation, and coping (Ussher, 2011).

Women's negotiation of negative premenstrual change

Women are not passive "sufferers" of premenstrual changes, despite their characterisation as such within biomedical and psychological discourse, which positions women as "having" or "not having" PMDs. A substantial number of women report positive aspects of premenstrual change if they are given the opportunity to do so, sometimes alongside negative changes (Alagna & Hamilton, 1986; Chaturvedi & Chandra, 1990; Lee, 2002; Stewart, 1989). Some self-identified PMS sufferers accept premenstrual changes as a normal part of experience, for example, by embracing their access to the "deeper energies" and emotions they experience at this time (Ussher & Perz, 2013a). There is also evidence that Western women can experience negative premenstrual changes in emotion, behaviour, or embodiment, but not discursively construct these as PMS and not experience distress associated with such changes (Cosgrove & Riddle, 2003). To position these women as "false negatives" who *really have* PMDs (Hamilton & Gallant, 1990) is to misinterpret the intrapsychic negotiation and resistance of dominant discourse in which they are engaged. Indeed, women who resist the label PMS could be seen to be "rewriting ideologies of gender" through creating "alternative" or "counter discourses" (Day, Johnson, Milnes, & Rickett, 2010, p. 238) that subvert the positioning of premenstrual change as pathology (Ussher & Perz, 2014).

Conversely, adopting the position "PMS sufferer" can be a positive strategy for women in dealing with negative premenstrual changes. In our research with Australian women, we found that many reported a consistent pattern of negotiation and management of "PMS" (Ussher & Perz, 2013b). This process typically began with self-awareness of negative premenstrual change, which facilitates acceptance that feelings are rarely constant and allows such change to be positioned as a normal part of women's experience, rather than something that is pathological and necessitates psychiatric diagnosis or "cure." As one woman told us, "this is how I'm feeling. That's okay" (p. 919). For many women, making an attribution of mood or behaviour change to "PMS" was positive, as, "it's almost as though it's a relief there's a reason for it" (p. 920). With this approach, women are less likely to engage in the cycle of guilt and self-blame associated with the experience or expression of premenstrual emotion that has been reported in previous research (e.g., Cosgrove & Riddle, 2003). In turn, this approach gave women permission to engage in proactive coping to avoid premenstrual distress, anticipatory coping to prepare for distress, and coping strategies to reduce premenstrual change or distress when it occurred (Ussher & Perz, 2013b).

Avoidance of stress, conflict, or responsibility during the premenstrual phase of the cycle was the most common management strategy reported by women (Ussher & Perz, 2013b). Avoidance has been described as "maladaptive" and a reflection of "trait anxiety" in previous research conducted with women who report PMS (Kuczmierczyk, Johnson, & Labrum, 1994, p. 304), which implicitly pathologises this style of coping. However, participants in our research described effectively diminishing negative emotional experiences through anticipatory awareness and subsequent avoidance of situations that might provoke anger or distress. Accounts of time-out to protect the self suggest that self-care was a strong motivation for self-regulation of both negative premenstrual change and the premenstrual self. These accounts are evocative of the 'room of one's own' that Virginia Woolf (1957) identified as so important to women's creativity, as well as their sanity, and described more recently as an essential 'health promoting resource for women' (Forssen & Carlstedt, 2006, p. 175). In accounts of coping with negative premenstrual change, women did not literally need a room of their own in order to take time-out from others; they could achieve solitude and divest themselves of responsibilities by engaging in gardening, watching television, reading a book, taking a long shower, or exercising. Whilst exercise has previously been acknowledged to be an effective coping strategy for premenstrual distress (Kirkpatrick, Brewer, & Stocks, 1990), our participants' accounts suggest that the absence of interaction with others, and the ability to focus on care of the self through exercise, also allows women to regulate negative premenstrual changes and avoid premenstrual distress. This is reminiscent of Figert's (2005, p. 110) comment that women need a "return to a menstrual hut ... and its monthly release from traditional women's roles of cooking, cleaning and family duties." This is a release that many of the women in our research gave themselves permission to take, as the discursive construction of "PMS" as a time when self-care is permissible legitimates women taking time-out from daily stress or responsibility. This demonstrates resistance to gendered discourse that emphasises women's self-renunciation (Jack, 1991) and positions women's self-care as selfish (O'Grady, 2005) and PMDs as a sign of the "monstrous feminine" (Ussher, 2006).

These findings provide explanations for why systematic review (Lustyk, Gerrish, Shaver, & Keys, 2009) and meta-analyses of randomised controlled trials (Busse, Montori, Krasnik, Patelis-Siotis, & Guyatt, 2009; Kleinstäuber, Witthöft, & Hiller, 2012) suggest that cognitive behaviour therapy (CBT) can reduce premenstrual anxiety and depression, have a beneficial impact on behavioural change, and reduce interference by negative premenstrual changes on daily living. Such interventions involve a combination of behavioural strategies, such as relaxation training, coping skills, social support, and anger management (Morse, Dennerstein, Farrell, & Varnavides, 1991; Pearlstein, Rivera Tovar, Frank, & Thoft, 1992; Slade, 1989), combined with cognitive restructuring to overcome the sense of helplessness associated with premenstrual distress and reframing of self-defeating cognitions (Blake, 1995; Ussher, Hunter, & Cariss, 2002). CBT has been demonstrated to be as effective as serotonin reuptake inhibitors (SSRIs) in reducing premenstrual distress in the short term, and at long-term follow-up to be more effective than SSRIs in reducing premenstrual distress and improving coping (Hunter et al., 2002; Kleinstäuber et al., 2012). We have found women-centred CBT to be effective in a one-to-one therapy mode (Hunter et al., 2002; Ussher, 2008), as well as a self-help modality (Ussher & Perz, 2006), in studies conducted in the UK and Australia.

In a recent randomised controlled trial, we found that including women's partners as part of a women-centred couple CBT was more effective than a one-to-one intervention and a wait-list control in reducing premenstrual distress and self-pathologisation and increasing women's coping ability (Ussher & Perz, 2017). This reinforces the importance of the role of partners in ameliorating premenstrual distress and suggests that PMDs need to be conceptualised as a relational experience. We found that the majority of women in the active conditions reported increased understanding and acceptance of embodied change, associated with marked decreases in negative conceptualisations of the premenstrual body (Ussher & Perz, 2017). Such women were also more likely to report engaging in self-care and coping strategies to deal with embodied change premenstrually, most notably in the couple condition. These findings suggest that self-perception of the body, rather than simple increase in weight or bloating, are central to women's feelings of negative premenstrual embodiment.

Conclusion

Premenstrual change is a normal part of experience for women of reproductive age, however a minority of women do experience moderate-to-severe premenstrual distress. Whether or not this distress is positioned as PMDs and results in self-pathologisation will influence women's experience of premenstrual change and their coping strategies. We have argued that PMDs need to be conceptualised as a material-discursive-intrapsychic phenomenon: a combination of the materiality of embodied change and the circumstances of a woman's life; discursive constructions of PMDs circulating in particular relational and cultural contexts; and women's strategies of intrapsychic and behavioural coping. Within this model, PMS is not positioned as an out-of-control illness, rather, as a label that makes sense of women's experience of psychological or embodied change in the premenstrual phase of the cycle (Ussher & Perz, 2014). Women-centred CBT can be effective in supporting women in the process of moving from a position of passivity beset with "raging hormones" to an agentic subject position, without denying her distress or positioning her body as an unruly vessel that needs to be medically managed (Ussher, 2008).

References

Alagna, S. W. & Hamilton, J. A. (1986). Social stimulus perception and self evaluation: Effects of menstrual cycle phase. *Psychology of Women Quarterly, 20,* 327–338.

American Psychiatric Association (2013). *Diagnostic and statistical manual of mental disorders, edition V.* Washington, DC: American Psychiatric Association.

Blake, F. (1995). Cognitive therapy for premenstrual syndrome. *Cognitive and Behavioral Practice, 2*(1), 167–185.

Bordo, S. (1993). *Unbearable weight: Feminism, culture and the body.* Berkeley, CA: University of California Press.

Brooks, J., Ruble, D. N., & Clarke, A. (1977). College women's attitudes and expectations concerning menstrual-related change. *Psychosomatic Medicine, 39,* 288–298.

Busse, J. W., Montori, V. M., Krasnik, C., Patelis-Siotis, I., & Guyatt, G. H. (2009). Psychological intervention for premenstrual syndrome: A meta-analysis of randomized controlled trials. *Psychotherapy and Psychosomatics, 78*(1), 6–15.

Chandraratne, N. K. & Gunawardena, N. K. (2011). Premenstrual syndrome: The experience from a sample of Sri Lankan adolescents. *Journal of Pediatric Adolescent Gynaecology, 24,* 304–311.

Chang, A. M., Holroyd, E., & Chau, J. P. (1995). Premenstrual syndrome in employed Chinese women in Hong Kong. *Health Care for Women International, 16,* 551–561.

Chaturvedi, S. K. & Chandra, P. S. (1990). Stress-protective functions of positive experiences during the premenstrual period. *Stress Medicine, 6,* 53–55.

Chaturvedi, S. K. & Chandra, P. S. (1991). Socio-cultural aspects of menstrual attitudes and premenstrual experiences in India. *Social Science & Medicine, 32,* 349–351.

Chrisler, J. C. (2004). PMS as a culture-bound syndrome. In J. C. Chrisler, C. Golden, & P. D. Rozee (Eds), *Lectures on the psychology of women* (3rd ed., pp. 110–127). Boston, MA: McGraw Hill.

Chrisler, J. C. (2008). 2007 presidential address: Fear of losing control: Power, perfectionism and the psychology of women. *Psychology of Women Quarterly, 32,* 1–12.

Chrisler, J. C. (2011). Leaks, lumps, and lines: Stigma and women's bodies. *Psychology of Women Quarterly, 35*(2), 202–214.

Chrisler, J. C. & Caplan, P. J. (2002). The strange case of Dr. Jekyll and Ms. Hyde: How PMS became a cultural phenomenon and a psychiatric disorder. *Annual Review of Sex Research, 13,* 274–306.

Chrisler, J. C., Johnston, I. K., Champagne, N. M., & Preston, K. E. (1994). Menstrual joy: The construct and its consequences. *Psychology of Women Quarterly, 18,* 375–387.

Chrisler, J. C. & Johnston-Robledo, I. (2002). Raging hormones? Feminist perspectives on premenstrual syndrome and postpartum depression. In M. Ballou & L. S. Brown (Eds), *Rethinking mental health and disorder: Feminist perspectives* (pp. 174–197). New York: Guilford Press.

Chrisler, J. C. & Levy, K. B. (1990). The media construct a menstrual monster: A content analysis of PMS articles in the popular press. *Women and Health, 16*(2), 89–104.

Clayton, A. H., Clavet, G. J., McGarvey, E. L., Warnock, J. K., & Weiss, K. (1999). Assessment of sexual functioning during the menstrual cycle. *Journal of Sex and Marital Therapy, 25,* 281–291.

Cortese, J. & Brown, M. A. (1989). Coping responses of men whose partners experience premenstrual symptomatology. *Journal of Obstetric, Gynecologic, & Neonatal Nursing, 18,* 405–412.

Cosgrove, L. & Caplan, P. J. (2004). Medicalizing menstrual distress. In P. J. Caplan & L. Cosgrove (Eds), *Bias in psychiatric diagnosis* (pp. 221–232). Northvale, NJ: Jason Aronson, Inc.

Cosgrove, L. & Riddle, B. (2003). Constructions of femininity and experiences of menstrual distress. *Women and Health*, *38*(3), 37–58.

Coughlin, P. C. (1990). Premenstrual syndrome: How marital satisfaction and role choice affect symptom severity. *Social Work*, *35*, 351–355.

Dalton, K. (1959). Menstruation and acute psychiatric illness. *British Medical Journal*, *1*, 148–149.

Day, K., Johnson, S., Milnes, K., & Rickett, B. (2010). Exploring women's agency and resistance in health-related contexts: Contributors' introduction. *Feminism & Psychology*, *20*(2), 238–241.

Dennerstein, L., Lehert, P., Bäckström, T. C., & Heinemann, K. (2009). Premenstrual symptoms – Severity, duration and typology: An international cross-sectional study. *Menopause International*, *15*(3), 120–126.

Dennerstein, L., Lehert, P., Keung, L. S., Pal, S. A., & Choi, D. (2010). Asian study of effects of premenstrual symptoms on activities of daily life. *Menopause International*, *16*(4), 146–151.

Figert, A. E. (1995). The three faces of PMS: The professional, gendered, and scientific structuring of a psychiatric disorder. *Social Problems*, *42*, 56–73.

Figert, A. E. (2005). Premenstrual syndrome as scientific and cultural artifact. *Integrative Physiological and Behavioral Science*, *40*, 102–113.

Forssen, A. S. K. & Carlstedt, G. (2006). "It's heavenly to be alone!" A room of one's own as a health promoting resource for women. Results from a qualitative study. *Scandinavian Journal of Public Health*, *34*, 175–181.

Frank, B., Dixon, D. N., & Grosz, H. J. (1993). Conjoint monitoring of symptoms of premenstrual syndrome: Impact on marital satisfaction. *Journal of Counseling Psychology*, *40*, 109–114.

Frank, R. (1931). The hormonal causes of premenstrual tension. *Archives of Neurological Psychiatry*, *26*, 1053.

Fredrickson, B. L. & Roberts, T.-A. (1997). Objectification theory: Toward understanding women's lived experiences and mental health risks. *Psychology of Women Quarterly*, *21*(2), 173–206.

Green, R. J., Bettinger, M., & Zacks, E. (1996). Are lesbian couples fused and gay male couples disengaged? Questioning gender straightjackets. In J. Laird & R.-J. Green (Eds), *Lesbians and gays in couples and families: A handbook for therapists* (pp. 185–230). San Francisco, CA: Jossey Bass.

Halbreich, U., Borenstein, J., Pearlstein, T., & Kahn, L. S. (2003). The prevalence, impairment, impact, and burden of premenstrual dysphoric disorder (PMS/PMDD). *Psychoneuroendocrinology*, *28*, 1–23.

Hamilton, J. A. & Gallant, S. (1990). Problematic aspects of diagnosing premenstrual phase dysphoria: Recommendations for psychological research and practice. *Professional Psychology: Research and Practice*, *21*(1), 60–68.

Hardy, C. & Hardie, J. (2017). Exploring premenstrual dysphoric disorder (PMDD) in the work context: A qualitative study. *Journal of Psychosomatic Obstetrics and Gynecology*, *38*(4), 292–300.

Hartlage, S., Freels, S., Gotman, N., & Yonkers, K. (2012). Criteria for premenstrual dysphoric disorder: Secondary analyses of relevant data sets. *Archives of General Psychiatry*, *69*(3), 300.

Haslam, N., Loughnan, S., & Sun, P. (2011). Beastly: What makes animal metaphors offensive?. *Journal of Language and Social Psychology*, *30*(3), 311–325.

Hoerster, K. D., Chrisler, J. C., & Gorman Rose, J. (2003). Attitudes toward and experience with menstruation in the U.S. and India. *Women and Health*, *38*, 77–95.

Hunter, M. S., Ussher, J. M., Cariss, M., Browne, S., Jelley, R., & Katz, M. (2002). Medical (fluoxetine) and psychological (cognitive-behavioural) treatment for premenstrual dysphoric disorder: A study of treatment process. *Journal of Psychosomatic Research*, *53*, 811–817.

Jack, D. C. (1991). *Silencing the self: Women and depression*. Cambridge, MA: Harvard University Press.

Jones, A., Theodos, V., Canar, W. J., Sher, T. G., & Young, M. (2000). Couples and premenstrual syndrome: Partners as moderators of symptoms? In K. B. Schmaling (Ed.), *The psychology of couples and illness: Theory, research, & practice* (pp. 217–239). Washington, DC: American Psychological Association.

Kaczmarek, M. & Trambacz-Oleszak, S. (2016). The association between menstrual cycle characteristics and perceived body image: A cross-sectional survey of Polish female adolescents. *Journal of Biosocial Science*, *48*(3), 374–390.

King, M. & Ussher, J. M. (2013). It's not all bad: Women's construction and lived experience of positive premenstrual change. *Feminism & Psychology*, *23*(3), 399–417.

King, M., Ussher, J. M., & Perz, J. (2014). Representations of PMS and premenstrual women in men's accounts: An analysis of online posts from PMSBuddy.com. *Women's Reproductive Health*, *1*(1), 3–20.

Kirkpatrick, M. K., Brewer, J. A., & Stocks, B. (1990). Efficacy of self-care measures for perimenstrual syndrome (PMS). *Journal of Advanced Nursing*, *15*(3), 281–285.

Kleinstäuber, M., Schmelzer, K., Ditzen, B., Andersson, G., Hiller, W., & Weise, C. (2016). Psychosocial profile of women with premenstrual syndrome and healthy controls: A comparative study. *International Journal of Behavioral Medicine*, *23*(6), 752–763.

Kleinstäuber, M., Witthöft, M., & Hiller, W. (2012). Cognitive-behavioral and pharmacological interventions for premenstrual syndrome or premenstrual dysphoric disorder: A meta-analysis. *Journal of Clinical Psychology in Medical Settings*, *19*(3), 308–319.

Koch, P. (2006). Women's bodies as a 'puzzle' for college men. *American Journal of Sexuality Education*, *1*, 51–72.

Kuczmierczyk, A. R., Johnson, C. C., & Labrum, A. H. (1994). Coping styles in women with premenstrual syndrome. *Acta Psychiatrica Scandinavica*, *89*(5), 301–305.

Kuczmierczyk, A. R., Labrum, A. H., & Johnson, C. C. (1992). Perception of family and work environments in women with premenstrual syndrome. *Journal of Psychosomatic Research*, *36*, 787–795.

Kurdek, L. A. (1987). Sex-role self schema and psychological adjustment in coupled homosexual and heterosexual men and women. *Sex Roles*, *17*, 549–562.

Laws, S. (1983). The sexual politics of pre-menstrual tension. *Women's Studies International Forum*, *6*, 19–31.

Lee, S. (2002). Health and sickness: The meaning of menstruation and premenstrual syndrome in women's lives. *Sex Roles*, *46*, 25–35.

Lorenz, T. K., Gesselman, A. N., & Vitzthum, V. J. (2017). Variance in mood symptoms across menstrual cycles: Implications for premenstrual dysphoric disorder. *Women's Reproductive Health*, *4*(2), 77–88.

Lupton, D. (2013). *Fat*. Abingdon, UK: Routledge.

Lustyk, M. B. K., Gerrish, W. G., Shaver, S., & Keys, S. L. (2009). Cognitive-behavioral therapy for premenstrual syndrome and premenstrual dysphoric disorder: A systematic review. *Archives of Women's Mental Health*, *12*(2), 85–96.

Markens, S. (1996). The problematic of "experience": A political and cultural critique of PMS. *Gender and Society*, *10*, 42–58.

McDaniel, S. H. (1988). The interpersonal politics of premenstrual syndrome. *Family Systems Medicine*, *6*, 134–149.

Mencher, J. (1990). Intimacy in lesbian relationships: A critical re-examination of fusion. In J. V. Jordan (Ed.), *Women's growth in diversity: More writings from the stone center* (pp. 311–330). New York, NY: Guilford Press.

Mooney-Somers, J., Perz, J., & Ussher, J. M. (2008). A complex negotiation: Women's experiences of naming and not naming premenstrual distress in couple relationships. *Women and Health*, *47*(3), 57–77.

Morris, K. L., Goldenberg, J., & Boyd, P. (2018). Women as animals, women as objects: Evidence for two forms of objectification. *Personality and Social Psychology Bulletin*, *44*(9), 1302–1314.

Morse, C. A., Dennerstein, L., Farrell, E., & Varnavides, K. (1991). A comparison of hormone therapy, coping skills training, and relaxation for the relief of premenstrual syndrome. *Journal of Behavioral Medicine*, *14*(5), 469–489.

Muljat, A. M., Lustyk, M. K. B., & Miller, A. (2007). Stress moderates the effects of premenstrual symptomatology on body image reports in women. *Annals of Behavioral Medicine*, *33*, S157–S157.

Nevatte, T., O'Brien, P., Bäckström, T., Brown, C., Dennerstein, L., Endicott, J., Epperson, C., Eriksson, E., Freeman, E., Halbreich, U., Ismail, K., Panay, N., Pearlstein, T., Rapkin, A., Reid, R., Rubinow, D., Schmidt, P., Steiner, M., Studd, J., Yonkers, K., & Sundström-Poromaa, I. (2013). ISPMD consensus on the management of premenstrual disorders. *Archives of Women's Mental Health*, *16*(4), 279–291.

O'Grady, H. (2005). *Women's relationship with herself: Gender, Foucault, therapy*. Abingdon, UK: Routledge.

Pearlstein, T., Rivera Tovar, A., Frank, E., & Thoft, J. (1992). Nonmedical management of late luteal phase dysphoric disorder: A preliminary report. *Journal of Psychotherapy Practice and Research*, *1*(1), 49–55.

Perz, J. & Ussher, J. M. (2006). Women's experience of premenstrual syndrome: A case of silencing the self. *Journal of Reproductive and Infant Psychology*, *24*(4), 289–303.

Pilver, C. E., Kasl, S., Desai, R., & Levy, B. R. (2011). Exposure to American culture is associated with premenstrual dysphoric disorder among ethnic minority women. *Journal of Affective Disorders*, *130*(1–2), 334–341.

Rapkin, A. J. & Lewis, E. I. (2013). Treatment of premenstrual dysphoric disorder. *Women's Health*, *9*(6), 537–556.

Rittenhouse, C. A. (1991). The emergence of premenstrual syndrome as a social problem. *Social Problems*, *38*(3), 412–425.

Robinson, R. L. & Swindle, R. W. (2000). Premenstrual symptom severity: Impact on social functioning and treatment-seeking behaviors. *Journal of Women's Health and Gender Based Medicine*, *9*, 757–768.

Rodin, M. (1992). The social construction of premenstrual syndrome. *Social Science and Medicine*, *35*(1), 49–56.

Romans, S., Clarkson, R., Einstein, G., Petrovic, M., & Stewart, D. (2012). Mood and the menstrual cycle: A review of prospective data studies. *Gender Medicine*, *9*(5), 361–384.

Ryser, R. & Feinauer, L. L. (1992). Premenstrual syndrome and the marital relationship. *American Journal of Family Therapy*, *20*, 179–190.

Sabin Farrell, R. & Slade, P. (1999). Reconceptualizing pre-menstrual emotional symptoms as phasic differential responsiveness to stressors. *Journal of Reproductive and Infant Psychology*, *17*(4), 381–390.

Schwartz, C. B. (2001). The relationship between partner social support and premenstrual symptoms. *Abstracts International: Section B: The Sciences & Engineering*, *61*(10-B), 5580.

Slade, P. (1989). Psychological therapy for premenstrual emotional symptoms. *Behavioural Psychotherapy*, *17*, 135–150.

Slade, P. & Jenner, F. A. (1980). Performance tests in different phases of the menstrual cycle. *Journal of Psychosomatic Research*, *24*, 5–8.

Smith, C. A. & Stillman, S. (2002). What do women want? The effects of gender and sexual orientation on the desirability of physical attributes in the personal ads of women. *Sex Roles*, *46*, 337–342.

Stewart, D. E. (1989). Positive changes in the premenstrual period. *Acta Psychiatrica Scandinavica*, *79*, 400–405.

Sveinsdottir, H., Lundman, B., & Norberg, A. (2002). Whose voice? Whose experiences? Women's qualitative accounts of general and private discussion of premenstrual syndrome. *Scandinavian Journal of Caring Sciences*, *16*, 414–423.

Teixeira, A. L. S., Dias, M. R. C., Damasceno, V. O., Lamounier, J. A., & Gardner, R. M. (2013). Association between different phases of menstrual cycle and body image measures of perceived size, ideal size, and body dissatisfaction. *Perceptual and Motor Skills*, *117*(3), 892–902.

Tipler, C. N. & Ruscher, J. B. (2017). Dehumanizing representations of women: The shaping of hostile sexist attitudes through animalistic metaphors★. *Journal of Gender Studies*, *28*(1), 109–118.

Tischner, I. (2013). *Fat lives: A feminist psychological exploration*. Abingdon, UK: Routledge.

Ussher, J. M. (1989). *The psychology of the female body*. New York: Routledge.

Ussher, J. M. (1999). Premenstrual syndrome: Reconciling disciplinary divides through the adoption of a material-discursive-intrapsychic approach. In A. Kolk, M. Bekker, & K. Van Vliet (Eds), *Advances in women and health research* (pp. 47–64). Amsterdam: Tilberg University Press.

Ussher, J. M. (2003a). The ongoing silencing of women in families: An analysis and rethinking of premenstrual syndrome and therapy. *Journal of Family Therapy*, *25*, 388–405.

Ussher, J. M. (2003b). The role of premenstrual dysphoric disorder in the subjectification of women. *Journal of Medical Humanities*, *24*(1/2), 131–146.

Ussher, J. M. (2004). Premenstrual syndrome and self-policing: Ruptures in self-silencing leading to increased self-surveillance and blaming of the body. *Social Theory & Health*, *2*, 254–272.

Ussher, J. M. (2006). *Managing the monstrous feminine: Regulating the reproductive body*. Abingdon, UK: Routledge.

Ussher, J. M. (2008). Challenging the positioning of premenstrual change as PMS: The impact of a psychological intervention on women's self-policing. *Qualitative Research in Psychology*, *5*(1), 33–44.

Ussher, J. M. (2011). *The madness of women: Myth and experience*. Abingdon, UK: Routledge.

Ussher, J. M., Hunter, M. S., & Browne, S. (2000). Good, bad or dangerous to know: Representations of femininity in narrative accounts of PMS. In C. Squire (Ed.), *Culture and psychology* (pp. 87–99). New York: Routledge.

Ussher, J. M., Hunter, M. S., & Cariss, M. (2002). A woman-centred psychological intervention for premenstrual symptoms, drawing on cognitive-behavioural and narrative therapy. *Clinical Psychology and Psychotherapy*, *9*, 319–331.

Ussher, J. M. & Perz, J. (2006). Evaluating the relative efficacy of a self-help and minimal psycho-educational intervention for moderate premenstrual distress conducted from a critical realist standpoint. *Journal of Reproductive and Infant Psychology*, *24*(2), 347–362.

Ussher, J. M. & Perz, J. (2008). Empathy, egalitarianism and emotion work in the relational negotiation of PMS: The experience of women in lesbian relationships. *Feminism and Psychology*, *18*(1), 87–111.

Ussher, J. M. & Perz, J. (2010). Disruption of the silenced-self: The case of pre-menstrual syndrome. In D. C. Jack & A. Ali (Eds), *The depression epidemic: International perspectives on women's self-silencing and psychological distress* (pp. 435–458). Oxford, UK: Oxford University Press.

Ussher, J. M. & Perz, J. (2013a). PMS as a gendered illness linked to the construction and relational experience of hetero-femininity. *Sex Roles, 68*(1–2), 132–150.

Ussher, J. M. & Perz, J. (2013b). PMS as a process of negotiation: Women's experience and management of premenstrual distress. *Psychology & Health, 28*(8), 909–927.

Ussher, J. M. & Perz, J. (2014). "I used to think I was going a little crazy": Women's resistance of the pathologization of premenstrual change. In S. McKenzie-Mohr & M. Lafrance (Eds), *Creating counterstories* (pp. 84–101). Abingdon, UK: Routledge.

Ussher, J. M. & Perz, J. (2017). Evaluation of the relative efficacy of a couple cognitive-behaviour therapy (CBT) for premenstrual disorders (PMDs), in comparison to one-to-one CBT and a wait list control: A randomized controlled trial. *Plos One, 12*(4), e0175068.

Ussher, J. M. & Perz, J. (2019). Resisting the mantle of the monstrous feminine: Women's construction and experience of premenstrual embodiment. In C. Bobel, B. Fahs, K. A. Hasson, E. Kissling, T. A. Roberts, & I. Winkler (Eds), *Palgrave critical menstrual studies handbook*. New York: Palgrave.

Ussher, J. M., Perz, J., Metusela, C., Hawkey, A. J., Morrow, M., Narchal, R., & Estoesta, J. (2017). Negotiating discourses of shame, secrecy, and silence: Migrant and refugee women's experiences of sexual embodiment. *Archives of Sexual Behavior, 46*(7), 1901–1921.

Ussher, J. M., Perz, J., & Mooney-Somers, J. (2007). The experience and positioning of affect in the context of intersubjectivity: The case of premenstrual syndrome. *Journal of Critical Psychology, 21*, 145–165.

Ussher, J. M., Rhyder-Obid, M., Perz, J., Rae, M., Wong, T. W. K., & Newman, P. (2012). Purity, privacy and procreation: Constructions and experiences of sexual and reproductive health in Assyrian and Karen women living in Australia. *Sexuality & Culture, 16*(4), 467–485.

Ussher, J. M. & Wilding, J. M. (1992). Interactions between stress and performance during the menstrual cycle in relation to the premenstrual syndrome. *Journal of Reproductive and Infant Psychology, 10*(2), 83–101.

Wong, L. & Khoo, E. (2011). Menstrual-related attitudes and symptoms among multi-racial Asian adolescent females. *International Journal of Behavioral Medicine, 18*(3), 246–253.

Yu, M., Zhu, X., Li, J., Oakley, D., & Reame, N. E. (1996). Perimenstrual symptoms among Chinese women in an urban area of China. *Health Care for Women International, 17*, 161–172.

Woolf, V. (1957). *A room of one's own*. New York, NY: Harcourt, Brace and World.

6

MENOPAUSE AND MIDLIFE

Psychosocial perspectives and interventions

Myra S. Hunter

This chapter concerns women's experience of midlife and the menopausal transition, with particular emphasis given to the impact of the psychological and social context. The main section describes a range of psychosocial interventions that have been developed to improve hot flushes and night sweats, mood, and sleep for midlife women. Psychosocial interventions are described, and the evidence from recent systematic and non-systematic reviews and meta-analyses are noted in evaluations of their effectiveness. In the final section, public health interventions, including prevention and work place initiatives, are discussed.

Women's experience of midlife and the menopause

The biomedical model of menopause tends to emphasize 'symptoms' (i.e., short and long term negative physical and psychological consequences, experience of 'loss and decline'; de Salis, Owen-Smith, Donovan, & Lawlor, 2017; Perz & Ussher, 2008), and hormonal therapy (HT) is recommended as the main pharmacological option for women with menopausal symptoms (National Institute for Health and Care Excellence [NICE], 2015; position statement of the North American Menopause Society [NAMS], 2017). However, in the promotion of HT, a broad range of physical and emotional reactions can too easily be seen as inevitable and attributed to biological causes. Although hormonal, menstrual, and vasomotor changes typically occur during the menopausal transition, the experience of the menopause as a whole is very much influenced by psychological and social factors, such as past experience, lifestyle, social and cultural meanings of menopause, and a woman's social and material circumstances. Meanings or narratives of menopause arise from the complex interaction between the biological and social, but the importance of psychosocial and cultural factors is often ignored.

Hot flushes and night sweats (i.e., vasomotor symptoms), sleep problems, and vaginal dryness are the main physical changes that are associated with stages of menopause in epidemiological studies in Western countries (Woods & Mitchell, 2005). Cross-cultural studies suggest wide variations in perceptions and reports of emotional and physical changes in women from different ethnic origins and living in different countries (Avis & Crawford, 2008). In general, Asian women tend to have more positive perceptions of the menopause (i.e., freedom from reproduction, access to higher social status, association of age with wisdom) compared with Middle-Eastern, North African, and Western women, who tend to have negative perceptions (i.e., associations with body decay and hormonal deficiency; Lock, 1994). Furthermore, women in Western countries tend to report more hot flushes than women in India, Japan, and China (Freeman & Sherif, 2007). Japanese women, for example, have been found to complain of shoulder stiffness and Taiwanese women of backache and tiredness, whereas there is evidence that Lebanese women mostly describe being fatigued and irritable (Obermeyer, 2000). Similarly, two multinational studies of Asian women showed that hot flushes were not the most commonly reported symptoms; body and joint aches, memory problems, sleeplessness, irritability, and migraines were (Haines, Xing, Park, Holinka, & Ausmanas, 2005; Huang, Xu, Nasri, & Jaisamrarn, 2010). In a more recent study comparing experiences of menopause amongst White Australian women and women in Laos, Australians reported higher rates of depression, as well as greater fears of ageing, weight gain, and cancer – fears not reported by Laotians who positioned menopause as a positive event (Sayakhot, Vincent, & Teede, 2012).

The results of the U.S. Study of Women's Health Across the Nation (SWAN) (Avis et al., 2001) highlight the diversity of experiences of the menopause in a sample of 14,906 women of European, African Chinese, Japanese, and Hispanic descent. Different patterns of menopausal symptoms were evident amongst women of different ethnicities living in the USA. In brief, African American women reported a high frequency of hot flushes, whereas East Asian women reported a low frequency; European American women reported more psychological and somatic symptoms than any other racial/ethnic group.

When women migrate from East to West they may need to negotiate contradictory meanings of menopause in their country of origin and their host country (Ussher, Hawkey, & Perz, 2019). The symbolic meanings attached to the menopause may change as a result of migration and modernization (Hall, Berry, & Matsumura, 2007; Richters, 1997). For example, women from the Indian sub-continent who had migrated to the U.K. reported vasomotor and psychological symptoms similar to those of White women living in the U.K., in contrast to women from the same cultural background who had remained in India, and who reported low levels of hot flushes and night sweats (Hunter et al., 2009b). Within the migrated group of women, poor general health, anxiety, and less acculturation were associated with more menopausal symptoms. This suggests that acculturation may affect the construction and experience of menopause for migrant women, but also that 'culture' is fluid and may not necessarily reflect national or ethnic demarcations.

Explanations of these cultural differences include social factors (marital/societal status and roles, education, and demographic characteristics), attitudes and meanings (cultural attitudes towards childrearing, women's roles, the end of reproductive life and ageing, including husband/partner's attitudes and mother's experience of the menopause), health (prior and current general and reproductive health, reproductive cycles), place of residence (rural versus urban, adaptation to seasonal variations in temperate climate), and lifestyle (smoking, diet, exercise, body mass) (Freeman & Sherif, 2007; Melby, Lock, & Kaufert, 2005). However, the interactions between biology and sociocultural factors are complex and poorly understood. Symptoms may not be reported due to social taboos surrounding the menopause in some cultures (Brown, Sievert, Morrison, Reza, & Mills, 2009), and results of studies have been found to vary depending on different methodologies used (Islam, Bell, Rizvi, & Davis, 2017).

There is also variation between women within ethnic groups, as well as variation across cohorts and generations (Utz, 2011). The way in which bodily changes are negotiated and constructed by individual women during menopause is likely to influence the degree to which such changes are distressing, and whether they are positioned as 'symptoms' (Hunter & Rendall, 2007). However, it is important not to overlook material and social influences; a fairly general finding is that women with poor health, less education, and low income are more likely to have more problematic experiences during the menopause (Delanoe et al., 2012; Im, Lee, Chee, Brown, & Dormire, 2010). A comprehensive understanding of menopause therefore needs to consider biological and psychosocial factors, with an awareness of the intersectional influences of gender, age, ethnicity, and class.

Qualitative studies provide examples of ways in which interpersonal, social, and cultural meanings impact upon women's experience of the menopause and the way in which women might challenge, endure, manage, or resist them (Hunter & O'Dea, 1997; Morris & Symonds, 2004; Perz & Ussher, 2008). For example, in a recent UK study, three inter-related narratives of menopause emerged from the accounts of 48 midlife women: menopause as a normal, biological process distinct from self, identity, and social transitions; menopause as a struggle provoking distress and a time of identity loss and social upheaval; menopause as a time of liberation and transformation (de Salis et al., 2017). Related themes (e.g., dealing with negative stereotypes of women's ageing; expectations and uncertainties about future physical and emotional 'decline'; taboos and silence; relief, reflection, and growth) have been previously reported (Hunter & O'Dea, 1997; Hvas, 2006; Rubinstein & Foster, 2012; Sergeant & Rizq, 2017). Women tend to draw on a range of different – positive, neutral, and negative – discourses when describing their experiences of menopause and midlife, and these tend to be context dependent.

The relational context is under-researched but, not surprisingly, there is evidence that social support is associated with a more positive experience. For example, in a recent study of Chinese women, higher family support was significantly associated with fewer menopausal symptoms (Zhao et al., 2018). Sexual interest and functioning tends to be affected by the quality of the relationship and partner's sexual functioning and attitudes, as well as by reductions in oestrogen that can cause vaginal dryness and pain during intercourse (Dennerstein, Lehert, & Burger, 2005). In general, sexual interest tends to lower with age, but this has been found to be associated with a range of factors, such as sexual functioning before the menopause, stress, ill-health, having problematic hot flushes and night sweats, low mood, relationship status (being in a relationship or having a new partner) and partner's sexual functioning, attitudes towards sex and ageing, and cultural background (including beliefs about the importance of sex) (Avis et al., 2005). Overall, previous sexual functioning and relationship factors seem to be more important influences on women's sex lives during the menopause than hormonal factors (Dennerstein et al., 2005; Ussher et al., 2015). Women in lesbian relationships have been reported to be more able than heterosexual couples to discuss the impact of bodily changes at midlife on their sexuality and to negotiate different ways of pleasuring each other, largely because they shared a broader definition of 'sex' that is not tied to penetration (Winterich, 2003).

Social meanings can influence the type and the number of physical and emotional changes (e.g., visual problems, mood swings, high blood pressure) that women attribute to the menopause (Hunter et al., 2009b). There is evidence that negative attitudes and expectations held *before* the menopause can predict symptom experience *during* the menopause (Ayers, Forshaw, & Hunter, 2010), and, interestingly, beliefs and attitudes toward menopause tend to be more positive in postmenopausal than in premenopausal women (Brown, Brown, Judd, & Bryant, 2017). Social discourses can therefore influence the meaning of the menopause for an individual woman and impact upon her experience of menopause. For example, negative cognitive and emotional appraisals of hot flushes (e.g., that they are embarrassing or shameful) and behavioural reactions to them (e.g., avoiding social situations) have been found to be associated with more problematic flushes and sweats (Hunter & Chilcot, 2013; Hunter & Mann, 2010; Reynolds, 2000). Hot flushes are often reported to be particularly distressing at work and lead to embarrassment and worry about potential stigmatisation (Griffiths & Hunter, 2015). Not surprisingly, if women think that they are viewed as 'unattractive', 'not needed', 'old' or 'unsuccessful' – thoughts that are associated with unduly negative stereotypes about menopause in general – they are more likely to feel distressed.

The available evidence from epidemiological and prospective studies suggests that the menopause is not necessarily associated with low mood or distress for most women (Avis et al., 2008; Brown, Bryant, & Judd, 2015; Guérin et al., 2017; Mishra & Kuh, 2012). In general, depression is more prevalent during midlife for both women and men, although women have a greater risk of depression than men at any age (Lang, Llewellyn, Hubbard, Langa, & Meltzer, 2011). Midlife is typically a life stage when men and women may be dealing with demanding life events and responsibilities, such as work, health problems, and caring roles. For example, according to the UK Health and Safety Executive, women aged 45–54 report more work-related stress than men or women of any other age group (Health and Safety Executive, 2018). Furthermore, evidence from a reanalysis of the Household Survey for England data shows that this midlife increase in depression is particularly evident amongst lower income groups for both women and men, thus emphasising the importance of social influences (Lang et al., 2011), and an intersectional perspective to understanding women's health.

Moreover, depressed mood should not be attributed automatically to a hormonal cause or to the menopause. An estimated 9–10% of women report an increase in psychological symptoms, including depressed mood, across the stages of menopause, but this increase tends to decrease post menopause, thus, for most, it is relatively transient (Almeida, Marsh, Flicker, & Hickey, 2016; Mishra & Kuh, 2012), and mood tends to improve after the menopausal transition (Campbell, Dennerstein, Finch, & Szoeke, 2017). Factors associated with anxiety and depressed mood for midlife women include past history, social factors (e.g., educational and occupational status), stressful life events (e.g., caring for children and parents, career and relationship shifts, ageing, body changes) and personal/family illness, surgical menopause, chronic or severe hot flushes and night sweats, attitudes toward menopause and ageing, and early life circumstances (Freeman et al., 2005; Mishra & Kuh, 2012; Vivian-Taylor & Hickey, 2014).

Clinical depression, or major depressive disorder (MDD), as opposed to depressive symptoms, tends to be associated with past depression, and existing treatments, such as cognitive behaviour therapy and antidepressants, are recommended (Maki et al., 2018). Overall, multiple factors including socioeconomic, individual psychological and social characteristics, and health factors are associated with risk for depressive symptoms and MDD during the menopause transition (Maki et al., 2018).

Timing of the menopause is also relevant since an early menopause can be distressing due to its impact on fertility and concerns about health. In addition, women often report fears of rapid ageing following early menopause, drawing upon the negative stereotypes described above (Mann et al., 2012; Singer et al., 2011). Early menopause can be particularly distressing when induced by breast cancer treatments and when physical symptoms associated with menopause and its social meanings are felt at a time when women are trying to get their lives back to normal (Hunter et al., 2009a; Parton, Ussher, & Perz, 2017).

There are complex and bidirectional relationships between hot flushes and low mood (Thurston et al., 2008; Worsley, Bell, Kulkarni, & Davis, 2014). Psychosocial factors such as poor health, low income, and stress are associated with troublesome menopausal symptoms and with low mood. Similarly, having persistent and/or troublesome hot flushes and sleep problems can make women feel depressed and irritable, and stress can in turn exacerbate menopausal symptoms. The relationships that have been found between hot flushes and low mood or depressive symptoms are not found to be significant for hot flushes and clinical depression (Maki et al., 2018).

The impact of psychosocial factors on experience of the menopause and midlife provides a clear rationale for the development and evaluation of non-medical interventions for women who have troublesome menopausal symptoms.

Psychosocial support and interventions

Most women do not seek medical attention for menopause, but, if they do, it is usually because they have problematic hot flushes and night sweats or they want information and advice (Hickey et al., 2017b). Many women prefer not to take HT, and it is not suitable for some women (e.g., women with a history of breast cancer) (European Menopause and Andropause Society Position Statement [EMAS] 2015; NICE, 2015). Concerns about side effects and safety of HT have contributed to an increased interest in non-hormonal treatments, informed choices for women, and self-management approaches.

The main outcomes that psychosocial interventions have targeted are hot flushes and night sweats, sleep, and mood. Measures of the impact (referred to as bother, problem-rating, and interference) of hot flushes and night sweats, as well as their frequency, are recommended because bother or interference is clinically meaningful and related to quality of life (Ayers & Hunter, 2013; Rand et al., 2011).

Lifestyle interventions

Smoking has been associated with an earlier menopause, as well as more frequent hot flushes (Archer et al., 2011), and caffeine use with more frequent flushes (Faubion et al., 2015), so modification of these behaviours is generally recommended, ideally before the menopause. Several reviews indicate that there is little consistent benefit for botanical or dietary supplements and that further studies are needed; moreover, some supplements can interact with medications (Drewe, Bucher, & Zahner, 2015; NICE, 2015).

Physically active women tend to report higher quality of life and fewer hot flushes than sedentary women (Vallance, Murray, Johnson, & Elavsky, 2010). However, when exercise (or physical activity) has been evaluated in randomized controlled trials as an intervention, it has not been found to be effective in alleviating hot flushes and night sweats, but may improve sleep and mood in postmenopausal women (Daley et al., 2014; NICE, 2015). In a recent prospective Canadian study, menopausal status was not associated with levels of stress, but participation in vigorous activity was associated with lower stress in a sample of midlife women (Guérin et al., 2017).

Weight tends to increase with age, and, whereas there is a redistribution of fat during the menopause to the abdomen, weight gain is not a necessary consequence of menopause. However, there is some evidence that weight loss, by means of exercise and a healthy diet, can lead to improvements in quality of life and also to reductions in hot flushes and night sweats (Davis et al., 2012).

Psychosocial interventions

A number of psychosocial or 'mind–body' interventions have been developed, including yoga, relaxation, paced breathing, clinical hypnosis, mindfulness, and cognitive behavioural therapies (CBT), and some of these are considered to have more effectiveness (EMAS, 2015; Hickey et al., 2017b; NAMS, 2015; Stefanopoulou & Grunfeld, 2017; van Driel, Stuursma, Schroevers, Mourits, & de Bock, 2018) than other non-medical approaches, such as herbal and complementary therapies, and such as reflexology and acupuncture (Borrelli & Ernst, 2010; Gentry-Maharaj et al., 2015).

Yoga, relaxation, and paced-breathing

Yoga typically involves breath control, simple meditation, and the adoption of specific bodily postures, and tends to be used for general health and relaxation. Styles of yoga vary in intensity, physical effort, and relaxation components. Overall, results have been inconsistent regarding its effectiveness in alleviating hot flushes and night sweats. However, a large randomized trial of 12 weekly 90-minute yoga classes with daily home practice (n=107) versus aerobic exercise training three times a week for 12 weeks (n=106) or usual activity (n=142) in women with hot flushes showed that neither yoga nor exercise reduced hot flushes, but both yoga and exercise improved sleep quality, and exercise also improved mood (Newton et al., 2014).

Relaxation has been used to moderate hot flushes and night sweats in a number of studies with mixed outcomes. Interventions typically lasted for 6–12 weeks and follow-up periods ranged from 3–6 months. Two systematic reviews of relaxation exercises for hot flushes and night sweats showed that there was insufficient evidence to recommend these treatments, although relaxation may well be beneficial to reduce stress and improve well-being (Saensak, Vutyavanich, Somboonporn, & Srisurapanont, 2014; Tremblay, Sheeran, & Aranda, 2008).

Paced-breathing tends to involve taking 6–8 slow deep breaths per minute while inhaling through the nose and exhaling through the mouth. The early work of Freedman and colleagues (Freedman, 2005; Freedman & Woodward, 1992) showed that hot flush frequency reduced following paced-breathing compared with relaxation and electroencephalographic biofeedback (control groups), using physiological measurement of hot flush frequency. However, these findings were not replicated for frequency nor severity of hot flushes in a later study by Carpenter and colleagues (2012), who compared paced-breathing, an attention control condition of fast shallow breathing, or usual-care, nor by Huang, Phillips, Schembri, Vittinghoff, and Grady (2015), who compared paced-breathing intervention (using a portable guided-breathing device) with recorded music. Consequently paced-breathing was not recommended as an effective treatment by NAMS.

Mindfulness and hypnosis

Mindfulness, and mindfulness-based stress reduction (MBSR), is a popular meditation-based intervention that focusses on self-regulation of emotions by emphasizing a moment-to-moment, non-judgemental, and non-reactive awareness of experiences; it is usually delivered in groups over eight weeks. Carmody et al. (2011) reported improvements in hot flush and night sweat frequency and bother compared with a wait-list control, but between-group differences were not statistically significant. Bower et al. (2015) used a similar design in a sample of breast cancer patients and found that the intervention led to significant short-term reduction in hot flushes, but the effects were not maintained at three-month follow-up. There is more evidence that mindfulness is effective in improving sleep, mood, and quality of life than specific menopausal symptoms, particularly in women who have had breast cancer (Bower et al., 2015; Carmody et al., 2011; Hoffman et al., 2012).

Hypnosis creates a deeply relaxed state using mental imagery and suggestions for changes in subjective sensations, emotions, thoughts, or behaviour. Elkins et al. (2008) showed that women who had menopausal symptoms following breast cancer treatment experienced fewer hot flushes and night sweats after receiving five weekly sessions of clinical hypnosis than a waitlist control group; this change represented a 69% reduction in hot flushes relative to baseline. In a second study with healthy women, hypnosis (five weekly sessions, each an hour long plus practise at home) resulted in significant reductions in both self-reported and physiologically measured HFNS compared with a structured control condition; findings remained significant at 12-week follow-up (Elkins, Fisher, Johnson, Carpenter, & Keith, 2013).

Overall, recent position statements, systematic reviews, and guidance indicate that there are insufficient or inconclusive data to recommend yoga, paced respiration, relaxation, or mindfulness as proven therapies for managing hot flushes and night sweats (EMAS, 2015; NAMS, 2015; NICE, 2015), although they may have other general benefits. However, the NAMS guideline recommends that two mind–body therapies have level I evidence showing efficacy in alleviating hot flushes and night sweats: clinical hypnosis according to the Elkin's protocol, and cognitive-behavioral therapy according to the MENOS1 and MENOS2 protocols.

Cognitive behaviour therapy (CBT)

A CBT approach was developed to help women to examine attitudes and beliefs about menopause, hot flushes and night sweats, (i.e., assumptions and beliefs about menopause and cognitive appraisal of hot flushes and night sweats), and behavioural reactions to them. The CBT approach is based on a cognitive model (Hunter & Chilcot, 2013; Hunter & Mann, 2010). It provides evidence-based information on exploration of attributions and social meanings and cognitive behavioural strategies to deal with stress, hot flushes, night sweats, and sleep. It can be delivered, with positive outcomes, in a self-help format and in groups of 6–8 women, over 4–6 weeks. The CBT interventions significantly reduced the impact (problem-rating) of hot flushes and night sweats in three randomized controlled trials including well women (MENOS2; Ayers, Smith, Hellier, Mann, & Hunter, 2012) and breast cancer patients (MENOS2; Duijts et al., 2012; Mann et al., 2012) with improvements maintained at a six-month follow-up. In the MENOS2 trial, the self-help format (book and CD) was found to be as effective as the group intervention, but group CBT resulted in greater improvement in quality of life than self-help CBT. Duijts et al. (2012) randomly assigned women to CBT, physical activity (PE), CBT and PE combined, or control group. The groups that included CBT showed a significant decrease in hot flush problem-rating at 12-week post-treatment and six-month follow-up. CBT also reduced subjective frequency of night sweats by an average of 39% and reduced objectively measured hot flushes (sternal skin conductance monitoring) in well women, but not in breast cancer patients (Stefanopoulou & Hunter, 2013). This may reflect differences in the meaning and nature of menopausal symptoms in breast cancer patients, which may be induced or exacerbated by cancer treatments.

Self-help CBT has also recently been evaluated in a work context and found to be effective in reducing hot flushes and night sweat frequency and problem-rating and in improving sleep quality and work and social adjustment (Hardy, Griffiths, Norton, & Hunter, 2018a) (see section on menopause and work).

Secondary mediation analyses of MENOS1 and MENOS2 suggest that CBT appears to work by changing cognitive appraisals (i.e., women's perceptions, attitudes, and beliefs about menopause and menopausal symptoms) and teaching helpful behavioural strategies, such as calm breathing (Chilcot, Norton, & Hunter, 2014; Norton, Chilcot, & Hunter, 2014). Qualitative interviews with participants at the end of MENOS1 and MENOS2 trials were conducted to explore women's views of the treatment. Women reported increased confidence and ability to cope with hot flushes and night sweats; key factors mentioned were acceptance and a restored sense of control (experienced on a number of different levels and often facilitated by calm breathing). Many women noticed that they attended differently to their hot flushes; for example, they may have had hot flushes but did not notice them. Perhaps reflecting the skills learned, the beneficial effects of the treatment, in some cases, extended beyond management of menopausal symptoms. Women also found the group context helpful in terms of normalizing their experiences, motivating them in homework tasks, and providing support (Balabanovic, Ayers, & Hunter, 2012, 2013).

CBT is also helpful for anxiety, low mood (NICE, 2015), and sleep problems (Espie, 2006). Telephone-based CBT has been shown to reduce sleep problems and insomnia reported by women during the menopausal transition and post menopause (McCurry et al., 2016). CBT for hot flushes and night sweats, including CBT for stress and sleep, is available as a self-help book (Hunter & Smith, 2014), and a group CBT manual for health professionals has been developed (Hunter & Smith, 2015).

Menopause and work

The employment rates for women are increasing, and more midlife and older women are working than ever before in most Western countries (Griffiths et al., 2016). More people in their 50s and 60s than any other age group are also unpaid carers for older relatives and for grandchildren (Yeandle, Bennett, Buckner, Fry, & Price, 2007). Women are more likely than men to be in low-paid, low-status jobs with less control and flexibility, working conditions known to be associated with the experience of stress (Health and Safety Executive, 2018).

Some women are concerned about the impact of menopause on their work, but the overall evidence is inconclusive (Jack et al., 2016). Two recent studies, conducted in Australia and the UK, showed that stage of menopause was unrelated to work outcomes such as perceived performance and absence (Hardy, Thorne, Griffiths, & Hunter, 2018b; Hickey et al., 2017a). Hardy et al. (2018b) found that work outcomes were mainly associated with work stress and aspects of the work environment. Certain work situations and physical working environments (e.g., aspects of work design, temperature) and work stress can increase the intensity of menopausal symptoms.

At work, hot flushes are reported as a source of distress and embarrassment for some women; concerns about the reactions of others are common (Smith, Mann, Mirza, & Hunter, 2011), and having to hide signs of menopause is often mentioned as an additional source of anxiety when at work (Sergeant & Rizq, 2017). Perhaps not surprisingly, some women prefer not to reveal age and gender-related matters at work, due to fear of stigmatization. Certain situations at work are reported to precipitate or exacerbate hot flushes, such as formal meetings, high visibility tasks (e.g., presentations), uniforms, and hot and poorly ventilated environments (Griffiths et al., 2016).

The UK Faculty of Occupational Medicine (2016) has published evidence-based advice about menopause and work for employers. Based upon what women say would be helpful, they advocated: (i) greater awareness for managers about menopause as a possible occupational health issue, (ii) increased flexibility of working hours and working arrangements, (iii) better access to informal and formal sources of support, and (iv) improvements in workplace temperature and ventilation.

In order to address (iii) above, a brief self-help CBT was evaluated in an RCT with 124 women working in eight UK organisations, who were experiencing troublesome or problematic hot flushes and night sweats (Hardy et al., 2018a). This brief intervention significantly reduced hot flush frequency and problem-ratings, and it improved sleep quality and work and social adjustment at 6 and 20 weeks follow-up, compared with a wait-list control group. It is also important for employers to foster a culture where it is acceptable to discuss menopausal symptoms (and any other health problem) that may impact on work life. In a recent study (Hardy, Griffiths, & Hunter, 2017), midlife women were asked how they wanted to be treated at work. They emphasized that menopause is relatively transient and highly variable; that managers should not view menopause as an 'affliction' or generalize about it on the basis of someone they know or their own experience; and they wanted managers to communicate with empathy and sensitivity, to be aware of menopause, and to ask how they might make helpful changes in the work environment. Employers could also develop guidance and policies and provide training for all staff on menopause and other health issues relevant to the management of an age-diverse workforce (Griffiths & Hunter, 2015).

Public health

There is a need for increased public awareness to challenge negative images of menopausal and older women, as well as health promotion to provide evidence-based advice on lifestyle factors that can improve health and well-being during mid and later life, but also throughout the lifespan. The challenge is to develop approaches that can engage women who have a variety of experiences, values, and lifestyles that normalize the menopause as a process involving personal adjustments as well as physical and psychosocial changes, and, at the same time, that provide helpful and effective treatments and strategies for those women who need them.

Menopause is still considered a taboo topic and women typically report confusion, uncertainty, and the need for information as they approach menopause. This is despite the proliferation of media interest and social media sites that offer advice, support, and discussion groups on menopause. There is an abundance of information in the popular literature regarding menopause; for example, celebrities have described their difficult experiences on television and radio shows, the promotion of treatments and lists of numerous symptoms on websites, and even musicals have been performed. But media and medicine tend to provide inconsistent and often contradictory information to women, most of which reflects a negative view of menopause and supports a biomedical model (Marnocha & Bergstrom, 2011).

Morris and Symonds (2004) argued that public health research and practice overly relies on the medical model of the menopause and that this prevents the voices of women being heard and understood; they advocated the use of both quantitative and qualitative studies. Their study of a sample of women in south Wales illustrates how a qualitative approach enabled understanding of the social context and individual challenges faced by the women who grew up in the 1950s when men were the main breadwinners and women worked in the home. With the rise in male unemployment due to loss of heavy industries in the 1980s, women began working in paid employment while continuing to meet demands at home. During midlife the women described having to 'manage their bodies' in order to fit within their jobs' organizational structure. Women described having concealed evidence of menstruation all their lives, but felt they lost control of the ability to conceal menopausal effects (i.e., hot flushes). The contradiction between acceptance of a role in which they were constantly at the service of others (at home and at work), but at the same time resenting that role, was often resolved by shifting the blame for these feelings onto 'uncontrollable' hormonal changes. In other words, the lack of control of the body became the explanation for their anger towards lack of power and control over other aspects of their lives. Although the women expressed mixed views, the definition of the menopause as a pathological state remained extremely influential. The authors concluded that this generation of women do not necessarily share a negative view of the menopause but are struggling against mixed messages from their own cultural background, from promotion of medicalized 'solutions', and from contemporary pressures of work (Morris & Symonds, 2004).

Nevertheless, there is some evidence that women who participate in psychoeducational and health promotion programmes have more accurate knowledge regarding menopause, more positive attitudes toward it, less discomfort associated with changes at these stages, and more frequent engagement in healthy habits than women who do not participate in these programmes (Toral et al., 2014; Tremblay et al., 2008). Targeting premenopausal women ages 40–45 in preparation for group sessions about expectations, personal goals, and life contexts has been advocated (Liao & Hunter, 1998; Toral et al., 2014). Menopause, as a time when women often seek advice from their doctors, is also arguably an opportunity to encourage positive health-related behaviours, such as stress reduction, smoking cessation, nutritional intake, and increased physical activity. NICE (2015) recommended individualized care and lifestyle advice along these lines. Such changes might benefit women going through the menopausal transition, as well as offer prevention of longer-term health problems. Women often want information and discussion about what might be expected as well as options available to them.

Community projects and support groups can also reach specific groups of women who may not access services or where there are gaps in services that meet the needs of midlife women. An example is Reclaim the Menopause, a community-based course developed by the charity Hands Inc., in the London borough of Hackney, in the UK. The 12-week course provides evidence-based education, CBT (based on Hunter & Smith, 2015), and psychosocial support to promote menopause awareness, challenge stigma, and increase self-management amongst menopausal women. Ethnicity was an important aspect of the work, as Hands Inc. was keen to reach women who might not otherwise access interventions. A pilot evaluation (Bellot et al., 2018) used questionnaires and focus groups to compare 13 women who attended the course with 15 who received only written information. At the end of the course attendees reported reduced menopausal symptoms, as well as improvements in mood and the quality of their lives. They described the group atmosphere as enabling them to speak openly and use humour to lighten the conversation within a culturally relevant setting. All of the course participants were Black British, as were two of the three course facilitators. The course was co-facilitated by a psychosexual therapist, a CBT therapist, and a Women's Health practitioner.

In conclusion, there is a need for increased public awareness to challenge overly negative expectations of and attitudes toward midlife and older women. This would ideally involve women and men, teachers, health care professionals, and other stakeholders such as employers and the media. Women tend to want balanced, evidence-based information that acknowledges diversity of values, experience, and social context. There are effective psychosocial interventions that can be offered as non-medical options for women who have troublesome hot flushes, night sweats, sleep problems, and low mood during midlife. This chapter highlights the psychosocial and cultural factors that influence women's experience of the menopause, but also the limitations of current research, which tends to view menopause from a Western context. Nevertheless, the consistent finding, across cultures, that social inequalities in education and socioeconomic status affect women's experience during midlife suggests that social change is needed to achieve lasting improvements to women's health.

References

Almeida, O. P., Marsh, K., Flicker, L., & Hickey, M. (2016). Depressive symptoms in midlife: The role of reproductive stage. *Menopause, 23*, 669–675.

Archer, D. F., Sturdee, D. W., Baber, R., De Villiers, T. J., Pines, A., Freedman, R. R., Gompel, A., Hickey, M., Hunter, M. S., Lobo, R. A., Lumsden, M. A., MacLennan, A. H., Maki, P., Palacios, S., Shah, D., Villaseca, P., & Warren, M. (2011). Menopausal hot flushes and night sweats: Where are we now?. *Climacteric, 14*, 515–528.

Avis, N. E. & Crawford, S. (2008). Cultural differences in symptoms and attitudes towards menopause. *Menopause Management, 17*(3), 8–13.

Avis, N. E., Stellato, R., Crawford, S., Bromberger, J., Ganz, P., Cain, V., & Kagawa-Singer, M. (2001). Is there a menopausal syndrome? Menopausal status and symptoms across racial/ethnic groups. *Social Science & Medicine, 52*(3), 345–356.

Avis, N. E., Zhao, X., Johannes, C., Ory, M., Brockwell, S., & Greendale, G. (2005). Correlates of sexual function among multi-ethnic middle-aged women: Results from the Study of Women's Health Across the Nation (SWAN). *Menopause, 12*(4), 385–398.

Ayers, B., Forshaw, M., & Hunter, M. S. (2010). The impact of attitudes towards the menopause on women's symptom experience: A systematic review. *Maturitas, 65*(1), 28–36.

Ayers, B. & Hunter, M. S. (2013). Health-related quality of life of women with menopausal hot flushes and night sweats. *Climacteric, 16*, 235–239.

Ayers, B., Smith, M., Hellier, J., Mann, E., & Hunter, M. S. (2012). Effectiveness of group and self-help cognitive behavior therapy in reducing problematic menopausal hot flushes and night sweats (MENOS 2): A randomized controlled trial. *Menopause, 19*, 749–759.

Balabanovic, J., Ayers, B., & Hunter, M. S. (2012). Women's experiences of group cognitive behaviour therapy for hot flushes and night sweats following breast cancer treatment: An interpretative phenomenological analysis. *Maturitas, 72*, 236–242.

Balabanovic, J., Ayers, B., & Hunter, M. S. (2013). Cognitive behaviour therapy for menopausal hot flushes and night sweats: A qualitative analysis of women's experiences of group and self-help CBT. *Behavioural and Cognitive Psychotherapy, 41*, 441–457.

Bellot, E., Rouse, N., & Hunter, M. S. (2018). Reclaim the menopause: A pilot study of an evidence based menopause course for symptom management and resilience building. *Post Reproductive Health, 24*(2), 79–81.

Borrelli, F. & Ernst, E. (2010). Alternative and complementary therapies for the menopause. *Maturitas, 66*, 333–343.

Bower, J. E., Crosswell, A. D., Stanton, A. L., Crespi, C. M., Winston, D., Arevalo, J., Ma, J., Cole, S. W., & Ganz, P. A. (2015). Mindfulness meditation for younger breast cancer survivors: A randomized controlled trial. *Cancer, 121*, 1231–1240.

Brown, D., Sievert, L. L., Morrison, L. A., Reza, A. M., & Mills, P. S. (2009). Do Japanese American women really have fewer hot flashes than European Americans? The Hilo Women's Health Study. *Menopause, 16*(5), 870–876.

Brown, L., Brown, V., Judd, F., & Bryant, C. (2017). It's not as bad as you think: Menopausal representations are more positive in postmenopausal women. *Journal of Psychosomatic Obstetrics & Gynecology, 39*(4), 81–288.

Brown, L. C., Bryant, C., & Judd, F. K. (2015). Positive well-being during the menopausal transition: A systematic review. *Climacteric, 18*, 456–469.

Campbell, K. E., Dennerstein, L., Finch, S., & Szoeke, C. E. (2017). Impact of menopausal status on negative mood and depressive symptoms in a longitudinal sample spanning 20 years. *Menopause, 24*, 490–496.

Carmody, J., Crawford, S., Salmoirago-Blotcher, E., Leung, K., Churchill, L., & Olendzki, N. (2011). Mindfulness training for coping with hot flashes: Results of a randomized trial. *Menopause, 18*, 611–620.

Carpenter, J. S., Burns, D. S., Wu, J., Otte, J. L., Schneider, B., Ryker, K., Tallman, E., & Yu, M. (2012). Paced respiration for vasomotor and other menopausal symptoms: A randomized, controlled trial. *Journal of General Internal Medicine, 28*, 193–200.

Chilcot, J., Norton, S., & Hunter, M. S. (2014). Cognitive behaviour therapy for menopausal symptoms following breast cancer treatment: Who benefits and how does it work? *Maturitas, 78*(1), 56–61.

Daley, A., Stokes-Lampard, H., & MacArthur, C. (2014). Exercise for vasomotor menopausal symptoms. *Cochrane Database Systematic Review*, (11), CD006108.

Davis, S. R., Castelo-Branco, C., Chedraui, P., Lumsden, M. A., Nappi, R. E., & Shah, D. (2012). Understanding weight gain at menopause. *Climacteric, 15*, 419–429.

Delanoe, D., Hajri, S., Bachelot, A., Draoui, D. M., Hassoun, D., Marsicano, E., & Ringa, V. (2012). Class, gender and culture in the experience of menopause: A comparative survey in Tunisia and France. *Social Science & Medicine, 75*, 401–409.

Dennerstein, L., Lehert, P., & Burger, H. (2005). The relative effects of hormones and relationship factors on sexual function of women through the natural menopausal transition. *Fertility and Sterility, 84*(10), 174–180.

de Salis, I., Owen-Smith, A., Donovan, J. L., & Lawlor, D. A. (2017). Experiencing menopause in the UK: The interrelated narratives of normality, distress, and transformation. *Journal of Women & Aging, 30*(6), 520–540.

Drewe, J., Bucher, K. A., & Zahner, C. (2015). A systematic review of non-hormonal treatments of vasomotor symptoms in climacteric and cancer patients. *SpringerOpen, 4*(1), 65.

Duijts, S. F., van Beurden, M., Oldenburg, H. S., Hunter, M. S., Kieffer, J. M., Stuiver, M. M., Gerritsma, M. A., Menke-Pluymers, M. B. E., Plaisier, P. W., Rijna, H., Cardozo, A. M. F. L., Timmers, G., van der Meij, S., van der Veen, H., Bijker, N., de Widt-Levert, L. M., Geenen, M. M., Heuff, G., van Dulken, E. J., Boven, E., & Aaronson, N. K. (2012). Efficacy of cognitive behavioral therapy and physical exercise in alleviating treatment-induced menopausal symptoms in patients with breast cancer: Results of a randomized, controlled, multicenter trial. *Journal of Clinical Oncology, 30*, 4124–4133.

Elkins, G., Marcus, J., Stearns, V., Perfect, M., Rajab, M. H., Ruud, C., Palamara, L., & Keith, T. (2008). Randomized trial of a hypnosis intervention for treatment of hot flashes among breast cancer survivors. *Journal of Clinical Oncology, 26*, 5022–5026.

Elkins, G. R., Fisher, W. I., Johnson, A. K., Carpenter, J. S., & Keith, T. Z. (2013). Clinical hypnosis in the treatment of postmenopausal hot flashes: A randomized controlled trial. *Menopause, 20*, 291–298.

Espie, C. A. (2006). *Overcoming insomnia and sleep problems*. London, UK: Constable and Robinson.

European Menopause and Andropause Society (EMAS) (2015). Position statement: Non-hormonal management of menopausal vasomotor symptoms. *Maturitas, 81*, 410–413.

Faculty of Occupational Medicine (FOM) (2016). *Guidance on menopause and the workplace*. London, UK. Retrieved from www.fom.ac.uk/health-at-work-2/information-for-employers/dealing-with-health-problems-in-the-workplace/advice-on-the-menopause.

Faubion, S. S., Sood, R., Thielen, J. M., & Shuster, L. T. (2015). Caffeine and menopausal symptoms: What is the association? *Menopause, 22*, 155–158.

Freedman, R. R. (2005). Hot flashes: Behavioral treatments, mechanisms, and relation to sleep. *American Journal of Medicine, 118*(12), 124–130.

Freedman, R. R. & Woodward, S. (1992). Behavioral treatment of menopausal hot flushes: Evaluation by ambulatory monitoring. *American Journal of Obstetrics and Gynecology, 167*, 436–439.

Freeman, E. W., Sammel, M. D., Lin, H., Gracia, C. R., Kapoor, S., & Ferdousi, T. (2005). The role of anxiety and hormonal changes in menopausal hot flashes. *Menopause, 12*, 258–266.

Freeman, E. W. & Sherif, K. (2007). Prevalence of hot flushes and night sweats around the world: A systematic review. *Climacteric, 10*, 197–214.

Gentry-Maharaj, A., Karpinskyj, C., Glazer, C., Burnell, M., Ryan, A., Fraser, L., Lanceley, A., Jacobs, I., Hunter, M. S., & Menon, U. (2015). Use and perceived efficacy of complementary and alternative medicines after discontinuation of hormone therapy: A nested United Kingdom collaborative trial of ovarian cancer screening cohort study. *Menopause, 22*(4), 384–390.

Griffiths, A., Ceausu, I., Depypere, H., Lambrinoudaki, I., Mueck, A., Pérez-López, F. R., Van der Schouw, Y. T., Senturk, L. M., Simoncini, T., Stevenson, J. C., Stute, P., & Rees, M. (2016). EMAS recommendations for conditions in the workplace for menopausal women. *Maturitas, 85*, 79–81.

Griffiths, A. & Hunter, M. S. (2015). Psychosocial factors and menopause: The impact of menopause on personal and working life. In S. C. Davies (Ed.), *Annual report of the Chief Medical Officer 2014: The health of 51%* (pp. 109–120). London, UK: Department of Health.

Guérin, E., Biagé, A., Goldfield, G., & Prud'homme, D. (2017). Physical activity and perceptions of stress during the menopause transition: A longitudinal study. *Journal of Health Psychology, 24*(6), 799–811.

Haines, C. J., Xing, S.-M., Park, K.-H., Holinka, C. F., & Ausmanas, M. K. (2005). Prevalence of menopausal symptoms in different ethnic groups of Asian women and responsiveness to therapy with three doses of conjugated estrogens/medroxyprogesterone acetate: The Pan-Asia Menopause (PAM) study. *Maturitas, 52*(3), 264–276.

Hall, L., Berry, J., & Matsumura, G. (2007). Meanings of menopause: Cultural influences on perception and management of menopause. *Journal of Holistic Nursing, 25*(2), 106–118.

Hardy, C., Griffiths, A., & Hunter, M. S. (2017). What do working menopausal women want? A qualitative investigation into women's perspectives on employer and line manager support. *Maturitas, 101*, 37–41.

Hardy, C., Griffiths, A., Norton, S., & Hunter, M. S. (2018a). Self-help cognitive behavior therapy for working women with problematic hot flushes and night sweats (MENOS@ Work): A multicenter randomized controlled trial. *Menopause, 25*, 508–519.

Hardy, C., Thorne, E., Griffiths, A., & Hunter, M. S. (2018b). Work outcomes in midlife women: The impact of menopause, work stress and working environment. *Women's Midlife Health, 4*, 3.

Health and Safety Executive (HSE) (2018). *Work related stress, depression or anxiety.* Retrived from www. hse.gov.uk/statistics/causdis/stress/stress.pdf, accessed 16 April 2018.

Hickey, M., Riach, K., Kachouie, R., & Jack, G. (2017a). No sweat: Managing menopausal symptoms at work. *Journal of Psychosomatic Obstetrics & Gynaecology, 22*, 1–8.

Hickey, M., Szabo, R. A., & Hunter, M. S. (2017b). Non-hormonal treatments for menopausal symptoms. *British Medical Journal, 359*, j5101.

Hoffman, C. J., Ersser, S. J., Hopkinson, J. B., Nicholls, P. G., Harrington, J. E., & Thomas, P. W. (2012). Effectiveness of mindfulness-based stress reduction in mood, breast- and endocrine-related quality of life, and well-being in stage 0 to III breast cancer: A randomized, controlled trial. *Journal of Clinical Oncology, 30*, 1335–1342.

Huang, A. J., Phillips, S., Schembri, M., Vittinghoff, E., & Grady, D. (2015). Device-guided slow-paced respiration for menopausal hot flushes: A randomized controlled trial. *Obstetrics & Gynecology, 125*, 1130–1138.

Huang, K.-E., Xu, L., Nasri, N., & Jaisamrarn, U. (2010). The Asian Menopause Survey: Knowledge, perceptions, hormone treatment and sexual function. *Maturitas, 65*(3), 276–283.

Hunter, M. S. & Chilcot, J. (2013). Testing a cognitive model of menopausal hot flushes and night sweats. *Journal of Psychosomatic Research, 74*, 307–312.

Hunter, M. S., Coventry, S., Mendes, N., & Grunfeld, A. E. (2009a). Menopausal symptoms following breast cancer treatment: A qualitative investigation of cognitive and behavioural responses. *Maturitas, 63*, 336–340.

Hunter, M. S., Gupta, P., Papitsch-Clarke, A., & Sturdee, D. (2009b). Mid-aged health in women from the Indian subcontinent (MAHWIS): A quantitative and qualitative study of experience of menopause in UK Asian women, compared to UK Caucasian and women living in Delhi. *Climacteric, 12*, 26–37.

Hunter, M. S. & Mann, E. (2010). A cognitive model of menopausal hot flushes and night sweats. *Journal of Psychosomatic Research, 69*, 491–501.

Hunter, M. S. & O'Dea, I. (1997). Bodily changes and multiple meanings. In J. M. Ussher (Ed.), *Body talk: The material and discursive regulation of sexuality, madness and reproduction* (pp. 199–222). Abingdon, UK: Routledge.

Hunter, M. S. & Rendall, M. J. (2007). Bio-psycho-socio-cultural perspectives on menopause. *Best Practice Research Clinical Obstetrics and Gynaecology, 21*(2), 261–274.

Hunter, M. S. & Smith, M. (2014). *Managing hot flushes and night sweats: A cognitive behavioural self-help guide to the menopause.* Abingdon, UK: Routledge.

Hunter, M. S. & Smith, M. (2015). *Managing hot flushes and night sweats: A manual for health professionals.* Abingdon, UK: Routledge.

Hvas, L. (2006). Menopausal women's positive experience of growing older. *Maturitas, 54,* 245–251.

Im, E.-O., Lee, B., Chee, W., Brown, A., & Dormire, S. (2010). Menopausal symptoms among four major ethnic groups in the U.S. *Western Journal of Nursing Research, 32,* 540–565.

Islam, R. M., Bell, R. J., Rizvi, F., & Davis, R. S. (2017). Vasomotor symptoms in women in Asia appear comparable with women in Western countries: A systematic review. *Menopause, 24*(11), 1313–1322.

Jack, G., Riach, K., Bariola, E., Pitts, M., Schapper, J., & Sarrel, P. (2016). Menopause in the workplace: What employers should be doing. *Maturitas, 85,* 88–95.

Lang, I. A., Llewellyn, D. J., Hubbard, R. E., Langa, K. M., & Meltzer, D. (2011). Income and midlife peak in common mental disorder prevalence. *Psychological Medicine, 41,* 1365–1372.

Liao, K. L. M. & Hunter, M. S. (1998). Preparation for the menopause: Prospective evaluation of a health education intervention for mid-aged women. *Maturitas, 29,* 215–224.

Lock, M. (1994). Menopause in cultural context. *Experimental Gerontology, 29*(3/4), 307–317.

Maki, P. M., Kornstein, S. G., Joffe, H., Bromberger, J. T., Freeman, E. W., Athappilly, G., Bobo, W. V., Rubin, L. H., Koleva, H. K., Cohen, L. S., & Soares, C. N. (2018). Guidelines for the evaluation and treatment of perimenopausal depression: Summary and recommendations. *Journal of Women's Health, 28*(2), 117–134.

Mann, E., Smith, M. J., Hellier, J., Balabanovic, J. A., Hamed, H., Grunfeld, E. A., & Hunter, M. S. (2012). Cognitive behavioural treatment for women who have menopausal symptoms after breast cancer treatment (MENOS 1): A randomised controlled trial. *Lancet Oncology, 13,* 309–318.

Marnocha, S. K. & Bergstrom, M. (2011). The lived experience of perimenopause and menopause. *Contemporary Nurse, 37,* 229–240.

McCurry, S. M., Guthrie, K. A., Morin, C. M., Woods, N. F., Landis, C. A., Ensrud, K. E., Larson, J. C., Joffe, H., Cohen, L. S., Hunt, J. R., Newton, K. M., Otte, J. L., Reed, S. D., Sternfield, B., Tinker, L. F., & LaCroix, A. Z. (2016). Telephone-based cognitive behavioral therapy for insomnia in perimenopausal and postmenopausal women with vasomotor symptoms: A MsFLASH randomized clinical trial. *Journal of the American Medical Association Internal Medicine, 176,* 913–920.

Melby, M. K., Lock, M., & Kaufert, P. (2005). Culture and symptom reporting at menopause. *Human Reproduction Update, 11*(5), 495–512.

Mishra, G. D. & Kuh, D. (2012). Health symptoms during midlife in relation to menopausal transition: British prospective cohort study. *British Medical Journal, 344,* e402.

Morris, M. E. & Symonds, A. (2004). 'We've been trained to put up with it': Real women and the menopause. *Critical Public Health, 14,* 311–323.

National Institute for Health and Care Excellence (NICE) (2015). *Diagnosis and management of menopause guideline.* Retrieved from www.nice.org.uk/guidance/ng23.

Newton, K. M., Reed, S. D., Guthrie, K. A., Sherman, K. J., Booth-LaForce, C., Caan, B., Sternfield, B., & Carpenter, J. S. (2014). Efficacy of yoga for vasomotor symptoms: A randomized controlled trial. *Menopause, 21,* 339–346.

The North American Menopause Society (NAMS) (2015). Position statement: Non-hormonal management of menopause-associated vasomotor symptoms. *Menopause, 22,* 1–20.

The North American Menopause Society (NAMS) (2017). Position statement: Hormone therapy. *Menopause, 24,* 728–753.

Norton, S., Chilcot, J., & Hunter, M. S. (2014). Cognitive behaviour therapy for menopausal symptoms (hot flushes and night sweats): Moderators and mediators of treatment effects. *Menopause, 21,* 574–578.

Obermeyer, C. M. (2000). Menopause across cultures: A review of the evidence. *Menopause, 7*(3), 184–192.

Parton, C., Ussher, J. M., & Perz, J. (2017). Experiencing menopause in the context of cancer: Women's constructions of gendered subjectivities. *Psychology and Health, 32*(9), 1109–1126.

Perz, J. & Ussher, J. M. (2008). "The horror of this living decay": Women's negotiation and resistance of medical discourses around menopause and midlife. *Women's Studies International Forum, 31,* 293–299.

Rand, K. L., Otte, J. L., Flockhart, D., Hayes, D., Storniolo, A. M., & Stearns, V. (2011). Modelling hot flushes and quality of life in breast cancer survivors. *Climacteric, 14,* 171–180.

Reynolds, F. (2000). Relationships between catastrophic thoughts, perceived control and distress during menopausal hot flushes: Exploring the correlates of a questionnaire measure. *Maturitas, 36*, 113–122.

Richters, J. M. A. (1997). Menopause in different cultures. *Journal of Psychosomatic Obstetrics and Gynaecology, 18*(2), 73–80.

Rubinstein, H. R. & Foster, J. L. H. (2012). 'I don't know whether it is to do with age or to do with hormones and whether it is to do with a stage in your life': Making sense of menopause and the body. *Journal of Health Psychology, 18*, 292–307.

Saensak, S., Vutyavanich, T., Somboonporn, W., & Srisurapanont, M. (2014). Relaxation for perimenopausal and postmenopausal symptoms. *Cochrane Database Systematic Review, 7*, CD008582.

Sayakhot, P., Vincent, A., & Teede, H. (2012). Cross-cultural study: Experience, understanding of menopause, and related therapies in Australian and Laotian women. *Menopause, 19*(12), 1300–1308.

Sergeant, J. & Rizq, R. (2017). 'Its all part of the big CHANGE': A grounded theory study of women's identity during menopause. *Psychosomatic Obstetrics & Gynecology, 38*, 189–201.

Singer, D., Mann, E., Hunter, M.S., Pitkin, J., & Panay, N. (2011). The silent grief: Psychosocial aspects of premature ovarian failure. *Climacteric, 14*(4), 428–437.

Smith, M. J., Mann, E., Mirza, A., & Hunter, M. S. (2011). Men and women's perceptions of hot flushes within social situations: Are menopausal women's negative beliefs valid? *Maturitas, 69*(1), 57–62.

Stefanopoulou, E. & Grunfeld, E. A. (2017). Mind–body interventions for vasomotor symptoms in healthy menopausal women and breast cancer survivors. A systematic review. *Psychosomatic Obstetrics and Gynecology, 38*, 210–225.

Stefanopoulou, E. & Hunter, M. S. (2013). Does pattern recognition software using the Bahr monitor improve sensitivity, specificity and concordance of ambulatory skin conductance monitoring of hot flushes? *Menopause, 20*, 1133–1138.

Thurston, R. C., Bromberger, J. T., Joffe, H., Avis, N. E., Hess, R., Crandall, C. J., Chang, Y., Green, R., & Matthews, K. A. (2008). Beyond frequency: Who is most bothered by vasomotor symptoms? *Menopause, 15*, 841–847.

Toral, M. V., Godoy-Izquierdo, D., García, A. P., Moreno, R. L., de Guevara, N. M. L., Ballesteros, A. S., Teresa Galván, C., & Godoy García, J. F. (2014). Psychosocial interventions in perimenopausal and postmenopausal women: A systematic review of randomised and non-randomised trials and non-controlled studies. *Maturitas, 77*, 93–110.

Tremblay, A., Sheeran, L., & Aranda, S. K. (2008). Psychoeducational interventions to alleviate hot flashes: A systematic review. *Menopause, 15*, 193–202.

Ussher, J., Perz, J., & Parton, C. (2015). Sex and the menopausal woman: A review and critical analysis. *Feminism & Psychology, 25*(4), 449–468.

Ussher, J. M., Hawkey, A., & Perz, J. (2019). "Age of despair", or "when life starts": Migrant and refugee women negotiate constructions of menopause. *Culture, Health and Sexuality, 21*(7), 741–756.

Utz, R. L. (2011). Like mother, (not) like daughter: The social construction of menopause and aging. *Journal of Aging Studies, 25*, 143–154.

Vallance, J. K., Murray, T. C., Johnson, S. T., & Elavsky, S. (2010). Quality of life and psychosocial health in postmenopausal women achieving public health guidelines for physical activity. *Menopause, 17*, 64–71.

van Driel, C. M. G., Stuursma, A. S., Schroevers, M. J., Mourits, M. J. E., & de Bock, G. H. (2018). Mindfulness, cognitive behavioural and behaviour-based therapy for natural and treatment-induced menopausal symptoms: A systematic review and meta-analysis. *British Journal of Obstetrics & Gynaecology, 126*(3), 330–339.

Vivian-Taylor, J. & Hickey, M. (2014). Menopause and depression: Is there a link? *Maturitas, 79*, 142–146.

Winterich, J. A. (2003). Sex, menopause, and culture: Sexual orientation and the meaning of menopause for women's sex lives. *Gender & Society, 17*(4), 627–642.

Woods, N. F. & Mitchell, E. S. (2005). Symptoms during the perimenopause: Prevalence, severity, trajectory, and significance in women's lives. *American Journal of Medicine, 118*(12), 14–24.

Worsley, R., Bell, R., Kulkarni, J., & Davis, S. R. (2014). The association between vasomotor symptoms and depression during perimenopause: A systematic review. *Maturitas, 77*, 111–117.

Yeandle, S., Bennett, C., Buckner, L., Fry, G., & Price, C. (2007). *Managing caring and employment* [Carers, Employment and Services Report Series]. London, UK: Carers UK.

Zhao, D., Liu, C., Feng, X., Hou, F., Xu, X., & Li, P. (2018). Menopausal symptoms in different sub-stages of perimenopause and their relationships with social support and resilience. *Menopause, 26*(3), 233–239.

PART II

Reproductive and gynecological disorders

7

MENSTRUAL-CYCLE-RELATED DISORDERS

Polycystic ovary syndrome, dysmenorrhea and menstrual migraine

Nancy Fugate Woods and Nancy J. Kenney

The purpose of this chapter is to review three menstrual-cycle-related health concerns: Polycystic ovary syndrome, dysmenorrhea, and menstrual migraine. These are each characterized by symptoms that are temporally associated with the menstrual cycle and related endocrine fluctuations that may affect women's experiences of the menstrual cycle. Each of these disorders will be described from a biomedical perspective (including diagnostic criteria and usual therapies) and then contrasted with women's reports of their experiences.

Polycystic ovary syndrome

Biomedical perspectives: diagnosis and treatment

Polycystic ovary syndrome (PCOS) is a heterogeneous endocrine disorder characterized by a combination of signs and symptoms of androgen excess and ovarian dysfunctions (Escobar-Morreale, 2018). A recent systematic review revealed that PCOS affects an estimated 6 to 10% of reproductive-aged women, depending on the criteria used for diagnosis (Bozdag, Mumusoglu, Zengin, Karabulut, & Yildiz, 2016). Moreover, the prevalence of PCOS varies by ethnicity and geography, with lowest reports for Chinese women, followed by White, Middle Eastern, and Black women (Bozdag et al., 2016; Ding et al., 2017).

Diagnosis of PCOS is based on criteria that are currently being debated. In 1990 the U.S. National Institutes of Health established criteria that include clinical hyperandrogenism (either hirsutism [excess facial or body hair] and/or testosterone levels) and ovarian dysfunction (oligomenorrhea, defined as fewer than eight menstrual periods per year, or chronic anovulation). Recent studies and clinical practice guidelines have employed the Rotterdam Criteria, which require the presence of two of three PCOS diagnostic criteria (i.e., androgen excess, ovulatory dysfunction, PCOS morphology of the ovary denoted by numbers of follicles 2–9 mm or increased ovarian volume), such that PCOS is defined by a heterogeneous set of criteria and androgen excess may not be required for a diagnosis. In response to these proposed criteria, the European Society of Endocrinology and the American Society of Reproductive Medicine have proposed that hyperandrogenemia be a required criterion for diagnosis of PCOS (Dunaif & Fauser, 2013). Until recently the prevalence of PCOS based on these different criteria in a community-based population has been unknown. March and colleagues (2010) studied a well-defined birth cohort of Australian women using a combination of interviews with health history, assays, and clinical exams (i.e., ultrasound). They compared prevalence estimates using the NIH, Rotterdam, and Androgen Excess Society criteria, and estimated that the prevalence of PCOS was 9%, 12–18%, and 10–12%, respectively.

Recent efforts have focused on identifying phenotypes of PCOS: Features that distinguish the different physical presentation of PCOS based on biomarkers such as blood tests for a variety of androgens as well as physical findings from clinical examination. Given recent thinking about the consequences of PCOS (reproductive or metabolic), multiple phenotypes have been proposed (Dunaif & Fauser, 2013). Women may demonstrate hyperandrogen-emia, ovulatory dysfunction, polycystic ovarian morphology, or a combination of any two of these. Different phenotypes are associated with different health consequences. For example, the NIH phenotype (hyperandrogenemia and oligo/anovulation) predicts meta-bolic syndrome and appears to identify risk for insulin resistance and type-2 diabetes. In contrast, a phenotype that emphasizes reproductive effects and risk of ovarian hyperstimula-tion, a potentially fatal consequence of ovulation induction therapy, includes ovarian morph-ology determined by ultrasound to obtain follicle counts as well as history of oligomenorrhea or amenorrhea (Dunaif & Fauser, 2013). An NIH expert panel recom-mended further research to identify biological and clinical markers that indicate different phenotypes of PCOS and improved measures of circulating androgens; additional research on causes, predictors, and long-term metabolic consequences of PCOS; and methods of pre-vention and treatment (Dunaif, 2012).

Assessment of PCOS ovarian morphology requires transvaginal ultrasonography to iden-tify 12 or more follicles that measure 2–9 mm in diameter in each ovary or increased ovar-ian volume in the absence of a dominant follicle (>10 mm). In adolescents, diagnosis of PCOS is based on clinical and/or biochemical evidence of hyperandrogenism in the pres-ence of infrequent menses; a pelvic exam and vaginal ultrasonography are not required for those who are not yet sexually active.

Ovulatory dysfunction usually results in infrequent menses, although many women with irregular ovulation may have regular menses. Because oligomenorrhea and periods of amen-orrhea are common during the first two years after menarche, these are not reliable indica-tors of ovulatory dysfunction as an indicator of PCOS for all adolescents. In perimenopause the diagnosis is made based on history of infrequent menses and hyperandrogenism during the reproductive years (Setji & Brown, 2014).

In women, androgens are produced in the adrenal cortex, adipose tissue, and skin, as well as the ovaries. Androgen can be converted from precursors in peripheral tissues (e.g., androstenedione, which is produced in the ovarian theca cells and the adrenal cortex) (Pas-quali & Gambineri, 2018). Androgen excess is assessed by measuring total testosterone, but recent evidence supports the importance of considering delta-4-androstenedione, free andro-gen index (FAI), and 5-alpha dihydrotestosterone because of their role in predicting meta-bolic risk. The adrenals produce androgens, and they also contribute to hyperandrogenemia: 11-oxygenated C-19 steroid metabolism products are significantly greater in women with PCOS than in other women, and these may play an important role in metabolic risk. More-over, women with normal levels of total testosterone who have ovarian dysfunction (OD-PCOm – PCO morphology) phenotype may have elevated delta-4-androstenedione or free androgen index (Pasquali, 2018).

Another physical finding is hirsutism (i.e., excess hair growth on the face, trunk, and other body areas). Hirsutism is measured with a standardized procedure to estimate the amount of body hair (Freeman-Galloway scale), although these estimates are not deemed highly reliable.

Current thinking is that PCOS is a complex multigenic disorder in which predisposing and protective genetic variants interact with environmental influences, including prenatal exposures and diet and lifestyle patterns, to result in different phenotypes. Familial aggregation of PCOS may be related to both heritable phenotypes and shared environments. Epigenetic initiators might include environmental exposure during fetal life and childhood. Exposure to environmental influences during pregnancy (e.g., maternal diabetes, smoking, hypertension) may contribute to intrauterine growth retardation, which in turn may predispose infants to a thrifty phenotype, such as being small for gestational age and at risk of insulin resistance and childhood overweight (Escobar-Morreale, 2018).

Given that two of three Rotterdam criteria must be met for PCOS diagnosis, it is possible that some women may present with hyperandrogenemia and ovulatory dysfunction and PCO (polycystic ovarian) morphology, some with hyperandrogenism and ovulatory dysfunction, some with hyperandrogenemia and PCO morphology, and some with ovulatory dysfunction and PCO morphology. With use of genomic technologies, the relationship between gene polymorphisms and PCOS phenotypes may become increasingly clear (Escobar-Morreale, 2018).

Symptoms

Symptoms of PCOS typically begin in adolescence and progress gradually. Androgen excess symptoms include hirsutism, acne, alopecia, and seborrhea; approximately 60% of women diagnosed with PCOS experience these. Ovarian dysfunction symptoms include menstrual dysfunction, such as oligomenorrhea or periods of amenorrhea, subfertility, and endometrial hyperplasia, which are experienced by approximately 17–33% of women with PCOS. Together, androgen excess and ovarian dysfunction symptoms are associated with insulin resistance and metabolic comorbidities. Weight gain is another common symptom among women with PCOS; it can exacerbate anovulation and hirsutism, and weight loss in overweight or obese women can increase the frequency of ovulation in those with and without PCOS (Dunaif & Fauser, 2013).

Pathophysiology

Polycystic ovary syndrome has been shown to be related to androgen excess, which stimulates abdominal adipose tissue development and visceral adiposity by inducing insulin resistance (inability to metabolize insulin effectively) and compensation by overproducing insulin (hyperinsulinemia). Evidence suggests that a defect in post-receptor insulin signal transduction is responsible for insulin resistance, which is found in 60–80% of women with PCOS and 95% of obese women with PCOS (Barthelmess & Naz, 2015). Insulin resistance and hyperinsulinemia, in turn, stimulate androgen secretion by the ovaries and adrenal glands (Escobar-Morreale, 2018). Although obesity may trigger androgen excess, lean women may also experience PCOS without evidence of visceral adiposity or insulin resistance.

Health consequences of PCOS

Polycystic ovary syndrome is increasingly recognized as a condition with reproductive as well as widespread metabolic consequences, including inflammatory and immune processes.

Some of the conditions associated with PCOS include: Cutaneous signs such as hirsutism, acne, alopecia (hair loss), and acanthosis nigricans (darkening of the skin at body folds such as armpits, groin, and neck); infertility; pregnancy complications such as gestational diabetes, pre-eclampsia, and preterm childbirth; endometrial cancer; depression and anxiety; sleep-disordered breathing/obstructive sleep apnea; nonalcoholic fatty liver disease and nonalcoholic steatohepatitis; type-2 diabetes mellitus; and cardiovascular disease risk factors such as hypertension, dyslipidemia, and obesity (Setji & Brown, 2014).

Fertility is a major concern for young reproductive-age women. Infertility is common: 30% of infertility is due to anovulation, an estimated 90% of which is due to PCOS (Barthelmess & Naz, 2015). An excess of insulin in the ovaries may enhance granulosa cell response to LH and stimulate androgen production. Higher LH levels can also cause granulosa cells to mature early in the ovarian cycle (Barthelmess & Naz, 2015).

Although research on menopause in women with PCOS is limited, one study revealed that age at menopause was 1–2 years later than average for women with PCOS (Minooee, Tehrani, Rahmati, Mansournia, & Azizi, 2018). Hyperandrogenism of ovarian and adrenal origin and insulin resistance persist after menopause in women with PCOS. Although androgen levels tend to decrease in women over 70 years of age, lower levels of sex hormone binding globulin (SHBG) and FSH persist. Markopoulos and colleagues (2011) found that postmenopausal women with PCOS demonstrated higher than average levels of total testosterone and adrenal androgens (androstenedione, dehydroepiandrosterone sulfate [DHEAS]), 17-hydroxyprogesterone, and free androgen index. SHBG levels were significantly lower among women with PCOS. In a prospective study of women diagnosed with PCOS based on ovarian histology from ovarian wedge resection for PCOS and subsequently re-studied in their 70s, the PCOS group had higher free androgen index (FAI) and lower FSH and SHBG levels than those without PCOS. In addition, DHEAS, total testosterone, and androstenedione levels were higher in premenopausal women with PCOS than those without, but similar after menopause, which suggests that differences became less marked among women in their 80s (Schmidt, Brannstrom, Landin-Wilhelmsen, & Dahlgren, 2011). Endometrial cancer risk is elevated among women with PCOS (attributed to hyperestrogenic anovulation), which results in exposure to estrogen in the absence of progesterone and menses in which endometrial cells are shed (Azziz et al., 2016).

In addition to fertility and reproductive concerns, cardiovascular disease, type-2 diabetes, and other health problems related to metabolism represent major concerns for women living with PCOS as they age. Women from a nationwide Danish population registry of patients diagnosed with PCOS had a higher prevalence of diabetes, dyslipidemia, and hypertension, as well as increased risk of stroke and thrombosis, than did a comparison group of women without PCOS. Thyroid disease, asthma, migraine, and depression also were more prevalent among women with PCOS, but fractures were rare. Infertility was also increased, but number of births was higher among women with PCOS, which might reflect women's attempts at pregnancy at a younger age owing to their fertility concerns. Women who had irregular menses and polycystic ovaries had a more adverse metabolic risk profile, including more frequent diagnosis of diabetes, due to insulin resistance among women with PCOS (Glintborg, Rubin, Nybo, Abranhamsen, & Andersen, 2015). Women 23–35 years of age from this same cohort were followed for an average of 11 years. Those with PCOS were more likely to develop cardiovascular disease, with a median age at diagnosis of 35 years for women with PCOS versus 36 years for women without PCOS. Hypertension was the most common cardiovascular diagnosis among the women studied. Obesity, diabetes, infertility, and prior use of oral contraceptives, as well as age and signs of metabolic syndrome (i.e., higher blood pressure, greater BMI, lipid status, glycemic status) were associated with greater risk of CVD among women with PCOS (Glintborg, Rubin, Nubo, Abrahamsen, & Andersen, 2018).

Although women with PCOS appear to have increased risk for CVD based on surrogate markers for CVD, such as flow-mediated dilation (measure of vascular dysfunction), carotid intima-media thickness (a non-invasive measure of atherosclerosis), and coronary artery calcium (an indicator of atherosclerosis), it is unclear whether U.S. women with PCOS have an actual increased risk for CVD mortality. PCOS is commonly diagnosed during women's reproductive years, but cardiovascular disease manifests 3–4 decades later. Because there have been few longitudinal studies of women with PCOS as they age, the U.S. Study of Women's Health Across the Nation (SWAN) cohort was evaluated for hyperandrogenic oligomenorrhea, and subsequently assessed for development of metabolic syndrome, self-reported stroke, and myocardial infarction. After they were followed for over 12 years, women with hyperandrogenemia and oligomenorrhea developed metabolic syndrome at a rate similar to their counterparts who were eumenorrheic and normoandrogenic, oligomenorrheic and normoandrogenic, and eumenorrheic and hyperandrogenic. Smoking and obesity were strong predictors of metabolic syndrome development. There were no differences in incidence of self-reported stroke or myocardial infarction among the groups studied (Polotsky et al., 2014). Another U.S. effort to evaluate CVD mortality in postmenopausal women with clinical features of PCOS involved participants in the Women's Ischemia Syndrome Evaluation Study (WISE). Although women with PCOS had an earlier menopause, were more likely to smoke, and had more angiographic coronary artery disease than women without the PCOS features of irregular menses and current high androgen levels, cumulative 10-year mortality was not significantly different between the groups (Merz et al., 2016). Studies of large cohorts of women carefully phenotyped for PCOS with standardized long-term follow-up are essential to resolve whether PCOS increases the risk of cardiovascular mortality (Gunning & Fauser, 2017).

Women with PCOS also experience an increased prevalence of obstructive sleep apnea (OSA) independent of obesity. Androgen levels and insulin resistance were related to obstructive sleep apnea in women with PCOS, as found in other populations with OSA (Tasall, Chapotot, Leproult, Whitmore, & Ehrmann, 2011).

Treatment of PCOS

Treatment of PCOS is directed at managing the reproductive and metabolic disorders that comprise the PCO syndrome. Strategies to treat ovarian dysfunction are based on interrupting the cyclic interrelationship of hyperandrogenism, insulin resistance, hyperinsulinemia, and obesity or excess weight by managing comorbid conditions (e.g., obesity, insulin resistance). Although estrogen/progestins (EPs) have been a mainstay of treatment to reduce hyperandrogenism, their use is reserved for late adolescents and adults. Metformin is beneficial in adolescents as an approach to managing symptoms related to insulin resistance and treating menstrual dysfunction in adults. For women with obesity and insulin resistance, weight loss lifestyle interventions (i.e., physical activity, diet change) are recommended. In addition, metformin and clomiphene citrate (CC) may be used together to induce ovulation. CC (a synthetic estrogen receptor modulator) has both estrogenic and anti-estrogenic properties and has a long history of use in ovulation induction; metformin has been used effectively to improve menstrual cyclicity and ovulation rates in women with PCOS (Pasquali, 2018).

Strategies for managing hirsutism include reducing endogenous production of androgens and non-hormonal treatment. Although androgen is produced in hair follicles, little attention has been given to exploring this source and developing appropriate treatment options. Other approaches are often recommended, including prescribed estrogen-progestins (EPs) emphasizing use of progestins with anti-androgenic properties, ethinyl estradiol, anti-androgens such as spironolactone or 5-alpha-reductase inhibitors such as finasteride insulin sensitizers such as metformin. In addition, hair removal by laser and other approaches such as electrolysis are cosmetic options often not covered by health insurance. Although metformin has shown modest effects on hyperandrogenism, its effects on hirsutism are limited (Pasquali, 2018).

Young women with PCOS are often advised to use oral contraceptives to manage their symptoms. Long-term use of hormonal contraception can reduce androgen production and prevent symptoms of hyperandrogenism, thus women who desire pregnancy are faced with difficult decisions about treatment that manages their symptoms but prevents pregnancy. Many women with PCOS use assisted reproductive technologies for conception, including ovulation induction of multiple follicles with clomiphene citrate. After three cycles of treatment, approximately one half of women with infrequent menstruation experience pregnancy, and approximately three quarters of women do after nine cycles (Barthelmess & Naz, 2015).

A recent narrative review of lifestyle and behavioral management interventions for women with PCOS indicated that outcomes of weight management programs are likely to benefit from inclusion of behavioral and psychological strategies (e.g., goal setting, self-monitoring, cognitive restructuring, problem solving, relapse prevention). Brennan and colleagues also noted that behavioral strategies that target motivation, social support, and psychological well-being are of value and can be applied to women living with PCOS at different reproductive stages of the lifespan (Brennan et al., 2017).

A recent systematic review and meta-analysis of the role of exercise training in women with PCOS revealed insufficient published data to describe the effect of exercise on ovulation, but there was a suggestion of improvement of menstrual regularity, pregnancy, and ovulation rates. Exercise interventions did improve lipid profiles and reduced waist circumference, systolic blood pressure, and fasting insulin (Benham et al., 2018).

Research about the type of dietary modification most effective for weight loss and metabolic outcomes for women with PCOS has not yet indicated which are optimal for women with various PCOS phenotypes (Moran et al., 2013). Considerations for dietary modifications focus on insulin resistance as well as weight loss. Consequently, many researchers have studied effects of limiting not only caloric intake but carbohydrate intake as well. Moran and colleagues' review indicated that greater weight loss occurred with a monounsaturated fat-enriched diet; greater menstrual regularity with a low-glycemic index diet; increased free androgen index with high-carbohydrate diets; greater reductions in insulin resistance, fibrinogen, total and high-density lipoprotein cholesterol with a low-carbohydrate or low-glycemic index diet; improved quality of life with a low-glycemic index diet; and improved depression and self-esteem with a high-protein diet.

Gower and Goss (2015) found that a lower-carbohydrate, higher-fat diet reduced abdominal and intermuscular fat and increased insulin sensitivity in adults at risk of type-2 diabetes. Among women with PCOS, the lower carbohydrate diet was associated with lower fasting insulin and glucose levels and increased insulin sensitivity and dynamic beta cell response. With this diet, women lost both intraabdominal adipose tissue and intermuscular fat, but, with a lower fat diet, women lost lean mass. Interest in the therapeutic use of very-low-carbohydrate (ketogenic) diets for women with PCOS is increasing (Paoli, Rubini, Volek, & Grimaldi, 2013).

Treating women with OSA with continuous positive airway pressure resulted in modest improvement in insulin sensitivity as well as a decrease in norepinephrine levels, which suggests that the decrease in insulin sensitivity was mediated by sympathetic nervous system activation (Tasall et al., 2011).

Although lifestyle changes, including those related to obesity, may have positive effects on health overall, it also is important to consider that genetic factors in the etiology of PCOS may limit the effectiveness of some interventions. Moreover, interventions that emphasize empowerment of women and support for the challenges they face in managing their symptoms are needed (Brennan et al., 2017).

Women's experiences of PCOS

In contrast to the majority of research conducted from a biomedical or psychiatric perspective, Kitzinger and Willmott (2002) studied women's experience of PCOS by interviewing women recruited through Verity, a British national self-help organization. Women reported feeling "freakish," "abnormal," and not "proper" women (p. 352), experiences related to three commonly experienced symptoms: Excess hair growth; irregular, absent, or disrupted menstrual periods; and infertility. Women's feelings of freakishness were linked to their notions of what normal or proper women are: Free of body/facial hair, menstruating regularly, and able to bear a child. Failing to be sufficiently womanly because of body and facial hair prompted a need to remove it, which required complex daily routines. In addition, avoiding communal bathing, showering, or changing facilities was important to protect their hairiness from discovery. At the same time, women experienced conflicted emotions about taking steps to resemble a feminine ideal: One feminist expressed shame for using electrolysis. Irregular menses were also a source of concern because women perceived menses as a sign of womanhood or fertility: Some concerned about infertility kept this secret from others, and some expressed that infertility defeated the purpose of being a woman. Kitzinger and Willmott concluded that PCOS is a "deeply stigmatizing condition" (p. 359), a "theft of womanhood" (p. 349).

Of all the symptoms associated with PCOS, hirsutism has been noted as most troublesome by many women, yet few studies have focused specifically on how hirsutism is experienced. Participants in these studies described experiencing their bodies as a yoke, a freak, a disgrace, and a prison (Ekback, Wijma, & Benzein, 2009). Those who described the body as a yoke were sorrowful and preoccupied with their hair growth, whereas those who saw their body as a freak described living with an invaded body, a forced identity, and an altered self, which reflects their experience as a person for whom hairiness had become the prominent aspect. Women who experienced their body as a disgrace described living with shame and guilt and being outside the female body norm. Those who described their body as a prison felt trapped in their bodies; they worked to remove hair and cover their bodies, used imagination to transcend their bodies, and some even contemplated suicide.

Women with hirsutism coped with unwanted hair growth by covering their bodies or isolating themselves from people, removing the unwanted hair, and finding ways of living with hair growth, such as through use of humor. Women also described difficulties hirsutism created in their sexual relations with men. For these women, "doing gender" meant developing ways of living with a visible sign of PCOS in a social context in which their bodies were not aligned with dominant norms of femininity (Pfister & Rømer, 2017). These experiences underscore women's alienation from their bodies (e.g., viewing hair as disgusting, masculine, or a sign of a body that was not well managed in relation to prevalent constructions of the female body).

In addition to feminine identity issues related to cosmetic/body image (e.g., weight, hairiness, acne) and reproductive identity issues related to menstruation and childbirth (e.g., irregular periods, amenorrhea, fear of infertility, infertility, uncertainty), women described an ill-health identity (Tomlinson et al., 2017). One aspect of the ill- health identity involved dealing with a lengthy time to diagnosis, uncertainty, bothersome symptoms, lack of physicians' empathy, medication side effects, and feeling like a guinea pig (i.e., a research subject). Another aspect of ill-health identity is related to the long-term implications of PCOS (e.g., risk of type-2 diabetes and endometrial cancer) (Tomlinson et al., 2017).

Women with PCOS often experienced prolonged delays in getting treatment, barriers to diagnosis, lack of empathy, and dismissal by health professionals for their concerns about hirsutism and weight gain. Once they were able to access care, women commonly described being disappointed by receiving limited information: Many did not get adequate explanations of their diagnosis or information on treatments that could alter their symptoms. Some women diagnosed their own conditions by searching for explanations in popular media (Snyder, 2006). Women found themselves searching for answers to questions about the causes of their symptoms and were frustrated by needing to see multiple physicians in order to get a diagnosis. With a diagnosis came devastation for some women. Little information was provided about the long-term health consequences of PCOS, although they acknowledged that often their primary concerns were fertility-related. Disparate understandings of the consequences of PCOS by women and their health care providers left women dissatisfied with their health care (Tomlinson et al., 2017).

Medications also proved challenging. Despite their anxiety about their fertility, women were prescribed oral contraceptives, often without an explanation of the rationale for their use. Other challenges in obtaining treatment included lack of health insurance coverage for body hair removal (e.g., laser therapy, electrolysis). Gaining control was achieved for some by finding a health care provider who explained PCOS and its treatment, including the progression of treatment. Some were able to let go of guilt about being overweight after they learned that weight gain was not their fault, an important consequence of diagnosis and treatment. Others reported negative experiences with health professionals who trivialized their symptoms of hirsutism or acne or were unaware of the symptoms' connection to PCOS (Snyder, 2006).

Not surprisingly, many women with PCOS felt isolated and marginalized and longed to be "normal," but, in some instances, health care professionals reinforced their feelings of abnormality (Snyder, 2006). Although most women attempted to maintain a positive outlook, many tried not to think about PCOS and its symptoms. Destigmatizing PCOS and its symptoms is an important part of giving voice to and supporting women who feel marginalized, stigmatized, and silenced about their condition. For example, health professionals' emphasis on androgens (sometimes described as "masculine" hormones) may not only be an inaccurate explanation of PCOS etiology, but also may reinforce the construction of women with PCOS as abnormal.

Quality of life and PCOS

Studies of women living with PCOS have focused on global quality of life, a general reflection of one's beliefs about functioning and achievements in various aspects of life, as well as on health-related quality of life, which emphasizes perceptions of the dimensions of life most likely to be affected by changes in health status (Avis et al., 2003). Women living with PCOS report lower quality of life in multiple domains (physical, psychological, environmental, social), as well as lower life satisfaction than those without PCOS (Rzonca, Bien, Wdowiak, Szymanski, & Iwanowicz-Palus, 2018). Overall, women with higher socioeconomic status (SES), shorter length of time since PCOS diagnosis, lower BMI, younger age, and having experienced motherhood reported higher quality of life and life satisfaction.

Studies of health-related quality of life of women with PCOS have focused on symptoms and their effects on women's lives. Women screened for PCOS reported their most common quality of life concerns were weight, followed by menstrual problems, infertility, emotions, and body hair (McCook et al., 2005). In a web-based survey, women with PCOS reported higher anxiety than those without PCOS (Barnard et al., 2007). Similar reports of anxiety and depression were found in a study of the North Finland Birth Cohort at ages 31 and 46 years. Women with PCOS or hirsutism experienced greater anxiety and depression symptoms than women without these symptoms; hirsutism alone was associated with a greater prevalence of depression. Neither BMI nor hyperandrogenism were related to either anxiety or depression scores. These findings suggest the importance of clinicians providing supportive health care for women with PCOS (Karjula et al., 2017).

Quality of life also has been linked to challenges women experience in managing their symptoms. In one study women rated quality of life lowest in relation to weight management followed by menstrual problems, menstrual predictability, infertility, hirsutism, emotional disturbance, and acne (Barnard et al., 2007).

Concept elicitation interviews with women diagnosed with PCOS and clinicians with expertise in PCOS revealed differences in perspectives (Martin, Halling, Eek, Krohe, & Paty, 2017). Although the highest proportion of patient-expressed symptoms were pain and discomfort (70% reported cramping), hair loss and growth (facial hair 75%), menstruation and bleeding (heavy bleeding 70%, infertility 70%), and bloating (60%), the clinicians did not consider cramping pain, heavy bleeding, or bloating to be important to patients with PCOS.

Impacts of PCOS reported by patients were related to emotional well-being (e.g., stress), coping behaviors, sleep and energy restrictions, and social/lifestyle limitations and restrictions. Their most frequently reported concerns were shaving, embarrassment, and impacts on sex and leisure, followed by with mood swings, frustration, and impaired relationships. Women also mentioned worry, anxiety/stress, impaired exercise, irritability, tiredness, and depression.

Women's dissatisfaction with their health care surfaced in many of the qualitative studies reported above, including discrepancies between symptoms women considered important and those clinicians identified. In a recent web-based study of 1,385 women with reported diagnoses of PCOS who resided in North America, Europe, and other regions of the world, few women reported satisfaction with their diagnosis experience or with the information they had received. Many reported having seen multiple health professionals over more than a two-year period to obtain a diagnosis. Addressing gaps in early diagnosis, education, and support was recommended (Gibson-Helm, Teede, Dunaif, & Dokras, 2017).

Dysmenorrhea

Biomedical perspectives

Dysmenorrhea is a painful condition characterized by severe cramping in the lower abdomen or pelvic area that occurs just prior to and during the first 1–2 days of menses. An estimated

16–91% of U.S. women of reproductive age experience dysmenorrhea, and 2–29% rate their pain as severe (Iacovides, Avidon, & Baker, 2015; Ju, Jones, & Mishra, 2014a). *Primary dysmenorrhea* refers to pain in the absence of pelvic pathology; it first occurs within 6–24 months of menarche (Iacovides et al., 2015). *Secondary dysmenorrhea* is associated with underlying pelvic conditions such as endometriosis, adenomyosis, fibroids, and pelvic inflammatory disease; it usually begins more than two years after menarche (Iacovides et al., 2015). Dysmenorrhea often is accompanied by other painful conditions such as irritable bowel syndrome, non-cyclic pelvic pain (Giamberardino et al., 2010), and a variety of symptoms such as gastrointestinal symptoms and others discussed in greater detail below. Evidence supports a relationship between dysmenorrhea and increased risk for future chronic pain conditions (Berkley, 2013; Iacovides et al., 2015; Westling et al., 2013).

Etiology

Over-production of uterine prostaglandins has been the most widely accepted etiologic explanation for dysmenorrhea (Dawood, 2006). Endometrial cells are sloughed during menstruation, and their disintegration releases arachidonic acid, which is a precursor for prostaglandin synthesis. In turn, prostaglandins stimulate myometrial hyper-contractility, which produces ischemia and hypoxic effects in the myometrium that induce pain. Prostaglandin production can be stimulated by epinephrine, peptide and steroid hormones, mechanical stimulation, and tissue trauma. In women with dysmenorrhea, falling levels of progesterone prior to menses initiate a process by which endometrial lysosomes liberate arachidonic acid, which, in turn, increases prostaglandin production. Women with dysmenorrhea have higher levels of prostaglandins in the luteal phase of their menstrual cycles than at other times and higher levels than do women without dysmenorrhea. PGF2-alpha (prostaglandin F2-alpha) has potent effects on vasoconstriction of the uterine blood vessels and enhances myometrial contraction. Although evidence supports contraction of an ischemic uterus as the cause of pain, it has also been suggested that prostaglandins sensitize nerve endings to pain (Iacovides et al., 2015). In addition, women with primary dysmenorrhea, as compared with women without, exhibit greater expression of genes that regulate pro-inflammatory cytokines and transform growth factor-beta, which are related to inflammation and may account for some of the symptoms women experience with dysmenorrhea (Iacovides et al., 2015).

In a recent review of 15 primary studies and three systematic reviews, Ju and colleagues (2014b) examined risk factors associated with dysmenorrhea. Both age and parity were associated inversely with the prevalence of dysmenorrhea. Mechanisms responsible for the relationship of both age and greater number of births with a lower incidence of dysmenorrhea remain unclear. Although there is a strong relationship between family history and dysmenorrhea, it is unclear whether the relationship is due to genetic predisposition or to learned behavior in one's family. Use of oral contraceptive pills was associated with a lower prevalence of dysmenorrhea. Lower SES and higher levels of stress also were associated with greater prevalence of dysmenorrhea. Although the biological mechanism responsible for the relationship between stress and dysmenorrhea is not known, stress initiates a neuroendocrine cascade that disrupts follicular development and progesterone synthesis as well as the production and release of cortisol and epinephrine, which influence prostaglandin synthesis and binding in the myometrium (Wang et al., 2004). Evidence for effects of smoking and being overweight was mixed across studies reviewed by Ju et al. Future research is needed to evaluate the environmental and genetic factors associated with dysmenorrhea (Iacovides et al., 2015; Ju et al., 2014b).

Women experience a variety of patterns of dysmenorrhea across the lifespan. Four different dysmenorrhea symptom trajectories were identified among young adult women in the Australian Longitudinal Study on Women's Health over a 13-year period (Ju et al., 2014a). The "normative" group included 38% of the total sample of 9,671 women who had no or few symptoms. A "low" group (28%) experienced increased prevalence of dysmenorrhea over time, from 20% to nearly 40%. A "recovering" group (17%) experienced decreased prevalence from 50% at ages 22–27 to only 10% at ages 34–39. A "chronic" group (17%) experienced a high prevalence of dysmenorrhea that varied between 70 and 80% throughout the study. Although these data support an overall declining prevalence of dysmenorrhea as women age, they also illustrate the different trajectories of symptoms women experience during young adult years. The trajectories reported here are consistent with Chen et al.'s (2018) findings that dysmenorrhea symptom experiences vary among women, ranging widely in severity from woman to woman and also over time within the same women. Thus, the symptom experience is dynamic as well as heterogeneous.

Diagnosis

Diagnosis of dysmenorrhea is based on a woman's description of her symptoms and their timing. Women with primary dysmenorrhea describe cramping as having begun around the time of menarche. Some women liken their cramps to labor pains. Symptom onset with menstruation is a key element of diagnosis. In general, symptoms start within hours before or at the beginning of menses and last 2–3 days (Dawood, 2006).

Secondary dysmenorrhea varies in its clinical presentation due to its relationship to a variety of underlying pathologies. Diagnosis of secondary dysmenorrhea usually involves a pelvic examination to identify pathologies, such as endometriosis, pelvic inflammatory disease, uterine fibroids, and pelvic adhesions (Dawood, 2006; Mannix, 2008).

Symptom phenotypes

Although dysmenorrhea co-occurs with other symptoms, symptom phenotypes were not identified until recently. Symptom ratings from 762 U.S. women with dysmenorrhea who responded to a web-based survey revealed three different phenotypes: Mild localized pain, severe localized pain, and severe multiple symptoms. Women with the mild localized pain phenotype rated abdominal cramps and dull abdominal pain or discomfort as mild, whereas women with the severe localized pain phenotype rated their abdominal cramps as severe. Women with the severe multiple symptom phenotype rated the following symptoms as severe: Abdominal cramps, dull abdominal pain or discomfort, low back pain, headache or migraine, aches all over, bloating, nausea, diarrhea, more bowel movements than usual (Chen, Ofner, Bakoyannis, Kwekkeboom, & Carpenter, 2017). Several characteristics differentiated women with the three different dysmenorrhea phenotypes. Women with the severe localized pain phenotype were more likely than those with the mild localized pain phenotype to have migraine or nonmigraine headaches. Women with the multiple severe symptoms phenotype were more likely than those with the mild or the severe localized pain phenotype to be older, Black, Hispanic, have experienced dysmenorrhea for fewer years, have migraine or nonmigraine headaches, have neck pain, or have pelvic pain other than dysmenorrhea.

The women in Chen et al.'s study (2017) also identified several factors that exacerbated their symptoms. Among these were heavy periods, menstrual irregularity, and underlying health conditions. Others' dysmenorrhea symptoms were influenced by genetics, dietary habits, and recent removal of intrauterine devices.

Not only is dysmenorrhea a heterogeneous condition, it is also linked to other chronic pain conditions, which raises the possibility of persistent central sensitization (Woolf, 2016). A recent review by Iacovides and colleagues (2015) established that greater pain sensitivity in women with dysmenorrhea occurs throughout the menstrual cycle. In addition, hyperalgesia was evident in women with dysmenorrhea when they were experiencing menstrual pain as well as at other times, and hyperalgesia was present in muscles both inside and outside the areas where menstrual pain was experienced. These findings led to the hypothesis that central sensitization occurs with dysmenorrhea, similar to other pain conditions (e.g., fibromyalgia). An abnormal augmentation of pain occurs by means of increased excitability of somato-visceral convergent neurons in the spinal cord and increased pain perception. Studies of cerebral structure and metabolism have revealed consequences of dysmenorrhea, including the role of viscero-visceral hyperalgesia, or cross-organ sensitization to pain input to the central nervous system. Evidence supports that effective treatment of one painful condition decreases pain from the other (Giamberardino et al., 2010).

Treatment of primary dysmenorrhea

Awareness of the consequences of untreated dysmenorrhea pain for future pain conditions has prompted a search for treatments. The most commonly used pharmacotherapeutic approach for primary dysmenorrhea is based on its prostaglandin-based etiology. Non-steroidal anti-inflammatory drugs (NSAIDS) (e.g., ibuprofen, sodium naproxen, ketoprofen) are prostaglandin (PG) synthetase inhibitors, several forms of which have been demonstrated to have comparable efficacy (Dawood, 2006; Iacovides et al., 2015; Mannix, 2008; Marjoribanks, Ayeleke, Farquhar, & Proctor, 2015). Nonetheless, some women do not respond to or cannot tolerate the PG inhibitors due to gastrointestinal or neurological side effects (Marjoribanks et al., 2015). Often oral contraceptives (OC) are used as a second choice treatment for these women (Wong, Farquhar, Roberts, & Proctor, 2009). Suppression of ovulation with reduction of the thickness of the endometrium and consequent reduced volume of menses reduces PG synthesis and, in turn, reduces menstrual pain. Some women who use OC experience adverse effects of nausea, headaches, and weight gain. Venous thromboembolism is a contraindication to oral contraceptive use for women at risk. Hormonal intrauterine devices provide another option for some women. In addition, some less frequently used pharmacologic approaches for managing dysmenorrhea pain include glycerol trinitrate or nitroglycerin, which suppresses uterine contractions through nitric oxide activity, and nifedipine, which reduces myometrial contractility through blocking calcium channels (Dawood, 2006; Mannix, 2008).

Surgical treatments, such as laparoscopic uterosacral nerve ablation (LUNA) and presacral neurectomy (PSN), have been reviewed. However, there was insufficient evidence to support use of nerve interruption in the management of dysmenorrhea (Proctor, Latthe, Farquhar, Khan, & Johnson, 2005).

Another treatment option is high-frequency transcutaneous electric nerve stimulation (TENS), which interferes with the ability to receive or perceive pain signals (Proctor, Smith, Farquhar, & Stones, 2002). Acupuncture and acupressure have been used to treat dysmenorrhea, but there is insufficient evidence to determine whether or not either of these is effective in treating primary dysmenorrhea, and few data are available on adverse events (Smith et al., 2016). Spinal manipulation has also been explored; high velocity, low amplitude manipulation did not appear more effective than sham manipulation in a Cochrane review (Proctor, Hing, Johnson, & Murphy, 2006).

Women have reported using dietary supplements including magnesium, thiamin, vitamins B and E, and herbal remedies, such as rose tea, but evidence of the efficacy of these therapies is needed (Proctor & Murphy, 2001). A recent systematic review of physical activity indicated that it may be an effective treatment for primary dysmenorrhea, but additional trials are needed to confirm efficacy (Matthewman, Lee, Kaur, & Daley, 2018). Heat has been shown to improve dysmenorrhea symptoms when applied to the back or abdomen (Iacovides et al., 2015). Use of herbal preparations, including Chinese medicine, has been reviewed, but there remains a need for strong clinical trials to support use of various preparations (Zhu, Proctor, Bensoussan, Wu, & Smith, 2008). The role of therapies that target central sensitization (e.g., gabapentin, tricyclic antidepressants) remains unclear. Behavioral interventions for primary and secondary dysmenorrhea have been explored, including studies of relaxation and pain management training, but better evidence for the efficacy of behavioral interventions is needed (Proctor, Murphy, Pattison, Suckling, & Farquhar, 2007).

Self-management of dysmenorrhea

Women's approaches to self-management of dysmenorrhea are symptom driven and include prescription pain medications (e.g., opioids) and hormonal contraceptives. In addition, they use over-the-counter pain medications (e.g., NSAIDS, acetaminophen) and medications for gastrointestinal symptoms. In addition, many use complementary health approaches, most commonly relaxation, natural products or dietary supplements, yoga, special dietary modification, massage from a therapist, nerve stimulation such as TENS, and acupressure. Other non-drug therapies include rest, heat, distraction such as watching television, and self-massage of abdomen (Chen, Kwekkeboom, & Ward, 2016).

Women's experiences of dysmenorrhea

Beliefs about dysmenorrhea and self-management

Chen and colleagues (2016) used Leventhal's Common Sense Model to guide data collection from over 700 women in an Internet survey. Women's representations of dysmenorrhea included commonly endorsed causes such as stress, physiology/menstruation, hormonal changes, diet/eating habits, unknown causes, heredity, aging, disease and disorders, and overweight. Most women agreed that dysmenorrhea is a normal part of a woman's life. On average, these women believed their symptoms are moderately severe with moderate effects on their daily life and that the symptoms would persist until menopause. They also believed that they had a moderate level of personal control and treatment control of their symptoms, but their beliefs about the dangers of medications and the value of complementary health care were neutral. Women also believed they had a moderately clear understanding of dysmenorrhea symptoms, thought dysmenorrhea affected them emotionally, but 20% were embarrassed to talk about their symptoms.

Women's representations of dysmenorrhea and self-management behaviors were related: Those who sought care from a conventional health care provider believed that dysmenorrhea negatively affected their daily life and had a clear understanding of dysmenorrhea, and those less likely to seek health care from a conventional provider believed that dysmenorrhea would continue until menopause and that symptoms are normal. Use of medications was associated with women's beliefs about the dangers of medications. Use of complementary health approaches was more likely among women with beliefs about negative consequences of dysmenorrhea, treatment control, and the value of complementary health approaches, but less likely among those with beliefs that symptoms are normal. Women who used other non-drug approaches were those with strong beliefs about treatment control and that pain would continue until menopause.

Health care experiences

Although there are efficacious therapies for primary dysmenorrhea, the majority of over 500 women in Chen and colleagues' (2018) study did not seek health care for dysmenorrhea. The most common reasons given by over 30% of women were that they assumed dysmenorrhea symptoms are normal and do not require treatment and a preference for managing their own symptoms using a variety of methods, including over-the-counter medications, complementary health approaches, and other coping strategies such as toughing it out or ignoring the symptoms. Fewer than 10% of women indicated that they lacked financial resources to access health care, believed health care providers would not offer to help them because they would think dysmenorrhea is not a disease, did not know about treatment options, felt wary about treatments and their effects, believed their symptoms are tolerable, felt embarrassed or afraid to seek health care, or did not use health care in general. Based on these findings, Chen and colleagues recommended that health professionals should: Provide screening for dysmenorrhea routinely; avoid trivializing or dismissing dysmenorrhea symptoms; initiate discussion and education about dysmenorrhea; consider women's preferences when offering treatment options; and raise public consciousness of dysmenorrhea and its consequences in women's lives.

Quality of life

The impact of dysmenorrhea on quality of life has been evaluated by how it affects family relationships, friendships, school and work performance, and social and recreational activities. Some women who responded to an Internet survey reported that dysmenorrhea had a negative impact on their lives, rendering them unable to sit, walk, or stand, so that they had to stay in bed or curl up in a ball. Some missed school or work and were unable to attend recreational activities or participate in family responsibilities, such as childcare. A few experienced negative effects of treatment (e.g., taking too much pain medication, getting abdominal burns from heating pads) (Chen et al. (2018). These findings are consistent with results of other studies in which women reported lost work and study time (e.g., Unsal, Ayranci, Tozun, Arslan, & Calik, 2010) with economic consequences for women and their families.

University students (average age 20 years) who experience dysmenorrhea have reported worse physical function, role functioning related to physical functioning, bodily pain, general health, and vitality than those without dysmenorrhea (Unsal et al., 2010). Likewise, menstruating U.S. Veterans' Affairs patients (average age 35 years) with dysmenorrhea have reported lower quality of life, including reduced physical and social functioning and worse bodily pain, and general health perceptions (Barnard, Frayne, Skinner, & Sullivan, 2003).

Interference of dysmenorrhea pain with sleep results in reduced sleep quality and efficiency and greater fatigue, which, in turn, are associated with negative mood, lower daytime functioning, and enhanced pain (Iacovides et al., 2015). Thus, a cycle exists in which dysmenorrhea, as well as other types of pain, is perpetuated through sleep disruption.

Although dysmenorrhea has been linked to anxiety and depression, it remains unclear whether women with dysmenorrhea are more likely to develop anxiety and/or depression or whether women with symptoms of depression or anxiety are more likely to experience dysmenorrhea. In a systematic review Bajalan and colleagues (2019) found few studies with data about the comorbidity of dysmenorrhea and psychological disorders. Effects of dysmenorrhea on anxiety and depression or effects of depression and anxiety on dysmenorrhea were inconsistent among the prospective studies.

A cross-sectional study of girls 11–17 years of age revealed that more severe depressive symptoms were associated with more severe menstrual symptoms, including dysmenorrhea and affective and somatic complaints (Dorn et al., 2009). A longitudinal study of a community sample of 262 girls aged 11–17 years over a three-year period revealed that menstrual symptom severity increased with age and then plateaued in later adolescence. Baseline menstrual symptoms (including menstrual pain, affect, and somatic symptoms), depressive symptoms, and somatic complaints were all related such that girls who reported higher depressive symptoms at baseline were also more likely to report more abdominal pain, somatic symptoms, and back pain at baseline. Girls who reported more depressive symptoms at baseline did not report more menstrual symptoms over subsequent years, except for those who reported low severity of menstrual symptoms at baseline. Those who reported more somatic menstrual symptoms at baseline were more likely to report greater menstrual symptoms, abdominal pain, and somatic symptoms at subsequent occasions. These results suggest that, although depressive symptoms are associated with dysmenorrhea symptoms at baseline, they do not appear to be associated with future dysmenorrhea symptoms. Nonetheless, the significant number of girls with higher depressive symptoms and complaints warrants further investigation and assessment of interventions to reduce their future risk of mood as well as somatic symptoms (Beal et al., 2014).

Menstrual migraine

Biomedical perspectives

Migraine headaches are among the most prevalent neurological health conditions. Migraine is an inherited central pain dysfunction, which involves a complex interplay between neurotransmitters, vasoactive inflammatory peptides such as calcitonin gene-related peptide (CGRP), and portions of the trigeminal nerve that innervate blood vessels in the brain. The end result is pain, nausea, and pain reactions to stimuli that are not typically painful (e.g., light and sound; i.e., allodynia) (Broner, Bobker, & Klebanoff, 2017). Migraines without aura (common migraines) occur more frequently, often last longer, and are more disabling than migraine with aura (Headache Classification Committee, 2018). Approximately one quarter of adults with migraine experience migraine with aura, which is characterized by visual and/or sensory and/or speech symptoms that develop gradually and last about one hour before the onset of a migraine headache.

The condition is not unique to the Western or industrialized world. An international survey conducted by WHO (2011) showed that approximately 10% of the population in the Americas, Europe, southeast Asia, and the western Pacific between the ages of 18 and 65 reported migraine headaches. Only Africa and the eastern Mediterranean regions reported lower migraine prevalence.

Girls and boys are equally likely to be affected by migraine prior to puberty (Pavlovic, Akcali, Bolay, Bernstein, & Maleki, 2017). Following puberty, the incidence of migraine increases for both girls and boys, but women are three times as likely as men to experience migraine at all points after puberty (Pavlovic et al., 2017; Stovner et al., 2007). Between the ages of 30 and 39, nearly one quarter of all U.S. women are reported to experience migraine (Pavlovic et al., 2017; Stewart, Lipton, Celentano, & Reed, 1992; Stovner et al., 2007). The fact that migraines are experienced by both women and men reduces some of the stigma women often experience when seeking help for conditions only experienced by women (e.g., dysmenorrhea, PCOS). The fact that practitioners who diagnose and treat migraines are more likely than the general population to be migraine suffers themselves (Evans, Lipton, & Silberstein, 2003; Schroeder et al., 2018) may make it easier for migraineurs who seek help to have their symptoms understood. Women are more likely than men to report migraine symptoms to their provider and are more likely than men to take prescription medications for their condition (Buse et al., 2013).

Etiology

Research indicates that migraines and the sex difference in migraine incidence are influenced by genetic, neurological, and hormonal factors. Recent research has identified a number of mutations that may underlie genetic transmission of susceptibility to migraine in humans (van den Maagdenberg, 2016). However, the research remains preliminary, and the relationship between genes and hormones is complex and does not account for all group differences in the experience of migraine.

Mice that carry a monogentic mutation associated with human migraines have been studied to assess sex differences in and the effects of sex hormones on cortical spreading depolarization, which typically occurs with migraine (Eikermann-Haerter et al., 2009b). Female mutant mice were more likely than males to experience cortical spreading depolarization, and depolarization was found to last longer in the females. Reduction of estrogen through ovariectomy reduced, and estrogen replacement post ovariectomy increased, the frequency and length of spreading cortical depolarization in female mutant mice. Orchiectomy and androgen replacement in male mutant mice had the opposite effects (Eikermann-Haerter et al., 2009a).

Functional brain imaging studies have indicated differences in brain structures and connectivity between structures in men and women with migraines. The insular cortex is thicker in female than in male migraineurs or male or female non-migraineurs (Maleki et al., 2012). It is unclear whether this and other differences in brain structures or pathways that related to sensory experience or emotional response are the cause or the outcome of migraine. Researchers who have looked at brain structures in relationship to migraine in women have not assessed the influence of hormonal changes across the monthly cycle or across the lifespan.

Differences in genes or brain morphology may account in part for sex differences in the experience of migraine, but they cannot easily account for women's experience of migraines in relationship to the monthly cycle of ovarian hormone production. The vast majority of regularly cycling women with migraine experience migraines during the perimenstrual phase (i.e., the two days before the onset of menses and the first three days of menses), a time of falling estrogen production. These menstrual migraines may last longer, be more resistant to treatment, and be more debilitating than migraines unrelated to menstruation (Guven, Guven, & Comoglu, 2017; MacGregor et al., 2010).

Menstrual migraine (MM) has been attributed to the more rapid decline in estrogen that occurs after the luteal peak (estrogen withdrawal hypothesis; MacGregor & Hackshaw,

2004; MacGregor et al., 2006; Pavlovic et al., 2016; Somerville, 1972). Pavlovic and colleagues have suggested that the more rapid rate of decline of estrogen is not the proximal cause of migraine but rather indicates a vulnerability through which migraine may be initiated by common triggers such as stress or lack of sleep.

Other factors may also underlie the experience of menstrual migraine. Trigeminal response to stimulation occurs at a shorter latency in women with MM during the perimenstrual period than during the follicular phase, a difference not observed with women without MM (Varlibas & Erdemoglu, 2009). Women's pain perception increases during the late luteal phase, regardless of whether they experience migraine (de Tommaso, 2011). This may be why migraines that occur in the perimenstruum are rated as more painful and debilitating than migraines at other times of the menstrual cycle (de Tommaso et al., 2009). Elevated prostaglandin (Silberstein & Merriam, 1993) and/or low serotonin (Chauvel, Multon, & Schoenen, 2018) levels may also play a role in the experience of migraine pain.

Women with migraines report reduced headache frequency and intensity across pregnancy and during the early postpartum period (Allais et al., 2013; Kvisvik, Stovner, Helde, Bovim, & Linde, 2011; Petrovski, Vetvik, Lundqvist, & Eberhard-Gran, 2018). Intensity, duration, and/or frequency increases again after childbirth (Kvisvik et al., 2011; Petrovski et al., 2018).

The relationship between menopause and migraine is complex. Onset of migraine during the peri- or post-menopausal periods is rare in women who have never experienced migraine before. Surgical menopause is generally associated with an increase or no change in migraine frequency compared with premenopause (Neri et al., 1993; Wang, Fuh, Lu, Juang, & Wang, 2003). After physiological menopause, many women report a decrease in migraine frequency (Lipton, Stewart, Diamond, Diamond, & Reed, 2001; Neri et al., 1993). Migraine with and without aura may be differentially affected by the menopause transition; the risk of migraine without aura appears to be significantly reduced post-menopause, whereas the risk of migraine with aura is unrelated to hormonal changes of menopause (Mattsson, 2003; Ripa et al., 2015).

Additional risk factors

Girls who experience menarche at an earlier age are at greater risk for migraine (but not non-migraine) headaches. Maleki and colleagues (2016, 2017) reported that each year that menarche is delayed is associated with a 7% decrease in the odds of experiencing migraine headaches. Although girls whose mothers experienced migraines were more likely to report migraine than those whose mothers did not, the effect of age of menarche remains even after accounting for familial history.

Sociocultural stress factors, many of which are more likely to occur in women or girls, are also associated with increased risk of migraine. Both women and men who report having experienced physical or sexual abuse or witnessed parental domestic violence as children are more likely to experience migraines as adults (Brennenstuhl & Fuller-Thomson, 2015; Tietjen et al., 2015). Women are more likely than men to report a history of childhood or adult sexual abuse and are more likely than men to experience intimate partner violence (Black et al., 2011; Lev-Wiesel & First, 2018; WHO, 2013).

Migraine often coexists with dysmenorrhea and endometriosis (Mannix, 2008; Tietjen, Conway, Utley, Gunning, & Herial, 2006; Tietjen et al., 2007). Migraineurs with endometriosis reported more frequent and disabling headaches than did migraineurs without endometriosis (Ferrero et al., 2004; Tietjen et al., 2007). Many studies suggest commonalities in the etiology and treatment of menstrual migraine and dysmenorrhea (see below, as well as the previous section on dysmenorrhea).

Treatment

Diagnosis of menstrual migraine relies on patients' notation of symptoms in daily diaries, which report both pain levels and monthly cycle data. There are no specific treatments approved to alleviate migraines that occur in relationship to menstruation (Allais, Chiarle, Sinigaglia, & Benedetto, 2018). Individuals with fewer headaches per month can be treated with triptans (Hu, Guan, Fan, & Jin, 2013) or NSAIDS (Allais et al., 2018). These drugs can be used to alleviate headache pain as well as to prevent MM. Triptans should not be used by individuals with hypertension or cardiovascular disease. Triptans need to be taken at the first warning signs of migraine onset. NSAIDS can be taken even after symptom onset, but most have more side effects and contraindications than triptans (Allais et al., 2018).

Prophylactic or preventative treatment involves the use of triptans or NSAIDS during the days leading up to menses and during menstrual bleeding (Hu et al., 2013). Triptans stimulate the production of the serotonin in the brain. Serotonin, in turn, reduces the inflammation and the vasodilation related to pain in migraine. This can reduce the duration and intensity of the MM. Cyclic prophylactic treatment with triptans is more effective in women with regular and predictable menses. Women with irregular cycles may have to use daily prophylactic treatment.

The relationship between calcitonin gene-related peptide (CGRP) and migraine has long been investigated. CGRP does not trigger migraine, but levels of the peptide increase during migraine attacks, and CGRP receptor antagonists have been found to treat acute migraine attacks effectively (Edvinsson, Haanes, Warfvinge, & Krause, 2018). In 2018, the U.S. Food and Drug Administration (FDA) approved the use of an injectable CGRP antagonist, erenumb (Aimovig), for treatment of migraine. A number of other drugs that are designed to reduce migraine frequency by blocking the actions of CGRP are in various stages of clinical trials prior to FDA approval.

Migraine and hormonal contraception

Migraine, in general, is associated with increased risk of cardiovascular disease and stroke for both women and men (Sacco, Ornello, Ripa, Pistoia, & Carolei, 2013; Spector et al., 2010). These risks are stronger in migraineurs with aura and higher in women than in men (Adelborg et al., 2018; Kurth et al., 2016). Because of the increased risk of cardiovascular disease and stroke, the World Health Organization (2004), the American College of Obstetricians and Gynecologists (ACOG, 2006), and the European Headache Federation (Sacco, Merki-Feld, Aelig-gidius, Bitzer, & Canonico, 2018) recommend that estrogen-containing medications not be prescribed for women with migraine with aura. A review of research on the use of estrogen-containing contraceptives by women with migraine concluded that the increase in stroke risk associated with migraine and the risk associated with estrogen-containing contraceptives are additive. The increased risk is clear with higher estrogen contraceptives (50 µg or more), but the data are less clear when contraceptives with lower doses of estrogen are involved (35 µg or less). But the overall stroke risk, although higher than that of women without migraine and women not using estrogen-containing contraceptives, remains low even when both factors are present (Sheikh, Pavlovic, Loder, & Burch, 2018). All sources agree that the quality of available data on the additivity of stroke risk of migraine and estrogen consumption is poor and that better studies are required.

Progestin-only contraceptives, including pills, subdermal implants, depot injections, and progestin-releasing IUDs, do not add to the cardiovascular risk of migraine and should be considered preferred contraceptive options (Brant, Ye, Teng, & Lotke, 2017). Progestin-only pills that contain 75 mcg/day desogestrel (a formulation not often used in the U.S.) have been shown to decrease the duration of menstrual migraines (Merki-Feld, Imthurn, Langner, Seifert, & Gantenbein, 2015; Nappi et al., 2011; Warhurst et al., 2018). One relatively small study suggested that progestin-only contraceptives that result in amenorrhea, including the progestin IUD, may reduce menstrual migraine incidence (Vetvik, MacGregor, Lundqvist, & Russell, 2014).

Menopausal hormone therapy (HT) and migraine

The effect of HT on the migraine experience of postmenopausal women is complex, and data are far from conclusive. A survey of experiences of members of the Migraine Action Association (a lay organization) showed that women using transdermal estrogen and oral progestogen (n=26) were more likely to report an improvement of headache symptoms than were women using oral estrogen and oral progestogen (n=52) (MacGregor, 1999). A larger study that used data from the Women's Health Study (17,107 postmenopausal women who either had never used or were current users of estrogen or HT) showed that current use of HT was associated with an increased risk of migraine (odds ratio 1.42, 95% confidence interval 1.24–1.62) compared with the never-used condition (Misakian et al., 2003). These data are particularly frustrating given the fact that women undergoing surgical menopause are more likely to be prescribed HT to reduce risks associated with early menopause and are also more likely to experience an increase in migraine symptomatology postmenopause.

Quality of life

Migraines can have serious deleterious effects on women's lives. Italian researchers used the Migraine Disability Assessment questionnaire (MIDAS) to determine the effects of pure MMs and menstrual-related migraines on the lives of 91 migraine sufferers and 83 controls (Nicodemo et al., 2008). Over one half of the migraineurs reported severe disability related to migraines, and approximately one quarter reported minimal or mild interference. Migraineurs reported missing approximately 6.5 days per month from household work and family/leisure activities. Absence from work/school was reported much less often (~2 days per month), although work/school performance may be limited for more days per month. Migraineurs also reported significantly lower physical functioning, general health, vitality, and social functioning than did controls, but migraineurs did not differ from controls in role limitations due to mental or emotional health problems (Nicodemo et al., 2008). Swedish women interviewed about their experience of living with migraine reported that they felt impelled to work during migraine attacks and feared that friends and co-workers would judge them as weak and/or lazy if they withdrew from activities during migraine attacks (Rutberg & Öhrling, 2012). Pavlovic and colleagues (2015) reported that women whose migraines were always or most associated with menstruation reported their headaches to be more severe than did women whose migraines were unrelated to menses. Menstrual migraines were found to have a greater impact on work, school, and household roles than migraines that occurred at other times in the menstrual cycle.

Conclusions

Polycystic ovary syndrome, dysmenorrhea, and menstrual migraine are costly medical conditions that can have serious deleterious effects on women's lives. Women who experience these conditions often find it difficult to get a definitive diagnosis or may not even seek medical assistance as the symptoms, though debilitating, are often viewed as "just a woman's lot in life." Practitioners may downplay the seriousness of the complaints or ignore aspects of the condition that are critically important to patients. Although there are very solid bodies of research addressing these conditions, there is a lot more that needs to be understood. There is also a need for further research outside of the context of developed Western countries, as cultural constructions of menstruation may impact upon women's experience of menstrual disorders. Equally, little attention has been paid to the ways in which the culturally determined gender roles of women interplay with the etiology of the conditions, with the willingness or ability of women to seek help, and with the response of medical professionals when women do seek help. Separation of the impact of gender role from the biological state of being female is not possible given the current state of research. All studies we reviewed appeared to assume that all study participants were cisgender individuals with both biological structures and hormones typically identified as female and gender identities as women. Future work needs to parse out the effects of female physiology from feminine gender roles and identity. Studies of female-bodied individuals who do not perform culturally and socially mandated gender scripts could broaden and finesse our understandings of the causes and consequences of these disorders. Transmen whose bodies have female physiology and anatomy but who do not have the feminine gender role may experience these conditions differently than cisgender women. Menstruating transmen face the increased pressure to keep their condition private in public places (Chrisler et al., 2016) and may face even more difficulty in seeking help for dysmenorrhea or menstrual migraine. Their concerns about the symptoms related to masculinizing symptoms of PCOS are likely to be different than those of cisgender women, but their concerns about metabolic and/or weight effects might be similar. Some, but not all, transgender individuals seek hormone treatments so that their bodies reflect their gender identity. Research on the incidence and consequences of endocrine-related conditions such as those discussed in this chapter can be fruitfully studied in biologically transitioning individuals.

References

ACOG Committee on Practice Bulletins – Gynecology (2006). The use of hormonal contraception in women with coexisting medical conditions. *Obstetrics and Gynecology, 107*, 1453–1472.

Adelborg, K., Szepligeti, S. K., Holland-Bill, L., Ehrenstein, V., Horvath-Puho, E., Henderson, V. W., & Sorensen, H. T. (2018). Migraine and risk of cardiovascular diseases: Danish population based matched cohort study. *British Medical Journal, 360*:k96.

Allais, G., Chiarle, G., Sinigaglia, S., & Benedetto, C. (2018). Menstrual migraine: A review of current and developing pharmacotherapies for women. *Expert Opinion on Pharmacotherapy, 19*(2), 123–136.

Allais, G., Rolando, S., De Lorenzo, C., Manzoni, G. C., Messina, P., Benedetto, C., & Bussone, G. (2013). Migraine and pregnancy: An internet survey. *Neurological Sciences, 34*(1), S93–S99.

Avis, N. E., Ory, M., Matthews, K. A., Shocken, M., Bromberger, J., & Colvin, A. (2003). Health-related quality of life in a multiethnic sample of middle-aged women: Study of Women's Health Across the Nation (SWAN). *Medical Care, 41*, 1262–1276.

Azziz, R., Carmina, E., ZiJang, C., Dunall, A., Laven, J. S. E., Legro, R. S., Lizneval, D., Natterson-Horowtiz, B., Teede, H. J., & Yildiz, B. O. (2016). Polycyst ovary syndrome. *Nature Reviews: Disease Primers, 2*, 16057.

Bajalan, Z., Moafi, F., Maradi-Baglooei, M., & Alimoradi, Z. (2019). Mental health and primary dysmenorrhea: A systematic review. *Journal of Psychosomatic Obstetrics and Gynaecology, 40*(3), 185–194.

Barnard, K., Frayne, S. M., Skinner, K. M., & Sullivan, L. M. (2003). Health status among women with menstrual symptoms. *Journal of Women's Health, 12*, 911–919.

Barnard, L., Ferriday, D., Guenther, N., Strauss, B., Balen, A. H., & Dye, L. (2007). Quality of life and psychological wellbeing in polycystic ovary syndrome. *Human Reproduction, 22*, 2279–2286.

Barthelmess, E. K. & Naz, R. K. (2015). Polycystic ovary syndrome: Current status and future perspective. *Frontiers in Bioscience, 6*, 104–119.

Beal, S. J., Dorn, L. D., Sucharew, H. J., Sontag-Padilla, L., Pabst, S., & Hillman, J. (2014). Characterizing the longitudinal relations between depressive and menstrual symptoms in adolescent girls. *Psychosomatic Medicine, 76*, 547–554.

Benham, J. L., Yamamoto, J. M., Friedenreich, C. M., Rabi, D. M., & Sigal, R. J. (2018). Role of exercise training in polycystic ovary syndrome: A systematic review and meta-analysis. *Clinical Obesity, 8*(4), 275–285.

Berkley, K. J. (2013). Primary dysmenorrhea: An urgent mandate. *Pain, 21*(3), 1–8.

Black, M. C., Basile, K. C., Breiding, M. J., Smith, S. G., Walters, M. L., Merrick, M. T., Chen, J., & Stevens, M. R. (2011). *The National Intimate Partner and Sexual Violence Survey (NISVS): 2010 summary report*. Atlanta, GA: National Center for Injury Prevention and Control, Centers for Disease Control and Prevention.

Bozdag, G., Mumusoglu, S., Zengin, D., Karabulut, E., & Yildiz, B. O. (2016). The prevalence and phenotypic features of polycystic ovary syndrome: A systematic review and meta-analysis. *Human Reproduction, 31*(12), 2841–2855.

Brant, A. R., Ye, P. P., Teng, S. J., & Lotke, P. S. (2017). Non-contraceptive benefits of hormonal contraception: Established benefits and new findings. *Current Obstetrics and Gynecology Reports, 6*(2), 109–117.

Brennan, L., Teede, H., Skouteris, H., Linardon, J., Hill, B., & Moran, L. (2017). Lifestyle and behavioral management of polycystic ovary syndrome. *Journal of Women's Health, 36*, 836–848.

Brennenstuhl, S. & Fuller-Thomson, E. (2015). The painful legacy of childhood violence: Migraine headaches among adult survivors of adverse childhood experiences. *Headache, 55*(7), 973–983.

Broner, S. W., Bobker, S., & Klebanoff, L. (2017). Migraine in women. *Seminars in Neurology, 37*, 601–610.

Buse, D. C., Loder, E. W., Gorman, J. A., Stewart, W. F., Reed, M. L., Fanning, K. M., Serrano, D., & Lipton, R. B. (2013). Sex differences in the prevalence, symptoms, and associated features of migraine, probable migraine, and other severe headache: Results of the American Migraine Prevalence and Prevention (AMPP) Study. *Headache, 53*(8), 1278–1299.

Chauvel, V., Multon, S., & Schoenen, J. (2018). Estrogen-dependent effects of 5-hydroxytryptophan on cortical spreading depression in rat: Modelling the serotonin-ovarian hormone interaction in migraine aura. *Cephalalgia, 38*(3), 427–436.

Chen, C. X., Kwekkeboom, K. L., & Ward, S. E. (2016). Beliefs about dysmenorrhea and their relationship to self-management. *Research in Nursing and Health, 39*, 263–276.

Chen, C. X., Ofner, S., Bakoyannis, G., Kwekkeboom, K. L., & Carpenter, J. S. (2017). Symptoms-based phenotypes among women with dysmenorrhea: A latent class analysis. *Western Journal of Nursing Research, 40*, 1–17.

Chen, C. X., Shieh, C., Draucker, C. B., & Carpenter, J. S. (2018). Reasons women do not seek health care for dysmenorrhea. *Journal of Clinical Nursing, 27*, e301–e308.

Chrisler, J. C., Gorman, J. A., Manion, J., Barney, A., Murgo, M., Adams-Clark, A., Newton, J., & McGrath, M. (2016). Queer periods: Experiences with menstruation in the masculine of center and transgender community. *Culture, Health, and Sexuality, 18*, 1238–1250.

Dawood, M. Y. (2006). Primary dysmenorrhea: Advances in pathogenesis and management. *Obstetrics and Gynecology, 108*, 428–441.

de Tommaso, M. (2011). Pain perception during menstrual cycle. *Current Pain and Headache Reports, 15*(5), 400–406.

de Tommaso, M., Valeriani, M., Sardaro, M., Serpino, C., Di Fruscolo, O., Vecchio, E., Cerbo, R., & Livrea, P. (2009). Pain perception and laser evoked potentials during menstrual cycle in migraine. *Journal of Headache and Pain, 10*(6), 423–429.

Ding, T., Hardiman, P. J., Petersen, I., Wang, F. F., Qu, F., & Baio, G. (2017). The prevalence of polycystic ovary syndrome in reproductive-aged women of different ethnicity: A systematic review and meta-analysis. *Oncotarget, 8*(56), 96351–96358.

Dorn, L. D., Negriff, S., Huang, B., Pabst, S., Hillman, J., Braverman, P., & Susman, E. J. (2009). Menstrual symptoms in adolescent girls: Association with smoking, depressive symptoms, and anxiety. *Journal of Adolescent Health, 44*, 237–243.

Dunaif, A. (2012). Genes, aging, and sleep apnea in polycystic ovary syndrome. *Nature Reviews/Endocrinology, 8*, 72–74.

Dunaif, A. & Fauser, B. C. J. M. (2013). Renaming PCOS: A two-state solution. *Journal of Clinical Endocrinology and Metabolism, 98*(11), 4325–4328.

Edvinsson, L., Haanes, K. A., Warfvinge, K., & Krause, D. N. (2018). CGRP as the target of new migraine therapies: Successful translation from bench to clinic. *Nature Reviews Neurology, 14*(6), 338–350.

Eikermann-Haerter, K., Baum, M. J., Ferrari, M. D., van den Maagdenberg, A., Moskowitz, M. A., & Ayata, C. (2009a). Androgenic suppression of spreading depression in familial hemiplegic migraine type-1 mutant mice. *Annals of Neurology, 66*(4), 564–568.

Eikermann-Haerter, K., Dilekoz, E., Kudo, C., Savitz, S. I., Waeber, C., Baum, M. J., Ferrari, M. D., van den Maagdenberg, A. M., Moskowitz, M. A., & Ayata, C. (2009b). Genetic and hormonal factors modulate spreading depression and transient hemiparesis in mouse models of familial hemiplegic migraine type 1. *Journal of Clinical Investigation, 119*(1), 99–109.

Ekback, M., Wijma, K., & Benzein, E. (2009). "It is always on my mind": Women's experiences of their bodies when living with hirsutism. *Health Care for Women International, 30,* 358–372.

Escobar-Morreale, H. F. (2018). Polycystic ovary syndrome: Definition, aetiology, diagnosis, and treatment. *Nature Reviews: Endocrinology, 14,* 270–284.

Evans, R. W., Lipton, R. B., & Silberstein, S. D. (2003). The prevalence of migraine in neurologists. *Neurology, 61*(9), 1271–1272.

Ferrero, S., Pretta, S., Bertoldi, S., Anserini, P., Remorgida, V., Del Sette, M., Gandolfo, C., & Ragni, N. (2004). Increased frequency of migraine among women with endometriosis. *Human Reproduction, 19*(12), 2927–2932.

Giamberardino, M. A., Constantini, R., Affaitati, G., Fabrizio, A., Lapenna, D., Tafuri, E., & Mezzetti, A. (2010). Viscero-visceral hyperalgesia: Characterization in different clinical models. *Pain, 15,* 307–322.

Gibson-Helm, M., Teede, H., Dunaif, A., & Dokras, A. (2017). Delayed diagnosis and a lack of information associated with dissatisfaction in women with polycystic ovary syndrome. *Journal of Clinical Endocrinology and Metabolism, 102,* 604–610.

Glintborg, D., Rubin, K. H., Nubo, M., Abrahamsen, B., & Andersen, M. (2018). Cardiovascular disease in a nationwide population of Danish women with polycystic ovary syndrome. *Cardiovascular Diabetology, 17,* 37.

Glintborg, D., Rubin, K. H., Nybo, M., Abranhamsen, B., & Andersen, M. (2015). Morbidity and medicine prescriptions in a nationwide Danish population of patients diagnosed with polycystic ovary syndrome. *European Journal of Endocrinology, 172,* 627–638.

Gower, B. A. & Goss, A. M. (2015). A lower-carbohydrate, higher-fat diet reduces abdominal and intermuscular fat and increases insulin sensitivity in adults at risk of type 2 diabetes. *Journal of Nutrition, 145,* 177S–183S.

Gunning, M. N. & Fauser, B. C. J. M. (2017). Are women with polycystic ovary syndrome at increased cardiovascular disease risk later in life?. *Climacteric, 20*(3), 222–227.

Guven, B., Guven, H., & Comoglu, S. (2017). Clinical characteristics of menstrually related and non-menstrual migraine. *Acta Neurologica Belgica, 117*(3), 671–676.

Headache Classification Committee of the International Headache Society (2018). The international classification of headache disorders. *Cephalalgia* (3rd ed.), *38,* 1–211.

Hu, Y., Guan, X. F., Fan, L., & Jin, L. J. (2013). Triptans in prevention of menstrual migraine: A systematic review with meta-analysis. *Journal of Headache and Pain, 14,* 7.

Iacovides, S., Avidon, I., & Baker, F. C. (2015). What we know about primary dysmenorrhea today: A critical review. *Human Reproduction Update, 31,* 762–778.

Ju, H., Jones, M., & Mishra, G. (2014b). The prevalence and risk factors of dysmenorrhea. *Epidemiologic Reviews, 36,* 104–113.

Ju, H., Jones, M., & Mishra, G. D. (2014a). Premenstrual syndrome and dysmenorrhea: Symptom trajectories over 13 years in young adults. *Maturitas, 78,* 99–105.

Karjula, S., Papunen, L. M., Auvinen, J., Ruokonen, A., Puukka, K., Franks, S., Jarvelin, M. R., Tapanainen, J. S., Jokelainen, J., Miettunen, J., & Piltonen, T. T. (2017). Psychological distress is more prevalent in fertile age and premenopausal women with PCOS symptoms: 15 year follow up. *Journal of Clinical Endocrinology and Metabolism, 102,* 1861–1869.

Kitzinger, C. & Willmott, J. (2002). "The thief of womanhood": Women's experience of polycystic ovarian syndrome. *Social Science and Medicine, 54,* 349–361.

Kurth, T., Winter, A. C., Eliassen, A. H., Dushkes, R., Mukamal, K. J., Rimm, E. B., Willett, W. C., Manson, J. E., & Rexrode, K. M. (2016). Migraine and risk of cardiovascular disease in women: Prospective cohort study. *British Medical Journal, 353*, 12610.

Kvisvik, E. V., Stovner, L. J., Helde, G., Bovim, G., & Linde, M. (2011). Headache and migraine during pregnancy and puerperium: The MIGRA-study. *Journal of Headache and Pain, 12*(4), 443–451.

Lev-Wiesel, R. & First, M. (2018). Willingness to disclose child maltreatment: CSA vs other forms of child abuse in relation to gender. *Child Abuse & Neglect, 79*, 183–191.

Lipton, R. B., Stewart, W. F., Diamond, S., Diamond, M. L., & Reed, M. (2001). Prevalence and burden of migraine in the United States: Data from the American Migraine Study II. *Headache, 41*(7), 646–657.

MacGregor, A. (1999). Effects of oral and transdermal estrogen replacement on migraine. *Cephalalgia, 19*(2), 124–125.

MacGregor, E. A., Frith, A., Ellis, J., Aspinall, L., & Hackshaw, A. (2006). Incidence of migraine relative to menstrual cycle phases of rising and falling estrogen. *Neurology, 67*(12), 2154–2158.

MacGregor, E. A. & Hackshaw, A. (2004). Prevalence of migraine on each day of the natural menstrual cycle. *Neurology, 63*(2), 351–353.

MacGregor, E. A., Victor, T. W., Hu, X. J., Xiang, Q. F., Puenpatom, R. A., Chen, W., & Campbell, J. C. (2010). Characteristics of menstrual vs nonmenstrual migraine: A post hoc, within-woman analysis of the usual-care phase of a nonrandomized menstrual migraine clinical trial. *Headache, 50*(4), 528–538.

Maleki, N., Field, A., & Kurth, T. (2016). Earlier age at menarche predicts increased risk of developing migraine, but not non-migraine headaches. *Headache, 56*, 4.

Maleki, N., Kurth, T., & Field, A. E. (2017). Age at menarche and risk of developing migraine or non-migraine headaches by young adulthood: A prospective cohort study. *Cephalalgia, 37*(13), 1257–1263.

Maleki, N., Linnman, C., Brawn, J., Burstein, R., Becerra, L., & Borsook, D. (2012). Her versus his migraine: Multiple sex differences in brain function and structure. *Brain, 135*, 2546–2559.

Mannix, L. K. (2008). Menstrual-related pain conditions: Dysmenorrhea and migraine. *Journal of Women's Health, 17*(5), 879–891.

March, W. A., Moore, V. M., Willson, K. J., Phillips, D. I. W., Norman, R. J., & Davies, M. J. (2010). The prevalence of polycystic ovary syndrome in a community sample assessed under contrasting diagnostic criteria. *Human Reproduction, 25*(2), 544–551.

Marjoribanks, J., Ayeleke, R. O., Farquhar, C., & Proctor, M. (2015). Nonsteroidal anti-inflammatory drugs for dysmenorrhea. *Cochrane Database*, CD001751.

Markopoulos, M. C., Rizos, D., Valsamakis, G., Deligeoroglou, E., Grigoriou, O., Chrousos, G. P., Creatsas, G., & Mastorakos, G. (2011). Hyperadrogenism in women with polycystic ovary syndrome persists after menopause. *Journal of Clinical Endocrinology and Metabolism, 96*, 623–631.

Martin, M. L., Halling, K., Eek, D., Krohe, M., & Paty, J. (2017). Understanding polycystic ovary syndrome from the patient perspective: A concept elicitation patient interview study. *Health and Quality of Life Outcomes, 15*, 162.

Matthewman, G., Lee, A., Kaur, J. G., & Daley, A. J. (2018). Physical activity for primary dysmenorrhea: A systematic review and meta-analysis of randomized controlled trials. *American Journal of Obstetrics and Gynecology, 219*(3), 255.

Mattsson, P. (2003). Hormonal factors in migraine: A population-based study of women aged 40 to 74 years. *Headache, 43*(1), 27–35.

McCook, J. D., Reame, N. E., & Thatcher, S. S. (2005). Health-related quality of life issues in women with polycystic ovary syndrome. *Journal of Obstetric, Gynecologic, and Neonatal Nursing, 34*, 12–20.

Merki-Feld, G. S., Imthurn, B., Langner, R., Seifert, B., & Gantenbein, A. R. (2015). Positive effects of the progestin desogestrel 75 mu g on migraine frequency and use of acute medication are sustained over a treatment period of 180 days. *Journal of Headache and Pain, 16*, 39.

Merz, C. N. B., Shaw, L. J., Azziz, R., Stanczyk, F. Z., Sopko, G., Raunstein, G. D., Kelsey, S. F., Kip, K. E., Cooper-Dehoff, R. M., Johnson, B. D., Vaccarino, V., Reis, S. E., Hodgson, T. K., Rogers, W., & Pepine, C. J. (2016). Cardiovascular disease and 10-year mortality in postmenopausal women with clinical features of polycystic ovary syndrome. *Journal of Women's Health, 25*(9), 875–881.

Minooee, S., Tehrani, F. T., Rahmati, M., Mansournia, M. A., & Azizi, F. (2018). Prediction of age at menopause in women with polycystic ovary syndrome. *Climacteric, 21*, 29–34.

Misakian, A. L., Langer, R. D., Bensenor, I. M., Cook, N. R., Manson, J. E., Buring, J. E., & Rexrode, K. M. (2003). Postmenopausal hormone therapy and migraine headache. *Journal of Women's Health, 12*(10), 1027–1036.

Moran, L. J., Ko, H., Misso, M., Marsh, K., Noakes, M., Talbot, M., Frearson, M., Thondan, M., Stepto, N., & Teede, H. J. (2013). Dietary composition in the treatment of polycystic ovary syndrome: A systematic review to inform evidence-based guidelines. *Journal of the Academy of Nutrition and Dietetics, 113*, 520–545.

Nappi, R. E., Sances, G., Allais, G., Terreno, E., Benedetto, C., Vaccaro, V., Polatti, F., & Facchinetti, F. (2011). Effects of an estrogen-free, desogestrel-containing oral contraceptive in women with migraine with aura: A prospective diary-based pilot study. *Contraception, 83*(3), 223–228.

Neri, I., Granella, F., Nappi, R., Manzoni, G. C., Facchinetti, F., & Genazzani, A. R. (1993). Characteristics of headache at menopause: A clinico-epidemiologic study. *Maturitas, 17*(1), 31–37.

Nicodemo, M., Vignatelli, L., Grimaldi, D., Sancisi, E., Fares, J. E., Zanigni, S., Pierangeli, G., Cortelli, P., Montagna, P., & Cevoli, S. (2008). Quality of life, eating, and mood disorders in menstrual migraine: A case-control study. *Neurological Sciences, 29*, S155–S157.

Paoli, A., Rubini, A., Volek, J. S., & Grimaldi, K. A. (2013). Beyond weight loss: A review of the therapeutic uses of very-low carbohydrate (ketogenic) diets. *European Journal of Clinical Nutrition, 67*, 789–796.

Pasquali, R. (2018). Contemporary approaches to the management of polycystic ovary syndrome. *Therapeutic Advances in Endocrinology and Metabolism, 9*(4), 123–136.

Pasquali, R. & Gambineri, A. (2018). New perspectives on the definition and management of polycystic ovary syndrome. *Journal of Endocrinological Investigation, 41*(10), 1123–1135.

Pavlovic, J. M., Akcali, D., Bolay, H., Bernstein, C., & Maleki, N. (2017). Sex-related influences in migraine. *Journal of Neuroscience Research, 95*(1–2), 587–593.

Pavlovic, J. M., Allshouse, A. A., Santoro, N. F., Crawford, S. L., Thurston, R. C., Neal-Perry, G. S., Lipton, R. B., & Derby, C. A. (2016). Sex hormones in women with and without migraine: Evidence of migraine-specific hormone profiles. *Neurology, 87*(1), 49–56.

Pavlovic, J. M., Stewart, W. F., Bruce, C. A., Gorman, J. A., Sun, H., Buse, D. C., & Lipton, R. B. (2015). Burden of migraine related to menses: Results from the AMPP study. *Journal of Headache and Pain, 16*, 24.

Petrovski, B. E., Vetvik, K. G., Lundqvist, C., & Eberhard-Gran, M. (2018). Characteristics of menstrual versus non-menstrual migraine during pregnancy: A longitudinal population-based study. *Journal of Headache and Pain, 19*, 27.

Pfister, G. & Rømer, K. (2017). "It's not very feminine to have a mustache": Experiences of Danish women with polycystic ovary syndrome. *Health Care for Women International, 38*(2), 167–186.

Polotsky, A. J., Allshouse, A. A., Crawford, S. L., Harlow, S. D., Khalil, N., Kazlauskaite, R., Santoro, N., & Legro, R. S. (2014). Hyperandrogenic oligomenorrhea and metabolic risks across menopausal transition. *Journal of Clinical Endocrinology and Metabolism, 99*(6), 2120–2127.

Proctor, M. L., Hing, W., Johnson, T. C., & Murphy, P. A. (2006). Spinal manipulation for primary and secondary dysmenorrhea. *Cochrane Database Systematic Reviews*, CD002119.

Proctor, M. L., Latthe, P. M., Farquhar, C. M., Khan, K. S., & Johnson, N. P. (2005). Surgical interruption of pelvic nerve pathways for primary and secondary dysmenorrhea. *Cochrane Database Systematic Reviews*, CD001896.

Proctor, M. L. & Murphy, P. A. (2001). Herbal and dietary therapies for primary and secondary dysmenorrhea. *Cochrane Database Systematic Reviews, 3*, CD002124.

Proctor, M. L., Murphy, P. A., Pattison, H. M., Suckling, J., & Farquhar, C. M. (2007). Behavioral interventions for primary and secondary dysmenorrhea. *Cochrane Database Systematic Reviews*, CD002248.

Proctor, M. L., Smith, C. A., Farquhar, C. M., & Stones, R. W. (2002). Transcutaneous electrical nerve stimulation and acupuncture for primary dysmenorrhea. *Cochrane Database Systematic Reviews*, CD002123.

Ripa, P., Ornello, R., Degan, D., Tiseo, C., Stewart, J., Pistoia, F., Carolea, A., & Sacco, S. (2015). Migraine in menopausal women: A systematic review. *International Journal of Women's Health, 7*, 773–782.

Rutberg, S. & Öhrling, K. (2012). Migraine – more than a headache: Women's experiences of living with migraine. *Disability and Rehabilitation, 34*(4), 329–336.

Rzonca, E., Bien, A., Wdowiak, A., Szymanski, R., & Iwanowicz-Palus, G. (2018). Determinants of quality of life and satisfaction with life in women with polycystic ovary syndrome. *International Journal of Environmental Research and Public Health, 15*, 376.

Sacco, S., Merki-Feld, G. S., Aelig-gidius, K. L., Bitzer, J., Canonico, M., Kurth, T., Lampi, B., Lidegaard, O., MacGregor, E. A., MassenVanDenBrink, A., Mitsikostas, D.-D., Nappi, R. E., Ntaios, G., Sandset, P. M., Martelletti, P., & European Society for Contraception and Reproductive Health (2018). Hormonal contraceptives and risk of ischemic stroke in women with migraine: A consensus statement from the European Headache Federation (EHF) and the European Society of Contraception and Reproductive Health (ESC). *Journal of Headache and Pain, 18*(No. 108).

Sacco, S., Ornello, R., Ripa, P., Pistoia, F., & Carolei, A. (2013). Migraine and hemorrhagic stroke a meta-analysis. *Stroke, 44*(11), 3032–3038.

Schmidt, J., Brannstrom, M., Landin-Wilhelmsen, K., & Dahlgren, E. (2011). Reproductive hormone levels and anthropometry in postmenopausal women with polycystic ovary syndrome (PCOS): A 21 year follow-up study of women diagnosed with PCOS around 50 years ago and their age-matched controls. *Journal of Clinical Endocrinology and Metabolism, 96*, 2178–2185.

Schroeder, R. A., Brandes, J., Buse, D. C., Calhoun, A., Eikermann-Haerter, K., Golden, K., & Nebel, R. A. (2018). Sex and gender differences in migraine: Evaluating knowledge gaps. *Journal of Women's Health, 27*(8), 965–973.

Setji, T. L. & Brown, A. J. (2014). Polycystic ovary syndrome: Update on diagnosis and treatment. *American Journal of Medicine, 127*, 912–919.

Sheikh, H. U., Pavlovic, J., Loder, E., & Burch, R. (2018). Risk of stroke associated with use of estrogen containing contraceptives in women with migraine: A systematic review. *Headache, 58*(1), 5–21.

Silberstein, S. D. & Merriam, G. R. (1993). Sex-hormones and headache. *Journal of Pain and Symptom Management, 8*(2), 98–114.

Smith, C. A., Armour, M., Zhu, X., Li, X., Lu, Z. Y., & Song, J. (2016). Acupuncture for dysmenorrhea. *Cochrane Database Systematic Reviews*, CD007854.

Snyder, B. S. (2006). The lived experience of women diagnosed with polycystic ovary syndrome. *Journal of Obstetric, Gynecologic & Neonatal Nursing, 35*, 385–392.

Somerville, B. W. (1972). Influence of progesterone and estradiol upon migraine. *Headache, 12*(3), 93–133.

Spector, J. T., Kahn, S. R., Jones, M. R., Jayakumar, M., Dalal, D., & Nazarian, S. (2010). Migraine headache and ischemic stroke risk: An updated meta-analysis. *American Journal of Medicine, 123*(7), 612–624.

Stewart, W. F., Lipton, R. B., Celentano, D. D., & Reed, M. L. (1992). Prevalence of migraine headache in the United States: Relation to age, income, race, and other sociodemographic factors. *Journal of the American Medical Association, 267*(1), 64–69.

Stovner, L. J., Hagen, K., Jensen, R., Katsarava, Z., Lipton, R. B., Scher, A. I., Steiner, T. J., & Zwart, J. A. (2007). The global burden of headache: A documentation of headache prevalence and disability worldwide. *Cephalalgia, 27*(3), 193–210.

Tasall, E., Chapotot, F., Leproult, R., Whitmore, H., & Ehrmann, D. A. (2011). Treatment of obstructive sleep apnea improves cardiometabolic function in young obese women with polycystic ovary syndrome. *Journal of Clinical Endocrinology and Metabolism, 96*, 365–374.

Tietjen, G. E., Buse, D. C., Fanning, K. M., Serrano, D., Reed, M. L., & Lipton, R. B. (2015). Recalled maltreatment, migraine, and tension-type headache results of the AMPP Study. *Neurology, 84*(2), 132–140.

Tietjen, G. E., Bushnell, C. D., Herial, N. A., Utley, C., White, L., & Hafeez, F. (2007). Endometriosis is associated with prevalence of comorbid conditions in migraine. *Headache, 47*(7), 1069–1078.

Tietjen, G. E., Conway, A., Utley, C., Gunning, W. T., & Herial, N. A. (2006). Migraine is associated with menorrhagia and endometriosis. *Headache, 46*(3), 422–428.

Tomlinson, J., Pinkney, J., Adams, L., Stenhouse, E., Bendall, A., Corrigan, O., & Letherby, G. (2017). The diagnosis and lived experience of polycystic ovary syndrome: A qualitative study. *Journal of Advanced Nursing, 73*(10), 1–24.

Unsal, A., Ayranci, U., Tozun, M., Arslan, G., & Calik, E. (2010). Prevalence of dysmenorrhea and its effect on quality of life among a group of female university students. *Upsala Journal of Medical Sciences, 115*, 138–145.

Van den Maagdenberg, A. (2016). Migraine genetics: New opportunities, new challenges. *Cephalalgia, 36*, 601–603.

Varlibas, A. & Erdemoglu, A. K. (2009). Altered trigeminal system excitability in menstrual migraine patients. *Journal of Headache and Pain, 10*(4), 277–282.

Vetvik, K. G., MacGregor, E. A., Lundqvist, C., & Russell, M. B. (2014). Contraceptive-induced amenorrhoea leads to reduced migraine frequency in women with menstrual migraine without aura. *Journal of Headache and Pain, 15*, 1–5.

Wang, I., Wang, X., Wang, W., Chen, C., Ronnennberg, A. G., Guang, W., Huang, A., Fang, Z., Zang, T., Wang, L., & Xu, X. (2004). Stress and dysmenorrhea: A population based prospective study. *Occupational and Environmental Medicine, 61*, 1021–1026.

Wang, S. J., Fuh, J. L., Lu, S. R., Juang, K. D., & Wang, P. H. (2003). Migraine prevalence during menopausal transition. *Headache, 43*(5), 470–478.

Warhurst, S., Rofe, C. J., Brew, B. J., Bateson, D., McGeechan, K., Merki-Feld, G. S., Garrick, R., & Tomlinson, S. E. (2018). Effectiveness of the progestin-only pill for migraine treatment in women: A systematic review and meta-analysis. *Cephalalgia, 38*(4), 754–764.

Westling, A. M., Tu, F. F., Griffith, J. W., & Hellman, K. M. (2013). The association of dysmenorrhea with noncyclic pelvic pain accounting for psychological factors. *American Journal of Obstetrics and Gynecology, 209*, 422e1–422e10.

Wong, C. L., Farquhar, C., Roberts, H., & Proctor, M. (2009). Oral contraceptive pill for primary dysmenorrhea. *Cochrane Database Systematic Review*, CD002120.

Woolf, C. J. (2016). Central sensitization: Implications for the diagnosis and treatment of pain. *Pain, 152*, S2–15.

World Health Organization (2004). *Medical eligibility criteria for contraceptive use.* (2nd ed.). Geneva: World Health Organization.

World Health Organization (2011). *Atlas of headache disorders and resources in the world 2011.* Geneva: World Health Organization, www.who.int/iris/handle/10665/44571.

World Health Organization (2013). *Global and regional estimates of violence against women: Prevalence and health effects of intimate partner violence and non-partner sexual violence.* Geneva: World Health Organization, www.who.int/reproductivehealth/publications/violence/9789241564625/en.

Zhu, X., Proctor, M., Bensoussan, A., Wu, E., & Smith, C. A. (2008). Chinese herbal medicine for primary dysmenorrhea. *Cochrane Database Systematic Reviews*, CD005288.

8

WOMEN'S EXPERIENCE OF ENDOMETRIOSIS

Elaine Denny and Annalise Weckesser

Endometriosis is usually thought of as a gynaecological condition caused by endometrial-like tissue found outside of the uterus, where it produces an inflammatory response influenced by hormonal fluctuations. It is generally found in women of reproductive age and is characterised by chronic pelvic pain (CPP) often around the time of menstruation, deep dyspareunia (pain on sexual intercourse), and dysmenorrhoea (pain associated with menstrual bleeding) (De Nardi & Ferrrari, 2011). However, some women with severe endometriosis experience no symptoms, and its existence is often only discovered opportunistically, for example during investigation or treatment for other conditions. As severity of symptoms do not always correlate with extent of endometrial plaques and as the aetiology is uncertain, endometriosis has been called an 'enigmatic disease' (Valle & Sciarra, 2003). Its definition is contested. Due to the fact that some women have a family history or may also suffer from autoimmune diseases, and because endometriosis has been associated with exposure to toxins such as dioxin, it is now sometimes classified within biomedicine as an autoimmune, environmental, hormonal, or genetic disorder (Seear, 2014). There is no definitive treatment, so interventions are focussed towards alleviation of symptoms, although any relief is often temporary, and many women will endure multiple courses of treatment over many years.

The prevalence rate in the general population is unknown because of a well-documented delay in diagnosis (Abbas, Ihle, Köster, & Schubert, 2012; Ballard, Lawton, & Wright, 2006); estimates vary between 2 and 15% of women of reproductive age and between 30 and 50% of women reporting the symptoms listed above. Delays in diagnosis of many years are common, and, although some studies define 'delay' as from first symptoms to diagnosis, whereas in others it is from first seeking health care to diagnosis, all agree that many women suffer long periods of pain before the cause is discovered. These discrepancies in reported incidence may be explained by participants recruited from high-risk populations; a recent population-based study of unselected low-risk women yielded a population incidence of around 1% in the general female population aged between 15 and 55 years (Goodman & Franasiak, 2018). It is also the case that most research into endometriosis has been conducted with White women in Europe, the USA, and Australia and therefore may not adequately reflect the position in other countries.

Endometriosis may impact on all aspects of life. A large ten-country study of women about to undergo laparoscopy for various reasons showed that those who were subsequently diagnosed with endometriosis had lower quality of life scores and lower work productivity than symptomatic women without endometriosis and the control group of women undergoing sterilisation (Nnoaham et al., 2011); the main drivers for the difference were the severity of pelvic pain and the disease itself. A systematic review showed that, despite large national differences, the direct costs (treatment) and indirect costs (unemployment, missed work days) of endometriosis constituted a considerable economic burden (Soliman, Yang, Du, Kelley, & Winkel, 2016).

Unpacking the complexities of endometriosis and demonstrating how they are bound up with a disease that is both contested and gendered will form the purpose of this chapter and help to explain the real life experience of women living with the disease. We begin by exploring endometriosis as a contested disease and the difficulties posed by trying to differentiate 'normal' and 'abnormal' menstruation. We move on to viewing it as gendered and considering how constructions of menstruation, fertility, and womanhood lead to the stigmatisation of those who do not conform to the feminine ideal. These sections provide a lens through which to make sense of the reality of living with endometriosis and the impact it has on lives and relationships.

Endometriosis as a contested condition

A contested disease or condition is one where there is no general consensus about the nature of its cause, its progression and treatment, or indeed whether it exists at all. A number of things may lead to a disease being contested, one of which is debate about where the parameters between 'normal' and 'abnormal' lie. In his work on chronic illness (CI) Bury (1991) argued that symptoms that are widely found throughout the general population are frequently the same presenting symptoms, albeit much more severe in CI, and this makes legitimation problematic. For women with endometriosis this raises two related problems. First, the ubiquitous nature of dysmenorrhoea means that women with endometriosis find that they have their symptoms trivialised and disbelieved by health professionals and by those around them (Ballard et al., 2006; Marcovic, Manderson, & Warren, 2008). Women will often report that they have been told that painful menstruation is part and parcel of the female condition, and, by not managing it as other women do, they are at fault and demonstrate a personal failing. The novelist Hilary Mantel, for example, was told that she must have a low pain threshold when she sought help for painful periods. This will often lead to women doubting their bodily experiences and delaying seeking help for their pain (Marcovic et al., 2008) or struggling to distinguish between 'normal' and 'abnormal' pelvic pain (Toye, Seers, & Barker, 2014). However, Seear (2009a) questioned the idea that somehow defining 'normal' and 'abnormal' menstrual pain will lead to better diagnosis and legitimation as the whole notion of menstrual irregularity is located within a context of shame and stigma. Far from blaming individual women for lack of awareness, the social context in which speaking of menstruation is taboo needs to be addressed in order for more open discussion about women's reproductive health. This will be explored further in the following section. Second, in order to be believed, illness needs to be sanctioned, and in Western industrial societies this responsibility lies with the medical profession, who will often display a scepticism towards menstrual problems and perpetuate myths, such as the notions that pregnancy 'cures' endometriosis and that some women are 'too young' for their pain to be caused by endometriosis (Denny & Mann, 2008).

When women do consult health professionals they may experience further delay to diagnosis by being dismissed as suffering from 'women's problems'. Menstrual problems are of low status within the medical profession, and there is therefore little interest in them. This is common at the primary care level with resistance to referral for specialist assessment, which leaves women with a feeling of being 'fobbed off' or disbelieved (Culley et al., 2013). Misdiagnosis is also common; inflammatory bowel disease (IBD) or inflammatory pelvic disease (IPD) is the most common initial diagnosis (Jones, Jenkinson, & Kennedy, 2004). A diagnosis provides legitimation of illness, allows entry to the sick role, and opens up a pathway to interventions and treatment. However, receiving a diagnosis of endometriosis does not necessarily provide a satisfactory end to a woman's problems. Rhodes and colleagues (2002) have noted the power of the visible in legitimating symptoms. Their research with people with low back pain demonstrated how a visible back lesion seen on an X-ray or scan provided the 'proof' that was needed to gain credibility. Women in particular feel that they need to be seen as credible patients in order to be taken seriously, and they work at presenting themselves to health professionals in a way that maintains their self-esteem and dignity (Werner & Malterud, 2003). Visible 'proof' of endometriosis is achieved via laparoscopy when endometriotic lesions can be visualised and photographed. However, as the extent of disease does not necessarily conform to the severity of symptoms, diagnosis will not always lead to satisfactory treatment. This is partly because of the trial and error nature of treatments for endometriosis and partly because women with few lesions may experience severe pain yet still find themselves disbelieved. The contested nature of endometriosis is characterised by uncertainty at the levels of diagnosis and symptomology, which in turn leads to uncertainty for the future (trajectory uncertainty) (Williams, 2000). As stated above, there is no definitive cure for endometriosis, and treatments depend on the preferred option and the clinical leanings (medicine or surgery) of the specialist. Women will often be prescribed various hormonal medications (with or without a confirmed diagnosis), many of which will affect fertility, albeit temporarily (see below for the impact of this on decision making). When these do not provide a permanent solution, surgery (from lasering of lesions to complete excision) will usually be offered. Radical surgery involves total hysterectomy with or without removal of ovaries. Endometriosis can reoccur despite any of these treatments, so women have to make decisions about accepting non-reversible treatments or enduring unpleasant side effects with the knowledge that they may not see any lasting improvement. However, following interventions, women may be viewed as having used up their share of attention and are expected to show gratitude for the clinician's skill by returning to normal functioning. Failure to do so may result in loss of professional and personal support mechanisms. However, for all of the uncertainty, modern medicine provides a fixed point of reference for dealing with long-term illness (Bury, 1982), and many women will not view their lack of acceptable and effective treatments as a problem of biomedicine, but as the failing of individual doctors (Denny, 2009).

Endometriosis as gendered

Gender, pain, and treatment

Hoffmann and Tarzian (2001) established that, although women and men may experience and respond to pain differently, determining whether such differences are rooted in biology or psychosocial factors is challenging given the complexity and multi-causal nature of pain experiences. Women are more likely than men to seek treatment for chronic pain, however they are also more likely to receive inadequate and poor care, as health care practitioners often initially discount women's verbal accounts of pain (Hoffmann & Tarzian, 2001). Such biases stem from a gendered moral evaluation of pain, in which the 'dominance of a somatic ideology inherent in medicine tends to define emotional expression in experiences of pain as socially undesirable, whereas suppression through stoicism tends to be highly valued' (Bendelow, 2000, p. 40). Whereas men are socialised and perceived to be more stoical when in pain (and thus should be 'believed' when they do seek care for pain), women are perceived to be more likely to report pain experiences as they are thought not to fear appearing vulnerable for doing so; thus the experiences of pain come to be seen as 'natural' for women, but 'abnormal' for men (Bendelow & Williams, 2002). Furthermore, women are believed to have a higher pain threshold and greater ability to cope with pain due to their reproductive capacity and everyday experiences of pain that accompany menstruation and childbirth (Bendelow, 2000; Hoffmann & Tarzian, 2001).

In women's interactions with health care professionals, they are often not asked about the qualitative nature of their pain (Denny, 2004, 2009), and many feel unheard and unseen when health care practitioners focus more narrowly on capturing pain levels through numeric scales or identifying the precise location of pain. Indeed, it is often only when women present with infertility, rather than with chronic pain or other endometriosis symptoms, that they come to receive a diagnosis (Denny, Culley, Papadopoulos, & Apenteng, 2011; Griffith, 2017). This failure to adequately listen to, and take seriously, women's reports of endometriosis-related pain led to the unprecedented step by the National Institute of Health and Care Excellence (NICE) in the UK to issue guidelines to health professionals to 'listen to patients' as an important factor in reducing diagnostic delays (Boseley, 2017). In Australia a National Action Plan for endometriosis has been announced by the Health Minister, who commented that women have suffered in silence for too long (Han, 2018). Such failures are not peculiar to those suffering with endometriosis pain, but rather are part of the wider historical, societal, and cultural context of gendered practices that surround pain and its treatment (Bendelow, 2000; Griffith, 2017).

Gendered biases in treatment are reflected in women's accounts of encounters with health care professionals and the challenges they face as they work towards credibility – and having their experiences of endometriosis-related pain recognised, believed, and ultimately diagnosed (as discussed above). Endometriosis is not only treated in highly gendered ways, but the condition itself is gendered as it concerns problems with women's reproductive health (specifically menstruation, dyspareunia, and infertility). Such problems are compounded by the secrecy and revulsion surrounding female genitalia (Labuski, 2015; Seear, 2009a).

Menstruation and stigma

Communication taboos that surround menstruation also shape these patient–health practitioner encounters. A common explanation for diagnostic delay is that doctors normalise women's menstrual pain and women delay seeking medical advice due to lack of knowledge concerning what constitutes 'normal' versus 'abnormal' menstrual experience. Although these are likely factors in diagnostic delays, women's reluctance to disclose menstrual pain and irregularities is also a factor and possibly a more significant one (Seear, 2009a). Seear (2009a) argued that menstruation is a 'discrediting attribute' (Goffman, 1968) and that speaking about it renders women vulnerable to stigmatisation. However, from a young age women and girls receive mixed messages about menstruation. On the one hand, they learn that it is shameful and embarrassing, and, on the other, that it is a normal and natural event (Britton, 1996; Fahs, 2016).

Women actively hide menstrual irregularities through practices of 'menstrual etiquette' (Laws, 1990), which involve the active concealment of any evidence of menstruation. An Australian study showed that women living with endometriosis anticipated social sanctioning if they disclosed their menstrual problems and felt reprimanded when they did so. For example, they thought that revealing menstrual problems may lead to difficulties with male partners who see such disclosures as 'excuse[s] to get out of duties that they believe women owe them' (Seear, 2009a, p. 1124). Therefore, to guard themselves from gendered ostracisation and stigma, women come to follow practices of concealment and silence around menstruation. Women living with endometriosis also follow these codes of menstrual etiquette in their interactions with health care practitioners (Cox, Henderson, Wood, & Cagliarini, 2003; Griffith, 2017).

'It's a woman's lot to suffer' is a sentiment often expressed regarding women's shared experiences of menstrual pain that reflects gendered stigma related to endometriosis. Statements such as 'because you're a woman you're just meant to put up with it' (Griffith, 2017, p. 50) are common in women's accounts of having their symptoms dismissed not only by medical professionals, but also by their family members and others.

Dyspareunia and stigma

Stigma also impedes open discussions of sex and sexual relationships, which are considered highly intimate and private matters in many cultures. Research with migrant women from various cultures and religions in Australia and Canada showed that shame and secrecy begins at menarche and sets the boundaries for, and mediates, discussion of sexuality and sexual relationships throughout life (Hawkey, Ussher, Perz, & Metusela, 2017). Dyspareunia, or pain during or after sex, is a common and stress-inducing symptom of endometriosis (Butt & Chesla, 2007; De Graaff et al., 2013; Hummelshoj, De Graaff, Dunselman, & Vercellini, 2014). Communication taboos regarding dyspareunia have been found to prevent women from seeking medical advice for such symptoms. Heterosexual women with endometriosis report sometimes having penetrative sex despite the pain and discomfort as they believe they must put their partners' pleasure and sexual needs before their own (Fritzer et al., 2013); they may feign enjoyment to fulfil notions of ideal womanhood (Elmerstig, Wijma, & Bertö, 2008). Hudson et al. (2016) found that gendered expectations about femininity and sex within heterosexual relationships shaped women's accounts of the disruption to their sexual relationships caused by endometriosis. Some women endured dyspareunia because of the desire for a pregnancy, which outweighed bodily discomfort; others compared their sexual relationship and intimacy unfavourably with what they considered 'normal' and assumed other couples had, which caused guilt and a sense of loss.

Infertility and stigma

The impact of endometriosis on fertility is not fully clear, but it has been estimated that nearly one half (47%) of infertile women may have the condition (Meuleman et al., 2009). Although communication taboos around menstruation and dyspareunia (Denny & Mann, 2007; Fritzer et al., 2013; Seear, 2009a) have been discussed within the endometriosis literature, stigma related to childlessness has yet to be considered fully (Griffith, 2017). Similar stigmas operate around their experiences of infertility and voluntary or involuntary childlessness for women with and without endometriosis, as they struggle or fail or refuse to meet normative cultural expectations for women to become (biological) mothers.

Ethnographic research undertaken with British women with endometriosis showed that women discussed both voluntary and involuntary childlessness (Griffith, 2017). Those who chose not to have children said that their biomedical treatment had been primarily based on assumptions that they would one day want (biological) children and on the beliefs of medical professionals that they would eventually change their minds in the future. Women believed their symptoms were taken more seriously by health care professionals when they said that they wanted to get pregnant. In addition, women viewed health care professionals as mistrusting their decision not to have (biological) children, as evidenced by being denied access to surgical treatments that could relieve their endometriosis symptoms but would also result in sterilisation (Griffith, 2017).

Those who experience involuntary childlessness report feelings of loss, grief, distress, and isolation (Culley et al., 2013; Hudson et al., 2016). Women with endometriosis feel unable to talk about their infertility with most people and generally speak only with their partners, mothers, and, to a lesser extent, their extended families (Griffith, 2017). Denny et al. (2011) have shown endometriosis-related infertility to be a particular concern for women from certain minority ethnic communities within the UK, due to cultural expectations and the status of motherhood, together with community and family pressure for married women to produce children. British Asian women in a study of couples living with endometriosis expressed concerns that their marriages would end if they were unable to have children. One woman stated: '[a]mongst Asian couples if you can't have a child, it's almost like you're a waste of space, they don't want to have you as a daughter-in-law or a wife who can't have a baby' (Hudson et al., 2016, p. 727). Infertility caused women to have feelings of guilt, failure, and personal responsibility.

Childlessness (both voluntary and involuntary) represents 'failed femininity' (Gillespie, 2001) in the context of socially constructed and globally hegemonic notions of womanhood. For women who experience infertility but want to give birth to biological children, there is also the association of the 'failed body' (Whitehead, 2014). In biomedical discourse, infertility is framed as disease, something to be diagnosed and treated, and also a source of stigma for women with endometriosis.

Pathologising women with endometriosis

Medical professionals frequently pathologise women with endometriosis, rather than the symptoms from which they suffer. Women report having been called hypochondriacs or psychosomatics, and have described feelings of vindication when endometriosis was finally diagnosed (Denny, 2004). A small, and rare, study of clinicians on their views of women's experiences with endometriosis and their psychosocial care needs indicated that some clinicians believed endometriosis was caused by poor mental health. One gynaecologist stated: 'Do mad people get endo or does endo make you mad? It's probably a bit of both' (Young, Fisher, & Kirkman, 2017, p. 90). Within the medical literature, women with endometriosis have been depicted as nervous, irrational, and/or hypochondriacs (Whelan, 1997, 2003).

Women resist medical professionals' attempts to ascribe psychological labels to them; instead they want their symptoms to receive medical labels so that they can receive medical or surgical treatment (Denny, 2009). Bullo's (2018) linguistic analysis of women's '(dis) empowerment accounts' of endometriosis traced how women were made to feel 'abnormal' when health care practitioners dismissed their symptoms as 'normal to womanhood'. Similarly, Seear (2014) found that women's accounts of endometriosis are dominated by a sense that they are 'inherently dysfunctional, irrational and disordered, ideas closely associated with menstruation and the feminine as monstrous' (p. 170). The construction of the reproductive female body as monstrous centres on the 'ambivalence associated with the power and danger perceived to be inherent in woman's fecund flesh, her seeping, leaking and bleeding womb standing for as a site of pollution and a source of dread' (Ussher, 2006, p. 1). Many endometriosis symptoms elicit notions of the feminine uncontrolled, unbounded (the antithesis of the masculine) body. Thus, a central paradox within the lived experience of women with endometriosis is that they feel they must fix the problematic aspects of their (monstrous) body/self, however by doing so they further reproduce their position as devalued feminine subjects (Seear, 2014).

The experience of endometriosis

Over the years, numerous clinical researchers have studied the efficacy of various medical and surgical treatments for endometriosis, but they have tended to use quantitative methodologies, and although they sometimes included a quality of life index or pain scale, they failed to capture the reality of life for women with the disease. By considering endometriosis as contested and gendered, and by focussing on qualitative studies that give women some control over reporting what is of importance to them, we can gain an insight into how the disease impacts on all aspects of women's lives.

The experience of endometriosis is best understood through the narratives of those women who live with the disease, yet patients' narratives have had an ambiguous status within biomedicine, with subjective stories treated as less reliable than supposedly objective investigations that produce signs of pathology (Hydén, 1997). However, within the social sciences, giving voice to those who too often are not heard is a valued goal.

In interviews women have described the pain of endometriosis as being 'like a knife', 'sharp', 'tearing', and 'breath catching' (see, for example, Moradi, Parker, Sneddon, Lopez, & Ellwood, 2014). Their descriptions centre on the pain's (at times) incapacitating intensity, which women have described as 'horrific', 'stabbing', and overwhelming (Denny, 2004; Huntington & Gilmour, 2005; Jones et al., 2004). Using a pre-operative questionnaire, Ballard, Lane, Hudelist, Banerjee, and Wright (2010) demonstrated that women who were subsequently diagnosed with endometriosis following diagnostic laparoscopy were more likely to report stabbing, gnawing, and dragging pain than were those with other types of pelvic pain or with dyschezia (pain on opening the bowels). Many experience this pain as something that takes over and controls their lives, although others actively resist this.

Frank (1995) delineated between restitution, quest, and chaos in his typology of narrative. Restitution narratives describe moving from health to illness and, after treatment, or just with time, moving back to health. Because of the long term and uncertain nature of endometriosis this is not the reality for many women with the condition, who conform more to quest or chaos narratives at various points in their lives. Quest narratives are prevalent in self-help groups, online communities, and patient charities, where people try to gain insight into their condition, share stories of their lives, and provide mutual support. In a personal narrative Kalia Wright (2019) explained how, after many years of pain, which was trivialised and treated as 'normal' by health care professionals, the word 'endometriosis' was finally mentioned by the fourth gynecologist she consulted. An online search led her to believe that the symptoms exactly matched her own. Armed with information about the timing, length, and quality of her pain, she returned to the gynecologist's office to demand a laparoscopy, which would provide visible proof of the disease. Despite biomedicine having failed her for many years, Wright still needed the medical diagnosis in order to feel vindicated in her quest and validated as a patient.

Many women speak about their time seeking a diagnosis as a 'battle' or a 'struggle' to be believed (Denny & Mann, 2008), and they consult many doctors and try various treatments in order to alleviate their pain. Cox, Henderson, Andersen, Cagliarini, and Ski (2003) have called this the 'medical merry-go-round', and it may include the use of complementary and alternative therapies, self-management, or disengagement (either temporarily or permanently) with conventional medical services. This resonates with Frank's chaos narrative, which is captured by many of the stories of women with endometriosis. Here there is no restitution, and the progress of the disease moves in uncertain and unpredictable ways. A participant in Huntington and Gilmour's (2005, p. 1129) study commented:

> You know you go into everything feeling positive so you start taking this drug feeling this is going to be it. You pick a particular surgery and you think right I will do this and it will be better, you wake up and you feel dreadful and you think okay that's fine and it will pass. After two months you start feeling as bad as you did before and after three months you are as bad as you were before and you think what's the point of doing it?

A new crisis of credibility (Bury, 1991) may result as women continue to experience symptoms, or symptoms return even after seemingly successful treatment. Supplies of goodwill and social support may dry up as suspicions grow that the woman may be exaggerating the extent of her illness. Women with cyclical symptoms only around menstruation may be able to plan their lives and activities around endometriosis, but for others, the randomness and unpredictable nature of symptoms make life difficult and chaotic. As one woman reported, 'life [becomes] permanently on hold' (Denny, 2009, p. 992) when she is unable to work, attend school, or participate in social and family life.

Impact of endometriosis on women's lives

Women in long-term relationships see endometriosis as a major factor in the relationship, yet few studies have included partners, and their experience is generally reported vicariously during interviews with women. From narrative interviews with women, their male partners, and dyadic interviews, Butt and Chesla (2007) described a typology of relational patterns that couples employed in order to cope with the woman's endometriosis, although these were not fixed and could shift. Some couples were seen as going through endometriosis together, or involved in caregiving either to or by the woman; some were described as being together but alone, as if, although living together as a unit, each partner existed in a separate world. For example, in one couple the man was very self-reliant and saw health as coming from within and achieved from the discipline of a good diet and plenty of exercise, whereas the woman valued companionship and emotional support. She would also listen to her body and rest during times of pain or fatigue, whereas her partner felt she should be more active at these times.

Endometriosis is a disease that mainly occurs during the reproductive years, and so current or future fertility is a major concern for many women, as described above. Although some women have no difficulty in conceiving, endometriosis is a factor in infertility, and women worry that their future fertility may be compromised, upsetting taken-for-granted assumptions about control over reproduction. This is exacerbated when the male and female partner have different priorities; women are more likely than their male partner to want to put off treatment, with the implication for continued pain, in order to prioritise pregnancy

(Hudson et al., 2016). In their study of the impact of endometriosis on couple dyads through the prism of biographical disruption (Bury, 1982), Hudson et al. (2016) found that disruption of sex and intimacy is caused not only by painful intercourse but also by other symptoms and factors associated with endometriosis. These include fatigue, reduced sex-drive as a result of medication, stress caused by infertility experiences, and generally feeling unattractive or unfeminine.

> 'I just felt I wasn't doing my wifely duties and just being abnormal' stated one participant, reflecting the guilt felt when unable to fulfil normative expectations of sex within a heterosexual relationship.
>
> *(p. 725)*

Many women experience disruption to education or employment because of their pain, which may be exacerbated when colleagues are reluctant to cover for sickness absence and make their feelings known: 'Somebody said to me "look, people really got the hump when you were off cos they were having to do your job as well"' (Denny, 2004, p. 42). In most countries endometriosis is not accepted as a disability in a legal sense (although individual women may obtain this categorisation), and so there is no obligation to make school or workplace adjustments for women in pain due to endometriosis. There is great variation in the extent to which employers are willing to accommodate women, and this may affect life chances, such as promotion, and indeed the ability to work at all. Women feel guilty (or are made to feel guilty) by their inability to contribute fully in the workplace. This is exacerbated by the stigma of menstruation, which makes it difficult to discuss symptoms of endometriosis with colleagues and managers; some women prefer to suffer in silence or attribute absences to another health problem. Thus women can find themselves in a secret little world (Gilmour, Huntington, & Wilson, 2008) and feel they are on their own because 'you don't talk about things "down there"' (Denny, 2004, p. 42).

A little reported effect of endometriosis is fatigue, which may exacerbate the problems discussed above, but is also debilitating in its own right (Gilmour et al., 2008), impacting on work and social life. Some women have found that this is treated as secondary to pain by clinicians and not given the importance that it merits. Similarly in research it is an issue that is frequently raised by women, but has not been the primary purpose of any study. However, it may be as important as pain in affecting the lived reality of women with endometriosis, and more research is needed into its impact on daily life.

Over time women may find that they need to work only part-time or move to a less stressful or physically demanding job. This may have financial implications, such as causing household budgets to be strained and increasing women's dependence on their partners (Hudson et al., 2016). These stresses can also cause relationships to break down.

> The relationship that I was in at that time broke up. I mean there were other things going on, but the stress of the health problems and stuff, so not only was my business sold, my house was sold, my relationship broke up all at the same time, as when I was really acutely ill.
>
> *(Huntington & Gilmour, 2005, p. 1128)*

Similarly women have described missing out on other goals in their lives, such as sport (Moradi et al., 2014), travel, or hobbies. Social life is frequently affected, with planned outings cancelled or missed, and women have reported losing friends and alienating relatives who do not understand why this keeps occurring. Women with fairly predictable symptoms may be more able to plan around their 'bad days', thereby minimising disruption to a normal life.

Resistance and endometriosis communities

> It is not a woman's lot to suffer, even if we've been raised that way. It is not OK to miss a part of your life because of pain and excessive bleeding. It is not OK to be bed-ridden for two-to-three days a month. It is not OK to [have] pain during sex.
>
> *(Attributed to actress Susan Sarandon, cited in Griffith, 2017, p. 52)*

As discussed above, endometriosis is a contentious illness due to its status as a condition often dismissed as illegitimate. 'Contestation' in relation to illness, however, 'also manifests in *practices of critical engagement*' by those who have been diagnosed with and/or experience the condition themselves (Moss & Teghtsoonian, 2008, p. 7, authors' emphasis). Women living with endometriosis engage in such critical practices, as they are not solely passive victims of medical discourses that dismiss their symptoms and/or pathologise them as patients.

In response to the failure of biomedical models to fully recognise and adequately treat the disease, many women seek to 'take control' over the management of their endometriosis. In this process, many come to acquire knowledge and expertise about the condition and/or seek out alternative therapies as a means of reclaiming control over their bodies and lives (Cox et al., 2003). Seear (2009b) warned that the responsibility to become an 'expert endometriosis patient' constitutes a 'third shift' for such women, compounding the existing stresses of living with the condition. Further, the 'self-help' logics underlying alternative therapy approaches place the burden of disease management and treatment on individual women. If a woman's symptoms do not subside, blame for this becomes individualised as the woman could be said not to have adequately undertaken the self-help/alternative therapy regimens properly (Seear, 2014).

Endometriosis operates both as a shared social identity and as a site of resistance, forming the basis of multiple national and transnational support, advocacy, and cyberspace groups (including Endo Warriors, Endo Invisible, and The Endometriosis Coalition) that now exist. The quote (above) attributed to Susan Sarandon, who has endometriosis, is widely shared online in such communities and is representative of the themes of resistance to the dismissal of women's endometriosis pain and symptoms by health professionals and the invisibility of endometriosis in wider public discourse. Other celebrities, including Lena Dunham, Hilary Mantel, and Padma Lakshmi, have publically stepped forward to disclose their personal stories as 'endo sufferers' to raise awareness and advocate for public spending on endometriosis research and treatment.

According to Whelan (2007), endometriosis patients constitute an epistemological community in which communal (and not individual) illness experience is held to be the most legitimate form of knowledge. Within this community, clinical knowledge is challenged, questioned, and seen as less valid because (the majority of) health professionals do not have the experiential knowledge that comes from living with the condition and because they are believed not to have the information, ability, or skill necessary to provide adequate care. Thus, Whelan argued, endometriosis communities not only constitute a form of political resistance, but they move beyond this to challenge dominant hierarchies of knowledge about the disease.

Conclusion

By viewing endometriosis through the dual prisms of gender and contest, we have brought into sharp relief the tensions that are inherent in the experience of the condition. First, in most cultures women are brought up to view menstruation as something secretive and shameful. Yet the pain of endometriosis and its impact on all aspects of life requires menstrual pain to be openly discussed in the workplace and among social contacts, thereby breaking the taboo of silence. The ubiquitous nature of dysmenorrhoea, and gendered notions about women's experience and reporting of pain, lead to women whose pain is indicative of endometriosis finding themselves disbelieved and needing to struggle for credibility. Ideas that there is some quantifiable measure of 'normal' that would act as a yardstick to a diagnosis is illusionary when considered in the context of a patriarchal medical profession who will continue to act as gatekeepers to services. Many health practitioners as well as friends and family display a scepticism about women's pain and make judgements about 'correct' levels of pain, which contradict the reality of the lives of women with endometriosis. Yet women need the legitimation of a diagnosis, an answer to why they have this pain. As women's traditional role and status has been (and for many remains) through reproduction, the pain of endometriosis is frequently given more credence when it is associated with infertility. Women for whom this is not an issue may find that they, rather than their condition, are pathologised and treated as dysfunctional and hypochondriac. Despite these tensions, there is resistance; women are taking control of their disease and their lives. In this chapter we have cited literature from the 1990s up to 2018. What is very noticeable is how little has changed; findings from recently published studies are interchangeable with those of earlier research. It seems that giving women with endometriosis a voice has not yet ended their struggle.

References

Abbas, S., Ihle, P., Köster, I., & Schubert, I. (2012). Prevalence and incidence of diagnosed endometriosis and risk of endometriosis in patients with endometriosis-related symptoms: Findings from a statutory health insurance-based cohort in Germany. *European Journal of Obstetrics and Gynecology and Reproductive Biology*, *160*(1), 79–83.

Ballard, K., Lane, H., Hudelist, G., Banerjee, S., & Wright, J. (2010). Can specific pain symptoms help in the diagnosis of endometriosis? A cohort study of women with chronic pelvic pain. *Fertility and Sterility*, *94*(1), 20–27.

Ballard, K., Lawton, K., & Wright, J. (2006). What's the delay? A qualitative study of women's experience of reaching a diagnosis of endometriosis. *Fertility and Sterility*, *5*, 1296–1301.

Bendelow, G. A. (2000). *Pain and gender*. Harlow, UK: Prentice Hall.

Bendelow, G. A. & Williams, S. J. (2002). Natural for women, abnormal for men: Beliefs about pain and gender. In S. Nettleton & J. Watson (Eds), *The body in everyday life* (pp. 199–217). London, UK: Routledge.

Boseley, S. (2017, September 6). "Listen to women": UK doctors issued with first guidance on endometriosis. *Guardian*. Retrieved from www.theguardian.com/society/2017/sep/06/listen-to-women-uk-doctors-issued-with-first-guidance-on-endometriosis.

Britton, C. J. (1996). Learning about "the curse": An anthropological perspective on experiences of menstruation. *Women's Studies International Forum*, *19*, 645–653.

Bullo, S. (2018). Exploring disempowerment in women's accounts of endometriosis experiences. *Discourse & Communication*, *12*, 569–586.

Bury, M. (1982). Chronic illness as biographical disruption. *Sociology of Health & Illness*, *4*, 167–182.

Bury, M. (1991). The sociology of chronic illness: A review of research and prospects. *Sociology of Health and Illness*, *13*, 451–468.

Butt, F. S. & Chesla, C. (2007). Relational patterns of couples living with chronic pelvic pain from endometriosis. *Qualitative Health Research*, *17*(5), 571–585.

Cox, H., Henderson, L., Andersen, N., Cagliarini, G., & Ski, C. (2003). Focus group study of endometriosis: Struggle, loss and the medical merry-go-round. *International Journal of Nursing Practice*, *9*(1), 2–9.

Cox, H., Henderson, L., Wood, R., & Cagliarini, G. (2003). Learning to take charge: Women's experiences of living with endometriosis. *Complementary Therapies in Nursing & Midwifery*, *9*(2), 62–68.

Culley, L., Hudson, N., Law, C., Denny, E., Mitchell, H., Baumgarten, M., & Raine-Fenning, N. (2013). The social and psychological impact of endometriosis on women's lives: A critical narrative review. *Human Reproduction Update*, *19*(6), 625–639, doi:10.1093/humupd/dmt027.

De Graaff, A., D'hooghe, T., Dunselman, G., Dirksen, C., Hummelshoj, L., WERF EndoCost Consortium, & Simoens S. (2013). The significant effect of endometriosis on physical, mental and social wellbeing: Results from an international cross-sectional survey. *Human Reproduction*, *28*(10), 2677–2685.

De Nardi, P. & Ferrrari, S. (2011). *Deep pelvic endometriosis: A multidisciplinary approach*. Milan: Springer Science.

Denny, E. (2004). 'You are one of the unlucky ones': Delay in the diagnosis of endometriosis. *Diversity in Health & Social Care*, *1*(1), 39–44.

Denny, E. (2009). 'I never know from one day to another how I will feel': Pain and uncertainty in women with endometriosis. *Qualitative Health Research*, *19*(7), 985–995.

Denny, E., Culley, L., Papadoupolos, I., & Apenteng, P. (2011). From womanhood to endometriosis: Findings from focus groups with women from different ethnic groups. *Diversity in Health & Care*, *8*(3), 167–180.

Denny, E. & Mann, C. H. (2007). Endometriosis-associated dyspareunia: The impact on women's lives. *Journal of Family Planning and Reproductive Health Care*, *33*(3), 189–193.

Denny, E. & Mann, C. H. (2008). Endometriosis and the primary care consultation. *European Journal of Obstetrics, Gynecology, and Reproductive Biology*, *139*(1), 111–115.

Elmerstig, E., Wijma, B., & Berterö, C. (2008). Why do young women continue to have sexual intercourse despite pain?. *Journal of Adolescent Health*, *43*(4), 357–363.

Fahs, B. (2016). *Out for blood: Essays on menstruation and resistance*. Albany, NY: State University of New York Press.

Frank, A. (1995). *The wounded storyteller: Body, illness, and ethics*. Chicago, IL: University of Chicago Press.

Fritzer, N., Haas, D., Oppelt, P., Hornung, D., Wölfler, M., Ulrich, U., Fischerlehner, G., & Hudelist, G. (2013). More than just bad sex: Sexual dysfunction and distress in patients with endometriosis. *European Journal of Obstetrics and Gynecology and Reproductive Biology*, *169*(2), 392–396.

Gillespie, R. (2001). Contextualizing voluntary childlessness within a postmodern model of reproduction: Implications for health and social needs. *Critical Social Policy*, *21*, 139–159.

Gilmour, J. A., Huntington, A., & Wilson, H. V. (2008). The impact of endometriosis on work and social participation. *International Journal of Nursing Practice*, *14*(6), 443–448.

Goffman, E. (1968). *Stigma: Notes on the management of a spoiled identity*. Harmondsworth, UK: Penguin.

Goodman, L. R. & Franasiak, J. M. (2018). Efforts to redefine endometriosis prevalence in low risk patients. *British Journal of Obstetrics & Gynaecology*, *125*, 63–68.

Griffith, V. A. (2017). The syndemic of endometriosis, stress, and stigma. In B. Ostrach, S. Lerman, & M. Singer (Eds), *Stigma syndemics: New directions in biosocial health* (pp. 35–60). New York, NY: Lexington Press.

Han, E. (2018). 700,000 women with endometriosis no longer have to suffer in silence. *Sydney Morning Herald*. Retrieved from www.smh.com.au/healthcare/700-000-women-with-endometriosis-no-longer-have-to-suffer-in-silence-20180723-p4zt3y.html.

Hawkey, A. J., Ussher, J. M., Perz, J., & Metusela, C. (2017). Experiences and constructions of menarche and menstruation among migrant and refugee women. *Qualitative Health Research*, *27*, 1473–1490.

Hoffmann, D. E. & Tarzian, A. J. (2001). The girl who cried pain: A bias against women in the treatment of pain. *Journal of Law, Medicine & Ethics*, *28*(s4), 13–27.

Hudson, N., Culley, L., Law, C., Mitchell, H., Denny, E., & Raine-Fenning, N. (2016). 'We needed to change the mission statement of the marriage': Biographical disruptions, appraisals, and revisions among couples living with endometriosis. *Sociology of Health & Illness*, *38*(5), 721–735.

Hummelshoj, L., De Graaff, A., Dunselman, G., & Vercellini, P. (2014). Let's talk about sex and endometriosis. *Journal of Family Planning and Reproductive Health Care*, *40*(1), 8–10.

Huntington, A. & Gilmour, J. A. (2005). A life shaped by pain: Women and endometriosis. *Journal of Clinical Nursing*, *14*(9), 1124–1132.

Hydén, L. C. (1997). Illness and narrative. *Sociology of Health & Illness*, *19*(1), 48–69.

Jones, G. L., Jenkinson, C., & Kennedy, S. (2004). The impact of endometriosis on quality of life: A qualitative analysis. *Journal of Psychosomatic Obstetrics and Gynecology*, *2*, 123–133.

Labuski, C. (2015). *It hurts down there: The bodily imaginaries of female genital pain.* Albany, NY: State University of New York Press.

Laws, S. (1990). *Issues of blood: The politics of menstruation.* Basingstoke, UK: Macmillan.

Marcovic, M., Manderson, L., & Warren, N. (2008). Endurance and contest: Women's narratives of endometriosis. *Health, 12*(3), 349–367.

Meuleman, C., Vandenabeele, B., Fieuws, S., Spiessens, C., Timmerman, D., & D'Hooghe, T. (2009). High prevalence of endometriosis in infertile women with normal ovulation and normospermic partners. *Fertility and Sterility, 92*(1), 68–74.

Moradi, M., Parker, M., Sneddon, A., Lopez, V., & Ellwood, D. (2014). Impact of endometriosis on women's lives: A qualitative study. *BMC Women's Health, 14*(1), 123.

Moss, P. & Teghtsoonian, K. (Eds) (2008). *Contesting illness: Process and practices.* Toronto, Canada: University of Toronto Press.

Nnoaham, K. E., Hummelshoj, L., Webster, P., d'Hooghe, T., de Cicco Nardone, F., de Cicco Nardone, C., & Zondervan, K. T. (2011). Impact of endometriosis on quality of life and work productivity: A multicenter study across ten countries. *Fertility and Sterility, 96*(2), 366–373.

Rhodes, L. A., McPhillips-Tangum, C. A., Markham, C., & Klenk, R. (2002). The power of the visible: The meaning of diagnostic tests in chronic back pain. In S. Nettleton & U. Gustafsson (Eds), *The sociology of health and illness reader* (pp. 35–47). Cambridge, UK: Polity.

Seear, K. (2009a). The etiquette of endometriosis: Stigmatisation, menstrual concealment and the diagnostic delay. *Social Science & Medicine, 69*(8), 1220–1277.

Seear, K. (2009b). The third shift: Health, work and expertise among women with endometriosis. *Health Sociology Review, 18*(2), 194–206.

Seear, K. (2014). *The makings of a modern epidemic: Endometriosis, gender and politics.* London, UK: Routledge.

Soliman, A. M., Yang, H., Du, E. X., Kelley, C., & Winkel, C. (2016). The direct and indirect costs associated with endometriosis: A systematic literature review. *Human Reproduction, 31*(4), 712–722.

Toye, F., Seers, K., & Barker, K. (2014). A meta-ethnography of patients' experiences of chronic pelvic pain: Struggling to construct chronic pelvic pain as 'real'. *Journal of Advanced Nursing, 70*(12), 2713–2727.

Ussher, J. (2006). *Managing the monstrous feminine: Regulating the reproductive body.* Abingdon, UK: Routledge.

Valle, R. F. & Sciarra, J. J. (2003). Endometriosis: Treatment strategies. *Annals of the New York Academy of Sciences, 997*(1), 229–239.

Werner, A. & Malterud, K. (2003). 'It is hard work behaving as a credible patient': Encounters between women with chronic pain and their doctors. *Social Science & Medicine, 57*(8), 1409–1419.

Whelan, E. (1997). Staging and profiling: The constitution of the endometriotic subject in gynecological discourse. *Alternate Routes: A Journal of Critical Social Research, 14.*

Whelan, E. (2003). Putting pain to paper: Endometriosis and the documentation of suffering. *Health, 7*(4), 463–482.

Whelan, E. (2007). 'No one agrees except for those of us who have it': Endometriosis patients as an epistemological community. *Sociology of Health & Illness, 29*(7), 957–982.

Whitehead, K. L. (2014). *Great expectations: Maternal ideation, injustice and entitlement in the online infertility community* (Doctoral dissertation). University of Toronto, Canada. Retrieved from https://tspace.library.utoronto.ca/bitstream/1807/43749/1/Krista_Whitehead_201311_PhD_thesis.pdf.

Williams, S. J. (2000). Chronic illness as biographical disruption or biographical disruption as chronic illness? Reflections on a core concept. *Sociology of Health and Illness, 22*(1), 40–67.

Wright, K. O. (2019). "You have endometriosis": Making menstruation-related pain legitimate in a biomedical world. *Health Communication, 34*, 912–915.

Young, K., Fisher, J., & Kirkman, M. (2017). Clinicians' perceptions of women's experiences of endometriosis and of psychosocial care for endometriosis. *Australian and New Zealand Journal of Obstetrics and Gynaecology, 57*(1), 87–92.

9

BREAST AND REPRODUCTIVE CANCERS

Genomics and risks

Cheryl B. Travis

This chapter describes the biochemistry and molecular biology of reproductive cancer, links these to cancer risks, and highlights two recent treatment options based on this science. Sections one and two supply context regarding cancer prevalence and survival as well as a synopsis of disparities in treatment and access to care. Section three provides an overview of cell biochemistry and genomics that increasingly inform the understanding of cancer risks covered in section four. Treatment innovations are covered in section five. The conclusion reminds readers of the importance of patient-centered care and shared decision making.

Prevalence, survival, and screening

Reproductive cancers

Reproductive cancers include cancers of the cervix, ovary, uterus, vulva, fallopian tubes, and vagina. Common warning signs of reproductive cancer include atypical bleeding, unusual discharge, or pain in the pelvic area. A search of the Global Cancer Observatory (GCO)[1] five-year prevalence of new and existing cases of reproductive[2] cancers provides a small hint of the lives affected (e.g., eastern Asia 871,802; North America 418,729; central and eastern Europe 396,268; eastern Africa 123,635) (International Agency for Research on Cancer (IARC), 2018b).

International data gathered by the American Cancer Society indicate that in the US and other developed countries, the five-year survival rate is favorable for cervical (73%) and uterine (83%) cancer (American Cancer Society, 2018). However, related data indicate that survival is consistently lower in less developed countries where screening is infrequent (Torre, Islami, Siegel, Ward, & Jemal, 2017). Variations in prevalence and survival by socio-economic class, race, and ethnicity are discussed in section three.

Causal factors vary. Some ovarian cancers are rooted in a group of heritable mutations known as Lynch syndrome, which was first identified in hereditary, non-polyposis, colorectal cancer (Shrader, 2017). Individuals with one or more of the Lynch syndrome mutations have a 24% increased risk for ovarian cancer and a 16–54% increased risk for endometrial cancer (Bonadona et al., 2011). More detail on mutations is provided in section four. For these and other cancers, early detection is critical for successful treatment and quality of life in survival.

Many reproductive cancers are most closely associated with human papillomavirus (HPV), including cancers of the cervix, vagina, and vulva. HPV is estimated to account globally for virtually all of cervical cancer (de Martel, Plummer, Vignat, & Franceschi, 2017; IARC, 2018a). Men also are vulnerable to HPV, with a potential for genital warts and cancer of the penis, anus, throat, tonsils, and tongue. Approximately 79 million Americans, most in their late teens and early 20s, are infected with HPV, and nearly all sexually active people are at risk for it (CDC, 2017). In developed countries, effective screening tests are readily available for cervical and endometrial cancer. For US women, screening is recommended every three years with cervical cytology (Pap test) (US Preventive Services Task Force, 2018).

Unfortunately, HPV encompasses a large family of related viruses, and many are not detected by the standard Pap test. Other, more comprehensive tests rely on liquid storage of the cervical specimen in a solution that preserves cell morphology (e.g., the cobas human papillomavirus test, developed by Roche pharmaceuticals; Rao et al., 2013). Nonetheless, high technology tests may not be available in lower income countries. An alternative testing regimen recognized by the World Health Organization (WHO) relies on visual inspection with ascetic acid (VIA) (Shah et al., 2016). This has the benefit of providing nearly instantaneous results, but also produces more false positives and unnecessary treatment.

Vaccination programs represent another growing approach to the elimination of HPV-related diseases. Two vaccines now are available that target HPV strains 16 and 18: Gardasil (US FDA approved in 2006 and marketed by Merck)[3] and Ceravix (approved in 2009 and marketed by GlaxoSmithKline). A third vaccine, Gardasil 9 (approved in 2014), targets nine HPV strains. Vaccines are administered in a two or three injection protocol spaced over several months. All vaccines initially were recommended for girls and women aged 9–26, but eventually were expanded to include boys and men.

HPV vaccination is now part of the national immunization programs in 82 countries (Kane & Giuliano, 2018). Estimates are that approximately 118 million women have been included in HPV vaccination programs. Scotland implemented a program to reduce three HPV types among 12–13-year-old girls, with 79–94% efficacy at seven-year follow-up (Kavanagh et al., 2017). The HPV-FASTER consortium of 11 European countries currently is testing a three-dose HPV vaccination program among women aged 25–45 (Bosch et al., 2015). However, the vast majority of these programs are in more developed regions (Bruni et al., 2016; Kane & Giuliano, 2018). Projects in Bhutan, Bolivia, Cambodia, Haiti, and Lesotho were initiated in 2009 (Ladner et al., 2012).

Many vaccination programs are seriously limited in effective prevention because they do not include men. Globally, only 1% of countries have programs that treat men, a limitation among even high-income countries (Kane & Giuliano, 2018). Australia was one of the first countries (2007) to introduce a publicly funded HPV vaccination program for both sexes, and now appears to be on track to eliminate cervical cancer (Hall et al., 2019).

Breast cancer

Worldwide, there is a vast range in the rate of breast cancer. Countries in the top quintile of breast cancer (e.g., Argentina, Australia, Belgium, US) have an average five-year prevalence of 334 per 100,000, whereas countries in the second quintile (e.g., France, Japan, Poland, Venezuela) have a five-year prevalence of 222 per 100,000 (IARC, 2018b).

Countries in lower quintiles have dramatically lower rates, but also tend to be countries with fewer resources by which to screen or detect cancer (e.g., Afghanistan, Chad, Honduras, Nepal) (IARC, 2018c).

Although breast cancer can be, and often is fatal, survival rates have improved. In the US, approximately three million women are alive today who have a history of breast cancer, including those currently in treatment and those who have completed treatment (BreastCancer.org, 2018). Overall survival in the US has increased substantially, including among women with metastatic cancer (Sundquist, Brudin, & Tejler, 2016). Several factors contribute to these survival gains: consistent screening, earlier detection and intervention, improved approaches to primary treatments, and longer follow-up with adjuvant treatments. However, women with low income or in developing countries may not have access to these treatments. Despite increased screening availability, barriers continue to exist for diverse groups of women (e.g., immigrant or non-native speakers) (Hulme et al., 2016). Canadian data indicate this is true for older, low-income, and immigrant women, particularly Asian immigrants (Lofters, Moineddin, Hwang, & Glazier, 2010; Xiong, Murphy, Mathews, Gadag, & Wang, 2010).

The prognosis and treatment options for breast cancer depend heavily on early detection. Professional reviews regarding screening guidelines have resulted in three different US recommendations. The US Preventive Services Task Force now recommends that screening begin at age 50 and be performed biannually, but might be done earlier and more often depending on risk factors for the individual woman. The American Cancer Society recommends that screening begin at age 45, whereas the American College of Obstetrics and Gynecology recommends that screening begin at age 40. These entities also have slightly different recommendations on at what age to stop mammography screening.

Disparities

Vast country disparities in health outcomes are clearly linked to economic standing. Breast cancer mortality and morbidity provide one example. I integrated data from the Global Cancer Observatory (GCO) and World Bank economic rankings and compared the median age-standardized mortality/morbidity ratio for breast cancer in 180 nations, from Afghanistan to Zimbabwe. A lower ratio indicates relatively lower mortality and overall better survival. When grouped according to their World Bank designation of country economy, the median mortality/morbidity ratio aligned perfectly with economic standing. Countries with economic classifications of high, upper-middle, lower-middle, and low had mortality/morbidity ratios of .197, .309, .427, and .554, respectively. Countries with lower-middle and low economic classifications had more than twice the age-adjusted mortality of high-income countries and substantially more than countries with an upper-middle income classification.

Other disparities in burden of disease, access to care, and health outcomes occur with respect to race and ethnicity, as well as indigenous, and immigrant status. Within the US, race/ethnicity disparities regarding breast and reproductive cancers are extensive and occur with respect to screening, stage at diagnosis, and death and survival rates (Lofters et al., 2010; NCI, 2018). Some of this disparity relates to differences in patterns of genetic mutations. Testing has identified a greater frequency of certain mutations, few instances of other mutations, and overall higher prevalence of triple-negative cancers among African American women (Keenan et al., 2015).

Screening for cervical, uterine, and breast cancer is a critical area of disparity. Women of minority race/ethnicity are less likely to have regular Pap tests (AHRQ, 2017). Infrequent

Pap testing in the US undoubtedly contributes to the higher cervical cancer mortality rates among non-Hispanic Black women, especially in southern states (Yoo et al., 2017). The true incidence of cervical cancer among Black women is probably underestimated because these women have a high rate of hysterectomy, which may disguise initial detection of cervical cancer (Beavis, Gravitt, & Rositch, 2017).

Treatment also varies with respect to race/ethnicity, but it is difficult to pinpoint mechanisms and pathways that sustain these disparities. One four-year study of US women with cervical cancer illustrates this complexity. After controlling for insurance coverage, treatment medications, and treatment protocol, Bandera, Lee, Rodriguez-Rodriguez, Powell, and Kushi (2016) found that Black women were more likely to have dose reductions,[4] delays in the weekly treatment schedule, or early discontinuation. Hispanic women also had more dose reductions, but not early discontinuation. However, when variations in day-to-day treatment protocols were controlled, Black and Hispanic women continued to have shorter survival time than White women.

Disparities in survival are informative about the overall effectiveness of the diagnosis, coordination among providers, and treatment plans. There is a longstanding pattern that US White women have a survival advantage relative to Black women with respect to breast (Miller, Smith, Ryerson, Tucker, & Allemani, 2017) and ovarian cancers (Stewart et al., 2017). The disparity in breast cancer survival in the US has been observed even when women received a diagnosis of ductal carcinoma *in situ* (DCIS), the most favorable prognosis (Narod, Iqbal, Giannakeas, Sopik, & Sun, 2015). For cervical and uterine cancers, survival among White women also is higher than among American Indian/Native Alaskan (AINA), Hispanic, and Asian/Pacific Islander (API) women (NCI, 2018).

Carcinogenesis and genomics

All cancers develop, change, and are sustained by mutations in specific genes and gene clusters. This was definitively established by The Cancer Genome Atlas (TCGA), a project begun in 2005 and finalized in 2018, administered by the National Cancer Institute within the US National Institutes of Health. The project included multiple research sites with the goal of sequencing the critical genes of an extensive list of cancers (e.g., breast, colon, lung, kidney, ovary, prostate, thyroid). The Human Genome project on breast cancer identified four basic genetic profiles with different implications for prognosis and further treatment research (The Cancer Genome Atlas et al., 2012).

Carcinogenesis is basically a process of genetic mutations. Although not all mutations lead to cancer, all cancers develop by a process of mutation. Since the human genome was sequenced in 2001, extensive gene sequencing has revealed specific mutations in a wide range of human cancers. However, a single mutation, inherited or otherwise, is rarely sufficient to produce cancer. There is general agreement that 2–8 mutations are necessary to produce cancer (Vogelstein et al., 2013).

The source of mutations may be classified broadly as germline or somatic. Germline mutations are inherited at conception from one or both parents who also carry the mutation. Cancers with germline mutations convey increased risk beginning at conception, tend to appear at an earlier age, and are more likely to metastasize (Osman, 2014). Germline mutations have been linked to breast, ovarian, prostate, and colon cancers. Germline mutations to BRCA1[5] or BRCA2 genes are particularly relevant to breast cancer.

Somatic mutations are by far the more common and emerge during ordinary cell division. This is not surprising, given that cell division occurs millions of times a day and requires the disassembly and reassembly of the thousands of elements in the human genome that are packed into every cell. However, not all somatic mutations are simply random errors of duplication. For example, the mutation process in cervical and several other reproductive cancers is set in motion by exposure to HPV.

In addition, somatic mutations may be acquired by exposure to chemical agents, pharmaceuticals, and environmental toxins. Examples of environmental carcinogens include asbestos, DDT, diethylstilbestrol,[6] steroidal estrogens, heavy metals such as lead, industrial solvents such as benzene and trichloroethylene, and byproducts of industrial activities such as waste incineration or herbicide applications. Industrial and agricultural waste products released into civic waterways are another hazard. Many, but not all, of these substances have been banned in the US and other developed countries. Other carcinogens are associated with lifestyle exposures (e.g., tobacco smoke, ultraviolet light).

Regardless of the source, cancer mutations often produce exaggerated rates of cell proliferation (mitosis) as well as resistance to normal anti-growth signals. Once present, a mutation is duplicated in all future copies of the cell. Even after cancer is diagnosed, additional mutations continue to emerge over time. Mutations in yet other genes may promote distant migration (metastasis) and support the ability of tumors to develop their own dedicated blood supply (angiogenesis). Late stage mutations also may impede natural aging of cancer cells (senescence) and obstruct internal signals involved in ordinary cell death (apoptosis), with the result that cancer cells resist chemotherapy and tend to persist and multiply in an immortal fashion. This is why regular screening, early diagnosis, and early treatment are so important.

Mutations in two classes of genes (i.e., tumor oncogenes, suppressor genes) have important roles in carcinogenesis. Mutations to oncogenes often amplify gene function and release restraints (e.g., exaggerated cell proliferation). For example, mutations of the Myc oncogene are associated with increased cell proliferation, whereas mutations in the Fas oncogene impair aging and death of cancer cells, effectively making them immortal. Some oncogene mutations are more destructive than others. An amplified expression of the oncogene RTKs promotes tumor growth and metastasis, as well as the ability to recruit a dedicated blood supply (Cell Signaling Technology, 2018). The Pik3CA oncogene is one of those commonly associated with breast cancer. Pik3CA mutations are associated with hormone-positive breast cancers and also may predict a poorer tumor response to trastuzumab-based therapies (Mukohara, 2015).

In contrast to oncogenes that may be amplified by mutations, tumor suppressor genes are often attenuated or silenced (deleted) by mutations. Some research suggests that accumulated damage to tumor suppressor genes may be more problematic than oncogene mutations (Hussain, Hofseth, & Harris, 2001; Romero-Laorden & Castro, 2017). For example, silencing of the tumor suppressor gene p53 has been associated with evasion of cell death (loss of apoptosis) in a wide range of advanced cancers, including cancers of the colon, lung, esophagus, breast, liver, and brain (Hollstein, Sidransky, Vogelstein, & Harris, 1991).

Mutations in tumor suppressor genes BRCA1 and BRCA2 typically attenuate repair functions and increase risk for breast and other cancers. Most BRCA mutations are germline (inherited), but estimates are that at least 10% are somatic (Dougherty et al., 2017). Although BRCA1/2 mutations account for only 5–10% of breast or reproductive cancers (Peshkin, Alabek, & Isaacs, 2011), these mutations have serious consequences for those who do carry them. Kuchenbaecker et al. (2017) searched databases from 16 countries[7] to track 6,036 BRCA1 and 3,820 BRCA2 carriers and followed them for a decade. They estimated a cumulative breast cancer risk of 72% for BRCA1 and 69% for BRCA2 carriers. These

BRCA mutations also increased the likelihood of developing cancer in the contralateral breast. Cumulative ovarian cancer risk was 44% for BRCA1 and 17% for BRCA2 carriers. A mutated BRCA1 is also associated with increased risk for ovarian and prostate cancers, whereas a mutated BRCA2 also imparts increased risks for prostate and colon cancers. Other studies have determined that men with inherited mutations in BRCA2 have a 100-fold increased risk of breast cancer, as well as an increased risk for prostate and pancreatic cancer (Childers, Maggard-Gibbons, Macinko, & Childers, 2018).

Risk factors

Many risk factors for breast and gynecological cancers have been identified (Binder et al., 2018; Tamimi et al., 2016). Key factors discussed here include breast density, obesity, age at menarche and menopause, age at first full-term pregnancy, and menopausal hormone therapy.

Breast density

Breasts may be classed as dense when there is relatively more functional breast tissue than adipose or connective tissue. A number of longitudinal studies have reported a greater incidence of cancer among women with dense breasts (for a review see Boyd et al., 2010). A four-fold increase in breast cancer risk has been reported for women in the top 25% of breast density compared with those in the lowest 25% (Boyd et al., 2007; Ho, Jafferjee, Covarrubias, Ghesani, & Handler, 2014). This increased risk is the basis for guidelines in more than 30 US states that require women be notified if their mammogram indicates high breast density and that they be informed of additional screening options (e.g., ultrasound, MRI, 3-D mammography).

Menarche and menopause

As with many types of cancer, an extended period of cell division and proliferation ultimately increases the possibility of mutations and eventual transformation to cancer cells. This is facilitated by early and/or extended exposure to reproductive hormones. Early age at menarche (≤12 yrs) or later age at menopause produce a higher lifetime dose of reproductive hormones, more cell division and proliferation, and more opportunities for gene mutation (Bernstein, 2002). The collaborative meta-analysis study of hormonal factors in breast cancer showed a 5% increase in the risk of breast cancer for every year of younger age at menarche and that these women were more likely to have estrogen-positive cancer (Collaborative Group on Hormonal Factors in Breast Cancer, 2012). The same study (2012) indicated that, compared with those who were post-menopausal, pre-menopausal women had a significantly greater likelihood of breast cancer at every year in the normal range of menopause (45–54), a finding that has been replicated (Day et al., 2015). The authors of these studies concluded that increased risk is due to longer exposure to reproductive hormones.

Age at First Full-Term (FFT) pregnancy

A relationship between early age at FFT pregnancy and lower rates of breast cancer has been documented for many decades. Initial reports defined early first pregnancy as 20 or younger, and generally indicated that lower lifetime risk accrued to mothers who had a first pregnancy ≤20 and who often had a higher number of pregnancies in their lifetime (Bain et al., 1981; Bernstein, 2002). Some current websites do not report age data, but instead give the misleading suggestion that "early" applies to pregnancy at age 25 or younger, whereas others imply it is age 30 or younger.

Newer technologies in genetics and molecular biology now provide some indication about causal pathways for early pregnancy and lower rates of cancer. In essence, it seems that early pregnancy lowers a woman's lifetime dose of estrogen by decreasing the proportion of breast cells that are estrogen receptor-positive and by decreasing proliferation of breast stem (progenitor) cells (Meier-Abt & Bentires-Alj, 2014). Further, during pregnancy, breast stem cells are genetically changed, are better able to repair DNA damage, and thus may be more effective in the process of tumor suppression (Russo, 2016).

Obesity

Observational studies have linked obesity[8] to breast, endometrial, ovarian, colorectal, esophageal, and pancreatic cancers (Kyrgiou et al., 2017). Data from the Nurses Health Study, based on thousands of US nurses followed over 20 years, are compelling. Weight gain post menopause was strongly associated with increased risk of breast cancer, in a linear dose-response pattern (Eliassen, Colditz, Rosner, Willett, & Hankinson, 2006). The focus here is not on risk due to lifestyle but on the biochemistry of adipose tissue. A clue to the biology that might drive this risk begins with the recognition that adipose tissue is not inert. Adipose tissue can function as part of the endocrine system[9] to produce estrogenic hormones (Kershaw & Flier, 2004; Nelson & Bulun, 2001). That is, the functional cancer link is through increased exposure to estrogens produced by adipose tissue.

Menopausal Hormone Therapy (HT)

Risks of menopausal HT are made more obvious by current practices in the treatment of breast and gynecological cancers. Approximately 75% of breast cancers are estrogen positive (Nadji, Gomez-Fernandez, Ganjei-Azar, & Morales, 2005; The Cancer Genome Atlas Network, 2012). That is, the growth of these tumors is accelerated by the action of estrogens as tumor promoters. For several decades, a standard treatment for estrogen+ breast cancer has included strategies to reduce circulating estrogen. Traditionally prescribed following chemotherapy, these drugs can operate in several ways. One common variation is designed to *block* cell uptake of circulating estrogen. These drugs also are known as selective estrogen receptor modulators or SERM (e.g., tamoxifen, fulvestrant). Another common variation is designed to *inhibit* the production of estrogens by treatment with aromatase inhibitors; these include anastrozole (marketed as Arimidex) and letrozole (marketed as Femara). An extensive meta-analysis funded by the UK Breast Cancer Research Council provides relevant comparisons of these two approaches. The study examined individual data on 31,920 postmenopausal women with estrogen-receptor-positive early breast cancer in the randomized trials of outcomes with tamoxifen compared with aromatase inhibitors and concluded that, in early intervention years, aromatase inhibitors reduced recurrence rates by about 30% (proportionately) compared with tamoxifen alone (Early Breast Trialists' Collaborative Group, 2015).

Many of the risk factors discussed in this chapter involve tumors with receptors for reproductive hormones (HR+). The vast majority (75%) of breast cancers are classified as estrogen positive, and a significant percentage of these are also progesterone positive (55%). Estrogens (estradiol, estrone, and estriol) and progesterone are essential in normal reproductive function, including breast development, ovulation, endometrial and uterine function, and sustaining pregnancy. In and of themselves, estrogens and progesterone do not appear to be carcinogens; they do not *initiate* mutations in normal cells. However, they may contribute to the proliferation of precancerous or cancerous cells that do contain mutations. That is, estrogens and progesterone may function as tumor promoters in carcinogenesis. Nonetheless, menopausal HT has been prescribed on the grounds of protecting older women from dementia, heart disease, stroke, osteoporosis, general diseases of aging, menopausal symptoms, and emotional agitation.

The primary forms of HT have been Premarin (estrogen alone) or Prempro (estrogen+progestin). Hormones in these drugs are produced from the urine of mares kept artificially pregnant, continuously fitted with a urine-catching harness, and housed in tightly confined spaces. Introduced in 1941 by the Canadian pharmaceutical firm Wyeth, the formula for horse-urine-derived hormones was later acquired by and marketed by Pfizer Inc.[10]

In 2000, 46 million women in the US were receiving Premarin and 22 million were receiving Prempro (Fletcher & Colditz, 2002). For these prescription practices to be medically justified, benefits must be reliable and nontrivial; furthermore, benefits must outweigh risks of harm. It has become increasingly apparent that neither of these stipulations can be fully met.

Evidence of the potential role of menopausal HT estrogens in breast cancer comes from observational (epidemiological) studies and from clinical trials. In order to answer the many questions concerning the role of menopausal HT, studies need to include thousands of women and must be of sufficient duration to detect carcinogenic mutations and cell proliferation associated with breast cancer.

The US Women's Health Initiative (WHI) remains the largest (16,608 post-menopausal women) and longest[11] clinical trial of menopausal HT and health. Women were randomly assigned to one of two treatment regimens: estrogen alone among women without a uterus[12] or a combined treatment of estrogen plus progestin for those with an intact uterus. Women not assigned to some form of HT received a placebo. After five years, the trial of estrogen+progestin was stopped for safety reasons. Compared with women who received a placebo, women who received estrogen+progestin had a 26% higher incidence of breast cancer (Writing Group for the Women's Health Initiative Investigators, 2002). This pattern remained consistent during all years of follow-up. In addition, women in the estrogen+progestin treatment group tended to have more advanced breast cancers than those in the control group.

Although the main goal of the WHI study was to explore potential benefits of HT estrogens in reducing heart disease, there was an ironic increase of myocardial infarction, blood clots, stroke, probable dementia, gallbladder disease, and death from cardiovascular disease among women who received either estrogen alone or estrogen+progestin (Manson, 2013; Manson et al., 2003; Writing Group for the Women's Health Initiative Investigators, 2002). Women who received combined therapy had a 29% increase in coronary heart disease (CHD), a pattern that emerged dramatically in the first year of treatment. Younger women suffered slightly fewer infarctions, but the difference was not statistically significant. Regardless of age, all women in the treatment arm experienced more strokes. WHI researchers concluded emphatically that HT should not be prescribed as prevention for CHD (Manson et al., 2003, 2013; Writing Group for the Women's Health Initiative Investigators, 2002).

In more recent years, secondary analyses of the WHI data have been designed to determine conditions where HT might be beneficial, despite other harms and risks. One proposition, known as the timing hypothesis, is based on the idea that younger women, relatively closer to the typical age of menopause, might benefit from hormone therapy, whereas it might not be beneficial for women aged 60 or older. However, these secondary analyses disclosed no significant benefit for younger women (Rossouw et al., 2007). A larger secondary analysis combined results from the WHI controlled trial with the WHI observational component that simply asked women to report their health practices and ongoing or new health conditions. This recombination allowed researchers to compare outcomes among larger numbers of users versus non-users (Prentice et al., 2008). However, the combined secondary analysis indicated even greater risk for breast cancer. Compared with non-users, women who *started HT early* in menopause had approximately a 50% increase in breast cancer risk when HT was in place for up to five years and double the risk if the regimen was in place for as long as ten years (Prentice et al., 2008). Regardless of age at which HT was begun, users of estrogen alone or combined estrogen+progestin had consistently more cases of stroke than non-users.

Independent data regarding the timing hypothesis come from a study of one million women in the UK. Researchers reported that, when HT began early (within five years of menopause), breast cancer risk increased by more than 40% for women taking estrogen-only supplements and by 53% for those taking estrogen-progestin supplements (Beral, Reeves, Bull, & Green, 2011). Smaller or shorter duration studies may show somewhat different results, but the WHI and the Million Woman studies are the largest, longest, and most comprehensive endeavors to date.

Once it became apparent that the timing hypothesis was not supported by the data, yet another proposition was suggested regarding possible benefits of HT. The essence of this proposition was that continued prescription of estrogens (alone or in combination) might be warranted if small benefits were aggregated across several chronic diseases (e.g., lower rates of diabetes, bone fracture, gallbladder disease). Perhaps a combined benefit would merit support for HT, notwithstanding risks of breast cancer, deep vein thrombosis, and stroke. Several studies were published along this line, but none of these potential benefits were confirmed (Gartlehner et al., 2017). After review of these studies, the US Preventive Services Task Force (2017) issued a formal statement that combined estrogen and progestin or estrogen alone has no net benefit for the primary prevention of chronic conditions.

Given the increased risk of breast cancer, with little counterbalancing benefit to cardiovascular health or chronic diseases, one would expect that physicians and women would avoid the risks of HT. In fact, several thousand US women who had used HT sued Pfizer and received settlements totaling approximately $1 billion (Compton, 2018). After settling major lawsuits, Pfizer withdrew Prempro from the market (Compton, 2018; Singer & Wilson, 2009). However, with slight variations, prescription of menopausal HT continues. US doctors continue to prescribe estrogen for vasomotor symptoms, but the costs, benefits, and trade-offs are seldom fully explained. Recall that most breast cancers are driven by estrogenic hormones, and even short-term or early HT come with an increased risk of initiating a potentially fatal cancer. Bothersome as they are, the cost of living with vasomotor symptoms pales in comparison with the burden of planning one's next round of chemotherapy. Taking estrogen supplements to minimize hot flashes is like women who smoke as a form of weight control—they may weigh less, but at what cost?

Emerging approaches to treatment

Increased utilization of gene assays and applied cell biochemistry are the most notable recent developments for cancer treatment. Two examples are especially noteworthy. Gene assays of cancer cells provide dramatically more detail about gene activity than standard classifications based on estrogen, progesterone, and HER2 receptors. For example, Oncotype DX gene assay uses applied genomics to inform treatment of early stage breast cancer. The second involves cyclin-dependent kinase inhibitors (CDK4/6), and applies biochemistry to interrupt cell mitosis at the molecular level in advanced stage breast cancer.

Gene profiling and assay

Genetic profiling provides information that can suggest the most optimal forms of treatment. Genomic assays may represent a useful, perhaps critical, tool in making treatment decisions in early stage breast cancer. Early stage is defined as small tumor size (T1–2), cells that are well-formed,[13] with no node involvement (N0),[14] and hormone positive (HR+) and HER2-negative. These cancer types have a relatively low (15%) likelihood of later metastasis (Paik et al., 2004). This means that approximately 85% of women with this cancer type who receive chemotherapy may be treated unnecessarily and struggle needlessly with side effects of chemotherapy.

The objective of a gene assay is to use information about genes that may have been silenced or amplified in order to distinguish those women who might safely bypass chemotherapy from those for whom chemotherapy is essential. Instead of chemotherapy, alternative treatments include estrogen blocking drugs (e.g., tamoxifen) or estrogen inhibiting drugs, otherwise known as aromatase inhibitors (e.g., anastrazole [Arimidex] or letrozole [Femara]).[15]

Three gene assays are currently available: Mammaprint, Oncotype DX, and uPA/PAI-1 (Duffy, O'Donovan, McDermott, & Crown, 2016). All assess the extent and nature of gene mutations in cancer cells and produce a score reflecting the likelihood of future metastasis. Cases with a sufficiently low score have the option of bypassing chemotherapy and using estrogen blocking or estrogen inhibiting treatment alone. Mammaprint targets 70 genes (Cardoso et al., 2016), whereas Oncotype DX and uPa/PAI-1 focus on 21 genes. Both Mammaprint and Oncotype DX assays are relevant to early cases that may or may not have positive lymph nodes. The uPA/PAI-1 assay was designed only for early cases that have no lymph node involvement.

For the sake of space, I focus here on the Oncotype DX. The Oncotype DX 21 gene assay provides information on the activity of 21 genes and assigns weights ranging from 0–100 to each marker with respect to the likelihood of cancer metastasis. The markers indicate gene mutations involving elements discussed in section one (e.g., increased cell proliferation, inhibition of cell aging or loss of apoptosis among cancer cells, the ability of cancer cells to migrate via metastasis). Lower scores on the Oncotype DX indicate less carcinogenic activity and a lower likelihood of later metastasis.

Developed by Genomic Health and launched in 2004, early work on the Oncotype DX verified the usefulness of low, middle, and high recurrence scores in forecasting ten-year survival for women aged ≥50 (Paik et al., 2004). In a related study, Paik et al. (2006) demonstrated that patients with high recurrence scores (RS >31) gained a definite benefit from chemotherapy, as reflected by a 27% reduction in ten-year cancer recurrence rate among those who received chemotherapy compared with those who did not. Alternatively, among patients with low recurrence scores (≤18), there was almost no difference in ten-year recurrence rates for those who received chemotherapy and those who received tamoxifen alone.

After observational studies, Oncotype DX testing was approved for phase-III randomized clinical trials. Separate studies assessed the potential usefulness among patients with very low recurrence scores <10 (Sparano et al., 2015) or slightly higher recurrence scores of <18 (Sparano et al., 2018). The emerging judgment appears to be that, given a sufficiently low Oncotype DX recurrence score, it may be reasonable to forego chemotherapy entirely and instead begin endocrine therapy as the first-line of treatment. Initial trends suggest that since the 21 gene recurrence score was developed, there has been a 15% drop in oncologists' recommendations for chemotherapy among node-negative and node-positive patients (Kurian et al., 2018). Application among younger pre-menopausal women is not recommended, as their cancers tend to involve inherited mutations and to be more aggressive.

Controlling cell proliferation: CDK4/6

Fundamental elements of carcinogenesis feature mutations that involve accelerated cell mitosis and proliferation. In cases of advanced cancer, these are often combined with attenuated cell senescence (aging) and delayed apoptosis (death) of cancer cells. However, new clinical applications can effectively inhibit mitosis of cancer cells. This science is based on work conducted independently by Lee Hartwell, Paul Nurse, and Tim Hunt in the 1970s and 1980s, for which they jointly received the Nobel Prize in 2001.

These new treatments target kinase molecules (a kind of enzyme in the cell) that must pair with cyclins (a kind of protein in the cell) in order to drive cell mitosis. Kinase molecules 4 and 6 are dependent on a particular type of cyclin: cyclin D. When there is over activation of CDK4/6, cell senescence is attenuated (Hortobagyi et al., 2016) and it becomes harder to kill or de-activate cancer cells. New treatments were designed to disrupt the pairing of these kinase with their preferred cyclin; hence the nomenclature cyclin-dependent kinase inhibitors or CDK4/6 inhibitors (see Cadoo, Gucalp, & Traina, 2014; Nature Education, 2014; Wolff, 2016).

These treatment options are specific to hormone-positive, HER2-negative breast cancer that has advanced and acquired additional mutations that make it resistant to endocrine therapy by estrogen blockers (e.g., tamoxifen) or estrogen inhibitors (e.g., fulvestrant [Faslodex]). The FDA approved clinical use of three drug formulations based on this biochemistry: Ibrance (palbociclib) marketed by Pfizer, Kisqali (ribociclib) marketed by Novartis, and Verzenio (abemaciclib) marketed by Eli Lilly. The FDA published notice of approval in early 2017 for Ibrance and Kisqali; Verzenio received its approval in early 2018. Each inhibits cancer cell mitosis and is prescribed in conjunction with estrogen blockers or inhibitors as part of treatment following chemotherapy. All were developed under the FDA expedited approval system for serious conditions.

FDA expedited approval requires that: the condition is serious, there is an unmet need, and research protocols incorporate a risk evaluation and mitigation strategy to assure safe use. Requirements for evidence of efficacy are lenient compared with requirements for other drugs. Expedited approval requires evidence of surrogate or intermediate markers of efficacy that are *reasonably likely* to predict clinical benefit beyond outcomes available with existing treatments.

Protocols of the clinical trials and effectiveness of the relevant drugs have been published for each: palbociclib (Cristofanilli et al., 2016; Turner et al., 2015), ribociclib (Hortobagyi et al., 2016), and abemaciclib (Sledge et al., 2017). Typically, several endpoints are monitored; progression-free survival is one of the more important outcomes. Clinical trials for each drug indicate some incremental addition of progression-free-survival compared with patients who received standard care. Follow-up information continues to be collected (e.g., tumor biomarkers of further mutations, overall survival, side effects). All have similar side effects, including potentially serious impairment of the immune system.

Trials were conducted and funded largely by the pharmaceutical firms that now market them. Depending on the brand and milligram dose, a prescription cost in the US may range from $5,000–$10,000 per month. In the first three quarters of 2017, palboclib (Ibrance) corporate sales reached $2.4 billion, making it one of the top ten bestselling cancer drugs (Philippidis, 2018). In light of the cost and the short time they have been available, these drugs are less likely to be included in the formulary of many for-profit health insurance plans, but in other countries they may be available through national health coverage.

Summary and concluding thoughts

Five major points shape this chapter. First, hundreds of thousands of women around the world have survived or are living with breast and reproductive cancer, and quality of life and survival are getting better, at least in developed nations. Second, there are substantial disparities linked to economic conditions as well as race and ethnicity. In particular, the record is not as favorable for women of color who are less likely to benefit from regular screening, early detection, or access to the most effective treatments. Third, cancer is a process of stepwise genetic change and changes to biochemistry, with continual change and alteration after diagnosis. Biochemistry and molecular biology are central to the natural history and eventual trajectory of every cancer. Fourth, the most common risk factors can be better understood in the context of this molecular biology, particularly the role of estrogens. Fifth, the growing science in these areas has become integral to most treatment plans.

My final point is to caution that biochemistry and molecular biology are not the complete story. There are a number of behaviors that substantially lower cancer risks. Regular screening is one of the best health behaviors women can adopt. Other beneficial behaviors include a healthy diet, exercise, weight maintenance, and avoidance of tobacco. The fact that the majority of breast cancers are estrogen and progesterone positive should put decision making about post-menopausal HT in a broader context.

Patient-centered care, relationships between providers and patients, and shared decision making are also critical elements. These ideas have been increasingly recognized as part of professional competence and as ultimately contributing to better outcomes. The Women's Health movement of the 1960s and 1970s promoted principles based on these broad goals. For example, women's groups called for clarity in diagnoses, full disclosure of risks and benefits of treatment, and active patient participation in decision making. Three decades later, the US Institute of Medicine endeavored to formally establish patient-centered care and shared decision making as standards of professional practice (IOM, 2001). Among the ten principles in the IOM report are six that focus on patients' interests and participation. The first of these defines patient-centered care as compassion, empathy, and responsiveness to the values and preferences of individual patients. In this context, care is customized according to patients' needs and values. The patient is the source of control and is entitled to unfettered access to her medical records, to the clinical knowledge base, and to any information relevant to making an informed decision. These principles are essential to the informed consent required by medical ethics and by law in some (but not all) countries. However, pervasive gender bias often means disregarding the voices of women who attempt to speak authoritatively about their own judgment and preferences. Sometimes this is obvious misogyny (Anderson, 2018) but also may appear as a kind of benevolence (Glick & Raberg, 2018).

Shared decision making includes information exchange—in both directions. Care providers should not intuit patient preferences. Patients should be invited not only to ask questions but also to state their preferences and to have their concerns and fears candidly addressed. The

Commonwealth Fund estimated that $1 billion could be saved annually in the US if patients received information about alternatives and full disclosure regarding risks of more invasive procedures (Schoen et al., 2007). Finally, it is well to remember that shared decision making should not be a one-time event. Habits of asking questions and information sharing will make it easier to engage in more complex or more sensitive issues throughout care and recovery.

Notes

1 The Global Cancer Observatory (GCO) is a searchable database managed by the International Agency for Research on Cancer (IARC) incorporating population-based cancer registries from the Association of Cancer Registries and the World Health Organization.
2 Including cervix, ovary, uterus, vagina, and vulva.
3 Food and Drug Administration clinical reviews and approval notices are available at www.fda.gov/Bio logicsBloodVaccines/Vaccines/ApprovedProducts/ucm093833.htm.
4 Lower doses typically occur in order to manage side effects (e.g., low hemoglobin in blood chemistry).
5 Genes are typically labeled by a combination of letters and numbers (e.g., BRCA1 or p53).
6 A source of birth defects.
7 Drawn from the Cancer in Five Continents registry and the NORDCAN Nordic country registry.
8 Obesity is defined as a body mass index of 30 or higher.
9 Endocrine organs include the hypothalamus, pituitary, thyroid, adrenal gland, pancreas, ovaries, and testes.
10 Pfizer Inc. includes Wyeth and Upjohn.
11 Seven years of treatment interventions, with 17 years of follow-up.
12 Unopposed estrogen causes uterine cancer, hence the need for a hysterectomy among these women.
13 Low-grade tumors have a cell histology that is well formed and similar in appearance to normal cells, whereas advanced grade tumor cells typically are misshapen and have a nucleus that appears scattered and disorganized.
14 If there is no lymph node involvement, a distant metastasis is less likely.
15 At times, tamoxifen is referred to as hormone treatment, which blocks the *uptake* of estrogens by individual cells in the body, while the entire *cessation* of estrogen *production* is sometimes referred to ovarian suppression.

References

Agency for Healthcare Research and Quality (AHRQ) (2017). *National healthcare quality and disparities report 2016 (and appendices)*. Rockville, MD: Author. Retrieved from www.ahrq.gov/research/find ings/nhqrdr/nhqdr16/index.html.
American Cancer Society (2018). *Cancer facts & figures*. Atlanta, GA: Author.
Anderson, K. J. (2018). Modern misogyny and backlash. In C. B. Travis & J. W. White (Eds), *APA handbook of the psychology of women* (Vol. 1, pp. 27–46). Washington, DC: American Psychological Association.
Bain, C., Willett, W., Rosner, B., Speizer, F. E., Belanger, C., & Hennekens, C. H. (1981). Early age at first birth and decreased risk of breast cancer. *American Journal of Epidemiology, 114*(5), 705–709.
Bandera, E. V., Lee, V. S., Rodriguez-Rodriguez, L., Powell, C. B., & Kushi, L. H. (2016). Racial/ethnic disparities in ovarian cancer treatment and survival. *Clinical Cancer Research, 22*(23), 5909–5914.
Beavis, A. L., Gravitt, P. E., & Rositch, A. F. (2017). Hysterectomy-corrected cervical cancer mortality rates reveal a larger racial disparity in the United States. *Cancer, 123*(6), 1044–1050.
Beral, V., Reeves, G., Bull, D., & Green, J. (2011). Breast cancer risk in relation to the interval between menopause and starting hormone therapy. *JNCI: Journal of the National Cancer Institute, 103*(4), 296–305.
Bernstein, L. (2002). Epidemiology of endocrine-related risk factors for breast cancer. *Journal of Mammary Gland Biology and Neoplasia, 7*(1, 1083–3021 (Print)), 3–15.
Binder, A. M., Corvalan, C., Mericq, V., Pereira, A., Santos, J. L., Horvath, S., Shepherd, J., & Michels, K. B. (2018). Faster ticking rate of the epigenetic clock is associated with faster pubertal development in girls. *Epigenetics, 13*(1), 85–94.
Bonadona, V., Bonaïti, B., Olschwang, S., Grandjouan, S., Huiart, L., & Longy, M., for the French Cancer Genetics Network (2011). Cancer risks associated with germline mutations in mlh1, msh2, and msh6 genes in Lynch syndrome. *JAMA: The Journal of the American Medical Association, 305*(22), 2304–2310.

Bosch, F. X., Robles, C., Díaz, M., Arbyn, M., Baussano, I., Clavel, C., Ronco, G., Dillner, J., Lehtinen, M., Petry, K.-U., Poljak, M., Kjaer, S. K., Meijer, C. J. L. M., Garland, S. M., Salmeron, J., Castellsague, X., Bruni, L., de Sanjose, S., & Cuzick, J. (2015). HPV-FASTER: Broadening the scope for prevention of HPV-related cancer. *Nature Reviews Clinical Oncology, 13*, 119.

Boyd, N. F., Guo, H., Martin, L. J., Sun, L., Stone, J., Fishell, E., Jong, R. A., Hislop, G., Chiarelli, A., Minkin, S., & Yaffe, M. J. (2007). Mammographic density and the risk and detection of breast cancer. *New England Journal of Medicine, 356*(3), 227–236.

Boyd, N. F., Martin, L. J., Bronskill, M., Yaffe, M. J., Duric, N., & Minkin, S. (2010). Breast tissue composition and susceptibility to breast cancer. *Journal of the National Cancer Institute, 102*(16), 1224–1237.

BreastCancer.org (2018). *U.S. breast cancer statistics.* Retrieved from www.breastcancer.org/symptoms/understand_bc/statistics.

Bruni, L., Diaz, M., Barrionuevo-Rosas, L., Herrero, R., Bray, F., Bosch, F. X., de Sanjose, S. & Castellsagué, X. (2016). Global estimates of human papillomavirus vaccination coverage by region and income level: A pooled analysis. *The Lancet Global Health, 4*(7), e453–e463.

Cadoo, K. A., Gucalp, A., & Traina, T. A. (2014). Palbociclib: An evidence-based review of its potential in the treatment of breast cancer. *Breast Cancer: Targets and Therapy, 6*, 123–133.

Cardoso, F., Van't Veer, L. J., Bogaerts, J., Slaets, L., Viale, G., Delaloge, S., Pierga, J.-Y., Brain, E., Causeret, S., DeLorenzi, M., Glas, A. M., Golfinopoulos, V., Goulioti, T., Knox, S., Matos, E., Meulemans, B., Neijenhuis, P. A., Nitz, U., Passalacqua, R., Ravdin, P., Rubio, I. T., Saghatchian, M., Smile, T. J., Sotiriou, C., Stork, L., Straehle, C., Thomas, G., Thompson, A. M., van der Hoeven, J. M., Vuylsteke, P., Bernards, R., Tryfondis, K., Rutgers, E., & Piccart, M. (2016). 70-Gene signature as an aid to treatment decisions in early-stage breast cancer. *New England Journal of Medicine, 375*(8), 717–729.

Cell Signaling Technology (2018). *Human oncogenes & tumor suppressor genes.* Danvers, MA: Author. Retrieved from www.cellsignal.com/contents/resources-reference-tables/human-oncogenes-amp-tumor-suppressor-genes/science-tables-oncogene.

Centers for Disease Control (CDC) (2017). *HPV and men.* Atlanta, GA: Author. Retrieved from www.cdc.gov/std/hpv/stdfact-hpv-and-men.htm.

Childers, K. K., Maggard-Gibbons, M., Macinko, J., & Childers, C. P. (2018). National distribution of cancer genetic testing in the United States: Evidence for a gender disparity in hereditary breast and ovarian cancer. *JAMA Oncology, 4*(6), 876–879.

Collaborative Group on Hormonal Factors in Breast Cancer (2012). Menarche, menopause, and breast cancer risk: Individual participant meta-analysis, including 118 964 women with breast cancer from 117 epidemiological studies. *The Lancet Oncology, 13*(11), 1141–1151.

Compton, K. (2018). Pfizer lawsuits and settlements. *DrugWatch.* Retrieved from www.drugwatch.com/manufacturers/pfizer.

Cristofanilli, M., Turner, N. C., Bondarenko, I., Ro, J., Im, S.-A., Masuda, N., Colleoni, M., DeMichele, A., Loi, S., Verma, S., Iwata, H., Harbeck, N., Zhang, K., Theall, K. P., Jiang, Y., Bartlett, C. H., Koehler, M., & Slamon, D. (2016). Fulvestrant plus palbociclib versus fulvestrant plus placebo for treatment of hormone-receptor-positive, HER2-negative metastatic breast cancer that progressed on previous endocrine therapy (PALOMA-3): Final analysis of the multicentre, double-blind, phase 3 randomised controlled trial. *The Lancet Oncology, 17*(4), 425–439.

Day, F. R., Ruth, K. S., Thompson, D. J., Lunetta, K. L., Pervjakova, N., Chasman, D. I., Stolk, L., Finucane, H. K., Sulem, P., Bulik-Sullivan, B., Esko, T., Johnson, A. D., Elks, C. E., Franceschini, N., He, C., Altmair, E., Brody, J. A., Franke, L. L., Huffman, J. E., Keller, M. F., McArdle, P. F., Nutile, T., Porcu, E., Robino, A., Rose, L. M., Schick, U. M., Smith, J. A., Teumer, A., Tragila, M., Vuckovic, D., Yao, J., Zhao, W., Albrecht, E., Amin, N., Corre, T., Hottenga, J.-J., Mangino, M., Smith, A. V., Tanaka, T., Abecasis, G. R., Andrulis, I. L., Anton-Culver, H., Antoniou, A. C., Arndt, V., Arnold, A. M., Barvieri, C., Beckman, M. W., Beeghly-Fadiel, A., Nenitez, L., Bernstein, L., Bielinski, S. J., Blomqvist, C., Boerinkle, E.., Bogdanova, N. V., Bojesen, S. E., Bolla, M. K., Borresen-Dale, A.-L., Boutin, T. S., Brauch, H., Brenner, H., Bruning, T., Burwinkel, B., Campbell, A., Campbell, H., Chanock, S. J., Chapman, J. R., Chen, Y.-D. I., Chenevix-Trench, G., Couch, F. J., Coviello, A. D., Cox, A., Czene, K., Darabi, H., DeVivo, I., Demerath, E. W., Dennis, J., Devilee, P., Dork, T., dos-Santos-Silva, I., Dunning, A. M., Eicher, J. D., Fasching, P. A., Faul, J. D., Figueroa, J., Flesch-Janys, D., Gandin, I., Garcia, M. E., Garcia-Closas, M., Giles, G. G., Girotto, G. G., Goldberg, M. S., Gonzalez-Neira, A., Goodarzi, M. O., Grove, M. L., Gudbjartsson, D. F., Guenel, P., Guo, X., Haiman, C. A., Hall, P., Hamann, U., Henderson, B. E., Hocking, L. J., Hofman, A.,

Homuth, G., Hooning, M. J., Hopper, J. L., Hu, J. B., Huang, J., Humphreys, K., Hunter, D. J., Jakubowska, A., Jones, S. E., Kabisch, M., Karasik, D., Knight, J. A., Kolcic, I., Kooperberg, C., Kosma, V.-M., Kriebel, J., Kristensne, V., Lambrechts, D., Langenberg, C., Li, J., Li, X., Lindstrom, S., Liu, Y., Luan, J., Lubinski, J., Magi, R., Mannermaa, A., Manz, J., Margolin, S., Marten, J., Martin, N. G., Masciullo, C., Meindi, A., Michailidou, K., Mihailov, E., Milani, L., Milne, R. L., Muller-Nurasyid, M., Nalls, M., Neale, B. M., Nevanlinna, H., Neven, P., Newman, A. B., Nordestgaard, B. G., Olson, J. E., Padmanabhan, S., Peterlongo, P., Peters, U., Petersman, A., Peto, J., Pharoah, P. D. P., Piratsu, N. N., Pirie, A., Pistis, O., Porteous, D., Psaty, B. M., Pylkas, K., Radice, P., Raffel, L. J., Rivadeneira, F., Rudan, I., Rudolph, A., Ruggiero, D., Sla, C. F., Sanna, S., Sawyer, E. J., Schlessinger, D., Schmidt, M. K., Schmidt, F., Schmutzler, R. K., Schoemaker, M. J., Scott, R. A., Seynaeve, C. M., Simard, J., Sorice, R., Southey, M. C., Stockl, D., Strauch, K., Swerdlow, A., Taylor, K. D., Thorsteinsdottir, U., Toland, A. E., Tomlinson, I., Truong, T., Tryggvadottir, L., Turner, S. T., Vozzi, D., Wang, Q., Wellons, M., Willemsen, G., Wilson, J. F., Winqvist, R., Wolffenbuttel, B. B. H. R., Wright, A. F., Yannoukakos, D., Zemunik, T., Zheng, W., Zygmut, M., Bergmann, S., Boomsma, D. I., Buring, J. E., Ferrucci, L., Montgomery, G. W., Gudnason, V., Spector, T. D., van Dujin, C. M., Alizadeh, B. Z., Ciullo, M., Crisponi, L., Easton, D. F., Gasparini, P. P., Gieger, C., Harris, T. B., Hayward, C., Kardia, S. L. R., Kraft, P., McKnight, B., Metsplu, A., Morrison, A. C., Reiner, A. P., Ridker, P. M., Rotter, J. I., Toniolo, D., Uitterlinden, A. G., Ulivi, S., Volzke, H., Wareham, N. J., Weir, D. R., Yerges-Armstron, L., Price, A. L., Stefansson, K., Visser, J. A., Ong, K. K., Chang-Clause, J., Murabito, J. M., Perry, J. R. B., & Murray, A. (2015). Large-scale genomic analyses link reproductive aging to hypothalamic signaling, breast cancer susceptibility and BRCA1-mediated DNA repair. *Nature Genetics, 47,* 1294.

de Martel, C., Plummer, M., Vignat, J., & Franceschi, S. (2017). Worldwide burden of cancer attributable to HPV by site, country and HPV type. *International Journal of Cancer, 141*(4), 664–670.

Dougherty, B. A., Lai, Z., Hodgson, D. R., Orr, M. C. M., Hawryluk, M., Sun, J., Yelensky, R., Spencer, S. K., Robertson, J. D., Ho, T. W., Fielding, A., Ledermann, J. A., & Barrett, J. C. (2017). Biological and clinical evidence for somatic mutations in BRCA1 and BRCA2 as predictive markers for olaparib response in high-grade serous ovarian cancers in the maintenance setting. *Oncotarget, 8*(27), 43653–43661.

Duffy, M. J., O'Donovan, N., McDermott, E., & Crown, J. (2016). Validated biomarkers: The key to precision treatment in patients with breast cancer. *Breast, 29*(2016), 192–201.

Early Breast Cancer Trialists' Collaborative Group (EBCTCG) (2015). Aromatase inhibitors versus tamoxifen in early breast cancer: Patient-level meta-analysis of the randomised trials. *The Lancet, 386*(10001), 1341–1352.

Eliassen, A. H., Colditz, G. A., Rosner, B., Willett, W. C., & Hankinson, S. E. (2006). Adult weight change and risk of postmenopausal breast cancer. *JAMA: The Journal of the American Medical Association, 296*(2), 193–201.

Fletcher, S. W. & Colditz, G. A. (2002). Failure of estrogen plus progestin therapy for prevention. *JAMA: The Journal of the American Medical Association, 288*(3), 366–368.

Gartlehner, G., Patel, S. V., Feltner, C., Weber, R. P., Long, R., Mullican, K., Boland, E., Lux, L., & Viswanathan, M. (2017). Hormone therapy for the primary prevention of chronic conditions in postmenopausal women: Evidence report and systematic review for the US Preventive Services Task Force. *JAMA: The Journal of the American Medical Association, 318*(22), 2234–2249.

Glick, P. & Raberg, L. (2018). Benevolent sexism and the status of women. In C. B. Travis & J. W. White (Eds), *APA handbook of the psychology of women* (Vol. 1, pp. 363–380). Washington, DC: American Psychological Association.

Hall, M. T., Simms, K. T., Lew, J.-B., Smith, M. A., Brotherton, J. M. L., Saville, M., Frazer, I. H., & Canfell, K. (2019). The projected timeframe until cervical cancer elimination in Australia: A modelling study. *The Lancet Public Health, 4*(10), e19–e27.

Ho, J. M., Jafferjee, N., Covarrubias, G. M., Ghesani, M., & Handler, B. (2014). Dense breasts: A review of reporting legislation and available supplemental screening options. *American Journal of Roentgenology, 203*(2), 449–456.

Hollstein, M., Sidransky, D., Vogelstein, B., & Harris, C. C. (1991). p53 mutations in human cancers. *Science, 253*(5015), 49–53.

Hortobagyi, G. N., Stemmer, S. M., Burris, H. A., Yap, Y.-S., Sonke, G. S., Paluch-Shimon, S., Campone, M., Blackwell, K. L., André, F., Winer, E. P., Janni, W., Verma, S., Conte, P., Arteaga, C. L.,

Cameron, D. A., Petrakova, K., Hart, L. L., Villanueva, C., Chan, A., Jakobsen, E., Nusch, A., Burdaeva, O., Grischke, E. M., Alba, E., Wist, E., Marschner, N., Favret, A. M., Yardley, D., Bachelot, T., Tseng, L. M., Blau, S., Xuan, F., Souami, F., Miller, M., Germa, C., Hirawat, S., & O'Shaughnessy, J. (2016). Ribociclib as first-line therapy for hr-positive, advanced breast cancer. *New England Journal of Medicine, 375*(18), 1738–1748.

Hulme, J., Moravac, C., Ahmad, F., Cleverly, S., Lofters, A., Ginsburg, O., & Dunn, S. (2016). "I want to save my life": Conceptions of cervical and breast cancer screening among urban immigrant women of South Asian and Chinese origin. *BioMed Central Public Health, 16*(No. 1077).

Hussain, S. P., Hofseth, L. J., & Harris, C. C. (2001). Tumor suppressor genes: At the crossroads of molecular carcinogenesis, molecular epidemiology and human risk assessment. *Lung Cancer, 34*, S7–S15.

Institute of Medicine (IOM): Committee on Quality of Health Care in America (2001). *Crossing the quality chasm: A new health system for the 21st century.* Washington, DC: National Academy Press.

International Agency for Research on Cancer (2018a). *Estimated age-standardized incidence rates (World) in 2018, vulva, vagina, corpus uteri, ovary, cervix uteri, females, all ages.* Lyon, France: Gobal Cancer Observatory. Retrieved from http://gco.iarc.fr/today/explore.

International Agency for Research on Cancer (2018b). *Estimated number of prevalent cases (5-year) as a proportion in 2018, breast, females, all ages (by country).* Lyon, France: Gobal Cancer Observatory. Retrieved from http://gco.iarc.fr/today/explore.

International Agency for Research on Cancer (2018c). *Estimated number of prevalent cases in 2018, breast, females, all ages.* Lyon, France: Global Cancer Observatory. Retrieved from http://gco.iarc.fr/today/explore.

Kane, M. A. & Giuliano, A. R. (2018). Eliminating HPV-related diseases as a public health problem: Let's start with cervical cancer. In X. F. Bosch (Ed.), *HPV world* (Vols 27–37, pp. 42–49). Barcelona, Spain: VEGA.

Kavanagh, K., Pollock, K. G., Cuschieri, K., Palmer, T., Cameron, R. L., Watt, C., Bhatia, R., Moore, C., Cubie, H., Cruickshank, M., & Robertson, C. (2017). Changes in the prevalence of human papillomavirus following a national bivalent human papillomavirus vaccination programme in Scotland: A 7-year cross-sectional study. *The Lancet Infectious Diseases, 17*(12), 1293–1302.

Keenan, T., Moy, B., Mroz, E. A., Ross, K., Niemierko, A., Rocco, J. W., Isakoff, S., Ellisen, L.W., & Bardia, A. (2015). Comparison of the genomic landscape between primary breast cancer in African American versus White women and the association of racial differences with tumor recurrence. *Journal of Clinical Oncology, 33*(31), 3621–3627.

Kershaw, E. E. & Flier, J. S. (2004). Adipose tissue as an endocrine organ. *The Journal of Clinical Endocrinology & Metabolism, 89*(6), 2548–2556.

Kuchenbaecker, K. B., Hopper, J. L., Barnes, D. R., Phillips, K.-A., Mooij, T. M., Roos-Blom, M.-J., Jervis, S., van Leeuwen, F. E., Milne, R. L., Andrieu, N., Goldgar, D. E., Terry, M. B., Rookus, M. A., Easton, D. F., & Antoniou, A. C. (2017). Risks of breast, ovarian, and contralateral breast cancer for BRAC1 and BRAC2 mutation carriers. *JAMA: The Journal of the American Medical Association, 317*(23), 2402–2416.

Kurian, A. W., Bondarenko, I., Jagsi, R., Friese, C. R., McLeod, M. C., Hawley, S. T., Hamilton, A. S., Ward, K. C., Hofer, T. P., & Katz, S. J. (2018). Recent trends in chemotherapy use and oncologists treatment recommendations for early stage breast cancer. *Journal of the National Cancer Institute, 110*(5), 493–500.

Kyrgiou, M., Kalliala, I., Markozannes, G., Gunter, M. J., Paraskevaidis, E., Gabra, H., Martin-Hirsch, P., & Tsilidis, K. K. (2017). Adiposity and cancer at major anatomical sites: Umbrella review of the literature. *British Medical Journal, 356*(j477).

Ladner, J., Besson, M.-H., Hampshire, R., Tapert, L., Chirenje, M., & Saba, J. (2012). Assessment of eight HPV vaccination programs implemented in lowest income countries. *BMC Public Health, 12*(1), 370.

Lofters, A., Moineddin, R., Hwang, S., & Glazier, R. (2010). Low rates of cervical cancer screening among urban immigrants: A population-based study in Ontario, Canada. *Medical Care, 48*(7), 611–618.

Manson, J. E. (2013). *Menopausal hormone therapy and health outcomes during the intervention and extended post-stopping phase of the women's health initiative randomized trials: Executive summary questions & answers.* Bethesda, MA: U.S. National Institutes of Health. Retrieved from www.whi.org/Documents/Global%20Paper%20Q%20and%20A.pdf.

Manson, J. E., Chlebowski, R. T., Stefanick, M. L., Aragaki, A. K., Rossouw, J. E., Prentice, R. L., Anderson, G., Howard, B. V., Thomson, C. A., LaCroix, A. Z., Wactawski-Wende, J., Jackson, R. D., Limacher, M., Margolis, K. L., Wassertheil-Smoller, S., Beresford, S. A., Cauley, J. A., Eaton, C. B.,

Gass, M., Hsia, J., Johnson, K. C., Kooperberg, C. B., Kuller, L. H., Lewis, C. E., Liu, S., Martin, L. W., Ockene, J. K., O'Sullivan, M. J., Powell, L. H., Simon, M. S., Van Horn, L., Vitolinis, M. Z., & Wallace, R. B. (2013). Menopausal hormone therapy and health outcomes during the intervention and extended poststopping phases of the women's health initiative randomized trials. *JAMA: The Journal of the American Medical Association, 310*(13), 1353–1368.

Manson, J. E., Hsia, J., Johnson, K. C., Rossouw, J. E., Assaf, A. R., Lasser, N. L., Trevisan, M., Black, H. R., Heckbert, S. R., Detrano, R., Strickland, O. L., Wong, N. D., Crouse, J. R., & Cushman, M. (2003). Estrogen plus progestin and the risk of coronary heart disease. *New England Journal of Medicine, 349*(6), 523–534.

Meier-Abt, F. & Bentires-Alj, M. (2014). How pregnancy at early age protects against breast cancer. *Trends in Molecular Medicine, 20*(3), 143–153.

Miller, J. W., Smith, J. L., Ryerson, A. B., Tucker, T. C., & Allemani, C. (2017). Disparities in breast cancer survival in the United States (2001–2009): Findings from the CONCORD-2 study. *Cancer, 123*, 5100–5118.

Mukohara, T. (2015). PI3K mutations in breast cancer: Prognostic and therapeutic implications. *Breast Cancer: Targets and Therapy, 7*, 111–123.

Nadji, M., Gomez-Fernandez, C., Ganjei-Azar, P., & Morales, A. R. (2005). Immunohistochemistry of estrogen and progesterone receptors reconsidered experience with 5,993 breast cancers. *American Journal of Clinical Pathology, 123*(1), 21–27.

Narod, S. A., Iqbal, J., Giannakeas, V., Sopik, V., & Sun, P. (2015). Breast cancer mortality after a diagnosis of ductal carcinoma in situ. *JAMA: The Journal of the American Medical Association: Oncology, 1*(7), 888–896.

National Cancer Institute (NCI) (2018). Surveillance, epidemiology, and end results program. *Cancer Stat Facts*. Bethesda, MD: Author. Retrieved from https://seer.cancer.gov/statfacts/html/ovary.html.

Nature Education (2014). CDK. *Scitable*. Cambridge, MA: Author. Retrieved from www.nature.com/scitable/topicpage/cdk-14046166.

Nelson, L. R. & Bulun, S. E. (2001). Estrogen production and action. *Journal of the American Academy of Dermatology, 45*(3, Supplement), S116–S124.

Osman, M. A. (2014). Genetic cancer ovary. *Clinical Ovarian and Other Gynecologic Cancer, 7*(1), 1–7.

Paik, S., Shak, S., Tang, G., Kim, C., Baker, J., Cronin, M., Baehner, F. L., Walker, M. G., Watson, D., Park, T., Hiller, W., Fisher, E. R., Wickerham, L., Bryant, J., & Wolmark, N. (2004). A multigene assay to predict recurrence of tamoxifen-treated, node-negative breast cancer. *New England Journal of Medicine, 351*(27), 2817–2826.

Paik, S., Tang, G., Shak, S., Kim, C., Baker, J., Kim, W., Cronin, M., Baehner, F. L., Watson, D., Bryant, J., Costantino, J. P., Geyer, C. E. Jr, Wickerham, D. L., & Wolmark, N. (2006). Gene expression and benefit of chemotherapy in women with node-negative, estrogen receptor–positive breast cancer. *Journal of Clinical Oncology, 24*(23), 3726–3734.

Peshkin, B. N., Alabek, M. L., & Isaacs, C. (2011). BRCA1/2 mutations and triple negative breast cancers. *Breast Disease, 32*(1/2), 25–33.

Philippidis, A. (2018). Top 10 best-selling cancer drugs, Q1–Q3 2017. *Genetic Engineering & Biotechnology News*: The lists. Retrieved from www.genengnews.com/the-lists/top-10-best-selling-cancer-drugs-q1q3-2017/77901033.

Prentice, R. L., Chlebowski, R. T., Stefanick, M. L., Manson, J. E., Pettinger, M., Hendrix, S. L., Hubbell, F. A., Kooperberg, C., Kuller, L. H., Lane, D. S., McTiernan, A., O'Sullivan, M. J., Rossouw, J. E., & Anderson, G. L. (2008). Estrogen plus progestin therapy and breast cancer in recently postmenopausal women. *American Journal of Epidemiolgy, 167*(10), 1207–1216.

Rao, A., Young, S., Erlich, H., Boyle, S., Krevolin, M., Sun, R., Apple, R., & Behrens, C. (2013). Development and characterization of the cobas human papillomavirus test. *Journal of Clinical Microbiology, 51*(5), 1478–1484.

Romero-Laorden, N. & Castro, E. (2017). Inherited mutations in DNA repair genes and cancer risk. *Current Problems in Cancer, 41*(4), 251–264.

Rossouw, J. E., Prentice, R. L., Manson, J. E., Wu, L., Barad, D., Barnabei, V. M., Ko, M., LaCroix, A. Z., Margolis, K. L., & Stefanick, M. L. (2007). Postmenopausal hormone therapy and risk of cardiovascular disease by age and years since menopause. *JAMA: The Journal of the American Medical Association, 297*(13), 1465–1477.

Russo, J. (2016). Reproductive history and breast cancer prevention. *Hormone Molecular Biology and Clinical Investigation, 27*(1), 3–10.

Schoen, C., Guterman, S., Shih, A., Lau, J., Kasimow, S., Gauthier, A., & Davis, K. (2007). *Bending the curve: Options for achieving savings and improving value in U.S. health spending.* Washington, DC: The Commonwealth Fund, pub. no. 1080. Retrieved from www.commonwealthfund.org/publications/ fund-reports/2007/dec/bending-the-curve–options-for-achieving-savings-and-improving-value-in-u-s–health-spending.

Shah, S. S., Senapati, S., Klacsmann, F., Miller, D. L., Johnson, J. J., Chang, H.-C., & Stack, M. S. (2016). Current technologies and recent developments for screening of HPV-associated cervical and oropharyngeal cancers. *Cancers, 8*(9), 85.

Shrader, K. A. (2017). The role of hereditary factors in ovarian carcinoma. *Clinical Obstetrics & Gynecology, 60*(4), 728–737.

Singer, N. & Wilson, D. (2009). Menopause as brought to you by big pharma. *New York Times.* Retrieved from www.nytimes.com/2009/12/13/business/13drug.html.

Sledge, G. W., Toi, M., Neven, P., Sohn, J., Inoue, K., Pivot, X., Burdaeva, O., Okera, M., Masuda, N., Kaufman, P. A., Koh, H., Grischke, E.-M., Frenzel, M., Lin, Y., Barringa, S., Smith, I. C., Bourayou, N., & Llombart-Cussac, A. (2017). MONARCH 2: Abemaciclib in combination with fulvestrant in women with HR+/HER2− advanced breast cancer who had progressed while receiving endocrine therapy. *Journal of Clinical Oncology, 35*(25), 2875–2884.

Sparano, J. A., Gray, R. J., Makower, D. F., Pritchard, K. I., Albain, K. S., Hayes, D. F., Geyer, C. E., Dees, E. C., Perez, E. A., Olson, J. A., Zujewski, J., Lively, T., Badve, S. S., Saphner, T. J., Wagner, L. I., Whelan, T. J., Ellis, M. J., Paik, S., Woods, P., Keene, M. M., Moreno, H. L. G., Reddy, P. S., Goggins, T. F., Mayer, I. A., Brufsky, A. M., Toppmeyer, D. L., Kaklamani, V. G., Atkins, J. N., Berenberg, J. L., & Sledge, G. W. (2015). Prospective validation of a 21-gene expression assay in breast cancer. *New England Journal of Medicine, 373*(21), 2005–2014.

Sparano, J. A., Gray, R. J., Makower, D. F., Pritchard, K. I., Albain, K. S., Hayes, D. F., Geyer, C. G., Dees, E. C., Goetz, M. P., Olson, J. A., Lively, T., Badve, S. S., Saphner, T. J., Wagner, L. I., Whelen, T. J., Ellis, M. J., Paik, S., Wood, W. C., Ravdin, P. M., Keane, M. M., Moreno, H. L. G., Reddy, P. S., Goggins, T. F., Mayer, I. A., Brufsky, A. M., Toppmeyer, D. L., Kaklamani, V. G., Berenberg, J. L., Abrams, J., & Sledge, G. W. (2018). Adjuvant chemotherapy guided by a 21-gene expression assay in breast cancer. *New England Journal of Medicine, 379*, 111–121.

Stewart, S. L., Harewood, R., Matz, M., Rim, S. H., Sabatino, S. A., Ward, K. C., & Weir, H. K. (2017). Disparities in ovarian cancer survival in the United States (2001–2009): Findings from the CONCORD-2 study. *Cancer, 123*, 5138–5159.

Sundquist, M., Brudin, L., & Tejler, G. (2016). Improved survival in metastatic breast cancer 1985–2016. *The Breast, 31*, 46–50.

Tamimi, R. M., Spiegelman, D., Smith-Warner, S. A., Wang, M., Pazaris, M., Willett, W. C., Eliassen, A. H., & Hunter, D. J. (2016). Population attributable risk of modifiable and nonmodifiable breast cancer risk factors in postmenopausal breast cancer. *American Journal of Epidemiology, 184*(12), 884–893.

The Cancer Genome Atlas Network, Koboldt, D. C., Fulton, R. S., McLellan, M. D., Schmidt, H., Kalicki-Veizer, J., & Palchik, J. D. (2012). Comprehensive molecular portraits of human breast tumours. *Nature, 490*, 61. Retrieved from www.nature.com/articles/nature11412#supplementary-information.

The Cancer Genome Atlas Network (2012). Comprehensive molecular portraits of human breast tumours. *Nature, 490*, 61, doi:10.1038/nature11412.

Torre, L. A., Islami, F., Siegel, R. L., Ward, E. M., & Jemal, A. (2017). Global cancer in women: Burden and trends. *Cancer Epidemiology Biomarkers & Prevention, 26*, 444–457.

Turner, N. C., Ro, J., André, F., Loi, S., Verma, S., Iwata, H., Harbeck, N., Loibl, S., Bartlett, C. H., Zhang, K., Giorgetti, C., Randolph, S., Koehler, M., & Cristofanilli, M. (2015). Palbociclib in hormone-receptor–positive advanced breast cancer. *New England Journal of Medicine, 373*(3), 209–219.

US Preventive Services Task Force (2017). *Hormone therapy for the primary prevention of chronic conditions in postmenopausal women*: US Preventive Services Task Force recommendation statement. *JAMA: The Journal of the American Medical Association, 318*(22), 2224–2233.

U.S. Preventive Services Task Force (2018). *Screening for cervical cancer*: US Preventive Services Task Force recommendation statement. *JAMA: The Journal of the American Medical Association, 320*(7), 674–686.

Vogelstein, B., Papadopoulos, N., Velculescu, V. E., Zhou, S., Diaz, L. A., & Kinzler, K. W. (2013). Cancer genome landscapes. *Science, 339*(6127), 1546–1558.

Wolff, A. C. (2016). CDK4 and CDK6 inhibition in breast cancer — A new standard. *New England Journal of Medicine, 375*(20), 1993–1994.

Writing Group for the Women's Health Initiative Investigators (2002). Risks and benefits of estrogen plus progestin in healthy postmenopausal women: Principal results from the women's health initiative randomized control trial. *JAMA: The Journal of the American Medical Association, 2002*(3), 321–333.

Xiong, H., Murphy, M., Mathews, M., Gadag, V., & Wang, P. P. (2010). Cervical cancer screening among Asian Canadian immigrant and nonimmigrant women. *American Journal of Health Behavior, 34*(2), 131–143.

Yoo, W., Kim, S., Huh, W., Dilley, S., Coughlin, S., Partridge, E., Chung, Y., Dicks, V., Lee, J.-K., & Bae, S. (2017). Recent trends in racial and regional disparities in cervical cancer incidence and mortality in United States. *Plos One, 12*(2), e0172548.

10

PSYCHOSOCIAL ASPECTS OF WOMEN'S SEXUAL AND REPRODUCTIVE WELL-BEING AFTER CANCER

Chloe Parton

Cancer is a significant health issue for women everywhere in the world (Gibberd, 2000). As survivorship rates rise in developed countries, quality of life research has been prioritised (Duffy & Allen, 2009). Regardless of the type of cancer, many women report a range of body changes that directly influence reproductive and sexual health, including premature menopause, vaginal dryness, vaginal shortening and narrowing, scarring of vaginal tissue, pain during intercourse, and changed physiological sexual responses that can diminish sexual desire and impair arousal and orgasm (Aerts, Enzlin, Verhaeghe, Vergote, & Amant, 2009; Donovan et al., 2007). Additional body changes (e.g., scarring, disfigurement, weight loss or gain, fatigue, impaired bladder and bowel functioning) are associated with reduced feelings of sexual attractiveness (Gilbert, Ussher, & Perz, 2011). Sexual and reproductive changes can persist long after the conclusion of treatment, with detrimental consequences for women's psychological well-being (Carter et al., 2010), intimate relationships, and sense of feminine identity (Perz, Ussher, & Gilbert, 2014).

Existing research in women's sexual and reproductive health after cancer has focussed on breast and gynecological cancers, primarily through a biomedical or psychological lens (Gilbert, Ussher, & Perz, 2010, 2011). However, women can experience disruption to sexual and reproductive well-being following treatment for a wide range of tumor types (Ussher, Perz, & Gilbert, 2015), and it is equally important to acknowledge the sociocultural context and role of cultural discourse in understanding women's cancer experiences (Gilbert et al., 2010).

In this chapter we provide a review of psychosocial aspects and adjustment to diagnosis and treatment of reproductive cancer, with a focus on body dissatisfaction and sexual embodiment. We draw on interviews we have conducted with women and include discussion of the impact of a broader range of cancers on sexual and reproductive well-being, where relevant. The context of women's lives is considered in a review of the influence of life stage and couple relationships on adjustment. Finally, a review of the implications of sociocultural context and the role of cultural discourse on current cancer research is also provided.

Women's experiences of body dissatisfaction after cancer

It does take a little bit of getting used to being lopsided, and coping with a horrible scar ... It does make a difference to the way you feel about yourself (62 years, breast and throat cancers).

One of the most widespread psychological consequences of cancer treatment is a change in women's feelings about their bodies, manifested as negative body image (Avis, Crawford, & Manuel, 2004; Moreira et al., 2011) and decreased feelings of sexual attractiveness (Beckjord & Compas, 2007; Reich, Lesur, & Perdrizet-Chevallier, 2008). The majority of studies in this area have focussed on body dissatisfaction in women with breast cancer (Gilbert et al., 2010). However, women with gynaecological (Hawighorst-Knapstein et al., 2004), colorectal (Manderson, 2005), and rectal (Benedict et al., 2016) cancers have also reported diminished body image. Body dissatisfaction following cancer is associated with lower emotional well-being and higher psychological distress (Mattsson et al., 2018; Moreira et al., 2011), loss of femininity (Archibald, Lemieux, Byers, Tamlyn, & Worth, 2006), and alterations to the sexual self (Wilmoth, 2001). A number of factors that increase the likelihood of distress associated with body dissatisfaction following cancer have been identified, including the impact of surgical treatments for breast cancer, hair loss due to chemotherapy, and individual psychological factors, which are outlined in detail below.

Common surgical treatments for breast cancer include breast conserving treatment (lumpectomy and radiation treatment) and mastectomy with or without reconstruction. Breasts are positioned as such a significant part of women's sense of self that having one breast is associated with being 'half a woman' (Manderson & Stirling, 2007, p. 82). This is reflected in findings that women who have had a mastectomy report greater body dissatisfaction than do those who have had breast conserving surgery, both immediately after surgery (Markopoulos et al., 2009) and at longer term follow-up (Lee, Sunu, & Pignone, 2009). Some women report body satisfaction following breast reconstruction (Nicholson, Leinster, & Sassoon, 2007; Rubino, Figus, Lorettu, & Sechi, 2007), whereas other women who experience reconstruction are not more satisfied than those who have had mastectomy alone (Avis et al., 2004). Breast reconstruction can assist in creating a physical appearance that appears 'normal' under clothing (Lee et al., 2009); however, it does not remove the psychological perception of having 'abnormal' breasts. For example, the absence of sensation, cold skin, and coming to terms with a new 'artificial' part of the body can be difficult for women (Snell et al., 2010).

Chemotherapy-induced hair loss has been examined as a significant source of body dissatisfaction amongst women. Hair signifies feminine identity, defines facial features, and is a visible identifier of cancer (Trusson & Pilnick, 2017); 52% of women with breast cancer report fear of negative judgement from others following hair loss (Pierrisnard et al., 2018). In this vein, hair loss has been associated with greater body dissatisfaction for women (Lemieux, Maunsell, & Provencher, 2008), and it is reported to be one of the most traumatic aspects of cancer treatment (Trusson & Pilnick, 2017). One qualitative study showed that women were more likely than men to talk about hair loss on their heads than on other parts of their body and to be encouraged by others to cover up their hair loss (with scarves, wigs, or hats) (Hilton, Hunt, Emslie, Salinas, & Ziebland, 2008). Some women have reported cutting their hair off before losing it through chemotherapy, as a way of coping by taking control back from cancer and its treatment (Frith, Harcourt, & Fussell, 2007).

In an attempt to understand the psychological factors that contribute to body dissatisfaction following cancer, some researchers have examined women's investment in body appearance. Results show that women who place greater importance on physical appearance report lower psychosocial adjustment and appearance satisfaction and higher body shame and self-consciousness following cancer (Moreira, Silva, & Canavarro, 2010). In contrast, self-compassion (Sherman, Woon, French, & Elder, 2017) and greater effort taken to feel attractive are associated with higher levels of psychosocial adjustment and lower psychological distress post cancer (Moreira et al., 2010). The majority of this research has been conducted with heterosexual women and reflects the relative invisibility of lesbian, bisexual, and queer women in cancer research (Quinn et al., 2015). However, there is some evidence that lesbians with breast cancer report less concern about their appearance following cancer (Fish, 2010) than heterosexual women do, and some lesbians have described themselves as 'better off' than heterosexual women, due to their partner's empathy and less focus on bodily appearance within their relationships (Boehmer, Miao, & Ozonoff, 2011, p. x). There is some evidence that African American women are less likely than European women to undergo breast-reconstruction, and more likely to accept a changed body, following breast cancer (Rubin, Chavez, Alderman, & Pusic, 2013). In combination, such findings suggest that intrapsychic factors (e.g., self-compassion, a sense of agency associated with embodiment), as well as sexual and cultural identities, can act to buffer women from detrimental psychological outcomes as a result of embodied changes following cancer.

Women's experiences of sexual well-being after cancer

I lost my libido completely and that was really hard … it became not a sexual relationship at all (20 years, acute myeloid leukaemia).

I used to be keen on having lots of sex and I still am, the thoughts there. It just seems so, so horrifying and an awful thing to do to my poor partner cause I'm just not the right shape and up to scratch anymore (47 years, colorectal cancer).

Changes in sexual desire, satisfaction, and activity are common consequences of cancer treatment for both women and men, across both reproductive and non-reproductive cancers (Perz et al., 2014). The focus has often been on coital sexual activity, but many women report that non-coital sexual activities (e.g., kissing, caressing, sexual fantasy) are also reduced (Tang, Lai, & Chung, 2010; Ussher et al., 2015). Some women resume sexual activity following treatment and into recovery (Préau, Bouhnik, Rey, & Mancini, 2011), but, for others, sexual pleasure and overall quality and satisfaction of their sexual relationship is reduced long-term post-cancer (Stafford & Judd, 2010). Furthermore, coital sex can remain problematic for heterosexual women, and, in some cases, is no longer possible due to physiological and anatomical changes or loss of sexual desire (Ussher, Perz, Gilbert, Wong, & Hobbs, 2013).

A bi-directional relationship between psychological distress and sexual functioning after cancer has been identified. Women who report sexual problems after cancer also report higher rates of psychological distress (Perz et al., 2014; Ussher, Perz, & Gilbert, 2012); distress is also a risk factor for impaired sexual functioning (Levin et al., 2010) and reduced sexual satisfaction post-cancer (Webber et al., 2011). In non-cancer studies, women's body image concerns have been shown to contribute to difficulties with sexual functioning (Woertman & van Den Brink, 2012). Specifically, cultural pressures to be sexually attractive inform the likelihood of women engaging in self-objectification with resultant increased monitoring and consciousness of the body, rather than attending to pleasurable sensory experiences during sex. Subsequently, physiological sexual responses are impaired (Sanchez

& Kiefer, 2007). In this vein, women with cancer who are dissatisfied with their bodies are more likely than others to report disrupted sexual functioning, reduced sexual interest (Donovan et al., 2007), sexual discomfort (Liavaag et al., 2008), and conscious monitoring of their bodies during sex (Parton, Ussher, & Perz, 2017b).

Changes to sexual functioning and psychological distress may be associated with onset of early menopause after cancer (Mann, Singer, Pitkin, Panay, & Hunter, 2012); higher levels of psychological distress are associated with greater incidence and severity of menopausal symptoms (Carter et al., 2010). Psychological distress has been linked to the threat posed by premature menopause to women's gendered identity, including fertility, femininity, and sexual functioning (Howard-Anderson, Ganz, Bower, & Stanton, 2012). For example, women who experience infertility after cancer report a sense of biographical disruption (Ussher, Perz, & The Australian Cancer and Fertility Study Team, 2018), which is associated with psychological distress and lowered quality of life, particularly if women have not already had a child at the time of diagnosis (Canada & Schover, 2012). Furthermore, many women report sexual changes following menopause-inducing cancer treatment, including vaginal dryness, pain on intercourse, and diminished sexual desire, which impact their intimate relationships and sense of feminine identity (Rogers & Kristjanson, 2002). Especially when accompanied by changes to body hair, weight, and mood, early menopause has been described by cancer survivors as 'devastating', and 'unexpected', and leading to a feeling of being old before their time (Ussher, Perz, & Parton, 2015).

The influence of life-stage and relational context on women's sexual and reproductive well-being after cancer

I was single before and I was running around doing a million things in life … then I was sort of confronted with the fertility at the time and I'm like, 'Holy moly, okay, yes, this is something that I wanted to think about in 5 years' (25 years, Hodgkin's lymphoma).

He doesn't even notice that you're lopsided, he doesn't notice that you've only got one breast anymore. And he made me to start to feel more comfortable with my body (71 years, breast cancer).

Life stage is one factor that may influence a woman's ability to adjust to changes to sexual embodiment following cancer. A number of studies suggest that younger pre-menopausal women do not cope as well psychologically as older post-menopausal women. For example, younger women report higher levels of psychological distress following cancer, both in general and in relation to impaired sexual functioning (Schmidt, Bestmann, Küchler, Longo, & Kremer, 2005). Furthermore, adolescents and young adult women who are diagnosed with cancer may experience challenges to their body image and sexuality at a time in life when identity and confidence are still developing, which can contribute to concerns about future relationships (Soanes & White, 2018). In contrast, older post-menopausal women report more general physical symptoms and slower recovery from cancer (Arndt et al., 2004). However, they also report lower cancer-related anxiety and general psychological distress and greater body satisfaction (Parker et al., 2007), despite lower sexual functioning (Likes, Stegbauer, Tillmanns, & Pruett, 2007).

A woman's relational context may also influence her adjustment to cancer. The range of physical, psychological, and relational challenges that result from cancer can create complex dynamics within couples, regardless of existing relationship quality (Sprung, Janotha, & Steckel, 2011; Ussher, Wong, & Perz, 2011). Both partners have been found to influence each other's coping strategies and distress (Badr, Carmack, Kashy, Cristofanilli, & Revenson, 2010), which suggests that cancer can be conceptualised as a 'we' disease (Kayser, Watson, & Andrade, 2007, p. 404). The experience of cancer may result in a woman's intimate part- ner viewing her differently; for example, there may be a shift from a sexual/romantic dynamic to a parent–child or patient–carer dynamic (Gilbert, Ussher, & Hawkins, 2009). Subsequently, the partner may assume a protective role, where the focus of the relationship is on caring for the woman with cancer (Fergus & Gray, 2009), rather than on the carer's needs, including sexual concerns. These changes may serve to de-sexualise women with cancer and disrupt sexual dynamics within intimate relationships, which has consequences for both partners (Hawkins et al., 2009).

In addition to a decline in sexual activity, many couples experience a decrease in intim- acy following cancer (Ussher et al., 2011), which can threaten attachment within the rela- tionship (Abbott-Anderson & Kwekkeboom, 2012). Couples who are more flexible with their sexual practices and notions of 'sexual functioning' (Reese, 2011), and who engage in non-coital sexual practices (Ussher et al., 2013), are able to renegotiate their sexual relation- ship with more success than couples who adhere to the notion of non-coital sexual practices as not 'real' sex or as only a precursor to sex. There is some evidence that lesbian and queer women experience less disruption to sexual functioning after cancer (Boehmer, Potter, & Bowen, 2009; Ussher, Perz, & Gilbert, 2014) as a consequence of sexual repertoires posi- tioned outside of the coital imperative, as well as a supportive relational context. In general, couples who place a stronger emphasis on intimacy through non-sexual physical touch and communication show stronger relational adjustment following cancer (Reese, 2011). For some couples, maintaining their sexual relationship, despite complications, can be a way of maintaining normalcy during cancer (Lindau, Surawska, Paice, & Baron, 2011).

The quality of the couple relationship can act as a buffer against detrimental psychological affects and sexual changes for women with cancer (Moreira et al., 2011; Tang et al., 2010). For example, women who report higher levels of relationship quality and intimacy also report higher levels of physical quality of life and fewer body image concerns (Moreira et al., 2011). Partner initiation of sex is associated with greater relationship satisfaction fol- lowing breast cancer, whereas adverse partner reactions to surgery scars predict reduced rela- tionship satisfaction (Wimberly, Carver, Laurenceau, Harris, & Antoni, 2005). Similarly, women's higher perceptions of men's relationship satisfaction predict those women's higher levels of self-acceptance better body image (Zimmermann, Scott, & Heinrichs, 2010). In one study, partner support was considered important by women who were adjusting to an ostomy prosthetic bag (Altschuler et al., 2009). The women described 'good' partner support as giving assurances about their body, femininity, and sexual desirability; using language that was comforting; and normalising the ostomy (Altschuler et al., 2009). Similar findings have been reported in relation to partner normalisation of mastectomy or breast reconstruction (Ussher et al., 2012). In combination, these findings suggest that women's perceptions of their bodies and identities as 'desirable' and 'sexual' are shaped by their relational context.

Compared with women in a relationship, women without long-term partners have reported greater feelings of embarrassment, concern about sexual attractiveness and weight loss or gain (Fobair et al., 2006), and psychological distress post-cancer (Ates et al., 2016; Klügel et al., 2017). Single women may be particularly vulnerable following cancer without an intim- ate partner to provide social support (Leung, Smith, & McLaughlin, 2016). Many unpartnered women encounter barriers to entering a relationship including fears regarding initiating a sexual relationship, uncertainty about when to disclose their cancer to a new partner, worry about the possibility of rejection (Ramirez et al., 2010), and concerns about a future partner's reaction to the possibility of infertility (Ussher, 2018). Such findings suggest that unpartnered women face additional challenges when adjusting to the impact of cancer on sexual and reproductive embodiment compared with women with a supportive partner.

Acknowledging the discursive context of women's sexual embodiment after cancer

It is important to acknowledge the discursive context within which women make sense of changes to sexual embodiment after cancer and the ways in which such embodied change has been discursively constructed in research. Discourses, as shared cultural meanings that are organised within socio-cultural contexts, shape the meanings that are available to women to make sense of their lived experiences, and some discourses occupy a privileged or 'taken-for-granted' position over others (Foucault, 1980). Discourses of femininity and cancer in Western societies stipulate particular ideals for women's identities, life-stage development, heterosexual relationships, and cancer survivorship, which can have implications for how women experience their sexual and reproductive bodies, as well as psychosocial adjustment, after cancer. In the main, research on changes to sexual functioning after cancer has adopted normative discourses of heterosexuality, in which coital sex is the taken-for-granted focus (Ussher et al., 2013; White, Faithfull, & Allan, 2013). This discourse can be viewed as part of the coital imperative, where acts of penile–vaginal penetration are viewed as 'real' sex and non-coital sexual activities are viewed as alternatives or precursors to sex (Potts, 2002). By implication, women risk being pathologised with a diagnosis of sexual dysfunction following cancer-related sexual changes as a result of a physical inability to engage in coital sex (Hyde, 2007). Conceptualising 'sex' outside of the coital imperative allows for the inclusion and validation of a greater diversity of sexual practices and also has implications for the development of health education and supportive interventions to facilitate renegotiation of sex after cancer (Schover et al., 2011; Ussher et al., 2013).

Feminine identities are strongly associated with cultural expectations that are attached to heterosexual relationships. However, few researchers have critically addressed how gendered power relations influence heterosexual relational dynamics and sexual practices following cancer (Hyde, 2007). For example, one study showed that the majority of women had resumed sexual activity one year after treatment, despite also reporting ongoing problems with lack of sexual interest, pain during intercourse, and vaginal lubrication (Jensen et al., 2004). Although some researchers might interpret this finding as an example of sexual resilience (e.g., Greenwald & McCorkle, 2008), further questions could be asked about why women are engaging in coital sex despite such difficulties. Coital sex is an expectation in heterosexual relationships (Potts, 2002), and many women in long-term heterosexual relationships report having sex for relational (rather than sexual) reasons (Hayfield & Clarke, 2012). In this context, not participating in coital sex with a male partner following cancer may be conceptualised as a failure as both a heterosexual partner and as a woman (Ussher et al., 2015), and thus serve as an identity threat.

Body dissatisfaction after cancer is associated with Western feminine ideals that place a high degree of value on the body's appearance and sexual attractiveness (Bordo, 2003). Women, particularly younger women, are considered at higher 'risk' of body image concerns within the general population (Nelson, Kling, Wängqvist, Frisén, & Syed, 2018). Lower body image scores following cancer indicate detrimental change that occurs after cancer treatment, beyond existing experiences. However, the 'risk' of body dissatisfaction is largely positioned as a product of individual women's psychology. Acknowledgement of discursive context includes recognition of the role of feminine cultural ideals in shaping women's embodied experience with cancer, as well as the ways that women negotiate these ideals.

Discursive constructions of cancer identities and women's embodied sexuality

It did have an effect on how probably I perceived myself as a woman, because I didn't feel whole anymore (60 years, breast and endometrial cancers).

Cancer has been described as 'disrupting' the sense of self through problematic body functioning, changes to social roles, and greater awareness of mortality (Little, Paul, Jordens, & Sayers, 2002; Ussher & Perz, 2018). In this vein, accounts of cancer tend to be characterised by experiences of uncertainty, risk, and loss of control, which can continue after the conclusion of medical treatment (Kaiser, 2008). As a disruptive life event, cancer can challenge continuity between past and present selves. Researchers have examined how women's identities are constructed and exposed variations in how women make sense of the self in relation to dominant discourses of cancer survivorship. For example, culturally privileged identities are those where people with cancer take up the 'fight' against cancer by complying with medical treatments while drawing on inner resources, adopting a positive attitude, and believing they can overcome the threat of cancer (Davis, 2008). According to this discourse, cancer is an opportunity for self-transformation (Bell, 2012). Some women who adopt such discourses are able to use them to make sense of their own experience. However, it is common for women to report experiences of cancer that are considerably more chaotic due to ongoing and significant physical and psychological consequences, including those related to reproductive and sexual well-being (Parton, Ussher, & Perz, 2017a; Thomas-MacLean, 2004). This can create difficulty for women trying to make sense of their identities in relation to dominant discourses of cancer survivorship and contribute to experiences of social isolation, which has led some researchers to conceptualise such identities as liminal (Little, Jordens, Paul, Montgomery, & Philipson, 1998).

In addition to cancer identities, discursive approaches have been used to examine the meanings that women ascribe to cancer-related body changes. Much of this research has detailed challenges to 'normal', 'healthy', 'feminine', and 'sexual' meanings that would usually be associated with women's bodies prior to cancer. For example, women with gynaecological cancer have reported difficulties reconciling 'private' and 'sexual' meanings usually associated with the vagina and vulva with biomedical meanings attributed during cancer treatment (White et al., 2013; Wray, Markovic, & Manderson, 2007). Discourses associated with a loss of control over the body have also been identified in response to embodied change constructed by women as 'unfeminine', 'abnormal', 'strange', or 'grotesque' (Manderson, 2005; Parton, Ussher, & Perz, 2016; Waskul & van der Riet, 2002). In these accounts, cancer-related changes are identified as breaching the body's boundaries both materially, in the case of bowel dysfunction, or symbolically through a failure to conform to cultural ideas of what an acceptable feminine body *should* be, as in the case of premature menopause, weight gain or hair loss, scarring, or disfigurement (Parton et al., 2016). Women with cancer can experience difficulties naming aspects of their bodies that do not easily fit within normal or feminine cultural constructions, due to a lack of culturally legitimate ways that they can talk about their embodied experience (Parton et al., 2016). Body changes associated with a loss of control are constructed as abject; can challenge feminine, sexual, and adult identities; and are associated with greater self-consciousness and reduced sexual confidence (Parton et al., 2016; Rozmovits & Ziebland, 2004).

Women have adopted a number of discursive and practical strategies to manage body changes and their associated consequences for identity. For example, women have been encouraged to move between speaking of their bodies as 'self' and 'other' to manage aspects of embodied change that are threatening to their feminine or sexual identity (Manderson & Stirling, 2007; Parton et al., 2016). In one study of mastectomy, this practice was suggested as a response to difficulties related to the 'presence' of a 'bodily absence' following surgery (Manderson & Stirling, 2007, p. 82). Women have also reported adopting strategies such as using humour to talk about their bodies (Waskul & van der Riet, 2002) or engaging in efforts to contain their bodies from public view by using clothing, wigs, make-up, or prostheses (Parton et al., 2016). In the context of sexual relationships, such practices extend to protecting aspects of the body constructed by women as 'abject', 'unfeminine', and 'unsexual' from being seen or touched during sex by a partner (Parton et al., 2017b). These practices can be interpreted as measures taken by women to manage or repair their identities as feminine and sexual. However, ongoing difficulties often remain due to long-term physical and psychological conse-quences of cancer.

Conclusion

Compromised sexual and reproductive well-being due to body concerns and sexual change can form a significant and distressing loss for many women. These consequences of cancer can continue long into survivorship. The lived experiences of body concerns, cancer-related menopause, and sexual changes occur within a sociocultural context, which women make sense of through cultural discourses of femininity, gender, and cancer. Physical changes from cancer and restrictive idealised cultural discourses of fem-ininity and cancer survivorship can have consequences for women's identities and the coping strategies employed to negotiate change. It is important for policy makers, health care practitioners, and researchers to acknowledge the sociocultural context of women's experiences with cancer. This means avoiding language and actions that might patholo-gise individual women for gendered experiences after cancer and acknowledging the loss to sexual and reproductive health, while also normalising the changes women commonly experience after cancer.

Despite widespread recognition amongst health care professionals that women experience distress associated with sexual and reproductive changes in the context of cancer, there is consistent evidence that such concerns are rarely addressed (Gilbert, Perz, & Ussher, 2016; Hordern & Street, 2007). There is some evidence that women who are considered to be 'older', do not have reproductive cancers, are not in a relationship, are in the later stages of cancer, or are in same-sex relationships are less likely to receive information about sexual changes from a cancer health care professional (Ussher et al., 2013). This absence of infor-mation or communication can leave women with cancer and their partners struggling to cope with changes to sexuality, feeling 'let down' by health care professionals, or thinking that their sexual needs and concerns are not legitimate (Landmark, Bøhler, Loberg, & Wahl, 2008). Thus, health professionals should actively provide information about sexual well-being and routinely discuss sexuality in a holistic manner (McKee & Schover, 2001). This could include specific suggestions related to sexual positioning, the use of sexual enhance-ment products, adjustment to changes, and expansion of sexual repertoires (Archibald et al.,

2006); information should also be provided to patients' partners. Health care professionals can also directly challenge the misconception that changes to the sexual and reproductive body are 'frivolous' during cancer, thus 'giving permission' for couples to talk about sex and to be sexually intimate (Schwartz & Plawecki, 2002, p. 3).

References

Abbott-Anderson, K. & Kwekkeboom, K. L. (2012). A systematic review of sexual concerns reported by gynecological cancer survivors. *Gynecologic Oncology, 124*(3), 477–489.

Aerts, L., Enzlin, P., Verhaeghe, J., Vergote, I., & Amant, F. (2009). Sexual and psychological functioning in women after pelvic surgery for gynaecological cancer. *European Journal of Gynaecological Oncology, 30*(6), 652–656.

Altschuler, A., Ramirez, M., Grant, M., Wendel, C., Hornbrook, M. C., Herrinton, L., & Krouse, R. (2009). The influence of husbands' or male partners' support on women's psychosocial adjustment to having an ostomy resulting from colorectal cancer. *Journal of Wound Ostomy & Continence Nursing, 36*(3), 299–305.

Archibald, S., Lemieux, S., Byers, E. S., Tamlyn, K., & Worth, J. (2006). Chemically-induced menopause and the sexual functioning of breast cancer survivors. *Women & Therapy, 29*(1/2), 83–106.

Arndt, V., Merx, H., Sturmer, T., Stegmaier, C., Ziegler, H., & Brenner, H. (2004). Age-specific detriments to quality of life among breast cancer patients one year after diagnosis. *European Journal of Cancer, 40*(5), 673–680.

Ates, O., Soylu, C., Babacan, T., Sarici, F., Kertmen, N., Allen, D., Sever, A., & Altundag, K. (2016). Assessment of psychosocial factors and distress in women having adjuvant endocrine therapy for breast cancer: The relationship among emotional distress and patient and treatment-related factors. *SpringerPlus, 5*(1), 1–7.

Avis, N., Crawford, S., & Manuel, J. (2004). Psychosocial problems among younger women with breast cancer. *Psycho-Oncology, 13*(5), 295–308.

Badr, H., Carmack, C. L., Kashy, D. A., Cristofanilli, M., & Revenson, T. A. (2010). Dyadic coping in metastatic breast cancer. *Health Psychology, 29*(2), 169–180.

Beckjord, E. & Compas, B. E. (2007). Sexual quality of life in women with newly diagnosed breast cancer. *Journal of Psychosocial Oncology, 25*(2), 19–36.

Bell, K. (2012). Remaking the self: Trauma, teachable moments, and the biopolitics of cancer survivorship. *Culture, Medicine, and Psychiatry, 36*(4), 584–6000.

Benedict, C., Philip, E. J., Baser, R. E., Carter, J., Schuler, T. A., Jandorf, L., Duhamel, K., & Nelson, C. (2016). Body image and sexual function in women after treatment for anal and rectal cancer. *Psycho-Oncology, 25*(3), 316–323.

Boehmer, U., Miao, X., & Ozonoff, A. (2011). Cancer survivorship and sexual orientation. *Cancer, 117*(16), 3796–3804.

Boehmer, U., Potter, J., & Bowen, D. J. (2009). Sexual functioning after cancer in sexual minority women. *Cancer Journal, 15*(1), 65–69.

Bordo, S. (2003). *Unbearable weight: Feminism, Western culture, and the body* (10th anniv. ed.). Berkeley, CA: University of California Press.

Canada, A. L. & Schover, L. R. (2012). The psychosocial impact of interrupted childbearing in long-term female cancer survivors. *Psycho-Oncology, 21*(2), 134–143.

Carter, J., Chi, D. S., Brown, C. L., Abu-Rustum, N. R., Sonoda, Y., Aghajanian, C., Levine, D. A., Baser, R. E., Raviv, L., & Barakat, R. R. (2010). Cancer-related infertility in survivorship. *International Journal of Gynecological Cancer, 20*(1), 2–8.

Davis, E. (2008). Risky business: Medical discourse, breast cancer, and narrative. *Qualitative Health Research, 18*(1), 65–76.

Donovan, K. A., Taliaferro, L. A., Alvarez, E. M., Jacobsen, P. B., Roetzheim, R. G., & Wenheim, R. M. (2007). Sexual health in women treated for cervical cancer: Characteristics and correlates. *Gynecologic Oncology, 104*(2), 428–434.

Duffy, C. & Allen, S. (2009). Medical and psychosocial aspects of fertility after cancer. *Cancer Journal, 15*(1), 27–33.

Fergus, K. D. & Gray, R. E. (2009). Relationship vulnerabilities during breast cancer: Patient and partner perspectives. *Psycho-Oncology, 18*(12), 1311–1322.

Fish, J. (2010). *Coming out about breast cancer in lesbian and bisexual women*. Health Policy Research Unit, De Montfort University, funded by the NHS National Cancer Action Team (pp. 1–28).

Fobair, P., Stewart, S. L., Chang, S., D'Onofrio, C., Banks, P. J., & Bloom, J. R. (2006). Body image and sexual problems in young women with breast cancer. *Psycho-Oncology, 15*(7), 579–594.

Foucault, M. (1980). *Power/knowledge: Selected interviews and other writings, 1972–1977*. Brighton, UK: Harvester Press.

Frith, H., Harcourt, D. M., & Fussell, A. (2007). Anticipating an altered appearance: Women undergoing chemotherapy treatment for breast cancer. *European Journal of Oncology Nursing, 11*(5), 385–391.

Gibberd, R. (2000). "Globocan 1: Cancer Incidence and Mortality Worldwide. J. Ferlay, D.M. Parkin and P. Pisani, IARC Press, Lyon, 1999. Price: $90 [review]. *Statistics in Medicine, 19*(19), 2714–2715.

Gilbert, E., Perz, J., & Ussher, J. M. (2016). Talking about sex with health professionals: The experience of people with cancer and their partners. *European Journal of Cancer Care, 25*, 280–293.

Gilbert, E., Ussher, J. M., & Hawkins, Y. (2009). Accounts of disruptions to sexuality following cancer: The perspective of informal carers who are partners of a person with cancer. *Health, 13*(5), 523–541.

Gilbert, E., Ussher, J. M., & Perz, J. (2010). Sexuality after breast cancer: A review. *Maturitas, 66*(4), 397–407.

Gilbert, E., Ussher, J. M., & Perz, J. (2011). Sexuality after gynaecological cancer: A review of the material, intrapsychic, and discursive aspects of treatment on women's sexual-wellbeing. *Maturitas, 70*(1), 42–57.

Greenwald, H. & McCorkle, R. (2008). Sexuality and sexual function in long-term survivors of cervical cancer. *Journal of Women's Health, 17*(6), 955–963.

Hawighorst-Knapstein, S., Fusshoeller, C., Franz, C., Trautmann, K., Schmidt, M., Pilch, H., Schoenefuss, G., Georg Knapstein, P., Koelbl, H., Kelleher, D. K., & Vaupel, P. (2004). The impact of treatment for genital cancer on quality of life and body image: Results of a prospective longitudinal 10-year study. *Gynecologic Oncology, 94*(2), 398–403.

Hawkins, Y., Ussher, J., Gilbert, E., Perz, J., Sandoval, M., & Sundquist, K. (2009). Changes in sexuality and intimacy after the diagnosis and treatment of cancer: The experience of partners in a sexual relationship with a person with cancer. *Cancer Nursing, 32*(4), 271–280.

Hayfield, N. & Clarke, V. (2012). "I'd be just as happy with a cup of tea": Women's accounts of sex and affection in long-term heterosexual relationships. *Women's Studies International Forum, 35*(2), 67–74.

Hilton, S., Hunt, K., Emslie, C., Salinas, M., & Ziebland, S. (2008). Have men been overlooked? A comparison of young men and women's experiences of chemotherapy-induced alopecia. *Psycho-Oncology, 17*(6), 577–583.

Hordern, A. J. & Street, A. F. (2007). Communicating about patient sexuality and intimacy after cancer: Mismatched expectations and unmet needs. *Medical Journal of Australia, 186*(5), 224–227.

Howard-Anderson, J., Ganz, P. A., Bower, J. E., & Stanton, A. L. (2012). Quality of life, fertility concerns, and behavioral health outcomes in younger breast cancer survivors: A systematic review. *Journal of the National Cancer Institute, 104*(5), 386–405.

Hyde, A. (2007). The politics of heterosexuality: A missing discourse in cancer nursing literature on sexuality. *International Journal of Nursing Studies, 44*(2), 315–325.

Jensen, P. T., Groenvold, M., Klee, M., Thranov, I., Petersen, M., & Machin, D. (2004). Early-stage cervical carcinoma, radical hysterectomy, and sexual function: A longitudinal study. *Cancer, 100*(1), 97–106.

Kaiser, K. (2008). The meaning of the survivor identity for women with breast cancer. *Social Science & Medicine, 67*(1), 79–87.

Kayser, K., Watson, L. E., & Andrade, J. T. (2007). Cancer as a "we-disease": Examining the process of coping from a relational perspective. *Families, Systems and Health, 25*(4), 404–418.

Klügel, S., Lücke, C., Meta, A., Schild-Suhren, M., Malik, E., Philipsen, A., & Müller, H. H. O. (2017). Concomitant psychiatric symptoms and impaired quality of life in women with cervical cancer: A critical review. *International Journal of Women's Health, 9*, 795–805.

Landmark, B. T., Bøhler, A., Loberg, K., & Wahl, A. K. (2008). Women with newly diagnosed breast cancer and their perceptions of needs in a health-care context. *Journal of Clinical Nursing, 17*(7b), 192–200.

Lee, C., Sunu, C., & Pignone, M. (2009). Patient-reported outcomes of breast reconstruction after mastectomy: A systematic review. *Journal of the American College of Surgeons, 209*(1), 123–133.

Lemieux, J., Maunsell, E., & Provencher, L. (2008). Chemotherapy-induced alopecia and effects on quality of life among women with breast cancer: A literature review. *Psycho-Oncology*, *17*(4), 317–328.

Leung, J., Smith, M. D., & McLaughlin, D. (2016). Inequalities in long term health-related quality of life between partnered and not partnered breast cancer survivors through the mediation effect of social support. *Psycho-Oncology*, *25*(10), 1222–1228.

Levin, A. O., Carpenter, K. M., Fowler, J. M., Brothers, B. M., Andersen, B. L., & Maxwell, G. L. (2010). Sexual morbidity associated with poorer psychological adjustment among gynecological cancer survivors. *International Journal of Gynecological Cancer*, *20*(3), 461–470.

Liavaag, A. H., Dørum, A., Bjøro, T., Oksefjell, H., Fosså, S. D., Tropé, C., & Dahl, A. A. (2008). A controlled study of sexual activity and functioning in epithelial ovarian cancer survivors. A therapeutic approach. *Gynecologic Oncology*, *108*(2), 348–354.

Likes, W. M., Stegbauer, C., Tillmanns, T., & Pruett, J. (2007). Correlates of sexual function following vulvar excision. *Gynecologic Oncology*, *105*(3), 600–603.

Lindau, S. T., Surawska, H., Paice, J., & Baron, S. R. (2011). Communication about sexuality and intimacy in couples affected by lung cancer and their clinical-care providers. *Psycho-Oncology*, *20*(2), 179–185.

Little, M., Jordens, C. F. C., Paul, K., Montgomery, K., & Philipson, B. (1998). Liminality: A major category of the experience of cancer illness. *Social Science & Medicine*, *47*(10), 1485–1494.

Little, M., Paul, K., Jordens, C. F. C., & Sayers, E. J. (2002). Survivorship and discourses of identity. *Psycho-Oncology*, *11*(2), 170–178.

Manderson, L. (2005). Boundary breaches: The body, sex and sexuality after stoma surgery. *Social Science & Medicine*, *61*(2), 405–415.

Manderson, L. & Stirling, L. (2007). The absent breast: Speaking of the mastectomied body. *Feminism & Psychology*, *17*(1), 75–92.

Mann, E., Singer, D., Pitkin, J., Panay, N., & Hunter, M. S. (2012). Psychosocial adjustment in women with premature menopause: A cross-sectional survey. *Climacteric*, *15*(5), 481–489.

Markopoulos, C., Tsaroucha, A. K., Kouskos, E., Mantas, D., Antonopoulou, Z., & Karvelis, S. (2009). Impact of breast cancer surgery on the self-esteem and sexual life of female patients. *Journal of International Medical Research*, *37*(1), 182–188.

Mattsson, E., Einhorn, K., Ljungman, L., Sundström-Poromaa, I., Stålberg, K., & Wikman, A. (2018). Women treated for gynaecological cancer during young adulthood: A mixed-methods study of perceived psychological distress and experiences of support from health care following end-of-treatment. *Gynecologic Oncology*, *149*(3), 464–469.

McKee, J. A. L. & Schover, L. R. (2001). Sexuality rehabilitation. *Cancer*, *92*(4 Suppl), 1008–1012.

Moreira, H., Crespo, C., Paredes, T., Silva, S., Canavarro, M. C., & Dattilio, F. (2011). Marital relationship, body image and psychological quality of life among breast cancer patients: The moderating role of the disease's phases. *Contemporary Family Therapy*, *33*(2), 161–178.

Moreira, H., Silva, S., & Canavarro, M. C. (2010). The role of appearance investment of women with breast cancer. *Psycho-Oncology*, *19*(9), 959–966.

Nelson, S. C., Kling, J., Wängqvist, M., Frisén, A., & Syed, M. (2018). Identity and the body: Trajectories of body esteem from adolescence to emerging adulthood. *Developmental Psychology*, *54*(6), 1159–1171.

Nicholson, R. M., Leinster, S., & Sassoon, E. M. (2007). A comparison of the cosmetic and psychological outcome of breast reconstruction, breast conserving surgery, and mastectomy without reconstruction. *Breast*, *16*(4), 396–410.

Parker, P., Youssef, A., Walker, S., Basen-Engquist, K., Cohen, L., Gritz, E., Wei, Q., & Robb, G. (2007). Short-term and long-term psychosocial adjustment and quality of life in women undergoing different surgical procedures for breast cancer. *Annals of Surgical Oncology*, *14*(11), 3078–3089.

Parton, C., Ussher, J. M., & Perz, J. (2017a). Experiencing menopause in the context of constructions of cancer: Women's gendered subjectivities. *Psychology and Health*, *32*(9), 1109–1126.

Parton, C., Ussher, J. M., & Perz, J. (2017b). Women's constructions of heterosex and sexual embodiment after cancer. *Feminism & Psychology*, *27*(3), 298–317.

Parton, C. M., Ussher, J. M., & Perz, J. (2016). Women's construction of embodiment and the abject sexual body after cancer. *Qualitative Health Research*, *26*(4), 490–503.

Perz, J., Ussher, J. M., & Gilbert, E. (2014). Feeling well and talking about sex: Psycho-social predictors of sexual functioning after cancer. *BMC Cancer*, *14*(1), 228–247.

Pierrisnard, C., Baciuchka, M., Mancini, J., Rathelot, P., Vanelle, P., & Montana, M. (2018). Body image and psychological distress in women with breast cancer: A French online survey on patients' perceptions and expectations. *Breast Cancer, 25*(3), 303–308.

Potts, A. (2002). *The science/fiction of sex: Feminist deconstruction and the vocabularies of heterosex.* New York: Routledge.

Préau, M., Bouhnik, A. D., Rey, D., & Mancini, J. (2011). Two years after cancer diagnosis, which couples become closer? *European Journal of Cancer Care, 20*(3), 380–388.

Quinn, G. P., Sanchez, J. A., Sutton, S. K., Vadaparampil, S. T., Nguyen, G. T., Green, B. L., Kanetsky, P. A., & Schabath, M. B. (2015). Cancer and lesbian, gay, bisexual, transgender/ transsexual, and queer/questioning (LGBTQ) populations. *CA: A Cancer Journal for Clinicians, 65*, 384–400.

Ramirez, M., McMullen, C., Grant, M., Altschuler, A., Hornbrook, M. C., & Krouse, R. (2010). Figuring out sex in a reconfigured body: Experiences of female colorectal cancer survivors with ostomies. *Women & Health, 49*(8), 608–624.

Reese, J. B. (2011). Coping with sexual concerns after cancer. *Current Opinion in Oncology, 23*(4), 313–321.

Reich, M., Lesur, A., & Perdrizet-Chevallier, C. (2008). Depression, quality of life and breast cancer: A review of the literature. *Breast Cancer Research and Treatment, 110*(1), 9–17.

Rogers, M. & Kristjanson, L. J. (2002). The impact on sexual functioning of chemotherapy-induced menopause in women with breast cancer. *Cancer Nursing, 25*(1), 57–65.

Rozmovits, L. & Ziebland, S. (2004). Expressions of loss of adulthood in the narratives of people with colorectal cancer. *Qualitative Health Research, 14*(2), 187–203.

Rubin, L., Chavez, J., Alderman, A., & Pusic, A. L. (2013). "Use what God has given me": Difference and disparity in breast reconstruction. *Psychology and Health, 28*(10), 1099–1120.

Rubino, C., Figus, A., Lorettu, L., & Sechi, G. (2007). Post-mastectomy reconstruction: A comparative analysis on psychosocial and psychopathological outcomes. *Journal of Plastic, Reconstructive & Aesthetic Surgery, 60*(5), 509–518.

Sanchez, D. & Kiefer, A. (2007). Body concerns in and out of the bedroom: Implications for sexual pleasure and problems. *Archives of Sexual Behavior, 36*(6), 808–820.

Schmidt, C. E., Bestmann, B., Küchler, T., Longo, W. E., & Kremer, B. (2005). Ten-year historic cohort of quality of life and sexuality in patients with rectal cancer. *Diseases of the Colon & Rectum, 48*(3), 483–492.

Schover, L. R., Rhodes, M. M., Baum, G., Adams, J. H., Jenkins, R., Lewis, P., & Jackson, K. E. (2011). Sisters peer counseling in reproductive issues after treatment (SPIRIT): A peer counseling program to improve reproductive health among African American breast cancer survivors. *Cancer, 117*(21), 4983–4992.

Schwartz, S. & Plawecki, H. M. (2002). Consequences of chemotherapy on the sexuality of patients with lung cancer. *Clinical Journal of Oncology Nursing, 6*(4), 212–216.

Sherman, K. A., Woon, S., French, J., & Elder, E. (2017). Body image and psychological distress in nipple-sparing mastectomy: The roles of self-compassion and appearance investment. *Psycho-Oncology, 26*(3), 337–345.

Snell, L., McCarthy, C., Klassen, A., Cano, S., Rubin, L., Hurley, K., Montgomery, G. H., Cordeiro, P. G., & Pusic, A. (2010). Clarifying the expectations of patients undergoing implant breast reconstruction: A qualitative study. *Plastic and Reconstructive Surgery, 126*(6), 1825–1830.

Soanes, L. & White, I. D. (2018). Sexuality and cancer: The experience of adolescents and young adults. *Pediatric Oncology, 65*(12), e27376.

Sprung, B. R., Janotha, B. L., & Steckel, A. J. (2011). The lived experience of breast cancer patients and couple distress. *Journal of the American Academy of Nurse Practitioners, 23*(11), 619–627.

Stafford, L. & Judd, F. (2010). Partners of long-term gynaecological cancer survivors: Psychiatric morbidity, psychosexual outcomes, and supportive care needs. *Gynecologic Oncology, 118*(3), 268–273.

Tang, C. S., Lai, B. P., & Chung, T. K. (2010). Influences of mastery, spousal support, and adaptive coping on sexual drive and satisfaction among Chinese gynecological cancer survivors. *Archives of Sexual Behaviour, 39*(5), 1191–1200.

Thomas-MacLean, R. (2004). Understanding breast cancer stories via Frank's narrative types. *Social Science & Medicine, 58*(9), 1647–1657.

Trusson, D. & Pilnick, A. (2017). The role of hair loss in cancer identity: Perceptions of chemotherapy-induced alopecia among women treated for early-stage breast cancer or ductal carcinoma in situ. *Cancer Nursing, 40*(2), E9–E16.

Ussher, J. M., Perz, J., & The Australian Cancer and Fertility Study Team (2018). Threat of biographical disruption: The construction and experience of infertility following cancer for women and men. *BMC Cancer, 18*(1), 250.

Ussher, J. M., Perz, J., & Gilbert, E. (2012). Changes to sexual well-being and intimacy after breast cancer. *Cancer Nursing, 35*(6), 456–464.

Ussher, J. M., Perz, J., & Gilbert, E. (2014). Women's sexuality after cancer: A qualitative analysis of sexual changes and renegotiation. *Women & Therapy, 37*, 205–221.

Ussher, J. M., Perz, J., & Gilbert, E. (2015). Perceived causes and consequences of sexual changes after cancer for women and men: A mixed method study. *BMC Cancer, 15*(268), 2–15.

Ussher, J. M., Perz, J., & The Australian Cancer and Fertility Study Team (2018). Threat of biographical disruption: The construction and experience of infertility following cancer for women and men. *BMC Cancer, 18*(250), 1–17.

Ussher, J. M., Perz, J., Gilbert, E., Wong, W. K., Mason, C., Hobbs, K., & Kirsten, L. (2013). Talking about sex after cancer: A discourse analytic study of health care professional accounts of sexual communication with patients. *Psychology and Health, 28*(12), 1370–1390.

Ussher, J. M., Perz, J., Gilbert, E., Wong, W. K. T., & Hobbs, K. (2013). Renegotiating sex and intimacy after cancer: Resisting the coital imperative. *Cancer Nursing, 36*(6), 454–462.

Ussher, J. M., Perz, J., & Parton, C. (2015). Sex and the menopausal woman: A critical review and analysis. *Feminism & Psychology, 25*(4), 449–468.

Ussher, J. M., Wong, W. K. T., & Perz, J. (2011). A qualitative analysis of changes in relationship dynamics and roles between people with cancer and their primary informal carer. *Health, 15*(6), 650–667.

Waskul, D. & van der Riet, P. (2002). The abject embodiment of cancer patients: Dignity, selfhood, and the grotesque body. *Symbolic Interaction, 25*(4), 487–513.

Webber, K., Mok, K., Bennett, B., Lloyd, A. R., Friedlander, M., Juraskova, I., & Goldstein, D. (2011). If I am in the mood, I enjoy it: An exploration of cancer-related fatigue and sexual functioning in women with breast cancer. *Oncologist, 16*(9), 1333–1344.

White, I. D., Faithfull, S., & Allan, H. (2013). The re-construction of women's sexual lives after pelvic radiotherapy: A critique of social constructionist and biomedical perspectives on the study of female sexuality after cancer treatment. *Social Science & Medicine, 76*, 186–196.

Wilmoth, M. C. (2001). The aftermath of breast cancer: An altered sexual self. *Cancer Nursing, 24*(4), 278–286.

Wimberly, S. R., Carver, C. S., Laurenceau, J. P., Harris, S. D., & Antoni, M. H. (2005). Perceived partner reactions to diagnosis and treatment of breast cancer: Impact on psychosocial and psychosexual adjustment. *Journal of Consulting and Clinical Psychology, 73*(2), 300–311.

Woertman, L. & van Den Brink, F. (2012). Body image and female sexual functioning and behavior: A review. *Journal of Sex Research, 49*(2), 184–211.

Wray, N., Markovic, M., & Manderson, L. (2007). Discourses of normality and difference: Responses to diagnosis and treatment of gynaecological cancer of Australian women. *Social Science & Medicine, 64*(11), 2260–2271.

Zimmermann, T., Scott, J. L., & Heinrichs, N. (2010). Individual and dyadic predictors of body image in women with breast cancer. *Psycho-Oncology, 19*(10), 1061–1068.

PART III

Contraception and infertility

11

CONTRACEPTION ACROSS THE REPRODUCTIVE LIFE-COURSE

Deborah Bateson

Women's ability to control if and when to have children is a fundamental human right, and contraception is therefore a keystone of reproductive justice (United Nations Population Fund, 1994). It is essential to women's well-being, health, and economic empowerment, and enables women to complete their education, join the workforce, and earn money for themselves and their households. It prevents poor neonatal outcomes, maternal deaths, debilitating chronic illness that can be caused by pregnancies that occur too soon or close together, and unwanted pregnancies that can lead women in desperation to seek out unsafe abortions. And it also allows women to enjoy a pleasurable sex life free from worries about unintended pregnancy – an aspect often neglected or avoided because of community or professional reluctance to discuss intimate issues.

Contraception is central to empowering women, but it has also been used to disempower. Forced sterilisations or contraceptive injections given without consent to women living in institutions or in Indigenous communities across the globe must never be forgotten. More recently, coercion by partners who may confiscate a woman's pills or refuse to use a condom has been of increasing concern (American College of Obstetricians and Gynecologists, 2013). And today's overwhelming range of internet commentators (some informed, some uninformed) can make it difficult for women to navigate their way to contraceptive choices that best suit their specific circumstances.

In this chapter I explore contraception as the keystone of reproductive justice. I examine the role of contraception in society from adolescence through to midlife and the perimenopause, particularly in relation to marginalised populations, in order to enhance our understanding of the complex nature of fertility control and contribute to the improvement of reproductive health for women across the world.

A brief history of contraception

Until the mid-nineteenth century, contraceptive methods were mostly male-controlled. Women had to rely on their partners 'pulling out' or using penile sheaths fashioned out of unsavoury materials such as animal intestines. Although ancient classical writings describe various pregnancy-preventing concoctions, most likely these acted to induce abortion rather than as contraceptives. Vaginal pessaries made from elephant or crocodile dung were among

175

the first female-controlled methods. The vulcanisation of rubber in the 1830s led to the creation of the cervical cap and diaphragm. Revolutionary as these new barrier methods may have been, they were unfortunately not always very reliable.

The most significant landmark in women's emancipation was the arrival of the contraceptive pill in the early 1960s. For the first time women could control their fertility independently. Moral panic ensued. In some countries, such as Australia, only married women were initially able to access the pill; family planning clinics kept a stash of wedding rings on hand for those in need of disguise. The 27.5% luxury goods tax (National Museum of Australia, n.d.) placed on the pill in Australia (finally removed in 1972) is one example of the censorious political attitudes toward the pill in that period. The early pill's high doses of hormones led to a significant risk of side-effects, and pharmaceutical companies have, ever since, sought to lower the dose of hormones and develop new formulations so as to reduce its negative side-effects and risks while retaining its effectiveness (Liao & Dollin, 2012).

By the mid-1960s intrauterine devices (IUDs) began to enter the market. The earliest types, such as the Lippes loop, were made of inert materials. Copper-releasing devices were introduced in the 1970s and hormonal devices in the 1990s. IUDs suffered a significant setback in the 1970s and 1980s due to a device called the Dalkon Shield whose unsealed multifilament thread was prone to harbour bacteria that could cause dangerous pelvic infections and even deaths (Christian, 1974). This resulted in mass class-action lawsuits and the eventual bankruptcy of the company that manufactured the device. Today, regulatory authorities across the world require large-scale multinational trials of new contraceptives. These have led to renewed recognition of the effectiveness of Long Acting Reversible Contraception (LARC) methods, which include IUDs as well as the contraceptive implants introduced in the early 2000s. Much of the evidence for the benefits of LARC comes from the CHOICE project (Secura, Allsworth, Madden, Mullersman, & Peipert, 2010) in the city of St. Louis (in the US) where the provision of free IUDs and implants to women aged 14–45 resulted in a significant reduction of adolescent pregnancy and abortion rates (Peipert, Madden, Allsworth, & Secura, 2012; Washington University Dept. of Obstetrics and Gynecology, n.d.). Increased access to LARC also played a significant role in the success of a multipronged ten-year strategy to reduce adolescent pregnancy in the UK (Hadley, Ingham, & Chandra-Mouli, 2016).

Global trends suggest a move away from the pill and increasing uptake of LARC, as negative perceptions about hormonal methods, especially among well-informed, educated younger women, become more common. In family planning clinics young women increasingly request 'more natural' methods such as copper rather than hormonal IUDs, and there is a growing community and media interest in 'natural family planning' or fertility awareness methods (Carey, 2017; Freilich et al., 2017). Fertility awareness methods require diligent daily recording of fertility indicators and, as a result, can be less effective than other methods, especially LARC, yet many of the women for whom such methods have 'failed' still stand by their choice as one that provides them with autonomy over their body (Turula, 2018). However, such autonomy may be a luxury for financially disadvantaged women whose choices, including the ability to access an abortion in case of failure, may be limited. Ironically this move to the 'natural' is also taken up by conservative US groups who promote 'natural family planning' by trying to restrict reproductive rights and limit access to other effective methods of contraception (Hasstedt, 2018).

Family planning programs have at times been used by governments to control population growth and prevent women from reproducing, rather than to promote women's reproductive rights. For example, the one child policy in China, initiated in 1979 and not phased out until 2015, contributed to a gender imbalance of 118 boys to every 100 girls (UNICEF, NWCCW, & NBS, 2014); certain population groups were allowed to conceive additional children, but others were forced to undergo sterilisation or have stringless IUDs ('Chinese rings') inserted and never removed. The contraceptive injection Depo Provera, given every three months, has had a particularly poor history of institutionalised abuse. Women with physical or cognitive disabilities, and young women in orphanages or 'homes for unmarried' mothers, have been injected without consent, even while the injection was still unlicensed and in the experimental stage. Indigenous women around the world, including Australian Aboriginal and Torres Strait Islander women, have been subject to coerced family planning practices (Arabena, 2006). Such practices continue unabated. Fifteen women in India recently died from complications of unsafe sterilisations performed in mass 'camps' they were paid to attend (Mohanty & Bhalla, 2016).

Throughout history, religion has influenced attitudes toward contraception and contraceptive practices (FPA UK, 2016; Pinter et al., 2016). Liberal Protestant churches tend to view contraception as acceptable so long as it does not encourage 'promiscuous behaviour', but less liberal churches only approve its use within marriage. The Roman Catholic Church only permits natural family planning, although many Catholics do not follow church teaching in this respect. Judaism has had a largely positive attitude toward sex, although male condoms and vasectomy are not permitted, as it is forbidden to 'waste seed'. In addition, orthodox women must abstain from intercourse during menstruation (and for seven days after); thus methods that cause irregular bleeding are unacceptable (Weisberg & Kern, 2009). Islam is strongly pro-family and, although the Qur'an does not explicitly refer to contraception, sexual ethics forbid sex outside marriage and sterilisation methods are unacceptable. More conservative Islamic leaders campaign against condoms and contraceptive methods other than withdrawal. Although Hinduism is strongly pro-family, there is no ban on any forms of contraception. This contrasts with Buddhism, which sees contraception as acceptable so long as it is used for family planning purposes rather than the pursuit of sexual pleasure (Srikanthan & Reid, 2008).

It is increasingly recognised that not only state institutions and religions, but also partners, family members, and health care professionals may exercise contraceptive coercion (Gold, 2014). Contraceptive pills may be discarded or a woman's IUD deliberately removed. Although doctors will always welcome men who accompany their partners to discuss contraception, they should ensure that women are also seen on their own. Women who feel unsafe with a method that could be detected by their partner, for instance, may wish to choose an injection or an IUD with the threads cut short at the cervix to ensure it is not felt during intercourse.

Overview of contraceptive methods

Contraception can be classified in a number of ways. From the perspective of reproductive justice, it is important to distinguish between male-controlled and female-controlled methods. Female-controlled methods have increased women's autonomy, but there is an argument for men sharing contraceptive responsibility. One of the most useful ways to classify contraception is how often a woman, or her partner, has to 'do something' to make the method work. In general, the less frequently an action needs to be remembered, the more effective the method is.

Permanent methods include vasectomy, usually under local anaesthetic, and tubal sterilisation, usually under general anaesthetic (Faculty of Sexual & Reproductive Healthcare, 2014a). Both are over 99% effective (fewer than 1 woman in 100 will become pregnant in the first year of use) but practically irreversible (Trussell, 2011). Expensive microsurgery offers the potential to reverse vasectomy, but success cannot be guaranteed, and consideration of hypothetical situations (e.g., meeting a new partner who wants children, the death of children in the family) is important during counselling to minimise the chance of future regret. In some countries women seeking sterilisation must gain the consent of their partner; although men of any age generally have little difficulty accessing vasectomy, women may be denied the option of tubal ligation by doctors who may believe it is not in their best interest. An alternative irreversible method – placement of small inserts into each fallopian tube to promote scar tissue formation – was recently withdrawn in several countries following reports of failure and chronic pain, which led to class-action litigation (Dyer, 2018).

Long Acting Reversible Contraception methods are over 99% effective (Trussell, 2011) but immediately reversible if a woman wants to become pregnant or wants to discontinue because of side-effects. IUDs and implants need to be inserted and removed by a trained doctor or nurse, usually under local anaesthetic, which can limit their accessibility. Contraceptive implants take the form of one or two matchstick-sized flexible rods placed under the skin of the upper inner arm, which slowly release a progestogen hormone over three or five years to prevent ovulation (Faculty of Sexual & Reproductive Healthcare, 2014b). Hormonal IUDs are plastic T-shaped devices placed in the uterus that release a low dose of a progestogen hormone called levonorgestrel for up to five years; copper IUDs last for five or ten years depending on the type (Faculty of Sexual & Reproductive Healthcare, 2015a). IUDs prevent fertilisation by stopping sperm movement and survival of the egg, and may also prevent implantation of a fertilised egg in the uterus. Hormonal IUDs reduce or even eliminate menstrual bleeding, which makes them an important option for women with heavy bleeding and anaemia, whereas copper IUDs tend to make bleeding longer and heavier. Copper IUDs are inexpensive, and implants are becoming increasingly more affordable and available in low-income countries, but the more expensive hormonal IUDs remain out of reach for many women. Pharmaceutical companies and governments should make efforts to provide these highly effective devices at low or no cost to the women who most need them.

The contraceptive injection must be given every three months, which reduces its effectiveness due to the need for frequent clinic visits (Faculty of Sexual & Reproductive Healthcare, 2015b). However, recent advances in self-administered injections (Spieler, 2014) potentially provide increased autonomy for women. Although injectables are very inexpensive and widely used in many low-income countries, they have some disadvantages, including a delay in return to fertility of up to one year, weight gain, and reduction in bone density. Studies are currently underway in sub-Saharan Africa to determine whether the Depo Provera injection is associated with an increased risk of HIV acquisition (WHO, 2017). As the injection is so prevalent in countries where young women are also most at risk of HIV, if such a link is proven, major policy changes will be needed.

Shorter-acting methods include the combined hormonal pill, the patch, and the vaginal ring, which contain oestrogen as well as a progestogen to prevent ovulation (Faculty of Sexual & Reproductive Healthcare, 2011). They are rated as over 99% effective (Trussell, 2011) but, because pills can be forgotten and packs can run out, 92% may be a more realistic estimate. There are many different pills on the market with potentially different side effects and additional benefits (e.g., improving skin, reducing vaginal bleeding). However, family planning organisations all recommend the tried and tested levonorgestrel-containing pills, which are generally the cheapest and also offer the lowest risk of serious side-effects such as blood clots (de Bastos et al., 2014). The patch, applied each week, and the vaginal ring, inserted for three weeks and then removed for one week, release hormones similar to the combined pill. The development of a cost-effective ring that lasts 12 months and combines contraceptive hormones and antiretroviral therapy to prevent HIV would make this option highly attractive for women in low-income countries with a high HIV risk (Population Council, 2018; Smith et al., 2017).

The progestogen-only pill comes as either a low-dose pill that must be taken in a very narrow three-hour time frame or a higher-dose formulation that can be taken in a more flexible time frame. It is generally reserved for women who are breastfeeding or who, due to medical conditions such as heart disease, are unable to use a method that contains oestrogen (Faculty of Sexual & Reproductive Healthcare, 2015c).

Barrier methods need to be used each time with sex. The diaphragm still has a role, albeit small, for women who accept its relatively high failure rate (around 84%) or are ambivalent about pregnancy (Faculty of Sexual & Reproductive Health Care, 2012, 2014; Trussell, 2011). Condoms offer the advantage of preventing sexually transmitted infections (STIs), but they are not as effective in preventing pregnancy as some other methods. Thus it is recommended that women combine condoms with another effective contraceptive. Female condoms are widely heralded for their potential to provide woman-controlled protection, but their promise has not yet been fulfilled due to a combination of low awareness, low availability, and high cost; in addition, women must have sufficient power within the relationship to negotiate their use (Martin, de Lora, Rochat, & Andes, 2016). Efforts to develop new types with features that enhance sexual pleasure should be encouraged (Joelving, 2008).

Fertility awareness methods, based on fertility signs and/or the days of the menstrual cycle, require dedication and vigilance as well as the cooperation of a partner, due to the many days in the cycle when unprotected sex is not permitted. Their effectiveness varies from 75% to 99% (Trussell, 2011), but some methods have not been well researched (Faculty of Sexual & Reproductive Healthcare, 2015a). The role of smartphone technology needs further investigation, and women who choose fertility awareness methods should seek out coaching and mentoring to optimise their effectiveness.

Breastfeeding ('lactational amenorrhoea method') is a globally important method of contraception. It can be used up to the first six months after childbirth and before the first menstrual period, but strict attention must be paid to breastfeeding frequency to ensure intervals of less than four hours (six hours at night) between feeds (Vekemans, 1997). Withdrawal is widely used across the globe and, although it appears to be successful, long-term users require control and commitment by the male partner, and it can fail if sperm are present in the pre-ejaculate.

Emergency contraception, used after unprotected sex to prevent pregnancy, plays an important role. There are two main types of emergency contraceptive pills (aka 'morning-after' pills), both of which work by preventing ovulation (Faculty of Sexual & Reproductive Healthcare, 2017c). The copper IUD can also be used to prevent pregnancy if it is inserted within five days of unprotected sex. Emergency contraception is subject to many myths, such as the mistaken belief that it is actually an abortion pill or that it is harmful to health or future fertility. Emergency contraceptive pills are available at pharmacies without a prescription in many countries, and even at supermarkets and vending machines in some high schools, but moral concern that increasing accessibility will lead to reckless sexual behaviour continues to curb its availability across the globe.

Access to contraception

Although there is now a wide range of contraceptive methods available, this does not mean that women have equal access to contraception and contraceptive services. Women in rural and remote areas may need to travel large distances and take time from work to find clinics that offer IUDs or implant insertion. Women from culturally and linguistically diverse migrant and refugee backgrounds can also find it difficult to access services. Access to interpreters may be limited and, in small minority groups, interpreters may be known to women, which could inhibit them from speaking freely. Women from some cultural backgrounds may be deterred from seeking contraception if only male practitioners are available, whereas others may consider contraception forbidden, dangerous, or at odds with the belief that having children is central to a woman's identity (Hawkey, Ussher, & Perz, 2018). In such cases, cultural context plays an essential role, and healthcare practitioners must ensure they provide culturally safe medical care. In Australia, for instance, a history of coerced contraception has led to mistrust among Aboriginal elders (Arabena, 2006). Provision of services to Aboriginal and Torres Strait Islander women requires the active inclusion of elders and other community members who can advise on women's business in relation to intimate issues. The recently documented high uptake and acceptability of contraceptive implants by women in three remote Aboriginal communities in Western Australia resulted from a community-driven approach that engaged elders as well as young people (Griffiths, Marley, Friello, & Atkinson, 2016).

The cost of contraception can also play a role in limiting access. Government subsidies vary across countries, as does remuneration for providers (who may then pass additional costs on to women). In some countries contraception is free either for all women or for young women, whereas in others subsidies only exist for those deemed eligible for financial support (Brekke, 2014).

Women with disabilities can find physical access to services difficult or impossible. Accessing contraception can also be challenging for women with cognitive disability (Family Planning Victoria, 2016), and data suggest that women with disabilities are less likely to receive comprehensive healthcare (Taouk, Fialkow, & Schulkin, 2018). Given the history of coerced contraception and the prevalence of sexual abuse in institutions, laws to protect women with cognitive disabilities have been developed, but they can be interpreted in overly cautious ways, resulting in a loss of autonomy for women who, with the right support, could make informed decisions about contraception for themselves (McCarthy, 2009). For women who cannot provide consent to contraception, even with appropriate support, a substitute decision-maker – often a parent – is required, except for sterilisation. The sterilisation of children and adults without their free and informed consent is prohibited in international law, has been banned in many countries, but still occurs, for instance, in Australia with the consent of the courts or relevant tribunals (Elliott, 2017). As mentioned above, consent to sterilisation remains a highly contentious issue across the world, and women who are capable of deciding for themselves still need their husbands' consent in some countries before doctors will proceed (EngenderHealth, 2002).

Provider bias may exist against lesbians who may be perceived as not at risk of pregnancy; their needs for the additional benefits of hormonal contraception (e.g., reducing menstrual blood loss or perimenopausal symptoms) may be overlooked, misunderstood, or dismissed. Transgender men with the capacity for pregnancy also need information and advice about options that will not counteract the masculinising effects of testosterone or cause undesirable side effects such as unpredictable vaginal bleeding (Faculty of Sexual & Reproductive Healthcare, 2017d). Finally, access issues also exist for women with complex medical conditions (e.g., hormonally-dependent cancers, heart disease, autoimmune conditions) in part because doctors may not be confident about which methods are safe for particular conditions (Faculty of Sexual & Reproductive Healthcare, 2016). This issue is all the more important because pregnancy could have serious health effects for such women.

Access to contraception information

Equally important is access to accurate information about contraception. School-based education has historically focussed on how to use contraception rather than on decision-making and positive choices in relationships. The 'abstinence-only' before marriage programs, recently rebranded as 'sexual risk avoidance' in the US, are harmful; there is evidence that such programs increase rather than decrease unintended pregnancies and STIs (Boyer, 2018; Santelli et al., 2017). By contrast, the school-based, age-appropriate, and sexuality-positive information provided for young people in the Netherlands has resulted in one of the lowest rates of adolescent pregnancy and STIs in the world (Weaver, Smith, & Kippax, 2005).

The availability of translated and culturally appropriate information about contraception poses another challenge, and many health professionals are still insufficiently trained in understanding the different ways contraception is perceived in diverse sociocultural settings. The media have long played a significant role in influencing contraceptive choice – sometimes for better, sometimes for worse. A 1995 UK media scare, triggered by an announcement about the increased risk of blood clots with third-generation pills, was estimated to have led to 10,000 more abortions and 30,000 more pregnancies than expected (Mills, 1997), and a 2014 *Daily Mail* story reported that more than 600,000 women had discontinued the pill due to health fears (Manning & Adams, 2014). Media stories should present risks meaningfully. Although a doubling of clotting risk sounds alarming, it actually amounts to four to six cases in every 10,000 women using the pill in one year (Bitzer et al., 2013; de Bastos et al., 2014). Both pregnancy and childbirth have significantly higher risks of blood clots than any contraceptive pill (Melbourne Haematology, 2012; Reid et al., 2011). More recent media stories have associated hormonal contraception with depression, based on a national Danish study in which women, especially adolescents, who had used a pill, implant, or hormonal IUD had a greater risk of receiving a first anti-depressant prescription than those who had not (Skovlund, Mørch, Kessing, & Lidegaard, 2016). The researchers conceded that other factors associated with adolescents' mental health had not been taken into account, but this information was not always included in media reports of the study. By contrast, evidence about the benefits of contraception (e.g., reduction in the risk of ovarian, uterine, and bowel cancer with use of the combined pill) are less commonly the focus of media stories (Wentzensen & de Gonzalez, 2015).

Women's experiences of contraception

Doctors tend to focus on the effectiveness and risks of different methods of contraception. However, these attributes may not match those that women prioritise. It is important for doctors to understand that what women seek in contraception is to a large extent motivated by their bodily experience, which has its cultural as well as personal aspects. The effect of contraception on vaginal bleeding is a prime example, as the salience and significance of menstrual bleeding varies significantly between cultures. A study of contraceptive implant use in Papua New Guinea showed high levels of satisfaction with few removals for bleeding problems 12 months after insertion (Gupta et al., 2017), in contrast to a study in Australia in which 30% of women had discontinued their implant by 12 months, mainly due to troublesome bleeding (Weisberg, Bateson, McGeechan, & Mohapatra, 2013).

Hormonal contraception can result in heavier bleeding, lighter or absent bleeding, or irregular spotting or bleeding; the latter is generally least desirable. The contraceptive pill was developed with a seven-day hormone-free break to mimic the natural menstrual cycle and guarantee a regular bleeding pattern in order to reassure women and their partners that this intervention was 'natural'. Ironically, this places women at great risk of breakthrough ovulation if even a single pill is missed, so today's pill packs have shorter breaks, and some have no breaks at all. These extended or continuous pill regimens (also referred to as 'menstrual suppression') mean that women can continue their active hormone pills for three months, 12 months, or even longer without any bleeding. Clinical trials of up to 12 months continuous pill use have not given rise to any safety issues but some researchers have documented their concerns about the implications of this practice in young women, at the time of development and before a first pregnancy, for bone density as well as a potential effect of increased hormonal exposure on risks such as blood clots (Hitchcock, 2008). Ongoing post-marketing regulatory surveillance is therefore essential for all hormonal contraceptives in order to capture safety signals for rare events that cannot be captured in relatively small trials. Progestogen-only injections, implants, and hormonal IUDs can also all result in an absence of bleeding for the entire time they are used, but only the injections have been associated with bone loss. Although women may worry about blood building up inside the uterus or perceive it to be unnatural, the lining of the uterus in fact thins out over time to reduce the amount of blood loss. This reduction can be beneficial for women with heavy menstrual bleeding with flooding and passage of blood clots that can cause anaemia and impact on relationships, work, and quality of life (Karlsson, Marions, & Edlund, 2014). The hormonal IUD and the combined hormonal contraceptive pill can therefore be useful choices for regulating heavy bleeding. Despite these advantages some women prefer a regular monthly bleeding pattern and should be supported to find a method of contraception that provides this. It is important that women are well informed and empowered to choose a method that accords with their bodily experience and preferences.

Another factor that is both medical and experiential is the effect of contraception on sexuality, in particular libido. Until recently this has been given little attention, perhaps in part because it is a difficult area to study given the multitude of factors that can affect sexual desire, and because of society's continuing discomfort in discussing women's expressions of sexuality. Women's own attitudes have often concerned (or at least been perceived to concern) the effect of contraceptive methods on the male partner's sexual pleasure rather than on their own, including concerns about condoms affecting his enjoyment or IUD threads causing him discomfort. Should contraceptives designed to enhance women's libido and sexual pleasure ever reach the market, it would be interesting to see the reaction of the pharmaceutical companies in their promotional campaigns, which so far have tended to focus on non-contraceptive benefits for acne or heavy bleeding rather than any links to sexuality (van Leeuwen et al., 2018).

Women's bodily experience of contraception plays out most intensely in relation to devices inserted into the body, including implants and IUDs. Medical devices have had a chequered history, including the recent recall of the hysteroscopic transvaginal sterilisation method (called Essure in Australia) related in part to complications such as failure and pain (Therapeutic Goods Administration, 2017). Again, women differ in their attitudes toward contraceptive devices, as shown in a recent qualitative study of the implant, where some praised it, and others rejected it (Inoue et al., 2016). Here too, informed choice is essential; all women should have access to reliable information and be empowered to make their own choices, in accordance with their own experiences and values.

Contraception across the life course

Adolescence

Providing contraception to adolescents to prevent unintended pregnancy is a global priority, given that their fertility is high and contraception access is often denied. Fears about adolescent sexuality, anxiety about the loss of parental control and protection, misinformation about the effects of contraception on young women's health and development, and concerns about the legality of providing contraception to minors hamper access.

In England and Wales as well as Australia, Canada, and New Zealand, contraception (with the exception of sterilisation) can be provided to young women of any age assessed as 'Gillick competent', a term that comes from a 1984 legal case, heard in the House of Lords, with Lord Fraser presiding (*Gillick* v *West Norfolk and Wisbech Area Health Authority and the DHSS*, 1985). Victoria Gillick, a mother of five adolescent girls, had sought to prevent the Department of Health and Social Security from advising doctors they could provide contraception to girls under 16 without parental consent. Famously, she lost the case. Lord Fraser set out criteria for assessing young women's functional ability to make decisions with regard to contraception (and indeed other areas of medicine) and to weigh its risks and benefits (Columbia Law School, 2008). Many parents find the transition from childhood through to adolescence and independent adulthood challenging and, as a family planning doctor, I have received many an angry phone call from mothers who simply cannot believe that their daughters have been provided with contraception without their knowledge; most eventually accept the situation. Although adolescents should always be encouraged to talk with their parents about contraception, this may not always be feasible or even safe, particularly for those from cultural backgrounds that do not allow sex before marriage. An assurance of confidentiality and privacy is fundamental in gaining the trust of girls who come to a clinic, and all staff must know how to respond when parents demand to know whether their daughter has visited the clinic. However, adolescents also need to be aware of the limits of confidentiality, as the law in most jurisdictions requires health care professionals to report young people at risk of harm to the relevant authorities to ensure their safety (Faculty of Sexual & Reproductive Healthcare, 2010). So, although it is essential to determine the capacity of girls under 16 to consent to contraception, we also need to assess whether they are at risk of harm by inquiring about the age of their partner, whether the relationship is consensual, and whether it involves someone in a position of power (e.g., a teacher), and by asking about their home situation, schooling, drug and alcohol use, mental state, and suicidality (HEADSS assessment; Cohen, Mackenzie, & Yates, 1991). Young women in the care of the state may be particularly disadvantaged with regard to their right either to access or to stop contraception and their right to privacy and confidentiality, both of which can be undermined by well-meaning but intrusive authorities, just as adolescents are at a critical stage in developing into an independent adult.

There are no medical reasons why adolescents cannot use any method of contraception, including emergency contraception and LARC, although Depo Provera injections are generally not first-line due to their effect on bone density at a time when peak bone mass has not yet been attained (Faculty of Sexual & Reproductive Healthcare, 2010). All young women need to be aware of the importance of condoms for preventing STIs and the need to combine them with another effective method of contraception, as condoms may not be available or used in the heat of the moment, or may be used incorrectly, or tear, break, or slip off. Adolescents also need to be aware about the availability of emergency contraception and about the most effective LARC methods. Although adolescents have generally used the pill, this appears to be changing and increasingly young women across the globe are making an informed choice about using an implant or an IUD (Pazol, Daniels, Romero, Warner, & Barfield, 2016).

Use after childbirth or abortion

Women who stop contraception to become pregnant may find it does not happen as quickly as planned, although there is no evidence that contraception causes a delay in the return of fertility except in the case of injectable progestogens. Hormonal contraception may provide a false sense of security with regular withdrawal bleeds on the pill for instance. When the pill is stopped the woman's cycle will return to what is 'normal' for her, which, in some cases, may be irregular ovulations and a reduced chance of pregnancy. Women sometimes say they feel 'cheated' by having put up with the side effects of contraception for many years only to find that, when they stop it, becoming pregnant requires assistance or a change of plan.

Although many pregnancies are planned, a nationally representative survey of Australians showed that 40% of those who had ever been pregnant (or a partner in a pregnancy) had experienced an unintended pregnancy (Rowe et al., 2016). A recent US study showed that almost one half of women who had experienced an unintended pregnancy reported having used contraception at the time (Finer & Henshaw, 2006). Contraception after childbirth is therefore a global priority as pregnancies that occur less than 18 months after childbirth are associated with poor outcomes for both the child and the mother, including premature birth, neonatal death, and maternal anaemia (Conde-Agudelo, Rosas-Bermudez, Castano, & Norton, 2012; WHO, 2013). Conception can occur much sooner after childbirth than is often thought possible. Ovulation can occur in women who are not breastfeeding 28 days after childbirth, and a pregnancy is possible from three weeks postpartum due to the survival of the sperm in the upper genital tract (Faculty of Sexual & Reproductive Healthcare, 2017a). Resumption of sexual activity after childbirth is variable, but studies suggest that almost one half of women have sex within six weeks (McDonald & Brown, 2013), which means they should not wait to discuss contraception until the traditional six-week postpartum check-up.

Breastfeeding delays ovulation, and can be used as an effective method of contraception before the baby is six months old, as long as menstruation has not restarted and the criteria of frequent feeding during the day and through the night are followed strictly. The Lactational Amenorrhoea Method (LAM) is both accessible and free, but experts recommend that it be combined with other contraceptive methods that are compatible with breastfeeding where possible – especially as the first ovulation can be unpredictable and will precede the first menstrual period. Methods with oestrogen are avoided in the early weeks after childbirth because of the elevated risk of blood clots. They are also not generally recommended during breastfeeding because of a possible effect on breastmilk supply. But methods without oestrogen can all be used by breastfeeding women, and the low dose progestogen-only pill has been particularly often prescribed, though the three-hour time frame for taking it each day is challenging, especially at a time when women's daily schedules are likely to be disrupted.

Long Acting Reversible Contraception methods are increasingly recognised as an effective and acceptable alternative for all women postpartum. Enhancing access to implants and IUDs even before a woman leaves the birthing facility is supported by the World Health

Organization (2013) as an effective strategy for optimising birth-spacing, as women are more likely to continue their method with immediate rather than delayed insertion. Traditional medical hierarchies are being broken down in many countries as nurses and midwives are trained, and remunerated, to deliver LARC. According to clinical guidelines (Faculty of Sexual & Reproductive Healthcare, 2016), IUDs can be inserted either within the first 48 hours after childbirth or from four-weeks postpartum, although in my family planning setting we generally wait for around eight weeks after a vaginal birth and 12 weeks following a caesarean-section due to the higher risks of perforation of the uterus, particularly if the woman is breastfeeding. Research is ongoing into the immediate insertion of IUDs, including placement of an IUD into the uterus at the time of caesarean-section; although it is associated with a higher chance of expulsion, this practice is acceptable to women and has many benefits (The American College of Obstetricians and Gynecologists, 2016). The challenge now is to ensure that these LARC methods are available and affordable in the low-income countries where they are needed most. But even in countries such as Australia significant policy changes are required to include LARC within hospital formularies and to ensure that trained midwives are available across the country. As the immediate postnatal period is a busy time with many competing priorities for the new mother, discussions about contraception should ideally occur prior to childbirth in order to support informed choice.

Provision of effective contraception after a surgical or medical abortion is also essential, and abortion services should ensure that women have the opportunity to leave with a method of contraception as well as information about emergency contraception and the need for condoms for those at risk of STIs (WHO, 2015). Surgical abortion is usually performed under sedation in a clinic or hospital, and women can choose to have an implant or IUD inserted at the same time. Medical abortion usually occurs in a woman's home following a medical consultation. It involves taking the drug mifepristone followed 24 to 48 hours later by misoprostol, which causes the uterus to expel the pregnancy. For medical abortions, contraception can potentially be started on the day the first medication is taken, except for the IUD, which can be inserted after the abortion is complete (Faculty of Sexual & Reproductive Healthcare, 2017a). Integrated services are essential; it is crucial to remember that women may have other priorities when they present for an abortion and to ensure that contraceptive choices are freely made.

Perimenopause

Conception is possible up to 12 months after the last menstrual period for women over 50. Although the chance of pregnancy is less than 1% (Faculty of Sexual & Reproductive Healthcare, 2017b), for that 1 individual in 100, an unintended pregnancy can become a personal crisis. Pregnancy at a later age is associated with an increased chance of chromosomal abnormalities and complications (e.g., gestational diabetes), and raising a child at an older age can be tiring and hard to combine with other demands such as ageing parents, adolescent children, and work challenges. Contraception is therefore important for perimenopausal women, but their needs may be overlooked by health care professionals who incorrectly assume the women are no longer sexually active. Women themselves may underestimate their fertility and stop contraception prematurely. The changing pattern of relationships and the ever increasing array of internet dating sites aimed at women in their 40s and 50s mean that now more than ever women are likely to meet new partners later in life and need information both about their contraceptive choices and about STI prevention (Bateson, Weisberg, McCaffery, & Luscombe, 2012). Some contraceptives are not recommended for women over 50, including the oestrogen-containing methods due to an increased age-related risk of blood clots, but these methods can be useful for women in their 40s who are experiencing hot flushes or night sweats and for women with heavy menstrual bleeding. The hormonal IUD is another useful option for perimenopausal women who are comfortable with the idea of a device in the uterus, as it combines effective contraception with treatment for heavy bleeding.

Empowering women through information at a time when a woman can feel 'invisible' is essential. Because some contraceptives such as the implant or hormonal IUD can suppress bleeding, it can be difficult to determine if menopause has occurred and whether contraception can be stopped, although a hormonal blood test can be a useful guide. The decision to stop contraception is highly personal and individual and must be respected by health professionals.

Conclusion

The importance of contraception to women's lives is now recognized within the United Nations Sustainable Development Goals; it was largely ignored in the previous Millennium Development Goals. The challenge now is to empower every woman of reproductive age, regardless of her background, to access the most up-to-date contraceptive choices, free of coercion. There is no cause for complacency here. Access to contraception and contraceptive services is still unequal, globally as well as locally in developed countries, for a variety of reasons, including availability of reliable information and trained health professionals, cost, and cultural and religious barriers of various kinds.

The concept of choice is fundamental. Increasing concern about side effects is creating a need for lower-dose hormonal methods as well as innovative non-hormonal methods, including methods for men, which must be affordable to both governments and individuals. A desire for autonomy and control over one's body with few visits to a healthcare provider means that researchers need to focus their efforts on longer-acting methods that women can potentially control themselves. Multipurpose prevention technologies (MPTs) that simultaneously combine contraception with medications to prevent HIV and other STIs, and more methods that can enhance sexual pleasure, are needed (Lusti-Narasimhan, Khosla, Temmerman, & Young Holt, 2014). Reproductive justice will only be achieved when women of all backgrounds can equally access high quality sexuality education, contraceptive information, and health services, which will require vocal as well as material support from the non-profit sector and from governments and communities across the world.

References

Gillick v West Norfolk and Wisbech Health Authority and the DHSS, No. [1985] 3 All E.R. 402 (House of Lords 1985).

The American College of Obstetricians and Gynecologists (2013). *Reproductive and sexual coercion.* Committee opinion no. 554. Washington, DC: Author. Retrieved from www.acog.org/-/media/Committee-Opinions/Committee-on-Health-Care-for-Underserved-Women/co554.pdf?dmc=1&ts=20180621T0356180254.

The American College of Obstetricians and Gynecologists (2016). *Immediate postpartum long-acting reversible contraception*, Committee opinion no. 670. Washington, DC: Author. Retrieved from www.acog.org/Clinical-Guidance-and-Publications/Committee-Opinions/Committee-on-Obstetric-Practice/Immediate-Postpartum-Long-Acting-Reversible-Contraception.

Arabena, K. (2006). Preachers, policies and power: The reproductive health of adolescent Aboriginal and Torres Strait Islander peoples in Australia. *Health Promotion Journal of Australia, 17,* 1036–1073.

Bateson, D. J., Weisberg, E., McCaffery, K. J., & Luscombe, G. M. (2012). When online becomes off-line: Attitudes to safer sex practices in older and younger women using an Australian internet dating service. *Sex Health, 9,* 152–159.

Bitzer, J., Amy, -J.-J., Beerthuizen, R., Birkhäuser, M., Bombas, T., Creinin, M., Darney, P. D., Vicente, L. F., Gemzell-Danielsson, K. Imthurn, B., Jensen, J. T. Kaunitz, A. M., Kubba, A., Lech, M. M., Mansour, D., Merki, G., Rabe, T., Sedlecki, K., Serfaty, D., Seydoux, J., Shulman, L. P., Sitruk-Ware, R., Skouby, S. O., Szarewski, A., Trussell, J., & Westhoff, C. (2013). Statement on combined hormonal contraceptives containing third- or fourth-generation progestogens or cyproterone acetate, and the associated risk of thromboembolism. *The European Journal of Contraception & Reproductive Health Care, 18,* 143–147.

Boyer, J. (2018). New name, same harm: Rebranding of federal abstience-only programs. *Guttmacher Policy Review, 21,* 11–16.

Brekke, K. (2014). U.S. falls behind other countries that provide free contraception. *Huffington Post.* Retrieved from www.huffingtonpost.com.au/entry/countries-free-birth-control_n_5553037.

Carey, P. (2017). Birth control: Natural methods of contraception on the rise in Australia. Retrieved from www.abc.net.au/news/health/2017-07-22/natural-methods-of-contraception-on-the-rise-in-australia/8683346.

Christian, C. D. (1974). Maternal deaths associated with an intrauterine device. *American Journal of Obstetrics and Gynecology, 119,* 441–444.

Cohen, E., Mackenzie, R. G., & Yates, G. L. (1991). HEADSS, a psychosocial risk assessment instrument: Implications for designing effective intervention programs for runaway youth. *Journal of Adolescent Health, 12,* 539–544.

Columbia Law School (2008). *Human & constitutional rights.* Retrieved from www.hrcr.org/safrica/childrens_rights/Gillick_WestNorfolk.htm.

Conde-Agudelo, A., Rosas-Bermudez, A., Castano, F., & Norton, M. H. (2012). Effects of birth spacing on maternal, perinatal, infant, and child health: A systematic review of causal mechanisms. *Studies in Family Planning, 43,* 93–114.

de Bastos, M., Stegeman, B. H., Rosendaal, F. R., Van Hylckama Vlieg, A., Helmerhorst, F. M., Stijnen, T., & Dekkers, O. M. (2014). Combined oral contraceptives: Venous thrombosis. *Cochrane Database of Systematic Reviews, 3,* 1–54.

Dyer, C. (2018). UK women launch legal action against Bayer over Essure sterilisation device. *British Medical Journal, 360,* k271.

Elliott, L. (2017). Victims of violence: The forced sterilisation of women and girls with disabilities in Australia. *Laws, 6,* 8–26.

EngenderHealth (2002). *Contraceptive sterilization: Global issues and trends.* New York, NY: Author. Retrieved from www.engenderhealth.org/pubs/family-planning/contraceptive-sterilization-factbook.

Faculty of Sexual & Reproductive Health Care (2014). *New product review from the clinical effectiveness unit – One size contraceptive diaphragm (Caya®).* London, UK: Author. Retrieved from www.fsrh.org/standards-and-guidance/documents/cec-ceu-newproductreview-caya-aug-2014.

Faculty of Sexual & Reproductive Healthcare (2010). *Contraceptive choices for young people.* London, UK: Author. Retrieved from www.fsrh.org/documents/cec-ceu-guidance-young-people-mar-2010.

Faculty of Sexual & Reproductive Healthcare (2011). *Combined hormonal contraception.* London, UK: Author. Retrieved from www.fsrh.org/documents/combined-hormonal-contraception.

Faculty of Sexual & Reproductive Healthcare (2012). *Barrier methods for contraception and STI prevention.* London, UK: Author. Retrieved from www.fsrh.org/documents/ceuguidancebarriermethods contraceptionsdi.

Faculty of Sexual & Reproductive Healthcare (2014a). *Male and female sterilisation.* London, UK: Author. Retrieved from www.fsrh.org/documents/cec-ceu-guidance-sterilisation-cpd-sep-2014.

Faculty of Sexual & Reproductive Healthcare (2014b). *Progestogen-only implants.* London, UK: Author. Retrieved from www.fsrh.org/documents/cec-ceu-guidance-implants-feb-2014.

Faculty of Sexual & Reproductive Healthcare (2015a). *Fertility awareness methods.* London, UK: Author. Retrieved from www.fsrh.org/standards-and-guidance/documents/ceuguidancefertilityawareness methods.

Faculty of Sexual & Reproductive Healthcare (2015b). *Progestogen-only injectable contraception.* London, UK: Author. Retrieved from www.fsrh.org/documents/cec-ceu-guidance-injectables-dec-2014.

Faculty of Sexual & Reproductive Healthcare (2015c). *Progestogen-only pills.* London, UK: Author. Retrieved from www.fsrh.org/documents/ceuguidanceprogestogenonlypills.

Faculty of Sexual & Reproductive Healthcare (2016). *UK medical eligibility criteria for contraceptive use (UKMEC)*. London, UK: Author. Retrieved from www.fsrh.org/standards-and-guidance/uk-medical-eligibility-criteria-for-contraceptive-use.

Faculty of Sexual & Reproductive Healthcare (2017a). *Contraception after pregnancy*. London, UK: Author. Retrieved from www.fsrh.org/standards-and-guidance/documents/contraception-after-pregnancy-guideline-january-2017.

Faculty of Sexual & Reproductive Healthcare (2017b). *Contraception for women aged over 40 years*. London, UK: Author. Retrieved from www.fsrh.org/standards-and-guidance/documents/fsrh-guidance-contraception-for-women-aged-over-40-years-2017.

Faculty of Sexual & Reproductive Healthcare (2017c). *Emergency contraception*. London, UK: Author: Author. Retrieved from www.fsrh.org/documents/ceu-clinical-guidance-emergency-contraception-march-2017.

Faculty of Sexual & Reproductive Healthcare (2017d). *FSRH CEU statement: Contraceptive choices and sexual health for transgender and non-binary people*. London, UK: Author. Retrieved from www.fsrh.org/documents/fsrh-ceu-statement-contraceptive-choices-and-sexual-health-for.

Family Planning Association (FPA UK) (2016). *Religion, contraception and abortion factsheet*. Derby, UK: Author. Retrieved from www.fpa.org.uk/factsheets/religion-contraception-abortion.

Family Planning Victoria (2016). Cognitive disability and sexuality. Melbourne, VIC, Australia: Author. Retrieved from www.fpv.org.au/for-you/people-with-a-disability/cognitive-disability-and-sexuality.

Finer, L. B. & Henshaw, S. K. (2006). Disparities in rates of unintended pregnancy in the United States, 1994 and 2001. *Perspectives on Sexual and Reproductive Health, 38*, 90–96.

Freilich, K., Holton, S., Rowe, H., Kirkman, M., Jordan, L., McNamee, K., Bayly, C., Mcbain, J., Sinnott, V., & Fisher, J. (2017). Sociodemographic characteristics associated with the use of effective and less effective contraceptive methods: Findings from the understanding fertility management in contemporary Australia survey. *The European Journal of Contraception & Reproductive Health Care, 22*, 212–221.

Gold, R. B. (2014). Guarding against coercion while ensuring access: A delicate balance. *Guttmacher Policy Review, 17*, 8–14.

Griffiths, E. K., Marley, J. V., Friello, D., & Atkinson, D. N. (2016). Uptake of long-acting, reversible contraception in three remote Aboriginal communities: A population-based study. *Medical Journal of Australia, 205*, 21–25.

Gupta, S., Mola, G., Ramsay, P., Jenkins, G., Stein, W., Bolnga, J., & Black, K. (2017). Twelve month follow-up of a contraceptive implant outreach service in rural Papua New Guinea. *Australian and New Zealand Journal of Obstetrics and Gynaecology, 57*, 213–218.

Hadley, A., Ingham, R., & Chandra-Mouli, V. (2016). Implementing the United Kingdom's ten-year teenage pregnancy strategy for England (1999–2010): How was this done and what did it achieve? *Reproductive Health, 13*, 139.

Hasstedt, K. (2018, June 18). Four big threats to the Title X family planning program: Examining the administration's new funding opportunity announcement. *HealthAffairs*. Retrieved from www.healthaffairs.org/do/10.1377/hblog20180614.838675/full.

Hawkey, A. J., Ussher, J. M., & Perz, J. (2018). "If you don't have a baby, you can't be in our culture": Migrant and refugee women's experiences and constructions of fertility and fertility control. *Women's Reproductive Health, 5*, 75–98.

Hitchcock, C. L. (2008). Elements of the menstrual suppression debate. *Health Care for Women International, 29*, 702–719.

Inoue, K., Kelly, M., Barratt, A., Bateson, D., Rutherford, A., Black, K. I., Stewart, M., & Richters, J. (2016). Australian women's experiences of the subdermal contraceptive implant: A qualitative perspective. *Australian Family Physician, 45*, 734–739.

Joelving, F. (2008, November 19). Sexing up the Pill. *Scienceline*. Retrieved from http://scienceline.org/2008/11/health-joelving-birth-control-pill-plus-testosterone.

Karlsson, T. S., Marions, L. B., & Edlund, M. G. (2014). Heavy menstrual bleeding significantly affects quality of life. *Acta Obstetricia Et Gynecologica Scandinavica, 93*, 52–57.

Liao, P. V. & Dollin, J. (2012). Half a century of the oral contraceptive pill: Historical review and view to the future. *Canadian Family Physician, 58*, e757–e760.

Lusti-Narasimhan, M., Khosla, R., Temmerman, M., & Young Holt, B. (2014). Advancing the sexual and reproductive health and human rights of women beyond 2015. *BJOG: an International Journal of Obstetrics & Gynaecology, 121*(1–2), 9.

Manning, S. & Adams, S. (2014, February 2). Deadly risk of pill used by 1m women: Every GP in Britain told to warn about threat from popular contraceptive. *Daily Mail*. Retrieved from www.dailymail.co.uk/news/article-2550216/Deadly-risk-pill-used-1m-women-Every-GP-Britain-told-warn-threat-popular-contraceptive.html.

Martin, J., de Lora, P., Rochat, R., & Andes, K. L. (2016). Understanding female condom use and negotiation among young women in Cape Town, South Africa. *International Perspectives on Sexual and Reproductive Health, 42*, 13–20.

McCarthy, M. (2009). 'I have the jab so I can't be blamed for getting pregnant': Contraception and women with learning disabilities. *Women's Studies International Forum, 32*, 198–208.

McDonald, E. A. & Brown, S. J. (2013). Does method of birth make a difference to when women resume sex after childbirth? *BJOG: An International Journal of Obstetrics & Gynaecology, 120*, 823–830.

Melbourne Haematology (2012). *Factor V (five) Leiden Mutation.* Coburg, VIC, Australia: Author. Retrieved from www.melbournehaematology.com.au/pdfs/factsheets/melbourne-haematology-factor-v.pdf.

Mills, A. (1997). Combined oral contraception and the risk of venous thromboembolism. *Human Reproduction, 12*, 2595–2598, doi:10.1093/humrep/12.12.2595.

Mohanty, S. & Bhalla, N. (2016, September 16). Indian activists welcome top court ban on 'sterilization camps' after women's deaths. *Reuters*. Retrieved from www.reuters.com/article/us-india-women-sterilisation/indian-activists-welcome-top-court-ban-on-sterilization-camps-after-womens-deaths-idUSKCN11M1YT.

The National Museum of Australia. (n.d.). *Defining moments in A. History – The Pill.* Retrieved from www.nma.gov.au/online_features/defining_moments/featured/the_pill.

Pazol, K., Daniels, K., Romero, L., Warner, L., & Barfield, W. (2016). Trends in long-acting reversible contraception use in adolescents and young adults: New estimates accounting for sexual experience. *Journal of Adolescent Health, 59*, 438–442.

Peipert, J. F., Madden, T., Allsworth, J. E., & Secura, G. M. (2012). Preventing unintended pregnancies by providing no-cost contraception. *Obstetrics & Gynecology, 120*, 1291–1297.

Pinter, B., Hakim, M., Seidman, D. S., Kubba, A., Kishen, M., & Di Carlo, C. (2016). Religion and family planning. *The European Journal of Contraception & Reproductive Health Care, 21*, 486–495.

Population Council (2018). *Population Council's one-year contraceptive ring advances to FDA review* [Press release]. New York, NY: Author. Retrieved from www.popcouncil.org/news/population-councils-one-year-contraceptive-ring-advances-to-fda-review.

Reid, R., Leyland, N., Wolfman, W., Allaire, C., Awadalla, A., Best, C., Dunn, S., Lemyre, M., Marcoux, V., Menard, C., Potestio, F., Rittenberg, D., Singh, S., & Senikas, V. (2011). Oral contraceptives and the risk of venous thromboembolism: An update. *International Journal of Gynecology & Obstetrics, 112*, 252–256.

Rowe, H., Holton, S., Kirkman, M., Bayly, C., Jordan, L., McNamee, K., McBain, J., Sinnott, V., & Fisher, J. (2016). Prevalence and distribution of unintended pregnancy: The understanding fertility management in Australia national survey. *Australian and New Zealand Journal of Public Health, 40*, 104–109.

Santelli, J. S., Kantor, L. M., Grilo, S. A., Speizer, I. S., Lindberg, L. D., Heitel, J., Schalet, A. T., Lyon, M. E., Mason-Jones, A. J., McGovern, T., Heck, C. J., Rogers, J., & Ott, M. A. (2017). Abstinence-only-until-marriage: An updated review of U.S. policies and programs and their impact. *Journal of Adolescent Health, 61*, 273–280.

Secura, G. M., Allsworth, J. E., Madden, T., Mullersman, J. L., & Peipert, J. F. (2010). The Contraceptive CHOICE project: Reducing barriers to long-acting reversible contraception. *American Journal of Obstetrics and Gynecology, 203*, 1–7.

Skovlund, C. W., Mørch, L., Kessing, L., & Lidegaard, Ø. (2016). Association of hormonal contraception with depression. *JAMA Psychiatry, 73*, 1154–1162.

Smith, J. M., Moss, J. A., Srinivasan, P., Butkyavichene, I., Gunawardana, M., Fanter, R., Miller, C. S., Sanchez, D., Yang, F., Ellis, S., Zhang, J., Marzinke, M. A., Hendrix, C. W., Kapoor, A., & Baum, M. M. (2017). Novel multipurpose pod-intravaginal ring for the prevention of HIV, HSV, and unintended pregnancy: Pharmacokinetic evaluation in a macaque model. *PLoS ONE, 12*, e0185946.

Spieler, J. (2014). Sayana® Press: Can it be a "game changer" for reducing unmet need for family planning? *Contraception, 89*, 335–338, doi:10.1016/j.contraception.2014.02.010.

Srikanthan, A. & Reid, R. L. (2008). Religious and cultural influences on contraception. *Journal of Obstetrics and Gynecology Canada, 30*, 129–137.

Taouk, L. H., Fialkow, M. F., & Schulkin, J. A. (2018). Provision of reproductive healthcare to women with disabilities: A survey of obstetrician-gynecologist's training, practices, and perceived barriers. *Health Equity, 2,* 207–215.

Therapeutic Goods Administration (2017). *Essure contraceptive device: Hazard alert – labelling update relating to potential risks* [Press release]. Symonston ACT, Australia: Author. Retrieved from www.tga.gov.au/node/764052.

Trussell, J. (2011). Contraceptive failure in the United States. *Contraception, 83,* 397–404.

Turula, T. (2018). Hyped birth control app natural cycles has been reported to the authorities – after 37 unwanted pregnancies. *Business Insider Nordic.* Retrieved from https://nordic.businessinsider.com/a-swedish-hospital-is-reporting-birth-control-app-natural-cycles-to-the-authorities–after-37-of-its-patients-got-pregnant–/.

UNICEF, NWCCW, & NBS (2014). *Children in China: An atlas of social indicators.* Beijing, People's Republic of China: Author. Retrieved from www.unicef.cn/en/uploadfile/2015/0114/20150114094309619.pdf.

United Nations Population Fund (1994). *Programme of Action of the International Conference on Population and Development.* New York, NY: Author. Retrieved from www.unfpa.org/sites/default/files/event-pdf/PoA_en.pdf.

Van Leeuwen, T., Bateson, D.J., Le Hunte, B., Barratt, A., Black, K.I., Kelly, M., Inoue, K., Rutherford, A., Stewart, M. Richter, J. (2018) Contraceptive Advertising - A Critical Multimodal Analysis. *Journal of Applied Linguistics and Professional Practice,* 13 (1–3): 321–342.

Vekemans, M. (1997). Postpartum contraception: The lactational amenorrhea method. *The European Journal of Contraception & Reproductive Health Care, 2,* 105–111.

Washington University Dept. of Obstetrics and Gynecology (n.d.). *The choice project.* St. Louis, MO: Author. Retrieved from www.choiceproject.wustl.edu.

Weaver, H., Smith, G., & Kippax, S. (2005). School-based sex education policies and indicators of sexual health among young people: A comparison of the Netherlands, France, Australia and the United States. *Sex Education, 5,* 171–188.

Weisberg, E., Bateson, D., McGeechan, K., & Mohapatra, L. (2013). A three-year comparative study of continuation rates, bleeding patterns and satisfaction in Australian women using a subdermal contraceptive implant or progestogen releasing-intrauterine system. *The European Journal of Contraception & Reproductive Health Care, 19,* 5–14.

Weisberg, E. & Kern, I. (2009). Judaism and women's health. *Journal of Family Planning and Reproductive Health Care, 35,* 53–55.

Wentzensen, N. & de Gonzalez, A. B. (2015). The Pill's gestation: From birth control to cancer prevention. *The Lancet Oncology, 16,* 1004–1006.

World Health Organization (WHO) (2013). Programming strategies for postpartum family planning. Geneva: Author. Retrieved from www.who.int/reproductivehealth/publications/family_planning/ppfp_strategies/en.

World Health Organization (WHO) (2015). Health worker roles in providing safe abortion care and post abortion contraception. Geneva: Author. Retrieved from www.who.int/reproductivehealth/publications/unsafe_abortion/abortion-task-shifting/en.

World Health Organization (WHO) (2017). Hormonal contraceptive eligibility for women at high risk of HIV: Guidance statement. Geneva: Author. Retrieved from www.who.int/reproductivehealth/publications/family_planning/HC-and-HIV-2017/en.

12

ABORTION IN CONTEXT

Jeanne Marecek

Worldwide, abortion is one of the commonest gynecological procedures (Sedgh et al., 2012). The common occurrence of induced abortion belies considerable diversity in the social, political, and medical contexts in which abortions are performed, as well as the diverse social and cultural meanings surrounding abortion. It also belies that range of ethical stances that induced abortion has brought forward in some locales and at some points in history.

Abortion figures importantly in the gender order. Controlling women's sexuality and reproduction is key to keeping women in a subordinated position (Angell, 2017). Gender relations necessarily shift when women gain the capacity to determine when they will bear children and the size of their completed families. Furthermore, when the state compels women to undergo abortions they do not want, their self-determination, privacy, and bodily autonomy are compromised. It is perhaps not surprising that treatises on the history of struggles over women's access to abortion often use terms like "war" and "battlefield."

I write this as a woman, a feminist, and a pro-choice advocate living in the United States. I am a cultural psychologist, with an interdisciplinary background in both Gender Studies and South Asia Studies. I have worked in South Asia (specifically, Sri Lanka) for years, so I draw many examples from experiences there.

In this chapter, I survey trends, patterns, and technologies of abortion and women's experiences of terminating pregnancies. Then I turn to questions about the personal experiences of women as they seek and obtain abortions. There is, of course, no single experience of abortion or response to it. Abortions are always embedded in sociocultural and political contexts, as well as in a matrix of local relationships. Moreover, emerging medical practices of abortion (e.g., medication abortion) offer new possibilities for women seeking abortions and for those who provide them. I begin by briefly recounting the history of abortion and women's access to abortion in different parts of the world.

Abortion in historical context

People have always desired to control the number of their offspring and the timing of births. The anthropologist George Devereux (1967) reviewed the available evidence from 350 pre-industrial societies and concluded that abortion appeared to be an "absolutely universal phenomenon" (p. 98). Devereux commented that it would be impossible "even to construct an imaginary social system in which no woman would ever feel at least compelled to abort" (quoted in Joffe & Reich, 2015, p. 45).

We can surmise that in pre-industrial societies women gained knowledge of substances and techniques for terminating a pregnancy by trial and error. There are records of a variety of botanicals (either ingested or inserted into the vagina) that could induce an abortion. There are also records of a variety of practices, such as bloodletting, strenuous physical exertion, fasting, ingesting certain plants, and massage, that were used to induce an abortion. Some of these measures, such as massage and the use of botanical preparations, remain in use in parts of the world such as Thailand and Myanmar (Whittaker, 2002).

Induced abortion was not particularly controversial until the latter part of the 19th century. For instance, when the U.S. enacted a law that prohibited abortion in 1821, the motivation was not to condemn abortion, but to protect women from being poisoned or injured at the hands of unqualified practitioners. In 1869, the Roman Catholic Pope Pius IX issued an edict declaring that a fetus is infused with a soul (*ensoulment*) at the moment of conception. This edict contradicted the longstanding theological distinction between an "animated" and "unanimated" fetus (Gilbert & Pinto-Correia, 2017). That is, for many centuries prior to the edict, Catholic doctrine did not regard a fetus as separate from the pregnant woman until "quickening," the moment when the woman felt the fetus move. Pius IX's edict, which became canon law in the Catholic Church, made abortion at any time during gestation a sin punishable by excommunication from the church. During the final years of the 19th century, a number of countries instituted civil laws against any induced termination of pregnancy. In the U.S., for example, the Comstock Act (1873) banned access to information about both abortion and birth control; in 1890, the U.S. passed another law that limited abortion to cases in which it was necessary to preserve the woman's life (Joffe, 1995). By the end of the 19th century, abortion was illegal or highly restricted in most countries in the global North (Berer, 2016).

Beginning around 1950, many countries in the global North relaxed the legal restrictions on abortion. This easing occurred in the context of the broad social movement toward gender equality and expanded rights for women. The active engagement of feminists was an important factor in this liberalization; other institutions (e.g., medical associations, some churches, and other religious organizations) also supported the liberalization of abortion laws. By the end of the 20th century, many countries in South and East Asia had also loosened legal restrictions on abortion (Center for Reproductive Rights, 2014). The liberalization of abortion laws, however, does not mean that an abortion is freely available to any woman who desires one. As I note below, there may be numerous barriers (notably, cost and difficulty in locating a provider) that block women's access to abortion.

Despite the trend toward liberalization, roughly 25% of the world's population currently resides in countries with laws that generally prohibit abortion (Center for Reproductive Rights, 2014). These countries, many of which are in Latin America and Africa, also account for roughly 80% of the world's unsafe abortions. Making abortions illegal does not prevent women from seeking them; rather, criminalizing abortion compels women to seek illegal abortions, which are often unsafe (Sedgh, Ashford, & Hussain, 2016).

At present, the circumstances under which abortion is legal vary widely across the world. At one extreme are countries (e.g., Chile, Malta, Nicaragua, the Philippines) in which abortion is prohibited altogether. At the other extreme is China, which is the only country in the world that imposes no restrictions on abortion at any stage of pregnancy. The majority of the world's population (roughly 60%) lived in countries with generally permissive abortion laws. That is, abortions are legally permitted either without restriction or under a broad range of circumstances. Nonetheless, apart from China, all countries set gestational age limits that prohibit abortion in the advanced stages of a pregnancy (Center for Reproductive Rights, 2014).

In some times and places, abortion has served as a means of birth control, sometimes because effective means of contraception were unavailable. This was true, for example, in the former USSR, in some post-Soviet societies, and in Cuba. Abortions have been and remain very common in Japan as well, where abortion is regarded as an unexceptional way of ending a pregnancy, and a woman might have a number of abortions in her lifetime. Such countries sometimes are said to have an "abortion culture" (Bélanger & Flynn, 2009; Karpov & Kaumläriäinen, 2005). There are also instances in which the state forces women to abort pregnancies. For example, the People's Republic of China, which will be discussed below, compelled women to terminate pregnancies as part of its stringent program of population control. Moreover, in some countries, forced abortions have been part of ethnic cleansing campaigns designed to eliminate members of minoritized groups.

Abortion technologies

Carried out properly, abortion is one of the safest procedures in Western biomedicine. Indeed, abortion is many times safer than childbirth. Abortions done early in a pregnancy (i.e., within the first 12 weeks after the woman's last menstrual period) are carried out either by medication or by a procedure called vacuum aspiration or suction aspiration. Vacuum aspiration, which takes 5–10 minutes, was invented in the early 1960s, and it came into widespread use soon thereafter (Joffe & Reich, 2015). Medication abortion (popularly termed a "pill abortion") involves taking medicines that induce an abortion. Medication abortions were first introduced in 2000 and involved mifepristone (then called RU-486). Currently, the protocol for a medication abortion involves either two different medications (mifepristone and misoprostol) or multiple doses of misoprostol. The pills are taken in sequence over the course of several days. This sets in motion a physical process akin to a miscarriage. According to current World Health Organization (WHO) standards, medication abortions can be provided up to 12 weeks after the first day of the women's last menstrual period (WHO, 2014). After 12 weeks, termination of a pregnancy requires a surgical procedure. The most common procedure, called dilation and extraction (D&E), is an outpatient procedure that requires clinic visits on two successive days.

In some parts of the world, medical systems other than Western biomedicine, such as Ayurveda and Unani (sometimes called Hikmat), are in wide use. These medical systems have methods of terminating pregnancies. Two such methods are massage and the use of "hot" medicines (Thoradeniya, personal communication, July 2016; Whittaker & Edwards, 2009).

When other means of terminating a pregnancy are unavailable, women often attempt to self-induce an abortion. They do so in a number of ways: Ingesting certain substances; inserting pointed objects or fluids into the uterus; engaging in strenuous exertion; or subjecting themselves to extremes of heat or cold. Such practices often present a serious threat to the health of the woman, and they can lead to death. Moreover, if the pregnancy is not ended, serious injury to the fetus can also occur.

A final technology worthy of mention, though it is not, strictly speaking, an abortion technology, is the Internet. The Internet has opened new possibilities for electronic communication and telemedicine. For example, a woman can have a video consultation with a physician who can then prescribe a medication abortion (Galewitz, 2016). The Internet has also enabled women in countries that prohibit abortion to obtain abortifacient pills by mail. Women on Web (www.womenonweb.org), for example, provided over 1,000 medication abortions a year to women in Ireland (i.e., the Republic of Ireland and Northern Ireland), during the time period when the legal grounds for abortion were very restrictive (Aiken, Gomperts, & Trussell, 2017). (Abortion became legally available in the Republic of Ireland on 1 January 2019.) Women on Web also provided medication abortions to pregnant women in Latin American countries during the Zika epidemic of 2016 (Aiken et al., 2016). Indeed, even in countries in which abortions are legal, women may decide to obtain pills and instructions from grassroots women's organizations, enabling them to self-manage their abortions (Baker & Bellanca, 2018). However, some jurisdictions prosecute women who self-manage their own abortions.

Unsafe abortion

Unsafe abortions are a significant cause of maternal mortality. The World Health Organization (2018) has estimated that 25 million unsafe abortions—roughly one out of three abortions—take place every year. Nearly all of these unsafe abortions take place in the global South. Three out of four abortions in Africa and in Latin America are unsafe.

The World Health Organization defines an abortion as "unsafe" if it is performed by a provider who lacks the necessary training or if it takes place in a setting that does not meet minimal medical standards. However, there may be other aspects of clandestine abortions that render women unsafe. For example, in Sri Lanka, some women have told researchers that they were forced to have sex with the abortionist before he would carry out the procedure; others reported that they were blackmailed by the abortionist, who demanded additional money following the procedure in order to guarantee secrecy (T. Munasinghe, personal communication, August 2017). Not infrequently, women delayed obtaining medical care for complications of an illegal abortion because they feared criminal prosecution (Thalagala, 2010). There may also be psychological and relational repercussions of searching out and undergoing a clandestine abortion (Chiweshe, Mavuso, & Macleod, 2017). Unsafe abortion, which is largely unstudied, is a key issue for social scientists and psychologists to address.

It is often assumed that abortions performed illegally are *de facto* unsafe, and those that are legal are safe. However, although legality and safety are often strongly related, one does not presume the other. A dramatic example of illegal but safe abortion is "Jane," an underground feminist collective in Chicago. The collective (officially known as the Abortion Counseling Service of Women's Liberation) performed over 11,000 safe abortions between 1969 and 1973, prior to the legalization of abortion in the U.S. (Joffe, Weitz, & Stacey, 2004; Kaplan, 1995). Jane's workers did not have professional medical qualifications, and they worked as unpaid volunteers. Most of Jane's clients were women from low-income neighborhoods in Chicago; many were African American. The fee that Jane charged was about $100, however, no woman was turned away because she could not pay.

A dramatic example of legal abortion that was unsafe is the case of Dr. Kermit Gosnell, a licensed physician practicing in Philadelphia. For decades, Gosnell operated an abortion clinic in a low-income neighborhood with a predominantly African American and immigrant population. Gosnell promised low fees and took dangerous shortcuts in order to cut costs. For example, he employed adolescents in lieu of trained staff, and his clinic was unsanitary. Also, Gosnell performed abortions beyond the 24-week limit on gestational age mandated by law. Gosnell was eventually charged with causing the death of one of his patients, as well as with deliberately killing some infants born live (Greasley, 2014). He was ultimately sentenced to life in prison without parole.

Regulating abortion: legal, social, and cultural practices

Beyond permitting or prohibiting abortion, governments also regulate abortions. Such regulations set the parameters for those who seek legal abortions and for medical personnel who provide them. Three important dimensions of legal regulation are: 1) the stage of a pregnancy (or gestational age) at which abortions are permitted or prohibited; 2) the circumstances under which abortion is permitted; and 3) the locus of decision-making regarding the abortion. In nearly every country in the world, the state sets an upper limit on the gestational age at which an abortion can be performed. This age limit is often contested, as opponents of abortion press for more stringent limits. Restrictions regarding the circumstances under which abortion is permitted vary widely. At one extreme, there are countries in which there are no circumstances under which abortion is permitted. At the other end of the spectrum are countries in which abortion within gestational time limits is available more or less at a woman's request. In some countries (e.g., the UK, Australia, Aotearoa/New Zealand), a woman's request for an abortion must be certified by one or more medical practitioners. Feminists have criticized the practice of vesting decision-making power in physicians rather than in the woman herself. However, this practice typically has not blocked women's access to abortion (Lee, 2004; Sheldon, 2016).

More recently, legal statutes have been proposed that would grant to medical personnel the right of conscientious refusal of care. (Such a right could be extended not only to physicians and nurses, but also to other hospital workers, ambulance drivers, and pharmacists.) Such statutes, of course, jeopardize women's access to abortion (Berer, 2008; Council of Europe, 2010; De Zordo, 2017). That, of course, is the intention of those who propose them. Such refusals may reflect genuine moral or ethical reservations, but they may also serve as a way to avoid the stigma associated with providing abortions, as well as the harassment, intimidation, and potential physical danger faced by abortion providers in some locales.

Formal legal regulations are only part of the picture. Laws may be open to loose interpretation, allowing providers and patients considerable latitude in applying them. For example, statutes that limit abortion to cases in which a woman's life is in danger can be interpreted loosely to include possible suicide. Also, laws are sometimes widely—though not openly—flouted, enabling hundreds of thousands of extralegal abortions. Reports suggest this is true in, for example, Sri Lanka, Zimbabwe, and Thailand (Arambepola & Rajapaksa, 2014; Chiweshe, 2015; Whittaker & Edwards, 2009). Moreover, in some instances, although abortion is illegal, "establishing a nonpregnancy" is not. In Bangladesh, for example, despite restrictive abortion laws, government health clinics routinely offer "menstrual regulation," using vacuum aspiration or medications for several weeks after a missed menstrual period (Whittaker, 2010).

Compulsory abortion

The discussion thus far has focused on whether women who want abortions can obtain them. This is, of course, the main bone of contention in present-day abortion politics in most parts of the world. But from a reproductive justice perspective, securing women's access to abortion is not the only issue. What about women who are forced to have abortions they do not want? Such forced abortions too violate the human right to bodily autonomy.

China's draconian program of population control offers a stark example of this human rights violation. In the early 1970s, the central government of China imposed mandatory birth limits. The specific allotments shifted somewhat between 1970 and 2015, and they differed for different sectors of the population (Rigdon, 1996). However, by and large, the state controlled women's reproductive bodies by intrusive surveillance practices, including mandatory pregnancy checks (e.g., a woman had to give evidence of her menstrual period) and mandatory IUD checks. Forced IUD insertions and forced sterilizations also took place (Whyte, Feng, & Cai, 2015). If a woman became pregnant, there was considerable psychological pressure, and possibly physical coercion, to abort the pregnancy (Rigdon, 1996). The Chinese state also resorted to compulsory abortions (and sterilizations) to prevent couples from having children if one partner was deemed to have "hereditary deformities," "mental retardation," or "eugenic defects" (Rigdon, 1996, p. 552).

Social contexts of abortion

Women who seek to terminate a pregnancy must navigate social institutions, norms, and societal structures in addition to legal constraints. Some religions (e.g., Catholicism) have raised moral objections to abortion under all but extraordinary circumstances. Devout women faced with an unsupportable pregnancy may experience considerable strain in weighing their possible courses of action. Some women may face religious or moral objections from their spouses or partners and their family members. Beyond the personal struggles that religious condemnation of abortion may engender, institutionalized religions can erect significant societal barriers to women's access to abortion. In the U.S., for example, the leadership of the Catholic Church has proscribed abortion, as well as artificial birth control, sterilization, fertility treatments, and surrogacy. Furthermore, the U.S. Catholic leadership has financed campaigns to elect anti-abortion candidates to local and national office. The goal is to restrict access to abortion to everyone, whether Catholic or not (Miller, 2014).

Cultural and social factors other than religious beliefs can also influence abortion practice. For example, pressures to bear sons rather than daughters have led to the practice of sex-selection abortion in India, Pakistan, Nepal, and China (Marecek, 2019). The desire to restrict the number of girls in a family has been sufficiently intense to produce noticeable imbalances in the sex ratios of the populations of these countries. The economist Amartya Sen (1990, p. 1) called attention to this in his 1990 assertion that "100 million women" were "missing" from Asia and North Africa. Although the exact figures have since been contested, there is no doubt as to the prevalence of sex-selection abortion (and in some instances, the selective neglect of infant girls and outright female infanticide). India, Pakistan, and Nepal all have passed legislation intended to halt the practice of sex-selection abortion, though few would argue that these legal prohibitions have been entirely successful.

Sex-selection abortion has generated a good deal of ethical debate, including among feminists. For some feminists, a pregnant woman's "right to choose" to terminate a pregnancy is paramount, irrespective of the reason for her choice. For others, sex-selection abortion is morally repugnant. Instead of joining the debate on these terms, more fine-grained accounts of so-called son preference offer other ways to frame the issues. Eklund and Purewal (2017), for example, pointed out that son preference is not solely based on a primordial tradition of male supremacy. Social, cultural, and economic arrangements at least partly drive the desire for sons rather than daughters. In India, Pakistan, and Nepal, for example, these arrangements include discriminatory practices such as exorbitant dowry demands and gender-biased inheritance laws. Were these practices to be abolished, the selective abortion of females might diminish.

Liberal individualism and abortion rights

In most Western high-income countries, the "right to choose" and the rights to bodily auton-omy, self-determination, and privacy have been the central principles of arguments for women's access to abortion (Marecek, Macleod, & Hoggart, 2017). These principles flow from the ethos of liberal individualism common to most of these countries and they remain the core of feminist advocacy for abortion in Western high-income countries (Ferree, 2003).

The ethos of liberal individualism is, however, far from universal. In much of the world, the idea of a self that is wholly independent and master of its fate makes little sense. Instead, the self is construed as embedded in a web of familial and community relations and inter-dependent. In such societies, those who advocate for abortion usually do so not in terms of individual freedom or women's "right to choose." Instead, they argue that abortion is a necessary element of women's reproductive health care. That is, without access to safe abortions, women resort to procedures that jeopardize their health and well-being. It flows from this logic that the provision of safe and legal abortion is a matter of gender equity and reproductive justice.

In the high-income countries of the global North, there has been a dramatic growth in scien-tific knowledge regarding prenatal development, genetic manipulation, and embryology. Along with this new knowledge has come an array of new technologies that dramatically expand the options for conception, pregnancy, and childbirth, at least for those who can pay for them (Gil-bert & Pinto-Correia, 2017). These technologies include prenatal screening, visualization tech-nologies, and obstetric ultrasound. As the capacity to identify genetic anomalies and potential disabilities increases, so too do pressures to abort fetuses that fall short of perfect. Feminist ethi-cists thus are challenged to develop a pro-choice stance that is sensitive to disability rights. Suf-fice it to say that feminist thinkers have long been mindful of the need to address the philosophical, moral, and ethical complexities at the nexus of abortion and disability rights (Hubbard, 1990/2008). Other advances in medical technology, such as fetal surgery and neo-natal intensive care, offer other challenges. As such technologies come into wide use, they work to transform an embryo or fetus into a patient—a bio-political subject entitled to health care (Morgan, 2009; Morgan & Roberts, 2012; Stephenson, Mills, & McLeod, 2017). This new con-figuration of the fetus and its social relations has implications for pro-choice advocates.

Ethical stances regarding termination of pregnancy cannot be disentangled from claims about when human life begins. As described above, the notion that human life begins at conception was asserted only in the late 1800s, in contradiction to longstanding views. It is far from universally held. The assertion is a theological one, not a conclusion based on sci-entific evidence. As the eminent developmental biologist Scott Gilbert (2008) has discussed, there is not, and cannot be, a scientific consensus on this matter. As Gilbert noted, the ques-tion of when life begins is framed within the religious perspective of "ensoulment;" it has no scientific answer.

If we look beyond the global North, we can see societies and religious traditions with quite different views of the fetus, personhood, and human life, as well as varied views on abortion. Moreover, there is neither a consensus among the various strains of particular religious tradi-tions nor consistency across historical time. Also, different societies seem to embrace different ideas about the point at which human life begins. For example, although Bangladesh and Sri Lanka strictly prohibit abortion, both allow "menstrual regulation" (using methods that are, to adopt the parlance of Western biomedicine, tantamount to a first-trimester abortion). This suggests that these societies embrace a definition of the beginning of life that does not rest on *ensoulment*. Another example is Japan, where abortion has been legal since 1949. As described earlier, abortions are not exceptional, and many women have more than one abortion during their reproductive years. In an important treatise on contemporary Japanese Buddhism, La Fleur (1992) described its view of prenatal development in terms of a liquid that flowed slowly into a fetus over the course of gestation. Arresting the flow of this liquid through abortion does not destroy life; it sends the incomplete fetus back to the divine world to await a future birth. If the construct of the "beginning of life" does not admit to a scientific or biological definition, then we might turn our attention to understanding the array of alternate definitions and meanings.

Anti-abortion activism

In some locales, abortion is an unexceptional aspect of women's health care. However, in other locales, opposition to abortion is formidable. For example, the opponents of abortion in the U.S. have played a prominent role in public discourse, electoral politics, legal debates, and health care. They have succeeded in mounting a wide range of barriers to abortion, along with an array of regulations, requirements, and restrictions on abortion procedures and the medical personnel who provide them. Some examples are regulations that require an obligatory waiting period before a patient can receive an abortion; statutes that block public funding for medical training in abortion care; bureaucratic procedures that impede doctors' and patients' access to pill abortions; and regulations that require physicians to give patients false information about the risks of undergoing an abortion.

Anti-abortion activists have also engaged in verbal harassment, threats of violence, and economic boycotts of physicians who provide abortions. Some providers have been murdered (Joffe, 2011). Other tactics aim directly at women seeking an abortion. These include online sales of fake abortion pills, fake "crisis pregnancy" services, and shrill confrontations at the entryways of clinics (Joffe, 2011). These activities and the resulting atmosphere of threat, stigma, and danger are part and parcel of the socioemotional landscape of abortion in the U.S. Moreover, in conservative states in the U.S., there has been an increasing trend toward indirect criminalization, such as prosecuting women who self-induce an abortion (and sometimes those who miscarry) with "child neglect" or "fetal assault" (Rowan, 2015).

Outside the U.S., the Central American countries of Nicaragua, Dominican Republic, and El Salvador, where abortion is illegal, provide stark instances of criminal prosecutions of abortion providers and of women who undergo abortions (Amnesty International, 2018).

Abortion in psychosocial perspective

There are many reasons why a woman may decide that she cannot continue a pregnancy. She may be informed by her physician that carrying the pregnancy will jeopardize her health and urged to end the pregnancy. Or medical tests may reveal that the fetus has severe abnormalities. Moreover, a woman may judge that her capacities, finances, emotional resources, or life circumstances do not enable her to bear and raise a child.

For some women, the decision to obtain an abortion is an easy one; for others, it is agonizing. The evidence suggests that in both the global North and the global South, most abortions are sought by women who are married or in long-term relationships and who already have children (Ban, Kim, & DeSilva, 2002; Beckman, 2017). Adding another child to their families may be economically or practically impossible. In other instances, women may seek to terminate a pregnancy because an out-of-wedlock pregnancy and single motherhood are stigmatized in the communities in which they live, or because their current life circumstances preclude raising a child.

In considering decision-making about abortion, we need to distinguish between pregnancies that are unintended and pregnancies that are unwanted. Unintended pregnancies occur for many reasons. Some may result from coerced or nonconsensual intercourse. Others may result from unprotected intercourse or from contraceptive failure. In many cases, such occurrences do not involve carelessness or irresponsibility on the part of the woman, but rather larger social or cultural problems. In Sri Lanka, for example, where sex education is minimal and sexual matters are seldom spoken of, many unintended pregnancies take place because women were uninformed or misinformed about fertility control. (A common false belief is that a woman cannot become pregnant while she is breastfeeding.) So-called modern methods of birth control are not widely used (even by married couples); couples rely on such failure-prone methods as abstinence, condoms, and withdrawal. Further, some women have reported that their husbands refused to use condoms or withdrawal (Thalagala, 2010).

Unintended pregnancies are common in Western high-income countries as well as in the countries of the global South. For instance, in North America and Australia, roughly half of all pregnancies are unintended (Guttmacher Institute, 2014).

When a woman discovers she is pregnant and did not intend to be, she faces the choice of whether or not to continue the pregnancy. In some cases, women can easily reach a decision. In other cases, however, the decision-making process is difficult and emotionally fraught, especially because a decision to end the pregnancy must be reached quickly.

A good number of unintended pregnancies are wanted. According to a study carried out in 2012, roughly 40% of unintended pregnancies were wanted and ended in births (Guttmacher Institute, 2014). Sometimes, however, a woman may come to realize that she cannot continue a wanted pregnancy. For instance, she may receive medical advice that carrying the pregnancy to term will imperil her health or that the fetus has severe abnormalities. Or a woman may want to continue the pregnancy, but her partner or family members may be strongly opposed. For example, in a study of urban teenagers in the U.S., my colleagues and I found that although many young teenagers wished to carry an unintended pregnancy to term, their mothers were vehemently opposed. They recognized that early childbearing was likely to disrupt their daughters' secondary school education (Flaherty, Marecek, Olsen, & Wilcove, 1983). In other instances, a marriage or relationship dissolves over the course of the pregnancy (oftentimes as a result of conflicts related to the pregnancy), and the woman may come to realize that she is not able to raise the child on her own (Purcell, 2015).

Women's experiences in securing abortions are varied, however the period between deciding to have an abortion and obtaining one is usually marked by anxiety. Time is of the essence: If the abortion is delayed beyond a certain point, the procedure that is necessary is medically more complicated, considerably more expensive, and perhaps harder to arrange. And, if the delay is too long, an abortion cannot be performed at all. When abortions are not covered by medical insurance, women must find the funds to cover the costs, which may include the medical expenses and also travel, childcare, and unpaid absences from work.

The difficulties of securing an abortion are multiplied when abortions are illegal and a clandestine provider must be found. Women of limited means likely have more limited options and may be forced to take more risks both medical and personal. Sri Lanka affords an example from the global South. Although abortion is illegal, it is estimated that nearly half (45%) are done on the sly in private clinics by qualified medical personnel (Arambepola & Rajapaksa, 2014). Affluent urban women are referred to these providers by their private doctors, and they can pay the price. Anecdotal evidence suggests that poor women face more perilous situations (Kumar, 2013; T. Munasinghe, personal communication, August 2017). There are stories of abortionists who were drunk, wearing a mask, operating in a darkened room, as well as of abortionists who forced women to perform oral sex following the procedure.

A final topic concerns the possible mental health consequences of abortion, a topic that has garnered a disproportionate amount of attention and interest among those who oppose abortion. Opponents of abortion repeatedly have put forward claims that abortion leads to prolonged and severe psychological distress among women. Some have invented terms such as "Post Abortion Trauma Syndrome," "Abortion PTSD," and "Post Abortion Stress Syndrome" to convey the notion that abortions lead to psychiatric disorder. None of these terms appear in professional diagnostic manuals such as the DSM (*Diagnostic and Statistical Manual of Mental Disorders*) in the U.S. and the ICD (*International Statistical Classification of Diseases and Related Health Problems of Diseases*). Indeed, given the wide array of contexts, motives, experiences, and personal backgrounds of women who have abortions, the notion of one uniform psychological reaction is implausible. Boyle (1997) offered an important analysis of this issue. Moreover, 25–30% of women in the U.S. have an abortion during their lifetime. If abortions led to psychiatric disorders, signs of an epidemic would be evident.

Because claims of psychological harm have been so insistent, social scientists and mental health researchers have expended considerable effort gathering empirical data on the actual psychological consequences of abortion. Comprehensive reviews of these studies show little evidence to support claims of far-reaching and pervasive distress (Adler et al., 1990; Major et al., 2009). Furthermore, a widely publicized study purporting to show an association between abortion history and mental health was debunked by researchers who carried out a proper re-analysis of the data (Steinberg & Finer, 2010).

Perhaps the most ambitious and well-designed study of women's experiences following abortion is the Turnaway Study, carried out in the U.S. by a team of researchers at the University of California-San Francisco. The Turnaway Study is a large-scale longitudinal investigation employing a quasi-experimental design to compare women who requested and received an abortion and women who requested an abortion but had been turned away (typically because the legal time limit had passed). Participants were re-contacted at six-month intervals for five years. The initial findings showed that, as one might expect, women who wanted abortions but were denied them initially reported more anger, regret, and anxiety. However, for both groups of women, negative emotions typically resolved quickly. Further, the mental health outcomes of women who had received abortions and women who were denied abortions did not differ (Biggs, Upadhyay, McCulloch, & Foster, 2017).

Of course, refuting claims of wholesale psychiatric disorder as a result of abortion does not mean that no women experience psychological difficulties following an abortion. One study suggests, unsurprisingly, that women with pre-existing psychiatric conditions constitute a group at risk for psychological difficulties (Gilchrist, Hannaford, Frank, & Kay, 1995). Detailing the specific experiences—both in a woman's personal history and in the circumstances surrounding the pregnancy and abortion—that lead to distress remains an important topic for psychological research.

In contrast to the extensive literature on the psychological consequences of safe and legal abortion, little is known about the psychological consequences of either unsafe abortions or illegal abortions. Common sense suggests that such abortions will lead to more psychological distress. Given the high incidence of both unsafe abortion and illegal abortion, this is a high priority area for future research (Chiweshe et al., 2017).

Conclusion

In this chapter, I have pointed to several ways in which women's experiences of terminating a pregnancy are embedded in the legal, social, and cultural contexts in which they live. Context makes a difference. The questions that researchers, health providers, and activists ask, as well as the answers they offer, need to be framed within the broader contexts of women's lives. In this brief conclusion, I take a step back to consider some broad themes, as well as to highlight priorities for future research. These themes are relevant as well to counselors who assist women who must make a decision about abortion and then find a way to implement it.

First, although the technologies for controlling fertility continue to improve, we cannot expect that effective contraception will entirely eliminate the need for abortion. Even affluent women in high-income countries where the best contraceptive technologies are on offer can experience an unplanned pregnancy.

Second, making abortions illegal does not prevent women from obtaining them. There is strong evidence that when safe abortions are criminalized, women turn to unsafe ones. Moreover, women of means have more and safer options than poor and minoritized women do. This disparity in access to abortions (which is mirrored in disparities in access to contraception) is a crucial matter of reproductive justice. Class, racial/ethnic, and locational inequities create stark inequities in access to abortion care.

Third, it is women in the global South who are most often forced to resort to illegal abortions, many of which are unsafe. Although some 25 million women undergo unsafe abortions every year, knowledge about such abortions and about the women who are forced to seek them is scant. Evidence suggests that such abortions contribute significantly to maternal mortality. Understanding more about unsafe abortion is an urgent priority, as is activism to eliminate them.

Fourth, although the immediate circumstances of women's lives play an important part in their decisions about childbearing, state policies form the backdrop. Perhaps the most obvious example is China's program of population control, in which state workers coerced couples to use IUDs, sterilization, and abortion to limit the size of their families. More broadly, however, the political economy of every state sets the conditions of possibility for family formation and childrearing. The Nordic countries, for example, provide a broad array of supports for children and parents, including generous parental leave, subsidized childcare, free health care, and free education. The U.S., in which there are few supports for children and families, little assistance to working parents, and limited and contested state health care, offers a contrasting example.

Fifth, women's experiences of abortion are intimately tied to other elements of reproductive health. One such element is access to reliable contraception. In China, for example, the IUDs that the state provided were failure-prone and led to unanticipated pregnancies (Rigdon, 1996). Another such element is the availability of accurate knowledge about fertility and reproduction. In Sri Lanka, for example, many women who sought abortions believed that they had been using adequate contraceptive measures (Thalagala, 2010). In Pakistan, some Muslim clerics preached that breastfeeding and withdrawal were the only methods of birth control that Islamic doctrine allowed (Bowen, 2004).

Sixth and finally, the abortion politics of the global North can have drastic impacts on the global South. In the U.S., for example, when a conservative government comes to power, the state cuts off funding to the United Nations Population Fund (UNFPA), claiming falsely that the UNFPA funds abortion services. In fact, UNFPA provides funds for a wide range of sexual and reproductive health care, including contraceptive supplies, family planning education and services, prenatal and obstetric care, and HIV services, to countries of the global South. Although the intent of the conservative U.S. governments has been to suppress abortions, cutting off funds for reproductive health care seems likely to increase unplanned pregnancies and, in turn, to increase the need for abortions (Bendavid, Avila, & Miller, 2011). This is a particularly ironic example of the global repercussions of so-called "pro-life" abortion politics of the U.S.

References

Adler, N. E., David, H. P., Major, B. N., Roth, S. H., Russo, N. F., & Wyatt, G. E. (1990). Psychological responses after abortion. *Science, 248*(4951), 41–44.

Aiken, A. R. A., Gomperts, R., & Trussell, J. (2017). Experiences and characteristics of women seeking and completing at-home medical termination of pregnancy through online telemedicine in Ireland and Northern Ireland: A population-based analysis. *British Journal of Obstetrics & Gynaecology, 124*, 1208–1215.

Aiken, A. R. A., Scott, J. G., Gomperts, R., Trussell, J., Worrell, M., & Aiken, C. E. (2016, July 28). Requests for abortion in Latin America related to concern about Zika Virus exposure. *New England Journal of Medicine, 375*, 396–398.

Amnesty International (2018). *Body politics*. London: Author.

Angell, M. (2017). The abortion battlefield. *New York Review of Books, 8*(10), June 22, 12.

Arambepola, C. & Rajapaksa, L. C. (2014). Decision making on unsafe abortions in Sri Lanka: A case-control study. *Reproductive Health, 11*, 91–99.

Baker, C. & Bellanca, E. (2018, January 26). Safe and supported: Inside the DIY abortion movement. Retrieved from http://msmagazine.com/blog/2018/01/26/safe-supported-inside-the-diy-abortion-movement.

Ban, D. J., Kim, J., & DeSilva, W. I. (2002). Induced abortion in Sri Lanka: Who goes to providers for pregnancy termination? *Journal of Biosocial Science, 34*, 202–315.

Beckman, L. J. (2017). Abortion in the United States: The continuing controversy. *Feminism & Psychology, 27*, 101–113.

Bélanger, D. & Flynn, A. (2009). The persistence of induced abortion in Cuba: Exploring the notion of an 'abortion culture'. *Studies in Family Planning, 40*, 13–26.

Bendavid, E., Avila, P., & Miller, G. (2011). United States aid policy and induced abortion in sub-Saharan Africa. *Bulletin of the World Health Organization, 889*, 873–880C.

Berer, M. (2008). A critical appraisal of laws on second trimester abortion. *Reproductive Health Matters, 16*(31-Supplement), 3–13.

Berer, M. (2016, October). *Decriminalisation*. Presentation at 12th FIAPAC Conference, Lisbon, Portugal: Improving Women's Journeys Through Abortion.

Biggs, M. A., Upadhyay, U., McCulloch, C. E., & Foster, D. G. (2017). Women's mental health and well-being 5 years after receiving or being denied an abortion: A prospective, longitudinal cohort study. *Journal of the American Medical Association Psychiatry, 74*, 169–178.

Bowen, D. L. (2004). *Islamic law and family planning, in Islam and social policy*. Nashville, TN: Vanderbilt University Press.

Boyle, M. (1997). *Re-thinking abortion: Psychology, gender, power, and the law*. London, UK: Routledge.

Center for Reproductive Rights (2014). *The world's abortion laws 2014*. New York, NY: Author. Retrieved from www.reproductiverights.org/sites/crr.civicactions.net/files/documents/Abortion Map2014.PDF.

Chiweshe, M. (2015). A narrative-discursive analysis of abortion decision-making in Zimbabwe (Unpublished Doctoral Dissertation). Rhodes University, South Africa.

Chiweshe, M., Mavuso, J., & Macleod, C. (2017). Reproductive justice in context: South African and Zimbabwean women's narratives of their abortion decision. *Feminism & Psychology, 27*, 203–224.

Council of Europe, Parliamentary Assembly (2010). *Resolution 1763: The right to conscientious objection in lawful medical care*. Brussels: Council of Europe.

De Zordo, S. (2017). "Good doctors do not object": Obstetricians-gynaecologists' perspectives on conscientious objection to abortion care and their engagement with pro-abortion rights protests in

Italy. In S. De Zordo, J. Mishtal, & L. Anton (Eds), *Fragmented landscapes: Abortion governance and associated protest logics in Europe* (pp. 147–168). Oxford, UK: Berghahn Books.

Devereux, G. (1967). A typological study of abortion in 350 primitive, ancient, and pre-industrial societies. In H. Rosen (Ed.), *Abortion in America: Medical, psychiatric, legal, anthropological, and religious considerations* (pp. 97–120). Boston, MA: Beacon Press.

Eklund, L. & Purewal, N. (2017). The bio-politics of population control and sex selective abortion in China and India. *Feminism & Psychology*, *27*, 34–55.

Ferree, M. M. (2003). Resonance and radicalism: Feminist framing in the abortion debates of the United States and Germany. *American Journal of Sociology*, *109*, 304–344.

Flaherty, E. W., Marecek, J., Olsen, K., & Wilcove, G. (1983). Preventing adolescent pregnancy: An interpersonal problem-solving approach. *Prevention in Human Services*, *2*(3), 49–64.

Galewitz, P. (2016, November 10). A study tests the safety of women using abortion pills sent by mail. *New York Times*, p. A13.

Gilbert, S. F. (2008). When 'personhood' begins in the embryo: Avoiding a syllabus of errors. *Birth Defects Research C: Embryo Today: Reviews*, *84*, 164–173.

Gilbert, S. F. & Pinto-Correia, C. (2017). *Fear, wonder, and science in the new age of reproductive biotechnology*. New York, NY: Columbia University Press.

Gilchrist, A. C., Hannaford, P. C., Frank, P., & Kay, C. R. (1995). Termination of pregnancy and psychiatric morbidity. *British Journal of Psychiatry*, *167*, 243–248.

Greasley, K. (2014). The pearl of the 'Pro-Life' movement? Reflections on the Kermit Gosnell controversy. *Journal of Medical Ethics*, *40*, 419–423.

Guttmacher Institute (2014, September). *New study finds that 40% of pregnancies worldwide are unintended*. New York, NY: Author. Retrieved from www.guttmacher.org/news-release/2014/new-study-finds-40-pregnancies-worldwide-are-unintended.

Hubbard, R. (1990/2008). Abortion and disability: Who should and who should not inhabit the world? In L. J. Davis (Ed.), *The disability studies reader* (2nd ed., pp. 93–103). New York, NY: Routledge.

Joffe, C. (1995). *Doctors of conscience: The struggle to provide abortion before and after Roe v. Wade*. Boston, MA: Beacon Press.

Joffe, C. (2011). *Dispatches from the abortion wars: The costs of fanaticism to doctors, patients and the rest of us*. Boston, MA: Beacon Press.

Joffe, C. E. & Reich, J. (2015). *Reproduction and society: Interdisciplinary readings*. New York, NY: Routledge.

Joffe, C. E., Weitz, T. A., & Stacey, C. L. (2004). Uneasy allies: Pro-choice physicians, feminist health activists, and the struggle for abortion rights. *Sociology of Health & Illness*, *26*, 775–796.

Kaplan, L. (1995). *The story of Jane: The legendary underground feminist abortion service*. Chicago, IL: University of Chicago Press.

Karpov, V. & Kaumläriäinen, K. (2005). 'Abortion culture' in Russia: Its origins, scope, and challenge to social development. *Journal of Applied Sociology*, *22*, 13–33.

Kumar, R. (2013). Abortion in Sri Lanka: The double standard. *American Journal of Public Health*, *103*, 400–404.

La Fleur, W. R. (1992). *Liquid life: abortion and Buddhism in Japan*. Princeton, NJ: Princeton University Press.

Lee, E. (2004). Young women, pregnancy, and abortion in Britain: A discussion of law 'in practice'. *International Journal of Law, Policy and the Family*, *18*, 283–304, doi:10.1093/lawfam/18.3.283.

Major, B., Appelbaum, M., Beckman, L., Dutton, M. A., Russo, N. F., & West, C. (2009). Abortion and mental health: Evaluating the evidence. *American Psychologist*, *64*, 863–890.

Marecek, J. (2019). Toward a transnational feminist psychology of women's reproductive experiences. In L. H. Collins, J. K. Rice, & S. Michikawa (Eds), *Towards a transnational psychology of women* (pp. 185–210). Washington, DC: American Psychological Association.

Marecek, J., Macleod, C. I., & Hoggart, L. (2017). Abortion in social, legal and healthcare contexts. *Feminism & Psychology*, *27*, 4–14.

Miller, P. (2014). *Good Catholics: The battle over abortion in the Catholic Church*. Berkeley, CA: University of California Press.

Morgan, L. (2009). *Icons of life: A cultural history of human embryos*. Berkeley, CA: University of California Press.

Morgan, L. M. & Roberts, E. F. (2012). Reproductive governance in Latin America. *Anthropology & Medicine*, *19*, 241–254.

Purcell, C. (2015). The sociology of women's abortion experience: Recent research and future directions. *Social Psychology Compass*, *5*, 585–596.

Rigdon, S. M. (1996). Abortion law and practice in China: An overview with comparisons to the United States. *Social Science & Medicine, 42*, 543–560.

Rowan, A. (2015). Prosecuting women for self-inducing abortion: Counterproductive and lacking compassion. *Guttmacher Policy Review, 18*, Summer. Retrieved from www.guttmacher.org/gpr/2015/09/prosecuting-women-self-inducing-abortion-counterproductive-and-lacking-compassion.

Sedgh, G., Ashford, L. S., & Hussain, R. (2016). Unmet need for contraception in developing countries: Examining women's reasons for not using a method (unpublished report). New York, NY: Guttmacher Institute. Retrieved from www.guttmacher.org/report/unmet-need-for-contraception-in-developingcountries.

Sedgh, G., Singh, S., Henshaw, S. K., Bankole, A., Shah, I. H., & Åhman, M. A. (2012). Induced abortion: Incidence and trends worldwide from 1995 to 2008. *Lancet, 379*(9816), 625–632.

Sen, A. (1990, December 20). More than 100 million women are missing. *New York Review of Books.* Retrieved from nybooks.com/articles/1990/12/20/more-than-100-million-women-are-missing/?printpage=true.

Sheldon, S. (2016). The decriminalisation of abortion: An argument for modernisation. *Oxford Journal of Legal Studies, 36*, 334–365.

Steinberg, J. & Finer, L. (2010). Examining the association of abortion history and current mental health: A reanalysis of the National Comorbidity Survey using a common-risk-factors model. *Social Science & Medicine, 72*, 72–82.

Stephenson, N., Mills, C., & McLeod, K. (2017). "Simply providing information": Negotiating the ethical dilemmas of pregnancy termination as they arise in the obstetric ultrasound clinic. *Feminism & Psychology, 27*, 72–91.

Thalagala, N. (2010). *Process, determinants and impact of unsafe abortions in Sri Lanka.* Colombo, Sri Lanka: Family Planning Association of Sri Lanka.

Whittaker, A. (2002). "The truth of our day by day lives": Abortion decision making in rural Thailand. *Culture, Health & Sexuality, 4*, 1–20.

Whittaker, A. (2010). *Abortion in Asia: Local dilemmas, global politics.* Oxford, UK: Berghahn Books.

Whittaker, A. & Edwards, L. (2009). *Abortion, sin, and the state in Thailand.* London, UK: Routledge.

Whyte, M. K., Feng, W., & Cai, Y. (2015). Challenging myths about China's one child policy. *The China Journal, 74*, 144–159.

World Health Organization (WHO) (2014). *Clinical practice handbook for safe abortion.* Geneva: Author. Retrieved from www.who.int/reproductivehealth/publications/unsafe_abortion/clinical-practice-safe-abortion/en.

World Health Organization (WHO) (2018). *Preventing unsafe abortion.* Geneva: Author. Retrieved from who.int/news-room/fact-sheets/detail/preventing-unsafe-abortion.

13

WOMEN'S EXPERIENCES OF INFERTILITY

Jessica L. Barnack-Tavlaris

Say a woman is more than the sum of her parts and I'll listen. Say that she is more than fruit and blossom and branch and I'll nod my head yes. But say the body does not want and I will fall to the floor under the weight of a world that does not heed the sweet talk of a heartbeat.

Sonja Livingston (2015, p. 78)

No two women's experience of infertility is exactly the same. It can consume someone's life; where some experience hope and resilience and others experience shame and despair. There are complex biopsychosocial factors that determine the impact of infertility on one's identity, well-being, and relationships. This chapter provides a review of the recent literature that has examined women's experiences of infertility, summarizes the limitations of the literature, and makes recommendations for future directions.

Infertility defined

In 2017, experts from around the world developed the International Glossary on Infertility and Fertility Care, in order to provide global consistency in communication and research reports (Zegers-Hochschild et al., 2017). In this glossary of 283 terms, infertility is defined as:

> A disease characterized by the failure to establish a clinical pregnancy after 12 months of regular, unprotected sexual intercourse or due to an impairment of a person's capacity to reproduce either as an individual or with his/her partner. Fertility interventions may be initiated in less than 1 year based on medical, sexual and reproductive history, age, physical findings and diagnostic testing. Infertility is a disease, which generates disability as an impairment of function.
>
> *(Zegers-Hochschild et al., 2017, p. 401)*

A woman who meets these criteria and has never previously had a clinical pregnancy (i. e., ultrasound confirmation of gestational sac or heartbeat along with high level of pregnancy hormone) is considered to have primary infertility, whereas a woman who is experiencing infertility but has previously had a pregnancy is diagnosed with secondary infertility. Global estimates of infertility prevalence are difficult to obtain due to differences in how data are collected across countries, the definitions of infertility used in the studies, and differential access to infertility screening and diagnosis. In addition, clinical definitions, such as the one from the international glossary, are heteronormative, which affects the accuracy of infertility rates for lesbian women.

In a systematic analysis of health surveys from 190 different countries and territories, Mascarenhas and colleagues (2012) estimated infertility prevalence among women who were in a heterosexual union (marriage or cohabitation) and unable to have a live birth after a five-year period. With this definition, they found that, in 2010, 1.9% of women between 20 and 44 years of age were experiencing primary, and 10.5% of women were experiencing secondary, infertility. Prevalence was highest in south Asia, sub-Saharan Africa, north Africa/Middle East, central/eastern Europe, and central Asia. Gerais and Rushwan (1992) estimated primary infertility rates of 10.1% in Africa, with rates as high as 32% in some regions. In another study of 12-month prevalence rates from population surveys, current infertility rates ranged from 3.5% to 16.7% in more developed countries and from 6.9% to 9.3% in less developed countries; overall median prevalence was estimated to be 9% (Boivin, Bunting, Collins, & Nygren, 2007). Stephen and Chandra (1998) predicted that approximately 6.5 million women in the U.S. will experience infertility by the year 2025; therefore, infertility seems to be a growing problem that warrants continued attention across the globe.

Causes of infertility

There are a number of factors that may contribute to infertility, each with different implications for prevention and treatment. Biological explanations for infertility can be attributed to male factors, female factors, or both. However, approximately 20% of infertility cases have no known biomedical cause (Greil, Schmidt, & Peterson, 2016). Ovulatory problems (e.g., polycystic ovarian syndrome [PCOS]) are the most frequent causes of female infertility, and most can be treated with hormones (Blundell, 2007; Greil et al., 2016). Other common female factors include endometriosis (uterine lining grows outside the uterus and causes scarring), uterine fibroids (benign tumors that can prevent implantation), and pelvic inflammatory disease (causes scarring that blocks the fallopian tubes).

Age is another significant risk factor because fertility decreases with normal age-related changes in the ovaries. A woman's fertility gradually declines after age 30, with significant decline after age 35 (American Society for Reproductive Medicine, 2012). The average age of motherhood in developed countries is higher than in developing countries (Central Intelligence Agency, 2016), and in many developed countries the average age of motherhood has been steadily increasing (Mathews & Hamilton, 2016). For example, the average age at first birth for women in the U.S., UK, and Australia is 26.4, 28.5, and 28.7 years respectively, compared with the age at first birth for women in Bangladesh (18.5 years) and Zimbabwe (20 years) (Central Intelligence Agency, 2016). Delaying pregnancy until later in life inevitably increases risk for infertility. Additional risk factors for infertility include both active and passive smoking, weight (underweight or overweight), sexually transmitted infections (STIs), exposure to toxins, and treatments for cancer and HIV (Blundell, 2007; Greil et al., 2016; Prince & Domar, 2013). Although age is a significant risk factor in developed countries, the primary risk factors in developing countries are STIs and infections during pregnancy (Ombelet, 2011).

When it comes to male factors, semen quantity and quality (shape and motility) are the most likely causes. Semen quality can be affected by congenital malformations, undescended testicles, vericocele (enlarged veins in the testicles), and exposure to environmental toxins

(Greil et al., 2016; Prince & Domar, 2013). Other male factors may include heavy weight, smoking, sexual dysfunction (the relation can be reciprocal; Berger, Messore, Pastuszak, & Ramasamy, 2016), and treatments for cancer. Proper evaluation of both partners in hetero-sexual couples is needed in order to provide the most appropriate treatment options.

Infertility treatments

Infertility is a medicalized condition for which there are complex treatment options. Regardless of the infertility's cause, it is primarily the woman's body that has to endure treatment. Advances in technology have increased the number of treatment options; how-ever, the existence of the possibilities can create pressure on women to pursue treatment, some of which are financially, physically, and emotionally invasive and taxing. Further, there are significant barriers to treatment, and there is wide variability in the extent to which insurance companies or national health services cover infertility treatments. In the U.S., some states have laws that require employers to cover infertility diagnosis and treat-ment (depending on the number of employees), some require employers to offer (but not necessarily to cover) services, and some states have no laws regarding infertility diagnosis or treatment (see Resolve: The National Infertility Association, 2018, for a current list of U.S. state laws). In countries where healthcare is universal (e.g., Canada, the U.K., Austra-lia), there is variability in infertility treatment coverage (Infertility Network, 2016). Despite high infertility rates, treatment options for individuals in the global South are extremely limited due to treatment's high cost and inaccessibility (Ombelet, 2011).

Depending on the diagnosis, infertility treatments can involve lifestyle changes (e.g., smoking cessation, changes in nutrition, physical activity), psychological and mind/body interventions (e.g., psychotherapy, yoga, acupuncture, meditation), surgery (e.g., to remove fibroids, treat endometriosis, repair tubal damage), and other medical treatments (e.g., ovula-tion induction, hormone treatment, assisted reproductive technology [ART], artificial insemination). In vitro fertilization (IVF) is the most common form of ART, and it is typic-ally used to treat infertility caused by damaged fallopian tubes, endometriosis, some male factors, premature ovarian failure, and sometimes unexplained infertility that has been unre-sponsive to other treatments (American College of Obstetricians and Gynecologists [ACOG], 2017). IVF typically involves drug therapy to trigger ovulation, followed by a procedure to retrieve the eggs from the ovaries and then fertilize them with the partner's or a donor's sperm. In some cases, donor eggs are also used. Several days later, the viable embryo(s) is(are) transferred to the uterus. Additional viable embryos can be frozen and transferred later (ACOG, 2017).

Success rates of ART are difficult to estimate because they depend on factors such as age, diagnosis, egg quality, and sperm quality. The Society for Assisted Reproductive Technology (SART, 2016) collects and publishes data on ART success rates in the U.S. The preliminary 2016 data revealed that 242,618 treatment cycles resulted in 71,296 births (ASRM, 2018). The live birth rates per egg retrieval cycle with the patient's own eggs ranged from 3.3% (for women older than 42 years) to 47.6% (for women younger than 35 years), which shows the importance of age in treatment success. An increased risk of multiple births is associated with IVF, especially if more than one embryo is transferred to the uterus. For example, 8.3% of the 47.6% mentioned previously were multiple births (8.1% twins, 0.2% triplets or more) (SART, 2016). As the IVF success rates demonstrate, a substantial number of women may not achieve a live birth following their first (and maybe last) treatment. In a prospective study of women in the U.K., prognosis-adjusted estimates revealed a cumulative live-birth rate of 65.3% after six cycles of IVF; thus, there is reason to continue treatment past three or four cycles, which is when IVF is more commonly discontinued (Smith, Tilling, Nelson, & Lawlor, 2015).

Many women across the globe lack access to treatment, which means there are disparities in who is able to achieve a live birth. Chambers and colleagues (2009) reviewed the economic impact of ART in developed countries and found the U.S. and U.K. to have the highest cost of IVF per live birth ($41,132USD and $40,364USD, respectively), whereas Scandinavia and Japan had the lowest ($24,485USD and $24,329USD, respectively). In the U.S., women of color and women of lower socioeconomic status have higher rates of infertility, but are less likely to receive treatment (Greil, McQuillan, Shreffler, Johnson, & Slauson-Blevins, 2011) because of the expense involved. In addition, although same-sex couples and transgender individuals rely on ART to have children, they often do not qualify for insurance coverage (when it's available) due to discrimination in the definitions of infertility that exist within some policies (Eyler, Pang, & Clark, 2014).

In developing countries, there are significant financial barriers to infertility treatment. It is estimated that the cost of an IVF cycle is at least one-half of an individual's annual income in every developing country (Nachtigall, 2006). Ombelet (2011) called for more research with simplified ART diagnostic and treatment procedures in order to improve access in developing countries. In addition to cost, there are social and cultural barriers to infertility treatment in some countries. For example, some religious beliefs prevent individuals from seeking infertility treatment, and in developing countries with growing populations that are working to encourage contraception, some practitioners do not consider infertility a public health priority (Nachtigall, 2006). The experience of infertility in many developing countries is highly stigmatized with significant social consequences such as blame, isolation, and violence (Nachtigall, 2006). However, the psychological and physical burden that women endure during treatment, as well as the expense incurred with each cycle, can result in avoidance or discontinuation of ART (Boivin et al., 2012). Thus, the process of receiving an infertility diagnosis, seeking treatment, and awaiting the outcome all have significant implications for women's physical and psychological well-being.

Psychosocial impact

The definition of infertility presented previously illustrates the biomedicalization of infertility, which is, in part, necessary to garner support for treatments and health care coverage. However, the words *failure* and *disability* suggest a deficit of the body (largely the woman's body), which can have psychological implications for how women cope with their diagnosis. In the last decade, more research has focused on understanding the psychosocial context that shapes the experience of infertility (Greil, Slauson-Blevins, & McQuillan, 2010). The psychosocial impact of infertility has been found to vary by gender in that women report more psychological distress and employ different coping strategies than men do (Greil et al., 2010). Some of the interconnected themes that have emerged from the recent multidisciplinary literature include the implications of an infertility diagnosis on women's identity, the complex relationship between psychological distress and infertility, and the impact of infertility on relationships.

Implications of an infertility diagnosis on women's identity

Sociocultural expectations for women (primarily heterosexual women) include the ability to nurture and care for others, to become a mother, and to have a strong maternal instinct. These expectations are heteronormative, and may not necessarily be applied to sexual and gender minority women (Donovan, 2008). The motherhood mandate (Russo, 1976) holds true for heterosexual women in general, but is particularly strong in societies where pronatalism is especially high (Benyamini, Gozlan, & Weissman, 2017). For example, in a study of migrant and refugee women from developing countries who were living in Australia and Canada, participants discussed a "motherhood imperative" and described motherhood as "synonymous with womanhood" (Hawkey, Ussher, & Perz, 2018, p. 80).

Many societies socialize girls to seek and achieve motherhood, and it is often assumed that they will want and be able to do so without intervention. The desire to become a mother is viewed in many cultures as biological, and thus those who do not feel or express that desire are viewed negatively (e.g., deviant, cold, selfish). Donovan (2008) pointed out that lesbian women do not always experience the same social pressure to become mothers, which provides support for the social constructivist viewpoint of a woman's desire to mother. These sociocultural pressures can affect the way women respond to and cope with an infertility diagnosis. When women experience social pressure to become mothers, infertility can threaten their identity (McCarthy, 2008) and may cause them to question their purpose in life (Devereaux & Hammerman, 1998), which is detrimental to their self-esteem and well-being. Infertility can be especially problematic for women who live in cultures where motherhood is the core of one's identity, yet reproductive agency is limited (Hawkey et al., 2018).

There is some evidence for the negative effects of sociocultural expectations on women's experience of distress during infertility. In a study conducted with women undergoing IVF, participants who reported having experienced more social pressure to become a mother were more likely to perceive their infertility as stressful than were those who report no or less pressure (Miles, Keitel, Jackson, Harris, & Licciardi, 2009). Sociocultural expectations for motherhood (or parenthood) can be particularly concerning for those whose fertility is compromised by a traumatic illness such as cancer. Cancer-related infertility can contribute to the biographical disruption that cancer survivors face, in that it disrupts their expected life course and identity (Ussher, Perz, & The Australian Cancer and Fertility Study Team, 2018). From a young age, so much of a woman's life focuses on her reproductive capacity. For example, the beginning of menstruation brings the possibility of conception, along with the pressure to prevent unplanned pregnancy. When someone wants and expects to be able to become a parent easily and without intervention, it can come as a shock and disappointment to have to conceptualize a different life plan.

An intersectional lens shows that the impact of infertility on one's sense of identity can vary depending on one's other socially constructed and dynamic identities (Ceballo, Graham, & Hart, 2015). The typical discourse of motherhood can exclude people with marginalized identities, such as women with low SES, lesbian women, and transgender men, and the paucity of research with diverse samples limits our knowledge of how sociocultural expectations interact with diverse identities and how that affects their experience of infertility. Transgender men who experience a gestational pregnancy may experience the ART and healthcare systems as exclusionary, which contributes to feelings of isolation (Charter, Ussher, Perz, & Robinson, 2018). Lesbian women also report significant barriers to ART access because of the heteronormative narrative on which infertility diagnosis and treatment are based (Donovan, 2008).

When individuals who want to become parents do not have access to, or do not experience success with, ART or adoption, or if they lack the resources to be what their society considers an *ideal* parent, they may seek to fulfill their desire to parent in other ways such as taking on the role of step-mother or caretaking of others in their social networks (Bell, 2009; Ussher & Perz, 2018).

Complex relationship between psychological distress and infertility

Infertility is a chronic stressor that impacts all aspects of a woman's life, and, for some, infertility has been associated with significant psychological distress and even clinical outcomes, such as anxiety and depression (e.g., Khodarahimi, Hosseinmirzaei, & Bruna, 2014; Miles et al., 2009; Shani, Yelena, Reut, Adrian, & Sami, 2016; Sultan & Tahir, 2011). However, it is unclear whether it is infertility itself, infertility treatment, or both that are responsible for increased psychological distress, and studies of the extent to which psychological distress affects treatment outcomes yield mixed evidence.

Greil and colleagues used the National Survey of Fertility Barriers to conduct a longitudinal study with U.S. women in order to tease apart the psychological distress that results from infertility treatment versus infertility itself (Greil, McQuillan, Lowry, & Shreffler, 2011). Women who had received infertility treatment reported more fertility-specific distress, and increased distress over time, than infertile women who had not received treatment. These findings suggest an association between infertility treatment and psychological well-being; however, the findings do not reveal the direction of causation. It is possible that women who experience the most distress from their infertility diagnosis are those who seek treatment. Longitudinal studies that measure fertility-related distress before treatment are needed to help clarify the direction of the association.

It is quite possible that infertility treatment alone would impact distress above and beyond an infertility diagnosis, given the significant physical, psychological, and financial burden of treatment. Infertility treatment is a consuming process in which individuals feel uncertainty and little control. Diagnostic and treatment procedures can be uncomfortable, painful, and interfere with work and daily life. Relational and sexual satisfaction can also be affected because sex becomes routinized rather than spontaneous. Boivin and colleagues (2012) proposed various ways in which medical professionals can alleviate the burden of treatment and prevent discontinuation. They described techniques that target patient, clinic, and treatment factors, some of which include tailoring educational materials to reduce patients' fear and negative attitudes toward treatment, improving communication strategies to reduce negative staff–patient interactions, and simplifying treatment protocols to reduce the physical burden on patients.

Given the strong desire (and, for many, social pressure) many women have to resolve their infertility, researchers have examined women's psychosocial experiences post-unsuccessful infertility treatment. The findings of these studies reveal both significant challenges and profound resilience. For example, McCarthy (2008) conducted an interview study that resulted in a rich exploration of the lived experience of 22 women with infertility. The women, who were, on average, four years out of unsuccessful medical treatment,

> revealed an experience of intense suffering coupled with an introspective effort to rediscover a sense of self and a feeling of balance, purpose, and meaning in their lives. Their stories were characterized as a paradox, the entertaining of two opposing perceptions that cancel each other. They struggled to reconcile their opposing identities of self, views of the world, and images of an anticipated future. They experienced loss and opportunity, emptiness and gratitude, and infertility as a 'present absence.'
>
> *(p. 320)*

Coping with fertility loss extends over one's lifetime, and the effects can reemerge later in life when women enter the phase in which they might have been a grandparent had their treatment been successful (Wirtberg, Möller, Hogström, Tronstad, & Lalos, 2007).

Less is known about how women who have experienced infertility adjust to life after treatment success. It is important to know more about how the trauma of infertility impacts the experience of pregnancy and parenthood. Adjusting to many new stressors and lack of sleep could exacerbate the pre-existing problems caused by years of infertility (Devereaux & Hammerman, 1998). Further, ART increases the risk of prematurity and congenital anomalies, which add complexity to the parenthood transition (McGrath, Samra, Zukowsky, & Baker, 2010). Women who conceive using ART are also more likely than other mothers to give birth to multiple infants. The transition to parenting multiples is stressful, and some research suggests that parents of multiples are more likely than parents of singletons to experience post-partum depression and anxiety (Baor & Soskolne, 2010; Klock, 2004; Vilska et al., 2009). Although the existing evidence is mixed and inconclusive (Gressier et al., 2015; Hammarberg, Fisher, & Wynter, 2008), some research suggests that women who experience infertility may be at greater risk for postpartum depression (Lee, Liu, Kuo, & Lee, 2011) and/or anxiety (Monti et al., 2008). Symptoms of postpartum depression or anxiety can be confusing for women who had such a strong desire to achieve pregnancy, which may make it more difficult for them to seek help. Postpartum depression itself is stigmatized, and women who have experienced infertility may feel even more stigmatized for having these symptoms.

Although some women experience clinical levels of anxiety and depression in response to an infertility diagnosis, it is important to point out that their rates of clinical psychopathology are similar to those of the general population of women. In addition, a limitation to this research is the variance in definitions of infertility and how researchers measure important variables, such as psychological distress, depression, anxiety, and treatment. More research is needed to understand the differences between women with infertility who report clinical levels of anxiety and depression and those who do not in order to understand how best to assist those who need support. In their review of the literature on infertility-related clinical anxiety, Peloquin and Lafontaine (2010) proposed a conceptual model that describes the intrapersonal, interpersonal, and contextual factors that correlate with clinical anxiety. Gender is a significant correlate, as women report more clinical anxiety than men do. Intrapersonal factors that may buffer clinical anxiety include problem-focused coping, satisfaction with social support networks, and secure attachment style. Preexisting anxiety and other comorbidities are intrapersonal factors that may be exacerbated by infertility, but more research is needed in this area (Peloquin & Lafontaine, 2010).

Interpersonal factors that predict clinical levels of anxiety include romantic attachment, dyadic adjustment, and dyadic coping strategies. Having an insecure romantic attachment, preexisting conflicts, and problems with communication can make it more difficult for couples to cope with the stress of infertility, which results in feelings of isolation (Peloquin & Lafontaine, 2010). Research with heterosexual couples experiencing infertility has also shown that dyadic coping strategies (in this case, cognitive appraisals) may be discordant, which can negatively impact women's adjustment and well-being (Thompson, Woodward, & Stanton, 2012). Dyadic coping strategies are understudied, especially in same-sex couples, and these could shed some light on the differences between those who develop clinical anxiety and those who do not.

The contextual factors identified by Peloquin and Lafontaine (2010) include medical factors (i.e., duration of infertility, type of diagnosis, number of treatment cycles) and sociocultural factors (e.g., high social pressure to conceive, high stigmatization of infertility or childlessness). Researchers who aim to identify clinical anxiety risk factors should consider these elements and study both members of the dyad at multiple time points along the duration of their experience with infertility. Knowledge of these risk factors can inform the development of programs of prevention and intervention that can prevent anxiety from reaching clinical levels.

Several studies of the effects of stress, anxiety, and depression on ART outcomes have yielded mixed results. In a meta-analysis of 31 prospective studies, researchers found small but significant negative correlations among stress, state and trait anxiety, and achieving a clinical pregnancy through ART; however, there were no significant correlations between state or trait anxiety and live birth rates following ART (Matthiesen, Frederiksen, Ingerslev, & Zachariae, 2011). The authors cautioned that there were significant methodological differences across the studies, and noted that several factors moderated the small but significant correlations, including age, the percentage of the sample who were using ART for the first time, and how long participants had been experiencing infertility. In another meta-analysis of 14 prospective studies that assessed emotional distress prior to ART, researchers found no significant effect of pre-infertility-treatment anxiety or depression on positive pregnancy test, positive fetal heart scan, or live birth (Boivin, Griffiths, & Venetis, 2011). Despite the mixed evidence regarding the effects of depression and anxiety on treatment outcomes, it is important to know how women cope effectively with the psychological distress associated with infertility.

Coping with infertility

The burden of infertility and the ways in which women cope can be understood in part by examining the sociocultural construction of women's bodies and reproduction. Pronatalist norms contribute to the stigma and negative stereotypes of infertile and childfree women, which can result in internalized oppression. Fertile women are considered normal and their experiences accepted and understood, whereas infertile (and childfree) women are considered other, presumed to be violating a group norm, and thus negatively evaluated by many people (Ashburn-Nardo, 2017; Whiteford & Gonzalez, 1995). Women who do not and/or cannot bear children may then experience guilt, isolation, and rejection. Chrisler and Johnston-Robledo (2018) used stereotype embodiment theory (Levy, 2009) to explain some of the negative effects of infertility on women's self-concept and well-being. The theory "proposes that stereotypes are embodied when their assimilation from the surrounding culture leads to self-definitions that, in turn, influence functioning and health" (Levy, 2009, p. 332). When women have assimilated cultural norms that shame and medicalize infertility, the experience of infertility may cause them to isolate themselves and avoid disclosing their stigmatized identity, which can lead to further isolation and even unintentionally reinforce negative stereotypes (Chrisler & Johnston-Robledo, 2018).

Some of the psychological distress experienced by women with infertility may also stem from their lack of control over treatment options and outcomes (Gourounti et al., 2012). Lack of control over health and health outcomes has been associated with poorer well-being in a variety of health-related contexts, and situations perceived to be out of one's control can cause individuals to engage in maladaptive coping strategies.

Cognitive appraisal is another theory that can inform our understanding of infertile women's coping and well-being (Lazarus & Folkman, 1984). According to this theory, a person appraises an event as stressful if it presents a challenge, is a source of harm, or can threaten well-being. Situational factors that contribute to the appraisal of an event as stressful include uncertainty, ambiguity, and prolonged duration (Lazarus & Folkman, 1984), all of which are relevant to the experience of infertility, and thus affect women's perceived control. For example, Joshi and colleagues (2009) found women with infertility had higher levels of psychological distress, engaged in less problem-focused coping, and were less able than fertile women to engage in cognitive avoidance (i.e., they were constantly thinking about their infertility). In addition, Shani and colleagues (2016) found that women with infertility who were at increased risk for suicide were more likely to engage in negative appraisal coping (i.e., denial, social withdrawal, self-blame), to have primary infertility, and to report depressive symptoms than were women with infertility who were not at risk for suicide. Finally, in a longitudinal study of women with primary ovarian insufficiency, avoidance coping mediated the relationship between psychological vulnerability at baseline and psychological distress 12 months later (Driscoll et al., 2016). It is important to note that some methodological limitations of these studies prevent conclusions about the direction of the relationship between the women's psychological distress and their coping. In addition, the effect of individuals' coping strategies on psychological outcomes is likely to be affected by their partner's coping strategies and the partners' compatibility with one another (Pasch & Sullivan, 2017). Coping strategies can help determine whether the experience of infertility has negative psychological effects or becomes an opportunity for growth.

Despite the documented negative effects of infertility, there is some evidence that post-traumatic growth (PTG; i.e., experiencing positive change after coping with a stressful event) can evolve from the experience of infertility (Tedeschi & Calhoun, 2004; Yu et al., 2014). In one study, women were surveyed about their social support, resilience, positive coping, and PTG; the relations between resilience and PTG, and between social support and PTG, were completely explained by positive coping (Yu et al., 2014). In other words, resilience and social support predicted more positive coping (e.g., thinking of different ways to solve a problem), which in turn predicted more PTG (Yu et al., 2014). Other positive coping strategies that have been reported in the literature include seeking emotional support, turning to spirituality, action-focused coping (Karaca & Unsal, 2015; Sexton, Byrd, & von Kluge, 2010), benefit finding, and finding other opportunities to nurture children (Bell, 2009; Peterson, Pirritano, Block, & Schmidt, 2011; Ussher & Perz, 2018).

Many women cope by turning to the Internet to find informational and emotional support. In the U.S. context, the National Infertility Association maintains a useful website (www.resolve.org) that provides individuals with a plethora of helpful information about infertility, coping, treatment, and options for making treatment affordable. In addition, the website connects people with local in-person support groups that meet regularly. Other less regulated infertility support groups and discussion forums can also be found on the Internet. Online infertility support groups offer self-help mechanisms such as empathy and the space to share personal experiences, exchange information, offer or receive advice, express gratitude, and reduce feelings of isolation (Malik & Coulson, 2010).

Researchers have investigated the effectiveness of various psychosocial interventions on infertility-related distress, including some web-based approaches. In a small study of women seeking infertility treatment, researchers randomly assigned participants to a cognitive-behavioral intervention (e.g., cognitive restructuring, relaxation, psychoeducational materials) that was delivered online or to a wait-list control condition (Sexton, Byrd, O'Donohue, & Jacobs, 2010). Although the intervention resulted in significant reductions in reports of general stress, there were no significant improvements in infertility-specific stress. In another study, a face-to-face mind-body intervention, which involved teaching women the relaxation response, positive stress appraisal and coping, and a focus on growth enhancement, resulted in increased perceived social support and decreased self-reported depressive symptoms (Psaros et al., 2015). There were no significant decreases in cortisol levels associated with the mind-body intervention.

Infertility counseling has become more integrated into the multidisciplinary treatment of people coping with infertility. Patients can benefit from processing their emotions and sharing their experiences in a safe environment. Van den Broeck and colleagues (2010) discussed common issues and interventions that serve as a framework for mental health professionals who are assisting individuals, couples, and groups with infertility. They offered many helpful suggestions for coping strategies that can be taught to patients, ways to empower patients to be active in their treatment, and how to improve communication between partners. One example includes teaching ART patients active coping techniques (e.g., distraction, relaxation) to use during the distressful waiting periods. In addition, couples can be asked to construct "roadmaps" to discuss alternative plans that each member of the dyad would be willing to explore if biological parenthood is no longer an option (Van den Broeck et al., 2010, p. 424).

Impact of infertility on relationships

Women coping with infertility need and seek support in a variety of ways; however, the experience of infertility can affect women's relationships with the exact people to whom they may turn for support. When women discuss their infertility, it is usually with their partners, close friends, or family. Some evidence suggests that women with primary infertility discuss their infertility with others more than do women with secondary infertility (Sormunen, Aanesen, Fossum, Karlgren, & Westerbotn, 2017). The process of infertility disclosure is complex because the experience can be painful and private. Partners may experience tension between wanting to keep their diagnosis private and wanting to seek support from friends and family (Bute, 2013; Steuber & Solomon, 2011). The persons experiencing infertility may intentionally initiate the disclosure to seek support; however, they may also disclose in an impromptu way, such as in response to frequent questions about when the couple plans to have children (Bute, 2013). Although disclosing can in some cases open up opportunities for support, it can also burden couples with having to educate others about infertility and force them to cope with unsupportive or insensitive remarks (Bute, 2013). Therefore, disclosure might be avoided, which contributes to feelings of isolation.

Individuals communicate about their infertility in interesting ways. Drawing on social determination theory (SDT; Deci & Ryan, 2000), Palmer-Wackerly and Krieger (2015) argued that the challenges of infertility (e.g., stress, uncertainty, loss, changing relationships) create a barrier to achieving the innate psychological needs of competence (i.e., ability to control their environment), autonomy (i.e., need for freedom), and relatedness (i.e., connection with others). As a result, people use metaphors to communicate and/or achieve those needs. Palmer-Wackerly and Krieger (2015) interviewed 22 individuals with infertility about their intra- and inter-personal experiences, and found that participants used various metaphors to communicate their needs for competence, autonomy, and relatedness. For example, they referred to infertility treatment as their "job," which helped them to communicate their competence by illustrating the amount of stress that accompanies treatment and the disappointment that accompanies treatment failure (despite one's best efforts) (p. 615). In a study of women's communication with practitioners during infertility treatment, participants commonly used metaphors to describe some of the negative aspects of treatment and their negative interactions with practitioners (e.g., "just a number"), whereas descriptions of positive experiences were more direct and even complimentary (Johnson, Quinlan, & Myers, 2017, p. 96). Metaphors allow individuals to take their complex experiences and emotions and put them into more concrete and understandable terms, which may be essential for communicating about this private and stigmatizing experience with family and friends.

Infertility can impact upon the relational and sexual satisfaction of the partners who are trying to conceive. The physical and emotional demands of treatment can negatively affect sexual functioning and satisfaction, at least temporarily. For example, correlational and observational studies have documented lower marital and sexual satisfaction (Sultan & Tahir, 2011) and higher sexual dysfunction (Khodarahimi et al., 2014) among couples experiencing infertility than among fertile couples. In an observational study, the impact on sexual satisfaction was found to be long-lasting (Wirtberg et al., 2007). Furthermore, better marital adjustment and greater perceived social support predict lower levels of psychological distress among women with infertility (Qadir, Khalid, & Medhin, 2015).

Despite findings that demonstrate the negative effects of infertility on a couple's relationship, there is also a study in which one-third of the couples who underwent unsuccessful infertility treatment over a five-year period reported that the experience of infertility had brought them closer together (Peterson et al., 2011). Pasch and Sullivan (2017) posited that the variability in how infertility affects relationship quality could be explained by the compatibility (or lack thereof) of the couple's coping strategies. They argued that traditional stress and coping models are inadequate to assess the interdependent nature of how each member of the dyad copes with the stress of infertility, and proposed a "stress and coping in couples model," which suggests that couples who have compatible stress appraisal and coping strategies also have better communication and thus better relationship outcomes (p. 132).

Given the difficulties infertility presents to them, couples have a strong need and desire for support; however, many do not seek it or feel that it is available to them. Read and colleagues (2014) interviewed heterosexual couples with infertility to explore their needs with regard to psychosocial support, and they found that from whom patients wanted support depended on why they needed support. For example, when experiencing difficulty coping with stress and relationship issues, participants preferred support from a psychologist, whereas online forums were preferred for seeking a shared experience and practical information. Barriers to seeking support included not being offered services, not having information about services, and negative attitudes toward psychological support (Read et al., 2014). These findings suggest that couples should be assessed for the type of support they desire and then provided with information about services that will fulfill those needs.

A limitation of the research on the impact of infertility on relationships is that often only one member of the dyad is interviewed. Researchers have emphasized the importance of studying both members of the dyad facing infertility, as relationship dynamics could differentially impact psychological outcomes. For some, the experience of infertility can cause relationship strain, whereas others experience increased closeness. More research that includes both members of the dyad could shed light on the factors that predict more positive outcomes.

Limitations of the extant literature and future directions

Although there is a great deal of recent literature on women's experience of infertility, there are limitations to these studies and unanswered questions remain. First, the lack of sociodemographic and cultural diversity within study samples limits the generalizability of the results and likely misrepresents and silences the experiences of women with marginalized identities

(Ceballo et al., 2015) and women from the global South. Diversity in the sexuality and relationship status of participants is also needed to develop theory and treatment recommendations that are not heteronormative. There are also methodological limitations to be considered. The majority of studies are descriptive, observational, and cross-sectional, which inhibits conclusions about cause and effect and the direction of the relations between statistically significant observations. There are some longitudinal studies, but they are generally conducted over a narrow time frame (Greil et al., 2010). Integration of qualitative and quantitative approaches would also enhance the existing literature, as most studies use just one of those methods (Greil et al., 2010). Finally, some methodologies may not be appropriate for every cultural context, which makes it difficult to compare findings across studies and cultures (Culley, Hudson, & Rapport, 2007).

Perhaps the most significant limitations are the bias in sampling methods, lack of fertile comparison groups, and assessment of just one member of the dyad facing infertility. Most studies recruit women from infertility clinics and are conducted with women seeking treatment, although there are a few exceptions (e.g., Bell, 2009, 2010; Greil et al., 2011a). Less is known about women who do not seek medical treatment for their infertility and how they differ from those who do seek treatment. The lack of fertile comparison groups in some studies limits the ability to understand the extent to which the findings differ from women in the general population (if at all). In addition, most of the research is focused on individuals who are not coping or adjusting well; it would be helpful to know more about those that are able to cope effectively with the experience of infertility.

Conclusion

Infertility has the potential to affect all aspects of a woman's life. Most women assume that they will be able to achieve pregnancy easily and quickly, and failure to do so can result in complex emotions and stigmatization. Infertility treatment itself can be difficult to access, may not always be successful, and comes with a heavy physical and psychological burden. The distress that results from infertility can be a barrier to resolving it or to achieving successful treatment outcomes. Informed health care providers can anticipate some of the struggles their infertility patients/clients may face, empower them to seek out all forms of social support, and teach adaptive coping strategies (e.g., relaxation techniques, emotional support, distraction, benefit finding). Adaptive coping strategies can buffer the effects of infertility-related stress on psychological well-being, which has implications for intervention development. Clinicians can also help raise women's awareness of the ways in which sociocultural expectations for womanhood and motherhood influence the experience of infertility and empower them to challenge these expectations. Finally, research that addresses the aforementioned limitations can improve our understanding of diverse women's experience of infertility and thus enhance the support they can receive from medical professionals and their own social support networks.

References

American College of Obstetricians and Gynecologists (2017). *Treating infertility*. Washington, DC: Author. Retrieved from www.acog.org/Patients/FAQs/Treating-Infertility#treatment.

American Society for Reproductive Medicine (2012). *Age and fertility: A guide for patients*. Retrieved from www.reproductivefacts.org/globalassets/rf/news-and-publications/bookletsfact-sheets/english-fact-sheets-and-info-booklets/Age_and_Fertility.pdf.

American Society for Reproductive Medicine (2018). *More than 71 thousand babies born from assisted reproductive technology cycles done in 2016.* Retrieved from www.sart.org/news-and-publications/news-and-research/press-releases-and-bulletins/more-than-71-thousand-babies-born-from-assisted-reproductive-technology-cycles-done-in-2016-latest-data.

Ashburn-Nardo, L. (2017). Parenthood as a moral imperative? Moral outrage and the stigmatization of voluntarily childfree women and men. *Sex Roles, 76,* 393–401.

Baor, L. & Soskolne, V. (2010). Mothers of IVF and spontaneously conceived twins: A comparison of prenatal maternal expectations, coping resources and maternal stress. *Human Reproduction, 25,* 1490–1496.

Bell, A. V. (2009). "It's way out of me league": Low-income women's experiences of medicalized infertility. *Gender & Society, 23,* 688–709.

Bell, A. V. (2010). Beyond (financial) accessibility: Inequalities within the medicalization of infertility. *Sociology of Health & Illness, 32,* 631–646.

Benyamini, Y., Gozlan, M., & Weissman, A. (2017). Normalization as a strategy for maintaining quality of life while coping with infertility in a pronatalist culture. *International Journal of Behavioral Medicine, 24,* 871–879.

Berger, M. H., Messore, M., Pastuszak, A. W., & Ramasamy, R. (2016). Association between infertility and sexual dysfunction in men and women. *Sexual Medicine Reviews, 4,* 353–365.

Blundell, R. (2007). Causes of infertility. *International Journal of Molecular Medicine and Advance Sciences, 3*(1), 63–65.

Boivin, J., Bunting, L., Collins, J. A., & Nygren, K. G. (2007). International estimates of infertility prevalence and treatment-seeking: Potential need and demand for infertility medical care. *Human Reproduction, 22,* 1506–1512.

Boivin, J., Domar, A. D., Shapiro, D. B., Wischmann, T. H., Fauser, B. C. J. M., & Verhaak, C. (2012). Tackling burden in ART: An integrated approach for medical staff. *Human Reproduction, 27,* 941–950.

Boivin, J., Griffiths, E., & Venetis, C. A. (2011). Emotional distress in infertile women and failure of assisted reproductive technologies: Meta-analysis of prospective psychosocial studies. *British Medical Journal, 342,* 1–9.

Bute, J. J. (2013). The discursive dynamics of disclosure and avoidance: Evidence from a study of infertility. *Western Journal of Communication, 77,* 164–185, doi:10.1080/10570314.2012.695425.

Ceballo, R., Graham, E. T., & Hart, J. (2015). Silent and infertile: An intersectional analysis of the experiences of socioeconomically diverse African American women with infertility. *Psychology of Women Quarterly, 39,* 497–511.

Central Intelligence Agency (2016). Mother's mean age at first birth. *World Factbook 2016.* Washington, DC: Author. Retrieved from www.cia.gov/library/publications/the-world-factbook/fields/2256.html.

Chambers, G. M., Sullivan, E. A., Ishihara, O., Chapman, M. G., & Adamson, G. D. (2009). The economic impact of assisted reproductive technology: A review of selected developed countries. *Fertility and Sterility, 91,* 2281–2294.

Charter, R., Ussher, J. M., Perz, J., & Robinson, K. (2018). The transgender parent: Experiences and constructions of pregnancy and parenthood for transgender men in Australia. *International Journal of Transgenderism, 19,* 64–77.

Chrisler, J. C. & Johnston-Robledo, I. (2018). *Women's embodied self: Feminist perspectives on identity and image.* Washington, DC: American Psychological Association.

Culley, L., Hudson, N., & Rapport, F. (2007). Using focus groups with minority ethnic communities: Researching infertility in British South Asian Communities. *Qualitative Health Research, 17*(1), 102–112.

Deci, E. L. & Ryan, R. M. (2000). The 'what' and 'why' of goal pursuits: Human needs and the self-determination of behavior. *Psychological Inquiry, 11,* 227–268.

Devereaux, L. L. & Hammerman, A. J. (1998). *Infertility and identity: New strategies for treatment.* Hoboken, NJ: Wiley.

Donovan, C. (2008). 'It's not really seen as an issue, you know, lesbian infertility it's kind of "what's that?"': Lesbians' unsuccessful experiences of medicalized donor insemination. *Medical Sociology Online, 3,* 15–24.

Driscoll, M. A., Davis, M. C., Aiken, L. S., Yeung, E. W., Sterline, E. W., Vanderhoof, V., & Nelson, L. M. (2016). Psychosocial vulnerability, resilience resources, and coping with infertility: A longitudinal model of adjustment to primary ovarian insufficiency. *Annals of Behavioral Medicine, 50,* 272–284.

Eyler, A. E., Pang, S. C., & Clark, A. (2014). LGBT assisted reproduction: Current practice and future possibilities. *LGBT Health, 1,* 151–156.

Gerais, A. S. & Rushwan, H. (1992). Infertility in Africa. *Population Sciences, 12,* 25–46.

Gourounti, K., Anagnostopoulos, F., Potamianos, G., Lykeridou, K., Schmidt, L., & Vaslamatzis, G. (2012). Perception of control, coping and psychological stress of infertile women undergoing IVF. *Reproductive BioMedicine Online, 24,* 670–679.

Greil, A. L., McQuillan, J., Lowry, M., & Shreffler, K. M. (2011a). Infertility treatment and fertility-specific distress: A longitudinal analysis of a population-based sample of U.S. women. *Social Science & Medicine, 73,* 87–94.

Greil, A. L., McQuillan, J., Shreffler, K. M., Johnson, K. M., & Slauson-Blevins, K. (2011b). Race-ethnicity and medical services for infertility: Stratified reproduction in a population-based sample of U.S. women. *Journal of Health and Social Behavior, 52,* 493–509.

Greil, A. L., Schmidt, L., & Peterson, B. D. (2016). Understanding and treating the psychosocial consequences of infertility. In A. Wenzel (Ed.), *The Oxford handbook of perinatal psychology* (pp. 524–547). New York, NY: Oxford University Press.

Greil, A. L., Slauson-Blevins, K., & McQuillan, J. (2010). The experience of infertility: A review of recent literature. *Sociology of Health & Illness, 32*(1), 140–162.

Gressier, F., Letranchant, A., Cazas, O., Sutter-Dallay, A. L., Falissard, B., & Hardy, P. (2015). Post-partum depressive symptoms and medically assisted conception: A systematic review and meta-analysis. *Human Reproduction, 30,* 2575–2586.

Hammarberg, K., Fisher, J. R. W., & Wynter, K. H. (2008). Psychological and social aspects of pregnancy, childbirth, and early parenting after assisted conception: A systematic review. *Human Reproduction Update, 14,* 395–414.

Hawkey, A. J., Ussher, J. M., & Perz, J. (2018). "If you don't have a baby, you can't be in our culture": Migrant and refugee women's experiences and constructions of fertility and fertility control. *Women's Reproductive Health, 5,* 75–98.

Infertility Network (2016). *Insurance/IVF funding.* Toronto, ON, Canada: Author. Retrieved from www. infertilitynetwork.org/insurance.

Johnson, B., Quinlan, M. M., & Myers, J. (2017). Commerce, industry, and security: Biomedicalization theory and the use of metaphor to describe practitioner-patient communication within Fertility, Inc. *Women's Reproductive Health, 4,* 89–105.

Joshi, H. L., Singh, R., & Bindu (2009). Psychological distress, coping and subjective well-being among infertile women. *Journal of the Indian Academy of Applied Psychology, 35,* 329–336.

Karaca, A. & Unsal, G. (2015). Psychosocial problems and coping strategies among Turkish women with infertility. *Asian Nursing Research, 9,* 243–250.

Khodarahimi, S., Hosseinmirzaei, S., & Bruna, M. M. O. (2014). The role of infertility in mental health, psychological distress and sexual dysfunction in a sample of Iranian women. *Women & Therapy, 37,* 178–194.

Klock, S. C. (2004). Psychological adjustment to twins after infertility. *Best Practice & Research Clinical Obstetrics Gynecology, 18,* 645–656.

Lazarus, R. S. & Folkman, S. (1984). *Stress, appraisal, and coping.* New York, NY: Springer.

Lee, S.-H., Liu, L.-C., Kuo, P.-C., & Lee, M.-S. (2011). Postpartum depression and correlated factors in women who received in vitro fertilization treatment. *Journal of Midwifery & Women's Health, 56,* 347–352.

Levy, B. (2009). Stereotype embodiment: A psychosocial approach to aging. *Current Directions in Psychological Science, 18,* 332–336.

Livingston, S. (2015). *Queen of the fall: A memoir of girls and goddesses.* Lincoln, NE: University of Nebraska Press.

Malik, S. H. & Coulson, N. S. (2010). Coping with infertility online: An examination of self-help mechanisms in an online infertility support group. *Patient Education & Counseling, 81,* 315–318.

Mascarenhas, M. N., Flaxman, S. R., Boerma, T., Vanderpoel, S., & Stevens, G. A. (2012). National, regional, and global trends in infertility prevalence since 1990: A systematic analysis of 277 health surveys. *PLoS Medicine, 9*(12), e1001356.

Mathews, T. J. & Hamilton, B. E. (2016). Mean age of mothers is on the rise: United States, 2000–2014. *National Center for Health Statistics Data Brief, 232,* 1–8. Retrieved from www.cdc.gov/nchs/data/datab riefs/db232.pdf.

Matthiesen, S. M. S., Frederiksen, Y., Ingerslev, H. J., & Zachariae, R. (2011). Stress, distress and outcome of assisted reproductive technology (ART): A meta-analysis. *Human Reproduction, 26,* 2763–2776.

McCarthy, M. P. (2008). Women's lived experience of infertility after unsuccessful medical intervention. *Journal of Midwifery and Women's Health, 53*, 319–324.

McGrath, J. M., Samra, H. A., Zukowsky, K., & Baker, B. (2010). Parenting after infertility: Issues for families and infants. *American Journal of Maternal Child Nursing, 35*(3), 156–164.

Miles, L. M., Keitel, M., Jackson, M., Harris, A., & Licciardi, F. (2009). Predictors of distress in women being treated for infertility. *Journal of Reproductive and Infant Psychology, 27*, 238–257.

Monti, F., Agostini, F., Fagandini, P., Paterlini, M., Battista La Sala, G., & Blickstein, I. (2008). Anxiety symptoms during late pregnancy and early parenthood following assisted reproductive technology. *Journal of Perinatal Medicine, 36*, 425–432.

Nachtigall, R. D. (2006). International disparities in access to infertility services. *Fertility and Sterility, 85*, 871–875.

Ombelet, W. (2011). Global access to infertility care in developing countries: A case of human rights, equity and social justice. *Facts, Views, & Vision in ObGyn, 3*, 257–266.

Palmer-Wackerly, A. L. & Krieger, J. L. (2015). Dancing around infertility: The use of metaphors in a complex medical situation. *Health Communication, 30*, 612–623.

Pasch, L. A. & Sullivan, K. T. (2017). Stress and coping in couples facing infertility. *Current Opinion in Psychology, 13*, 131–135.

Peloquin, K. & Lafontaine, M.-F. (2010). What are the correlates of infertility-related clinical anxiety? A literature review and the presentation of a conceptual model. *Marriage & Family Review, 46*, 580–620.

Peterson, B. D., Pirritano, M., Block, J. M., & Schmidt, L. (2011). Marital benefit and coping strategies in men and women undergoing unsuccessful fertility treatments over a 5-year period. *Fertility & Sterility, 95*, 1759–1763.

Prince, L. B. & Domar, A. D. (2013). The stress of infertility. In M. V. Spiers, P. A. Geller, & J. D. Kloss (Eds), *Women's health psychology* (pp. 328–354). Hoboken, NJ: Wiley.

Psaros, C., Kagan, L., Shifren, J. L., Willett, J., Jacquart, J., Alert, M. D., & Park, E. R. (2015). Mind-body group treatment for women coping with infertility: A pilot study. *Journal of Psychosomatic Obstetrics & Gynecology, 36*, 75–83.

Qadir, F., Khalid, A., & Medhin, G. (2015). Social support, marital adjustment, and psychological distress among women with primary infertility in Pakistan. *Women & Health, 55*, 432–446.

Read, S. C., Carrier, M.-E., Boucher, M.-E., Whitley, R., Bond, S., & Zelkowitz, P. (2014). Psychosocial services for couples in infertility treatment: What do couples really want? *Patient Education and Counseling, 94*, 390–395, doi:10.1016/j.pec.2013.10.025.

Resolve, the National Infertility Association (2018). *Coverage by state*. McLean, VA: Author. Retrieved from https://resolve.org/what-are-my-options/insurance-coverage/coverage-state.

Russo, N. F. (1976). The motherhood mandate. *Journal of Social Issues, 32*, 143–153.

Sexton, M. B., Byrd, M. R., O'Donohue, W. T., & Jacobs, N. M. (2010). Web-based treatment for infertility-related psychological distress. *Archives of Women's Mental Health, 13*, 347–358.

Sexton, M. B., Byrd, M. R., & von Kluge, S. (2010). Measuring resilience in women experiencing infertility using the CD-RISC: Examining infertility-related stress, general distress, and coping styles. *Journal of Psychiatric Research, 44*, 236–241.

Shani, C., Yelena, S., Reut, B. K., Adrian, S., & Sami, H. (2016). Suicidal risk among infertile women undergoing in-vitro fertilization: Incidence and risk factors. *Psychiatry Research, 240*, 53–59.

Smith, A. D. A. C., Tilling, K., Nelson, S. M., & Lawlor, D. A. (2015). Live-birth rate associated with repeat in vitro fertilization treatment cycles. *Journal of the American Medical Association, 314*, 2654–2662.

Society for Assisted Reproductive Technology (2016). *National summary report*. Birmingham, AL: Author. Retrieved from www.sartcorsonline.com/rptCSR_PublicMultYear.aspx?ClinicPKID=0#help.

Sormunen, T., Aanesen, A., Fossum, B., Karlgren, K., & Westerbotn, M. (2017). Infertility-related communication and coping strategies among women affected by primary or secondary infertility. *Journal of Clinical Nursing, 27*, e335–e344.

Stephen, E. H. & Chandra, A. (1998). Updated projections of infertility in the United States: 1995–2025. *Fertility and Sterility, 70*, 30–34.

Steuber, K. R. & Solomon, D. H. (2011). Factors that predict married partners' disclosures about infertility to social network members. *Journal of Applied Communication Research, 39*(3), 250–270.

Sultan, S. & Tahir, A. (2011). Psychological consequences of infertility. *Hellenic Journal of Psychology, 8*, 229–247.

Tedeschi, R. G. & Calhoun, L. G. (2004). Posttraumatic growth: Conceptual foundations and empirical evidence. *Psychological Inquiry, 15*, 1–18.

Thompson, E. H., Woodward, J. T., & Stanton, A. L. (2012). Dyadic goal appraisal during treatment for infertility: How do different perspectives relate to partners' adjustment? *International Journal of Behavioral Medicine, 19*, 252–259.

Ussher, J. M. & Perz, J., The Australian Cancer and Fertility Study Team (ACFST) (2018). Threat of biographical disruption: The gendered construction and experience of infertility following cancer for women and men. *BMC Cancer, 18*, 1–17.

Van den Broeck, U., Mery, M., Wischmann, T., & Thorn, P. (2010). Counselling in infertility: Individual, couple, and group interventions. *Patient Education and Counseling, 81*, 422–428.

Vilska, S., Unkila-Kallio, L., Punamäki, R.-L., Poikkeus, P., Repokari, L., Sinkkonen, J., & Tulppala, M. (2009). Mental health of mothers and fathers of twins conceived via assisted reproduction treatment: A 1-year prospective study. *Human Reproduction, 24*, 367–377.

Whiteford, L. M. & Gonzalez, L. (1995). Stigma: The hidden burden of infertility. *Social Science & Medicine, 40*, 27–36.

Wirtberg, I., Möller, A., Hogström, L., Tronstad, S.-E., & Lalos, A. (2007). Life 20 years after unsuccessful infertility treatment. *Human Reproduction, 22*, 598–604.

Yu, Y., Peng, L., Chen, L., Long, L., He, W., Li, M., & Wang, T. (2014). Resilience and social support promote posttraumatic growth of women with infertility: The mediating role of positive coping. *Psychiatry Research, 215*, 401–405.

Zegers-Hochschild, F., Adamson, G. D., Dyer, S., Racowsky, C., de Mouzon, J., Sokol, R., & van der Poel, S. (2017). The international glossary on infertility and fertility care, 2017. *Fertility and Sterility, 108*, 393–406.

14

FERTILITY AND CANCER

Michelle Peate, Lesley Stafford and Yasmin Jayasinghe

As hard as the cancer treatment was, losing my fertility was the hardest thing.
(Graham, 2017)

The reproductive rights of women are a fundamental issue in human health and society. Embedded in this is the importance of autonomy: Women have the freedom to make their own decisions about childbearing and rearing roles and to live the life they choose. Although some women are childfree by choice, most young women wish to have children (Weston, Qu, & Parker, 2005) and the ability to have a child is considered a core social value that is an important part of adult development and identity (Cousineau & Domar, 2007; Lechner, Bolman, & van Dalen, 2007). Women are more likely than men to experience infertility and unplanned childlessness, and the impact of unwanted infertility can have damaging social and psychological consequences, such as depressive symptoms, risk of abuse, loss of control, ostracism, social stigma, self-blame, and mental distress (Cousineau & Domar, 2007; Dyer, Abrahams, Mokoena, Lombard, & van der Spuy, 2005; Fleetwood & Campo-Engelstein, 2010; Kirkman, 2008; Lechner et al., 2007; McLeod & Ponesse, 2008). This distress is often described as a complicated grief response for the loss of the child who has ceased to be a possible reality (Lechner et al., 2007). Additionally, women who desire a child but do not achieve this goal may reflect on the loss of possible benefits of having children, such as additional social interactions, support, and global well-being, particularly in old age (Grundy & Read, 2012).

The potential impacts of involuntary childlessness may be exacerbated for women with a health condition that may affect fertility, such as cancer. These women are facing the threat of infertility at a younger age than their peers (Barton et al., 2013). Women's fertility decisions at the time of cancer diagnosis have long-term impacts on the ability to achieve future parenting goals, and their choices can result in some of the negative consequences described above, particularly if their choices are not informed. Therefore, fertility values and options must be considered before commencing cancer treatment given that parenthood and infertility may have life-altering impacts on the course of a woman's life (Logan, Perz, Ussher, Peate, & Anazodo, 2018). In this chapter the impact of cancer treatment on fertility, cancer-related infertility distress, assessing fertility after cancer, the fertility options available to people with cancer, pregnancy and achieving parenthood after cancer, and the barriers and ethical issues associated with fertility in the context of cancer are discussed.

Cancer treatment and fertility

The social trend of later childbearing (Sonmezer & Oktay, 2006) has led to increasing numbers of premenopausal women without children, or who have not yet completed their families at the time of cancer diagnosis. Thus, cancer poses a threat to the life plans of women who wish to have children in the future (Ussher et al., 2018b). The likelihood of infertility ranges from 0% to 98% in young premenopausal women with cancer, as measured by the cessation of menstruation (i.e., amenorrhea) depending on the treatment received (Peate, Stafford, & Hickey, 2017; Stern et al., 2013). Cancer treatment typically comprises a combination of surgery, radiotherapy, chemotherapy, endocrine therapy, targeted therapy, and/or immunotherapy – depending on cancer type. Not all treatments will affect fertility. Scenarios where fertility may be directly affected include:

1   Surgery and/or radiotherapy of, or including, the pelvic region (i.e., damaging the reproductive organs) or areas of the brain that play a role in the reproductive cycle (e.g., damage to the hypothalamic-pituitary-gonadal [HPG] axis) (Wallace, Anderson, & Irvine, 2005).
2   Adjuvant chemotherapy regimens that are gonadotoxic to the ovaries and affect gonadal function, with alkylating agents classed as the most damaging (Anderson et al., 2015). Although modern chemotherapies appear to be less toxic than older therapies, women may still experience some ovarian dysfunction following treatment (e.g., premature menopause) (Chow et al., 2016).

In both scenarios, the exact mechanism for damage to the ovaries is unclear, however the prevalent theory is based upon the consensus that women are born with a finite number of ovarian follicles (i.e., immature eggs). Over a woman's life, the number of follicles stored in her ovaries (i.e., the ovarian reserve) diminishes through a continual process of follicular growth and degeneration. Menopause occurs when the number of follicles left in the ovary falls below a critical threshold (Wallace & Kelsey, 2010). Exposure to chemotherapy and radiotherapy can reduce the ovarian reserve by accelerating rates of follicular activation and atresia, damaging ovarian vasculature, and causing ovarian atrophy (Meirow, Biederman, Anderson, & Wallace, 2010). The extent of damage depends on a woman's age at diagnosis and the type, dose, and duration of treatment. The result can be acute or temporary ovarian failure, premature ovarian insufficiency (menopause by 40 years), and infertility (Meirow et al., 2010; Stern et al., 2013). Post cancer, even those women who recover menstrual function soon after treatment are more likely than their healthy peers to experience early menopause (Maltaris, Boehm, Dittrich, Seufert, & Koelbl, 2006). Advanced reproductive age and low pre-treatment ovarian reserve (ovarian follicle pool) are the most important risk factors (Jayasinghe, Wallace, & Anderson, 2018); younger women are less likely than women over 35 to become menopausal following treatment (Jung et al., 2010). Additional consideration needs to be given to the duration of treatment because natural age-related decline in fertility also occurs during treatment. For instance, a woman may be in her mid to late 40s when she completes cancer treatment, an age when rates of spontaneous conception are low. Furthermore, pelvic radiotherapy may lead to radiation injury to the uterus (uterine fibrosis), which can cause problems with implantation and uterine growth in pregnancy and result in poor obstetric outcomes, such as miscarriage, premature birth, and stillbirth (Anderson et al., 2015; Meirow et al., 2010). The combination of treatment-related and individual factors can make it difficult to predict the likelihood of infertility for any given individual.

Cancer-related infertility distress

Over 50% of young women 40 years or younger at diagnosis are concerned about future fertility, and over 75% of women aged 35 or younger at diagnosis wish to consider pregnancy following cancer treatment (Pagani et al., 2011; Schover, Rybicki, Martin, & Bringelsen, 1999). Concerns about infertility have been found to be greater in women who have yet to complete their families, those who have experienced prior difficulty in conceiving, and those younger than 40 years (Logan et al., 2018; Peate, Meiser, Hickey, & Friedlander, 2009). Although important to both men and women, risk of infertility is of greater concern to women (Crawshaw, 2013a; Gupta, Edelstein, Albert-Green, & D'Agostino, 2013). Unpartnered women report additional concerns about not knowing their fertility status until they try to become pregnant, and they may need to find a partner first (Connell, Patterson, & Newman, 2006). Concerns about potential infertility and the inability to conceive in the future often result in psychological distress and worse physical well-being (Carter et al., 2010; Howard-Anderson, Ganz, Bower, & Stanton, 2012; McQuillan, Greil, White, & Jacob, 2003).

For some women with cancer, treatment-induced infertility can be more distressing than the treatment itself (Graham, 2017). Women with cancer-related infertility have levels of depression twice that of the general population and reduced quality of life, specifically in areas of emotional well-being, identity, self-esteem, sexuality, and relationships (Absolom et al., 2008; Avis, Crawford, & Manuel, 2004; Crawshaw, 2013b; Duffy & Allen, 2009; Howard-Anderson et al., 2012). The patient, partner, and family may experience great distress, and the threat of infertility may result in anger and a sense of loss and grief (Hershberger, Finnegan, Pierce, & Scoccia, 2013). Women with cancer also report feeling more isolated compared with their age-matched peers (Anderson et al., 2011).

Fertility concerns may also influence a woman's cancer treatment decisions, with an impact on consequent health and survival outcomes. For example, in one study, 18% of women with breast cancer reported considering less effective cancer treatment due to fertility concerns; some women refused chemotherapy (1%) or endocrine therapy (3%) or reduced adherence to endocrine therapy (11%) (Ruddy et al., 2014).

Most of the available research assumes heterosexuality and there is very little about the impact of cancer-related infertility in sexual minorities (Quinn et al., 2015), and although intentions of fertility and aspirations of parenthood are likely different for sexual minority groups than for heterosexuals (Fantus et al., 2015), a proportion of women from sexual minority groups desire to be parents (D'Augelli, Rendina, Sinclair, & Grossman, 2007). An American study amongst LGB adolescents (15–19 years) found that 36% of females were extremely likely to raise children, 67% indicated some degree of likelihood, and 54% expected to raise their own biological children (D'Augelli et al., 2007). Whether this applies in the current context or in a cancer population is unknown. Evidence suggests that in a cancer context, differences exist between LGBTQ and heterosexual individuals with LGBTQ less likely to report fertility concerns as affecting romantic relationships; more open to raising non-biological children; more open to the likelihood of not becoming a parent (Russell, Galvin, Harper, & Clayman, 2016). Furthermore, when faced with infertility, LGBTQ patients' views on relationships, parenthood, and family building result in less distress and they are generally more satisfied with, or indifferent to, fertility information provided, in comparison with their heterosexual counterparts (Russell et al., 2016). These data need to be carefully interpreted in the context of cultural, institutional, and individual biases that may influence how sexual minorities may view their own intentions for parenthood (Fantus et al., 2015).

As there is currently no way to reverse the impacts of cancer and its treatment on fertility, consideration needs to be given to the significant psychological implications of potential infertility and fears associated with the impact of pregnancy on prognosis. Clinical practice guidelines, such as those published by the American Society of Clinical Oncology (ASCO) and those from the British Fertility Society, recommend discussion of the impact of cancer treatment on fertility and fertility preservation options as part of treatment planning for all patients prior to commencing gonadotoxic treatment (Oktay et al., 2018; Yasmin et al., 2018). For some women, this discussion may be about managing expectations about long-term effects of cancer and its treatment, and for others it may concern opportunities to achieve later parenting goals. Although there is no guarantee of future parenthood, fertility preservation gives women additional options if they become infertile following cancer.

Assessing fertility after cancer

Regular ovarian surveillance is recommended for cancer survivors to exclude premature ovarian insufficiency and assess ovarian reserve (European Society for Human Reproduction et al., 2016), particularly for those who want to consider preservation options during this period (Jayasinghe et al., 2018). The presence (or absence) of menstruation following cancer treatment does not precisely reflect ovarian reserve, as significant ovarian decline may be present despite regular menses and pregnancy occurs in 5–10% of women with primary ovarian insufficiency (the cessation of menses due to the loss of ovarian function before 40 years of age) (Pinelli, Simi, Maria, Cela, & Artini, 2017). There are no gold standard tests for fertility, therefore several predictors are used to "measure" reproductive potential. Age is the main predictor for future fertility (female fertility rapidly declines after age 35 in the general population). Excluding the scenario where women receive sterilising treatment for their cancer, age also is a risk factor for future infertility (Levine, Kelvin, Quinn, & Gracia, 2015). However, age alone is of limited value in predicting a successful pregnancy (Bancsi et al., 2002). Hormonal biomarkers, such as follicle stimulating hormone (FSH), lutenising hormone (LH), estradiol, inhibin B, antimullerian hormone (AMH), and ultrasound measurements, such as antral follicle count and ovarian volume, are used to assess ovarian function. The most promising proxy measure for ovarian function appears to be AMH because it reflects earlier stages of follicle development, which could more closely approximate the ovarian reserve and can be measured at any time of the menstrual cycle (Anderson & Cameron, 2011). It may also predict the potential for ovarian recovery (Anderson, Rosendahl, Kelsey, & Cameron, 2013). However, AMH is not without its disadvantages. Like other biomarkers, it is a proxy for the size of the primordial follicle pool. There is also enormous variability in AMH levels within age groups, and there are technical problems with AMH measurement (e.g., lack of standardisation) (Findlay, Hutt, Hickey, & Anderson, 2015). Notably, none of these biomarkers reliably predict pregnancy or menopause (Anderson, Nisenblat, & Norman, 2010).

Fertility preservation options for women with cancer

Whether a woman desires biological offspring in the future or not, the option of fertility preservation prior to cancer treatment provides opportunities to achieve parenthood goals, and it may ameliorate some of the negative impacts of unwanted infertility. There are three main fertility preservation options: cryopreservation of oocytes, embryos, or ovarian tissue. In addition to fertility preservation techniques, women may also consider ovarian protection during their cancer treatment.

Oocyte cryopreservation

The process for preserving oocytes typically involves hormonal stimulation for 10–14 days to promote follicle growth and oocyte maturation. Once the oocytes have matured, they are collected and cryopreserved (i.e., frozen). When the woman decides to use the stored oocytes, she will undergo further hormonal stimulation to prepare the uterus, and the oocyte will be thawed and fertilised with available sperm. If successful, the embryo formed will be transferred to the uterus. Ideally, the embryo will implant, grow, and result in a successful pregnancy.

The reported likelihood of success from oocyte cryopreservation is variable across studies; likelihood of live birth per oocyte collected ranges between 1 and 6% (Gnoth et al., 2011; Goldman, Noyes, Knopman, McCaffrey, & Grifo, 2013), and live births per embryo transfer range from 0 to 60% (Garcia-Velasco et al., 2013; Goldman et al., 2013). However, the live birth data from frozen oocytes are still relatively new, and most of the data are from older women (i.e., over 35 years) who are likely to have poorer success rates. A small but promising study shows better success in cancer than in non-cancer patients (25% versus 13% live births per embryo transfer), but this needs to be interpreted carefully due to the very small sample size (Garcia-Velasco et al., 2013).

There are some risks to oocyte cryopreservation. The two-week delay may not be appropriate for patients with aggressive malignancies (Stern et al., 2013). Hormonal stimulation is contraindicated for women with oestrogen-responsive cancers, and there is a very small risk of severe ovarian hyperstimulation syndrome (Stern et al., 2013).

Oocyte cryopreservation is ideal for post-pubertal women who do not have a partner or access to donor sperm, have a moral or ethical issue with preservation of embryos, and where there is enough time for ovarian stimulation. This procedure is not appropriate for prepubertal girls due to immaturity of the HPG axis and the inability to mature oocytes for collection (Stern et al., 2013).

Embryo cryopreservation

Embryo cryopreservation is the most established technique for fertility preservation in women (Anderson et al., 2015). Like oocyte cryopreservation, this starts with 10–14 days of ovarian stimulation. However, after mature oocytes have been collected, they are fertilised using sperm from a partner or donor. The embryos will then be cryopreserved for later use. When women decide to use the stored embryos later, they will require further hormonal stimulation to prepare the uterus. The embryo that survives the thawing process will be transferred to the uterus. Ideally, the embryo will implant, grow, and result in a successful pregnancy.

The reported likelihood of success from embryo cryopreservation ranges between 4 and 75% live births per embryo transfer (Rato, Gouveia-Oliveira, & Plancha, 2012; Shapiro et al., 2010). There is variability to these numbers depending on age at oocyte collection and the quality of the oocytes, sperm, and embryos. Also, these data should be interpreted with some caution, as these average live birth data come from older women without a previous history of cancer.

The risks of this procedure are similar to those of oocyte cryopreservation in regard to the two-week delay and exposure to hormones during ovarian stimulation (Stern et al., 2013). This process has the added challenge that women need to have access to partner or donor sperm. It is also inappropriate for prepubertal girls because of their hormonal immaturity and ethical concerns related to creating embryos for minors. Women considering this option also need to consider the legal implications regarding ownership of embryos created with a partner, as consent from both parties is required for use of the embryos.

Ovarian tissue cryopreservation

Cryopreservation of ovarian tissue is the only option available for prepubertal girls and women that require immediate gonadotoxic therapy. Cortical segments of the ovary or an entire ovary can be harvested via a laparoscopic procedure. The tissue is then frozen and later thawed and transplanted when needed. Orthotopic transplantation back to the original site allows for spontaneous conception with the restoration of fertility (Donnez & Dolmans, 2015). Heterotopic transplantation (e.g., to the abdominal cavity or elsewhere) is easier to perform, and provides easier access to oocytes if assisted reproduction is desired in the future, yet yields lower success rates of pregnancy (Stern et al., 2013). This procedure is transitioning from experimental to standard practice (Dolmans, & Manavella, 2018); about 130 babies have so far been born worldwide (Donnez & Dolmans, 2017). However, the data are promising, and a recent meta-analysis shows live birth and ongoing pregnancy rates of 38% (Pacheco & Oktay, 2017).

A key benefit of this procedure is the ability to act immediately without delaying cancer treatment because hormonal stimulation and sperm are not needed. It also allows for the possibility of resumption of hormone function, which has been reported in 90% of patients within 4–9 months after transplantation (Meirow, Roness, Kristensen, & Andersen, 2015). As this is a surgical procedure, there are well-documented anesthetic and surgical risks. Furthermore, reintroduction of cancer cells with the grafting of the (untreated) ovarian tissue is a major risk, and the technology for accurate detection of malignant cells is under current development (Yasmin et al., 2018).

Ovarian protection

There are methods targeted to reduce the impact of cancer treatment on fertility:

1 Ovarian transposition (oophoropexy) involves surgically moving one or both ovaries away from a radiation field, but it does not protect against chemotherapy. It may preserve ovarian function in 16 to 90% of women (Aubard, Piver, Pech, Galinat, & Teissier, 2001; Morice et al., 2000).
2 Gonadotrophin-releasing hormone agonists (GnRHa) suppress ovarian function to potentially reduce insult to the ovarian follicles (Lambertini et al., 2015).

Overall, evidence to support ovarian protection in preserving fertility remains limited, and it should not be used in place of more established fertility preservation methods.

Pregnancy after cancer

For some women, pregnancy may be central to achieving a sense of fulfillment, even with the use of donor eggs (Stuart-Smith, Smith, & Scott, 2011). A nested case-control study of physical and mental health correlates of pregnancy showed that mental health was marginally better in women who had had a child after breast cancer than those who did not (Gorman et al., 2010). Pursuing parenthood after cancer may help women to regain a sense of normalcy by reclaiming their lives and achieving the goals they had set prior to diagnosis (Duffy & Allen, 2009). More time since diagnosis appears to result in fewer pregnancy-related concerns (Avis et al., 2004). Reasons for not pursuing pregnancy following cancer include fear of recurrence and belief that it would be selfish to have a child when lifespan is potentially compromised; age or relationship status; clinician recommendation; poor understanding of the risks; insufficient counselling; and patient's preference (Connell et al., 2006; Del Mastro, Catzeddu, & Venturini, 2006; Ives, Saunders, Bulsara, & Semmens, 2007). There is also the fear that pregnancy and breastfeeding may adversely affect prognosis and impede detection of breast cancer in women with hormone receptor positive breast cancer (Connell et al., 2006).

Population-based or cohort and case-control studies can help in understanding the impact of pregnancy on cancer prognosis. Available data do not appear to show a worse outcome following pregnancy (Yasmin et al., 2018); in fact, pregnancy may even confer a survival benefit, as is seen in women with breast cancer (Azim et al., 2011). The British Fertility Society clinical guidelines state that women should be informed that there is no evidence of increased risk of cancer recurrence because of pregnancy (Yasmin et al., 2018).

Although there are little data about birth outcomes in women post cancer, overall it appears there is no increased risk to offspring of survivors compared with the general population (Lawrenz et al., 2011; Yasmin et al., 2018). These data need to be interpreted in the context of the high rate of induced abortion (20–44%) post cancer treatment, a likely reflection of the uncertainties about safety of pregnancy following cancer (Pagani et al., 2011). A few studies show increased risk of preterm delivery and low birth weight (Dalberg, Eriksson, & Holmberg, 2006). Results are mixed as to whether miscarriage rates are higher in survivors (Langagergaard, 2011; Velentgas et al., 1999). Women who have pelvic irradiation, particularly if exposure occurs before their first menstrual cycle, may have obstetric risks, such as early and late miscarriage, prematurity, stillbirth, low birth weight, neonatal and/or postpartum haemorrhage, and possibly uterine rupture and placental attachment disorders (Yasmin et al., 2018). There does not seem to be risk of malformations or infant death (Yasmin et al., 2018). Although most of the data are from women with breast cancer, outcomes for women who conceive after cancer are reassuring, and they should not be discouraged from pregnancy.

Achieving parenthood following cancer

Not all women want to have children after cancer treatment. However, if a woman decides she is ready to have children, her options will depend on her situation and whether she underwent a previous fertility preservation procedure.

Natural conception

If she is in a heterosexual relationship, a woman may opt to start by attempting a natural conception with a partner. If in a same sex relationship, a woman may wish to consider donor insemination. Infertility is defined as a 12-month period of unprotected intercourse that does not result in a pregnancy, after which it is recommended that couples seek assistance. Since women who have undergone treatment for cancer are likely to have reduced fertility, assessment of fertility using some of the methods described above to determine need for intervention and/or to reduce the time window of unprotected intercourse/

insemination without pregnancy to six months before considering intervention, is recommended (Peate et al., 2017).

Using assisted reproduction

Women who did not undergo fertility preservation prior to cancer treatment may wish to consider preserving fertility soon after cancer treatment to increase their chances of pregnancy later. Although chemotherapy may already have diminished ovarian reserve, the woman's ovarian reserve will continue to decrease with increasing age so there is some logic to pausing cancer treatment to preserve oocytes/embryos/tissue, provided enough time since chemotherapy has passed to minimise risk of toxic effects and under supervision of their treating oncologist and fertility specialist. After fertility preservation, women can resume endocrine treatment. After cancer treatment is complete or when women are ready to conceive, they may consider natural or assisted reproduction.

Women who cryopreserved oocytes, embryos, or ovarian tissue prior to cancer treatment will have an option to use this material. Embryos can be transferred, and oocytes fertilised and transferred, into a prepared uterus. There are limited data on live birth rates from frozen embryos or oocytes following cancer. Live birth rates per frozen embryo transfer are approximately 44.1% in women younger than 35 years and 35.8% in women aged 35–39 years (Kato et al., 2012), with rates up to 75% reported (Shapiro et al., 2010). Similar live birth per transfer rates of 50–55% in women younger than 36 years and 18–37% in women over 34 years have been reported (Chang et al., 2013; Goldman et al., 2013). Both procedures may require hormonal stimulation to stimulate oocyte maturation and prepare the uterus for embryo transfer and this is contraindicated in hormone responsive cancers; however, there are no data to suggest that hormonal stimulation for oocyte maturation impacts on prognosis or recurrence. With ovarian tissue cryopreservation there may be concerns about re-seeding the cancer (Donnez & Dolmans, 2015). Should these options be unsuccessful or unfeasible, it may be worth considering using donor eggs or embryos.

Donor eggs or embryos may also be a good option for women who are concerned about transmission of genetic susceptibility to cancer (e.g., BRCA1/2 genetic mutations). The chance of success from these options is largely dependent on the age of the oocytes, with younger oocytes more likely to result in a successful live birth (Cobo & García-Velasco, 2016). However, access to donor oocytes and embryos may be challenging.

Other options to achieve parenthood

Alternative options for becoming a parent without pregnancy include surrogacy (e.g., for cases where the uterus has been damaged), adoption or foster care (which have the advantage of not transmitting any cancer genes); however, these are not without challenges and can be difficult for people with a history of cancer to access.

Not having children after cancer

Some women will opt not to have children after cancer treatment. Concerns about how to best avoid pregnancy have been reported, with hormonal contraception considered unsafe and male sterilisation thought undesirable (Connell et al., 2006; Thewes, Butow, Girgis, &

Pendlebury, 2004). Failed contraception has been linked to anxiety and fear of recurrence (Connell et al., 2006). Hormonal contraception (e.g., the contraceptive pill or implants) is often contraindicated in women with hormone responsive cancers. Therefore, it is recommended that these women use non-hormonal forms of contraception such as barrier methods (e.g., condoms, diaphragms, intrauterine contraceptive devices), or male or female sterilisation.

Barriers to, and ethical considerations regarding, fertility preservation

There are several barriers to fertility preservation and associated ethical considerations that influence access to options. These will vary between clinics.

Established versus experimental procedures

Established procedures such as oocyte and embryo cryopreservation can be accessed from most fertility clinics. However, ovarian tissue preservation will only be available from some centres. *Ethical consideration*: Should cancer patients be offered procedures that are experimental?

Cost

Some countries will offer subsided services for cancer patients and/or fertility preservation may be included in health insurance coverage, however there is often an out-of-pocket cost that is incurred by the patient. Additionally, it is typical to have annual storage fees and there is also the future cost for using the stored material to achieve pregnancy. These may be limiting factors for patients. Additionally, clinicians may take patients' ability to pay into account when considering referrals (Logan, Perz, Ussher, Peate, & Anazodo, 2017). *Ethical considerations*: What is the impact of cost on equitable access to care? Does facilitating use of donor eggs and embryos promote reproductive tourism, particularly in situations where donors receive financial motivation (Lindheim, Chase, & Sauer, 2001)?

Fertility preservation success rates

The perception and understanding of the success of fertility preservation can influence discussions about fertility preservation (Logan et al., 2017). *Ethical considerations*: Do the benefits of fertility preservation outweigh the risks, especially considering there is no guarantee of success? Does offering fertility preservation give false hope?

Age limits

Some clinics may not offer fertility preservation based on the limited success in women above a certain age limit (e.g., 40 years). Clinicians may also be guarded about discussing fertility in prepubertal children due to limited outcome data (Logan et al., 2017). *Ethical considerations*: In a paediatric setting, are parents the right people to make the decision for their child? Can they separate their own desires from what is in their child's best interest? What if there is disagreement between the parents? What should the role of the child be in the decision-making process? Can young patients separate their lack of current desire from what their potential future desires for children may be? These issues may be compounded when the child is grappling with gender diversity issues.

Safety criteria

Access may be limited to those who pass safety criteria, such as criminal and child protection checks.

Partner and relationship criteria

Regulations may apply for who can donate or access sperm, specifically same-sex couples and single women (Rashedi et al., 2018). Clinics may require a minimum relationship time before an embryo can be created, or, conversely, if a woman is with a new partner her former divorce may need to be finalised.

Health

Clinics may turn away women with severe physical or mental illness, poor prognosis, or high risk of recurrence (Logan et al., 2017). *Ethical considerations*: Will failure to carry out fertility preservation cause the patient suffering, particularly in societies where women are abused and/or ostracised for being infertile? If a patient has very poor prognosis, there is a possibility that she will die before using her stored reproductive material so should fertility preservation be offered?

Storage

Facilities or regulations may limit the duration of storage of frozen material. *Ethical considerations*: Who has access to, and authority over, the material should the patient die? When should it be disposed of?

Gender

Adolescent boys are more likely to have fertility discussed than girls (Ussher, Cummings, Dryden, & Perz, 2016).

Time constraints

Concerns about delaying cancer treatment or concerns about overwhelming patients at a vulnerable and stressful time can hinder discussions (Logan et al., 2017).

Clinician knowledge and attitude

Clinicians are less likely to discuss infertility if they believe the patient is not at significant risk, have less knowledge of referral pathways and lack of awareness of clinical guidelines, have anxiety around the contraindication of fertility preservation with hormone-sensitive cancers (greater concern linked with being male, in a private clinic setting, and personal partner/parent status), or have a moral objection to the procedure (Logan et al., 2017; Shimizu et al., 2013; Ussher et al., 2016).

Parity

Mothers report fertility concerns being neglected by clinicians (Lee et al., 2011).

Discomfort

Some clinicians or patients may want to avoid discussion because of feelings of embarrassment (Logan et al., 2017).

Cultural, religious, and social norms

Women may not have full control of their reproductive preferences or assisted reproduction may be legislated against (Fleetwood & Campo-Engelstein, 2010). *Ethical consideration*: Does fertility preservation promote the idea that a female identity is tied to reproductive status?

Empowering women by facilitating timely fertility preservation decisions

Women with cancer need to be informed about all the risks of their treatments in order to make informed decisions. They must be made aware of the potential impact on their fertility, and they must be educated regarding their fertility preservation options before treatment and about achieving a pregnancy after treatment. Decisions to try to conceive following cancer are challenging: Women weigh up their desire for children against their fears of recurrence and potential inability to detect future cancers. Given the motivators and reasons for avoiding pregnancy, it is important that women are well informed about the risks and well supported in the decision-making process. Additionally, for some women fertility preservation prior to cancer treatment may not be a viable option, or assisted reproductive procedures may fail, and future parenthood may not be possible. How best to provide evidence-based information and psychosocial support to cancer patients who wish to conceive both before and after cancer treatment is an important clinical issue in need of greater attention.

However, despite clinical recommendations, fertility preservation is often inadequately discussed, which results in feelings of dissatisfaction, sadness, anger, and frustration (Logan et al., 2018). Many clinicians do not provide the recommended care to all eligible patients, and many patients feel inadequately informed and lack the support that they require (Logan et al., 2017, 2018; Ussher et al., 2016; Ussher, Parton, & Perz, 2018a). General psychological distress in women post cancer is related to perceptions of reproductive issues rather than actual fertility status (Sobota & Ozakinci, 2014). Fertility preservation has been regarded as one of the most difficult decisions women have to make (Hershberger et al., 2013), and it is considered to be a difficult decision by two-thirds of women (Mersereau et al., 2013). It should also be recognised that there is a heterosexual bias in fertility discussions – with an implication that fertility is only possible within a heteronormative cisgender opposite-sex relationship (Fantus et al., 2015). More research in gender diverse groups is needed. There is clearly a need for better fertility information and support that is tailored to an individual's needs, as improving the quality of decision-making could reduce long-term feelings of regret (Chan et al., 2014).

There is no right or wrong fertility preservation decision, but the impact on well-being can be profound. Decision support is needed in these complex scenarios. To address these needs, decision aids regarding fertility preservation prior to cancer treatment have been developed and found to be effective; they improve fertility-related knowledge, facilitate information retention, reduce decisional conflict and regret, and are almost as helpful as counselling (Garvelink et al., 2013; Hoff, Brandon, & Mersereau, 2015; Peate et al., 2012). It is crucial that all women are made aware of the risk of infertility and given options to maximise future opportunity to become a parent, manage expectations, and reduce regret.

It can be empowering for women to discuss the impact of cancer treatment on fertility and make decisions about protecting fertility. Fertility preservation may potentially give women the opportunity to delay motherhood and establish greater control over if, when, and how they reproduce. Conversely, there is also a need to manage expectations about the chances of future parenthood following cancer (with and without fertility preservation) as some will not achieve their goal of future parenthood. As described earlier in this chapter, unplanned infertility can be distressing, and the discussion needs to consider their desires, sexual orientation, cultural setting, and medical situation. In particular, it needs to also take into account that institutional and individual biases may influence the way in which different groups contemplate their fertility and the options available to them. Knowledge of and access to meaningful options in respect to their situation, and the ability to follow one's own preferences can promote and secure the positive social conditions that enhance a woman's autonomy and well-being.

References

Absolom, K., Eiser, C., Turner, L., Ledger, W., Ross, R., Davies, H., Coleman, R., Hancock, B., Snowden, J., & Greenfield, D. (2008). Ovarian failure following cancer treatment: Current management and quality of life. *Human Reproduction, 23*(11), 2506–2512.

Anderson, D. J., Yates, P., McCarthy, A., Lang, C. P., Hargraves, M., McCarthy, N., & Porter-Steele, J. (2011). Younger and older women's concerns about menopause after breast cancer. *European Journal of Cancer Care, 20*(6), 785–794.

Anderson, K., Nisenblat, V., & Norman, R. (2010). Lifestyle factors in people seeking infertility treatment: A review. *The Australian & New Zealand Journal of Obstetrics & Gynaecology, 50*(1), 8–20.

Anderson, R. A. & Cameron, D. A. (2011). Pretreatment serum anti-mullerian hormone predicts long-term ovarian function and bone mass after chemotherapy for early breast cancer. *The Journal of Clinical Endocrinology and Metabolism, 96*(5), 1336–1343.

Anderson, R. A., Mitchell, R. T., Kelsey, T. W., Spears, N., Telfer, E. E., & Wallace, W. H. (2015). Cancer treatment and gonadal function: Experimental and established strategies for fertility preservation in children and young adults. *The Lancet Diabetes & Endocrinology, 3*(7), 556–567.

Anderson, R. A., Rosendahl, M., Kelsey, T. W., & Cameron, D. A. (2013). Pretreatment anti-Mullerian hormone predicts for loss of ovarian function after chemotherapy for early breast cancer. *European Journal of Cancer, 49*(16), 3404–3411.

Aubard, Y., Piver, P., Pech, J. C., Galinat, S., & Teissier, M. P. (2001). Ovarian tissue cryopreservation and gynecologic oncology: A review. *European Journal of Obstetrics, Gynecology, and Reproductive Biology, 97*(1), 5–14.

Avis, N. E., Crawford, S., & Manuel, J. (2004). Psychosocial problems among younger women with breast cancer. *Psychooncology, 13*(5), 295–308.

Azim, Jr., H. A., Santoro, L., Pavlidis, N., Gelber, S., Kroman, N., Azim, H., & Peccatori, F. A. (2011). Safety of pregnancy following breast cancer diagnosis: A meta-analysis of 14 studies. *European Journal of Cancer, 47*(1), 74–83.

Bancsi, L. F., Broekmans, F. J., Eijkemans, M. J., de Jong, F. H., Habbema, J. D., & te Velde, E. R. (2002). Predictors of poor ovarian response in in vitro fertilization: A prospective study comparing basal markers of ovarian reserve. *Fertility and Sterility, 77*(2), 328–336.

Barton, S. E., Najita, J. S., Ginsburg, E. S., Leisenring, W. M., Stovall, M., Weathers, R. E., Sklar, C. A., Robison, L. L., & Diller, L. (2013). Infertility, infertility treatment, and achievement of pregnancy in female survivors of childhood cancer: A report from the Childhood Cancer Survivor Study cohort. *The Lancet Oncology, 14*(9), 873–881.

Carter, J., Raviv, L., Applegarth, L., Ford, J. S., Josephs, L., Grill, E., Sklar, C., Sonoda, Y., Baser, R., & Barakat, R. R. (2010). A cross-sectional study of the psychosexual impact of cancer-related infertility in women: Third-party reproductive assistance. *Journal of Cancer Survivorship, 4*(3), 236–246.

Chan, S. W., Cipres, D., Katz, A., Niemasik, E. E., Kao, C. N., & Rosen, M. P. (2014). Patient satisfaction is best predicted by low decisional regret among women with cancer seeking fertility preservation counseling (FPC). *Fertility and Sterility, 102*(3), e162.

Chang, C. C., Elliott, T. A., Wright, G., Shapiro, D. B., Toledo, A. A., & Nagy, Z. P. (2013). Prospective controlled study to evaluate laboratory and clinical outcomes of oocyte vitrification obtained in in vitro fertilization patients aged 30 to 39 years. *Fertility and Sterility, 99*(7), 1891–1897.

Chow, E. J., Stratton, K. L., Leisenring, W. M., Oeffinger, K. C., Sklar, C. A., Donaldson, S. S., Ginsberg, J. P., Kenney, L. B., Levine, J. M., Robison, L. L., Shnorhavorian, M., Stovall, M., Armstrong, G. T., & Green, D. M. (2016). Pregnancy after chemotherapy in male and female survivors of childhood cancer treated between 1970 and 1999: A report from the Childhood Cancer Survivor Study cohort. *The Lancet Oncology, 17*(5), 567–576.

Cobo, A. & García-Velasco, J. A. (2016). Why all women should freeze their eggs. *Current Opinion in Obstetrics & Gynecology, 28*(3), 206–210.

Connell, S., Patterson, C., & Newman, B. (2006). A qualitative analysis of reproductive issues raised by young Australian women with breast cancer. *Health Care for Women International, 27*(1), 94–110.

Cousineau, T. M. & Domar, A. D. (2007). Psychological impact of infertility. *Best Practice & Research Clinical Obstetrics & Gynaecology, 21*(2), 293–308.

Crawshaw, M. (2013a). Male coping with cancer-fertility issues: Putting the 'social' into biopsychosocial approaches. *Reproductive Biomedicine Online, 27*(3), 261–270.

Crawshaw, M. (2013b). Psychosocial oncofertility issues faced by adolescents and young adults over their lifetime: A review of the research. *Human Fertility, 16*(1), 59–63.

D'Augelli, A. R., Rendina, H. J., Sinclair, K. O., & Grossman, A. H. (2007). Lesbian and gay youth's aspirations for marriage and raising children. *Journal of LGBT Issues in Counseling, 1*(4), 77–98, doi:10.1300/J462v01n04_06.

Dalberg, K., Eriksson, J., & Holmberg, L. (2006). Birth outcome in women with previously treated breast cancer: A population-based cohort study from Sweden. *PLoS Medicine, 3*(9), e336.

Del Mastro, L., Catzeddu, T., & Venturini, M. (2006). Infertility and pregnancy after breast cancer: Current knowledge and future perspectives. *Cancer Treatment Reviews, 32*(6), 417–422.

Dolmans, M. M. & Manavella, D. D. (2018). Recent advances in fertility preservation. *Journal of Obstetrics and Gynaecology Research, 45*(2), 266–279.

Donnez, J. & Dolmans, M. M. (2015). Ovarian cortex transplantation: 60 reported live births brings the success and worldwide expansion of the technique towards routine clinical practice. *Journal of Assisted Reproduction and Genetics, 32*(8), 1167–1170.

Donnez, J. & Dolmans, M. M. (2017). Fertility preservation in women. *New England Journal of Medicine, 377*(17), 1657–1665.

Duffy, C. & Allen, S. (2009). Medical and psychosocial aspects of fertility after cancer. *Cancer Journal, 15*(1), 27–33.

Dyer, S. J., Abrahams, N., Mokoena, N. E., Lombard, C. J., & van der Spuy, Z. M. (2005). Psychological distress among women suffering from couple infertility in South Africa: A quantitative assessment. *Human Reproduction, 20*(7), 1938–1943.

European Society for Human Reproduction, Embryology Guideline Group on P. O. I., Webber, L., Davies, M., Anderson, R., Bartlett, J., & Vermeulen, N. (2016). ESHRE guideline: Management of women with premature ovarian insufficiency. *Human Reproduction, 31*(5), 926–937.

Fantus, S., Gupta, A. A., Lorenzo, A. J., Brownstone, D., Maloney, A. M., & Shaul, R. Z. (2015). Addressing fertility preservation for lesbian, gay, and bisexual adolescents and young adults with cancer. *Journal of Adolescent and Young Adult Oncology, 4*(4), 152–156.

Findlay, J. K., Hutt, K. J., Hickey, M., & Anderson, R. A. (2015). What is the "ovarian reserve"? *Fertility and Sterility, 103*(3), 628–630.

Fleetwood, A. & Campo-Engelstein, L. (2010). The impact of infertility: Why ART should be a higher priority for women in the global South. *Cancer Treatment and Research, 156*, 237–248.

Garcia-Velasco, J. A., Domingo, J., Cobo, A., Martinez, M., Carmona, L., & Pellicer, A. (2013). Five years' experience using oocyte vitrification to preserve fertility for medical and nonmedical indications. *Fertility and Sterility, 99*(7), 1994–1999.

Garvelink, M. M., ter Kuile, M. M., Fischer, M. J., Louwe, L. A., Hilders, C. G., Kroep, J. R., & Stiggelbout, A. M. (2013). Development of a decision aid about fertility preservation for women with breast cancer in the Netherlands. *Journal of Psychosomatic Obstetrics and Gynaecology, 34*(4), 170–178.

Gnoth, C., Maxrath, B., Skonieczny, T., Friol, K., Godehardt, E., & Tigges, J. (2011). Final ART success rates: A 10 years survey. *Human Reproduction, 26*(8), 2239–2246.

Goldman, K. N., Noyes, N. L., Knopman, J. M., McCaffrey, C., & Grifo, J. A. (2013). Oocyte efficiency: Does live birth rate differ when analyzing cryopreserved and fresh oocytes on a per-oocyte basis? *Fertility and Sterility, 100*(3), 712–717.

Gorman, J. R., Roesch, S. C., Parker, B. A., Madlensky, L., Saquib, N., Newman, V. A., & Pierce, J. P. (2010). Physical and mental health correlates of pregnancy following breast cancer. *Psychooncology, 19*(5), 517–524.

Graham, S. (2017, June 22). What it's like to be left infertile by cancer at the age of 23. *Cosmopolitan.* Retrieved from www.cosmopolitan.com/uk/body/health/a10201217/infertility-young-cancer-side-effects-infertile.

Grundy, E. & Read, S. (2012). Social contacts and receipt of help among older people in England: Are there benefits of having more children? *The Journals of Gerontology. Series B, Psychological Sciences and Social Sciences, 67*(6), 742–754.

Gupta, A. A., Edelstein, K., Albert-Green, A., & D'Agostino, N. (2013). Assessing information and service needs of young adults with cancer at a single institution: The importance of information on cancer diagnosis, fertility preservation, diet, and exercise. *Supportive Care in Cancer, 21*(9), 2477–2484.

Hershberger, P. E., Finnegan, L., Pierce, P. F., & Scoccia, B. (2013). The decision-making process of young adult women with cancer who considered fertility cryopreservation. *Journal of Obstetric, Gynecologic, and Neonatal Nursing, 42*(1), 59–69.

Hoff, H. S., Brandon, A., & Mersereau, J. E. (2015). Fertility preservation decision aid increases knowledge and decreases decision conflict. *Fertility and Sterility, 103*(2), e24–e25.

Howard-Anderson, J., Ganz, P. A., Bower, J. E., & Stanton, A. L. (2012). Quality of life, fertility concerns, and behavioral health outcomes in younger breast cancer survivors: A systematic review. *Journal of the National Cancer Institute, 104*(5), 386–405.

Ives, A., Saunders, C., Bulsara, M., & Semmens, J. (2007). Pregnancy after breast cancer: Population based study. *British Medical Journal, 334*(7586), 194–196.

Jayasinghe, Y. L., Wallace, W. H. B., & Anderson, R. A. (2018). Ovarian function, fertility and reproductive lifespan in cancer patients. *Expert Review of Endocrinology & Metabolism, 13*(3), 125–136.

Jung, M., Shin, H. J., Rha, S. Y., Jeung, H. C., Hong, S., Moon, Y. W., Kim, H., Oh, K., Yang, W., Roh, J., & Chung, H. C. (2010). The clinical outcome of chemotherapy-induced amenorrhea in premenopausal young patients with breast cancer with long-term follow-up. *Annals of Surgical Oncology, 17*(12), 3259–3268.

Kato, K., Takehara, Y., Segawa, T., Kawachiya, S., Okuno, T., Kobayashi, T., Bodri, D., & Kato, O. (2012). Minimal ovarian stimulation combined with elective single embryo transfer policy: Age-specific results of a large, single-centre, Japanese cohort. *Reproductive Biology and Endocrinology, 10*(1), 1–7.

Kirkman, M. (2008). Being a 'real' mum: Motherhood through donated eggs and embryos. *Women's Studies International Forum, 31*(4), 241–248.

Lambertini, M., Ceppi, M., Poggio, F., Peccatori, F. A., Azim, Jr., H. A., Ugolini, D., Pronzato, P., Loibl, S., Moore, H. C. F., Partridge, A. H., Bruzzi, P., & Del Mastro, L. (2015). Ovarian suppression using luteinizing hormone-releasing hormone agonists during chemotherapy to preserve ovarian function and fertility of breast cancer patients: A meta-analysis of randomized studies. *Annals of Oncology, 26*(12), 2408–2419.

Langagergaard, V. (2011). Birth outcome in women with breast cancer, cutaneous malignant melanoma, or Hodgkin's disease: A review. *Clinical Epidemiology, 3*, 7–19.

Lawrenz, B., Banys, M., Henes, M., Neunhoeffer, E., Grischke, E.-M., & Fehm, T. (2011). Pregnancy after breast cancer: Case report and review of the literature. *Archives of Gynecology and Obstetrics, 283*(4), 837–843.

Lechner, L., Bolman, C., & van Dalen, A. (2007). Definite involuntary childlessness: Associations between coping, social support and psychological distress. *Human Reproduction, 22*(1), 288–294.

Lee, R. J., Wakefield, A., Foy, S., Howell, S. J., Wardley, A. M., & Armstrong, A. C. (2011). Facilitating reproductive choices: The impact of health services on the experiences of young women with breast cancer. *Psychooncology, 20*(10), 1044–1052.

Levine, J. M., Kelvin, J. F., Quinn, G. P., & Gracia, C. R. (2015). Infertility in reproductive-age female cancer survivors. *Cancer, 121*(10), 1532–1539.

Lindheim, S. R., Chase, J., & Sauer, M. V. (2001). Assessing the influence of payment on motivations of women participating as oocyte donors. *Gynecologic and Obstetric Investigation, 52*(2), 89–92.

Logan, S., Perz, J., Ussher, J., Peate, M., & Anazodo, A. (2017). Clinician provision of oncofertility support in cancer patients of a reproductive age: A systematic review. *Psychooncology*, *27*(3), 748–756.

Logan, S., Perz, J., Ussher, J., Peate, M., & Anazodo, A. (2018). A systematic review of patient oncofertility support needs in reproductive cancer patients aged 14 to 45 years of age. *Psychooncology*, *27*(2), 401–409.

Maltaris, T., Boehm, D., Dittrich, R., Seufert, R., & Koelbl, H. (2006). Reproduction beyond cancer: A message of hope for young women. *Gynecologic Oncology*, *103*(3), 1109–1121.

McLeod, C. & Ponesse, J. (2008). Infertility and moral luck: The politics of women blaming themselves for infertility. *International Journal of Feminist Approaches to Bioethics*, *1*(1), 126–144.

McQuillan, J., Greil, A. L., White, L., & Jacob, M. C. (2003). Frustrated fertility: Infertility and psychological distress among women. *Journal of Marriage and Family*, *65*(4), 1007–1018.

Meirow, D., Biederman, H., Anderson, R. A., & Wallace, W. H. (2010). Toxicity of chemotherapy and radiation on female reproduction. *Clinical Obstetrics and Gynecology*, *53*(4), 727–739.

Meirow, D., Roness, H., Kristensen, S. G., & Andersen, C. Y. (2015). Optimizing outcomes from ovarian tissue cryopreservation and transplantation; activation versus preservation. *Human Reproduction*, *30*(11), 2453–2456.

Mersereau, J. E., Goodman, L. R., Deal, A. M., Gorman, J. R., Whitcomb, B. W., & Su, H. I. (2013). To preserve or not to preserve: How difficult is the decision about fertility preservation? *Cancer*, *119*(22), 4044–4050.

Morice, P., Juncker, L., Rey, A., El-Hassan, J., Haie-Meder, C., & Castaigne, D. (2000). Ovarian transposition for patients with cervical carcinoma treated by radiosurgical combination. *Fertility and Sterility*, *74*(4), 743–748.

Oktay, K., Harvey, B. E., Partridge, A. H., Quinn, G. P., Reinecke, J., Taylor, H. S., Wallace, W. H., Wang, E. T., & Loren, A. W. (2018). Fertility preservation in patients with cancer: ASCO clinical practice guideline update. *Journal of Clinical Oncology*, *36*(19), 1994–2001.

Pacheco, F. & Oktay, K. (2017). Current success and efficiency of autologous ovarian transplantation: A meta-analysis. *Reproductive Sciences*, *24*(8), 1111–1120.

Pagani, O., Partridge, A., Korde, L., Badve, S., Bartlett, J., Albain, K., Gelber, R., & Goldhirsch, A. (2011). Pregnancy after breast cancer: If you wish, ma'am. *Breast Cancer Research and Treatment*, *129*(2), 309–317.

Peate, M., Meiser, B., Cheah, B. C., Saunders, C., Butow, P., Thewes, B., Hart, R., Phillips, K.-A., Hickey, M., & Friedlander, M. (2012). Making hard choices easier: A prospective, multicentre study to assess the efficacy of a fertility-related decision aid in young women with early-stage breast cancer. *British Journal of Cancer*, *106*(6), 1053–1061.

Peate, M., Meiser, B., Hickey, M., & Friedlander, M. (2009). The fertility-related concerns, needs and preferences of younger women with breast cancer: A systematic review. *Breast Cancer Research and Treatment*, *116*(2), 215–223.

Peate, M., Stafford, L., & Hickey, M. (2017). Fertility after breast cancer and strategies to help women achieve pregnancy. *Cancer Forum*, *41*(1), 32–39.

Pinelli, S., Simi, G., Maria, E. R. O., Cela, V., & Artini, P. G. (2017). Premature ovarian insufficiency: Current progress and future prospectives. *Current Trends in Clinical Embryology*, *4*(1), 28–33.

Quinn, G. P., Sanchez, J. A., Sutton, S. K., Vadaparampil, S. T., Nguyen, G. T., Green, B. L., Kanetsky, P. A., & Schabath, M. B. (2015). Cancer and lesbian, gay, bisexual, transgender/transsexual, and queer/questioning (LGBTQ) populations. *CA: A Cancer Journal for Clinicians*, *65*(5), 384–400.

Rashedi, A. S., Roo, S. F. de, Ataman, L. M., Edmonds, M. E., Silva, A. A., Scarella, A., et al. (2018). Survey of third-party parenting options associated with fertility preservation available to patients with cancer around the globe. *Journal of Global Oncology*, *4*, 1–7.

Rato, M. L., Gouveia-Oliveira, A., & Plancha, C. E. (2012). Influence of post-thaw culture on the developmental potential of human frozen embryos. *Journal of Assisted Reproduction and Genetics*, *29*(8), 789–795.

Ruddy, K. J., Gelber, S. I., Tamimi, R. M., Ginsburg, E. S., Schapira, L., Come, S. E., Borges, V. F., Meyer, M. E., & Partridge, A. H. (2014). Prospective study of fertility concerns and preservation strategies in young women with breast cancer. *Journal of Clinical Oncology*, *32*(11), 1151–1156.

Russell, A. M., Galvin, K. M., Harper, M. M., & Clayman, M. L. (2016). A comparison of heterosexual and LGBTQ cancer survivors' outlooks on relationships, family building, possible infertility, and patient-doctor fertility risk communication. *Journal of Cancer Survivorship*, *10*(5), 935–942.

Schover, L. R., Rybicki, L., Martin, B. A., & Bringelsen, K. A. (1999). Having children after cancer. A pilot survey of survivors' attitudes and experiences. *Cancer, 86*(4), 697–709.

Shapiro, B. S., Daneshmand, S. T., Garner, F. C., Aguirre, M., Hudson, C., & Thomas, S. (2010). Similar ongoing pregnancy rates after blastocyst transfer in fresh donor cycles and autologous cycles using cryopreserved bipronuclear oocytes suggest similar viability of transferred blastocysts. *Fertility and Sterility, 93*(1), 319–321.

Shimizu, C., Bando, H., Kato, T., Mizota, Y., Yamamoto, S., & Fujiwara, Y. (2013). Physicians' knowledge, attitude, and behavior regarding fertility issues for young breast cancer patients: A national survey for breast care specialists. *Breast Cancer, 20*(3), 230–240.

Sobota, A. & Ozakinci, G. (2014). Fertility and parenthood issues in young female cancer patients: A systematic review. *Journal of Cancer Survivorship, 8*(4), 707–721.

Sonmezer, M. & Oktay, K. (2006). Fertility preservation in young women undergoing breast cancer therapy. *Oncologist, 11*(5), 422–434.

Stern, C., Conyers, R., Orme, L., Barak, S., Agresta, F., & Seymour, J. (2013). Reproductive concerns of children and adolescents with cancer: Challenges and potential solutions. *Clinical Oncology in Adolescents and Young Adults, 3*, 63–78.

Stern, C., Gook, D., Hale, L. G., Agresta, F., Oldham, J., Rozen, G., & Jobling, T. (2013). First reported clinical pregnancy following heterotopic grafting of cryopreserved ovarian tissue in a woman after a bilateral oophorectomy. *Human Reproduction, 28*(11), 2996–2999.

Stuart-Smith, S. J., Smith, J. A., & Scott, E. J. (2011). Treatment decision making in anonymous donor egg in-vitro fertilisation: A qualitative study of childless women and women with genetically related children. *Human Fertility, 14*(2), 97–105.

Thewes, B., Butow, P., Girgis, A., & Pendlebury, S. (2004). The psychosocial needs of breast cancer survivors; a qualitative study of the shared and unique needs of younger versus older survivors. *Psychooncology, 13*(3), 177–189.

Ussher, J. M., Cummings, J., Dryden, A., & Perz, J. (2016). Talking about fertility in the context of cancer: Health care professional perspectives. *European Journal of Cancer Care, 25*(1), 99–111.

Ussher, J. M., Parton, C., & Perz, J. (2018a). Need for information, honesty and respect: Patient perspectives on health care professionals communication about cancer and fertility. *Reproductive Health, 15*(1), 2.

Ussher, J. M., Perz, J., Miller, A., Patterson, P., Wain, G., & Hobbs, K., Fertility Study Team (2018b). Threat of biographical disruption: The gendered construction and experience of infertility following cancer for women and men. *BMC Cancer, 18*(1), 250.

Velentgas, P., Daling, J. R., Malone, K. E., Weiss, N. S., Williams, M. A., Self, S. G., & Mueller, B. A. (1999). Pregnancy after breast carcinoma: Outcomes and influence on mortality. *Cancer, 85*(11), 2424–2432.

Wallace, W. H., Anderson, R. A., & Irvine, D. S. (2005). Fertility preservation for young patients with cancer: Who is at risk and what can be offered? *The Lancet Oncology, 6*(4), 209–218.

Wallace, W. H. & Kelsey, T. W. (2010). Human ovarian reserve from conception to the menopause. *PLoS One, 5*(1), e8772.

Weston, R., Qu, L., & Parker, R. A. (2005). *"It's not for lack of wanting kids." A report on the fertility decision making project (Research Report No. 11)*. Southbank VIC, Australia: Australian Institute of Family Studies. Retrieved from https://aifs.gov.au/publications/its-not-lack-wanting-kids-report-fertility-decision-making/export.

Yasmin, E., Balachandren, N., Davies, M. C., Jones, G. L., Lane, S., Mathur, R., Webber, L., & Anderson, R. A. (2018). Fertility preservation for medical reasons in girls and women: British fertility society policy and practice guideline. *Human Fertility, 21*(1), 3–26.

15

ASSISTED CONCEPTION

Fertility preservation, surrogate motherhood, gamete/embryo donation and in vitro fertilization

Olga B. A. van den Akker

Most people across the world expect, and want, to become parents at some stage in their life (Lampic et al., 2006). However, 48 million couples experience infertility due to medical reasons (Mascarenhas et al., 2012), and these rates are rising. The rise in infertility (or involuntary childlessness) is also due in part to global changes in lifestyle factors, such as delayed childbearing (Mathews & Hamilton, 2016), same-sex partnerships, and women and men deciding to become solo parents (van den Akker, 2017a). These medical and lifestyle factors present biological challenges that can be treated with assisted conception (AC), including fertility preservation, surrogate motherhood, gamete or embryo donation, and in vitro fertilisation (IVF). In this chapter I explore the processes involved in overcoming barriers to parenthood and the psychological effects associated with these. The contexts in which the medical and lifestyle factors associated with involuntary childlessness occur, and overcoming these barriers, are also discussed from within the wider sociocultural, family, and work environments.

Whatever the underlying reasons, involuntary childlessness is often associated with feelings of personal failure because parenthood continues to be considered by many to be a necessary part of individuals' life time trajectories into adulthood (van den Akker, 2012). The impact of failing to complete this expected major life goal has been described as a life crisis (Ussher et al., 2018) that leaves the mental health of about 10% of the population seeking AC worldwide in crisis (Benyamini et al., 2009; Eugster & Vingerhoets, 1999; Payne et al., 2019). A recent systematic review and meta-analysis of the long-term mental health of infertile patients who failed to become parents has shown that their individual needs and their relationships improved over time, and that individuals who were able to accept their childlessness, and make meaning of their life by pursuing new goals, tended to adjust better than those who did not (Gameiro & Finnigan, 2017). There is therefore a real need for appropriately tailored psychosocial support for those who receive a diagnosis of infertility and for individuals who relinquish their parenthood goals but do not adjust.

Fertility treatment availability

Most developed countries consider infertility a medical condition and have national health policies to cover some or all infertility treatment, including IVF (e.g., Australia, Austria, Denmark, Finland, France, Germany, Iceland, the Netherlands, Norway, Sweden, the UK; Hughes & Giacomini, 2001), whereas other countries (e.g., the US) consider fertility treatment a socially constructed need (van den Akker, 2012) or a luxury to be financed by patients with the means to afford it. The uncertainties about costs, insurance, unclear cause-(s) of infertility, treatment length, and outcomes can cause substantial amounts of stress. Distress, anxiety, and depression are associated with the chances of a successful outcome (Purewal et al., 2018). This suggests that there is a circularity of broadly psychological and physiological factors impacting the AC process, which leaves many people on a never-ending treadmill of treatment distress followed by treatment failure followed by further distress and failure.

It has been estimated that less than one half of infertile women are able to pursue treatment; those who can tend to be White, older, heterosexual, and married with middle- to high-incomes (Datta et al., 2016). The others cannot afford private treatment or are excluded from treatment (i.e., same sex attracted or trans individuals; single women). Different policies have therefore led to inequities in access to AC, particularly third-party treatment, as costs can be prohibitive. However, even those who are able to pursue privately funded treatment face hardship. Moving house or getting into serious debt to fund the treatment have been reported (Cook, 2015), whilst others are known to feel caught in a job to secure the income necessary to pay the costs of treatment (van den Akker et al., 2017b), or end up making a decision about the costs and benefits of their 'desire' for a child versus the 'worth' of a child (Klitzman, 2017).

Schmidt et al. (1995) and Boivin et al. (2007) reported that the proportion of couples from the developed world seeking treatment to overcome their infertility averages just over 47% and 50%, respectively, but less than one half of them actually receive treatment. Some of this discrepancy may be because of unavailability of health care resources as described above, but there are also large numbers of people who desire parenthood but do not receive treatment, including many LGBT couples and single women and men, because not all countries treat their parenthood needs equally. The fate of those who do not seek treatment is less studied (Schmidt et al., 1995), but is likely to be of substantial additional concern as they appear to be less well educated and affluent than their treatment-seeking counterparts.

Assisted conception

Despite the discrepancy in treatment availability and the disparity within populations who access treatment, increasing infertility rates and more people reporting problems conceiving (Dhalwani et al., 2013) have led to increasing demands for AC worldwide (Farquhar et al., 2015). The latest statistics from the UK, for example (HFEA, 2016), show that in 2014, 52,288 women had 67,708 cycles of in vitro fertilisation (IVF) or intra cytoplasmic sperm injection (ICSI), a rise on previous years with no sign of abating. In addition to IVF/ICSI and related treatments involving a couple's own gametes, a large number of treatments involve donor gametes (Kupka et al., 2016), and surrogacy arrangements also have seen a rise in popularity (Crawshaw et al., 2012). Use of third-party input, such as gametes, embryos, and genetic or gestational surrogates in AC, although common, is proportionally less frequent (only 10% of fertility treatment cycles in Europe; Kupka et al., 2016) than use of IVF and associated techniques that use a couple's own gametes. The lack of frequency is partly because patients are dependent upon the supply of donors or surrogates, but is also because most patients prefer a full genetic link (Hendriks et al., 2017; van den Akker, 2000). Consequently, psychosocial and medical factors are again important in terms of AC treatment options.

Furthermore, AC is expensive and only sometimes funded by national health policies or insurance, but treatment with donated gametes and embryos add even more to those IVF/ICSI costs; (commercial) surrogacy is the most expensive. The reproductive landscape is therefore shifting (Cohen, 2015) from the relatively young heterosexual two-parent family with genetically related and gestated offspring produced at no cost to include families that consist of one or more (often older) women or men, and babies conceived in test tubes and genetically or gestationally related to other individuals at high costs and against biological and medical odds. These shifts from tradition have implications for families of the future and for society at large (van den Akker, 2016a). In addition, there are psychological costs associated with the physical and social effects of AC treatments, which are increasingly complex and varied, as is shown below.

Assisted reproductive technologies

Intra Uterine Insemination (IUI) and IVF/ICSI

Assisted reproductive technologies (known as ART or AC) can involve numerous different techniques, which vary in complexity and intensity of treatment, including IUI, IVF, and IVF with ICSI. In IUI, no conception outside the uterus is necessary, whereas in IVF, not only does conception take place in vitro (i.e., outside the uterus), but it also involves the removal of gametes from the female and male parents to create the desired embryo in a test tube. Finally, in ICSI, when the sperm is unable to penetrate the oocyte, it is injected directly into the oocyte in the hope of producing a viable embryo. Only about 70% of treatments for infertility are successful (Troude et al., 2016), which leaves the remaining 30% to try again (and again), or to give up hope of ever becoming a genetic parent.

Additional third-party AC treatments

Assisted conception not only circumvents obstacles to fertility, but it can also replace mitochondria or gametes from third-party donors to bypass genetic conditions. Social needs of involuntarily childless single individuals and same-sex couples also require the involvement of a third party, such as donated gametes (oocytes or sperm), embryos, surrogates, or a combination of these, which is legal in some (e.g., the UK) but not all (e.g., Italy) countries. Solo individuals, LGBT individuals or couples, and heterosexual couples with ovarian or sperm failures or absence of the uterus (e.g., previously treated cancer patients, women unable to sustain a pregnancy or born without a uterus) can use third-party assisted conception. Third-party assisted conception therefore fulfils a need for individuals who cannot produce a child without the assistance of the third-party donor or surrogate for medical or lifestyle reasons.

Unlike IVF, which is state funded for heterosexual couples in some countries (e.g., the UK), (unlimited) third-party AC is rarely fully supported by national health services (Israel is an exception that provides financial support to all), which leaves most of those in need of the more complex interventions to fund treatment themselves. This has created a further imbalance in solo/same-sex third-party AC routes to parenting compared with the majority of heterosexual IVF routes to parenting. In addition to these inequalities in access, there are further gestational and genetic link complexities associated with third-party assisted conception, including different amounts of genetic, gestational, and epigenetic contributions from the third party, that affect the parent status of individuals who use third-party treatment to conceive. Questions about who the child's parent, grandparent, uncle, niece, and other extended family are tend to be based on social not genetic roles, and can have far-reaching psychological effects on members of these recipient and donor families (Blyth et al., 2017; Frith et al., 2017).

Surrogate motherhood

In genetic surrogacy, the third-party contribution is the greatest contribution to the development and makeup of the child. The surrogate mother bears the child for another person, and has contributed her own oocyte to the baby. A female recipient does not contribute the oocyte or the gestational epigenetic environment to the baby, although a male recipient may have contributed his sperm (or a donor sperm can be used) (van den Akker, 2017a). Gestational surrogacy, on the other hand, refers to a surrogate who carries an embryo from a heterosexual couple, a donated embryo from yet another source, or an embryo created from the commissioning woman's oocyte and sperm from her partner or a donor. Either way, the surrogate does not contribute the oocyte, although the gestational and epigenetic influences are again contributed by her (van den Akker, 2017a). Within the genetic/gestational routes, there are also differences in the manner in which surrogacy is offered in different countries, such as altruistic versus commercial, which makes cross-border surrogacy particularly complex (van den Akker, 2017a). In commercial surrogacy, the recipient or commissioning parent(s) pay for a surrogate, a clinic, and embryos or gametes. This has been interpreted as 'baby buying'. In altruistic surrogacy, a surrogate tends to receive expenses for her part in conceiving, carrying, birthing, and relinquishing the baby. The former model is accepted across many countries that legalise or do not object to surrogacy as a commercial business practice, including India and some American states, whereas the latter model is legalised in, for example, the UK and Australia. In addition to these distinctions, commercial surrogacy is often anonymous, whereas altruistic surrogacy rarely is. The psychosocial outcomes for both families (surrogate and recipient) in altruistic and commercial surrogacy have been shown to be relatively problem free (van den Akker, 2005, 2007, 2017a), although accurate record keeping and accuracy of genetic information is critical, particularly for the welfare and human rights perspectives of the child (Crawshaw et al., 2012, 2016; UN CRC, 1989). Research on couples or individuals who commission surrogacy overseas, and of surrogates in such arrangements, has shown that both parties have coped well in some studies, whereas others have shown numerous problems, including stigma and issues with legal parentage and passports (for a full discussion, see van den Akker, 2017a).

Embryo donation

In embryo donation, a woman receives an embryo from another source, often from another infertile couple who had surplus embryos following their own successful treatment, and provides the epigenetic gestational environment herself. Embryo donation is not a popular option for donors because it means relinquishing a fully genetically related child, or full sibling to their existing children (de Lacey, 2005, 2007), but less is known about recipients of donated embryos. Australia reported its first successful embryo donation in the early 1980s (Trounson et al., 1983), which was, as in most countries, practiced under the laws of anonymity, with few exceptions (International Federation of Fertility Societies, 2016). Recent research on the relationships and boundaries proposed between embryo providers and their recipients (Frith et al., 2017) shows that early contact between donor and recipient families is favoured by both parties and allows for more open interpretations of parenthood and family belonging. This contact is based upon trust (similar to surrogacy), and, when broken, can lead to significant harm to the child(ren) concerned and the donors (*The New Daily*, 2017).

Gamete donation

Oocyte and sperm donation are much more common than surrogacy or embryo donation. Sperm donation is a relatively old technique as it does not need to involve technology. Oocyte or egg donation, on the other hand, involves all of the processes of IVF, as the oocytes are retrieved from the woman following follicular stimulation with hormones. This process can be painful, and the hormonal stimulation can have additional physical and psychological effects on the women who undergo this process. Once a sufficient number of adequate oocytes have been retrieved, they are either frozen (as in fertility preservation for the treatment of serious disease such as cancer or for age-related reasons) or fertilised in vitro for subsequent implantation in a recipient woman. Individuals who donate, or think about donating, gametes interpret a gamete differently than an embryo (Purewal & van den Akker, 2009) with less emphasis on a 'life' or a baby.

Nevertheless, donors and donor-conceived adults value knowing something about their true genetic relatives and origins, as evidenced by the increasing interest in ancestry profile building and in obtaining genetic health information. Research on donors has shown that they often want to find out the result of their donations (Blyth et al., 2017) and, like donor-conceived adult offspring (Frith et al., 2018), they have numerous reasons for contacting DNA-based linking registers to obtain information about their genetic children or siblings. Searches for donors by offspring (van den Akker et al., 2015) and searches for offspring by donors (Crawshaw et al., 2016) are becoming increasingly better understood; not finding those for whom they searched can have a significant impact on identity and lead to other psychological conflict (Crawshaw, 2017). As a consequence, anonymous donations are now increasingly no longer acceptable in many countries, although there are still some countries where the welfare of the child is put behind that of the prospective parents, and some parents still prefer to hide the fact that fertility treatment, and treatment with donor gametes in particular, were used in their child's conception

Mitochondrial donation

Mitochondrial donation involves routine IVF with the addition that a family's affected mitochondria (mitochondrial disease) are replaced with a donor's healthy mitochondria, so that the parents have the chance to give birth to a healthy child. Here, prior to the IVF, the DNA of a woman's oocyte that contains the faulty mitochondria are transferred to a donor egg with healthy mitochondria. In the UK, it is estimated that 1 in 200 children are born with faulty mitochondrial DNA, and a proportion of these develop more serious mitochondria-related disorders (Wellcome Trust, 2018). Mitochondrial disease can occur in young people and lead to disability and mortality because no treatment is currently available. The British Parliament was the first in the world to vote in support of mitochondrial donation in 2015. Since then, the technique has been licensed and regulated by the Human Fertilisation and Embryology Authority for clinical use (HFEA, 2017 –Guidance note 33, modification of Section 31ZA, 2A). Although progressive, the HFEA failed to agree that mitochondrial donors, like gamete and embryo donors, should be identifiable to the children born from these techniques and noted instead that mitochondrial donors would be anonymous as the amount of genetic contribution was small, although at age 16 they can find out if mitochondrial donation was used in their conception (Guidance note 33, modification of Section 31ZA).

Fertility preservation

Children, adolescents, and young adults who are preparing to receive treatment for serious disease (e.g., cancer) have the option to preserve their potential fertility by gamete cryopreservation (or freezing). Similarly, individuals who are at risk of late childbearing for lifestyle reasons, such as prioritising careers or education, or not being in a stable relationship, and transgender individuals who are transitioning through hormonal intervention, also have the opportunity to preserve their gametes for use at a later date, even one that is well beyond their natural reproductive capacity (Charter et al., 2018). Although sperm, oocyte, and embryo cryopreservation are standard practices and widely available, research with children and adolescents with cancer has considered the specific guideline needs for health care providers because of the sensitive nature of fertility preservation in these vulnerable populations (Loren et al., 2013).

In 2006, an American expert panel carried out a systematic review and reported that only a few randomised controlled trials existed on the impact of fertility preservation in cancer patients (Lee et al., 2006). Recommendations for guidelines included improving and providing informed consent before cancer therapy and providing education about the possibility of subsequent infertility and the fertility preservation options. An updated review concluded that no substantive revisions to the 2006 American Society of Clinical Oncology recommendations were necessary (Loren et al., 2013). However, additional recommendations were made, which included emphasising the possibility of infertility with all patients treated during their reproductive years because their initial focus may be on the cancer diagnosis and they might not think about this issue if it were not raised by their health care providers. However, more recent research has shown that guidelines are not always followed in practice (Logan et al., 2018; Ussher, Perz, & ACFST, 2018).

Although, in some countries, access to supportive services for people undergoing fertility preservation prior to treatment for diseases such as cancer is now well established in some (Atkin et al., 2014) but not all cases (Logan et al., 2018; Parton, Ussher, & Perz, 2019), these services are less established within other contexts, such as the transgender community (Charter et al., 2018; Riggs & Due, 2017). There is some evidence that researchers and health care providers are beginning to recognise the importance of fertility preservation beyond oncology patients (Wallace et al., 2014). The guidelines developed specifically for people who wish to modify their bodies and appearance in regard to sex traits extend to recommendations about fertility preservation (Hembree et al., 2009; WPATH, 2011). However, although all non-heterosexual family-building individuals requiring third-party AC are faced with a significant dilemma, assisted reproduction with fresh or frozen gametes does not always result in a successful outcome. Transgender individuals have the additional experience of high levels of distress when undergoing fertility preservation. In addition to experiencing gender dysphoria to a greater or lesser extent (discomfort or distress that is caused by a discrepancy between a person's gender identity and their sex assigned at birth, the associated gender role, and/or primary and secondary sex characteristics), healthcare needs to be tailored to each individual's needs (Charter et al., 2018).

Psychological effects of fertility preservation and treatment

For each individual seeking treatment to build a family, the physically and psychologically taxing experiences of many of the treatments are compounded by the financial demands on the state or on the individual bearing that economic burden. Many of the physical and psychological effects are more pronounced in women because, although both women and men undergoing treatment have been found to experience high levels of psychological distress, women report more distress than men do (Ying et al., 2016). Women undergo the most intrusive investigations and treatments, bear the brunt of failed pregnancies with the arrival of unwanted monthly menstrual periods, and anticipate another cycle of the same hormonal preparation, monitoring, and embryo transfer (ET) once their body is ready. Unfortunately, the psychological stress experienced by women during treatment may in itself negatively affect treatment outcomes (Matthiesen et al., 2011; Purewal et al., 2017, 2018), although the exact mechanisms are not known (Homan et al., 2007).

Other meta-analytic research and a critical review provide further evidence that psychological support or psychological treatment during ART (i.e., tailored to remove or reduce the psychological distress) may improve treatment outcomes (Frederiksen et al., 2015; Hämmerli et al., 2009). However, this is seldom offered routinely as part of the treatment process (Payne et al., 2019), particularly in the longer term when third-party treatment is used (Crawshaw et al., 2016). Women undergoing fertility treatment, whether successfully (Toscano & Montgomery, 2009) or unsuccessfully (Gameiro & Finnigan, 2017), report psychological distress, and their support needs are well known (Boivin et al., 2005). However, those who never succeed in becoming parents and relinquish their parenthood goals have continuing psychological needs (Gameiro & Finnigan, 2017), which tend to be ignored in research.

LGBT and solo family building

Psychological distress and lack of additional psychological support are also issues that affect most fertile couples in same-sex relationships and solo individuals attempting to build a family. Research on same-sex, bisexual, solo, and transgender family building is increasing, and poses additional complexities, although some of the third-party interventions and genetic link options also apply to heterosexual couples who cannot use their own gametes or uterus. Research on heterosexual couples has largely focussed on the psychosocial welfare of the parents, whereas research on LGB individuals tends to be focussed on child welfare and parent–child interactions. Reports of lesbian families who used sperm donation have generally shown good parent/child relationships, good parenting, and good child adjustment (e.g., Golombok et al., 2003). Research on the welfare of gay men and their families created with surrogate mothers (their preferred route to parenthood; Blake et al., 2017) also shows good psychosocial adjustment in the parents and their surrogate children, a greater closeness with their families of origin, and improved self-esteem (Bergman et al., 2010). Most gay fathers have a relationship with their surrogate, although not with an egg donor, and disclose the conception route to their children (Carone et al., 2018).

Research on the specific fertility needs of bisexual individuals and couples has shown that improvements in tailored, or at least non-heteronormative, services are necessary (Yager et al., 2010). Similarly, Ross and Epstein (2006) studied the experiences of lesbian and bisexual women and reported that additional support needs were necessary regarding donor insemination services. Recommendations for improvements in services include providing cues that the service is positive about lesbian and bisexual parenting, that specific infertility support is necessary for lesbian and bisexual couples, that opportunities are created for women to make informed choices about interventions that match their known fertility status, and that accessible services are offered to known sperm donors, including gay men.

Solo parenting is somewhat more complex as here only one parent takes on full responsibility for the child(ren), which presents those parents with a burden they cannot share, as they do not include a father (solo women) or mother (solo men) figure in the new family. Solo men, like women, tend to prefer a child with a genetic link, and often choose surrogacy to achieve this (Carone et al., 2017). According to Golombok et al. (1997), children raised in fatherless families are no different from those in other families; solo parents experienced greater warmth and interaction and children were more securely attached to their mother, although they did feel less cognitively and physically competent than their peers from families where a father was present (i.e., compared with heterosexual and same-sex two-parent families).

Transgender individuals can choose to preserve their fertility prior to hormone therapy to change their gender, and this option ensures that their own gametes (from their original gender) can be used in fertility treatment to build a family, as removal of testes or ovaries and hormonal treatment will make it impossible to have genetically related children later on. Counselling transgender individuals when they request body modifications about fertility preservation options is therefore crucially important. Counselling is also important in relation to the unconventional outcomes of fertility preservation and transgendering, as transgender men and women use their own ova and sperm, respectively, to function as a mother or father according to their gametic contribution, but function socially in reversed parental identities (Murphy, 2012). Research is therefore beginning to show the needs of heterosexual and LGBT individuals and couples for psychological and social support before, during, and following their treatment, regardless of the outcomes, and policies and practices are being developed to implement changes (see, for example, the UK HFEA, 2017).

The wider sociocultural context

Assisted conception treatment does not take place in a social vacuum. It affects women and men who are in contact with others around them, including family, friends, the communities in which they live, and their colleagues and employers. Fertility is associated with femininity and masculinity across different cultures world-wide, and not being able to reproduce has been stigmatised (Hawkey et al., 2018; Inhorn, 2003) with appalling consequences in some countries (van den Akker, 2017a). A person's social milieu also dictates ethical concerns. For example, Collins and Chan (2017) reported that women in the US were concerned about treatment if it increased twinning rates (54%) and involved third-party input (48–51%), although IVF (30%) and partner insemination (14%) were also ethically problematic to some. A number of sociocultural determinants (e.g., being Black) were associated with greater treatment concern, whereas being Hispanic was associated with concern about donor eggs, and religiosity predicted concerns about IVF and all third-party AC. Catholics and other Christians had additional concerns regarding IUI. These results suggest that ethical concerns about fertility treatments are prevalent, tend to be specific to the treatment option, and may explain some of the differences in help-seeking behaviours and treatment choices made. In addition to socioculturally determined ethical concerns, media framing is also likely to contribute to a population's attributions of stigma regarding AC options (see, e.g., van den Akker et al., 2016b, 2016c), in addition to limitations in resources to access funding.

The family environment

Given that a child with a full genetic link is preferred universally, and this is possible via IVF using one's own gametes and via gestational surrogacy (Freeman et al., 2014; van den Akker, 2000), it continues to be the desired choice for most couples undergoing fertility treatment (Hendriks et al., 2017). But, as many individuals seeking treatment do not succeed in conceiving a baby genetically related to one or both of them, they then need to make a choice that does not only affect the couple and the child, but also the immediate and extended family, as one half (or neither side) of the family has a continuation of their 'blood line' (i.e., the genetic link). Donors' (or genetic surrogates') extended families too face a continuation of their 'blood line' within another family, where parents, grandparents, and siblings have no means of contact with a full or partial genetic child elsewhere. These losses are generally under investigated. For recipient families where this lack of a genetic link represents an issue, secrecy and deception about the child's genetic origins are prevalent. These parents cannot bear the stigma they believe is associated with third-party AC. Deception about origins is also at the expense of the human rights of the child (UNCRC, 1989). Family, friends, and communities tend to find out or reveal the secrets surrounding the child, often with unhappy consequences (Crawshaw, 2017).

The work environment

A recent large-scale survey of people considering or going through AC in the UK showed that, in addition to absences for clinic appointments, physical and emotional problems resulted in more absences from work (Payne et al., forthcoming) than was previously reported in the Netherlands (Bouwmans et al., 2008). Taking time off from employment for treatment with no guarantee of success is potentially risky in a number of ways. First, if treatment cycles fail, they may be repeated, which increases the time off work. This in turn leads to the need to disclose to an employer, manager, or colleagues that they are having fertility treatment, which is known to be associated with stigma for both women and men (Inhorn, 2003). Because AC treatment to conceive is such a personal matter, and experiencing failures of treatment compound the already vulnerable position of those undergoing it, having to disclose it (often repeatedly) is intrusive, particularly if the person is single or LGBT and did not intend to share that information at work (van den Akker et al., 2017b).

An interesting cross-European study showed that 24% of women believed that work interfered with treatment (Domar et al., 2012), whereas in Britain, Payne et al. (forthcoming) found that women experienced bi-directional conflict or interference between the demands of work and the time and the emotional demands of treatment. This was influenced by the extent to which they shifted their identity and priorities away from career to becoming a mother during treatment, a finding that confirms Walker's (2017) research.

Career concerns may therefore be linked to attempts to conform to (gendered) ideal worker norms, although emotional and physical problems (e.g., side effects or complications associated with treatment) are also important and are likely to be relevant to work absenteeism. The stress associated with balancing these worker/potential parent concerns and conflicts may affect treatment outcomes (Matthiesen et al., 2011; Purewal et al., 2017), and, in extreme cases, may lead some prospective parents to give up on their career. Alternatively, the uncertainty associated with the treatment may encourage others to focus more on their career in case of treatment failure.

Conclusion

Assisted conception in all its forms presents many psychosocial as well as medical opportunities, challenges, and risks. Clearly AC involves rapid scientific and technological developments, and the future will no doubt continue to show more innovation in the creation and nurturing of embryos. Although the psychological, familial, social, cultural, and workplace environmental impacts of infertility and treatment success or failure apply to all people, individuals with specific ill health, or with gender or sexual or relationship fluidity, may experience additional issues when attempting to become parents, as they do when they are existing parents moving from one sexual or romantic preference or identity to another. The evidence so far has shown that, with increasing use of technology and innovation to assist individuals to achieve the goal of parenthood, accurate record keeping, monitoring, and human rights need to be at the forefront of these interventions. Perhaps most importantly, individuals who opt for AC need to be sure they are cognitively consonant with their behaviors and allow the resultant children their basic human right to accurate birth and genetic information. The experience of fertility, infertility (or involuntary childlessness), and treatment success and/or failures therefore straddle psychological, behavioral, sociocultural, physical, and medical domains. Each of these domains should therefore be weighted proportionally in research, policy, and practice.

References

Atkin, K., Chattoo, S., & Crawshaw, M. (2014). Clinical encounters and culturally competent practice: The challenges of providing cancer and infertility care. *Policy and Politics*, *42*, 581–596.

Benyamini, Y., Gozlan, M., & Kokia, E. (2009). Women's and men's perceptions of infertility and their associations with psychological adjustment: A dyadic approach. *British Journal of Health Psychology*, *14*, 1–16.

Bergman, K., Rubio, R., & Green, R. J. (2010). Gay men who become fathers via surrogacy: The transition to parenthood. *Journal of GLBT Family Studies*, *6*, 111–141.

Blake, L., Carone, N., Raffanello, E., Slutsky, J., & Ehrhardt, A. (2017). Gay fathers' motivations for and feelings about surrogacy as a path to parenthood. *Human Reproduction*, *32*, 860–867.

Blyth, E., Crawshaw, M., Frith, L., & van den Akker, O. (2017). Gamete donors' reasons for, and expectations and experiences of, registration with a voluntary donor linking register. *Human Fertility*, *21*, 1–11.

Boivin, J., Bunting, L., Collins, J., & Nygren, K. (2007). International estimates of infertility prevalence and treatment-seeking: Potential need and demand for infertility medical care. *Human Reproduction*, *22*, 1506–1512.

Boivin, J., Takefman, J., & Braverman, A. (2005). Giving bad news: 'It's time to stop'. In N. Macklon (Ed.), *IVF in the medically complicated patient: A guide to management* (pp. 233–240). London: Taylor & Francis.

Bouwmans, C., Lintsen, B., Verhaak, C., Eijkemans, R., Habbema, J., Braat, D., & Hakkaart-Van Roijen, L. (2008). Absence from work and emotional stress in women undergoing IVF or ICSI: An analysis of IVF-related absence from work in women and the contribution of general and emotional factors. *Acta Obstetrica et Gynecologica Scandinavica*, 87, 1169–1175.

Carone, N., Baiocco, R., & Lingiardi, V. (2017). Single fathers by choice using surrogacy: Why men decide to have a child as a single parent. *Human Reproduction*, 32, 1871–1879.

Carone, N., Baiocco, R., Manzi, D., Antoniucci, C., & Caricato, V. (2018). Surrogacy families headed by gay men: Relationships with surrogates and egg donors, fathers' decisions over disclosure, and children's views on their surrogacy origins. *Human Reproduction*, 33, 248–257.

Charter, R., Ussher, J. M., Perz, J., & Robinson, K. (2018). The transgender parent: Experiences and constructions of pregnancy and parenthood for transgender men in Australia. *International Journal of Transgenderism*, 19(1), 64–77.

Cohen, P. N. (2015). Divergent responses to family inequality. In P. R. Amato, A. Booth, S. M. McHale, & M. Van Hook (Eds), *Families in an era of increasing inequality* (pp. 25–33). New York, NY: Springer.

Collins, S. & Chan, E. (2017). Sociocultural determinants of US women's ethical views on various fertility treatments. *Reproductive BioMedicine Online*, 35, 669–677.

Cook, M. (2015, May 23). US women go into debt for IVF. *BioEdge*. Retrieved from www.bioedge.org/bioethics/us-women-go-into-debt-for-ivf1/11447, accessed 29 November 2017.

Crawshaw, M. (2017). Direct-to-consumer DNA testing: The fallout for individuals and their families unexpectedly learning of their donor conception origins. *Human Fertility*, 11, 1–4.

Crawshaw, M., Blyth, E., & van den Akker, O. (2012). The changing profile of surrogacy in the UK: Implications for policy and practice. *Journal of Social Welfare and Family Law*, 34(3), 1–11.

Crawshaw, M., Frith, L., van den Akker, O., & Blyth, E. (2016). Voluntary DNA-based information exchange and contact services following donor conception: An analysis of service users' needs. *New Genetics and Society*, 35, 372–392.

Datta, J., Palmer, M., Tanton, C., Gibson, L., Jones, K., Macdowall, W., Glasier, A., Sonnenberg, P., Field, N., Mercer, C., Johnson, A., & Wellings, K. (2016). Prevalence of infertility and help seeking among 15 000 women and men. *Human Reproduction*, 31, 2108–2118.

de Lacey, S. (2005). Parent identity and 'virtual' children: Why parents discard rather than donate unused embryos. *Human Reproduction*, 20, 1661–1669.

de Lacey, S. (2007). Decisions for the fate of frozen embryos: Fresh insights into patients' thinking and their rationales for donating or discarding embryos. *Human Reproduction*, 22, 1751–1758.

Dhalwani, N., Fiashi, L., West, J., & Tata, L. (2013). Occurrence of fertility problems presenting to primary care: Population level estimates of clinical burden and socioeconomic inequalities across the UK. *Human Reproduction*, 28, 960–968.

Domar, A., Gordon, K., Garcia-Velasco, J., & La Marca, A. (2012). Understanding the perceptions of and emotional barriers to infertility treatment: A survey in four European countries. *Human Reproduction*, 27, 1073–1079.

Eugster, A. & Vingerhoets, A. (1999). Psychological aspects of in vitro fertilization: A review. *Social Science & Medicine*, 48, 575–589.

Farquhar, C., Rishworth, J., Brown, J., Nelen, W., & Marjoribanks, J. (2015). Assisted reproductive technology: An overview of Cochrane reviews. *Cochrane Reviews*, 17, CD010537.

Frederiksen, Y., Farver-Vestergaard, I., Grønhøj Skovgård, N., Ingerslev, H., & Zachariae, R. (2015). Efficacy of psychosocial interventions for psychological and pregnancy outcomes in infertile women and men: A systematic review and meta-analysis. *British Medical Journal: Open*, 2015, e006592.

Freeman, T., Graham, S., Entehaj, F., & Richards, M. (2014). *Relatedness in assisted reproduction: Families, origins and identities*. Cambridge, UK: Cambridge University Press.

Frith, L., Blyth, E., Crawshaw, M., & van den Akker, O. (2018). Secrets and disclosure in donor conception. *Sociology of Health and Illness*, 40, 188–203.

Frith, L., Blyth, E., & Lui, S. (2017). Family building using embryo adoption: Relationships and contact arrangements between provider and recipient families: A mixed methods study. *Human Reproduction*, 32, 1092–1099.

Gameiro, S. & Finnigan, A. (2017). Long term adjustment to unmet parenthood goals following ART: A systematic review and meta-analysis. *Human Reproduction Update*, 23, 1–16.

Golombok, S., Perry, S., Burston, B., Murray, A., Mooney-Sommers, C., Stevens, J., & Golding, M. (2003). Children with lesbian parents: A community study. *Developmental Psychology*, 39, 20–33.

Golombok, S., Tasker, F., & Murray, C. (1997). Children raised in fatherless families from infancy: Family relationships and the socioemotional development of children of lesbian and single heterosexual mothers. *Journal of Child Psychology and Psychiatry, 38,* 783–791.

Hämmerli, K., Znoj, H., & Barth, J. (2009). The efficacy of psychological interventions for infertile patients: A meta-analysis examining mental health and pregnancy rate. *Human Reproduction Update, 15,* 279–295.

Hawkey, A., Ussher, J. M., & Perz, J. (2018). "If you don't have a baby, you can't be in our culture": Migrant and refugee women's experiences and constructions of fertility and fertility control. *Women's Reproductive Health, 5,* 75–78.

Hembree, W. C., Cohen-Kettenis, P., Determarre-van de Waal, H., Gooren, L. J., Meyer, W. J., Spack, N. P., Tangpricha, V., & Montori, V. M. (2009). Endocrine treatment of transsexual persons: An Endocrine Society clinical practice guideline. *Journal of Clinical Endocrinology and Metabolism, 94,* 3132–3154.

Hendriks, S., Peeraer, K., Bos, H., Repping, S., & Dancet, E. (2017). The importance of genetic parenthood for infertile men and women. *Human Reproduction, 39,* 2076–2087.

Homan, G., Davies, M., & Norman, R. (2007). The impact of lifestyle factors on reproductive performance in the general population and those undergoing infertility treatment: A review. *Human Reproduction Update, 13,* 209–223.

Hughes, E. & Giacomini, G. (2001). Funding in vitro fertilization treatment for persistent subfertility: The pain and the politics. *Fertility and Sterility, 76,* 431–442.

Human Fertilisation and Embryology Authority (2016). *Fertility treatment in 2014: Trends and figures.* London, UK: Author. Retrieved from www.hfea.gov.uk/docs/HFEA_Fertility_treatment_Trends_and_figures_2014.pdf, accessed 25 October 2017.

Human Fertilisation and Embryology Authority (2017, October). *Code of practice. 33. Mitochondrial donation (version 3.0).* London, UK: Author. Retrieved from www.hfea.gov.uk/code-of-practice/33#section-header, accessed 22 January 2018.

Inhorn, M. (2003). Global infertility and the globalization of new reproductive technologies: Illustrations from Egypt. *Social Science & Medicine, 56,* 1837–1851.

International Federation of Fertility Societies (2016). Mt. Royal, NJ: Author. Retrieved from www.iffs-reproduction.org/events/EventDetails.aspx?id=361015.

Klitzman, R. (2017). How much is a child worth? Providers' and patients' views and responses concerning ethical and policy challenges in paying for ART. *PLoS One, 12*(2), e0171939.

Kupka, M., D'Hooghe, T., Ferraretti, A., de Mouzon, J., Erb, K., Castilla, J., Calhaz-Jorge, C., De Geyter, C., & Goosens, V. (2016). Assisted reproductive technology in Europe, 2011: Results generated from European registers by ESHRE. *Human Reproduction, 6,* 233–248.

Lampic, C., Svanberg, A., Karlström, P., & Tyden, T. (2006). Fertility awareness, intentions concerning childbearing, and attitudes towards parenthood among female and male academics. *Human Reproduction, 21,* 558–564.

Lee, S., Schover, L., Partridge, A., Patrizio, P., Wallace, W., Hagerty, K., Beck, L., Brennan, L., & Oktay, K. (2006). American Society of Clinical Oncology recommendations on fertility preservation in cancer patients. *Journal of Clinical Oncology, 24,* 2917–2931.

Logan, S., Perz, J., Ussher, J. M., Peate, M., & Anazodo, A. A. (2018). Systematic review of patient oncofertility support needs in reproductive cancer patients aged 14 to 45 years of age. *Psycho-oncology, 27,* 401–409, doi:10.1002/pon.4502.

Loren, A., Mangu, P., Beck, L., Brennan, L., Magdalinski, A., Partridge, A., Quinn, G., Wallace, W., & Oktay, K. (2013). Fertility preservation for patients with cancer: American Society of Clinical Oncology clinical practice guideline update. *Journal of Clinical Oncology, 31,* 2500–2510.

Mascarenhas, M., Flaxman, S., Boerma, T., Vanderpoel, S., & Stevens, G. (2012). National, regional and global trends in infertility prevalence since 1990: A systematic analysis of 277 health surveys. *PLoS Medicine, 9,* e1001356.

Mathews, T. & Hamilton, B. (2016). *Mean age of mothers is on the rise: United States, 2000–2014* [NCHS Data Brief]. Hyattsville, MD: National Center for Health Statistics. Retrieved from www.cdc.gov/nchs/data/databriefs/db232.htm.

Matthiesen, S., Frederiksen, Y., Ingerslev, H., & Zachariae, R. (2011). Stress, distress, and outcomes of assisted reproductive technology (ART): A meta-analysis. *Human Reproduction, 26,* 2763–2776.

Murphy, T. (2012). The ethics of fertility preservation in transgender body modifications. *Journal of Bioethical Inquiry, 9,* 311–316.

Parton, C., Ussher, J. M., & Perz, J. (2019). Hope, burden or risk: a discourse analytic study of the construction and experience of fertility preservation in the context of cancer. *Psychology & Health*, *34*(4), 456–477.

Payne, N., Lewis, S., Constantinou, C., & van den Akker, O. (forthcoming). Experiences of combining work and fertility treatment: Personal meanings and conflicts. *Journal of Psychosomatic Obstetrics & Gynecology*, *40*(2), 1-10, DOI: 10.1080/0167482X.2018.1460351.

Payne, N., Seenan, S., & van den Akker, O. (2019). Experiences and psychological distress of fertility treatment and employment. *Journal of Psychosomatic Obstetrics & Gynecology*, *40*(2), 156–165, doi:10.1080/0167482X.2018.1460351.

Purewal, S., Chapman, S., & van den Akker, O. (2017). A systematic review and meta-analysis of psychological predictors of successful assisted reproductive technologies. *BMC Research Notes*, *10*, 711.

Purewal, S., Chapman, S., & van den Akker, O. (2018). Depression and state anxiety scores during assisted reproductive technologies (ART) treatment predict ART outcomes: A meta-analysis. *Reproductive BioMedicine Online*, *36*(6), 646–657, doi:10.1016/j.rbmo.2018.03.010.

Purewal, S. & van den Akker, O. (2009). 'I feel like they were mine and I should be looking after them': An exploration of non-patient women's attitudes towards oocyte donation. *Journal of Psychosomatic Obstetrics*, *30*, 215–222.

Riggs, D. & Due, C. (2017). *A critical approach to surrogacy: Reproductive desires and demands*. Abingdon, UK: Routledge.

Ross, L. & Epstein, D. (2006). Lesbian and bisexual women's recommendations for improving the provision of assisted reproductive technology services. *Fertility and Sterility*, *86*, 735–738.

Schmidt, L., Munster, K., & Helm, P. (1995). Infertility and the seeking of infertility treatment in a representative population. *British Journal of Obstetrics and Gynecology*, *102*, 978–984.

The New Daily (2017, November 26). Mother feeling 'robbed' of child after leftover embryos donated. Retrieved from https://thenewdaily.com.au/entertainment/tv/2017/11/26/embryo-donate-ivf-mother-fertility, accessed 26 September 2019.

(The United Nations Convention on the Rights of the Child UNCRC) (1989). *The United Nations Convention on the Rights of the Child*. London, UK: UNICEF. Retrieved from www.unicef.org.uk/Documents/Publication-dfs/UNCRC_PRESS200910web.pdf, accessed 1 December 2017.

Toscano, S. & Montgomery, R. (2009). The lived experience of women pregnant (including preconception) post in vitro fertilization through the lens of virtual communities. *Health Care for Women International*, *30*, 1014–1036.

Troude, P., Santin, G., Guibert, J., & de la Rochebrochard, E. (2016). Seven out of 10 couples treated by IVF achieve parenthood following either treatment, natural conception or adoption. *Reproductive Biomedicine Online*, *5*, 560–567.

Trounson, A., Leeton, J., Bescnko, M., Cood, C., & Conti, A. (1983). Pregnancy established in an infertile patient after transfer of a donated embryo fertilised in vitro. *British Medical Journal*, *286*, 835–838.

Ussher, J. M., Parton, C., & Perz, J. (2018). Need for information, honesty, and respect: Patient perspectives on health care professionals' communication about cancer and fertility. *Reproductive Health*, *15*, 2–16.

Ussher, J. M., Perz, J., & The Australian Cancer and Fertility Study Team (ACFST) (2018). Threat of biographical disruption: The construction and experience of infertility following cancer for women and men. *BMC Cancer*, *18*, 250.

van den Akker, O. (2000). The importance of a genetic link in mothers commissioning a surrogate baby in the UK. *Human Reproduction*, *15*, 1849–1855.

van den Akker, O. (2005). A longitudinal pre pregnancy to post delivery comparison of genetic and gestational surrogate and intended mothers: Confidence and gyneology. *Journal of Psychosomatic Obstetrics and Gynecology*, *26*, 277–284.

van den Akker, O. (2007). Psychosocial aspects of surrogate motherhood. *Human Reproduction Update*, *13*(1), 53–62.

van den Akker, O. (2012). *Reproductive health psychology*. Oxford: Wiley-Blackwell.

van den Akker, O. (2016a). Reproductive health matters. *Psychologist*, *29*(1), 2–5.

van den Akker, O. (2017a). *Surrogate motherhood families*. Cham, Switzerland: Palgrave Macmillan.

van den Akker, O., Camara, I., & Hunt, B. (2016b). 'Together ... for only a moment': British media construction of altruistic non-commercial surrogate motherhood. *Journal of Reproductive and Infant Psychology*, *34*, 271–281.

van den Akker, O., Crawshaw, M., Blyth, E., & Frith, L. (2015). Expectations and experiences of gamete donors and donor-conceived adults searching for genetic relatives using DNA linking through a voluntary register. *Human Reproduction*, *30*(1), 111–121.

van den Akker, O., Fronek, P., Blyth, E., & Frith, L. (2016c). 'This neo-natal ménage à trois': British media framing of transnational surrogacy. *Journal of Reproductive and Infant Psychology*, *34*, 15–27.

van den Akker, O., Payne, N., & Lewis, S. (2017b). Catch-22? Disclosing assisted reproductive technology treatment in the workplace. *International Journal of Workplace Health Management*, *10*, 364–375.

Walker, S. (2017). *The experience of combining fertility treatment and paid employment: Women's narratives*. Project submitted to the University of Auckland, New Zealand. Retrieved from http://aut.researchgateway.ac.nz/bitstream/handle/10292/4788/WalkerS.pdf?sequence=3, accessed 17 November 2017.

Wallace, S., Blough, K., & Kondapalli, L. (2014). Fertility preservation in the transgender patient: Expanding oncofertility care beyond cancer. *Journal of Gynecological Endocrinology*, *30*, 868–871.

Wellcome Trust (2018). *Mitochondrial donation*. London, UK: Author. Retrieved from https://wellcome.ac.uk/what-we-do/our-work/mitochondrial-donation, accessed 22 January 2018.

World Professional Association for Transgender Health (WPATH) (2011). *Standards of care for the health of transsexual, transgender, and gender nonconforming people*, 7th version. Retrieved from https://wpath.org/publications/soc, accessed 17 November 2017.

Yager, C., Brennan, D., Steele, L., Epstein, R., & Ross, L. (2010). Challenges and mental health experiences of lesbian and bisexual women who are trying to conceive. *Health & Social Work*, *35*, 191–200.

Ying, L., Har Wu, L., & Loke, A. Y. (2016). Gender differences in emotional reactions to in vitro fertilization treatment: A systematic review. *Journal of Assisted Reproductive Genetics*, *33*, 167–179.

PART IV

Pregnancy and childbirth

16

'ADOLESCENT PREGNANCY'[1]

Social problem, public health concern, or neither?

Catriona Ida Macleod and Tracey Feltham-King

There are a number of 'hot' reproductive health issues that invoke significant public interest. These issues feature prominently in policy documents, public health resources are designated to address them, and politicians are called to account for progress made. Amongst the obvious candidates for 'hot' issues (e.g., maternal mortality, abortion) stands, surprisingly for some, adolescent pregnancy. Pregnancy amongst young women evokes a range of responses from the public, school and health authorities, teachers and health service providers, and policy makers. These responses vary from outright hostility, moral outrage, and exclusion through to support and understanding. In the midst of these responses, a few, isolated, voices claim that the notion of 'adolescent pregnancy' is a historical artifact and a social construction that is used to regulate young women's sexuality, especially marginalized young women. These scholars and activists argue that both a moralistic and a (so-called) neutral public health response are complicit in normalizing particular gendered power relations.

Adolescent pregnancy rates have been found to be highly variable, as indicated in a review of 59 countries (Sedgh, Finer, Bankole, Eilers, & Singh, 2015). In that study, based on country data, the highest rate of pregnancies per 1,000 15–19-year-old women was 187 (Burkina Faso) and the lowest 8 (Switzerland). The percentage of these pregnancies that ended in abortion varies greatly as well. The highest is 67% in Denmark and the lowest is 4% in Albania. In the 16 countries in which data were available, the study showed that adolescent pregnancy rates have declined since the mid-1990s. These statistics alert us to the social and historical location of reproductive issues, as the common age of first pregnancy and the resolution of these pregnancies is vastly uneven across geographical and historical spaces.

In this chapter we outline three major approaches to adolescent pregnancy. The first is the 'social problem' approach, in which adolescent pregnancy is viewed as, for the most part, deleterious for the young woman, her offspring, and society. This position fuels public outrage when the numbers of pregnant adolescents (especially when they are school pupils) are revealed in newspapers. The second is a public health response, which is well established and which has much institutional kudos. Here the neutral language of population-wide health is used to underpin preventive efforts in relation to adolescent pregnancy. In the third approach, authors point to the problems underlying both of these positions, arguing that arbitrarily separating younger pregnant women from older pregnant women is premised on particular power relations.

Adolescent pregnancy as a 'social problem'

Although the rates of adolescent pregnancy have decreased in many countries, expert and social attention to the 'problem' has not (Wilson & Huntington, 2005). Media coverage inevitably constructs early reproduction as leading to social disintegration, personal tragedy, or both (Jaworski, 2009). In parallel, extensive research on the outcomes of adolescent pregnancy has been conducted. These outcomes, which are almost always cast in negative terms, cohere around two major themes: harm to self and child, and social disintegration. The emphasis on particular problems may differ across countries and contexts. Bonell (2004), for example, showed how health is the major issue in UK research, whereas in the USA adolescent pregnancy is viewed as problematic because of the associated welfare expenditure and intergenerational transmission of poverty. In general, however, a host of problems are associated with adolescent pregnancy.

Reports of harm to self (i.e., the young woman) include negative pregnancy and birth outcomes, educational disadvantage, poor socio-economic outcomes, and sub-optimal parenting practices. Harm to child is reported to include poor health and educational outcomes and negative psychological consequences. Social disintegration concerns refer to the perpetuation of poverty, contribution to over-population, and reliance on welfare (Macleod & Tracey, 2010). Each of these factors has been thoroughly researched in various contexts, and many studies have pointed to negative personal and social consequences.

Increasingly, however, there are points of contestation concerning the easy association of early reproduction with negative outcomes. Take, for example, the reported health and obstetric outcomes. On the one hand, Jeha, Usta, Ghulmiyyah, and Nassar's (2015) research showed increased risk of maternal anemia, infections, eclampsia and preeclampsia, emergency caesarean section, postpartum depression, premature birth, and low birth weight. Gupta, Kiran and Bhal (2008), on the other hand, found no significant perinatal outcomes between younger and older women, despite the higher incidence of preterm labour amongst the younger women.

In a World Health Organization multi-country study (of 29 countries), it was found that, compared with mothers 20–24 years old, those in the 10–19 year age bracket experienced a number of adverse pregnancy outcomes (Ganchimeg et al., 2014). However, as noted by the authors of this and other reviews, there is the possibility that the differences between pregnancy outcomes for older and younger women are due to confounding variables, such as the adequacy of antenatal care, marital status, maternal health behaviours (e.g., smoking), and socio-economic status (Chen et al., 2007). Amongst these factors, socio-economic status emerges as the major confounding variable, as some authors claim that it is not age *per se* that creates heightened risk for young pregnant women, but rather differences in socio-economic status (Macleod, 2011).

In addition, researchers have argued that categorizing the obstetric outcomes of pregnancies amongst those less than 15 years old with those older than 15 is misleading. Malabarey, Balayla, Klam, Shrim and Abenhaim (2012), in a population-based study of millions of births in the United States, found significant differences between births to 10–14 year-old and 15–19 year-old mothers. The former were less likely to have had adequate prenatal care and more likely not to have had any prenatal care. Intrauterine growth restriction was more common among the younger adolescents, as were premature births, stillbirths, and infant deaths. These contestations point to the difficulties attendant upon the overarching category of 'adolescent pregnancy' without the requisite attention being paid to social, socio-economic, healthcare, and educational contexts and to differences between very young and older teenagers.

Many researchers, in outlining the negative outcomes of early reproduction, use the results to advocate for better services for young people. The logic here is that if researchers can indicate that early reproduction leads to disadvantage, then it is contingent upon governments and healthcare practitioners to provide additional support to overcome these disadvantages. While this is a laudable goal, Shaw, Lawlor and Najman (2006) argued that nuance is needed in understanding the consequences of early reproduction. Their research showed that 'not *all* teenage mothers and their offspring have adverse outcomes, and that many if not the majority have good outcomes' (p. 2527). Indeed, many authors have argued that for certain young women early reproduction is a rational and advantageous choice within their socio-political circumstances (see later discussion).

In addition, as Smithbattle (2007) pointed out, race and social class are implicated in the long-term challenges that pregnant and mothering young women may face. The nuance suggested by these authors implies understanding the consequences of early reproduction from an intersectional perspective in which the determinants of ill-health are seen as socially located and as mutually reinforcing one another (Hankivsky & Christoffersen, 2008).

This kind of nuance – viewing adolescent pregnancy intersectionally and as something that varies from negative through to positive – clearly has implications in terms of how service providers approach young people's sexual and reproductive health. Without the automatic assumption that early reproduction leads to negative health, education, and parenting outcomes, and with an understanding of the complex and interweaving determinants of negative outcomes where they do occur, services can be adjusted to the particular social circumstances within which young women are located.

These arguments concerning the outcomes of early reproduction highlight the political nature of research on the outcomes of adolescent pregnancy. Indeed, as indicated by Macvarish (2010, p. 313), teenage parenthood has 'been amplified as a social problem' in contrast to the 'de-moralizing' (lessening of moral sanction) that has taken place, in many contexts, with regard to sex outside the confines of marriage. This amplification has potential social and political effects, in particular the creation of moral outrage, stigma, and stereotyping, which have material effects in the young women's lives (e.g., in terms of access to healthcare, employment, schooling). When these effects are paired with strict regulation of young women's sexuality as occurs in some communities (see, for example, Hawkey et al., 2018), a double stigmatization occurs.

In relation to this, Barcelos (2014, p. 486) posed the question: '[I]s it possible that the stigmatization and regulation of young women's reproduction reinforces and reproduces existing health and social inequalities?' In other words, are possible negative outcomes at least partially to do with the manner in which young women are perceived and interacted with when pregnant? A positive answer to the latter question was provided by the Birth to Twenty study conducted in South Africa. Richter, Norris, and Ginsburg (2006, p. 122) reported that 'young women, the fathers (18–22 years old), and their parents are locked into a silence of fear and shame preventing them from providing mutual support and from accessing available services'.

What is important to note is that the shame and silence attendant upon early reproduction is not static. Previously, in many countries, it was the marital status of the young women that was stigmatized. Unmarried, pregnant young women were 'morally' excluded from society, often being sent to homes for unmarried mothers, giving birth in secret, and putting the child up for adoption. However, with the rise of feminism and the increasing availability of contraception and abortion in many contexts, the moral taint of 'unwed mother' and 'illegitimate child' has waned. Instead, young women are judged by different standards – physical and social maturity, ability to mother, levels of poverty, contribution to society. These standards are, at least on the surface of it, not morally loaded, but nevertheless cast young women as irresponsible, immature, incapable, and contributing to continued cycles of poverty (Koffman, 2011).

Adolescent pregnancy as a public health concern

Public health is a discipline and practice premised on understanding population-wide health and illness trends and on the institution of prevention programs to improve health amongst the particular population under examination. Prevention generally takes the form of primary prevention (preventing the illness/health problem in the first place), secondary prevention (ensuring early diagnosis and treatment of an illness/health problem where it does occur), and tertiary prevention (preventing additional illnesses or disabling conditions associated with the illness/health problem).

Epidemiologically, rates of adolescent pregnancy may be measured according to the percentage of pregnancies amongst women below the age of 20 (usually 15–19 year olds), or as the number of pregnancies per 1,000 young women in a particular population. The latter is the most commonly used method. As indicated above, rates vary considerably both geographically and historically.

Within a public health approach, the focus of primary prevention of adolescent pregnancy consists of reducing the number of young women who conceive. In general, preventive efforts entail a form of sexuality education, delivered either within schools or through out-of-school programs. Given the nature of its content, however, sexuality education is highly disputed. One of the major rifts is whether it should promote abstinence only or should introduce wider discussion of risk-reducing strategies, including the use of contraception and of barrier methods to prevent HIV and STIs. In reviews of studies of the effectiveness of these two broad approaches, Chin et al. (2012) and the Preventive Community Services Task Force (2012) found that there was clear evidence that group-based comprehensive sexuality education reduces the risk of pregnancy, HIV, and STIs, but no conclusions can be drawn about the effectiveness of abstinence-only programs (given the methodological flaws of the studies and the varied results). Indeed, the decline in adolescent pregnancies in the United States has been shown to be related to increased contraceptive uptake and usage amongst teenagers rather than due to delayed sexual debut or reduced sexual activity (Boonstra, 2014).

In addition to sexuality education, peer counseling or peer education programs have been instituted in a number of countries. These programs are premised on the idea that young people are more likely to talk about sex and sexuality with their peers than with older people. Therefore, training is provided to a cohort of young women and men to enable them to conduct lay counseling or education programs with their peers. Despite the sound logic behind the programs, and the successes reported by some programs, Tolli (2012), in a review of programs conducted in Europe, concluded that, overall, there is no evidence that peer education significantly reduces the risk of pregnancy (or HIV and STIs).

Researchers have increasingly indicated that concentrating on the behavioural aspects of pregnancy prevention in sexuality education is insufficient. Instead they have argued for a concentration on the interactional space within which conception takes place rather than on the behaviours of young women (Rosen, 2004). For example, in South Africa, research shows that young women struggle to negotiate condom usage in age-disparate relationships, especially those that are transactional in nature (the classic 'sugar daddy' scenario) (Toska, Cluver, Boyes, Pantelic, & Kuo, 2015). In countries where child marriage is common (even if not legal), researchers have argued that interventions should be premised on an understanding of how transitions to adulthood, in the form of marriage, childbirth, and school leaving, are viewed and negotiated (Psaki, 2016). These findings point to the need to address systemic and social issues and for interventions to be informed by intersectional understandings of contextual power relations.

This is not to say that all systemic preventive programs have been met with enthusiasm. A controversial approach has been to provide young women, especially in global South countries, with incentives to stay in school on the basis that pregnancy often follows school dropout (Phillips & Mbizvo, 2016). There is injustice attendant upon incentivizing 'beating the odds' in the context of poor socio-economic circumstances, collapsing educational institutions, and limited income-generation opportunities. Avoiding rape, sexual violence, and coercion are no longer simply the responsibility assigned to young women, but are also turned into a competition where those fortunate enough to escape unscathed are rewarded.

Secondary prevention involves ensuring that young women who do become pregnant attend antenatal care early and regularly. This has been noted as a challenge, particularly when these young women are: unaware that they are pregnant; hiding their pregnancies as a result of stigma or fear of being excluded from schooling; or unsuccessfully attempting to seek a termination of pregnancy. Researchers have suggested that outreach programs should assist with early detection and care (Fleming, Tu, & Black, 2012), which would include encouraging autonomous decision-making regarding the outcome of a pregnancy.

Tertiary prevention implies providing care that is suitable to young pregnant women and that ensures the best outcomes for the pregnancy. Obviously, the quality of antenatal care in a country is key to this endeavor. Even within well-functioning clinics, however, healthcare workers may act as a barrier to care by 'failing to provide young people with supportive, nonjudgmental, youth-appropriate services' (Morris & Rushwan, 2015, p. S40). Nevertheless, guidelines specific to adolescent pregnancies have been developed in various countries (Fleming et al., 2015; Magness, 2012). Some alternative models of antenatal care, such as the Centering Pregnancy Prenatal Care (CPPC) model that provides risk assessment, health promotion, and support within a group setting (rather than the individual examination room), have been shown to be successful with young women (Trotman et al., 2015).

A key element in the public health model is an analysis of the costs and benefits of interventions, especially in the use of public funds. An example of this was provided by Eloundou-Enyegue and Stokes (2004). Noting the argument that early reproduction disrupts schooling and therefore contributes to gender inequity in schooling, these authors posed the following question: '[Would] policy efforts to reduce unintended pregnancy among teens … pay off in terms of narrowing national gender gaps in education?' (p. 305). Acknowledging that the association may well be the result of the socioeconomic disadvantage of poorer teenagers, rather than pregnancy *per se*, the authors answered their cost-benefit analysis with a tentative 'yes and no': Investing in adolescent fertility programs may have benefits in some countries, they suggested, but not in others.

Ironically, much of the investment in public health programs appears not to have paid off. For example, Hanson, Myers, and Ginsburg (2011), in their study of 10,000 young women in the sophomore cohort of a nationally representative High School and Beyond

Survey in the US, showed that exposure to sexuality education courses and knowledge of birth control had no effect on the chances that they would experience pregnancy as a teenager. What *was* significantly associated with avoiding early reproduction was the young women and their parents holding values that stress responsibility.

Alternative views

Given the contestations noted with regard to the first two approaches to early reproduction, it is not surprising that a number of alternative views have emerged. The first concentrates on the historical contingency of the notion of 'adolescent pregnancy'. Arney and Bergman (1984) first alluded to this when they showed how, during the 1960s in the United States, the morally loaded terms 'illegitimate child' and 'unwed mother' were collapsed into the (supposedly) scientifically neutral term 'teenage pregnancy'. This shift allowed for the deployment of scientific inquiry and surveillance concerning young women's bodies. Although part of a general movement to 'risk surveillance' regarding pregnancy, in which medical and social norms are inculcated in women's lives through healthcare interactions and media depictions, the shift to 'teenage pregnancy' foregrounded age specifically and allowed for the deployment of developmental psychology inquiry into the competence of young women to carry a pregnancy and parent a child.

More recently, Koffman (2011) demonstrated how, in the United Kingdom, a moral-Christian discourse initially held sway, in which a woman's character – and not her age or maturity – was of central concern. This shifted to a psychological discourse, in which the immaturity of teenagers and hence their inability to parent, was foregrounded. As noted by Koffman (2011), while a moral-Christian discourse is punitive, it still allows for the possibility of change: The 'fallen' woman may repent and live according to the prescribed tenets of a moral life. However, '[b]eing a teenager is not a subjectivity that one could alter at will. No amount of responsible behavior would disprove the proposition that a young person is emotionally immature and therefore ill-equipped to parent' (Koffman, 2011, p. 11). As a result, pregnancy and parenting amongst young people are rendered inherently problematic.

Second, researchers have argued that, for many young women, pregnancy is not the disaster that it is often portrayed to be. These authors, sometimes called revisionists, have pointed to the positive experiences many young people have of parenting (Arai, 2009): 'the experience of pregnancy and parenting is transformative and may invoke a positive refocusing of life aspirations for educational and career attainment' (O'Brien Cherry, Chumbler, Bute, & Huff, 2015. p. 1). In addition, early reproduction may make rational sense in disadvantaged circumstances where women may experience foreshortened healthy life expectancy and very few opportunities in the job market. For such women, having children while they are younger and healthy is an advantage, especially in depressed economic circumstances. In addition, these women are more likely while they are young to have extended family support for childcare (Geronimus, 2003).

Third, scholars have pointed to the power relations underpinning understandings of and approaches to adolescent pregnancy. Researchers who use Foucauldian approaches have argued that the risk discourses emanating from the public health attempt at preventing adolescent pregnancy act to shape the bodies of young women (in particular): 'Constructions of risk produce young women in a subjective state that envisions their bodies in a position of "pre-pregnancy" that must be regulated (through abstinence and contraceptive use) and monitored (through expert authorities such as health professionals)' (Barcelos, 2014, p. 483).

Young women's bodies are therefore always already unruly, with restraint and self-control touted as the measures required to tame the body. Young women cannot, however, be left to their own devices in exercising such restraint: The intervention of experts is needed. Professional intervention must be continual and constant as the risk is ongoing: The 'pre-pregnant' body is constantly at risk of becoming the pregnant body (Macleod, 2011).

The pregnant teenage body is used in these prevention efforts to demonstrate the calamitous outcomes of the lack of restraint and self-control. Pictures of a heavily pregnant young woman, most often displayed from the side with swollen stomach highly visible, abound in media depictions and health promotion programs. Sad stories, confessions, and 'troubling' statistics concerning the extent of the problem tend to accompany these images. Young mothers are, in some cases, brought into classrooms to provide an experiential account of the dangers of sex (Chabot, Shoveller, Johnson, & Prkachin, 2010). As such, the pregnant teen-aged body is 'abject and irresponsible, a failure to rational public health and a threat to the neoliberal state, the normative family, and the discipline of public health' (Barcelos, 2014, p. 483).

Researchers have argued, thus, that public health attempts to reduce adolescent pregnancy are far from neutral. Through the various preventive campaigns discussed above, public health 'demarcates (in)appropriate reproductive bodies, consolidates heterosexual power, produces ever-expanding at-risk populations, and calls on individuals and populations to work on their bodies in very specific ways' (Barcelos, 2014, p. 486). Childhood and innocence are utilized as a means through which the 'good' heteronormative relationships are constituted and governed (Robinson, 2012). In addition to the underlying assumptions about ideal family forms, beliefs about social class, the expected life course, and responsibility for making decisions concerning sexuality and reproductive health are perpetuated (Bute & Russell, 2012).

Fourth, researchers have started to grapple with alternative interventions. As indicated in Macleod (2014, p. 130), 'feminists need to advocate for care and interventions that speak to and overcome gender dynamics that are oppressive to young women (and men) and that empower women in exercising their sexual and reproductive rights'. This includes attuning interventions to local specifics, the prevention of unwanted and unsupportable pregnancies (rather than simply 'adolescent pregnancies'), promoting access to non-discriminatory and legal termination of pregnancy services, and provision of non-discriminatory health and education services.

Given the negativity surrounding early reproduction, interventions with young women, their partners, and their families require overcoming the stigma and 'spoiled identities' attached to early reproduction (Bennett & Assefi, 2005; Shaw, 2011). This implies working with the discursive and social practices deployed by educators and health service providers. For example, Breheny and Stephens (2007) found that, in talking about early reproduction in New Zealand/Aotearoa, doctors, midwives, and nurses drew upon 'Developmental' and 'Motherhood' discourses to position young mothers as problematic. Young mothers were depicted as naive, distracted, self-centered, and unable to mother 'correctly'. These characteristics were seen as at odds with the attributes of 'good' mothers. These discourses were drawn upon to illustrate how 'adolescence' cannot be reconciled with 'good' mothering. These discursive practices therefore provide little room for positive healthcare engagement with young mothers. Similarly, in their research on pregnancy in South African schools, Shefer, Bhana, and Morrell (2013) found that moralistic discourses on adolescence, normative gender roles, and female sexuality were drawn on by teachers to depict pregnancy amongst school pupils as leading to social decay.

An important aspect of feminist advocacy in relation to early reproduction is overcoming the idea that schooling and pregnancy/parenting are incompatible (Lall, 2007; Pillow, 2006). For example, authors have noted the positive effects of the school-based Early Childhood Centers for Children of Teen Parents Program in the United States (Crean, Hightower, & Allan, 2001). While this kind of support is essential, support for young women not to return to school, to attend school on a part-time basis, or to return to school later is also important (Austerberry & Wiggins, 2007).

Finally, as many teenaged parents continue to reside with their extended families, it is important to acknowledge the impact on, and provide support to, the multi-generational family. In addition, despite negative social stereotypes of adolescent fathers, research increasingly suggests that most fathers desire involvement with their children (Beers & Hollo, 2009; Swartz & Bhana, 2009). The alternative approaches discussed in this section, although they differ in focus, have in common a vision of social or reproductive justice, to which we turn now.

Reproductive justice and adolescent pregnancy

Adolescent pregnancy is common. However, adolescents' experiences of pregnancy and birth vary greatly around the world. It has been estimated that, worldwide, approximately 20,000 adolescents give birth every day; 95% of these adolescent pregnancies occur in low- to middle-income countries around the globe (Williamson, 2013). In these countries, pregnant adolescents who are from minority groups, are impoverished, poorly educated, live in rural areas, or are otherwise marginalized are more likely to become pregnant than are wealthier, better educated, urban adolescents. In addition, these at-risk adolescents are more likely to have unmet needs for contraception, less likely to use contraception of their choice, more likely to undergo unsafe abortion, and more likely to be infected by HIV (Chandra-Mouli, McCarraher, Phillips, Williamson, & Hainsworth, 2014).

In contexts (such as those described above) where multiple overlapping systemic and social failures are apparent, the continued focus on the behaviour of the individual pregnant adolescent functions as an injustice. This has fuelled calls for a shift from a public health approach to one in which reproductive rights and reproductive justice are foregrounded. The need for the shift is underpinned by evidence that young people's reproductive rights (e.g., access to contraception, non-discriminatory antenatal care, support during pregnancy and birth) have been undermined in many countries (Ganchimeg et al., 2014).

Reproductive justice advocates have argued, however, that while the promotion of reproductive rights is useful and necessary, it is insufficient to address the multiple oppressions experienced by young people. The reproductive justice framework goes further than the rights approach in that it highlights the continuation of reproductive inequities, gendered power relations, and the intersectionality of race, class, location, religion, ability, and sexual orientation in health outcomes, as well as deconstructs normative frameworks and taken-for-granted assumptions that underpin interventions (Macleod, 2017).

The reproductive justice approach has as its starting point the acknowledgement of the intertwining of the individual and the societal. The limitation of the 'social problem' approach to adolescent pregnancy is a very good illustration of this. Within that approach the social problem is limited to a very narrow focus on the individual adolescent, her 'problematic' pregnancy, and the assumed social degeneration that the pregnancy will induce. In this approach there is little acknowledgement of the pre-existing profoundly unresponsive and problematic context in which many pregnant young women experience their reproductive health. In these situations the amplification of adolescent pregnancy as a social problem can be read as an attempt to ignore the needs of the young woman herself and to deflect blame onto her for the dysfunctional context. Besides the fact that the approach to adolescent pregnancy as a 'social problem' is inaccurate (as discussed in the previous section), stigmatization exacerbates and reinforces existing health and social inequalities.

The concentration on individual behaviour change (which renders young women responsible for their own situations) is what critical scholars highlight as injustice. While the agency of young women needs to be acknowledged, these scholars have noted that pregnant adolescents are also located within particular intersecting power relations. These power relations are kept in place by normative assumptions constructed by classist, heteronormative, and gendered discourses and practices. These assumptions are deeply entrenched and construct not only understandings of pregnancy and motherhood but also adolescents' 'appropriate' aspirations and normative life trajectories (Macleod, 2011).

The potency of these discourses is evident in contexts where, despite the attainment of legislative sexual and reproductive rights for youth, reproductive injustice continues. This is clearly illustrated in post-Apartheid South Africa where rights have been prioritized in sexual and reproductive health policy in acknowledgement of the gross historical gendered injustices that occurred during Apartheid. However, despite improved access to schools and clinics and excellent progressive legislation and policy, educators and health service providers continue to operate in ways that exclude pregnant adolescents. The classist, heteronormative, and gendered discourses on which they draw in positioning young women as irresponsible patients and inadequate mothers are reinforced by the strictly hierarchical spaces in which healthcare and education are provided (Feltham-King, 2016; Shefer et al., 2013).

In contexts of scarcity, state institutions are frequently hard-pressed to deliver quality services to any citizens, not simply young people. In these locations, the burdens of service delivery are exacerbated by overcrowding and insufficient resources of all kinds (Müller, Röhrs, Hoffman-Wanderer, & Moult, 2016). Those expected to deliver services often resort to street-level bureaucracy, a process whereby health service providers develop their own, often authoritarian, day-to-day processes to manage and simplify their workloads and control untenable working conditions (Feltham-King, 2016). While young people experience the same injustices as older people in poorly functioning healthcare systems, they also, however, bear the burden of being viewed as personally responsible for any poor outcomes and for perpetuating social disintegration.

Within the complexity noted above, we argue for a focus on contextual healthcare inequities that fracture along multiple lines of differentiation and on what Macleod (2016) called the supportability of pregnancies. Macleod's (2016) supportability framework 'allows for an analysis of the intersection of individual cognitions, emotions, and behaviour with micro-level interactive spaces (e.g., partners, family, healthcare service providers) and macro-level issues (e.g., policy, cultural patterns)', where supportability is conceptualized as follows: the capacity of a woman to carry a pregnancy in such a way that she experiences positive health and welfare. "Supportability" is multifaceted, referring to the combination of a woman's physiological, emotional and cognitive capacities to carry a pregnancy, which are enabled or constrained through the micro-level and macro-level "support" that she receives.

In other words, 'supportability' is intricately interwoven with, and can never be separated from, 'support'. Attention is paid not only to the young woman and her personal needs or challenges, but also, and simultaneously, to the systemic, social, discursive, socio-economic, and healthcare context within which she experiences her pregnancy. An exclusive focus on the individual behaviour and cognitions of young people (e.g., whether they planned the pregnancy, whether they used contraception) is replaced with a broad-based focus on systemic issues, power relations, and social justice. The reality of inequities and multiple, fractured power relations that cohere around the supportability of young women's pregnancies must, we argue, be the starting point for establishing reproductive justice for pregnant adolescents.

Conclusions

In July 2017, the American Academy of Child & Adolescent Psychiatry posted the following on their web-page:

Children Having Children
No. 31; Updated July 2017

> Teenage pregnancy can be a crisis for the pregnant girl and her family. Common reactions include anger, guilt, and denial. If the father is young and involved, similar reactions can occur in his family. Babies born in the U.S. to teenage mothers are at risk for long-term problems in many major areas of life, including dropping out of school, health problems, incarceration, becoming teenage parents themselves, and underemployment. The teenage mothers themselves are also at risk for these problems.

This posting demonstrates how deep-seated the 'social problem' approach to adolescent pregnancy is. It is taken up in a range of spaces, including sites that draw on the legitimacy of psychiatric expertise. The 'social problem' approach complements the public health approach, particularly with regard to the ostensible negative health outcomes contingent upon early reproduction. Given the health problem status that is (almost automatically) ascribed to adolescent pregnancy, public health specialists are tasked with instituting primary, secondary, and tertiary preventive programs.

However, there are a number of contestations concerning the easy association of adolescent pregnancy with negative consequences. In particular, researchers have pointed to the multiple confounding factors that may well better account for observed negative outcomes, in particular disadvantaged socio-economic status and healthcare opportunities. A number of alternative approaches have arisen that highlight: the historical contingency and social construction of the signifier 'adolescent pregnancy'; the possibility that early reproduction is a rational choice and positive life trajectory; the gendered, class-based, racialised, and heteronormative power relations underpinning understandings of and interventions concerning adolescent pregnancy.

Researchers who take an alternative approach to the standard 'social problem' or public health approach have pointed out that, in eschewing these stances, they are not intimating that no support or interventions should be provided to young people. Instead, they advocate for interventions that recognise young people's reproductive rights, foster reproductive justice in overcoming the multiple and intertwining oppressive conditions that lead to health injustices, and foreground the supportability of the pregnancy as the key concern.

Acknowledgments

This work is based on research supported by the South African Research Chairs initiative of the Department of Science and Technology and National Research Foundation of South Africa (grant no. 87,582).

Notes

1 We have placed 'adolescent pregnancy' in scare quotes in the title of this chapter to highlight the historical contingency and social construction of the signifier (see Macleod, 2011, for more detail). For ease of reading, however, we do not continue this practice throughout the chapter. We refer to teenagers and adolescents interchangeably, noting, however, that neither of these terms is without problems, in particular the term 'adolescents' that has colonialist roots (Macleod, 2011).

References

Arai, L. (2009). What a difference a decade makes: Rethinking teenage pregnancy as a problem. *Social Policy and Society, 8*(2), 171.

Austerberry, H. & Wiggins, M. (2007). Taking a pro-choice perspective on promoting inclusion of teenage mothers: Lessons from an evaluation of the sure start plus programme. *Critical Public Health, 17*(1), 3–15. Retrieved from www.tandfonline.com/doi/pdf/10.1080/09581590601045246.

Barcelos, C. A. (2014). Producing (potentially) pregnant teen bodies: Biopower and adolescent pregnancy in the USA. *Critical Public Health, 24*(4), 476–488.

Beers, L. A. S. & Hollo, R. E. (2009). Approaching the adolescent-headed family: A review of teen parenting. *Current Problems in Pediatric and Adolescent Health Care, 39*(9), 216–233.

Bennett, S. E. & Assefi, N. P. (2005). School-based teenage pregnancy prevention programs: A systematic review of randomized controlled trials. *The Journal of Adolescent Health: Official Publication of the Society for Adolescent Medicine, 36*(1), 72–81.

Bonell, C. (2004). Why is teenage pregnancy conceptualized as a social problem? A review of quantitative research from the USA and UK. *Culture, Health & Sexuality, 6*(3), 255–272.

Boonstra, H. D. (2014). What is behind the declines in teen pregnancy rates? *Guttmacher Policy Review, 17*(3), 15–21. Retrieved from www.guttmacher.org/pubs/gpr/17/3/gpr170315.pdf.

Breheny, M. & Stephens, C. (2007). Irreconcilable differences: Health professionals' constructions of adolescence and motherhood. *Social Science & Medicine (1982), 64*(1), 112–124.

Bute, J. J. & Russell, L. D. (2012). Public discourses about teenage pregnancy: Disruption, restoration, and ideology. *Health Communication, 27*(7), 712–722.

Chabot, C., Shoveller, J. A., Johnson, J. L., & Prkachin, K. (2010). Morally problematic: Young mothers' lives as parables about the dangers of sex. *Sex Education, 10*(2), 201–215.

Chandra-Mouli, V., McCarraher, D. R., Phillips, S. J., Williamson, N. E., & Hainsworth, G. (2014). Contraception for adolescents in low and middle income countries: Needs, barriers, and access. *Reproductive Health, 11*(1), 1.

Chen, X.-K., Wen, S. W., Fleming, N., Demissie, K., Rhoads, G. G., & Walker, M. (2007). Teenage pregnancy and adverse birth outcomes: A large population based retrospective cohort study. *International Journal of Epidemiology, 36*(2), 368–373.

Chin, H. B., Sipe, T. A., Elder, R., Mercer, S. L., Chattopadhyay, S. K., Jacob, V., Wethington, H. R., Kirby, D., Elliston, D. B., Griffith, M., Chuke, S. O., Briss, S. C., Ericksen, I., Galbraith, J. S., Herbst, J. H., Johnson, R. L., Kraft, J. M., Noar, S. M., Romero, L. M., Santelli, J. & Community Preventive Services Task Force (2012). The effectiveness of group-based comprehensive risk-reduction and abstinence education interventions to prevent or reduce the risk of adolescent pregnancy, human immunodeficiency virus, and sexually transmitted infections: Two systematic reviews for the Guide to Community Preventive Services. *American Journal of Preventive Medicine, 42*(3), 272–294.

Crean, H. F., Hightower, A. D., & Allan, M. J. (2001). School-based child care for children of teen parents: Evaluation of an urban program designed to keep young mothers in school. *Evaluation and Program Planning, 24*(3), 267–275.

Eloundou-Enyegue, P. M. & Stokes, C. S. (2004). Teen fertility and gender inequality in education. *Demographic Research, 11*(11), 305–334.

Feltham-King, T. (2016). Risk and responsibility: The management of the teenaged pregnant women within the antenatal healthcare nexus. *Unpublished doctoral dissertation*, Rhodes University, Grahamstown, South Africa.

Fleming, N., O'Driscoll, T., Becker, G., Spitzer, R. F., & CANPAGO COMMITTEE (2015). Adolescent pregnancy guidelines. *Journal of Obstetrics and Gynaecology Canada, 37*(8), 740–756.

Fleming, N. A., Tu, X., & Black, A. Y. (2012). Improved obstetrical outcomes for adolescents in a community-based outreach program: A matched cohort study. *Journal of Obstetrics and Gynaecology Canada, 34*(12), 1134–1140.

Ganchimeg, T., Ota, E., Morisaki, N., Laopaiboon, M., Lumbiganon, P., & Zhang, J.; WHO Multi-country Survey on Maternal Newborn Health Research Network (2014). Pregnancy and childbirth outcomes among adolescent mothers: A World Health Organization multicountry study. *BJOG: An International Journal of Obstetrics and Gynaecology, 121*(Suppl), 40–48.

Geronimus, A. T. (2003). Damned if you do: Culture, identity, privilege, and teenage childbearing in the United States. *Social Science & Medicine, 57*(5), 881–893.

Gupta, N., Kiran, U., & Bhal, K. (2008). Teenage pregnancies: Obstetric characteristics and outcome. *European Journal of Obstetrics, Gynecology, and Reproductive Biology, 137*(2), 165–171.

Hankivsky, O. & Christoffersen, A. (2008). Intersectionality and the determinants of health: A Canadian perspective. *Critical Public Health, 18*(3), 271–283.

Hanson, S. L., Myers, D. E., & Ginsburg, A. L. (2011). The role of responsibility and knowledge in reducing teenage out-of-wedlock childbearing. *Journal of Marriage and the Family, 49*(2), 241–256.

Hawkey, A. J., Ussher, J. M., & Perz, J. (2018). Regulation and resistance: Negotiation of premarital sexuality in the context of migrant and refugee women. *The Journal of Sex Research, 55*(9), 1116–1133, doi:10.1080/00224499.2017.1336745.

Jaworski, B. K. (2009). Reproductive justice and media framing: A case-study analysis of problematic frames in the popular media. *Sex Education, 9*(1), 105–121.

Jeha, D., Usta, I., Ghulmiyyah, L., & Nassar, A. (2015). A review of the risks and consequences of adolescent pregnancy. *Journal of Neonatal-Perinatal Medicine, 8*(1), 1–8.

Koffman, O. (2011). Children having children? Religion, psychology and the birth of the teenage pregnancy problem. *History of the Human Sciences, 25*(1), 119–134.

Lall, M. (2007). Exclusion from school: Teenage pregnancy and the denial of education. *Sex Education, 7*(3), 219–237.

Macleod, C. (2011). *'Adolescence,' pregnancy, and abortion: Constructing a threat of degeneration.* Abingdon, UK: Routledge.

Macleod, C. (2014). 'Adolescent pregnancy': A feminist issue. In A. L. Cherry & M. E. Dillon (Eds), *International handbook of adolescent pregnancy: Medical, psychosocial, and public health responses* (pp. 129–145). New York, NY: Springer.

Macleod, C. I. (2016). Public reproductive health and "unintended" pregnancies: Introducing the construct "supportability". *Journal of Public Health (United Kingdom), 38*(3), e384–e391.

Macleod, C. I. (2017). "Adolescent" sexual and reproductive health: Controversies, rights, and justice. In A. L. Cherry, L. Baltag, & M. E. Dillon (Eds), *An international handbook on adolescent health and development: The public health response* (pp. 169–181). New York, NY: Springer.

Macleod, C. I. & Tracey, T. (2010). A decade later: Follow-up review of South African research on the consequences of and contributory factors in teen-aged pregnancy. *South African Journal of Psychology, 40*(1), 18–31.

Macvarish, J. (2010). The effect of "risk-thinking" on the contemporary construction of teenage motherhood. *Health, Risk & Society, 12*(4), 313–322.

Magness, J. (2012). Adolescent pregnancy: The role of the healthcare provider. *International Journal of Childbirth Education, 27*(4), 61–64. Retrieved from http://search.ebscohost.com/login.aspx?direct=true&db=cin20&AN=2011705071&site=ehost-live.

Malabarey, O. T., Balayla, J., Klam, S. L., Shrim, A., & Abenhaim, H. A. (2012). Pregnancies in young adolescent mothers: A population-based study on 37 million births. *Journal of Pediatric and Adolescent Gynecology, 25*(2), 98–102.

Morris, J. L. & Rushwan, H. (2015). Adolescent sexual and reproductive health: The global challenges. *International Journal of Gynecology & Obstetrics, 131*(S1), S40–S42.

Müller, A., Röhrs, S., Hoffman-Wanderer, Y., & Moult, K. (2016). "You have to make a judgment call". Morals, judgments and the provision of quality sexual and reproductive health services for adolescents in South Africa. *Social Science and Medicine, 148*, 71–78.

O'Brien Cherry, C., Chumbler, N., Bute, J., & Huff, A. (2015). Building a "better life". *SAGE Open, 5*(1), 215824401557163.

Phillips, S. J. & Mbizvo, M. T. (2016). Empowering adolescent girls in Sub-Saharan Africa to prevent unintended pregnancy and HIV: A critical research gap. *International Journal of Gynecology & Obstetrics, 132*(1), 1–3.

Pillow, W. (2006). Teen pregnancy and education: Politics of knowledge, research, and practice. *Educational Policy*, *20*(1), 59–84.

Preventive Community Services Task Force (2012). Recommendations for group-based behavioral interventions to prevent adolescent pregnancy, human immunodeficiency virus, and other sexually transmitted infections. *American Journal of Preventive Medicine*, *42*(3), 304–307.

Psaki, S. (2016). Addressing child marriage and adolescent pregnancy as barriers to gender parity and equality in education. *PROSPECTS*, *46*(1), 109–129.

Richter, L. M., Norris, S. A., & Ginsburg, C. (2006). The silent truth of teenage pregnancies – Birth to Twenty cohort's next generation. *Scientific Letters*, *96*(2), 13–14.

Robinson, K. H. (2012). "Difficult citizenship": The precarious relationships between childhood, sexuality and access to knowledge. *Sexualities*, *15*(3–4), 257–276.

Rosen, D. (2004). "I just let him have his way": Partner violence in the lives of low-income, teenage mothers. *Violence Against Women*, *10*(1), 6–28.

Sedgh, G., Finer, L. B., Bankole, A., Eilers, M. A., & Singh, S. (2015). Adolescent pregnancy, birth, and abortion rates across countries: Levels and recent trends. *Journal of Adolescent Health*, *56*(2), 223–230.

Shaw, M., Lawlor, D. A., & Najman, J. M. (2006). Teenage children of teenage mothers: Psychological, behavioural and health outcomes from an Australian prospective longitudinal study. *Social Science & Medicine (1982)*, *62*, 2526–2539.

Shaw, R. L. (2011). Women's experiential journey toward voluntary childlessness: An interpretative phenomenological analysis. *Journal of Community & Applied Social Psychology*, *21*(2), 151–163.

Shefer, T., Bhana, D., & Morrell, R. (2013). Teenage pregnancy and parenting at school in contemporary South African contexts: Deconstructing school narratives and understanding policy implementation. *Perspectives in Education*, *31*, 1–10.

Smithbattle, L. (2007). Legacies of advantage and disadvantage: The case of teen mothers. *Public Health Nursing*, *24*(5), 409–420.

Swartz, S. & Bhana, A. (2009). *Teenage tata: Voices of young fathers in South Africa*. Cape Town, South Africa: HSRC Press.

Tolli, M. V. (2012). Effectiveness of peer education interventions for HIV prevention, adolescent pregnancy prevention and sexual health promotion for young people: A systematic review of European studies. *Health Education Research*, *27*(5), 904–913.

Toska, E., Cluver, L. D., Boyes, M., Pantelic, M., & Kuo, C. (2015). From "sugar daddies" to "sugar babies": Exploring a pathway among age-disparate sexual relationships, condom use and adolescent pregnancy in South Africa. *Sexual Health*, *12*(1), 59.

Trotman, G., Chhatre, G., Darolia, R., Tefera, E., Damle, L., & Gomez-Lobo, V. (2015). The effect of centering pregnancy versus traditional prenatal care models on improved adolescent health behaviors in the perinatal period. *Journal of Pediatric and Adolescent Gynecology*, *28*(5), 395–401.

Williamson, N. (2013). *Motherhood in childhood: Facing the challenge of adolescent pregnancy*. New York, NY: UN Population Fund.

Wilson, H. & Huntington, A. (2005). Deviant (M)others: The construction of teenage motherhood in contemporary discourse. *Journal of Social Policy*, *35*(1), 59.

17

SMOKING AND PREGNANCY

Risk factors, women's experiences and interventions

Michael Ussher, Felix Naughton, Caitlin Notley and Linda Bauld

Maternal smoking is the main preventable cause of morbidity and death among pregnant women and their infants in high-income countries; this includes stillbirth, miscarriage, foetal growth restriction, prematurity, low birth weight, and perinatal mortality and morbidity (Källén, 2001; Rogers, 2009; Salihu & Wilson, 2007). There are also risks of long-term effects on infants, such as psychiatric adjustment (Fergusson, Woodward, & Horwood, 1998), attention deficit disorder (Thapar et al., 2003), and cancers (Schwartzbaum, George, Pratt, & Davis, 1991). Moreover, maternal smoking during pregnancy is associated with an increased risk of offspring smoking later in life (Roberts et al., 2005), thereby contributing to the continuation of smoking across generations.

Smoking in pregnancy is also associated with substantial health care costs. For example, in the UK the annual smoking-attributable maternal and infant health-care costs are estimated at £20–£87.5 million (Godfrey, Pickett, Parrott, Mdege, & Eapen, 2010). Besides financial savings, stopping smoking during pregnancy is associated with enormous health benefits for the mother and child, including improved birth outcomes (Chamberlain et al., 2017).

The global prevalence of smoking during pregnancy is estimated to be 2%, with the European region having the highest prevalence at 8%, with a prevalence of more than 10% in 29 (17%) of 174 countries and more than 20% in 12 (7%) countries (Lange, Probst, Rehm, & Popova, 2018). The prevalence of smoking in pregnancy is decreasing in many high-income countries (Lange et al., 2018); however, rates are declining more slowly among women of lower socio-economic status (Graham, Hawkins, & Law, 2010). While in some low- and middle-income countries the prevalence is not declining (Bloch et al., 2008; Dias-Dame & Cesar, 2015; Silveira et al., 2016). Cigarette smoking is overrepresented among economically disadvantaged women (Higgins & Chilcoat, 2009); therefore reducing smoking can also reduce health inequalities such as infant mortality (Gray et al., 2009). Besides social deprivation, failure to stop smoking in pregnancy is associated with lower level of education, not living with a partner/not married, members of the household who smoke, higher cigarette dependence, drinking alcohol, higher parity, not planning to breast-feed, depression, and stress (Riaz, Lewis, Naughton, & Ussher, 2018). Overall, this review by Riaz and colleagues indicates the importance of social factors in smoking cessation during pregnancy, and the potential intersection of different aspects of identity in women's experience of smoking (Triandafilidis, Ussher, Perz, & Hupputz, 2017). Moreover, another study reported that experts in the field consider smoking being a social norm, an acceptable behaviour in the women's close social network, to be the main barrier to smoking cessation during pregnancy (Campbell et al., 2018).

A higher proportion of women stop smoking during pregnancy than at other times in their lives; in high-income nations around one half of women smokers are likely to quit during pregnancy (Centers for Disease Control and Prevention, 2017). The majority of pregnant smokers who quit report doing so within a couple of days of becoming aware of their pregnancy, and many of these women quit without formal support (Heil et al., 2014). Unfortunately, around 40% of women who quit return to smoking within six months of childbirth (Jones, Lewis, Parrott, Wormall, & Coleman, 2016; Rockhill et al., 2016). Higher rates of return to smoking are found among women who are less educated, younger, multiparous, living with a partner or household member who smokes, overly stressed, depressed, anxious, not breastfeeding, intending to quit only for the duration of the pregnancy, and have low confidence that they can remain abstinent (Orton, Coleman, Coleman-Haynes, & Ussher, 2017).

In this chapter we review qualitative research on women's experience of smoking and cessation, both during pregnancy and postpartum. This research considers factors at the individual, interpersonal, and organisational level. We also consider the evidence for the effectiveness of interventions to aid smoking cessation during pregnancy with a focus on face-to-face behavioural support, financial incentives, self-help, pharmacotherapy, and population-level interventions.

Qualitative synthesis of factors that influence women's smoking and smoking cessation during pregnancy and postpartum

Qualitative studies, from a range of countries, of perceptions of smoking and of both barriers and facilitators of smoking cessation in pregnancy have been examined in two systematic reviews (Flemming, Graham, Heirs, Fox, & Sowden, 2013; Flemming, McCaughan, Angus, & Graham, 2015). The first review (Flemming et al., 2013) identified 27 papers published since 1990, and the second (Flemming et al., 2015), using the same searches, identified an additional 15 papers published by May 2013. These studies reported the experiences of 1,100+ women aged 15 to 49 years. Participants were pregnant or mothers with young babies who had smoked prior to pregnancy and went on either to quit or to continue smoking. In a further study, researchers interviewed 41 women in the UK who were pregnant or had recently been pregnant (Bauld et al., 2017).

Five broad themes were identified that are related to continued smoking, attempts to stop, and success of quit attempts. The themes are: psychological well-being; relationships with significant others; changing connections between the woman and infant; perceptions regarding the risks of smoking; and access to or use of support services to stop smoking. One approach to help understand these factors and how they operate at multiple levels is the social ecological framework (SEF) (Schneider & Stokols, 2009), which illustrates how factors that influence smoking and cessation operate at individual, interpersonal, and organisational levels. The papers in the two systematic reviews and the recent UK study provide data on women's experiences relevant to each level of the SEF.

Individual factors in smoking during pregnancy

(It) relieves stress psychologically at least. I have cut down, but I can't stop.
I smoke about 20 a day or maybe more, depending on my day or night.
(Hotham, Atkinson, & Gilbert, 2002, as cited in Flemming et al., 2015, p. 8)

Key among the individual factors is women's experience of disadvantage and its influence on smoking uptake and continued smoking. In developed countries especially, most women who continue to smoke in pregnancy are less affluent, as the challenges of limited resources can act as a barrier to cessation. Such women tend to express a lack of belief in their ability to stop smoking and a perception that smoking relieves stress, as illustrated above. Pregnant women often appear to be aware of some of the harms of smoking. Uncertainty about risks, or not accepting advice or information provided about risks, can contribute to continued smoking.

Interpersonal factors in pregnancy

> I found that I was judged as a disgusting, uneducated, gutter rat. I found this by the way people would look, question my motives, make comments on my parental ability, etc.
>
> *(Wigginton & Lee, 2013, as cited in Flemming et al., 2015, p. 9)*

Women's beliefs about smoking in pregnancy are influenced by close relationships with family and friends. Risk messages from social networks are often more accepted or understood than those delivered by health professionals such as midwives or doctors. However, in some studies, family and friends can serve as supporters for smoking cessation by offering advice and encouragement and adding to the woman's motivation to stop smoking. In a few studies, workplaces that do not permit smoking, or support from colleagues to quit, may also be important. Stigma surrounding smoking, as evidenced in the extract above, and women's attempts to hide their smoking from family or friends, or avoid smoking in public, can serve as barriers as well as motivators to move away from tobacco use. Continued smoking by the pregnant woman's partner can act as a serious barrier to cessation, as can criticism or, in some earlier studies, aggressive behaviour if a woman is not successful in stopping. Alternatively, partners can also act as an important source of support in some cases during a quit attempt:

> I don't know, I think I would have done a lot better if he had quit. Being at home and when you really wanted one, if he lit up then I would take one.
>
> (Edwards & Sims-Jones, 1998, as cited in Flemming et al., 2015, p. 9)

Organisational factors in pregnancy

There is a less well-developed qualitative literature on factors at the organisational level, including how services to support smoking cessation can help pregnant women to achieve abstinence. However, studies from several countries have shown an apparent lack of smoking-related discussion, advice, and support by healthcare professionals; for example:

> They sort of asked me if I was still smoking, that's all they said to me. I think to be fair the midwives … they are busy.
>
> *(Bauld et al., 2017, p. 40)*

Where smoking cessation interventions were available, support from a healthcare professional emerged as important, including how the risks of smoking were explained by that professional and how smoking cessation was integrated into maternity care. Cessation services that offer flexibility in service delivery, home appointments, and one-to-one support were well received, as was the offer of Nicotine Replacement Therapy (NRT) in pregnancy. Carbon monoxide (CO) screening can serve as a powerful motivational tool for cessation by providing feedback on reduced CO levels during quit attempts.

Postpartum return to smoking

A recent systematic review synthesised the qualitative evidence on women's experience of post-partum smoking relapse (Notley, Blyth, Craig, Edwards, & Holland, 2015); 22 papers based on 16 studies reported the views of 1,031 postpartum women. Factors that impacted relapse mapped to the SEF and were consistent with the experiences of women attempting to quit smoking in pregnancy, but were also related to the complexities of the postpartum period.

At the individual level, key themes were beliefs, motivation, and physiological factors. For example, women's beliefs about smoking as a means of coping with stress during pregnancy extended to influence reasons given for smoking relapse; this was presented by women as a strategy for coping with the stress of caring for a new-born. Loss of extrinsic motivation to quit during the pregnancy (for the health of the foetus) appeared to be a key factor in prompting relapse after childbirth: "I didn't think of myself when I quit smoking, I thought of the baby first and that is what motivated me" *(*Edwards & Sims-Jones, 1998, as cited in Notley et al., 2015, p. 1718).

During the immediate postpartum period women often felt that physiological changes influenced cigarette cravings; some reported an almost immediate return of cravings that had been absent during pregnancy. For example, one woman said: "It was basically the craving just came back" (Edwards & Sims-Jones, 1998, as cited in Notley et al., 2015, p. 1719).

At the interpersonal level, postpartum identity change (i.e., adjusting to a mothering identity) and social influences were critical. There was a strongly expressed need for social support in maintaining smoking abstinence, especially support from a partner. Partner's smoking status was a key facilitator of relapse prevention, but, conversely, acted as a barrier when the partner was a smoker.

> Although during pregnancy her husband encouraged her to quit—even reducing his own smoking to just one cigarette a day to offer support—after delivery they began to smoke together while drinking and after meals as a way of spending time together.
>
> *(author interpretation Nichter et al., 2008, as cited in Notley et al., 2015, p. 1720)*

Face-to-face behavioural support for smoking cessation

Evidence for effectiveness of interventions

Face-to-face behavioural support for smoking cessation is part of routine pregnancy care in many high-income countries (e.g., National Institute for Health and Care Excellence (NICE), 2010; Siu, 2015; World Health Organization [WHO], 2013). In this section we consider the evidence for smoking cessation during pregnancy as aided by individual face-to-face behavioural support, including counselling, health education, feedback, and social support from peers and/or partners. We focus on individual, rather than group, support as women who smoke in pregnancy have expressed a strong preference for individual support (Ussher, West, & Hibbs, 2004), most likely due to the embarrassment of being around other smokers. Furthermore, few group-based interventions have been tested. First, we consider the synthesis of evidence provided in a systematic review (Chamberlain et al., 2017), then we discuss the intervention components.

The review examined evidence from randomised controlled trials (RCTs), cluster-randomised trials, and quasi-RCTs to assess the effects of smoking cessation interventions during pregnancy on smoking and perinatal outcomes. Counselling had a strong effect on cessation compared with usual care (30 studies—most common type of study, average risk ratio [RR] 1.44, 95% CI 1.19 to 1.73), with a smaller effect when compared with active but less intensive interventions. There was no evidence that any particular type of counselling was better than others. However, some studies show that motivational interviewing does not appear to aid cessation in pregnancy or postpartum (Hayes et al., 2013; Heckman, Egleston, & Hofmann, 2010). This may be because these women are already highly motivated to quit to protect their baby. The review showed that health education was not effective when compared with usual care, possibly because women are already well aware of the harms of smoking. Feedback had a benefit when compared with usual care and when combined with other strategies, such as counselling, although not in comparison with active but less intensive interventions. Social support interventions were not effective when provided by peers or partners, but it is unclear why these interventions failed. One study showed that individual smoking cessation counselling combined with a physical activity intervention was no more effective than counselling alone for aiding smoking cessation at end-of-pregnancy, although it was not clear whether the women had raised their exercise levels sufficiently (Ussher et al., 2015).

Pooled results from the Chamberlain et al. (2017) review showed that the interventions were significantly associated with higher mean birthweight and reductions in low birthweight and neonatal intensive care admissions. There was no evidence for effects on preterm births or stillbirths. It is not clear whether these findings can be extended to women in low- and middle-income countries, adolescents, ethnic and minority populations, or to women with mental health problems or substance misuse. Other studies have focussed on preventing postpartum return to smoking and have so far had little success (Hajek et al., 2013; Levine, Cheng, Marcus, Kalarchian, & Emery, 2016; Su & Buttenheim, 2014).

Intervention components

The interventions covered in the above review by Chamberlain and colleagues involve a range of behaviour change techniques (BCTs). A BCT is the "observable, replicable and irreducible component of an intervention designed to alter or redirect causal processes that regulate behaviour" (e.g., goal setting, problem solving, action planning) (Michie et al., 2013, p. 5) and that address barriers against, or maximise facilitators towards, smoking cessation. As most interventions involve multiple BCTs, which may be tailored to individual women, in the review by Chamberlain et al. it is difficult to assess the independent effect of specific BCTs. With reference to a smoking-specific taxonomy (Michie, Churchill, & West, 2011), a review (Lorencatto, West, & Michie, 2012) showed that 11 BCTs were applied within interventions that showed a positive effect on smoking cessation, including the BCTs of goal setting, information about consequences of smoking/cessation, and relapse prevention. Lorencatto et al. reported that only 15% of treatment manuals used by UK Stop Smoking Services advocated all 11 BCTs.

A recent study showed that very few BCTs in effective RCTs addressed what experts considered to be the key barriers and facilitators to smoking cessation in pregnancy, such as smoking as a social norm, quitting not a priority, or desire to protect baby (Campbell et al., 2018). Additional research is needed to determine which BCTs, or combinations of these, are most effective in helping women to stop smoking during pregnancy. Also, such studies ought to include assessments of fidelity so that the actual BCTs delivered are clear. Finally, interventions need to include more BCTs that target the important barriers to and facilitators of smoking cessation in pregnancy, while also being implementable within existing healthcare structures.

Financial incentives

A systematic review identified 21 trials of financial incentives for smoking cessation (Cahill, Hartmann-Boyce, & Perera, 2015), including nine trials with pregnant smokers. A meta-analysis, with approximately 1,300 women, showed that, overall, incentives were effective for smoking cessation in pregnancy at longest follow-up (OR 3.60 95%, CI 2.39–5.43). Three trials showed a clear benefit of contingent rewards, where the incentives were dependent on biochemically validated smoking cessation. The largest trial was in the UK, involved around 600 women, and offered up to £400 of shopping vouchers for setting a quit date (£50), quitting at 4 weeks (£50), quitting at 12 weeks (£100), and quitting at end-of-pregnancy (£200) (Tappin et al., 2015). In the intervention arm incentives were combined with the offer of support from the National Health Service (NHS) stop smoking service and the control arm received the offer of this NHS support alone (i.e., without incentives). At the end of pregnancy, the quit rate was 15% in the incentives arm compared with 4% in the control arm. Additional analysis showed that incentives for smoking cessation in pregnancy were cost-effective (Boyd, Briggs, Bauld, Sinclair, & Tappin, 2016). A multi-centre UK trial of financial incentives for smoking in pregnancy, modelled on the study by Tappin and colleagues (2015), is underway.

Self-help

Self-help for smoking cessation is commonly defined as structured materials that assist the individual in making a quit attempt and sustaining abstinence without significant assistance from a health professional or group support (Lancaster & Stead, 2005; Naughton, Prevost, & Sutton, 2008). Self-help can be delivered by paper-based booklet or other print media, video or DVD, audio recording, Interactive Voice Response system, SMS text message, smartphone app, web browser on a smartphone, computer or tablet, or any other medium where support is not directly delivered by a person.

Smoking cessation self-help booklets are of interest to approximately one half of pregnant smokers who want to quit (Ussher et al., 2004). A cohort study that followed women through pregnancy and postpartum showed that, among smokers, the interest in cessation self-help increased more than other types of cessation support from early to late pregnancy and was the support type of most interest in late pregnancy (Naughton et al., 2018). This may be because, as a woman's pregnancy becomes easily noticeable, perceptions of social stigmatisation and shame regarding smoking in pregnancy increase (Abrahamsson, Springett, Karlsson, & Ottosson, 2005), as does actual stigmatisation (Wigginton & Lee, 2013). The appeal of self-help might be enhanced as it is often available with little if any contact with healthcare professionals, thereby minimising perceptions of judgement from others, which is a barrier to face-to-face support (Ussher, Etter, & West, 2006).

A systematic review of randomised controlled trials showed that self-help interventions almost double the chances of quitting smoking in pregnancy compared with usual care or no intervention (Naughton et al., 2008). The effect remained when restricted to the analysis of trials that only evaluated booklet or paper-based self-help materials. A recent systematic review of digital self-help interventions for smoking cessation in pregnancy showed that these interventions increase the chances of quitting by approximately 40%, compared with usual care or non-digital self-help (Griffiths et al., 2018). The most effective types of digital self-help identified in the review were SMS text message systems and computer programs. Fidelity of intervention delivery may be an important factor in determining effectiveness of digital self-help interventions. For example, the trials that evaluated computer interventions had supervised usage of the programs, which ensured high usage rates, and an evaluation of an SMS text message system showed that over 80% of women reported having read all the text messages they had received at least once (Naughton et al., 2017). In contrast, the only evaluation of a smartphone app for smoking cessation in pregnancy showed no evidence of an effect on smoking behaviour, most likely due to low engagement rates (Tombor et al., 2018).

Pharmacotherapies

There are three main smoking cessation medications generally available: NRT, Bupropion, and Varenicline. NRT is the only smoking cessation pharmacotherapy that is currently licenced for use during pregnancy, and it is provided by prescription in many countries to pregnant women with moderate to high nicotine dependence. NRT use has not, to date, been associated with pregnancy complications or abnormalities (Coleman, Chamberlain, Davey, Cooper, & Leonardi-Bee, 2015). NRT is effective outside of pregnancy, increasing the absolute abstinence rate from 10% (placebo/no NRT) to 16% (Stead et al., 2012), but its effectiveness during pregnancy remains unclear. A pooled analysis of NRT versus placebo among pregnant smokers in five trials does not support its effectiveness; NRT was associated with a non-statistically significant increase in abstinence of 3% (9% to 12%) (Coleman et al., 2015). A key question, therefore, is why NRT does not promote abstinence in pregnancy in the same way as it does outside of pregnancy. There are two key factors, one biological and one behavioural.

The biological problem

Studies have shown that nicotine metabolism, or clearance, is 60% higher among pregnant than among postpartum women (Dempsey, Jacob, & Benowitz, 2002). The increased clearance of nicotine, and its by-product cotinine, is present in early pregnancy; it may peak at around 18–22 weeks, and remain at that level until late pregnancy, before reducing postpartum (Bowker, Lewis, Coleman, & Cooper, 2015). This increased clearance rate means that pregnant smokers need nicotine more regularly and at higher doses than they needed pre-pregnancy to prevent withdrawal and cravings. Thus, pregnant smokers report more severe withdrawal and cravings than other smokers (Berlin, Singleton, & Heishman, 2016).

The behavioural problem

Pregnant women provided with NRT have demonstrated low adherence rates. Continuous use of NRT for the recommended treatment period is typically below 20% in pregnancy (Coleman et al., 2012; Fish et al., 2009; Wisborg, Henriksen, Jespersen, & Secher, 2000). A key factor is that many pregnant smokers significantly underestimate the risks of smoking (Ferguson & Hansen, 2012) and overestimate the risks of NRT (Hotham et al., 2002). Some women are concerned that NRT could increase their exposure to nicotine compared with smoking, and thereby increase foetal harm and nicotine dependence (Bowker et al., 2015). Women can also have low beliefs about the effectiveness of NRT, find standard doses of NRT unhelpful, and wish to test whether they can maintain abstinence without NRT (Fish et al., 2009), most likely to minimise medication use in pregnancy (Twigg, Lupattelli, & Nordeng, 2016). Some also report using NRT to reduce rather than to abstain from smoking as they think they cannot manage the cravings to smoke with NRT and see the need for some occasional smoking (Bowker et al., 2016). In addition, the perceived side effects of NRT account for about 10–20% of pregnant women stopping use (Coleman et al., 2012; Fish et al., 2009).

Increasing the effectiveness of nicotine replacement therapy

Improved adherence to NRT patches is associated with increased rates of smoking cessation in pregnancy, and this relationship is likely to be at least partially causal (Vaz et al., 2016). No interventions promoting adherence to NRT for pregnant women have been evaluated. However, an intervention, if generally effective at increasing adherence, is also likely to increase the effectiveness of NRT in pregnancy (Hollands et al., 2015), although it may need to be combined with dual therapy NRT to ensure that a sufficient dose of nicotine is provided to combat the increased metabolism of nicotine during pregnancy.

The role of electronic cigarettes

Electronic cigarettes (ECs) are increasingly used in many countries as an aid to smoking cessation (Delnevo et al., 2016; West, Beard, & Brown, 2018), including during pregnancy (Kurti et al., 2017). It has been argued that the potential benefits of ECs probably outweigh harms and that ECs may have an important role in harm reduction (Goniewicz et al., 2014; Hajek, Etter, Benowitz, Eissenberg, & McRobbie, 2014; McNeil, Brose, Calder, Bauld, & Robson, 2018). In the UK it is recommended that pregnant women should not be discouraged from using ECs to stop smoking if they have struggled to quit without a cessation aid (Smoking in Pregnancy Challenge Group, 2016). However, due to a lack of evidence on efficacy and safety, in Australia (Australian Medical Association, 2015) and the US (American Congress of Obstetricians and Gynecologists, 2015) women are advised not to use ECs in pregnancy. Also, pregnant women have reported concerns about ECs, mostly due to perceived potential harm and the perceived stigma of vaping during pregnancy (Bowker et al., 2016). In the UK, the first large trial of ECs for smoking cessation in pregnancy, underway at the time of writing, should provide evidence as to the efficacy and safety of this approach for pregnant women.

Population level interventions

There is good evidence that population-level tobacco control policies can reduce smoking rates in the general population (WHO, 2008), but limited evidence is available about pregnant women. In England, a national mass media campaign on smoking and pregnancy was shown to increase awareness of smoking dangers in pregnant women, as well as to increase calls to a pregnancy stop smoking helpline. However, there was no evidence of changes in smoking prevalence (Campion, Owen, McNeill, & McGuire, 1994). More recently, exposure to a US national anti-smoking campaign for a general audience was associated with smoking cessation in pregnant women (England et al., 2017), whereas in Australia pregnancy smoking rates did not appear to be related to anti-smoking advertisements (Havard et al., 2017). Cigarette labels that graphically depict pregnancy-related harm appear to be perceived as effective among women of reproductive age (Kollath-Cattano, Osman, & Thrasher, 2017) and would be expected to reduce smoking rates in pregnancy (Tauras, Peck, Cheng, & Chaloupka, 2017), but we could not find any studies that assessed perceptions of these labels or plain packaging by pregnant women. Emerging evidence suggests an association between bans on smoking in public places and reductions in smoking during pregnancy (Frazer et al., 2016). There is also evidence from US studies that raising cigarette prices reduces rates of smoking in pregnancy (Adams et al., 2012; Colman, Grossman, & Joyce, 2003; Levy & Meara, 2006; Ringel & Evans, 2001). Simulation models would suggest that further substantial price rises are needed if the impact on reducing smoking rates in pregnancy is to continue (Higgins et al., 2017).

Conclusions

Although rates of smoking during pregnancy are declining in high-income countries, smoking cessation support remains a public health priority due to the adverse effects on maternal, foetal, and child health and to rising smoking rates among women in low- and middle-income countries (World Health Organization, 2013). Women's experience of smoking and smoking cessation is influenced by individual, social, and organisational factors. This places women in a complex situation where they may struggle to reconcile health messages about the harms of smoking with social and cultural norms that make smoking acceptable within their communities. For women who succeed in stopping smoking during pregnancy, maintaining abstinence can be time limited—a sacrifice made for the health of the foetus. Both initial success in smoking cessation and the likelihood of relapse are influenced by multiple factors, including social identity of the woman, smoking status of her partner, and poor maternal mental health; these factors may need to be given greater consideration in the development of smoking cessation interventions. There is scarce evidence for interventions that prevent return to smoking after childbirth, an area that has been particularly under-researched. There is some evidence for effective smoking cessation interventions during pregnancy. Providing behavioural support is the most established of these interventions, but success rates are modest, and more work is needed to adapt generic interventions to the complex needs of pregnant women. NRT is effective in non-pregnant populations but has not been shown to be similarly effective during pregnancy, and studies are required to determine whether NRT can become effective with increased adherence and higher doses of nicotine. Electronic cigarettes are now commonly used in pregnancy in some countries, and work is needed to establish the relative safety and efficacy of these devices. A small number of studies have demonstrated that financial incentives show great promise for helping pregnant women to stop smoking, and this work needs to be generalised and extended to the postpartum period. Pregnant women tend to favour self-help interventions to aid cessation, and digital interventions, in particular, have shown benefits and are among the most cost-effective interventions for cessation in pregnancy. Finally, population-level intervention, such as plain tobacco packaging, could potentially have the greatest impact on smoking in pregnancy and postpartum, yet pregnancy-specific work in this area is in its infancy.

References

Abrahamsson, A., Springett, J., Karlsson, L., & Ottosson, T. (2005). Making sense of the challenge of smoking cessation during pregnancy: A phenomenographic approach. *Health Education Research*, 20, 367–378.

Adams, E. K., Markowitz, S., Kannan, V., Dietz, P. M., Tong, V. T., & Malarcher, A. M. (2012). Reducing prenatal smoking: The role of state policies. *American Journal of Preventive Medicine*, 43(1), 34–40.

American Congress of Obstetricians and Gynecologists (2015). *New fact sheet on E-cigarettes.* Washington, DC: Author. Retrieved from www.acog.org/About-ACOG/ACOG-Departments/Tobacco–Alcohol–and-Substance-Abuse/Tobacco/New-Fact-Sheet-on-E-Cigarettes.

Australian Medical Association (2015). Tobacco smoking and E-cigarettes – The AMA position. Barton, ACT, Australia: Author. Retrieved from https://ama.com.au/position-statement/tobacco-smoking-and-e-cigarettes-2015.

Bauld, L., Graham, H., Sinclair, L., Flemming, K., Naughton, F., Ford, A., McKell, J., McCaughan, D., Hopewell, S., Angus, K., Eadie, D., & Tappin, D. (2017). Barriers to and facilitators of smoking cessation in pregnancy and following childbirth: Literature review and qualitative study. *Health Technology Assessment, 21*(36), 1–158.

Berlin, I., Singleton, E. G., & Heishman, S. J. (2016). Craving and withdrawal symptoms during smoking cessation: Comparison of pregnant and non-pregnant smokers. *Journal of Substance Abuse Treatment, 63,* 18–24.

Bloch, M., Althabe, F., Onyamboko, M., Kaseba-Sata, C., Castilla, E. E., Freire, S., Garces, A. L., Parida, S., Goudar, S. S., Kadir, M. M., Goco, N., Thornberry, J., Daniels, M., Bartz, J., Hartwell, T., Moss, N., & Goldenberg, R. (2008). Tobacco use and secondhand smoke exposure during pregnancy: An investigative survey of women in 9 developing nations. *American Journal of Public Health, 98,* 1833–1840.

Bowker, K., Campbell, K. A., Coleman, T., Lewis, S., Naughton, F., & Cooper, S. (2016). Understanding pregnant smokers' adherence to nicotine replacement therapy during a quit attempt: A qualitative study. *Nicotine & Tobacco Research, 18,* 906–912, doi:10.1093/ntr/ntv205.

Bowker, K., Lewis, S., Coleman, T., & Cooper, S. (2015). Changes in the rate of nicotine metabolism across pregnancy: A longitudinal study. *Addiction, 110,* 1827–1832.

Boyd, K. A., Briggs, A. H., Bauld, L., Sinclair, L., & Tappin, D. (2016). Are financial incentives cost-effective to support smoking cessation during pregnancy? *Addiction, 111,* 360–370.

Cahill, K., Hartmann-Boyce, J., & Perera, R. (2015). Incentives for smoking cessation. *Cochrane Database of Systematic Reviews, 5,* CD004307.

Campbell, K. A., Fergie, L., Coleman-Haynes, T., Cooper, S., Lorencatto, F., Ussher, M., Dyas, J., & Coleman, T. (2018). Improving behavioral support for smoking cessation in pregnancy: What are the barriers to stopping and which behavior change techniques can influence these? Application of theoretical domains framework. *International Journal of Environmental Research and Public Health, 15,* ii: E359.

Campion, P., Owen, L., McNeill, A., & McGuire, C. (1994). Evaluation of a mass media campaign on smoking and pregnancy. *Addiction, 89,* 1245–1254.

Centers for Disease Control and Prevention (2017). *Tobacco use and pregnancy.* Atlanta, GA: Author. Retrieved from www.cdc.gov/reproductivehealth/MaternalInfantHealth/TobaccoUsePregnancy/index.htm.

Chamberlain, C., O'Mara-Eves, A., Porter, J., Coleman, T., Perlen, S. M., Thomas, J., & McKenzie, J. E. (2017). Psychosocial interventions for supporting women to stop smoking in pregnancy. *Cochrane Database of Systematic Reviews, 2,* CD001055.

Coleman, T., Chamberlain, C., Davey, M. A., Cooper, S. E., & Leonardi-Bee, J. (2015). Pharmacological interventions for promoting smoking cessation during pregnancy. *Cochrane Database of Systematic Reviews, 12,* CD010078.

Coleman, T., Cooper, S., Thornton, J. G., Grainge, M. J., Watts, K., & Britton, J., Smoking, Nicotine, and Pregnancy (SNAP) Trial Team (2012). A randomized trial of nicotine-replacement therapy patches in pregnancy. *New England Journal of Medicine, 366,* 808–818.

Colman, G., Grossman, M., & Joyce, T. (2003). The effect of cigarette excise taxes on smoking before, during and after pregnancy. *Journal of Health Economics, 22,* 1053–1072.

Delnevo, C. D., Giovenco, D. P., Steinberg, M. B., Villanti, A. C., Pearson, J. L., Niaura, R. S., & Abrams, D. B. (2016). Patterns of electronic cigarette use among adults in the United States. *Nicotine & Tobacco Research, 18,* 715–719.

Dempsey, D., Jacob, 3rd, P., & Benowitz, N. L. (2002). Accelerated metabolism of nicotine and cotinine in pregnant smokers. *Journal of Pharmacology and Experimental Therapeutics, 301,* 594–598.

Dias-Dame, J. L. & Cesar, J. A. (2015). Disparities in prevalence of smoking and smoking cessation during pregnancy: A population-based study. *BioMed Research International, 2015,* 345430.

Edwards, N. & Sims-Jones, N. (1998). Smoking and smoking relapse during pregnancy and postpartum: Results of a qualitative study. *Birth, 25,* 94–100.

England, L., Tong, V. T., Rockhill, K., Hsia, J., McAfee, T., Patel, D., Rupp, K., Conrey, E. J., Valdivieso, C., & Davis, K. C. (2017). Evaluation of a federally funded mass media campaign and smoking cessation in pregnant women: A population-based study in three states. *British Medical Journal: Open*, 7(12), e016826.

Ferguson, S. G. & Hansen, E. C. (2012). A preliminary examination of cognitive factors that influence interest in quitting during pregnancy. *Journal of Smoking Cessation*, 7, 100–104.

Fergusson, D. M., Woodward, L. J., & Horwood, L. J. (1998). Maternal smoking during pregnancy and psychiatric adjustment in late adolescence. *Archives of General Psychiatry*, 55, 721–727.

Fish, L. J., Peterson, B. L., Namenek Brouwer, R. J., Lyna, P., Oncken, C. A., Swamy, G. K., Myers, E. R., Pletsch, P. K., & Pollak, K. I. (2009). Adherence to nicotine replacement therapy among pregnant smokers. *Nicotine & Tobacco Research*, 11, 514–518.

Flemming, K., Graham, H., Heirs, M., Fox, D., & Sowden, A. (2013). Smoking in pregnancy: A systematic review of qualitative research of women who commence pregnancy as smokers. *Journal of Advanced Nursing*, 69, 1023–1036.

Flemming, K., McCaughan, D., Angus, K., & Graham, H. (2015). Qualitative systematic review: Barriers and facilitators to smoking cessation experienced by women in pregnancy and following childbirth. *Journal of Advanced Nursing*, 71, 1210–1226.

Frazer, K., Callinan, J. E., McHugh, J., van Baarsel, S., Clarke, A., Doherty, K., & Kelleher, C. (2016). Legislative smoking bans for reducing harms from secondhand smoke exposure, smoking prevalence and tobacco consumption. *Cochrane Database of Systematic Reviews*, 2, CD005992.

Godfrey, C., Pickett, K. E., Parrott, S., Mdege, N. D., & Eapen, D. (2010). *Estimating the costs to the NHS of smoking in pregnancy for pregnant women and infants*. York, UK: Public Health Research Consortium, University of York.

Goniewicz, M. L., Knysak, J., Gawron, M., Kosmider, L., Sobczak, A., Kurek, J., Prokopowicz, A., Jablonska-Czapla, M., Rosik-Dulewska, C., Havel, C., Jacob, P., & Benowitz, N. (2014). Levels of selected carcinogens and toxicants in vapour from electronic cigarettes. *Tobacco Control*, 23, 133–139.

Graham, H., Hawkins, S. S., & Law, C. (2010). Lifecourse influences on women's smoking before, during and after pregnancy. *Social Science & Medicine*, 70, 582–587.

Gray, R., Bonellie, S. R., Chalmers, J., Greer, I., Jarvis, S., Kurinczuk, J. J., & Williams, C. (2009). Contribution of smoking during pregnancy to inequalities in stillbirth and infant death in Scotland 1994–2003: Retrospective population based study using hospital maternity records. *British Medical Journal*, 339, b3754.

Griffiths, S. E., Parsons, J., Fulton, E. A., Naughton, F., Tombor, I., & Brown, K. E. (2018). Are digital interventions for smoking cessation in pregnancy effective? A systematic review and meta-analysis. *Health Psychology Review*, 12(4), 333–356.

Hajek, P., Etter, J. F., Benowitz, N., Eissenberg, T., & McRobbie, H. (2014). Electronic cigarettes: Review of use, content, safety, effects on smokers and potential for harm and benefit. *Addiction*, 109, 1801–1810.

Hajek, P., Stead, L. F., West, R., Jarvis, M., Hartmann-Boyce, J., & Lancaster, T. (2013). Relapse prevention interventions for smoking cessation. *Cochrane Database of Systematic Reviews*, 8, CD003999.

Havard, A., Tran, D. T., Kemp-Casey, A., Einarsdottir, K., Preen, D. B., & Jorm, L. R. (2017). Tobacco policy reform and population-wide antismoking activities in Australia: The impact on smoking during pregnancy. *Tobacco Control*. Advance online publication.

Hayes, C. B., Collins, C., O'Carroll, H., Wyse, E., Gunning, M., Geary, M., & Kelleher, C. C. (2013). Effectiveness of motivational interviewing in influencing smoking cessation in pregnant and postpartum disadvantaged women. *Nicotine & Tobacco Research*, 15, 969–977.

Heckman, C. J., Egleston, B. L., & Hofmann, M. T. (2010). Efficacy of motivational interviewing for smoking cessation: A systematic review and meta-analysis. *Tobacco Control*, 19, 410–416.

Heil, S. H., Herrmann, E. S., Badger, G. J., Solomon, L. J., Bernstein, I. M., & Higgins, S. T. (2014). Examining the timing of changes in cigarette smoking upon learning of pregnancy. *Preventive Medicine*, 68, 58–61.

Higgins, S. T. & Chilcoat, H. D. (2009). Women and smoking: An interdisciplinary examination of socioeconomic influences. *Drug and Alcohol Dependence*, 104(Suppl 1), S1–S5.

Higgins, S. T., Reed, D. D., Redner, R., Skelly, J. M., Zvorsky, I. A., & Kurti, A. N. (2017). Simulating demand for cigarettes among pregnant women: A low-risk method for studying vulnerable populations. *Journal of the Experimental Analysis of Behavior*, 107, 176–190.

Hollands, G. J., McDermott, M. S., Lindson-Hawley, N., Vogt, F., Farley, A., & Aveyard, P. (2015). Interventions to increase adherence to medications for tobacco dependence. *Cochrane Database of Systematic Reviews, 2,* CD009164.

Hotham, E. D., Atkinson, E. R., & Gilbert, A. L. (2002). Focus groups with pregnant smokers: Barriers to cessation, attitudes to nicotine patch use and perceptions of cessation counselling by care providers. *Drug and Alcohol Review, 21,* 163–168.

Jones, M., Lewis, S., Parrott, S., Wormall, S., & Coleman, T. (2016). Re-starting smoking in the postpartum period after receiving a smoking cessation intervention: A systematic review. *Addiction, 111,* 981–990.

Källén, K. (2001). The impact of maternal smoking during pregnancy on delivery outcome. *European Journal of Public Health, 11,* 329–333.

Kollath-Cattano, C., Osman, A., & Thrasher, J. F. (2017). Evaluating the perceived effectiveness of pregnancy-related cigarette package health warning labels among different gender/age groups. *Addictive Behaviors, 66,* 33–40.

Kurti, A. N., Redner, R., Lopez, A. A., Keith, D. R., Villanti, A. C., Stanton, C. A., Gaalema, D. E., Bunn, J. Y., Doogan, N. J., Cepeda-Benito, A., Roberts, M. E., Phillips, J., & Higgins, S. T. (2017). Tobacco and nicotine delivery product use in a national sample of pregnant women. *Preventive Medicine, 104,* 50–56.

Lancaster, T. & Stead, L. F. (2005). Self-help interventions for smoking cessation. *Cochrane Database of Systematic Reviews, 3,* CD001118.

Lange, S., Probst, C., Rehm, J., & Popova, S. (2018). National, regional, and global prevalence of smoking during pregnancy in the general population: A systematic review and meta-analysis. *The Lancet Global Health, 6,* e769–e776.

Levine, M. D., Cheng, Y., Marcus, M. D., Kalarchian, M. A., & Emery, R. L. (2016). Preventing postpartum smoking relapse: A randomized clinical trial. *JAMA Internal Medicine, 176,* 443–452.

Levy, D. E. & Meara, E. (2006). The effect of the 1998 master settlement agreement on prenatal smoking. *Journal of Health Economics, 25,* 276–294.

Lorencatto, F., West, R., & Michie, S. (2012). Specifying evidence-based behavior change techniques to aid smoking cessation in pregnancy. *Nicotine & Tobacco Research, 14,* 1019–1026.

McNeil, A. B., Brose, L. S., Calder, R., Bauld, L., & Robson, D. (2018). *Evidence review of e-cigarettes and heated tobacco products.* London, UK: Public Health England. Retrieved from www.gov.uk/govern ment/publications/e-cigarettes-and-heated-tobacco-products-evidence-review.

Michie, S., Churchill, S., & West, R. (2011). Identifying evidence-based competences required to deliver behavioural support for smoking cessation. *Annals of Behavioral Medicine, 41,* 59–70.

Michie, S., Richardson, M., Johnston, M., Abraham, C., Francis, J., Hardeman, W., Eccles, M., Cane, J., & Wood, C. E. (2013). The behavior change technique taxonomy (v1) of 93 hierarchically clustered techniques: Building an international consensus for the reporting of behavior change interventions. *Annals of Behavioral Medicine, 46,* 81–95.

National Institute for Health and Care Excellence (NICE) (2010). *Quitting smoking in pregnancy and following childbirth. Public health guidance 26.* London, UK: NICE. Retrieved from www.nice.org.uk/guid ance/ph26.

Naughton, F., Cooper, S., Foster, K., Emery, J., Leonardi-Bee, J., Sutton, S., Jones, M., Ussher, M., Whitemore, R., Leighton, Matthew ; Montgomery, Alan ; Parrott, Steve Coleman, T. (2017). Large multi-centre pilot randomized controlled trial testing a low-cost, tailored, self-help smoking cessation text message intervention for pregnant smokers (MiQuit). *Addiction, 112,* 1238–1249.

Naughton, F., Prevost, A. T., & Sutton, S. (2008). Self-help smoking cessation interventions in pregnancy: A systematic review and meta-analysis. *Addiction, 103,* 566–579.

Naughton, F., Vanderbloemen, L., Orton, S., Bowker, K., Coleman, T., Leonardi-Bee, J., … Ussher, M. (2018). Attitudes toward and use of smoking cessation support across pregnancy and after delivery. Manuscript submitted for publication.

Nichter, M., Nichter, M., Adrian, S., Goldade, K., Tesler, L., & Muramoto, M. (2008). Smoking and harm-reduction efforts among postpartum women. *Qualitative Health Research, 18,* 1184–1194.

Notley, C., Blyth, A., Craig, J., Edwards, A., & Holland, R. (2015). Postpartum smoking relapse: A thematic synthesis of qualitative studies. *Addiction, 110,* 1712–1723.

Orton, S., Coleman, T., Coleman-Haynes, T., & Ussher, M. (2017). Predictors of postpartum return to smoking: A systematic review. *Nicotine & Tobacco Research, 20,* 665–673.

Riaz, M., Lewis, S., Naughton, F., & Ussher, M. (2018). Predictors of smoking cessation during pregnancy: A systematic review and meta-analysis. *Addiction, 113*, 610–622.

Ringel, J. S. & Evans, W. N. (2001). Cigarette taxes and smoking during pregnancy. *American Journal of Public Health, 91*, 1851–1856.

Roberts, K. H., Munafo, M. R., Rodriguez, D., Drury, M., Murphy, M. F., Neale, R. E., & Nettle, D. (2005). Longitudinal analysis of the effect of prenatal nicotine exposure on subsequent smoking behavior of offspring. *Nicotine & Tobacco Research, 7*, 801–808.

Rockhill, K. M., Tong, V. T., Farr, S. L., Robbins, C. L., D'Angelo, D. V., & England, L. J. (2016). Postpartum smoking relapse after quitting during pregnancy: Pregnancy risk assessment monitoring system, 2000–2011. *Journal of Women's Health, 25*, 480–488.

Rogers, J. M. (2009). Tobacco and pregnancy. *Reproductive Toxicology, 28*, 152–160.

Salihu, H. M. & Wilson, R. E. (2007). Epidemiology of prenatal smoking and perinatal outcomes. *Early Human Development, 83*, 713–720.

Schneider, M. & Stokols, D. (2009). Multilevel theories of behavior change: A social ecological framework. In S. A. Shumaker, J. K. Ockene, & K. A. Riekert (Eds), *The handbook of health behavior change* (4th ed., pp. 85–105). New York, NY: Springer.

Schwartzbaum, J. A., George, S. L., Pratt, C. B., & Davis, B. (1991). An exploratory study of environmental and medical factors potentially related to childhood cancer. *Medical and Pediatric Oncology, 19*, 115–121.

Silveira, M. F., Matijasevich, A., Menezes, A. M., Horta, B. L., Santos, I. S., Barros, A. J., Barros, F. C., & Victora, C. G. (2016). Secular trends in smoking during pregnancy according to income and ethnic group: Four population-based perinatal surveys in a Brazilian city. *BMJ Open, 6*(2), e010127.

Siu, A. L. & U.S. Preventive Services Task Force (2015). Behavioral and pharmacotherapy interventions for tobacco smoking cessation in adults, including pregnant women: U.S. Preventive Services Task Force recommendation statement. *Annals of Internal Medicine, 163*, 622–634.

Smoking in Pregnancy Challenge Group, The (2016). *Use of electronic cigarettes in pregnancy: A guide for midwives and other healthcare professionals.* London, UK: The Smoking in Pregnancy Challenge Group.

Stead, L. F., Perera, R., Bullen, C., Mant, D., Hartmann-Boyce, J., Cahill, K., & Lancaster, T. (2012). Nicotine replacement therapy for smoking cessation. *Cochrane Database of Systematic Reviews, 11*, CD000146.

Su, A. & Buttenheim, A. M. (2014). Maintenance of smoking cessation in the postpartum period: Which interventions work best in the long-term? *Maternal and Child Health Journal, 18*, 714–728.

Tappin, D., Bauld, L., Purves, D., Boyd, K., Sinclair, L., & MacAskill, S.; Cessation in Pregnancy Incentives Trial Team (2015). Financial incentives for smoking cessation in pregnancy: Randomised controlled trial. *British Medical Journal, 350*, h134.

Tauras, J. A., Peck, R. M., Cheng, K. W., & Chaloupka, F. J. (2017). Graphic warning labels and the cost savings from reduced smoking among pregnant women. *International Journal of Environmental Research and Public Health, 14*, ii E164.

Thapar, A., Fowler, T., Rice, F., Scourfield, J., van Den Bree, M., Thomas, H., Harold, G., & Hay, D. (2003). Maternal smoking during pregnancy and attention deficit hyperactivity disorder symptoms in offspring. *American Journal of Psychiatry, 160*(1985–1989), 5.

Tombor, I., Beard, E., Brown, J., Shahab, L., Michie, S., & West, R. (2018). *Randomised factorial experiment of components of the SmokeFree Baby smartphone application to aid smoking cessation in pregnancy.* Manuscript submitted for publication.

Triandafilidis, Z., Ussher, J. M., Perz, J., & Hupputz, K. (2017). Doing and undoing femininities: An intersectional analysis of young women's smoking. *Feminism and Psychology, 27*(4), 465–488.

Twigg, M. J., Lupattelli, A., & Nordeng, H. (2016). Women's beliefs about medication use during their pregnancy: A UK perspective. *International Journal of Clinical Pharmacy, 38*, 968–976.

Ussher, M., Etter, J. F., & West, R. (2006). Perceived barriers to and benefits of attending a stop smoking course during pregnancy. *Patient Education and Counseling, 61*, 467–472.

Ussher, M., Lewis, S., Aveyard, P., Manyonda, I., West, R., & Lewis, B. (2015). Physical activity for smoking cessation in pregnancy: Randomised controlled trial. *British Medical Journal, 350*, h2145.

Ussher, M., West, R., & Hibbs, N. (2004). A survey of pregnant smokers' interest in different types of smoking cessation support. *Patient Education and Counseling, 54*(1), 67–72.

Vaz, L. R., Aveyard, P., Cooper, S., Leonardi-Bee, J., Coleman, T., & Trial Team, S. N. A. P. (2016). The association between treatment adherence to nicotine patches and smoking cessation in pregnancy: A secondary analysis of a randomized controlled trial. *Nicotine & Tobacco Research, 18*, 1952–1959.

West, R., Beard, B., & Brown, J. (2018). *Trends in electronic cigarette use in England: Smoking toolkit study*. London, UK: University College London. Retrieved from www.smokinginengland.info/latest-statistics.

Wigginton, B. & Lee, C. (2013). Stigma and hostility towards pregnant smokers: Does individuating information reduce the effect? *Psychology & Health, 28*, 862–873.

Wisborg, K., Henriksen, T. B., Jespersen, L. B., & Secher, N. J. (2000). Nicotine patches for pregnant smokers: A randomized controlled study. *Obstetrics and Gynecology, 96*, 967–971.

World Health Organization (WHO) (2008). *WHO report on the global tobacco epidemic, 2008: The MPOWER package*. Geneva: Author. Retrieved from http://apps.who.int/iris/bitstream/10665/43818/1/9789241596282_eng.pdf.

World Health Organization (WHO) (2013). *WHO recommendations for the prevention and management of tobacco use and second-hand smoke exposure in pregnancy*. Geneva: Author. Retrieved from www.who.int/tobacco/publications/pregnancy/guidelinestobaccosmokeexposure/en.

18

MEDICAL ASPECTS OF PREGNANCY

Annemarie Hennessy

Pregnancy holds a unique position in the health journey of a woman and her family. Every woman's contact with community health services and/or hospital services during her pregnancy is an opportunity to support health literacy and thus to measure and understand risks to her health. All available data suggest that childbirth should be attended by an assistant trained in the care of normal childbirth and in the anticipation of risk. While achieving optimal sexual and reproductive health touches on all aspects of a woman's life, a culturally appropriate and planned approach to pregnancy can ensure that normal pregnancy is supported as naturally as possible and childbirth is not treated as an illness. But as importantly, in the circumstances where common conditions and sometimes potentially dramatic medical complications do occur, a whole-of-health-system approach is required to ensure that childbirth can be the successful event that every woman wants.

Understanding the scope of the medical aspects of any individual pregnancy include learning of the full cycle of reproductive events. This includes a woman's pregnancy planning, conception events, her access to and journey through antenatal care, the childbirth process, immediate post-partum issues (e.g., feeding support and practices), and the impact of pregnancy events on her long-term health and well-being and that of her family. This chapter will focus on the medical aspects of pregnancy.

Considerable global effort is made to understand these aspects of the childbirth journey from an individual, regional and national perspective. Nations' league tables, which compare countries' maternal and perinatal outcomes, unintended pregnancies, and adolescents' childbearing, are available, and it is clear that these factor in the ambition to improve global health (expressed in United Nations Millennial Goals, and, recently, the Sustainable Development Goals) (United Nations 2018; WHO 2018). Globally, there were an estimated 385 maternal deaths per 100,000 live births in 1990 (WHO 2018) and 216 per 100,000 live births in 2015 (United Nations 2018), which indicates that significant advances are being made to reduce the scourge of "death in childbirth." The fact that these figures are collated annually in a rigorous fashion is a testament to the global importance of maternal and infant health and what the figures tell us about a population's health in general.

The focus on mortality as a marker is unfortunately still required to allow a focus on overall improvement in health system efficacy. Many countries now have so few deaths that a refocus on maternal illness in pregnancy, and then on long-term indicators of women's and babies' health after complicated pregnancy will occur in the next decade, as it should (Bellamy et al. 2007; Withagen et al. 2005). The slower impact on reducing unintended pregnancies in two thirds of countries surveyed in 2017 remains an issue of global concern (United Nations 2018). The younger and vulnerable members of the community where unintended pregnancy is more common may well have reduced access to the health care that they need.

Normal physiological changes in pregnancy

Part of the medical assessment of a pregnancy is dependent on whether normal physiological adaptations to pregnancy are occurring. These are commonly identified by a woman as amenorrhea, breast soreness, swelling, mood changes, "morning sickness," and changes in sleep pattern. Swelling is usually in the ankles and face and is a sign of retaining salt and fluid in order to support the growth and development of the fetus and the need for blood flow to the uterus and placenta (Tkachenko, Shchekochikhin, and Schrier 2014). These changes assist the mother's circulatory adaptation to pregnancy, but are not transferred to the fetus who has an independent circulation separated by the placenta. The rapid and dramatic increase in placental hormones causes the nausea associated with pregnancy (Niebyl 2010), which has become the focus of recent clinical guidelines to improve pregnancy care (Bulletins-Obstetrics, Committee on Practice 2018). These changes contribute to an intense dislike of noxious smells (Cameron 2014) and mood changes (Tyrlik, Konecny, and Kukla 2013). The factors involved in "pregnancy-related emotions" and the potential for mental health disorders in pregnancy include physical and social influences as well as the woman's health and social support. The impact of medical complications of a pregnancy cannot be underestimated (East et al. 2011).

Changes in sleep pattern are well known but have only recently been scientifically described (Izci-Balserak et al. 2018). Other common physical changes can include dizziness due to decreased blood pressure (Tkachenko, Shchekochikhin, and Schrier 2014), palpitations due to an increase in heart rate (Dietz et al. 2016), and joint aches and pains due to changes in hormone production (Ireland and Ott 2000). Changes in the immune response are necessary for the foreign tissue of the placenta and fetus to grow in the uterus without maternal immune attack (Hyde and Schust 2016). This "suppression" of the immune system is essential even though it leads to an increase in infection risk and severity.

Measurable changes determined through standard blood testing in pregnancy include changes in blood parameters (e.g., dilutional anaemia) (Roy and Pavord 2018), changes in kidney blood flow (Conrad and Davison 2014), changes in glucose (Banerjee 2018) and thyroid metabolism (Budenhofer et al. 2013), and changes in infection risk and rates (Kourtis, Read, and Jamieson 2014). The pregnant woman has an increased rate of breathing (Tan and Tan 2013). In fact, there are few body systems unchanged by the progression of pregnancy. The commonest complaints in pregnancy are "heartburn" and acid reflux into the oesophagus due to laxity between the oesophagus and stomach caused by pregnancy hormones (relaxin), and joint or back ache due to hormone effects on joints, especially those related to preparation for opening the pelvis to allow passage of the baby through the birth canal (Baccari and Calamai 2004). These changes are an increased burden on the mother's body, and having had multiple pregnancies is now seen as a cumulative risk factor for complications in a subsequent pregnancy (Haug et al. 2018) and also for later-life health issues (Bellamy et al. 2007).

The purpose of monitoring in pregnancy

The commonest high-level goal of maternal care is to reduce maternal mortality through increased rates of attended birth, and to decrease early childhood death (perinatal mortality rates, including stillbirth) (United Nations 2018). Maternal mortality is caused by obstetric complications such as sepsis, obstructed labour (where the baby does not survive the passage through the birth canal), or massive haemorrhage. Bleeding can be due to a low-lying placenta (placenta praevia) or placental separation from the uterine wall (placental abruption). Preterm labour (delivery before 37 weeks gestation) can be due to infection or abnormal positions of the fetus (e.g., transverse lying baby), both of which jeopardise the likelihood of a live-born child. Severe congenital abnormalities that indicate that a pregnancy will not lead to a live baby can be anticipated and allow a family time to make decisions about continuing the pregnancy. Considerable advances have been made in the early detection of conditions (e.g., Down Syndrome) from early risk scores and genetic testing (Deans et al. 2017); the application of these scores to an individual's decision depends on personal, religious, cultural, and legal considerations, which differ around the globe (March of Dimes 2006).

Monitoring for these structural issues of a pregnancy is factored into early pregnancy screening through early physical examination by an expert health care worker, midwife, or other maternity specifically trained nurse, doctor, or specialist obstetrician, as well as by an ultrasound assessment, the safe, gold standard in obstetric care (Papageorghiou et al. 2014). Monitoring for obstetric changes has now extended to include assessment for the "medical complications" of pregnancy as outlined below. Some of these are problems specific to pregnancy (e.g., gestational diabetes, preeclampsia) (Myers et al. 2013; Sweeting et al. 2018) and others are conditions (e.g., asthma) where treatment and monitoring need to be tailored for maternal and fetal safety.

Medical complications have a strong overlap with abnormal placental ("afterbirth") function, and measures of placental function should be part of the risk stratification, which is currently based on history, examination, basic blood tests, and ultrasound (Sweeting et al. 2018). Newer tests of placental function are being investigated in terms of their physiological changes in normal pregnancy (Myers et al. 2013). The use of these newer tests of placental function are specific to *an individual* pregnancy and therefore will potentially allow determination of the likely trajectory of that pregnancy when these tests are taken into account during routine antenatal care. Thus, we can start to bring "individualised" care to a given pregnancy and develop preventive strategies that are timely and safe.

Routine antenatal care

Routine antenatal care is specifically designed to anticipate risk, especially as pregnancy advances. In an optimal maternal care system, initial clinical reviews are undertaken monthly, then fortnightly from 28 to 36 weeks gestation, and then weekly from 36 weeks gestation until childbirth. These patterns of review differ around the world. The number of planned antenatal visits is a metric of health system success, and correlates with maternal and perinatal mortality. It is optimal that women be seen as close to 12 weeks gestation as possible (Neu, Duchon, and Zachariah 2015), as this sets the stage for anticipated risk and thus directs the need for community-based ongoing review and local medical review or tertiary care for complex conditions (e.g., rheumatic heart disease, history of recurrent miscarriage, management of severe congenital abnormality).

The early history of relevance to ascertaining risk is reproductive history including menstrual history, mode of pregnancy (including periods of infertility), medical history, surgical history, infection history, smoking, alcohol and illicit drug use, over-the-counter drug use, allergies, and mental health history. Family history relative to diabetes and hypertension, renal disease, bleeding or clotting tendency, pregnancy outcomes including diabetes and pre-eclampsia, and genetic diseases is critically important.

Apart from establishing the woman's medical and obstetric history and her family history, the early pregnancy visit includes a routine set of observations: blood pressure; urine testing for protein or signs of infection; weight; fetal assessment and fundal (uterine) height to establish or confirm gestational dates; checking for signs and symptoms of disease such as changes in thirst, breathlessness, palpitations, headache, lower leg swelling, vaginal bleeding, and fetal movements. Any of these positive signs or symptoms suggest a need for urgent referral for expert and/or medical review to exclude preeclampsia, diabetes, fetal growth restriction, sepsis, or other medical complications of pregnancy.

Regular fetal monitoring can include an ultrasound test at 12 weeks to determine the precise date of gestation. There is a marked uniformity of size of the early fetus in the early stages of a pregnancy that makes the anticipated date of delivery more accurate (Papageor-ghiou et al. 2014). Early ultrasound also assists with the assessment of pregnancy viability and fetal chromosomal abnormality (e.g., Down Syndrome). This is done through multiple measurements including the neck thickness of the fetus (nuchal translucency) and blood tests that indicate placental function. A glucose tolerance test may be useful in some situations for the early detection of gestational diabetes (Sweeting et al. 2018).

Regular blood tests are undertaken through pregnancy to determine infection risk to the fetus, the mother's blood count (haemoglobin, platelets, white cell count), and her iron levels. The TORCH tests are a world-wide standard for congenital infections where there is an increased risk of disability and growth restriction related to the mother carrying rubella (German measles), HIV (Human Immunodeficiency Virus), cytomegalovirus (CMV), syphilis, hepatitis B or C, or toxoplasmosis (Chung, Shin, and Lee 2018; Neu, Duchon, and Zachariah 2015).

The screening blood tests for congenital abnormalities and preeclampsia include placental growth factor (PlGF), pregnancy-associated placental protein -A (PAPP-A), and beta-human chorionic gonadotrophin (beta-HCG) (Myers et al. 2013; Sweeting et al. 2018). An individual assessment provides a risk score based on a mother's age, history, and the combination of ultra-sound and blood test results. Low-dose aspirin is now being recommended in order to reduce the chances of developing preeclampsia in a given pregnancy (Rolnik et al. 2017). Counselling women and families about the consequences of screening tests is needed. The decision to continue or terminate the pregnancy, as well as the level of care anticipated, can be based on interpretation of these measures and varies widely around the world (Chung, Shin, and Lee 2018). In places where there is a long distance between maternal care clinics and the family's home, risk assessment that allows for safe childbirth remotely would be very welcome. Given that only 78% of pregnancies around the world were attended by any health expertise in 2016, early assessment of risk is critical to improving maternal and perinatal outcomes (United Nations 2018). This rate has increased from 59% in 1990 and demonstrates that targeting health strategies can lead to improvements in outcome. "Ongoing work with the health systems in sub-Saharan Africa are required given that the rate in 2016 of skilled care was only 53 per cent of live births" (United Nations 2018).

Prevention and intervention

Early assessment of pregnancy allows health and medical staff to manage life style risks including overweight and smoking. Both have been shown to effect the rates of complications especially fetal size appropriate to the length of the pregnancy (gestational adjusted weight). Smoking has been shown to lead to reduced weight (small for gestational age, <10%ile [SGA], or intrauterine growth restriction, <3rd%ile [IUGR]) (Orzechowski and Miller 2012). Efforts to stop or reduce smoking in pregnancy are essential to improving outcomes. Alcohol can lead to fetal alcohol syndrome (FAS), whereby the baby has reduced intellectual capacity and characteristic facial features (Roozen et al. 2016). Public health interventions are targeted to reduce FAS by raising community awareness. Again there are striking differences around the globe in the effectiveness of these campaigns.

Being overweight or obese has been shown both to increase and decrease gestational adjusted baby weight (Kapadia et al. 2015), and can be related to the development of high blood pressure, diabetes, and obstructive sleep apnoea. Efforts to reduce maternal weight during pregnancy, however, are problematic and can lead to disturbances in fetal and placental growth if not managed carefully.

Vitamin supplementation has also been shown to improve outcomes and has a major health benefit. The global recommendation for folic acid to be given in the first 12 weeks of the pregnancy has rapidly and dramatically reduced the rates of spina bifida in many countries, but not all (Kancherla and Black 2018). Arguments for food fortification are still being made, and this strategy would further reduce the rates of neural tube defects (Wald, Morris, and Blakemore 2018). Inclusion of iodine in early pregnancy dietary management has been instigated to prevent developmental delay in newborns and infants (Zimmermann 2012). Advice to add vitamin D to a pregnancy diet regimen is designed to prevent complications including hypertension risk, but the benefits need to be fully elucidated (Wagner and Hollis 2018).

Calcium supplement is recommended because a low calcium diet has been associated with preeclampsia (Izumi et al. 1997). This has not been demonstrated in countries where there is adequate access to dairy, and the impact of supplemental calcium intake on future bone health is not proven (Hofmeyr and Manyame 2017).

Common medical complications of pregnancy

The commonest medical complications of pregnancy include preeclampsia, post-partum haemorrhage or clotting, and pregnancy-related bacterial infection (sepsis) (United Nations 2018). All of these conditions are common around the world and account for the majority of cases of direct maternal death and disability. Indirect deaths due to accident or suicide also figure significantly in world figures, whereby death is not caused by pregnancy *per se*, but the impact of being pregnant is a likely contributor to the event. Most of these conditions can be anticipated and, with appropriate risk management strategies including education of mothers and families, can be prevented or treated.

World figures of antenatal care and monitoring clearly demonstrate an improvement in maternal and perinatal outcome with increased pregnancy surveillance and skilled birth attendants. Thus, the majority of mortal conditions in pregnancy can be prevented. In 2015, the global maternal mortality ratio stood at 216 maternal deaths per 100,000 live births (United Nations 2018). Estonia boasts a maternal death rate of 2 per 100,000 live births, the lowest in the world, and sub-Saharan Africa (250 per 100,000 live births) still has rates well above millennial targets (WHO 2018). The pregnancy evaluation strategy also allows a global focus on birth outcomes. In 2015, the global neonatal mortality rate was 19 deaths per 1,000 live births, a decrease from 31 deaths per 1,000 live births in 2000. Neonatal mortality is highest in Central and Southern Asia and in sub-Saharan Africa, at 29 deaths per 1,000 live births in each of those regions in 2015 (United Nations 2018).

That effective action can be taken is best demonstrated by the improvements seen in 2013 when the maternal mortality rates declined to 50% of those seen in 2000 (WHO 2018) and by 44% for mortality of children under five years (United Nations 2018). One critical impact of improving perinatal survival is on number of pregnancies per woman. As the perinatal death rate declines, the fewer pregnancies a family needs to sustain its future (Parikh et al. 2010). Decreasing the number of pregnancies a woman has can positively impact her health and therefore her life and economic productivity.

Other maternal complications that are specific to pregnancy include iron deficiency anaemia, cholestasis (liver disease), and gestational diabetes. Diabetes can have great impact on preparation for childbirth, the outcomes of the pregnancy itself, the long-term development of the baby, and the long-term health of the mother. The commonest complications of pregnancy will now be discussed in some detail.

Hypertension in pregnancy

The commonest complication of pregnancy is high blood pressure in its various forms. The standard definitions include two conditions related purely to pregnancy (i.e., gestational hypertension and preeclampsia) and two related to long-term blood pressure elevation (i.e., chronic hypertension and superimposed preeclampsia in the setting of chronic hypertension) (Lowe et al. 2015).

From early in pregnancy, ideally before 12 weeks gestation, blood pressure is measured as part of routine antenatal care. The normal pattern of blood pressure is a decrease with a nadir at 24 weeks gestation (Tkachenko, Shchekochikhin, and Schrier 2014). This natural decline is a function of the hormone balance, which provides a high blood flow to the developing placental bed and thus enhances nutrient supply to the fetus via placental exchange. The decrease in blood pressure also facilitates increased renal blood flow, which enhances renal clearance of toxins from the blood stream. The increase in blood flow to the brain can lead to headaches, and to the skin, an increased sense of warmth. Another consequence of this decrease in blood pressure is an activation of salt and water retention whereby there is an expansion of plasma volume and activation of red cell production to provide increased improved oxygen-carrying capacity. These changes are a result of placental hormones and stimulation of maternal adrenal hormones, and are experienced by women as syncope (fainting spells) and dizziness.

Hypertension in pregnancy is largely asymptomatic, which is why blood pressure (BP) should be screened at each antenatal visit. The criteria for high BP in pregnancy are widely debated with the role of home monitoring, 24-hour monitoring, time-limited clinic readings (for 2–4 hours), and single clinic-visit readings still uncertain. The best agreed criteria are that, if the BP is above 140 and/or 90 mmHg on two readings four hours or more apart, the readings are then classified as hypertension in pregnancy. These numbers are substantially higher than the gestation-adjusted measures that reflect the natural vasodilation (decreased blood pressure) in normal pregnant women. The impact of any increase of 25 mmHg or more above the systolic BP and/or 15 mmHg above the diastolic BP should not be underestimated. It is important that the woman understands the numbers and the need for and impact of blood pressure readings. This impact might mean more frequent antenatal visits, commencing drug treatment, and overall, an escalation in the support needed to plan the delivery.

Severe hypertension, increased to above 160 mmHg in the systolic reading and >100 mmHg in the diastolic, constitutes a medical emergency. The woman should be reviewed immediately by the highest level of medical care available, which can include transfer to a tertiary hospital where medications (e.g., antihypertensives, magnesium sulphate) can be administered and where induced childbirth is possible and a premature baby supported if necessary.

To standardise BP readings in pregnancy, devices themselves are validated and considerable work is going into developing devices that are simple to use by women at home and that signal a problem with a traffic light system (Stergiou et al. 2018). Many devices that are cheap and purchasable on the open market are not valid or safe to use in pregnancy. Some current work has established the home normal readings and provides guidance about when to seek advice or medical help.

The risk factors for high blood pressure in pregnancy include chronic hypertension, renal disease, clotting disorders, congenitally abnormal fetus, autoimmune conditions (e.g., systemic lupus erythematosus, thyroid disease) (Lowe et al. 2015). Women with assisted reproductive technology pregnancies (IVF) and multiple gestations (twins, triplets) are at increased risk. Women are assessed at their first pregnancy review for any increased risk for preeclampsia. This includes a blood pressure reading and, in most countries, a urine test to exclude prior renal disease. The timing of the pregnancy is assessed against the first day of the last menstrual period and, if available, an ultrasound performed before 12 weeks gestation. The mother's personal and family history is important here, as any prior time of high BP, even if on the oral contraceptive pill, classifies a mother with chronic hypertension for the purpose of pregnancy monitoring and, therefore, as a high-risk pregnancy.

Women with short cohabitation time with her partner or a new partner are considered at risk for preeclampsia (Parikh et al. 2010). Some related factors could be considered targets for public health intervention, particularly in cultural contexts where younger women are expected or plan to have an immediate family after finding a partner (Hawkey, Ussher, and Perz 2018). The impact of age on risk for preeclampsia is variable; developed countries show no impact in adolescents (Garner et al. 2018), and others show an impact of maternal age on the likelihood of premature birth and or small for gestational age fetus. At the other end of the age spectrum, one study showed that women who wait ten years or more to have another pregnancy increase their risk to that of a first pregnancy (3–5%) (Cormick et al. 2016); the delay could be due to a possible change in partner, a known risk factor for preeclampsia.

For women who are already on medications to control for elevated BP, a change to medications that are safe and effective in pregnancy may need to occur (Webster et al. 2017). Medications are carefully monitored for safety to the growing fetus and are chosen depending on suitability for the mother. Most of these medication choices are relatively "old-fashioned" in order to have a body of evidence and experience that they are safe in human use. There is no perfect treatment, as some of the medications can make asthma worse or increase the chances of depression as side effects. Safe choices include alphamethyldopa, clonidine, hydralazine, and some of the non-selective beta-blockers. Researchers continue to monitor the types of medications that can be used and their safety in preventing complications of pregnancy (Magee et al. 2015). Safety and efficacy of BP medication treatment require a high degree of clinical precision.

Aspirin is increasingly used to prevent preeclampsia in women deemed at high risk. This is based on a recent large clinical trial in which women at higher risk were given aspirin 150 mg at night from before 16 weeks of gestation. This reduced the preeclampsia rate from 4.6% to 1.8% (Rolnik et al. 2017). Askie et al. (2007) analysed the data from multiple clinical trials and a benefit of aspirin was found in most groups (including women with kidney disease). The impact of prevention strategies had the strongest benefit in developing countries, where the frequency of preeclampsia is higher and where care is limited, and should be carefully considered in any analysis of a local response. Where some countries have only four antenatal visits per pregnancy (e.g., Malawi), the importance of that initial visit cannot be underestimated. However, if prior history of hypertension or renal disease and family history of hypertension are sufficiently robust, an argument for preventive treatment can be made. The decisions about medication use as a risk management strategy for pregnant women are complex and, in part, justify the assessment and resourcing of high risk clinics around the globe.

Women with increase in BP are screened for the development of preeclampsia, the hypertensive disorder of pregnancy with the worst outcomes. It is most usually identified by the appearance of protein in the urine, detected on a dipstick test or by boiling the urine. A one-off urine sample can be sent to the laboratory to measure the protein content (Waugh et al. 2017). There are also standardised blood tests that help decide who has preeclampsia and how urgently they need to be treated and/or give birth.

Eclampsia, or pregnancy seizure, occurs in around 1.5% of women with preeclampsia. Although preeclampsia rates are declining, the rate of seizure in those with preeclampsia is static or increasing in some countries (Thornton et al. 2013). Prevention of the seizure by the widespread use of magnesium sulphate was justified after completion of the MAGPIE study (Altman et al. 2002). That was one of the largest, multinational, clinical trials conducted on preeclampsia, with a major contribution from African countries; not only were seizures prevented, but the reduction in maternal mortality was powerfully demonstrated. This is now widespread common practice, as magnesium sulphate is a cheap drug, although its administration is not without complications and it requires careful and skilled monitoring (Saha et al. 2017).

The preventable complications of preeclampsia include: acute kidney injury; liver rupture; stroke (intracerebral haemorrhage); seizure (eclampsia); postpartum haemorrhage; small baby; extreme prematurity with its attendant risk of brain development, sight, and hearing; other prematurity with its risk of infection, jaundice, and respiratory failure, as well as intracerebral haemorrhage; death of the fetus *in utero*.

The impact of preeclampsia on a woman's future reproductive potential and plans has received little investigation. The dire consequences of maternal death and stroke is a family left without the mother of a newborn baby and altered ability to raise that child and their siblings. The impact of excessive bleeding (via disseminated intravascular coagulation, DIC), which can accompany preeclampsia, can include hysterectomy, thereby permanently limiting a woman's capacity for another pregnancy. Given that preeclampsia occurs in the first pregnancy in 75% of cases, the impact on decisions about planning future pregnancies can be profound.

The consequence of most preeclampsia after childbirth is immediate and total recovery from the events themselves. However, knowledge about the impact of preeclampsia on future cardiovascular health has started to be identified (Bellamy et al. 2007). The most severe cases, notably those women who give birth before 34 weeks of gestation because of features of severe preeclampsia, are the most likely to have future events, which include renal disease, stroke, and cardiac disease, and are related to earlier onset of hypertension than those women with a normotensive outcome. Women who have had preeclampsia are more likely to have hypertension in their mid-40s as compared with the mid-50s for women with a healthy pregnancy (Lind, Hennessy, and McLean 2014). This is tempered by other reproduction events including use of the oral contraceptive pill (OCP) (Chiu et al. 2012), breastfeeding (Lupton, Chiu, Lujic, et al. 2013), time at birth of the first child (Lind, Hennessy, and Chiu 2015), and the presence of any of the hypertensive disorders of pregnancy. These interactions can delay the onset of later-life hypertension for years. Studies by Lupton and colleagues of the blood vessels in the eye (retinal vessels) show a narrower vessel structure (arteries and veins) throughout pregnancy compared with healthy pregnant women (Lupton, Chiu, Hodgson, et al. 2013).

Post-Partum Haemorrhage (PPH)

The commonest cause of bleeding immediately after delivery relates to the shape and contraction of the uterus after childbirth. The raw inner surface of the uterus, especially from the site of the placenta, has the potential to bleed torrentially unless the uterus con-tracts down on itself. This process is facilitated in modern obstetric services by the injec-tion of syntocinon (a synthetic hormone), given in the upper thigh or vein, at the time of placental delivery (Adnan et al. 2018). Since the introduction of this agent in standard practice, the rate of PPH has reduced to ~20% of childbirths, with 5/1000 categorised as severe.

The uterus can be irritated into contraction by rubbing vigorously on the top surface through the abdominal wall, and attending staff are trained to undertake this manoeuvre. Injections directly into the uterus can help to control blood loss (Alalfy et al. 2018). In extreme cases, the blood vessels that supply the uterus need to be blocked, and, if the bleed-ing continues, the uterus may need to be removed by a trained surgeon or equivalent.

Medical causes of bleeding contribute to morbidity and mortality from post-partum haemorrhage (Kramer et al. 2013). This includes preeclampsia where women can develop disseminated intravascular coagulation (DIC). The mainstay of treatment of preeclampsia is with early birth before DIC develops to prevent this complication. When blood product replacement is required, there is a high degree of cost and monitoring. Other rare haemato-logical conditions such as idiopathic thrombocytopenic purpura (ITP) are autoimmune con-ditions that effect women of child-bearing age. Medical stabilisation and planning for childbirth are key requirements for a safe pregnancy outcome in these cases.

Clotting in pregnancy

The sudden and devastating effect of blood clot from the lower legs travelling to the lungs (pulmonary embolus) accounts for around 9% of all maternal deaths. These are generally more difficult to predict than other medical complications of pregnancy, but several risk factors have been identified: Being overweight or obese, prior pelvic surgery, including caesarean section, smoking, older age, and past history of clotting. Paradoxically, events that lead to early excessive bleeding, including pelvic surgery and blood product replace-ment, are risk factors for subsequent clots (Thurn, Wikman, and Lindqvist 2018). These risks are assessed and a plan to give injectable medication (low molecular weight heparin [LMWH]) to prevent a clot is now a standard of care for those in the highest risk groups (Fogerty 2018). LMWH is only active in the mother (it does not pass across the placenta), and thereby reduces the risk of clotting in the mother without an impact on the risk of bleeding in the fetus or the potential development of congenital malformations from drug treatment.

The other significant clotting complication of pregnancy is that associated with stroke risk in women with valvular heart disease. Anticoagulation medication is required through-out the pregnancy, and the timing and decisions about childbirth need to be carefully planned so as to diminish the impact of postpartum haemorrhage.

Pregnancy-related bacterial infection (sepsis)

International comparison of rates of pregnancy sepsis and sepsis mortality help us understand the impact of a health system focussed on its youngest and most vulnerable. This shows rates as high as 38% of maternal deaths in sub-Saharan Africa and the lowest rates in Europe as 1/100,000. These data refer to bacterial infections, which impact recovery from childbirth and termination of pregnancy. In Africa, these bacterial infections are comorbid with HIV/AIDS in 53% of cases. Other contributors are pneumonia (25%), tuberculosis (8.3%), and meningitis (6.3%) (Seale et al. 2009).

Prolonged ruptured membranes, prolonged labour (longer than 24 hours), lack of sterile technique in management, and poor access to antibiotics have long been seen as major preventable causes of maternal death. In fact, the germ theory of infection was discovered after the unintended infection of women after childbirth was identified as the commonest cause of their demise (Noakes et al. 2008). Hand washing has saved many lives by preventing the spread of life-threatening bacteria. Safe time in labour and duration of membrane rupture are critical to identifying those women who should be treated with antibiotics to prevent maternal death (Bonet et al. 2018).

The other common bacterial infection seen in pregnancy is urinary tract infection (Szweda and Marcin 2016). This is screened for in early pregnancy by dipstick testing and then, if necessary, culturing the urine. The presence of a strong history of previous infections in the mother should indicate a need for consideration of early childhood reflux renal disease (rates of 4–20/1000) and its associated renal injury (glomerular sclerosis), which are strong risk factors for preeclampsia. Antenatal screening for urinary tract infection identifies treatable organisms and their sensitivity to antibiotics, and the possibility of preventing premature contractions and birth as a consequence of bladder or kidney infection. The risk of a urinary tract infection is not measurably greater in pregnancy, but the likelihood of an upper tract infection (pyelonephritis) is increased 30-fold, and the complication of premature birth is real and can be prevented with early and appropriate treatment with an antibiotic. All antibiotics carry classifications of safety for the fetus (Category A: safest, Category B: probably safe in women, Category C: known to cause a reversible effect on the fetus, and Categories D and X: unsafe in pregnancy); the safest choices should be made in every event in every pregnancy.

Toward the end of the pregnancy, vaginal swabs are taken to identify those with Group B streptococcus colonisation. This can cause infections in the mother, but bacteria can also be transferred to the baby and lead to newborn meningitis and pneumonia. Antibiotics given at the time of childbirth dramatically decrease this risk (Darlow et al. 2015). The balance of arguments about maternal treatment and reduced risk need to be offset by the arguments about appropriate use of antibiotics with increasing global antibiotic resistance and better knowledge about the impact of antibiotic use on microbiome function and potential epigenetic effects.

Pregnancy-related viral infection

The common viral infections in pregnancy vary widely around the globe. Usual antenatal care screens for hepatitis B and C, toxoplasmosis, cytomegalovirus, syphilis, HIV, herpes, and rubella (German Measles). These are often referred to as TORCH screening (Chung, Shin, and Lee 2018; Neu, Duchon, and Zachariah 2015). New viral infections arise with dramatic effects on the fetus. Zika virus is one such example; it arose in Polynesia and gained penetration in northeast South America in 2013–2017 (Khaiboullina et al.). A worldwide effort to discover the cause of congenital microcephaly (small brain and head and associated mental retardation) and develop a vaccine for those women at risk was instigated, and the cause and treatments were discovered very quickly (Mehand et al. 2018).

The immune changes that result in the mother being able to grow the tissue foreign to her body (placenta and baby) are called immunosuppression. These changes are likely to contribute to increased susceptibility to some infections and, in the case of influenza, were no doubt contributing factors to the high rates of mortality due to the swine influenza (H1N1) epidemic in 2009 (Pebody et al. 2010). Other infections carry the risk of vertical transmission from mother to the baby (across the placenta) or through the birth process. Some of these can be treated (hepatitis C), some inform the mode of birth (e.g., active herpes infection requires caesarean delivery), and some require treatment of the baby after birth (HIV). Some are identifiable as population risks (hepatitis B) with consequences for the newborn's lifelong liver health (Sookoian 2006).

Diabetes in pregnancy

As obesity rates increase around the globe, the impact on pregnancy is manifest by gestational diabetes. Gestational diabetes is a metabolic condition whereby there is an increase in circulating glucose in the mother to provide caloric availability to the fetus due to insulin resistance created by the placenta. The increased glucose availability leads to bigger babies (macrosomia), which itself leads to complications in the childbirth process, and the possibility of later life metabolic complications including diabetes. Considerable work is being undertaken to determine the exact measures of sugar concentration in the mother's blood that should trigger a diagnosis of gestational diabetes and to what extent treatment should be offered (Martis et al. 2018). Treatment could include sensible dietary advice regarding intake of excess sugar-containing foods and drinks, but could also include insulin injections with very tight blood sugar targets and reporting, which can have a major impact on the pregnancy and its management. The risk of subsequent non-pregnancy-related type-2 diabetes is well described (Tobias 2018).

There are increasing numbers of women around the world with pre-existing diabetes, mostly type-2, who enter the pregnancy with diabetes management plans in place (Murphy 2018). This is largely due to pre-existing obesity and positive family history, and public health campaigns are increasingly addressing this global epidemic (Ali et al. 2017). Type-1 diabetes, or juvenile diabetes, is now easily survivable, and pregnancy planning is required and complicated. The use of continuous glucose monitoring and pump-delivered insulin are often necessary and provide a high level of medical complexity in managing these pregnancies. This management intensifies in the setting of other illnesses (e.g., infection), where the risk of diabetic ketoacidosis is increased in pregnancy and which can lead to maternal and fetal death. Exquisite management of glucose metabolism is required at the time of childbirth, to minimise maternal complications and decrease the risk to the newborn baby due to low or high blood sugar levels.

Overlap syndromes between diabetes and hypertension are implied by a common set of risk factors, such as obesity. Prediction strategies often work for both gestational-related conditions (Sweeting et al. 2018), and treatments such as metformin appear to diminish the complications of both conditions (Alqudah et al. 2018).

Heart disease in pregnancy

The commonest type of heart disease in pregnant women is rheumatic. This is a common disease in developing countries as a result of overcrowding, skin and throat infections, and poverty (Karthikeyan and Guilherme 2018). It is seen in indigenous populations where living conditions do not mirror those of more affluent sectors of society (Vaughan et al. 2018). This association underpins the principle of social determinants of health, where many social, economic, and historical factors contribute to poorer health outcomes (Vaughan et al. 2018). Rheumatic heart disease leads to valve problems, including valvular narrowing (stenosis), whereby there is limited capacity for the heart to adjust to the increasing volume demands of pregnancy. In the latter parts of pregnancy, heart failure (breathlessness) and arrhythmia (palpitations) occur and can lead to significant maternal ill health, stillbirth, and maternal death (Mocumbi et al. 2018). Considerable effort to identify and treat rheumatic fever (to prevent the heart disease consequences), to treat the social determinants of poor health (poverty and overcrowding), and to identify and treat early heart disease with close monitoring in pregnancy and early referral to a tertiary centre, will result in a decrease in the death and disability from heart disease in pregnancy.

Other common cardiac conditions seen in pregnancy include arrhythmias and cardiomyopathy. Postpartum cardiomyopathy is a rare but devastating condition that may lead to intractable heart failure and the need for a heart transplant (Asad et al. 2018).

Liver disease in pregnancy

Apart from the hepatitis infections described above, there are rare and life-threatening liver complications of pregnancy. These include cholestasis of pregnancy, which increases the rate of fetal loss (Mays 2010), and acute fatty liver of pregnancy, which increases risk of maternal death (Wu et al. 2018). These rare complications are best managed in a tertiary centre with expertise in complex medical management. The monitoring of liver disease in pregnancy requires frequent blood testing and monitoring of fetal growth and well-being. Timing of childbirth requires a strong multidisciplinary team.

Conclusion

Pregnancy brings a woman and her family in direct contact with their country's health system. Management of that pregnancy provides an opportunity to determine the immediate outcomes of the pregnancy for the family, the future health of the baby and the mother, and these events' impact on the health of families and communities. The infant's growth and development and the need for early medical or educational intervention can be determined by assessment of the events of the pregnancy. Similarly, the chance to offer families a safe and predictable outcome has health benefits across the whole family unit, as well as for society more generally.

Most maternal deaths can be prevented, and the impact of a focused approach to maternal health through the UN Sustainable Development Goals not only impacts the health and well-being of a family, but indicates the success and impact of a health system that is working well for all of its citizens. Taking account of and impacting the social determinants of health are critical for improving the health of all women wherever they live and work.

References

Adnan, N., Conlan-Trant, R., McCormick, C., Boland, F., and Murphy, D. J. 2018. "Intramuscular versus intravenous oxytocin to prevent postpartum haemorrhage at vaginal delivery: Randomised controlled trial." *British Medical Journal* 362:k3546.

Alalfy, M., Lasheen, Y., Hossam Elshenoufy, I. M., Elzahaby, H. W., Kaleem, H., Sawah, E., Azkalani, A., Saber, W., and Rashwan, A. S. S. A. 2018. "The efficacy of intrauterine misoprostol during cesarean section in prevention of primary PPH, a randomized controlled trial." *The Journal of Maternal-Fetal & Neonatal Medicine*: Sep 26:1–7, doi: 10.1080/14767058.2018.1519796.

Ali, M. K., Siegel, K. R., Chandrasekar, R., Tandon, R., Montoya, P. A., Mbanya, J. C., Chan, J., Zhang, P., and Narayan, K. M. 2017. "Diabetes: An update on the pandemic and potential solutions." In *Cardiovascular, respiratory, and related disorders*, edited by Prabhakaran, D., Anand, S., Gaziano, T. A., Mbanya, J. C., Wu, Y., and Nugent, R. Washington (DC): The International Bank for Reconstruction and Development/The World Bank.

Alqudah, A., McKinley, M. C., McNally, R., Graham, U., Watson, C. J., Lyons, T. J., and McClements, L. 2018. "Risk of pre-eclampsia in women taking metformin: A systematic review and meta-analysis." *Diabetic Medicine* 35 (2):160–172.

Altman, D., Carroli, G., Duley, L., Farrell, B., Moodley, J., Neilson, J., Smith, D., and Group Magpie Trial Collaboration 2002. "Do women with pre-eclampsia, and their babies, benefit from magnesium sulphate? The Magpie Trial: A randomised placebo-controlled trial." *Lancet* 359 (9321):1877–1890.

Asad, Z., Abideen, U., Maiwand, M., Farah, F., and Dasari, T. W. 2018. "Peripartum cardiomyopathy: A systematic review of the literature." *Clinical Cardiology* 41 (5):693–697.

Askie, L. M., Duley, L., Henderson-Smart, D. J., and Stewart, L. A. 2007. "Antiplatelet agents for prevention of pre-eclampsia: A meta-analysis of individual patient data." *The Lancet* 369 (9575):1791–1798.

Baccari, M. C. and Calamai, F. 2004. "Relaxin: New functions for an old peptide." *Current Protein and Peptide Science* 5 (1):9–18.

Banerjee, R. R. 2018. "Piecing together the puzzle of pancreatic islet adaptation in pregnancy." *Annals of the New York Academy of Sciences* 1411 (1):120–139.

Bellamy, L., Casas, J.-P., Hingorani, A. D., and Williams, D. J. 2007. "Pre-eclampsia and risk of cardiovascular disease and cancer in later life: Systematic review and meta-analysis." *British Medical Journal* 335 (7627):974.

Bonet, M., Souza, J. P., Abalos, E., Fawole, B., Knight, M., Kouanda, S., Lumbiganon, P., Nabhan, A., Nadisauskiene, R., Brizuela, V., and Metin Gülmezoglu, A. 2018. "The global maternal sepsis study and awareness campaign (GLOSS): Study protocol." *Reproductive Health* 15 (1):16.

Budenhofer, B. K., Ditsch, N., Jeschke, U., Gärtner, R., and Toth, B. 2013. "Thyroid (dys)function in normal and disturbed pregnancy." *Archives of Gynecology and Obstetrics* 287 (1):1–7.

Bulletins-Obstetrics, Committee on Practice 2018. "ACOG Practice Bulletin No. 189: Nausea and vomiting of pregnancy." *Obstetrics & Gynecology* 131 (1):e15–e30.

Cameron, E. L. 2014. "Pregnancy and olfaction: A review." *Frontiers in Psychology* 5 (67), doi:10.3389/fpsyg.2014.00067.

Chiu, C. L., Lujic, S., Thornton, C., O'Loughlin, A., Makris, A., Hennessy, A., and Lind, J. M. 2012. "Menopausal hormone therapy is associated with having high blood pressure in postmenopausal women: Observational cohort study." *PLOS ONE* 7 (7):e40260.

Chung, M. H., Shin, C. O., and Lee, J. 2018. "TORCH (toxoplasmosis, rubella, cytomegalovirus, and herpes simplex virus) screening of small for gestational age and intrauterine growth restricted neonates: Efficacy study in a single institute in Korea." *Korean Journal of Pediatrics* 61 (4):114–120.

Conrad, K. P. and Davison, J. M. 2014. "The renal circulation in normal pregnancy and preeclampsia: Is there a place for relaxin?" *American Journal of Physiology-Renal Physiology* 306 (10):F1121–F1135.

Cormick, G., Betrán, A. P., Ciapponi, A., Hall, D. R., and Hofmeyr, G. J., on behalf of the Calcium Pre-Eclampsia Study Group 2016. "Inter-pregnancy interval and risk of recurrent pre-eclampsia: Systematic review and meta-analysis." *Reproductive Health* 13 (1): 83.

Darlow, B., Campbell, N., Austin, N., Chin, A., Grigg, C., Skidmore, C., Voss, L., Walls, T., Wise, M., and Werno, A. 2015. "The prevention of early-onset neonatal group B streptococcus infection: New Zealand Consensus Guidelines 2014." *The New Zealand Medical Journal*, 128 (1425):69–76.

Deans, Z. C., Allen, S., Jenkins, L., Farrah Khawaja, R. J., Hastings, K. M., Patton, S. J., Sistermans, E. A., and Chitty, L. S. 2017. "Recommended practice for laboratory reporting of non-invasive prenatal testing of trisomies 13, 18 and 21: A consensus opinion." *Prenatal Diagnosis* 37 (7):699–704.

Dietz, P., Watson, E. D., Sattler, M. C., Ruf, W., Titze, S., and Mireille, V. P. 2016. "The influence of physical activity during pregnancy on maternal, fetal or infant heart rate variability: A systematic review." *BMC Pregnancy and Childbirth* 16 (1):326.

East, C., Conway, K., Pollock, W., Frawley, N., and Brennecke, S. 2011. "Women's experiences of pre-eclampsia: Australian action on preeclampsia survey of women and their confidants." *Journal of Pregnancy*, ID 375653, doi.org/10.1155/2011/375653.

Fogerty, A. E. 2018. "Management of venous thromboembolism in pregnancy." *Current Treatment Options in Cardiovascular Medicine* 20 (8):69.

Garner, A. J., Robertson, A., Thornton, C., Lee, G., Makris, A., Middleton, S., Sullivan, C., and Hennessy, A. 2018. "Adolescent perinatal outcomes in South West Sydney, Australia." *Mayo Clinic Proceedings: Innovations, Quality & Outcomes* 2 (1):10–15.

Haug, E. B., Horn, J., Markovitz, A. R., Fraser, A., Macdonald-Wallis, C., Tilling, K., Romundstad, P. R., Rich-Edwards, J. W., and Åsvold, B. O. 2018. "The impact of parity on life course blood pressure trajectories: The HUNT study in Norway." *European Journal of Epidemiology* 33 (8):751–761.

Hawkey, A., Ussher, J. M., and Perz, J. 2018. ""If you don't have a baby, you can't be in our culture": Migrant and refugee women's experiences and constructions of fertility and fertility control." *Women's Reproductive Health* 5 (2):75–98.

Hofmeyr, G. J. and Manyame, S. 2017. "Calcium supplementation commencing before or early in pregnancy, or food fortification with calcium, for preventing hypertensive disorders of pregnancy." *Cochrane Database of Systematic Reviews*, 9, CD011192, doi: 10.1002/14651858.CD011192.pub2.

Hyde, K. J. and Schust, D. J. 2016. "Immunologic challenges of human reproduction: An evolving story." *Fertility and Sterility* 106 (3):499–510.

Ireland, M. L. and Ott, S. M. 2000. "The effects of pregnancy on the musculoskeletal system." *Clinical Orthopaedics and Related Research®* 372:169–179.

Izci-Balserak, B., Keenan, B. T., Corbitt, C., Staley, B., Perlis, M., and Pien, G. W. 2018. "Changes in sleep characteristics and breathing parameters during sleep in early and late pregnancy." *Journal of Clinical Sleep Medicine* 14 (07):1161–1168.

Izumi, A., Minakami, H., Kuwata, T., and Sato, I. 1997. "Calcium-to-creatinine ratio in spot urine samples in early pregnancy and its relation to the development of preeclampsia." *Metabolism – Clinical and Experimental* 46 (10):1107–1108.

Kancherla, V. and Black, R. E. 2018. "Historical perspective on folic acid and challenges in estimating global prevalence of neural tube defects." *Annals of the New York Academy of Sciences* 1414 (1):20–30.

Kapadia, M. Z., Park, C. K., Beyene, J., Giglia, L., Maxwell, C., and McDonald, S. D. 2015. "Weight loss instead of weight gain within the guidelines in obese women during pregnancy: A systematic review and meta-analysis of maternal and infant outcomes." *PLOS ONE* 10 (7):e0132650.

Karthikeyan, G. and Guilherme, L. 2018. "Acute rheumatic fever." *The Lancet* 392 (10142):161–174.

Khaiboullina, S., Uppal, T., Martynova, E., Rizvanov, A., Baranwal, M., and Verma, S. C. 2018. "History of ZIKV infections in India and management of disease outbreaks." *Frontiers in Microbiology* 9 (2126), doi:10.3389/fmicb.2018.02126.

Kourtis, A. P., Read, J. S., and Jamieson, D. J. 2014. "Pregnancy and infection." *New England Journal of Medicine* 370 (23):2211–2218.

Kramer, M. S., Berg, C., Abenhaim, H., Dahhou, M., Rouleau, J., Mehrabadi, A., and Joseph, K. S. 2013. "Incidence, risk factors, and temporal trends in severe postpartum hemorrhage." *American Journal of Obstetrics and Gynecology* 209 (5):449.e1–449.e7.

Lind, J. M., Hennessy, A., and Chiu, C. L. 2015. "Association between a woman's age at first birth and high blood pressure." *Medicine* 94 (16):e697.

Lind, J. M., Hennessy, A., and Mark, M. 2014. "Cardiovascular disease in women: The significance of hypertension and gestational diabetes during pregnancy." *Current Opinion in Cardiology* 29 (5):447–453.

Lowe, S. A., Bowyer, L., Karin Lust, L. P., McMahon, M., Morton, R. A., North, M. P., and Said, J. M. 2015. "SOMANZ guidelines for the management of hypertensive disorders of pregnancy 2014." *Australian and New Zealand Journal of Obstetrics and Gynaecology* 55 (5):e1–e29.

Lupton, S. J., Chiu, C. L., Hodgson, L. A. B., Tooher, J., Lujic, S., Ogle, R., Wong, T. Y., Hennessy, A., and Lind, J. M. 2013. "Temporal changes in retinal microvascular caliber and blood pressure during pregnancy." *Hypertension* 61 (4):880–885.

Lupton, S. J., Chiu, C. L., Lujic, S., Hennessy, A., and Lind, J. M. 2013. "Association between parity and breastfeeding with maternal high blood pressure." *American Journal of Obstetrics and Gynecology* 208 (6):454.e1–7.

Magee, L. A., von Dadelszen, P., Rey, E., Ross, S., Asztalos, E., Murphy, K. E., Menzies, J., Sanchez, J., Singer, J., Gafni, A., Gruslin, A., Helewa, M., Hutton, E., Lee, S. K., Lee, T., Logan, A. G.,

Ganzevoort, W., Welch, R., Thornton, J. G., and Moutquin, J.-M. 2015. "Less-tight versus tight control of hypertension in pregnancy." *New England Journal of Medicine* 372 (5):407–417.

March of Dimes 2006. "Global report on birth defects: The hidden toll of dying and disabled children." White Plains, NY: Author. Retrieved from www.marchofdimes.org/materials/global-report-on-birth -defects-the-hidden-toll-of-dying-and-disabled-children-wall-chart.pdf.

Martis, R., Crowther, C. A., Shepherd, E., Alsweiler, J., Downie, M. R., and Brown, J. 2018. "Treatments for women with gestational diabetes mellitus: An overview of Cochrane systematic reviews." *Cochrane Database of Systematic Reviews* 8, CD012327, doi: 10.1002/14651858.CD012327.pub2.

Mays, J. K. 2010. "The active management of intrahepatic cholestasis of pregnancy." *Current Opinion in Obstetrics and Gynecology* 22 (2):100–103.

Mehand, M. S., Al-Shorbaji, F., Millett, P., and Murgue, B. 2018. "The WHO R&D Blueprint: 2018 review of emerging infectious diseases requiring urgent research and development efforts." *Antiviral Research* 159:63–67.

Mocumbi, A. O., Jamal, K. K. F., Mbakwem, A., Shung-King, M., and Sliwa, K. 2018. "The Pan-African Society of Cardiology position paper on reproductive healthcare for women with rheumatic heart." *Cardiovascular Journal of Africa* 29:1–10.

Murphy, H. R. 2018. "Intensive glycemic treatment during Type 1 diabetes pregnancy: A story of (mostly) sweet success!" *Diabetes Care* 41 (8):1563–1571.

Myers, J. E., Kenny, L. C., McCowan, L. M. E., Chan, E. H. Y., Dekker, G. A., Poston, L., Simpson, N. A. B., and North, R. A. 2013. "Angiogenic factors combined with clinical risk factors to predict preterm pre-eclampsia in nulliparous women: a predictive test accuracy study." *BJOG: An International Journal of Obstetrics and Gynaecology* 120 (10):1215–1223.

Neu, N., Duchon, J., and Zachariah, P. 2015. "TORCH Infections." *Clinics in Perinatology* 42 (1):77–103.

Niebyl, J. R. 2010. "Nausea and vomiting in pregnancy." *The New England Journal of Medicine* 363 (16):1544–1550.

Noakes, T. D., Borresen, J., Hew-Butler, T., Lambert, M. I., and Jordaan, E. 2008. "Semmelweis and the aetiology of puerperal sepsis 160 years on: An historical review." *Epidemiology and Infection* 136 (1):1–9.

Orzechowski, K. M., and Miller, R. C. 2012. "Common respiratory issues in ambulatory obstetrics." *Clinical Obstetrics and Gynecology* 55 (3):798–809.

Papageorghiou, A. T., Ohuma, E. O., Altman, D. G., Todros, T., Ismail, L. C., Ann Lambert, Y. A., Jaffer, E. B., Gravett, M. G., Manorama Purwar, J., Noble, A., Ruyan Pang, C. G., Victora, F. C., Barros, M. C., Salomon, L. J., Bhutta, Z. A., Kennedy, S. H., and Villar, J. 2014. "International standards for fetal growth based on serial ultrasound measurements: The Fetal Growth Longitudinal Study of the INTERGROWTH-21st Project." *The Lancet* 384 (9946):869–879.

Parikh, N. I., Cnattingius, S., Dickman, P. W., Mittleman, M. A., Ludvigsson, J. F., and Ingelsson, E. 2010. "Parity and risk of later-life maternal cardiovascular disease." *American Heart Journal* 159 (2):215–221.e6.

Pebody, R. G., McLean, E., Zhao, H., Cleary, P., Bracebridge, S., Foster, K., Charlett, A., Hardelid, P., Waight, P., Ellis, J., Bermingham, A., Zambon, M., Evans, B., Salmon, R., McMenamin, J., Smyth, B., Catchpole, M., and Watson, J. M. 2010. "Pandemic influenza A (H1N1) 2009 and mortality in the United Kingdom: Risk factors for death, April 2009 to March 2010." *Eurosurveillance* 15 (20):19571.

Rolnik, D. L., Wright, D., Poon, L. C., O'Gorman, N., Syngelaki, A., de Paco Matallana, C., Akolekar, R., Cicero, S., Janga, D., Singh, M., Molina, F. S., Persico, N., Jani, J. C., Plasencia, W., Papaioannou, G., Tenenbaum-Gavish, K., Meiri, H., Gizurarson, S., Maclagan, K., and Nicolaides, K. H. 2017. "Aspirin versus placebo in pregnancies at high risk for preterm preeclampsia." *New England Journal of Medicine* 377 (7):613–622.

Roozen, S., Peters, G.-J. Y., Kok, G., Townend, D., Nijhuis, J., and Curfs, L. 2016. "Worldwide prevalence of fetal alcohol spectrum disorders: A systematic literature review including meta-analysis." *Alcoholism: Clinical and Experimental Research* 40 (1):18–32.

Roy, N. B. A. and Pavord, S. 2018. "The management of anaemia and haematinic deficiencies in pregnancy and post-partum." *Transfusion Medicine* 28 (2):107–116.

Saha, P. K., Kaur, J., Goel, P., Kataria, S., Tandon, R., and Saha, L. 2017. "Safety and efficacy of low dose intramuscular magnesium sulphate (MgSO4) compared to intravenous regimen for treatment of eclampsia." *Journal of Obstetrics and Gynaecology Research* 43 (10):1543–1549.

Seale, A. C., Michael Mwaniki, C. R., Newton, J. C., and Berkley, J. A. 2009. "Maternal and early onset neonatal bacterial sepsis: Burden and strategies for prevention in sub-Saharan Africa." *The Lancet Infectious Diseases* 9 (7):428–438.

Sookoian, S. 2006. "Liver disease during pregnancy: Acute viral hepatitis." *Annals of Hepatology* 5 (3):231–236.

Stergiou, G. S., Dolan, E., Anastasios Kollias, N. R., Poulter, A. S., Staessen, J. A., Zhang, Z.-Y., and Weber, M. A. 2018. "Blood pressure measurement in special populations and circumstances." *The Journal of Clinical Hypertension* 20 (7):1122–1127.

Sweeting, A. N., Wong, J., Heidi Appelblom, G. P., Ross, H. K., Williams, P. F., Sairanen, M., and Hyett, J. A. 2018. "A first trimester prediction model for gestational diabetes utilizing aneuploidy and pre-eclampsia screening markers." *The Journal of Maternal-Fetal & Neonatal Medicine* 31 (16):2122–2130.

Szweda, H. and Marcin, J. 2016. "Urinary tract infections during pregnancy: An updated overview." *Development Period Medicine* 20:263–272.

Tan, E. K. and Tan, E. L. 2013. "Alterations in physiology and anatomy during pregnancy." *Best Practice & Research Clinical Obstetrics & Gynaecology* 27 (6):791–802.

Thornton, C., Dahlen, H., Korda, A., and Hennessy, A. 2013. "The incidence of preeclampsia and eclampsia and associated maternal mortality in Australia from population-linked datasets: 2000–2008." *American Journal of Obstetrics and Gynecology* 208 (6):476.e1–476.e5.

Thurn, L., Wikman, A., and Lindqvist, P. G. 2018. "Postpartum blood transfusion and hemorrhage as independent risk factors for venous thromboembolism." *Thrombosis Research* 165:54–60.

Tkachenko, O., Shchekochikhin, D., and Schrier, R. W. 2014. "Hormones and hemodynamics in pregnancy." *International Journal of Endocrinology and Metabolism* 12 (2): e14098.

Tobias, D. K. 2018. "Prediction and prevention of Type 2 diabetes in women with a history of GDM." *Current Diabetes Reports* 18 (10):78.

Tyrlik, M., Konecny, S., and Kukla, L. 2013. "Predictors of pregnancy-related emotions." *Journal of Clinical Medicine Research* 5 (2):112–120.

United Nations 2018. "About the sustainable development goals." Retrieved from www.un.org/sustainabledevelopment/sustainable-development-goals, accessed 22 October 2018.

Vaughan, G., Kylie Tune, M. J., Peek, L., Pulver, J., Remenyi, B., Belton, S., and Sullivan, E. A. 2018. "Rheumatic heart disease in pregnancy: Strategies and lessons learnt implementing a population-based study in Australia." *International Health*, 10(6):480–489, doi:10.1093/inthealth/ihy048.

Wagner, C. L. and Hollis, B. W. 2018. "The implications of vitamin D status during pregnancy on mother and her developing child." *Frontiers in Endocrinology* 9 (500):1–10.

Wald, N. J., Morris, J. K., and Blakemore, C. 2018. "Public health failure in the prevention of neural tube defects: Time to abandon the tolerable upper intake level of folate." *Public Health Reviews* 39 (1):2.

Waugh, J., Hooper, R., Lamb, E., Robson, S., Shennan, A., Milne, F., Price, C., Thangaratinam, S., Berdunov, V., and Bingham, J. 2017. "Spot protein-creatinine ratio and spot albumin-creatinine ratio in the assessment of pre-eclampsia: A diagnostic accuracy study with decision-analytic model-based economic evaluation and acceptability analysis." *Health Technology Assessment* 21 (61):1.

Webster, L. M., Conti-Ramsden, F., Seed, P. T., Webb, A. J., Nelson-Piercy, C., and Chappell, L. C. 2017. "Impact of antihypertensive treatment on maternal and perinatal outcomes in pregnancy complicated by chronic hypertension: A systematic review and meta-analysis." *Journal of the American Heart Association* 6 (5):e005526.

World Health Organization (WHO) 2018. *Millennium development goals.* Geneva: Author. Retrieved from www.who.int/topics/millennium_development_goals/about/en, accessed 8 October 2018.

Withagen, M. I. J., Wallenburg, H. C. S., Steegers, E. A. P., Hop, W. C. J., and Visser, W. 2005. "Morbidity and development in childhood of infants born after temporising treatment of early onset pre-eclampsia." *BJOG: An International Journal of Obstetrics and Gynaecology* 112 (7):910–914.

Wu, Z., Huang, P., Gong, Y., Wan, J., and Zou, W. 2018. "Treating acute fatty liver of pregnancy with artificial liver support therapy: Systematic review." *Medicine* 97 (38):e12473.

Zimmermann, M. B. 2012. "The effects of iodine deficiency in pregnancy and infancy." *Paediatric and Perinatal Epidemiology* 26 (s1):108–117.

19

MISCARRIAGE

Heather Rowe and Alexandra J. Hawkey

Miscarriage is a common complication of pregnancy. It is defined as the loss of pregnancy between conception and 24 weeks gestation, when the foetus reaches viability (Mitchell-Jones & Bottomley, 2017), although definitions of miscarriage may vary between countries. It is estimated that 20% of clinically recognised conceptions end spontaneously in miscarriage, most within the first three months of gestation (Avalos, Galindo, & Li, 2012). However, it is difficult to determine the actual prevalence of miscarriage, given that many are experienced before women know that they are pregnant, and because, in some countries where legal, safe abortion is unavailable, it is not always possible to make a clear clinical distinction between miscarriage and induced abortion (Vazquez, 2002). Common causes of miscarriage include maternal structural or endocrine abnormalities, chromosomal abnormalities, and infection (Rai & Regan, 2006), but many are medically unexplained (Regan & Rai, 2000). Specific risk factors for miscarriage are maternal underweight, overweight, and obesity (Balsells, García-Patterson, & Corcoy, 2016; Boots & Stephenson, 2011); active or passive smoking (Pineles, Park, & Samet, 2014); and older maternal age at conception (Avalos et al., 2012).

In this chapter we explore the psychosocial aspects of miscarriage. First, we describe women's experience of and treatments for miscarriage, sociocultural contexts of miscarriage, implications of miscarriage for women's mental health, and explanatory models of miscarriage grief. We also discuss sociodemographic and psychological risk factors for post-miscarriage psychological distress and the psychological support needs of women following miscarriage.

Miscarriage and its treatments

Depending on the gestational stage, miscarriage may be prolonged, painful, accompanied by large blood loss and perhaps the sight of the products of conception, and may be experienced as frightening or even traumatic (Bellhouse, Temple-Smith, Watson, & Bilardi, 2018; Wojnar, 2007). An "incomplete" miscarriage occurs when tissue is retained in the uterus that can lead to haemorrhage and infection. All miscarried pregnancies were once considered incomplete, and thus surgical curettage – evacuation of the uterus under general anaesthetic – was the treatment of choice. The procedure itself carries risks, including cervical trauma and subsequent cervical "incompetence," preterm birth, uterine perforation, haemorrhage, and intrauterine adhesions (Lemmers et al., 2016; Nanda, Lopez, Grimes, Peloggia, & Nanda, 2012). However, ultrasound examinations indicate that only a proportion of miscarriages are incomplete; thus pharmacological treatments for incomplete miscarriage aimed at minimizing morbidity, mortality, and unnecessary surgical intervention can be used (Blum et al., 2007; Neilson, Gyte, Hickey, Vazquez, & Dou, 2013).

Women motivated by a desire for a natural course of miscarriage or apprehension about anesthesia and surgery may elect medical treatment, whereas those who choose surgery value quick resolution and the fact that there is no possibility of seeing the foetus (Ogden & Maker, 2004; Olesen, Graungaard, & Husted, 2015; Schreiber et al., 2016). These different values confirm that women experiencing miscarriage should be offered an informed choice about active management where it is necessary. Little is known about differences in the long-term physical and psychological impact of medical and surgical treatments (Neilson et al., 2013).

A need for treatment for miscarriage brings women into contact with health care services. Factors that shape a women's experience of miscarriage include the attitudes of health care staff and the availability of counselling, support, and other follow-up services. Dissatisfaction with the health care system and health care professionals is common; many women report inadequate information and emotional support following a pregnancy loss (Bellhouse et al., 2018; deMontigny, Verdon, Meunier, & Dubeau, 2017). Women in high-income countries frequently report poor recognition by staff of the magnitude of the experience (Rowlands & Lee, 2010b), insensitive care (e.g., being cared for alongside women who are pregnant or in labour; Due, Obst, Riggs, & Collins, 2018), insufficient information about why their pregnancy miscarried and the implications for future pregnancies, and deficiencies in psychological or medical follow-up (Bellhouse et al., 2018; Edwards, Birks, Chapman, & Yates, 2018).

It has been suggested that unhelpful and insensitive attitudes among staff may reflect their own emotional responses to pregnancy loss (Brier, 1999). Primary care health professionals may recognize that women are likely to experience emotional distress after miscarriage that might be ameliorated by discussion of their feelings, but they do not necessarily feel confident that they can provide this for women in their care (Prettyman & Cordle, 1992). Staff education and training about how to provide psychologically informed care is needed, particularly because poor social support and a failure of practitioners to provide compassionate care can be associated with prolonged emotional distress (Wojnar, 2007).

Sociocultural context of miscarriage

The psychosocial repercussions of miscarriage for individual women are likely to be influenced by culturally-specific beliefs and practices regarding conception, inheritance and ideas about family identity, individual responsibility, and attribution of cause (Gerber-Epstein, Leichtentritt, & Benyamini, 2008; van der Sijpt, 2014). Blame for pregnancy loss is largely attributed to the woman. For instance, in western Kenya miscarriage has been said to occur due to a woman's infidelity to her husband or transgression of traditional taboos, such as becoming pregnant before her husband has paid the bride-price (Dellicour et al., 2013). Interviews with women from Qatar revealed that miscarriage is often attributed to the supernatural, including God's will, the "evil eye," or possession by *jinn* (i.e., supernatural creatures in Arabic and Islamic mythology; Kilshaw et al., 2017). In some societies pregnancy loss is grounds on which a man may divorce his wife (Vazquez, 2002), especially where having many children is accorded high social status.

Societies differ in the degree to which they permit, or even encourage, discussion of adverse pregnancy events. In high-income countries, contemporary discourse emphasizes the desirability of women's autonomy and control of their bodies during pregnancy and childbirth. Implicit in this is the notion that individuals have personal agency to ensure a happy, healthy pregnancy outcome, which can result in self-blame when pregnancy loss occurs (Bellhouse et al., 2018; Layne, 2003). Social conventions discourage disclosure of pregnancy until after 12-weeks gestation, when the risk of miscarriage declines (Bute, Brann, & Hernandez, 2017). Similarly, but for different reasons, migrant Latina women living in the U.S. describe silencing of discussion about their miscarriage and associated grief. This is because, in their culture, children are a source of status for women and essential to their partner's manhood. The silence results in women feeling abandoned and misunderstood (Leach, Wojnar, & Pettinato, 2014). In contrast, women in some settings (e.g., Yucatan, Mexico, Nepal) are able to speak candidly about all kinds of pregnancy loss, which is regarded as beneficial (Jordan, 1993; March, 2001). Similarly, discussion of miscarriage is not silenced among Qatari women, who view early pregnancy loss as "normal" because they are aware of other women who have miscarried (Kilshaw et al., 2017).

Rice (2000) described the beliefs of Hmong women living in Australia, for whom miscarriage creates considerable anxiety at the family and societal levels. This is because of a belief that miscarriage may portend the failure of the family to extend its lineage and because it is seen as a threat to the existence of the clan itself. Religious concerns are focussed on the loss of a place within the family for the rebirth of a soul. These reactions to miscarriage reflect anxiety about disruption to the harmony between the social and supernatural worlds, which is regarded as essential for health.

It has been argued (Layne, 2003; Reiheld, 2015) that in high-income countries, where adverse pregnancy and birth outcomes are rare and there are few social scripts for responding to or conceptualizing those outcomes, discussion of these events is discouraged. This means that women may suffer alone without appropriate acknowledgement or support from others (Harvey, Moyle, & Creedy, 2001; Rowlands & Lee, 2010b). However, there is a growing discourse in these settings that discouragement of open discussion about miscarriage may silence women and promote minimization of the physical and emotional effects of pregnancy loss (Harvey et al., 2001). Encouragement of public discussion may promote the open disclosure necessary to garner or access social support, though it is acknowledged that overcoming societal-level privacy rules for talking about miscarriage may be difficult for some women (Bute et al., 2017). Recently, the widespread use of social media has promoted a discourse that encourages disclosure and discussion of stigmatizing events including miscarriage, with the aim of educating women and reducing isolation among those experiencing them (Andalibi & Forte, 2018).

Miscarriage and mental health

Miscarriage is experienced by many women as a significant life crisis associated with negative emotions (Bellhouse et al., 2018; Radford & Hughes, 2015) that can persist for long periods, particularly if miscarriage is recurrent (Tavoli et al., 2018). Despite the frequency of miscarriage, there is a paucity of explicit theoretical frameworks to explain psychological reactions to it. There is generally an implicit assumption that the bereavement or loss model is appropriate (Slade, 1994), despite critique of this theoretical position (Murphy & Merrell, 2009).

There is good evidence that, even though a foetus may not legally qualify as a person, many women attribute personhood to their foetus and are emotionally invested in their pregnancy from the earliest weeks (Frost, Bradley, Levitas, Smith, & Garcia, 2007). Affective and behavioural reactions that occur following a miscarriage are thought to be similar to reactions that occur after other significant losses (Brier, 2008). Grief has been conceptualized as a normal adaptive response to loss, characterized by feelings of sadness, emptiness, angry protest, and yearning, which will normally resolve without intervention over time (Brier, 2008). Grief reactions to pregnancy loss include feelings of emptiness, guilt, shame, helplessness, and low self-esteem, which are exacerbated by the absence of an object for which to mourn (Adolfsson, Larsson, Wijma, & Bertero, 2004; Frost & Condon, 1996; Gerber-Epstein et al., 2008). Grief following miscarriage appears to be unique in that there is an emphasis on "times ahead rather than remembered times" (e.g., a focus on images of an anticipated future, hopes, dreams), rather than on negative past experiences (Brier, 2008, p. 460; Frost et al., 2007). When health professionals and communities minimize the degree of distress and assume that women will make a rapid and spontaneous recovery (Kong, Lok, Lam, Yip, & Chung, 2010; Rowlands & Lee, 2010b), healthy grieving and adaptation can be severely undermined (Rowlands & Lee, 2010b).

The range of emotional reactions to miscarriage may be transient for some women and prolonged for others (Magee, Macleod, Tata, & Regan, 2003; Simmons, Singh, Maconochie, Doyle, & Green, 2006). Not all women will experience miscarriage as a profound loss, and there appears to be a range of severity, from expressions of ambivalence, relative indifference, or relief at one end of the spectrum to the need for psychiatric care at the other (Farren et al., 2016; Flink-Bochacki et al., 2018). This range is likely to be associated with differences in personal circumstances, including the significance of the loss, as well as familial, social, and cultural meanings (Corbet-Owen & Kruger, 2001). Women's own descriptions of miscarriages have been interpreted as a process involving stages of turmoil, adjustment, and resolution rather than as psychological morbidity (Maker & Ogden, 2003).

As with other human loss, an appreciation of the relationship between grief and depression is essential to understanding the psychological implications of miscarriage (Ritsher & Neugebauer, 2002). Only a minority of women experience symptoms for more than six months, some of which may lead to "complicated grief," which is associated with depression or more severe psychiatric problems (Monk, Houck, & Shear, 2006). Neugebauer and Ritsher (2005) reported that the clinically significant symptoms of depression among women after miscarriage were unrelated to grief. Beutel, Deckardt, von Rad, and Weiner (1995) suggested that grief reactions are preceded by joyful anticipation of motherhood and are of relatively short duration, whereas depressive reactions are more likely with a history of depression, elevated distress in pregnancy, difficult personal relationships, and/or disadvantaged social circumstances.

Incidence and course of psychological symptomatology following miscarriage

There is a body of research on the incidence and course of psychological symptomatology following miscarriage (Farren et al., 2018). However, interpretation of these data is hampered by the variety of methodologies employed and measures used to assess symptoms. In addition, a number of methodological limitations restrict the conclusions that may be drawn from the studies. For example, differences between study and comparison groups may confound results, and there is variation in the extent to which the study methodology itself may act as a therapeutic intervention. There is also the question of the potential confounding effect on the assessment of psychological sequelae of miscarriage and of the provision of psychological care, such as counselling, during or after treatment. It is therefore surprising that very few researchers have reported details of any care that may have been offered to study participants or whether participants sought or received assistance from professional or lay support groups prior to psychological assessment.

In a recent review, Farren et al. (2018) estimated that 8–20% of women experience elevated depression symptoms suggestive of moderate depression, and 18–32% experience elevated anxiety, which resolves within one year after early pregnancy loss. Methodologically rigorous studies in high-income countries that included both standardized psychometric measures and comparison groups have consistently shown significantly elevated rates of depression, anxiety, and adjustment symptoms among women immediately following miscarriage, in comparison with women with uncomplicated pregnancy or women in the community who are not pregnant; their symptoms decline over time to levels comparable with women in control groups one year later (Farren et al., 2016; Jacob, Polly, Kalder, & Kostev, 2017). The most relevant comparison group is women with uncomplicated pregnancy rather than non-pregnant women; however, similar rates of depressive symptoms have been found in pregnant women and community samples of women of a similar age who are not pregnant (Llewellyn, Stowe, & Nemeroff, 1997).

There is some evidence that anxiety symptoms are more variable and persistent than depression (Farren et al., 2018) and may lead to other complex anxiety disorders, such as PTSD or obsessive-compulsive disorder, particularly among women with a history of this disorder (Brier, 2004). Prevalence estimates of PTSD following miscarriage vary considerably due to methods of assessment, from 28% (Farren et al., 2016) to 0.6% (Sham, Yiu, & Ho, 2010). This suggests both a need for more research and a model of care that meets the needs of women who present with symptoms of PTSD (Bowles et al., 2000; Lee & Slade, 1996). Some women have reported that continuing distress influences their decision to conceive again (Cordle & Prettyman, 1994).

Sociodemographic and psychological risk factors

There is inconsistent evidence of a relationship between sociodemographic factors, including age, occupation, and marital status, on psychological distress following miscarriage. Several factors have been identified as predictors of more intense emotional responses to early pregnancy loss, including prior miscarriages, a history of infertility or fertility treatment, no living children, social isolation, and a poor quality partner relationship (Nynas, Narang, Kolikonda, & Lippmann, 2015; Volgsten, Jansson, Svanberg, Darj, & Stavreus-Evers, 2018). Elevated rates of psychological morbidity, in particular depression and anxiety disorders (Farren et al., 2016; Lok & Neugebauer, 2007), may re-emerge in subsequent pregnancies, even after the birth of a healthy baby (Blackmore et al., 2011; Fertl, Bergner, Beyer, Klapp, & Rauchfuss, 2009).

Other studies, however, suggest that reproductive factors such as childlessness may not directly influence the risk of depression following miscarriage, although it may be associated with greater duration of perinatal distress (deMontigny et al., 2017). For example, two years following miscarriage, grief symptoms had declined among women who already had children, but not among women without existing children. There is also evidence to suggest that higher satisfaction with the health care provided to women who have miscarried is associated with more positive mental health outcomes (deMontigny et al., 2017; Rowlands & Lee, 2010a).

The impact of mental health history on emotional adaptation to pregnancy loss has been investigated. Neugebauer et al. (1997) assessed the risk of a first or recurrent episode of major depressive disorder among a large cohort in the six months following loss, and compared it with the risk in a population-based sample drawn from the community. The six-month total incidence rates for the miscarriage and the community samples were 10.9% and 4.3%, respectively. In both groups, the risk of an episode of major depressive disorder was substantially higher among women with a history of major depressive disorder. Similarly women with no history of anxiety or depression showed improvements in mental health over time after miscarriage, but women with a history of one or both diagnoses reported poorer adjustment and a decline in mental health over time (Rowlands & Lee, 2010a). This finding concurs with those from studies of mood disorders at other phases of reproductive life. For example, a personal history of mood disorder or psychiatric diagnosis has been consistently associated with depression during the postpartum period (Biaggi, Conroy, Pawlby, & Pariante, 2016).

In a large data-linkage study in the United States (Seng et al., 2001), women diagnosed with PTSD were twice as likely to have had a previous miscarriage and seven times more likely to have been a victim of violence than were women who had not miscarried. This raises the possibility of the causal misattribution of psychopathology to the miscarriage experience itself, when it might more accurately be described for some women as a re-arousal of prior trauma. The interaction between previous adverse life experiences, such as abuse and violence, and the experience of miscarriage warrants specific investigation.

It has been argued that sociodemographic factors contribute little to the understanding of the meaning of miscarriage to an individual woman (Lok & Neugebauer, 2007; Slade, 1994), therefore a more fruitful approach may be to investigate the role of thoughts and cognitions, in particular women's understanding of the medical explanations of the cause of the miscarriage (Nikčević, Kuczmierczyk, & Nicolaides, 2007; Tunaley, Slade, & Duncan, 1993). It is also possible that individual differences in attributional style (i.e., an individual's propensity to locate the cause of an adverse event either internally or to external factors over which she or he has less control) may be salient. However, studies of the role of cognition in psychological adaptation to miscarriage have produced inconsistent findings (Robinson, Stirtzinger, Stewart, & Ralevski, 1994; Tunaley et al., 1993).

Psychological support following miscarriage

Moulder (1994) described two models on which professional care for women who have had a miscarriage may be based. The "medical" model assumes that the miscarriage is a minor mishap that can be treated, whereas the "gestational" model recognizes the loss involved, but describes the magnitude of loss in terms of the stage of pregnancy at which it occurred: The later the miscarriage, the greater the loss. The medical model is commonly reflected in women's descriptions of an absence of empathy or support during their care following miscarriage (Rowlands & Lee, 2010b). However, Moulder argued that neither of these models accurately explains the diversity of women's responses to pregnancy loss and proposed a model with greater potential explanatory power. This is based on an understanding of maternal–foetal emotional attachment, loss, and the degree of individual investment in the pregnancy (Moulder, 1994).

In general, follow-up professional care after miscarriage is not provided, even though women commonly report a desire for it (Bellhouse et al., 2018; Due et al., 2018), attend when it is available, and report that it is helpful (Nikčević, Kuczmierczyk, & Nicolaides, 1998; Slade, 1994). Poor or lack of psychosocial care following miscarriage may limit the capacity of health care providers to identify psychological morbidity (Wong, Crawford, Gask, & Grinyer, 2003). Brier (2004) recommended post-miscarriage screening for anxiety and depressive symptoms and referral for professional assistance, but it is not known whether this approach results in improved psychological outcomes.

The specific features of miscarriage suggest that a broader conceptualization of a thera-peutic approach is needed. In particular, a combination of explanation of the medical reasons for miscarriage (if known) and psychological support may ameliorate the guilt reactions commonly experienced after miscarriage. Nikčević et al. (2007) found that medical investi-gations to determine the cause of foetal death and a subsequent consultation together with psychological counselling can be beneficial in reducing women's distress following miscar-riage. Post-treatment interventions aimed at reducing feelings of self-blame and enhancing self-esteem appear to be promising means of improving psychological adaptation to miscar-riage (Nikčević et al., 2007). A recent RCT in Hong Kong evaluated the efficacy of a supportive counselling program for women who had miscarried (Kong, Chung, & Lok, 2014). Not all women found the program beneficial, which suggests that the intervention should be reserved for women who express the need or who are more vulnerable or already experiencing distress. However, there are few high quality studies that consider effectiveness of interventions for women with specific vulnerabilities (Campillo, Meaney, McNamara, & Donoghue, 2017).

Women's responses to miscarriage are likely to be mediated by the reactions of others, including family members and the broader society in which they live (Abboud & Liamput-tong, 2005; Rowlands & Lee, 2010b). The extent to which the psychological reactions of the women's partners may limit their capacity to provide emotional support remains under-explored. Men also grieve the loss of a pregnancy (Conway & Russell, 2000), but their grief may be less intense and of shorter duration than that of women (Huffman, Schwartz, & Swanson, 2015; Volgsten et al., 2018). A small qualitative study revealed that men may experience confusion about how to behave socially or how to provide appropriate emo-tional support to their partners in the presence of their own feelings of loss after miscarriage (Puddifoot & Johnson, 1997). Women who were still depressed six months after spontan-eous pregnancy loss were significantly more likely than those who were not depressed to have partners who avoided talking about the loss and who were less supportive (Beutel, Willner, Deckardt, Von Rad, & Weiner, 1996). In common with other forms of bereave-ment, support from broader social networks, including local health services, may assist in the adaptation to pregnancy loss (Rajan & Oakley, 1993; Rowlands & Lee, 2010b). It is unlikely that a single approach to the psychological care of women after spontaneous preg-nancy loss will be effective in all settings and for all cultural groups. Specific religious or cultural beliefs about the cause of the miscarriage or the fate of the miscarried "child" could be taken into account in planning interventions (Brin, 2004).

Most women have reported needing some form of support following miscarriage. Researchers surveyed 205 European women about their needs and preferences (Séjourné, Callahan, & Chabrol, 2010). Participants disclosed that they desired an in-depth discussion with their doctor (87%), the opportunity to contact a health care professional at any time (e.g., Internet, telephone) (70%), improved medical follow-up (64%), and group therapy for women who had experienced miscarriage (64%). Less frequently requested were an informa-tional brochure (55%), systematic appointments as part of standard care with a psychologist or psychiatrist (48%), or a referral to a psychologist or psychiatrist (45%). More research and evaluation are needed to ensure that programs to support women and their families are tailored to their specific needs and are culturally appropriate.

Summary

There is general agreement that many women experience miscarriage as highly distressing and that subsequent psychopathology, including depression and anxiety, is higher than in community samples, but in most women resolves without professional intervention. Health care services are involved in preventing the potential medical complications of miscarriage through active treatment, but are generally not perceived to provide psychological support at the time of treatment or at follow-up, despite the fact that women commonly regard this as an important component of care. The particular factors that predispose some women to more intense psychological reactions have not yet been clearly identified, but vulnerability generated by a history of mental health problems and experiences of assisted conception, childlessness, and adverse life events appear salient and warrant additional investigation.

Most research in health services has been conducted in high-income countries, and less is known about other settings. There appears to be a role for psychological intervention, immediately after treatment or in the long term, for women with specific vulnerabilities, but there is little evidence of successful approaches. However, it is acknowledged that women who use health services after losing a pregnancy may benefit from a more psychologically informed model of care than currently exists in many settings. Even though it is common, miscarriage should not be regarded as a routine event in women's lives; policies for the delivery and assessment of short- and long-term psychological care for women who have experienced miscarriage should be developed. Health care services should ensure that staff members are attuned to women's psychological needs following miscarriage, and the education and training of health professionals should ensure that they are equipped to respond with empathy and sensitivity.

References

Abboud, L. & Liamputtong, P. (2005). When pregnancy fails: Coping strategies, support networks and experiences with health care of ethnic women and their partners. *Journal of Reproductive and Infant Psychology, 23*(1), 3–18.

Adolfsson, A., Larsson, P. G., Wijma, B., & Bertero, C. (2004). Guilt and emptiness: Women's experiences of miscarriage. *Health Care for Women International, 25*(6), 543–560.

Andalibi, N. & Forte, A. (2018, April). *Announcing pregnancy loss on Facebook: A decision-making framework for stigmatized disclosures on identified social network sites.* Paper presented at the CHI Conference on Human Factors in Computing Systems, Montreal QC, Canada.

Avalos, L., Galindo, C., & Li, D.-K. (2012). A systematic review to calculate background miscarriage rates using life table analysis. *Birth Defects Research Part A: Clinical and Molecular Teratology, 94*(6), 417–423.

Balsells, M., García-Patterson, A., & Corcoy, R. (2016). Systematic review and meta-analysis on the association of prepregnancy underweight and miscarriage. *European Journal of Obstetrics & Gynecology and Reproductive Biology, 207,* 73–79.

Bellhouse, C., Temple-Smith, M., Watson, S., & Bilardi, J. (2018). "The loss was traumatic ... some healthcare providers added to that": Women's experiences of miscarriage. *Women and Birth, 32*(2), 137–146.

Beutel, M., Deckardt, R., von Rad, M., & Weiner, H. (1995). Grief and depression after miscarriage: Their separation, antecedents, and course. *Psychosomatic Medicine, 57*(6), 517–526.

Beutel, M., Willner, H., Deckardt, R., Von Rad, M., & Weiner, H. (1996). Similarities and differences in couples' grief reactions following a miscarriage: Results from a longitudinal study. *Journal of Psychosomatic Research, 40*(3), 245–253.

Biaggi, A., Conroy, S., Pawlby, S., & Pariante, C. M. (2016). Identifying the women at risk of antenatal anxiety and depression: A systematic review. *Journal of Affective Disorders, 191*, 62–77.

Blackmore, E. R., Côté-Arsenault, D., Tang, W., Glover, V., Evans, J., Golding, J., & O'Connor, T. G. (2011). Previous prenatal loss as a predictor of perinatal depression and anxiety. *British Journal of Psychiatry, 198*(5), 373–378.

Blum, J., Winikoff, B., Gemzell-Danielsson, K., Ho, P. C., Schiavon, R., & Weeks, A. (2007). Treatment of incomplete abortion and miscarriage with misoprostol. *International Journal of Gynecology & Obstetrics, 99*(S2), S186–S189.

Boots, C. & Stephenson, M. D. (2011). Does obesity increase the risk of miscarriage in spontaneous conception: A systematic review. *Seminars in Reproductive Medicine, 29*(6), 507–513.

Bowles, S. V., James, L. C., Solursh, D. S., Yancey, M. K., Epperly, T. D., Folen, R. A., & Masone, M. (2000). Acute and post-traumatic stress disorder after spontaneous abortion. *American Family Physician, 61*(6), 1689–1696.

Brier, N. (1999). Understanding and managing the emotional reactions to a miscarriage. *Obstetrics & Gynecology, 93*(1), 151–155.

Brier, N. (2004). Anxiety after miscarriage: A review of the empirical literature and implications for clinical practice. *Birth, 31*(2), 138–142.

Brier, N. (2008). Grief following miscarriage: A comprehensive review of the literature. *Journal of Women's Health, 17*(3), 451–464.

Brin, D. (2004). The use of rituals in grieving for a miscarriage or stillbirth. *Women & Therapy, 27*(3–4), 123–132.

Bute, J. J., Brann, M., & Hernandez, R. (2017). Exploring societal-level privacy rules for talking about miscarriage. *Journal of Social and Personal Relationships, 36*, 379–399.

Campillo, S. L. I., Meaney, S., McNamara, K., & Donoghue, K. (2017). Psychological and support interventions to reduce levels of stress, anxiety or depression on women's subsequent pregnancy with a history of miscarriage: An empty systematic review. *British Medical Journal Open, 7*(9), E017802[web].

Conway, K. & Russell, G. (2000). Couples' grief and experience of support in the aftermath of miscarriage. *British Journal of Medical Psychology, 73*(4), 531–545.

Corbet-Owen, C. & Kruger, L. (2001). The health system and emotional care: Validating the many meanings of spontaneous pregnancy loss. *Families, Systems & Health, 19*(4), 411–427.

Cordle, C. J. & Prettyman, R. J. (1994). A 2-year follow-up of women who have experienced early miscarriage. *Journal of Reproductive and Infant Psychology, 12*(1), 37–43.

Dellicour, S., Desai, M., Mason, L., Odidi, B., Aol, G., Phillips-Howard, P. A., & ter Kuile, F. O. (2013). Exploring risk perception and attitudes to miscarriage and congenital anomaly in rural western Kenya. *Plos One, 8*(11), e80551.

deMontigny, F., Verdon, C., Meunier, S., & Dubeau, D. (2017). Women's persistent depressive and perinatal grief symptoms following a miscarriage: The role of childlessness and satisfaction with healthcare services. *Archives of Women's Mental Health, 20*(5), 655–662.

Due, C., Obst, K., Riggs, D. W., & Collins, C. (2018). Australian heterosexual women's experiences of healthcare provision following a pregnancy loss. *Women and Birth, 31*(4), 331–338.

Edwards, S., Birks, M., Chapman, Y., & Yates, K. (2018). Bringing together the 'threads of care' in possible miscarriage for women, their partners and nurses in non-metropolitan EDs. *Collegian, 25*(3), 293–301.

Farren, J., Jalmbrant, M., Ameye, L., Joash, K., Mitchell-Jones, N., Tapp, S., & Bourne, T. (2016). Post-traumatic stress, anxiety and depression following miscarriage or ectopic pregnancy: A prospective cohort study. *British Medical Journal Open, 6*(11), E011864[web].

Farren, J., Mitchell-Jones, N., Verbakel, J. Y., Timmerman, D., Jalmbrant, M., & Bourne, T. (2018). The psychological impact of early pregnancy loss. *Human Reproduction Update, 24*(6), 731–749.

Fertl, K. I., Bergner, A., Beyer, R., Klapp, B. F., & Rauchfuss, M. (2009). Levels and effects of different forms of anxiety during pregnancy after a prior miscarriage. *European Journal of Obstetrics & Gynecology and Reproductive Biology, 142*(1), 23–29.

Flink-Bochacki, R., Hamm, M. E., Borrero, S., Chen, B. A., Achilles, S. L., & Chang, J. C. (2018). Family planning and counseling desires of women who have experienced miscarriage. *Obstetrics & Gynecology, 131*(4), 625–631.

Frost, J., Bradley, H., Levitas, R., Smith, L., & Garcia, J. (2007). The loss of possibility: Scientisation of death and the special case of early miscarriage. *Sociology of Health & Illness, 29*(7), 1003–1022.

Frost, M. & Condon, J. T. (1996). The psychological sequelae of miscarriage: A critical review of the literature. *Australian and New Zealand Journal of Psychiatry, 30*(1), 54–62.

Gerber-Epstein, P., Leichtentritt, R. D., & Benyamini, Y. (2008). The experience of miscarriage in first pregnancy: The women's voices. *Death Studies, 33*(1), 1–29.

Harvey, J., Moyle, W., & Creedy, D. (2001). Women's experience of early miscarriage: A phenomenological study. *Royal Australian Nursing Federation, 19*(1), 8–14.

Huffman, C. S., Schwartz, T. A., & Swanson, K. M. (2015). Couples and miscarriage: The influence of gender and reproductive factors on the impact of miscarriage. *Women's Health Issues, 25*(5), 570–578.

Jacob, L., Polly, I., Kalder, M., & Kostev, K. (2017). Prevalence of depression, anxiety, and adjustment disorders in women with spontaneous abortion in Germany: A retrospective cohort study. *Psychiatry Research, 258*, 382–386.

Jordan, B. (1993). *Birth in four cultures. A crosscultural investigation of childbirth in Yucatan, Holland, Sweden, and the United States. Revised and expanded by Robbie Davis-Floyd.* Long Grove, IL: Waveland Press.

Kilshaw, S., Omar, N., Major, S., Mohsen, M., El Taher, F., Al Tamimi, H., & Miller, D. (2017). Causal explanations of miscarriage amongst Qataris. *BMC Pregnancy and Childbirth, 17*(1), 250.

Kong, G., Chung, T., & Lok, I. (2014). The impact of supportive counselling on women's psychological wellbeing after miscarriage – a randomised controlled trial. *Journal of Obstetrics & Gynaecology, 121*(10), 1253–1262.

Kong, G. W. S., Lok, I. H., Lam, P. M., Yip, A. S. K., & Chung, T. K. H. (2010). Conflicting perceptions between health care professionals and patients on the psychological morbidity following miscarriage. *Australian and New Zealand Journal of Obstetrics and Gynaecology, 50*(6), 562–567.

Layne, L. L. (2003). Unhappy endings: A feminist reappraisal of the women's health movement from the vantage of pregnancy loss. *Social Science & Medicine, 56*(9), 1881–1891.

Leach, S., Wojnar, D., & Pettinato, M. (2014). Lived experience of miscarriage for nine Latina immigrant women. *Journal of Theory Construction and Testing, 18*(1), 11–16.

Lee, C. & Slade, P. (1996). Miscarriage as a traumatic event: A review of the literature and new implications for intervention. *Journal of Psychosomatic Research, 40*(3), 235–244.

Lemmers, M., Verschoor, M. A. C., Hooker, A. B., Opmeer, B. C., Limpens, J., Huirne, J. A. F., & Mol, B. W. M. (2016). Dilatation and curettage increases the risk of subsequent preterm birth: A systematic review and meta-analysis. *Human Reproduction, 31*(1), 34–45.

Llewellyn, A. M., Stowe, Z. N., & Nemeroff, C. B. (1997). Depression during pregnancy and the puerperium. *Journal of Clinical Psychiatry, 58*(Suppl 15), 26–32.

Lok, I. H. & Neugebauer, R. (2007). Psychological morbidity following miscarriage. *Best Practice & Research Clinical Obstetrics & Gynaecology, 21*(2), 229–247.

Magee, P. L., Macleod, A. K., Tata, P., & Regan, L. (2003). Psychological distress in recurrent miscarriage: The role of prospective thinking and role and goal investment. *Journal of Reproductive and Infant Psychology, 21*(1), 35–47.

Maker, C. & Ogden, J. (2003). The miscarriage experience: More than just a trigger to psychological morbidity? *Psychology & Health, 18*(3), 403–415.

March, K. (2001). Childbirth with fear. In: S. Chase & M. Rogers (Eds), *Mothers and children: feminist analyses and personal narratives* (pp. 168–173). New Brunswick, NJ: Rutgers University Press.

Mitchell-Jones, N. & Bottomley, C. (2017). Diagnosis of miscarriage. In E. Kirk (Ed.), *Early pregnancy ultrasound: A practical guide* (pp. 17–22). Cambridge, UK: Cambridge University Press.

Monk, T. H., Houck, P. R., & Shear, M. K. (2006). The daily life of complicated grief patients: What gets missed, what gets added? *Death Studies, 30*(1), 77–85.

Moulder, C. (1994). Towards a preliminary framework for understanding pregnancy loss. *Journal of Reproductive and Infant Psychology, 12*(1), 65–67.

Murphy, F. & Merrell, J. (2009). Negotiating the transition: Caring for women through the experience of early miscarriage. *Journal of Clinical Nursing, 18*(11), 1583–1591.

Nanda, K., Lopez, L. M., Grimes, D. A., Peloggia, A., & Nanda, G. (2012). Expectant care versus surgical treatment for miscarriage. *Cochrane Database of Systematic Reviews, 3*(3), CD003518.

Neilson, J. P., Gyte, G. M. L., Hickey, M., Vazquez, J. C., & Dou, L. (2013). Medical treatments for incomplete miscarriage. *Cochrane Database of Systematic Reviews, 2013*(3), CD007223.

Neugebauer, R., Kline, J., Shrout, P., Skodol, A., O'Connor, P., Geller, P. A., Stein Z., & Susser, M. (1997). Major depressive disorder in the 6 months after miscarriage. *Journal of the American Medical Association, 277*(5), 383–388.

Neugebauer, R. & Ritsher, J. (2005). Depression and grief following early pregnancy loss. *International Journal of Childbirth Education, 20*(3), 21–23.

Nikčević, A. V., Kuczmierczyk, A. R., & Nicolaides, K. H. (1998). Personal coping resources, responsibility, anxiety, and depression after early pregnancy loss. *Journal of Psychosomatic Obstetrics & Gynecology, 19*(3), 145–154.

Nikčević, A. V., Kuczmierczyk, A. R., & Nicolaides, K. H. (2007). The influence of medical and psychological interventions on women's distress after miscarriage. *Journal of Psychosomatic Research, 63*(3), 283–290.

Nynas, J., Narang, P., Kolikonda, M. K., & Lippmann, S. (2015). Depression and anxiety following early pregnancy loss: Recommendations for primary care providers. *Primary Care Companion for CNS Disorders, 17*(1), doi: 10.4088/PCC.

Ogden, J. & Maker, C. (2004). Expectant or surgical management of miscarriage: A qualitative study. *British Journal of Obstetrics & Gynaecology, 111*(5), 463–467.

Olesen, M. L., Graungaard, A. H., & Husted, G. R. (2015). Deciding treatment for miscarriage – experiences of women and healthcare professionals. *Scandinavian Journal of Caring Sciences, 29*(2), 386–394.

Pineles, B. L., Park, E., & Samet, J. M. (2014). Systematic review and meta-analysis of miscarriage and maternal exposure to tobacco smoke during pregnancy. *American Journal of Epidemiology, 179*(7), 807–823.

Prettyman, R. J. & Cordle, C. (1992). Psychological aspects of miscarriage: Attitudes of the primary health care team. *British Journal of General Practice, 42*(356), 97–99.

Puddifoot, J. E. & Johnson, M. P. (1997). The legitimacy of grieving: The partner's experience at miscarriage. *Social Science & Medicine, 45*(6), 837–845.

Radford, E. J. & Hughes, M. (2015). Women's experiences of early miscarriage: Implications for nursing care. *Journal of Clinical Nursing, 24*(11–12), 1457–1465.

Rai, R. & Regan, L. (2006). Recurrent miscarriage. *Lancet, 368*(9535), 601–611.

Rajan, L. & Oakley, A. (1993). No pills for heartache: The importance of social support for women who suffer pregnancy loss. *Journal of Reproductive and Infant Psychology, 11*(2), 75–87.

Regan, L. & Rai, R. (2000). Epidemiology and the medical causes of miscarriage. *Best Practice & Research Clinical Obstetrics & Gynaecology, 14*(5), 839–854.

Reiheld, A. (2015). "The event that was nothing": Miscarriage as a liminal event. *Journal of Social Philosophy, 46*(1), 9–26.

Rice, P. L. (2000). When the baby falls: The cultural construction of miscarriage among Hmong women in Australia. *Women & Health, 30*(1), 85–103.

Ritsher, J. B. & Neugebauer, R. (2002). Perinatal bereavement grief scale: Distinguishing grief from depression following miscarriage. *Assessment, 9*(1), 31–40.

Robinson, G. E., Stirtzinger, R., Stewart, D. E., & Ralevski, E. (1994). Psychological reactions in women followed for 1 year after miscarriage. *Journal of Reproductive and Infant Psychology, 12*(1), 31–36.

Rowlands, I. & Lee, C. (2010a). Adjustment after miscarriage: Predicting positive mental health trajectories among young Australian women. *Psychology, Health & Medicine, 15*(1), 34–49.

Rowlands, I. & Lee, C. (2010b). 'The silence was deafening': Social and health service support after miscarriage. *Journal of Reproductive and Infant Psychology, 28*(3), 274–286.

Schreiber, C. A., Chavez, V., Whittaker, P. G., Ratcliffe, S. J., Easley, E., & Barg, F. K. (2016). Treatment decisions at the time of miscarriage diagnosis. *Obstetrics & Gynecology, 128*(6), 1347–1356.

Séjourné, N., Callahan, S., & Chabrol, H. (2010). The utility of a psychological intervention for coping with spontaneous abortion. *Journal of Reproductive and Infant Psychology, 28*(3), 287–296.

Seng, J. S., Oakley, D. J., Sampselle, C. M., Killion, C., Graham-Bermann, S., & Liberzon, I. (2001). Posttraumatic stress disorder and pregnancy complications. *Obstetrics & Gynecology, 97*(1), 17–22.

Sham, A. k.-h., Yiu, M. g.-c., & Ho, W. y.-b. (2010). Psychiatric morbidity following miscarriage in Hong Kong. *General Hospital Psychiatry, 32*(3), 284–293.

Simmons, R. K., Singh, G., Maconochie, N., Doyle, P., & Green, J. (2006). Experience of miscarriage in the UK: Qualitative findings from the National Women's Health Study. *Social Science & Medicine, 63*(7), 1934–1946.

Slade, P. (1994). Predicting the psychological impact of miscarriage. *Journal of Reproductive and Infant Psychology, 12*(1), 5–16.

Tavoli, Z., Mohammadi, M., Tavoli, A., Moini, A., Effatpanah, M., Khedmat, L., & Montazeri, A. (2018). Quality of life and psychological distress in women with recurrent miscarriage: A comparative study. *Health and Quality of Life Outcomes, 16*(1), 150.

Tunaley, J. R., Slade, P., & Duncan, S. B. (1993). Cognitive processes in psychological adaptation to miscarriage: A preliminary report. *Psychology & Health, 8*(5), 369–381.

van der Sijpt, E. (2014). The unfortunate sufferer: Discursive dynamics around pregnancy loss in Cameroon. *Medical Anthropology*, *33*(5), 395–410.

Vazquez, J. C., Hickey, M., & Neilson, J. P. (2002). Medical management for miscarriage (Protocol for a Cochrane Review). *The Cochrane Library*, Issue 4. Oxford, Update Software.

Volgsten, H., Jansson, C., Svanberg, A. S., Darj, E., & Stavreus-Evers, A. (2018). Longitudinal study of emotional experiences, grief and depressive symptoms in women and men after miscarriage. *Midwifery*, *64*, 23–28.

Wojnar, D. (2007). Miscarriage experiences of lesbian couples. *Journal of Midwifery & Women's Health, 52*(5), 479–485.

Wong, M. K., Crawford, T. J., Gask, L., & Grinyer, A. (2003). A qualitative investigation into women's experiences after a miscarriage: Implications for the primary healthcare team. *British Journal of General Practice*, *53*(494), 697–702.

20

THE ULTIMATE IN WOMEN'S LABOR

Stillbirth and grieving

Joanne Cacciatore and Jill Wieber Lens

A woman visits her obstetrician's office for what will be her final examination before the birth of her baby. She is excited, nervous, and impatient as she thinks about her baby's long awaited birth. The nursery is ready. Her breasts have already begun to produce small amounts of colostrum, an edge in immunizing her child from possible illness and infection during this most vulnerable period of development. During the routine examination, she learns that her cervix is 80% effaced and she is dilated to three centimeters. Her body is preparing; her baby is ready for birth. As her obstetrician listens for the baby's heartbeat, however, signs of life cannot be found. The woman naïvely, but patiently, waits as her physician leaves the room to get an ultrasound machine.

Within the next few minutes, she will learn that her baby has died but that she will still give birth: stillbirth. Within the next hours, she will experience the excruciatingly painful, sometimes terrifying, birth–death process. Five, 10, or sometimes 24 hours or more later, her baby will slip through her body, born into a silent delivery room, sounds interrupted only by her own labored breaths and perhaps tears of grief and terror. If she desires, she will hold her baby as she decides whether to bury or cremate. If she is too frightened or over-whelmed to hold her baby, she may lament that decision for the rest of her life. Days later, while negotiating plans for her child's funeral, her body will produce breast milk. Maternal hormones will flood her bloodstream, signaling attachment behaviors and emotions, but she will have no place to enact her feelings of maternity. Instead, she will lay her baby to rest while still in trauma and shock, and, along with her baby, she will say farewell to a future she had meticulously planned in the previous months. She had not expected any of this.

This mother will likely experience the effects of traumatic grief physically, cognitively, emotionally, existentially, and interpersonally (DeFrain, Martens, Stork, & Stork, 1990). This loss may impact many of her social relationships (Cacciatore, Froen, & Killian, 2014; Shreffler, Hill, & Cacciatore, 2012), and, if this was to be her first child, her identity as "mother" has been abruptly severed. She expected to be caring for her new baby and has instead been catapulted into a different role: a grieving mother. Years later, like many other parents who have lost a child, she may continue to experience grief symptoms such as tear-fulness and sadness, lack of motivation, and self-blame, sometimes misidentified in medicine as Major Depressive Disorder (MDD) (Cacciatore, Lacasse, Lietz, & McPherson, 2014; Surkan, Radestad, Cnattingius, Steineck, & Dickman, 2008). Life will never be what it was before her child's death (DeFrain et al., 1990). The value of her grief, and the worthiness of her baby's life, will have been challenged by social norms (evidenced in policy, language, and attitudes) that fail to comprehend her embodied encounter with the death of her baby.

Giving birth to a baby who has already died is a uniquely tragic experience of the female body, often followed by paternalistic judgments from others, including the medical community (Cacciatore & Bushfield, 2008). Reactions range from fatalism ("it was meant to be" or "bad luck") to blaming the mother, which create further shame and guilt (DeFrain et al., 1990). Still today, in some cultures, stillbirth is considered a punishment from the gods for women's transgressions (Frøen et al., 2011). Mothers of stillborn children have often been looked upon with suspicion as, historically, some claimed stillbirth to hide infanticide (Catalano, 2015). This history has persisted. Mothers in the United States may face prosecution, especially if they are poor and Black, and further victimized by allegations of substance use during pregnancy (Herbert, 2001; Layne, 2006). During prenatal healthcare visits in Western countries, women are often told that if they do the right things, eat the right foods, and follow their doctor's recommendations, they will give birth to a healthy baby. In the case of an unexplained stillbirth (the majority of cases), women are often left to blame themselves for having done "something wrong" (Cacciatore, Froen, & Killian, 2014).

The social implications of cultures' explicit silence on this tragic birth outcome are evident in everyday life and in medicine and midwifery. When examined through a feminist lens, it is apparent that the culture of social constraints around grief and the lack of recognition of these stillborn babies as *babies* can serve to retraumatize grieving mothers (Brin, 2004; Cosgrove, 2004). In addition, the medical community often masks the realities of stillbirth from the realm of possibility for pregnant women. Historically, this trend to overlook stillbirth has affected data collection and interventions. For example, the U.S. National Institutes of Health (NIH, 2018) began studying sudden infant death syndrome (SIDS) in the early 1970s, but it took another 30 years, until 2003, for the NIH to include stillbirth in its research funding agenda.

In this chapter we examine stillbirth using a feminist theoretical lens. We first describe the surprising frequency of stillbirth, of the millions of women worldwide who lose their babies in this way. We then discuss how these women's experiences are undermined by the cultural taboo of stillbirth, how their experiences are minimized culturally, and how this causes them to be further traumatized. The next part of the chapter describes changes to paternalistic medical care after stillbirth, but criticizes medical care before stillbirth as remaining paternalistic by refusing to educate women about the risks of stillbirth. The next part describes how stillbirth has been inadvertently relatively marginalized within a feminist agenda, and assures that recognition of stillbirth is consistent with that agenda. The chapter concludes with recommendations for the future.

The frequency of deaths due to stillbirth

Generally speaking, *stillbirth* refers to the death of a baby after a set number of weeks of gestation, but before birth. That number of weeks of pregnancy that defines stillbirth varies widely across geographical contexts (Frøen et al., 2011). For example, according to the World Health Organization (2018), stillbirth is an in utero death at 28 weeks gestation or later. In the U.S, the definition of "fetal death" (as opposed to stillbirth) varies by state; some states base it on the weight (usually more than 500 grams), others on estimated gestational age of 20 weeks or more, and others use a combination of both (MacDorman & Gregory, 2015). A significant number of stillbirths are late-term (after 37 weeks gestation), and many die on or near their due dates, often during labor (MacDorman & Gregory, 2015). The different definitions, between countries and even within the same country, make data collection difficult (Stanton, Lawn, Rahman, Wilczynska-Ketende, & Hill, 2006).

Stillbirth occurs globally to approximately 2.6 million women and their babies annually (Flenady et al., 2011). Based on 2015 data of stillbirths after 28 weeks of pregnancy, and with the caveat that data may be inaccurate, Pakistan had the highest rate of stillbirths: 43.1 stillbirths per 1,000 live births (Blencowe et al., 2016). Most of the other countries with the top ten highest stillbirth rates are in Africa, including Nigeria, Chad, Guinea-Bissau, Niger, and Somalia (Blencowe et al., 2016). These rates would be even higher if stillbirths before 28 weeks had been included. Women in developing countries are much more likely than women in developed countries to experience stillbirth; however, like many health disparities, the likelihood varies greatly according to ethnicity, socioeconomic class, and the quality of healthcare available (Frøen et al., 2011). Stillbirth still occurs in developed nations too often. Approximately 24,000 stillbirths occurred in the U.S. in 2013, more than 65 each day, at a rate of 5.96 stillbirths per 1,000 live births based on the 20-week definition (MacDorman & Gregory, 2015). Other developed countries have lower rates; Australia's stillbirth rate in 2015 was estimated at 2.7 and the United Kingdom's at 2.9 stillbirths per 1,000 live births (Lawn, Blencowe, Waiswa, Amouzou, & Mathers, 2016). Again though, these numbers would be higher if the 20-week definition of stillbirth had been used.

Exceptions may exist, but deaths due to stillbirth are usually not counted in infant mortality data. For example, the World Health Organization does not include stillbirths in its routine mortality data (Stanton et al., 2006). In the United States, none of the more than 20,000 deaths due to stillbirth each year are counted in infant mortality data. Any such death, regardless of gestational age or weight, is instead classified as a "fetal death." Policies regarding stillbirth are paradoxical: a baby who dies at 9 pounds and 42 weeks gestation, only seconds prior to birth, is a fetal death; whereas a baby who is born alive at 19 weeks gestation, weighs less than 1 pound, but takes a single breath, is classified an "infant death" and counted in infant mortality data. If the deaths of stillborn babies were counted in mortality statistics, stillbirth would be the 11th leading cause of all deaths internationally (Phillips & Millum, 2014). Stillbirth claims more lives in Western countries than all other causes of infant deaths combined and, as stated earlier, it is at least ten times more prevalent than SIDS (Frøen et al., 2011). The distinction between "fetal" and infant mortality is important, as there is public concern about infant mortality, but not about stillbirth (MacDorman & Gregory, 2015). Furthermore, the deficiencies in data collection strengthen common misconceptions about stillbirth. These misconceptions include stillbirth's believed obscurity due to medical advancements, the belief that proper prenatal care will prevent stillbirth (Kelley & Trinidad, 2012), and that stillbirth only happens in undeveloped countries because of poorer healthcare (Kelley & Trinidad, 2012).

The taboo and myths of stillbirth

Whatever is unnamed, undepicted in images, whatever is omitted from biography, censored in collections of letters, whatever is misnamed as something else, made difficult-to-come-by, whatever is buried in the memory by the collapse of meaning under an inadequate or lying language—this will become, not merely unspoken, but unspeakable.

Adrienne Rich (1995, p. 199)

Despite its commonality, stillbirth remains hidden culturally (Frøen et al., 2011). Researchers have described it as *invisible*: the outside world sees neither the life nor the death (DeFrain, Martens, Stork, & Stork, 1986). The mother knows that both birth and death occurred. She felt the baby grow in her womb, and she later learns that the baby also died there. She buries her child, not her pregnancy.

Public acknowledgment of any type of death before birth is rare (Lawn et al., 2009). In undeveloped nations, stillbirth is even more hidden as births occur at home; the family privately buries, and often does not publicly mourn, the child (Lawn et al., 2009). While death, or many types of deaths, remain taboo subjects, the death of an unborn baby, especially one who could have survived outside the mother's womb, is especially taboo (Maiorescu, 2015).

When stillbirth is acknowledged, it is to a limited extent. For example, stillbirth is often conflated with miscarriage, grouped together as "pregnancy losses" (CDC, 2017). It is true that before stillbirth, the woman was pregnant, and after, she is not. But the reason she is no longer pregnant is because she gave birth to her dead child. A unique and already loved individual has died.

That a child died should be obvious based on what happens after the mother gives birth to her stillborn baby. A mother should be offered the option to hold her deceased child, a measure that research demonstrates helps the mother to grieve (Erlandsson, Warland, Cacciatore, & Rådestad, 2013). It is not possible to hold a pregnancy loss, but mothers can hold their deceased babies. Similarly, a mother cannot bury a pregnancy, but she will need to decide to either cremate or bury her stillborn child, as she is likely legally obligated to do (Cacciatore, 2009). Her child's name will appear on the death certificate, possibly the only legal recognition that the child did exist (Cacciatore, 2009). The mother will wake up days later with her breasts full of milk, but no living baby to feed. Using the phrase "pregnancy loss" to describe stillbirth denies the traumatic reality of stillbirth: a child died.

The "pregnancy loss" characterization also conflates stillbirth with miscarriage. Miscarriage is the type of pregnancy loss that occurs before 20 weeks of gestation. The timing creates numerous differences in the two experiences. Miscarriages may involve medical treatment, such as a dilation and curettage, which is common in miscarriages before 12 weeks (Layne, 2006), but does not occur with stillbirth. Similarly, miscarriages do not necessitate cremation or burial, as often the fetus had not developed far enough to enable either. Parents may have already named their child, but that name will not appear on a death certificate, as death registration and final disposition laws do not exist for miscarriages.

Grouping stillbirth and miscarriage together as "pregnancy loss" has caused many to inappropriately attribute the same characteristics to each. The view that stillbirth is inevitable due to fetal abnormalities is widespread yet inaccurate (Lawn et al., 2016). Only around 7.4% of global annual stillbirths are due to abnormalities, some of which are neural tube defects, which are preventable (Lawn et al., 2016). A recent study of stillbirths in the United States demonstrated that, conservatively, at least one fourth of stillbirths could be prevented with proper medical care (Page et al., 2018). Risk factors for stillbirth are known; although some of those risk factors could perhaps be reduced or eliminated with proper medical care, the majority of stillbirths globally occur during childbirth. The fatalism of stillbirth is a myth that, if dispelled, might encourage further medical research.

The conflation of stillbirth with miscarriage minimizes stillbirth, as does another characterization of stillbirth: the use of the word "fetus" to describe the child that the mother buries. Fetus is a technical, medical term, denoting a baby developing in the mother's uterus. From the first heartbeat to birth, medically, the "baby" is a "fetus." And thus, under this technical characterization, only a fetus dies in stillbirth. The clinical formality required in the medical profession, however, is not required nor even common among laypersons. Taxonomical structures in medicine provide specific definitions and parameters for the developmental milestones of pregnancy. They do not, however, provide guidance for the use of the word *fetus* contextually (Sanger, 2017). That includes the context of stillbirth, in which medical language does not accurately reflect a woman's lived experience. As already mentioned, the mother holds a child, not a fetus; she buries her child, not a nameless, genderless fetus. Many stillborn babies are full-term, and some even die during childbirth. They are fully developed babies, who could have survived outside of the womb.

In the social context, medical technicality does not require that "fetus" be used to describe a not yet born baby. The best evidence of this is that doctors do not even use the term during a woman's pregnancy. In a desired pregnancy that is developing normally, "medical professionals are more likely to socially support the attribution of 'baby' or 'child' status to the fetus" (Petchesky, 1987, p. 277). Any eagerly pregnant woman who has had an ultrasound knows that the doctor points out the baby's hands, not the "fetus's" hands. "[B]ut when something goes wrong, the medical terminology is quickly redeployed" (Browne, 2016, p. 402). And thus, after stillbirth, the technical medical characterization of "fetus" appears.

It is true that doctors, like many other people, are uncomfortable with grief, particularly when it is traumatic. Doctors who deliver babies do not normally confront death, and they often fear that mothers will blame them for the death (Kelley & Trinidad, 2012). But her doctor's reaction, the care she receives after stillbirth, and the reaction of others have long-lasting consequences for mothers (Nuzum, Meaney, & O'Donoghue, 2014). Doctors must thus acknowledge the mother's loss: the same "baby" the doctor monitored for the past five or so months is now dead (Nuzum et al., 2014).

The taboo and minimizations have led to the dominant view that stillbirth is "a terrible loss," but not the same as losing "a child" (Kelley & Trinidad, 2012), a view incongruent with mothers' experiences. Grieving mothers say that they lost their baby, their child, or a member of their family, and "most [parents] refer to the loss as a baby" (PLIDA, 2016). To mothers, and parents generally, stillbirth is no different than infant death. Parents "describe the grief of stillbirth as being just as deep, painful, and significant as it would be to lose an infant who is born and survives a few weeks in intensive care" (Kelley & Trinidad, 2012, p. 10). Plainly, stillbirth is the death of a child who is real and will always be remembered as part of the family (DeFrain et al., 1990). When asked what "they most wanted the general public to know about stillbirth and how it affects families," parents overwhelmingly answered that "*a stillbirth is a death in the family*" (DeFrain et al., 1990, p. 128).

The lack of public acknowledgment of the devastation of stillbirth stigmatizes and retraumatizes families by minimizing the strength of their attachment and the significance of the relationship lost, particularly the mother–child relationship. Stillbirth is the death of the mother's child, but she may feel unable to grieve openly or to remind others of her child's birthday, a birthday that coincides with the day the child died (Kelley & Trinidad, 2012). Even friends and family may not recognize the child's existence (Littlewood, 1992). Mothers feel isolated. Many opt not to discuss their child because it makes others feel awkward and uncomfortable (Kelley & Trinidad, 2012). Mothers experience a traumatic grief in stillbirth, and then they feel marginalized when they realize that their child's life and death are unacknowledged (Murphy & Cacciatore, 2017). To understand the meaning of the death of a baby during or prior to birth, we must have a common language that is informed by the perspectives of grieving mothers as the relevant community, the experts in their own experiences (Kuhn, 1962), both colloquially and among scientists and health professionals.

Grieving mothers have too long allowed others, those who have not experienced the death of a child, to control both the nomenclature of and conversation about their emotional reactions. Yet, they are, and should be, recognized as authorities on stillbirth. They know first hand the loss and trauma they suffer. Both medical providers and the lay community should use language that takes into account these women's lived experience. That language should include the words *baby*, *child*, and the child's specific *name* to make them visible and to validate the mothers' connection to their child. Most grieving mothers are eager to discuss their children who died, but, aside from a support group, they lack a safe and accepting place to do so (DeFrain et al., 1986). Stillbirth is a tragedy, but mothers should not have to suffer it alone.

Compassionate and empowering medical care

The most significant changes to medical treatment of stillbirth have occurred in the psychosocial caregiving for mothers *after* stillbirth. In the mid-20th century, when mothers went to the hospital to give birth, they were often unconscious, sometimes for days, due to "twilight sleep," and, in Western nations, most babies were born with the use of forceps (Simkin, 1996). When babies died during birth, mothers often never saw them, let alone remembered their births. Their babies were whisked away by nurses, as it was thought to be "for the mother's own good" to quickly bury their children and act as if nothing had happened at all. One mother, who was never told where her stillborn daughter was buried, found her 40 years later when her children tracked down the grave and bought their sister a headstone. They took their mother there as a surprise, at which time she finally was able to grieve openly (Porter, 2011).

Eventually, the "pretend it didn't happen" standard of medical care changed. The changes were not prompted by medical providers, but instead by the efforts of grieving mothers in grassroots support groups who began to demand access to the child in the late 1970s (Murphy & Cacciatore, 2017). In the 1980s, doctors in the United States regularly started offering parents access to their stillborn child and encouraging parents to hold and spend time with their stillborn child. In the United Kingdom, hospitals routinely offer parents photographs and footprints, and also strongly encourage parents to hold their child (Kelley & Trinidad, 2012). Mothers do not want to forget their child, and this time with their child and the keepsakes help to ensure that they have memories (Kelley & Trinidad, 2012). Similarly, rituals, such as funerals or memorials, can also be helpful to mothers (Brin, 2004). These changes in health care practice have been shown to help parents grieve (Murphy & Cacciatore, 2017), and the keepsakes and rituals help parents recognize their children and create meaning, when they are ready (Brin, 2004).

Another type of caregiving created by grieving mothers emerged in the same timeframe. Support groups started emerging in the 1970s; their creation was led by women, most often by American women, and was linked to the empowerment of women (Layne, 2006). Support groups give grieving parents a space to talk openly about their children, an ability that does not exist in public given the cultural aversion to grief in general, but especially in relation to the death of a baby. Connecting with other grieving mothers in a support group setting has been shown to be beneficial and reduce significantly symptoms of traumatic stress (Cacciatore, 2007). Another similar form of support can be found in psychotherapy. Feminist scholars have explained how therapists can better help grieving mothers by recognizing that a mother's grief after stillbirth is often "disenfranchised," which therapists can help to diminish by providing a "place where a woman does not experience the social discomfort of the others to whom she tries to speak about her loss and pain" (Cosgrove, 2004, pp. 116–117).

Grieving mothers have significantly changed medical treatment and assistance for parents after stillbirth. But little has changed with respect to treatment for possible stillbirth *before* the child dies. The strategy seems to be just to hope that stillbirth will not happen. For most mothers, that hope is not enough, as one in 200 unborn children will die in stillbirth in developing nations (Cousens et al., 2011). Presumably because of the low risk and the anxiety it may cause the mother, there is little information about stillbirth in pregnancy books or pamphlets at doctors' offices. Even in the literature on the negative social and emotional outcomes in women who experience a loss before birth, stillbirth is addressed only as a type of "pregnancy loss" (Layne, 2003a, 2006), again inappropriately conflating stillbirth and miscarriage (Cacciatore & Bushfield, 2008). Doctors warn women about the risk of miscarriage, but not stillbirth. Parents' worries focus on miscarriage and premature birth, but not on stillbirth (Kelley & Trinidad, 2012).

Mothers typically do not know anything about stillbirth unless it happens to them. After stillbirth, parents surveyed explain that before it happened to them, they believed that stillbirth was extremely rare (Kelley & Trinidad, 2012). They believed that proper prenatal care would prevent it, only to learn later that they were wrong (Kelley & Trinidad, 2012). After their own child died, parents were surprised to learn the frequency of stillbirth worldwide (Kelley & Trinidad, 2012). "The distraught and bewildered parents" must then "come to terms with an outcome that affects one pregnancy in 200 (beyond 23 weeks of gestation); yet this event will often never have previously been mentioned in a conversation with any health professional" (Smith, 2011, p. 1307).

Current medical care remains paternalistic, similar to standard traditional medical practices after stillbirth; medical providers seem to think there is no need to educate mothers about such a low risk, even though the low risk is of the worst severity: the child's death. The lack of education about stillbirth is yet another example of what has been described as the benevolent sexism deeply embedded in the culture of pregnancy (Watson, 2014). Doctors believe that it is healthier for women not to know, that the anxiety women would experience worrying about stillbirth creates a more significant, perhaps psychological, risk than the actual risk of stillbirth (Kelley & Trinidad, 2012), another remnant of the "doctor knows best" medical standard.

The low risk alone, however, cannot explain the lack of information parents receive. Parents are well educated about other low risks of child death, such as SIDS, a risk ten times lower than the risk of stillbirth (Frøen et al., 2011), in part due to risk-reduction public health education campaigns in many countries (Hauck & Tanabe, 2008). The campaigns are focused on educating caregivers to put babies to sleep on their backs. France, for example, began its risk reduction campaign in 1994; its rate of SIDS deaths decreased 86% between 1990 and 2008 (Hauck & Tanabe, 2008). Ireland began its risk-reduction campaign in 1992 and decreased its rate of SIDS deaths by 73% between 1990 and 2007 (Hauck & Tanabe, 2008). In the United States, the "back to sleep" education campaign is on billboards, commercials, and posters in medical offices (Layne, 2006). Most of the countries that adopted a risk-reduction campaign saw an over 50% decline in the rates of deaths due to SIDS (Hauck & Tanabe, 2008). The success of these campaigns demonstrates the efficacy of education. Yet, there is scant information about the risk or prevention of stillbirth. Few mothers are educated about the known risk factors, which include obesity, maternal age over 35, and smoking (Flenady et al., 2011). Simple measures such as sleeping on one's left side and monitoring baby's movement, particularly during the final few weeks of pregnancy, can help to reduce the risk of stillbirth (Fretts, 2014). Some obstetricians may offer this advice to newly pregnant women, however they do not explain its role in preventing stillbirth. This simple acknowledgment may motivate behavioral changes and more diligent kick counting during pregnancy. One parent said it best: "If stillbirth really is ten times as common as cot death, we cannot be the only ones who had bought three sleep positioners but had never once considered the possibility of stillbirth" (Smith, 2011, p. 1307).

Feminist legal scholars have criticized the view within medical discourse and practice of the weak and emotional pregnant woman unable to make decisions (Madeira, 2012). We similarly need to revisit the view of the weak and emotional pregnant woman who may be dismayed at the low possibility her child could die before birth. The lack of education leaves women uninformed, with only questions after their child's death. Why did this happen to me? Why didn't anyone warn me about it? What could I have done to save my child? Why is there very little research in this area? Mothers spend much of their lives worrying about their children's safety and health, but current paternalistic medical care before a baby is born robs them of the awareness of stillbirth risk. Grieving mothers were the force behind enabling mothers to see and hold their babies after stillbirth (Murphy & Cacciatore, 2017) and the creation of support groups (Layne, 2006). They will also likely play an important role in educating pregnant women of the risks of stillbirth.

Protecting the mother's choice to have a baby

Feminism seeks to empower women, and feminist scholarship has discussed the theoretical meanings of what it means to be pregnant, to give birth to a child, and to be a mother (Browne, 2016). These theoretical discussions have, however, tended to neglect stillbirth; the norm in feminist literature, as elsewhere, is to "presume that pregnancy results in a living child" (Browne, 2016, p. 387; Layne, 2003b). Feminist literature has also, of course, discussed a woman's choice not to become a mother and consistently defended a woman's right to choose abortion. An emphasis on abortion has sometimes meant a minimization of a woman's experience in stillbirth (Lens, 2018). The fear among some feminists is that "if one were to acknowledge there was something of value lost" in stillbirth, "one would thereby automatically accede the inherent personhood of embryos/fetuses" (Layne, 1997, p. 305). Similarly, any equation of "fetal life with that of born persons" could be made part of efforts to restrict abortion rights (Sanger, 2012, p. 305).

In order to protect abortion rights in the United States, pro-choice groups have sometimes opposed legal recognition of stillbirth. One example is opposition to legal recourse for parents if stillbirth is due to someone else's conduct, such as medical malpractice. Some pro-choice groups have argued against "wrongful death" claims after stillbirth, the same type of claim available for the death of a living child (Siano, 1998). Another example is opposition to the creation of birth certificates for stillbirth, a movement spearheaded in the United States by a grassroots group led by grieving mothers, the MISS Foundation. This limited recognition would accompany the already available certificates of fetal death. Again, the pro-choice groups argued against this limited recognition for fear of encroachment on abortion rights (Sanger, 2012).

The protection of abortion rights, however, need not involve the minimization of stillbirth (Lens, 2019). Even the U.S. Supreme Court in *Roe v. Wade* (1973), the same case where it announced the right to abortion, explained how the parents' wrongful death claim for "unborn children" was consistent with the right to abortion. Similarly, within the New York state legislature's debate on stillborn birth certificates, the state's powerful pro-choice lobbying group explained its support for the certificates due to their recognition of the pain parents experience in the loss of their expected baby (Sanger, 2012).

Many women choose not to become mothers, some by successfully avoiding pregnancy, and some by choosing abortion. Some women may choose abortion earlier in life, and then later choose to become a mother, yet lose that child to stillbirth. An abortion in her past further complicates a woman's experience with stillbirth (DeFrain et al., 1990). Feminists need not forsake recognition of stillbirth to protect a woman's right to choose abortion (Browne, 2016). In addition to defending abortion, feminists can and should still "account for the value of intrauterine or fetal life, and to allow for the wide range of emotions and responses that can attend both the voluntary termination of a pregnancy and its involuntary loss" in stillbirth (Browne, 2016, p. 403).

Recommendations for a hopeful future: research and public health campaigns

Recognition of stillbirth has improved, as has care for mothers after stillbirth. Yet, as we have already intimated, more can be done. A first step to help reduce stillbirth is to improve data collection. Inconsistent definitions make it difficult to obtain good data, data that are necessary for research regarding the risk factors for and causes of stillbirth. The medical community must make stillbirth a priority, as more babies die in stillbirth than in the first year after birth. That progress is possible is undeniable as developed nations have varied stillbirth rates (Cousens et al., 2011).

Another important step to empower women is to inform mothers of the chance of still-birth. Doctors usually tell mothers to count their baby's movements, but rarely tell them the dire meaning of a change in movement. Proper warnings of the risk will better enable mothers to monitor their own babies, especially near the end of the pregnancies. The risk of stillbirth is low, but the consequence is ultimate, and mothers need to know.

It is of great import to adopt language and care that reflects the loss the mother suffers—not just of a pregnancy, not just of a fetus, but of her child, a child who was and is a member of the family. Sensitive language and appropriate concern are important not just from medical providers but also the community generally. We hope that, one day, grieving mothers will be able to talk openly about their children who died without fear of dismissal or minimization. Until then, community support groups give mothers a place to discuss the death of her child with others who understand how she feels. In the United States, recognition of the baby's birth, not just her or his death, can be obtained by parents who request a Certificate of Birth Resulting in Stillbirth (as it is most often called) from their office of vital records.

Medical providers should provide woman-focused care that empowers mothers to make choices about rituals such as seeing and holding her baby, naming her baby, and even taking photographs and collecting other mementos of her baby. Rituals, including funerals, should be encouraged (Brin, 2004). Validating the existence of the baby is akin to validating her as a mother, something that holds great meaning for most grieving women. Postpartum emotional support for both practical matters, such as tending to other surviving children and managing lactation, as well as psychological support, will be crucial for most.

Stillbirth is simultaneous birth and death, and the culmination of these two social transformations has led to the erasure of these much-wanted babies. The erasure makes these deaths, and the grief that follows them, invisible, and makes the work that these mothers do invisible (Daniels, 1987). It is long past time for this erasure to end. Grieving mothers, again, are leading the charge.

References

Blencowe, H., Cousens, S. C., Jassir, F. B., Say, L., Chou, D., Mathers, C., Hogan, D., Shiekh, S., Qureshi, Z. U., You, D., Lawn, J., & Lancet Stillbirth Epidemiology Investigator Group (2016). National, regional, and worldwide estimates of stillbirth rates in 2015, with trends from 2000: A systematic analysis. *Lancet, 4*(2), e104.

Brin, D. J. (2004). The use of rituals in grieving for a miscarriage or stillbirth. *Women & Therapy, 27* (3–4), 128–130.

Browne, V. (2016). Feminist philosophy and prenatal death: Relationality and the ethics of intimacy. *Signs, 41*(2), 387, 402–404.

Cacciatore, J. (2007). Effects of support groups on post traumatic stress responses in women experiencing stillbirth. *Omega, 55*(71), 83–84.

Cacciatore, J. (2009). The silent birth: A feminist perspective. *Social Work, 54*, 91–94.

Cacciatore, J. & Bushfield, S. (2008). Stillbirth: A sociopolitical issue. *Affilia, 23*, 378–387.

Cacciatore, J., Froen, F., & Killian, M. (2014). The effects of self-blame on anxiety and depression among grieving women. *Journal of Mental Health Counseling, 35*, 342–359.

Cacciatore, J., Lacasse, J., Lietz, C., & McPherson, J. (2014). A parent's TEARS: Primary results from the traumatic experiences and resiliency study. *Omega, 68*, 183–205.

Catalano, A. (2015). *A global history of child death: Mortality, burial, and parental attitudes.* New York, NY: Peter Lang.

Centers for Disease Control and Prevention (CDC) (2017). *Facts about stillbirth.* Retrieved from www.cdc.gov/ncbddd/stillbirth/facts.html.

Cosgrove, L. (2004). The aftermath of pregnancy loss: A feminist critique of the literature and implications for treatment. *Women & Therapy, 27*(3), 107–122.

Cousens, S., Blencowe, H., Stanton, C., Chou, D., Ahmed, S., Steinhardt, L., Creanga, A. A., Tunçalp, Ö., Balsara, Z. P., Gupta, S., Say, L., & Lawn, J. (2011). National, regional, and worldwide estimates of stillbirth rates in 2009 with trends since 1995: A systematic analysis. *Lancet, 377*, 1319–1330.

Daniels, A. K. (1987). Invisible work. *Social Problems, 34*, 403–414.

DeFrain, J., Martens, L., Stork, J., & Stork, W. (1986). *Stillborn: The invisible death.* New York, NY: Lexington Books.

DeFrain, J., Martens, L., Stork, J., & Stork, W. (1990). The psychological effects of a stillbirth on surviving family members. *Omega, 22*, 83–110.

Erlandsson, K., Warland, J., Cacciatore, J., & Rådestad, I. (2013). Seeing and holding a stillborn baby: Mothers' feelings in relation to how their babies were presented to them after birth –findings from an online questionnaire. *Midwifery, 29*(3), 246–250.

Flenady, V., Koopmans, L., Middleton, P., Frøen, J. F., Smith, G. C., Gibbons, K., Coory, M., Gordon, A., Ellwood, D., Mcintyre, H. D., Fretts, R., & Ezzati, M. (2011). Major risk factors for stillbirth in high-income countries: A systematic review and meta-analysis. *Lancet, 377*(9774), 1331–1340.

Fretts, R. C. (2014). The stillbirth 'scandal.' *BMC Pregnancy and Childbirth, 15*(supp.1), A11.

Frøen, J. F., Cacciatore, J., McClure, E. M., Kuti, O., Jokhio, A., Islam, M., & Shiffman, J. (2011). Stillbirths: Why they matter. *Lancet, 377*, 1353–1366.

Hauck, F. & Tanabe, K. (2008). International trends in sudden infant death syndrome: Stabilization of rates requires further action. *Pediatrics, 122*(3), 660–661.

Herbert, B. (2001, May 24). In America; stillborn justice. *New York Times.* Retrieved from www.nytimes.com/2001/05/24/opinion/in-america-stillborn-justice.html.

Kelley, M. C. & Trinidad, S. B. (2012). Silent loss and the clinical encounter: Parents' and physicians' experiences of stillbirth – a qualitative analysis. *BMC Pregnancy and Childbirth, 12*, 137.

Kuhn, T. S. (1962). *The structure of scientific revolutions.* (1st ed.). Chicago, IL: University of Chicago Press.

Lawn, J., Blencowe, H., Waiswa, P., Amouzou, A., & Mathers, C. (2016). Stillbirths: Rates, risk factors, and acceleration towards 2030. *Lancet, 387*(10018), 587–603.

Lawn, J., Yakoob, M. Y., Hawns, R. A., Soomro, T., Darmstadt, G., & Bhutta, Z. (2009). 3.2 million stillbirths: Epidemiology and overview of the evidence review. *BMC Pregnancy and Childbirth, 9*(1), 8.

Layne, L. (1997). Breaking the silence: An agenda for a feminist discourse of pregnancy loss. *Feminist Studies, 23*(2), 289–315.

Layne, L. (2003a). Unhappy endings: A feminist reappraisal of the women's health movement from the vantage of pregnancy loss. *Social Science and Medicine, 56*, 1881–1891.

Layne, L. (2003b). *Motherhood lost: A feminist account of pregnancy loss in America*. London, UK: Routledge.

Layne, L. (2006). Pregnancy and infant loss support: A new, feminist, American, patient movement? *Social Science and Medicine, 62*(3), 602–613.

Lens, J. W. (2018). Tort law's devaluation of stillbirth. *Nevada Law Journal, 18*. Advance online publication. Retrieved from https://ssrn.com/abstract=3235402.

Littlewood, J. (1992). *Aspects of grief: Bereavement in adult life*. London, UK: Taylor & Francis.

MacDorman, M. & Gregory, E. (2015). Fetal and perinatal mortality: United States, 2013. *National Vital Statistics Reports, 64*(8), 1–24. Retrieved from www.cdc.gov/nchs/data/nvsr/nvsr64/nvsr64_08.pdf.

Madeira, J. L. (2012). Woman scorned? Resurrecting infertile women's decision-making autonomy. *Maryland Law Review, 71*, 355.

Maiorescu, R. (2015). Public relations for the bereaved: Online interactions in a community for stillbirth and neonatal death charity. *Public Relations Review, 41*(2), 293–295.

Murphy, S. & Cacciatore, J. (2017). The multiple impact of stillbirth on families: A review of recent literature exploring the psychological, social, and economic ramifications of losing a baby. *Seminars in Fetal and Neonatal Medicine, 22*(3), 129–134.

National Institutes of Health (2018). NICHD SIDS research information. Retrieved July, 2018 from www.nichd.nih.gov/health/topics/sids/researchinfo.

Nuzum, D., Meaney, S., & O'Donoghue, K. (2014). The impact of stillbirth on consultant obstetrician gynaecologists: A qualitative study. *British Journal of Obstetrics and Gynaecology, 121*(8), 1020–1028.

Page, J. M., Thorsten, V., Reddy, U. M., Dudley, D. J., Hogue, C. J. R., Saade, G. R., Pinar, H., Parker, C. B., Conway, D., Stoll, B. J., Coustan, D., Bukowski, R., Varner, M. W., Goldenberg, R. L., Gibbins, K., & Silver, R. M. (2018). Potentially preventable stillbirth in a diverse U.S. cohort. *Obstetrics & Gynecology, 131*, 336–343.

Petchesky, R. P. (1987). Fetal images: The power of visual culture in the politics of reproduction. *Feminist Studies, 13*(2), 263–292.

Phillips, J. & Millum, J. (2014). Valuing stillbirths. *Bioethics, 29*, 413–423.

Porter, R. (2011, March 16). A chance to say goodbye: How heartbroken couples find the graves of their stillborn children. *Daily Mail*. Retrieved from www.dailymail.co.uk/femail/article-1366962/How-heartbroken-couples-secret-graves-long-lost-stillborn-children.html.

Pregnancy Loss and Infant Death Alliance (PLIDA) (2016). Bereaved parents' right to self-determination regarding their baby. Retrieved from www.plida.org/wp-content/uploads/2012/01/PLIDA_BereavedParentsRighttoSelf-Determination.pdf.

Rich, A. (1995). *Lies, secrets, and silence*. New York, NY: W.W. Norton.

Roe v. Wade (1973). 410 U.S. 113, 161.

Sanger, C. (2012). "The birth of death": Stillborn birth certificates and the problem for law. *University of California Law Review, 100*(269), 305.

Sanger, C. (2017). *About abortion*. Cambridge, MA: Harvard University Press.

Shreffler, K., Hill, T., & Cacciatore, J. (2012). The impact of infertility, miscarriage, stillbirth, and child death on marital dissolution. *Journal of Divorce and Remarriage, 53*, 91–107.

Siano, J. R. (1998). A woman's right to choose: Wrongful death statutes and abortion rights – consistent at last. *Women's Rights Law Reporter, 19*, 288.

Simkin, P. (1996). The experience of maternity in a woman's life. *Journal of Obstetric Gynecology and Neonatal Nursing, 25*, 247–252.

Smith, G. (2011). A bonfire of the tape measure. *Lancet, 377*, 1307.

Stanton, C., Lawn, J., Rahman, H., Wilczynska-Ketende, K., & Hill, K. (2006). Stillbirth rates: Delivering estimates in 190 countries. *Lancet, 367*, 1487–1488.

Surkan, P. J., Radestad, I., Cnattingius, S., Steineck, G., & Dickman, P. W. (2008). Events after stillbirth in relation to maternal depressive symptoms: A brief report. *Birth, 35*(2), 153–157.

Watson, H. (2014). Medicine still needs feminism. *British Medical Journal, 348*, 24.

World Health Organization (2018). Stillbirths. Retrieved from www.who.int/maternal_child_adolescent/epidemiology/stillbirth/en.

21

PSYCHOLOGICAL ASPECTS OF PREGNANCY AND PREGNANCY HEALTH CARE IN THEIR SOCIAL AND CULTURAL CONTEXTS

Jane R. W. Fisher and Karin Hammarberg

Safe motherhood is now more assured and pregnancy-related deaths are rare among women living in World-Bank-classified high-income countries. However, most women live in resource-constrained low- and lower-middle-income countries, where they have less access to preconception health information, family planning services, recommended antenatal care, skilled birth attendants, health care facilities in which to give birth, and basic and emergency obstetric care, than women have in high-income countries. They are less likely to have access to secondary schooling, to be able to generate an adequate and secure income, and to have had the sexual and reproductive health education that is essential to being able to make autonomous choices about when to have a child and how many children they wish to have. They are more likely to live in crowded circumstances and to be poorly nourished and, when pregnant, to carry a coincidental burden of infectious diseases. Their lives are more likely to be constrained by rigid gender stereotypes about appropriate roles and responsibilities for women. Gender-based violence is prevalent in all contexts, but especially in cultures in which women and girls are devalued and their rights ignored. They are also at greater risk of dying from pregnancy-related causes, to experience the maternal morbidities of haemorrhage and infection, to give birth to babies who are underweight and not to have access to the health care they need in these circumstances. As pregnancy and childbirth have become safer, awareness has grown in clinical, public health, and research communities of individual and contextual factors associated with health in pregnancy and the links to foetal health and development (Fisher, Cabral de Mello, & Isutzu, 2009). This chapter will discuss the psychological aspects of pregnancy health and pregnancy health care, in their social and cultural contexts, and describe how explanatory theories are shaped, historically, by prevailing stereotypes.

The social and cultural contexts of pregnancy

The total fertility rate is the estimated average number of children born to each woman if current population patterns prevail in her lifetime. The United Nations' most recent

World Population Prospects (2017) reveal that in 1955–1960, the total fertility rate among women in high-income nations was 3.0 children, in middle-income was 5.48 and in low-income was 6.54. Sixty years later, these had fallen across the world to 1.72 children per woman in high-income, 2.35 in middle-income and 4.62 in low-income nations. Nevertheless, they reveal the substantial disparities in numbers of children born to women who have greater opportunities for full social and economic participation than those who have fewer.

The United Nations Population Fund (2017) argues that there are two critical determinants of these disparities: gender inequality, and inequalities in realizing sexual and reproductive health and rights. Lacking access to contraception, living in a rural area, and having limited education increase the likelihood of unintended pregnancy or of pregnancy related to family expectations. Together these cement the health risks and economic limitations that can embed cycles of reduced capability, unrealized human rights, and poverty for women and their children.

The 1994 International Conference on Population and Development (United Nations Population Fund, 1994) concluded that elimination of disparities for women and girls in education, income-generating work, and political participation rely predominantly on their reproductive rights being realized. More than 20 years later in 2015, the 2030 Agenda for Sustainable Development (United Nations, 2016) explicitly identifies in Goal 5 that gender equality and gender empowerment are essential for achieving flourishing economies and dignity for every woman and every girl, everywhere, and in Target 5.6 that this can only be achieved by universal access to reproductive health and reproductive rights.

In high-income nations, the average age at which a woman first gives birth is increasing. For example, in Australia in 1970 it was in the early 20s, but by 2010 it had increased to the late 20s (Li, Zeki, Hilder, & Sullivan, 2013). The same pattern prevails elsewhere. In the USA it increased from 27.2 years in 2003 to 28.2 years in 2015. In 2016, in Tokyo, Japan it was 32.2 years and in Switzerland 30.2 years (Mathews & Hamilton, 2016; Worldatlas, 2017).

This change is commonly attributed to women electing to 'delay childbearing', because they are pursuing personal career ambitions, or activities like travel, or are seeking financial security (Fyfe & Davies, 2015). Holton, Fisher, and Rowe (2011) investigated the factors associated with having or not having children among 569 women aged 30–34 years who had been selected at random from the Australian Electoral Roll and completed a postal survey anonymously. In this group, 219 women (38%) had not (yet) had a child and the predominant reason for this was that they did not have a partner or a partner willing to commit to parenthood. Reasons relating to education and employment were less prominent, and wishing to establish a career before having children and not wanting to give up freedom were rarely provided as primary reasons. These data confirm those from other high-income nations that the most common reason for women to be childless by their mid-30s is the difficulty in finding a man who is willing to commit to partnership and parenthood. Few women wish to become intentional single parents using donor sperm (Hammarberg et al., 2017).

There is a growing disjunction in high-income nations which is contributing to these reproductive patterns. The largest group of un-partnered men are those who have limited education and are either not employed or doing unskilled work, and the largest group of single women are those with postgraduate qualifications and professional employment (2009). Given that people tend to partner across a small rather than a large social distance, the likelihood of these two groups of people meeting each other's preferences for characteristics desired in a life partner is low. Puur, Olah, Tazi-Preve, and Dorbritz (2008) investigated another potential contributing factor. They analyzed data contributed by men aged 20–44 years in eight European countries to the Population Policy Acceptance Study (Höhn, Avramov, & Kotowska, 2008). They concluded that while women's participation rates in higher education and income-generating work have increased dramatically, there have been 'few signs' of men increasing responsibilities for the work of caregiving and management of household tasks. This has led to 'incoherence in levels of gender equity' with more having been achieved in the public than the private sphere, and that fertility has declined as a consequence.

There is a copious social commentary about what have been described as impossible dilemmas for women. Anne-Marie Slaughter's (2012) essay 'Why women can't have it all' describes her situation as an academic seconded to a public policy role in another city, and concludes that the costs to dependent children of their mothers pursuing senior roles are prohibitive and constraining. British writer Shirley Conran (2001/2002) argues that 'the battle to have life and love', which young women assume was 'won by their mothers', is essentially unchanged, even intensified and that the 'bitter trade-off' between a dynamic career and a satisfying home life' remains. Conran asserts that women believe that by completing education and establishing a career before seeking to conceive they are serving the interests of future children, but are unaware that they are then placing in jeopardy the possibility of having a child at all. One of the consequences of this social change is that as age has an inevitable and inexorable adverse impact on female fertility, there are growing numbers of women experiencing age-related fertility difficulties (Schmidt, Sobotka, Bentzen, & Nyboe Andersen, 2011). It is not possible to distinguish at a population level whether women without children are voluntarily or involuntary childfree, but it is suggested on the basis of qualitative investigations that some women are 'childfree by choice', due to lack of desire to become a parent, personal health concerns, personal advancement, and a belief that it is not good to bring more children into the world (Agrillo & Nelini, 2008; Blackstone & Stewart, 2016).

Desire for motherhood

Most women want to have children, commonly at least two, but in high-income countries most have fewer children than they want, and many would have children, or more children, if their circumstances were different (Holton et al., 2011). It is in the context of assured maternal and infant health and survival that consciousness of the psychological aspects of pregnancy, childbirth and early parenthood has grown. In the past 50 years, there has been copious and increasingly sophisticated research into the psychological aspects, social needs and nature and determinants of mental health problems during reproductive life.

Considerations of the psychological aspects of pregnancy were first published by psychoanalysts in the mid- to late-twentieth century. These clinician theorists used conceptual frameworks that presumed health outcomes were governed entirely by individual factors. They asserted that for women, reproduction is the ultimate affirmation of femininity, and the only pathway to true psychosexual maturity. Freud construed pregnancy not as the choice of a mature and independent person, but as a woman's acting out of her unconscious desire to compensate for the penis she lacked (Astbury, 1986). Helen Deutsch (1945) described a quintessentially female biological state of motherliness. Benedek (1970) saw pregnancy not as a substitute for a penis, but rather as an expression of a hormonally generated instinct, a biologically motivated step in the maturation of the woman.

Subsequent psychological theories did not view the decision to have a child as a substitutive, unconscious process, and as reflecting broader, but nevertheless individual factors. Leifer (1977) concluded on the basis of interviews with 19 nulliparous pregnant women, that a wanted pregnancy is part of a planned process of embracing adult life, occurring at a time of emotional and practical readiness, in response to desires to intensify the relationship with an intimate partner, and to grow as an individual. Turrini (1980) concluded that there is also a strong influence from observing peers experiencing pregnancy, birth, and caring for a baby.

Psychological adjustment to pregnancy

Psychodynamic theories argue that there are inevitable maturational challenges experienced during pregnancy which require tolerance of disequilibrium and uncertainty, and a capacity to develop new solutions and strategies (Baraitser, 2009; Hall, 2016). For example, surveys of homogeneous cohorts of women who were pregnant, using psychoanalytically derived techniques of projective testing and interpretation of material provided by patients in clinical interviews, followed small-scale interview-based studies (Shereshefsky & Yarrow, 1973). They reached generally similar conclusions that profound psychological changes occur during pregnancy. These changes were construed as responses both to the physiological changes of pregnancy and to internal psychological processes. Pregnancy was characterized as including ambivalence and heightened psychological responsiveness, which could lead to disorganization (Breen, 1975). Wolkind and Zajicek (1981) preferred to describe these as a normal transition best understood as an accelerated developmental process.

While acknowledging individual differences in intensity, some elevation of anxiety was argued to be inevitable and probably pregnancy-specific (Grossman, Eichler, & Winickoff, 1980). Breen (1975) and Leifer (1977) concluded that for some pregnant women this elevated anxiety led to increased growth and maturation conferring increased self-confidence, a greater sense of completeness, and a perception of having advanced to another generation. Leifer (1977) observed that many women enjoy their pregnant appearance, feel proud of their fertility, are excited about sensations of foetal movements, and enjoy the increased regard of others. Some women did not display this increased maturation and Leifer (1977) concluded that adjustment to pregnancy and parenthood were linked to degree of 'personal stability' and that 'good adaptation during pregnancy is predictive of good mothering behaviour'.

Lubin, Gardener, and Roth (1975) conducted one of the few then available cohort studies; 93 'middle class' women completed self-report instruments in each trimester of pregnancy. They found that anxiety varied in a 'U-form', being highest in the first and third and lowest in the mid-trimester of pregnancy. Glazer (1980) conducted a similar study which included both more socioeconomically advantaged participants with private health insurance as well as those from recruited from public clinics. Both concluded that severity of anxiety in pregnancy reflected experiences of coincidental adverse life events and that as the physical demands increased, so did anxiety. Concerns were predominantly about the health of the baby and these outweighed anxieties about other experiences. These two authors were among the first to acknowledge that social circumstances influenced pregnancy anxiety, which was found to be higher among women who were younger and less well educated than among women occupying a higher socioeconomic position. Nevertheless, subsequent research, influenced by the psychoanalytic theorists, continued to focus on individual characteristics as vulnerabilities, without comprehensive consideration of the influence on their psychological functioning of social, cultural, and contextual factors.

Pregnancy and mental health problems

Landmark studies published in the 1960s stimulated a large body of research, which has sought to establish the prevalence and determinants of perinatal mental health problems among women. Less of this research has been specific to pregnancy and more has focussed on women's psychological functioning after childbirth.

There are descriptive historical accounts of disturbed behaviour associated with childbearing. Paffenbarger and Ralph (1964), in one of the first epidemiological investigations, reviewed medical records to report prevalence and some correlates of psychoses or 'psychoneurotic attacks' requiring hospital admission occurring among women who were pregnant or who had recently given birth. He concluded that, while rare (a rate of 5 per 10,000 pregnancies), the events occurring during pregnancy reflected 'prepartum conflict over unwanted pregnancy'.

The most serious pregnancy-related mental health problem is suicide. It has been argued that pregnant women are at lower risk of dying by suicide (Marzuk, Tardiff, Leon, & Hirsch, 1997) than non-pregnant women. Socially stigmatized causes of death are less reliably recorded and therefore probably under-ascertained (Graham, Filippi, & Ronsmans, 1996). Post-mortem examinations after suicide do not always include the uterine examination necessary to confirm pregnancy and examinations of obstetric records in addition to death certificates have identified significant under-ascertainment (Brockington, 2001). In high-income nations, rates of death by suicide during pregnancy have diminished over the past century, a change attributed to the increased availability of contraception, affordable and accessible services for the termination of pregnancy, and reduction in the stigma associated with ex-nuptial births (Frautschi, Cerulli, & Maine, 1994; Kendell, 1991). Nevertheless, as other causes diminish, deaths by suicide remain a significant contributor to pregnancy-related deaths in these settings. Khalifeh, Hunt, Appleby, and Howard (2016) reviewed all deaths by suicide among women who had received psychiatric care in the previous 12 months in a 15-year period (1997–2012) from the British National Health Service. Among the 4,785 women who died by suicide, 98 women were either pregnant or had given birth in the prior year. Deaths by suicide in the non-perinatal period diminished over the interval, but the rate in the perinatal period did not change. In many low-income countries vital registration systems are weak and population level data about causes of pregnancy-related deaths are unavailable. However, there are some specific investigations which have used verbal autopsies. In Vietnam, for example, of all pregnancy-related deaths in seven provinces (2000–2001) 8% overall, but in some provinces 16.5%, were by suicide, with problematic 'community behaviours towards women' a contributing factor (World Health Organization, 2005). In Nepal, the Department of Health Services examined maternal deaths 1998–2008 in eight districts and found that while there was an overall reduction from 539 to 229 per 100,000 live births, suicide was the leading cause, accounting for 16% of deaths (Karki, 2011).

Deaths by suicide in pregnancy are primarily associated with what have been termed the intolerable predicaments of unwanted pregnancy or entrapment in situations of sexual or physical abuse or poverty (Brockington, 2001; Frautschi et al., 1994). Suicide is disproportionately associated with adolescent pregnancies and appears to be the last resort for women with unwanted pregnancies in settings in which reproductive choice is limited; access to contraception by single women is prohibited, and legal pregnancy termination services are unavailable (Appleby, 1991; Frautschi et al., 1994). In low-income countries, young women who fear parental or social sanction, who lack the financial means to pay for an abortion, or who cannot obtain a legal abortion may attempt to induce abortion themselves. Women who do this by self-poisoning, use of instruments, self-inflicted trauma, or herbal and folk remedies are at increased risk of death by misadventure (Smith, 1998). In a population survey of mortality associated with abortion in Maharashtra, India, death rates from abortion-related complications were found to be disproportionately higher among adolescents, because they were more likely than older women to use untrained service providers. In addition, a number of adolescents had died by suicide to preserve the family honour without seeking abortion (Ganatra & Hirve, 2002).

Although deaths by suicide may be rare, suicidal behaviours, including thoughts of suicide and acts of self-harm, are more prevalent (Brockington, 2001). There is some evidence that suicidal behaviours are increased among women who have experienced pregnancy loss, including following ectopic pregnancy (which can carry loss of future fertility as well as loss of the foetus) and foetal death or still birth (Schiff & Grossman, 2006). In pregnancy, suicidal ideas and behaviours are more common among women with rather than without a history of childhood sexual abuse, and among those who have experienced gender-based violence (Stark & Flitcraft, 1995).

The predominant research focus in the field has been on the prevalence, determinants and course of depression and, to a lesser extent, anxiety, now often termed the perinatal common (non-psychotic) mental disorders (PCMD). Symptoms of depression, including appetite change, lowered energy, sleep disturbance, and reduced libido, are also normal symptoms of pregnancy, and their psychological significance might have been underestimated. Large cohort studies reveal that rates of depression are at least as high in late pregnancy as they are postpartum. Prevalence estimates are higher when self-report symptom checklists are used than when diagnoses are established by clinical interviews. In a systematic review and meta-analysis of 21 surveys Bennett, Einarson, Taddio, Koren, and Einarson (2004) found that first trimester prevalence was 7.4%, in the second 12.8%, and in the last trimester 12.0%.

Sustained elevated maternal anxiety in pregnancy has been associated with adverse effects on infant birthweight (Texiera, Fisk, & Glover, 1999), and later behavioural and emotional problems among children (Glover & O'Connor, 2002; O'Connor, Heron, Golding, Beveridge, & Glover, 2002). While the specific links between severity, duration, and trimester of exposure and these outcomes remain uncertain, Kinsella and Monk (Kinsella & Monk, 2009) conclude that alterations in intrauterine physiology attributable to maternal psychological state can influence health across the life course. However, the source of maternal anxiety was not investigated in these studies.

Investigations of the perinatal mental health of women living in low- and lower-middle-income countries has only been conducted more recently, most published since 2000 (Fisher et al., 2012a). This is in part because of competing health priorities, including obstetric emergencies, and coincidental burden of communicable diseases and malnutrition. Research attention was slowed by beliefs that traditional confinement and post-partum practices, including social seclusion, prescribed rest, increased practical support from female family members, provision of specific foods and herbal preparations, gift giving and an honoured status were protective (Fisher et al., 2012a). This is now known to be an oversimplification: the presumption that culturally prescribed supportive care is available to all does not reflect reality for many women (Fisher, Morrow, Ngoc, & Anh, 2004). A systematic review of the evidence from these settings revealed that the weighted mean average prevalence of antenatal mental disorders (15.6%, 95% CI 15.4%–15.9%) was substantially higher than in high-income countries (Fisher et al., 2012a). However, there is a significant difference in prevalence estimates by recruitment sites: the lowest were among relatively advantaged women recruited from urban tertiary teaching hospitals, and the highest from women in rural communities. This indicates a social gradient in which prevalence is highest amongst the most socially and economically disadvantaged women, especially those living in rural areas with little access to health services.

Risk and protective factors for perinatal mental health problems

Contrary to arguments that perinatal mental health problems are attributable to individual psychological vulnerabilities, the weight of evidence is that they are multifactorially determined by interactions among social, cultural, and contextual risk and protective factors. These factors are comparable between high- and low-income countries, but risks are more prevalent and access to protective factors more limited in the latter. Unwanted or unintended conception, being single, lacking income-generating work, having a low income or adverse early experiences within family of origin, increase the level of depressive symptoms (Fisher, Herrman, Cabral de Mello, & Chandra, 2013; Scottish Intercollegiate Guidelines Network, 2012).

A woman's perinatal mental health is protected by having better education, paid work, maternity leave, sexual and reproductive health services, including family planning, and supportive, non-judgemental relationships with her own parents, her partner, and her wider social network, in particular same-age peers (Berthiaume, David, Saucier, & Borgeat, 1996; Brugha et al., 1998; Pajulo, Savonlahti, Sourandera, Heleniusb, & Piha, 2001).

Physical, sexual, or emotional violence perpetrated by an intimate partner, neglected in investigations until about 2000, is a major risk factor. The systematic review by Howard, Oram, Galley, Trevillion, and Feder (2013) found that any lifetime experience of intimate partner violence doubled the risk of antenatal depression (see Table 21.1).

Table 21.1 Risk factors for perinatal common mental disorders in women.

Social:

- low socioeconomic position,
- exposure to interpersonal violence,
- income insecurity, lack of maternity benefits and pregnancy-related discrimination,
- criticism, coercion and lack of empathic support from the intimate partner,
- role restrictions regarding housework and infant care, and excessive unpaid workloads,
- insufficient access to social resources, including practical and emotional support,
- crowded housing,
- lack of access to family planning services to enable reproductive choice about when and how many children to have,
- in some settings, having a female fetus.

Psychological:

- cognitive capability and learning style,
- personality, including capacities for emotional regulation and adaptation to new experiences,
- interpersonal skills, including capacity to trust and form sustained relationships,
- past experience of neglect or sexual, physical, or emotional abuse,
- past mental health problems.

Biological:

- general health,
- nutritional status,

(Continued)

Table 21.1 (Cont.)

- coincidental burden of infectious or chronic disease,
- substance use,
- adverse obstetric events including life-threatening complications and perinatal loss.

Sources: Fisher, et al., 2012a; Flach et al., 2011; Fottrell et al., 2010; Scottish Intercollegiate Guidelines Network, 2012.

Vulnerable subgroups

Infertility and treatment with assisted reproductive technologies (ART) affect couples' psychological well-being, marital relationships, sexual relationships, and quality of life negatively (Gameiro et al., 2015; Luk & Loke, 2015). As most ART treatments are unsuccessful, many women who eventually conceive with ART have experienced the additional emotional burdens of previous treatment failure. Further, as some 20% of ART pregnancies miscarry, some have experienced pregnancy loss. They are also older and more likely to have a multiple pregnancy than women who conceive spontaneously (Dyer et al., 2016). Taken together, most women who conceive after infertility treatment have experienced significant emotional distress before achieving pregnancy.

There are two reviews of studies of the psychological aspects of pregnancy after infertility and assisted conception. These reported that, compared with women who conceive spontaneously, women who conceive with ART have more pregnancy-specific anxiety but are similar to other women on most other measures of psychological adjustment (Gourounti, 2016; Hammarberg, Fisher, & Wynter, 2008). Gourounti (2016) also found that women who had conceived with ART had more positive attitudes toward pregnancy demands, and higher levels of maternal–foetal attachment. Although not at higher risk of mental health problems, women who have conceived with ART (Gressier et al., 2015) are more likely to experience early parenting difficulties requiring hospital admission (Fisher, Rowe, & Hammarberg, 2012). The authors concluded that pregnancy and motherhood might be idealized after ART conception and that women may be underprepared for the social isolation, the repetitive and potentially isolating work of infant care, and the ambivalence and powerlessness that caring for an unsettled infant can arouse. Extreme gratitude that the treatment has enabled them to have a baby may constrain complaints or requests for help. Others might then underestimate their need for support and provide less assistance than might be given in other circumstances.

In addition to the contribution of social factors to pregnancy mental health, anxiety can be generated among women by prenatal genetic diagnosis and screening (Green, 1990). This occurs independently of test results and is worsened if there is a long interval between the test and the results becoming available (Green, 1990). It can be modified by skilled genetic counselling and psychosocial support, but may persist over time (Keenan, Basso, Goldkrand, & Butler, 1991). Although it is argued that genetic screening is beneficial, anxieties are aroused unnecessarily by false positive results for women whose foetuses are actually healthy (Marteau et al., 1992).

Terminating a pregnancy because of foetal abnormality can have lasting psychological sequelae (Green, 1990). Hunfeld, Taselaar-Kloos, Agterberg, Wladimiroff, and Passchier (1997) compared 27 women with a history of pregnancy termination after at least 20 weeks' gestation due to foetal abnormality who had a subsequent live birth, with 27 mothers of newborns without such a history. Those with prior pregnancy loss had significantly greater anxiety and depression than women without such a history, which was interpreted as re-evoked grief about the previous loss. They also perceived their infants to have more problems and were more anxious about infant care (Hunfeld et al., 1997; Hunfeld, Wladimiroff, & Passchier, 1994).

Pregnancy and body image

Investigations of the impact of natural pregnancy-related physiological changes on women's body image are inconclusive but most have found that negative body image in pregnancy is associated with symptoms of depression, low self-esteem and weight gain above recommended limits (Meireles, Neves, de Carvalho, & Ferreira, 2015). Negative body image and body dissatisfaction are common among women in high-income settings, attributed usually to the socially constructed ideal of thinness as the beauty standard for women (Malson, 2009).

A qualitative study of 19 pregnant women concluded that women's images of their bodies during pregnancy are complex and influenced by their recognition of the functionality of the pregnant body. Partner support and positive feedback about the pregnant body and open communication about weight and body image in antenatal care are valued and perceived as helpful (Watson, Broadbent, Skouteris, & Fuller-Tyszkiewicz, 2016; Loth, Bauer, Wall, Berge, & Neumark-Sztainer, 2011) compared body satisfaction between 68 pregnant women and 927 women who were not pregnant and found that those who were pregnant had higher mean scores on the Body Shape Satisfaction Scale, indicating more body satisfaction. As the pregnant women had also been assessed before pregnancy this study demonstrated that they experienced a significant increase in body satisfaction from pre-pregnancy, despite weight gain.

Investigating the impact of social media on body image during pregnancy Hicks and Brown (2016) explored the influence of Facebook on body image among 269 pregnant women who completed online questionnaires. Women with Facebook accounts had more body image concerns than women who did not have a Facebook account. Among Facebook users, 85% checked their account at least once every day, spending more than an hour on the site on average each day. Increased Facebook use was associated with more body image dissatisfaction and more than half of Facebook users reported that they frequently compared their bodies to those of other pregnant women (Hicks & Brown, 2016). As a modern phenomenon, the causal relationships between body dissatisfaction in pregnancy and psychological factors remain unclear (Fuller-Tyszkiewicz, Skouteris, Watson, & Hill, 2013).

Conclusion

Pregnancy health, including mental health, is influenced extensively by structural factors and social circumstances and not just by individual characteristics. Ensuring that women are able to choose when and how many pregnancies they wish to have, at the age they want to have them, and that their health needs are well met, requires consideration of these factors. Psychologically-informed pregnancy health services in which there is a rights-based approach to care can empower women and optimize mental health. However, protection and promotion of pregnancy-related psychological functioning will require social inequalities to be addressed through the realization of girls' and women's human rights to education, nutrition, gender-sensitive health care, equal social and economic participation, personal safety, individual autonomy and freedom from discrimination.

References

Agrillo, C. & Nelini, C. (2008). Childfree by choice: A review. *Journal of Cultural Geography, 25*(3), 347–363.

Appleby, L. (1991). Suicide during pregnancy and in the first postnatal year. *BMJ, 302*(6769), 137–140.

Astbury, J. (1986). Reproduction and femininity. *New Doctor, 41,* 28–31.

Baraitser, L. (2009). *Maternal encounters: The ethics of interruption.* London: Routledge.

Benedek, T. (1970). The psychobiology of pregnancy (Chapter 5). In E. Anthony & T. Benedek (Eds), *Parenthood, its psychology and psychopathology* (pp. 137–151). Boston: Little, Brown and Company.

Bennett, H. A., Einarson, A., Taddio, A., Koren, G., & Einarson, T. R. (2004). Prevalence of depression during pregnancy: Systematic review. *Obstetrics and Gynecology, 103*(4), 698–709.

Berthiaume, M., David, H., Saucier, J., & Borgeat, F. (1996). Correlates of gender role orientation during pregnancy and the postpartum. *Sex Roles, 35*(11/12), 781–800.

Blackstone, A. & Stewart, M. D. (2016). "There's more thinking to decide": How the childfree decide not to parent. *The Family Journal, 24*(3), 296–303.

Breen, D. (1975). *The birth of a first child. Towards an understanding of femininity.* London: Tavistock Publications.

Brockington, I. (2001). Suicide in women. *International Clinical Psychopharmacology, 16,* S7–S19.

Brugha, T. S., Sharp, H. M., Cooper, S.-A., Weisender, C., Britto, D., Shinkwin, R., Sherrif, T., & Kirwan, P. H. (1998). The Leicester 500 project: Social support and the development of postnatal depressive symptoms, a prospective, cohort survey. *Psychological Medicine, 28*(1), 63–79.

Conran, S. (2001/2002). *Guide to work-life balance.* London, UK: Work Life Balance Trust.

Deutsch, H. (1945). *The psychology of women. A psychoanalytic interpretation. vol 2: Motherhood.* New York: Grune and Stratton.

Dyer, S., Chambers, G. M., de Mouzon, J., Nygren, K. G., Zegers-Hochschild, F., Mansour, R., Ishihara, O., Banker, M., & Adamson, G. D. (2016). International committee for monitoring assisted reproductive technologies world report: Assisted reproductive technology 2008, 2009 and 2010. *Human Reproduction, 31*(7), 588–1609.

Fisher, J. R., Cabral de Mello, M., & Isutzu, T. (2009). Pregnancy, childbirth and the postpartum year. In J. Fisher, J. Astbury, M. Cabral de Mello, & S. Saxena (Eds), *Mental health aspects of women's reproductive health. A global review of the literature* (pp. 8–43). Geneva: World Health Organization and United Nations Population Fund.

Fisher, J. R., de Mello, M. C., Patel, V., Rahman, A., Tran, T., Holton, S., & Holmes, W. (2012a). Prevalence and determinants of common perinatal mental disorders in women in low- and lower-middle-income countries: A systematic review. *Bulletin of the World Health Organization, 90*(2), 139–149.

Fisher, J. R., Herrman, H., Cabral de Mello, M., & Chandra, P. (2013). Women's mental health. In V. Patel, A. Cohen, H. Minas, & M. J. Prince (Eds), *Global mental health: principles and practice 2013* (pp. 354–384). New York: Oxford University Press.

Fisher, J. R., Morrow, M. M., Ngoc, N. T., & Anh, L. T. (2004). Prevalence, nature, severity and correlates of postpartum depressive symptoms in Vietnam. *BJOG: An International Journal of Obstetrics and Gynaecology, 111*(12), 1353–1360.

Fisher, J. R., Rowe, H., & Hammarberg, K. (2012b). Admissions for early parenting difficulties among women with infants conceived by assisted reproductive technologies: A prospective cohort study. *Fertility and Sterility, 97*(6), 1410–1416.

Flach, C., Leese, M., Heron, J., Evans, J., Feder, G., Sharp, D., & Howard, L. M. (2011). Antenatal domestic violence, maternal mental health and subsequent child behaviour: A cohort study. *BJOG: An International Journal of Obstetrics and Gynaecology, 118*(11), 1383–1391.

Fottrell, E., Kanhonou, L., Goufodji, S., Behague, D. P., Marshall, T., Patel, V., & Filippi, V. (2010). Risk of psychological distress following severe obstetric complications in Benin: The role of economics, physical health and spousal abuse. *British Journal of Psychiatry, 196*(1), 18–25.

Frautschi, S., Cerulli, A., & Maine, D. (1994). Suicide during pregnancy and its neglect as a component of maternal mortality. *International Journal of Gynaecology and Obstetrics, 47,* 275–284.

Fuller-Tyszkiewicz, M., Skouteris, H., Watson, B. E., & Hill, B. (2013). Body dissatisfaction during pregnancy: A systematic review of cross-sectional and prospective correlates. *Journal of Health Psychology*, *18*(11), 1411–1421.

Fyfe, M. & Davies, J. (2015, June 4). Motherhood on ice. *Sydney Morning Herald*.

Gameiro, S., Boivin, J., Dancet, E., de Klerk, C., Emery, M., Lewis-Jones, C., Thorn, P., Van den Broeck, U., Venetis, C., Verhaak, C. M., Wischmann, T., Vermeulen, N. (2015). ESHRE guideline: Routine psychosocial care in infertility and medically assisted reproduction—a guide for fertility staff. *Human Reproduction*, *30*(11), 2476–2485.

Ganatra, B. & Hirve, S. (2002). Induced abortions among adolescent women in rural Maharashtra, India. *Reproductive Health Matters*, *10*(19), 76–85.

Glazer, G. (1980). Anxiety levels and concerns among pregnant women. *Research in Nursing & Health*, *3*(3), 107–113.

Glover, V. & O'Connor, T. G. (2002). Effects of antenatal stress and anxiety: Implications for development and psychiatry. *British Journal of Psychiatry*, *180*, 389–391.

Gourounti, K. (2016). Psychological stress and adjustment in pregnancy following assisted reproductive technology and spontaneous conception: A systematic review. *Women Health*, *56*(1), 98–118.

Graham, W., Filippi, V., & Ronsmans, C. (1996). Demonstrating programme impact on maternal mortality. *Health Policy and Planning*, *11*(1), 16–20.

Green, J. M. (1990). Prenatal screening and diagnosis: Some psychological and social issues. *BJOG: An International Journal of Obstetrics & Gynaecology*, *97*(12), 1074–1076.

Gressier, F., Letranchant, A., Cazas, O., Sutter-Dallay, A. L., Falissard, B., & Hardy, P. (2015). Postpartum depressive symptoms and medically assisted conception: A systematic review and meta-analysis. *Human Reproduction*, *30*(11), 2575–2586.

Grossman, F. K., Eichler, L. S., & Winickoff, S. A. (1980). *Pregnancy, birth, and parenthood*. San Francisco: Jossey-Bass.

Hall, C. (2016). Womanhood as experienced in childbirth: Psychoanalytic explorations of the body. *Psychoanalytic Social Work*, *23*(1), 42–59.

Hammarberg, K., Fisher, J. R., & Wynter, K. (2008). Psychological and social aspects of pregnancy, childbirth and the first postpartum year after ART: A systematic review. *Human Reproduction Update*, *14*, 395–414.

Hammarberg, K., Kirkman, M., Pritchard, N., Hickey, M., Peate, M., McBain, J., Agresta, F., Bayly, C., & Fisher, J. (2017). Reproductive experiences of women who cryopreserved oocytes for non-medical reasons. *Human Reproduction*, *32*(3), 575–581.

Hicks, S. & Brown, A. (2016). Higher Facebook use predicts greater body image dissatisfaction during pregnancy: The role of self-comparison. *Midwifery*, *40*, 132–140.

Höhn, C., Avramov, D., & Kotowska, I. E. (2008). *People, population change and policies: Lessons from the population policy acceptance study*. (Vol. 1–2). Berlin: Springer.

Holton, S., Fisher, J., & Rowe, H. (2011). To have or not to have? Australian women's childbearing desires, expectations and outcomes. *Journal of Population Research*, *28*(4), 353.

Howard, L. M., Oram, S., Galley, H., Trevillion, K., & Feder, G. (2013). Domestic violence and perinatal mental disorders: A systematic review and meta-analysis. *PLoS Medicine*, *10*(5), e1001452–e1001452.

Hunfeld, J. A. M., Taselaar-Kloos, A. K. G., Agterberg, G., Wladimiroff, J. W., & Passchier, J. (1997). Trait anxiety, negative emotions and the mothers' adaptation to an infant born subsequent to late pregnancy loss: A case-control study. *Prenatal Diagnosis*, *17*(9), 843–851.

Hunfeld, J. A. M., Wladimiroff, J. W., & Passchier, J. (1994). Pregnancy termination, perceived control, and perinatal grief. *Psychological Reports*, *74*(1), 217–218.

Karki, C. (2011). Suicide: Leading cause of death among women in Nepal. *Kathmandu University Medical Journal*, *9*(3), 157–158.

Keenan, K. L., Basso, D., Goldkrand, J., & Butler, W. J. (1991). Low level of maternal serum alpha-fetoprotein: Its associated anxiety and the effects of genetic counseling. *American Journal of Obstetrics and Gynecology*, *164*(1 Pt 1), 54–56.

Kendell, R. E. (1991). Suicide in pregnancy and the puerperium. *British Medical Journal*, *302*, 126–127.

Khalifeh, H., Hunt, I. M., Appleby, L., & Howard, L. M. (2016). Suicide in perinatal and non-perinatal women in contact with psychiatric services: 15 year findings from a UK national inquiry. *The Lancet Psychiatry*, *3*(3), 233–242.

Kinsella, M. T. & Monk, C. (2009). Impact of maternal stress, depression & anxiety on fetal neurobehavioral development. *Clinical Obstetrics and Gynecology, 52*(3), 425–440.

Leifer, M. (1977). Psychological changes accompanying pregnancy and motherhood. *Genetic Psychology Monographs, 95*, 55–96.

Li, Z., Zeki, R., Hilder, L., & Sullivan, E. (2013). *Australia's mothers and babies 2011.* Canberra: AIHW National Perinatal Epidemiology and Statistics Unit.

Loth, K. A., Bauer, K. W., Wall, M., Berge, J., & Neumark-Sztainer, D. (2011). Body satisfaction during pregnancy. *Body Image, 8*(3), 297–300.

Lubin, B., Gardener, S., & Roth, A. (1975). Mood and somatic symptoms during pregnancy. *Psychosomatic Medicine, 37*(2), 136–146.

Luk, B. H.-K. & Loke, A. Y. (2015). The impact of infertility on the psychological well-being, marital relationships, sexual relationships, and quality of life of couples: A systematic review. *Journal of Sex & Marital Therapy, 41*(6), 610–625.

Malson, H. (2009). Appearing to disappear. Postmodern femininities and self-starved subjectivities. In H. Malson & M. Burns (Eds), *Critical feminist approaches to eating disorders* (pp. 135–155). London: Routledge.

Marteau, T. M., Johnston, M., Kidd, J., Michie, S., Cook, R., Slack, J., & Shaw, R. W. (1992). Psychological models in predicting uptake of prenatal screening. *Psychology & Health, 6*(1–2), 13–22.

Marzuk, P. M., Tardiff, K., Leon, A., & Hirsch, C. S. (1997). Lower risk of suicide during pregnancy. *American Journal of Psychiatry, 154*(1), 122.

Mathews, T. J. & Hamilton, B. E. (2016). Mean age of mothers is on the rise: United States, 2000–2014. *NCHS Data Brief,* (232), 1–8.

Meireles, J. F., Neves, C. M., de Carvalho, P. H., & Ferreira, M. E. (2015). Body dissatisfaction among pregnant women: An integrative review of the literature. *Cien Saude Colet, 20*(7), 2091–2103.

O'Connor, T. G., Heron, J., Golding, J., Beveridge, M., & Glover, V. (2002). Maternal antenatal anxiety and children's behavioural/emotional problems at 4 years: Report from the Avon Longitudinal Study of Parents and Children. *British Journal of Psychiatry, 180*, 502–508.

Paffenbarger, J. & Ralph, S. (1964). Epidemiological aspects of parapartum mental illness. *British Journal of Preventive & Social Medicine, 18*(4), 189.

Pajulo, M., Savonlahti, E., Sourandera, A., Heleniusb, H., & Piha, J. (2001). Antenatal depression, substance dependency and social support. *Journal of Affective Disorders, 65*(1), 9–17.

Puur, A., Olah, L. S., Tazi-Preve, M. I., & Dorbritz, J. (2008). Men's childbearing desires and views of the male role in Europe at the dawn of the 21st century. *Demographic Research, 19*, 1883–1912.

Schiff, M. A. & Grossman, D. C. (2006). Adverse perinatal outcomes and risk for postpartum suicide attempt in Washington state, 1987–2001. *Pediatrics, 118*(3), e669–e675.

Schmidt, L., Sobotka, T., Bentzen, J. G., & Nyboe Andersen, A. (2011). Demographic and medical consequences of the postponement of parenthood. *Human Reproduction Update, 18*(1), 29–43.

Scottish Intercollegiate Guidelines Network (SIGN) (2012). Management of perinatal mood disorders. Edinburgh: *Scottish Intercollegiate Guidelines Network.*

Shereshefsky, P. M. & Yarrow, L. J. (1973). *Psychological aspects of a first pregnancy and early postnatal adaptation.* New York: Raven Pr.

Slaughter, A. (2012, July/August issue). Why women still can't have it all. *The Atlantic Magazine.*

Smith, J. P. (1998). Risky choices: The dangers of teens using self-induced abortion attempts. *Journal of Pediatric Health Care, 12*(3), 147–151.

Stark, E. & Flitcraft, A. (1995). Killing the beast within: Woman battering and female suicidality. *International Journal of Health Services, 25*(1), 43–64.

Texiera, J., Fisk, N., & Glover, V. (1999). Association between maternal anxiety in pregnancy and increased uterine artery resistance index: Cohort based study. *British Medical Journal, 318*(7177), 153–157.

The United Nations Population Fund (2017). *State of the world's population 2017.* New York: UNFPA.

Turrini, P. (1980). Psychological crises in normal pregnancy (Chapter 8). In B. Blum, J. Fosshage, K. Frank, H. Grayson, C. Loew, & H. Lowenheim (Eds), *Psychological aspects of pregnancy, birthing and bonding* (pp. 135–150). New York: Human Sciences Press.

United Nations (2016). *Sustainable development goals report 2016.* New York: United Nations.

United Nations Population Fund (1994*). Program of action adopted at the International Conference on Population and Development.* Cairo: UNFPA.

Watson, B., Broadbent, J., Skouteris, H., & Fuller-Tyszkiewicz, M. (2016). A qualitative exploration of body image experiences of women progressing through pregnancy. *Women Birth*, *29*(1), 72–79.

Wolkind, S. & Zajicek, E. (1981). *Pregnancy, a psychological and social study*. London: Academic Press.

World Health Organization (2005). *Maternal mortality in Vietnam, 2000-2001: An in-depth analysis of causes and determinants*. Manila: WHO Regional Office for the Western Pacific.

Worldatlas (2017). Countries with the oldest average mother's age at first birth. Retrieved from www.worldatlas.com/articles/countries-with-the-highest-mother-s-mean-age-at-first-birth.html.

22

CHILDBIRTH AND SEXUALITY

Hannah H. Dahlen and Sahar Sobhgol

Childbirth as a contested space

Throughout documented history and across cultures childbirth has been memorialized as both mystery and power, and those who attended women giving birth, mostly midwives, have been both revered and feared (Ehrenreich & English, 2010). It is only relatively recently that childbirth has been made public, its mysteries exposed through media and technologies like ultrasound and men have been permitted to enter the birth space. In many countries around the world midwives have been usurped as lead care providers at birth with a concerted attempt to eradicate them in some places; and this continues even today (Clifford, 2019; Greenfield, 2019).

The medicalization of childbirth has been written about extensively (Dahlen, Homer, Leap, & Tracy, 2011). There is a fascinating body of literature reporting on particular phases in childbirth history, such as the twilight era, where many women were sedated and restrained for birth. Some women actually requested twilight sleep in order to avoid the horrors of birth in medicalized environments (Hairston, 1996). The introduction of routine episiotomies (surgical cutting of the perineum) remained unquestioned until the 1980s. In 1984 Sleep and colleagues published the first large randomized controlled trial showing routine episiotomy caused even more harm than occurred naturally during birth (Kitzinger & Simkin, 1984; Sleep et al., 1984). There are still many countries around the world over 30 years later that continue to routinely use episiotomy during childbirth, often without consent (Hussein, Dahlen, Duff, & Schmied, 2016; Hussein, Dahlen, & Schmied, 2012). By the end of the 19th century women were made to give birth on uncomfortable obstetric beds with stirrups, handcuffs and shoulder restrainers used, despite having moved about and birthed upright throughout human history (Dahlen et al., 2011).

There is little doubt medicalization has played a role in reducing the maternal and perinatal mortality rate but these rates have remained unchanged in many developing nations for the past 10–20 years (FIGO, 2018). This is despite a significant escalation in interventions like caesarean section (FIGO, 2018). In some developed nations like the USA, the rate of mothers dying in childbirth has doubled in the past decade and it is now ranked 46th in the world in terms of maternal mortality (Wong & Kitsantas, 2019). In many countries, such as the USA, UK and Australia, women of colour, and in particular Indigenous women, have worse outcomes than the population as a whole. Black women in the USA and the UK die in higher numbers in childbirth than white women (American College of Obstetricians and Gynecologists, 2015). In Australia Aboriginal and Torres Strait Islander women and babies died at much higher rates than their non-Indigenous counterparts (Kildea, Tracy, Sherwood, Magick-Dennis, & Barclay, 2016). Kildea et al. (2016) state that the disparities in health outcomes for Aboriginal and Torres Strait Islander women are due to enduring effects of colonization, social exclusion, sustained institutional racism, and stark inequalities across many of the social determinants of health, including incomes, employment, education, access to good services and health care. The commencement of dedicated programs in Australia to enable Aboriginal women to give birth 'on country' and the efforts to increase the numbers of Indigenous midwives will hopefully address some of these disparities (Kildea et al., 2017; West et al., 2016). These programs also respect the fact that within Aboriginal culture childbirth is seen as a woman's mystery and woman's business (Kildea et al., 2017).

A systematic review on maternal health care among migrant populations in North America, Europe and Australia noted access to maternal health care is affected by unavailability of qualified interpreters and lack of appropriate professionals and facilities (Almeida, Caldas, Ayres-de-campos, Salcedo-Barrientos, & Dias, 2013). This brings to light the social inequality and embedded racism that impacts on care and maternity care provision and increasingly this is being exposed and addressed (American College of Obstetricians and Gynecologists, 2015; Villarosa, 2018). Women's sexual orientation also brings unique needs, with lesbian women reporting unfortunate attitudes and ignorance from health providers (Wilton, 2001). We thus cannot discuss childbirth without understanding that the position of women in society, their social status, ethnic background, colour of their skin and sexual orientation, can all impact on their treatment and outcomes. This overview sets the scene for understanding the broader context of childbirth discussed in this chapter.

Childbirth as a liminal state

Childbirth has been described as a liminal state. It is indeed the betwixt and between (Turner, 1969), a suspended state of chaos and order that separates that that was before and that that comes after. When a woman is having her first baby, two people are born: the new baby and the new mother. With the birth of these two new beings come new identities, the crossing of boundaries, and with this comes a state of both threat and vulnerability and power and growth. Liminality has been used to consider women's health issues in areas such as cervical screening (Forss, Tishelman, Widmark, & Sachs, 2004), infertility (Allen, 2007), childbirth rituals (Hogan, 2008), premature birth (Taylor, 2008) and breastfeeding (Dykes, 2006).

Reed, Barnes and Rowe (2016) interviewed women who had a physiological birth and presented the rite of passage as comprising three phases: separation, liminal and incorporation (Reed et al., 2016). The authors found that during birth women separated from the external world and sought to minimize both external and internal distractions. In the liminal phase they entered their own world and experienced what was described as a state of altered consciousness. Once the baby was born they reintegrated themselves with the external world and their birth experience was incorporated into their sense of self. Lupton and Schmied (2013) analyzed interviews with women who had recently given birth for the first time to explore how they described both their own embodiment and that of their babies. They used the term 'the body being born' to describe the liminality and fragmentation of the fetal/baby body as women experienced it when giving birth (Lupton & Schmied, 2012).

Women who gave birth vaginally without anesthesia experienced an intense physicality as the 'body being born as it forced its way out', whereas those experiencing caesarean section experienced both their own body and that of their baby as absent and alienated. While most women took time to come to terms with the baby when it was born, seeing it as strange and unknown, those who delivered by caesarean section had to work even harder to come to terms with the birth experience. The liminal state is a state of openness and vulnerability and it is easy to see how the way women are treated or the birth events they experience can lead to birth trauma. It is also enables some understanding around the importance of relationship-based care and trust in leading women to have more positive experiences when giving birth, discussed in greater depth later in this chapter.

The physicality of childbirth

Having a baby has intense psychological and sociological aspects, with many societies focussing on it as a dangerous physical event needing extensive intervention to protect the lives of the mother and her baby. Many health professionals hold a biomedical positioning about birth, seeing it through a lens of Cartesian mind–body separation and this contributes to a technocratic paradigm that predominates in obstetrics (Davis-Floyd, 1994). New models of care such as continuity of midwifery care are actually very old 'social models' that have now been re-discovered and have a social and relationship-based focus. Women (and their babies) who experience these models of care and receive care from midwives they know throughout the pregnancy, birth and postnatal continuum have significantly better outcomes than in standard fragmented medical models (Sandall, Soltani, Gates, Shennan, & Devane, 2016). For this reason, we have begun the chapter with the contested space that childbirth is embedded in and some of the psychological understandings of birth before we move into the physical aspect. As we are both midwives we take a holistic woman-centered approach and prioritizing these understandings fits with the paradigms we hold.

The hormones of childbirth

For most women, giving birth follows a nine- to ten-month period of conceiving and growing a baby. Once labour commences, most women embrace its arrival, though for some there is fear, and for some extreme fear (also known as tocophobia) (O'Connell, Leahy-Warren, Khashan, Kenny, & O'Neill, 2017). A growing belly and all the accompanying physical discomforts may be nature's way of making women grateful at the end when the contractions finally start. There is much focus in the medical literature, and in society as a whole, on the anatomical aspects of giving birth, but less focus on hormones involved in the whole process and in connecting the mother and baby during and after the birth (Buckley, 2015). Hormones like oxytocin which increase during labour, birth and following birth (colloquially termed the hormone of love) also play an important role in connection and sexual activity.

The hormones involved in labour and birth have evolved over millions of years and have been fine-tuned to optimize reproductive success, which has been important for the survival of the human race (Buckley, 2015). There are some central hormonal systems that operate during childbirth and these are: oxytocin; beta-endorphins; epinephrine-norepinephrine (adrenaline-noradrenaline) and related stress hormone systems; and prolactin. These hormones get the baby ready to be born, enhance labour effectiveness, help the woman cope with the physiological stress of labour and the pain, promote the transition of the woman to mother and the foetus to newborn, as well as optimize breastfeeding and maternal–infant attachment (Buckley, 2015). Lactation and maternal–infant attachment after birth are also critically dependent on the hormones cascading through a mother and baby's body. Having the baby on the mother's chest (skin to skin) straight after the birth regulates hormones such as oxytocin, and breastfeeding further activates hormones such as oxytocin and prolactin (Stevens, Schmied, Burns, & Dahlen, 2014).

The consequences of over-intervening in the ancient process of birth

There is much about the process of childbirth that still remains a mystery. Disturbing this process with unnecessary intervention and stress, or care that lacks compassion, can have serious ramifications for the mother and baby (Dahlen et al., 2014; Peters et al., 2018). For example, commonly used medical interventions, such as caesarean section and forceps, may impact on women's long-term physical health (Keag, Norman, & Stock, 2018; Polidano, Zhu, & Bornstein, 2017). A recent large systematic review (included 79 studies) found women who gave birth by caesarean section compared with vaginal birth had an increased risk in future pregnancies of miscarriage, ectopic pregnancy, stillbirth, placenta previa, placenta accrete, placental abruption, hysterectomy and antepartum haemorrhage. There was an increase in urinary incontinence and pelvic organ prolapse associated with vaginal birth compared with caesarean section (Keag et al., 2018).

Evidence is also mounting on the long-term health effects on children of common birth interventions, such as caesarean section (Keag et al., 2018; Polidano et al., 2017). Caesarean section has been associated with an increase in immune-related disorders, such as asthma, diabetes, obesity and inflammatory bowel disease (Cardwell et al., 2008; Huang et al., 2015; Hyde, Mostyn, Modi, & Kemp, 2012). The recent systematic review discussed above (Keag et al., 2018) also found that children born by caesarean section compared with vaginal birth had higher rates of asthma up until age 12 and obesity up until age 28.

A call to humanize maternity care

Today there are many childbirth interventions that disturb this ancient hormonal physiology, and while sometimes this is necessary to save lives, it is apparent we have gone too far without consideration of the potential short- and long-term consequences (Dahlen et al., 2013; FIGO, 2018; WHO, 2018). The recent *Lancet series on caesarean section* (FIGO, 2018), *Lancet series on midwifery* (Renfrew et al., 2014) and the *WHO recommendations: intrapartum care for a positive childbirth experience* (WHO, 2018) address this issue, calling for a reduction in unnecessary birth intervention and a move towards relationship-based models, in particular continuity of midwifery care. A call from leading researchers around the world to recognize the importance of positive experiences for women during pregnancy, birth and the postpartum period, that also reduce the incidence of adverse events, is leading to a critical change in the conversation and research prioritization in this space (Kennedy et al., 2018). Three inter-related research themes have been identified: examination and implementation of models of care that enhance both well-being and safety; investigating and optimizing physiological, psychological and social processes in pregnancy, childbirth and the postnatal period; and development and validation of outcome measures that capture short- and longer-term well-being (Kennedy et al., 2018). This means we are hopefully moving into a new era in childbirth research and policy that will improve care for women, babies and their families.

Sexuality and childbirth

Childbirth is a fundamental component of a woman's sexuality if she becomes a mother. Harel (2007) believes the mentioning of sexuality in the context of childbirth is considered taboo in Western society as it goes against the cultural and deeply held Judeo/Christian beliefs of pain in labour being something to be survived and even as punishment for women's sin; Eve's punishment in the Garden of Eden was to experience pain in labour (Harel, 2007). The sequence of events that encompass a woman's broader reproductive and sexual cycle, from menstruation through to ovulation and conception, followed by pregnancy, labour, birth and breastfeeding, are sexual events (Buckley, 2010). Most pregnancies result from a sexual act and the pregnant belly represents this act very publicly.

As has already been described, oxytocin, the 'hormone of love', is critical in many aspects of human connection, calmness, love, healing and belonging (Buckley, 2015). Giving birth has been described as akin to sex, with the same rush of hormones making the mind and body work in harmony, and the need for privacy and safety in both human experiences is very similar (Gaskin, 2002; Odent, 2014). Ina May Gaskin, the famous American midwife, has written about how sexual connection during labour and birth can help labour progress when it has stalled (Gaskin, 2002). However, many women would not necessarily agree that giving birth is a sexual event, and for good reason. In public birthing environments with strangers coming in and out of birth rooms, it is easy to see why many women do not feel giving birth has anything remotely sexual about it. In environments where privacy is maintained and the care provider is known, women have reported 'orgasmic births' (Davis, 2010; Mayberry & Daniel, 2016); though it is important to point out that the vast majority of women do not have orgasms when giving birth.

The sexuality of childbirth has thus lost meaning and recognition over the past century, as birth has moved from home to hospital (Tew, 1990). With this move has come the loss of privacy and reduced opportunity for intimacy during labour and birth, which Buckley (2010) argues widens the gap between sexuality and childbirth.

Birth trauma and sexuality

For partners viewing the sounds and movements women make during labour and birth (often like those made during intercourse) it can at times be confusing, as the act of birth and the very sexual nature of what they are witnessing coalesce. For some partners watching birth and the things that may be done to someone they love can be very traumatizing (Elmir & Schmied, 2016). Some men (there is very little research on same sex partners) describe the impact of the birth experience on the sexual relationship and feeling physically and emotionally distant from their partner (Elmir & Schmied, 2016). This led at times to fear or lack of desire in relation to physical intimacy after the birth (White, 2007). The Madonna/Whore Complex has been coined by authors to describe the conflicted perception partners can feel between seeing the woman as mother of their child versus their sexual partner (Mesch, 2009).

For women, especially those who have a past history of sexual abuse, labour and birth can also be a time when memories are triggered (for example, when vaginal examinations are undertaken) and trauma may be exacerbated (Leeners, Gorres, Block, & Hengartner, 2016; Simpson, Schmied, Dickson, & Dahlen, 2018). A study by Leeners et al. (2016) of 85 women who had given birth and had a history of childhood sexual abuse found that 41% described memories of the traumatic experiences intruding during childbirth and 58%

experienced dissociation. A recent systematic review also showed a higher number with past sexual abuse go on to develop post-traumatic stress disorder following childbirth (Simpson et al., 2018).

The pelvic floor and mode of birth

When a woman is pregnant and gives birth, pelvic floor muscles stretch to accommodate the growing/birthing baby. Vaginal birth, and in particular instrumental birth, can negatively affect pelvic organ support and sexual functioning in women (Elbegway, Elshamy, & Hanfy, 2010). However, women who have caesarean sections may also have pelvic floor damage (Keag et al., 2018). Around 70–80% of women will have some perineal injury during birth and so it is reasonable that women need some time to recover after the birth before intercourse recommences, in the case of heterosexual women (Dahlen & Priddis, 2018). The exhaustion that follows with a new baby can also have an impact on sexual resumption for all women (Dahlen & Priddis, 2018).

When it comes to discussing the impact of birth on sexual health, much of the focus is on the impact of vaginal birth compared with caesarean section and hence the focus is on the pelvic floor and perineum. However, if we look at the two largest randomized controlled trials that followed women up after childbirth and compared the two modes of birth (vaginal birth and caesarean section), then we find another picture emerges. In one study, which randomized 1,398 women to planned caesarean section and 1,406 women to planned vaginal birth, the mode of birth was not associated with problematic urinary incontinence or urinary incontinence that affected the quality of life. Partner relationships, including painful intercourse, were similar between the groups. In a study which randomized over 1,000 women with babies in a breech position to caesarean section or vaginal birth (Hannah et al., 2000), and followed those women up for two years, there were no differences between groups in pain, subsequent pregnancy, incontinence, depression, urinary, menstrual or sexual problems (Hannah et al., 2004). It is quite clear that instrumental birth (forceps and vacuum) is associated with significant pelvic floor and perineal morbidity for women compared with unassisted vaginal birth (Handa, Blomquist, McDermott, Friedman, & Muñoz, 2012).

Sexual intimacy during pregnancy and following birth

Pregnancy and sexual function

Pregnancy is associated with significant life changes that can interrupt physical and emotional connections of the couple. Some studies have found that sexual function worsens during pregnancy and is not fully recovered by six months postpartum (Pauls, Occhino, & Dryfhout, 2008). This may be due to the fact that the woman does not feel like having sexual contact with her partner or that physical changes alter her perception of her body. Women may also be experiencing physical discomfort which can impact on their desire for, and enjoyment of sexual activity. There may also be fears of harming the foetus which can be held by both partners despite the lack of evidence to support these fears.

Prospective studies about sexual function during pregnancy are limited. Despite the significant gains in knowledge about female sexuality in recent years, sexual function and sexual behaviour during pregnancy has received insufficient attention (Erol et al., 2007). This may well also reflect the belief systems held by society that pregnancy, despite clearly being evidence of sexual connection, is also considered to be a non-sexual state.

According to the evidence available, the prevalence of sexual dysfunction increases during pregnancy (Ribeiro et al., 2014; Yeniel & Petri, 2014; Yıldız, 2015). Sexual dysfunction is defined as the disturbance in sexual desire and psychophysiological changes that characterize the sexual response and cause interpersonal difficulty and marked distress (Pauls et al., 2008). For example, Bartellas, Crane, Daley, Bennett and Hutchens (2000), in a cross-sectional study, reported that vaginal intercourse and sexual activity overall decrease throughout pregnancy. Most women (58%) reported a decrease in sexual desire (Bartellas et al., 2000). Oruç et al. (1999) found that dyspareunia (painful intercourse) was common during pregnancy and pregnancy has a negative effect on orgasmic quality. This may be due to both physical and psychological reasons. Subsequently, dyspareunia and orgasmic quality influenced the frequency of sexual activity. They also found that sexual activity declined as the pregnancy advanced (Oruç et al., 1999). Leite et al. (2009) undertook a cohort study and reported that women's sexual activity showed a similar pattern during the first and second trimester, however there was a significant decrease in the third trimester. There was a significant difference in women's sexual function when comparing the second and third trimester, with a greater decline in the third trimester (Leite et al., 2009). Aslan, Aslan, Kızılyar, Ispahi and Esen (2005) also found that sexual function significantly decreased during pregnancy, particularly during the third trimester (Aslan et al., 2005). Gałązka, Droszdzol-Cop, Naworska, Czajkowska and Skrzypulec-Plinta (2015) reported that desire, arousal, orgasm and satisfaction decreased significantly with the progression of pregnancy, which affected couples' sexual satisfaction (Gałązka et al., 2015).

It is estimated that approximately 63% to 93% of all pregnant women experience sexual dysfunction (Ribeiro et al., 2014). The real prevalence of sexual dysfunction is largely unknown and is likely to be underreported (Pauls et al., 2008). It is important to note, however, that for some couples the lack of sexual contact during pregnancy and in the early postnatal period is accepted and not a cause of distress, but for others this is not the case.

Sexual function and activity during pregnancy is also influenced by cultural, religious and family beliefs (Jawed-Wessel & Sevick, 2017), though there is a preponderance of information regarding white heterosexual women. Employment and family issues, such as family violence, can also cause a decline in sexual function during pregnancy (Erol et al., 2007; Pauls et al., 2008). There are some conditions in which coital intercourse absolutely needs to be avoided and these may include; threatened miscarriage, preterm labour, placenta previa, vaginal bleeding and preterm premature rupture of membranes (Jones, Chan, & Farine, 2011). In contrast, there are some misconceptions and misbeliefs that need to be addressed by health care professionals and women need to be made aware of them. These include that sexual function during pregnancy harms the baby or causes preterm labour or miscarriage (Jones et al., 2011). In some cultures, there is a belief that sexual activity should be completely avoided during pregnancy (Erol et al., 2007; Yeniel & Petri, 2014).

Nature has found a partial solution to this in heterosexual populations, by reducing men's testosterone during late pregnancy and following the birth (Gettler, McDade, Feranil, & Kuzawa, 2011). The more the male partner interacts with the new baby the lower their testosterone (Gettler et al., 2011). Men with higher testosterone are more likely to mate, but then this declines rapidly after they become fathers (Gettler et al., 2011). Nature has worked out a tradeoff between mating and parenting, as is seen in other species where fathers care for their young. What happens in same sex couples is less clear.

338

Pelvic floor exercises and sexual function

Given the fact that sexual function declines during pregnancy, there is limited information available about treatment or support for women. The integrity and function of pelvic floor muscles are particularly relevant given that the role of this musculature is recognized as critical to sexual function. The importance of pelvic floor muscle function has been confirmed by studies using magnetic resonance imaging as well as surface electromyography during sexual arousal and sexual intercourse (Ferreira et al., 2015). During vaginal penetration, the pelvic floor muscle is slightly stretched and widened to allow intercourse to occur and it contracts during orgasm (Ferreira et al., 2015). Pelvic floor muscle exercises contribute to increased blood flow to the pelvis and enhanced vaginal and clitoral receptivity and responsiveness for pleasure during intercourse for both partners and for orgasmic muscular response. Some studies have shown that strong pelvic floor muscles may be associated with better orgasmic and arousal potentials, desire, excitement and vaginal lubrication (Ferreira et al., 2015).

Poor pelvic floor muscle strength after birth is one of the major factors that affect women's sexual function in the postpartum period (Golmakani, Zare, Khadem, Shareh, & Shakeri, 2015), along with the effect of sleep deprivation and breastfeeding. Instrumental vaginal birth, perineal trauma and episiotomy often negatively influence pelvic floor muscle strength leading to pelvic floor muscle damage and sexual dysfunction. Pelvic floor exercises after birth seem to have a positive effect on sexual function (Sobhgol, Priddis, Smith, & Dahlen, 2018). Psychological factors may be influential, confounding results, as improved self-acceptance, body awareness and satisfaction also have an impact (Rosenbaum, 2007). Other authors have suggested that there is a relationship between pelvic floor muscle strength and positive body self-perception (Sacomori, Cardoso, & Vanderlinde, 2010).

As the couple transition to parenthood, adjustments occur in their relationship and resumption of a physical sexual relationship is one of these adjustments. There are many factors that can affect sexual resumption and frequency after a baby is born, and some of these are sleep deprivation, a sore perineum and low libido. For example, in a study involving focus groups with 25 women, researchers found women's body image and sexual patterns change after giving birth, resulting in lowered sexual desire, which made their sexual needs discordant with those of their partner (Olsson, Lundqvist, Faxelid, & Nissen, 2005). Feeling unhappy about the changes to their body following the birth reduced women's confidence in this area. Sleep deprivation and less free time also impacted on how women felt towards sexual contact with their partner (Olsson et al., 2005). Women can feel guilty about these feelings and feel a failure so it is important that health professionals have conversations with the couple and are open and supportive about this.

Breastfeeding

Breastfeeding is recognized as the best source of nutrition for babies and it is associated with health benefits (both short and long term) for mother and baby, as well as having social, economic and environmental advantages (Horta, Bahl, Maritines, & Victora, 2007). The World Health Organization recommends that all babies are exclusively breastfed for the first six months of life and for up to two years of age (WHO, 2017). Despite this recommendation, breastfeeding rates remain low. For example, in Australia and New Zealand where most women initiate breastfeeding, only 15–18% are exclusively breastfeeding at six months (Australian Government Department of Health, 2019). A global breastfeeding scorecard put out by

WHO and UNICEF in collaboration with the Global Breastfeeding Collective found that out of 194 countries only 40% of children under six months are breastfed exclusively and only 23 countries had breastfeeding rates above 60% (all low-income countries) (UNICEF & WHO, 2018). An annual investment of under US$5 per newborn has been estimated as potentially increasing the global rate of exclusive breastfeeding among children under six months to 50% by the year 2025 (UNICEF & WHO, 2018). *Nurturing the health and wealth of nations: The investment case for breastfeeding* states that meeting this target could save the lives of 520,000 children under the age of five and could also generate US$300 billion in economic gains over ten years (Global Breastfeeding Collective, 2017). These gains would be due to a reduction in illness and health care costs and an increase in productivity. In five of the world's largest emerging economies (China, India, Indonesia, Mexico and Nigeria) a lack of investment in breastfeeding results in an estimated 236,000 children dying per year and US$119 billion in economic losses (Global Breastfeeding Collective, 2017).

Women also gain significant health benefits from breastfeeding with a lowered risk for breast cancer, ovarian cancer, type 2 diabetes and heart disease (Global Breastfeeding Collective, 2017). In countries where there is not ready access to contraception breastfeeding can also help with birth spacing (Global Breastfeeding Collective, 2017; UNICEF & WHO, 2018).

Women needing to return to work away from home at an earlier time tend to stop breastfeeding earlier than those who do not. The International Labour Organization recommends that countries should enact legislation that gives women the right to 18 weeks of paid maternity leave (International Labour Organization, 2019). Currently 12% of countries meet this target (UNICEF & WHO, 2018). Workplace barriers continue to have a major influence on breastfeeding as well. A review of 193 United Nations Member States found that 26.7% did not guarantee breastfeeding breaks in any form and 25% provided neither paid maternity leave nor paid breastfeeding breaks (Atabay et al., 2015). Those who do feed long term are frequently criticized and not supported (Dowling & Pontin, 2015). Women with unsupportive partners, family (Hall, McLelland, Gilmour, & Cant, 2014) and workplaces (Gatrell, 2007) are less likely to successfully breastfeed and pressure can be put on them to cease breastfeeding altogether.

Breastfeeding as a liminal state

Like childbirth, breastfeeding has also been described as a liminal experience (Mahon-Daly & Andrews, 2002) and a transition between states of being two individuals or one individual or neither (Dowling & Pontin, 2015). Women who breastfeed can feel themselves marked out as different and between social identities of woman and mother. They have moved from woman to mother in society's eyes and are in a space where their identity will shift again back to woman as they re-enter the workplace and their children grow older. Women who breastfeed long term have been described as 'betwixt and between' and their actions make their breastmilk and their bodies 'matter out of place' (Dowling & Pontin, 2015). With the rise of social media, there has been a re-claiming of women's ownership over their breasts and a development of a community of support to do this in. The rise of the 'brelfie' (selfies of women breastfeeding) is one good example of this (Locatelli, 2017; Mecinska, 2018).

Breastfeeding and sexuality

Breastfeeding, like pregnancy and birth, has an effect on women's perceptions of themselves as sexual beings. Most women identify a return of sexual interest soon after birth as important (Avery, Duckett, & Frantzich, 2000). For heterosexual women, average time to resuming intercourse is 5–8 weeks following the birth (Rowland, Foxcroft, Hopman, & Patel, 2005). Little is known about women in same sex relationships. Breastfeeding can impact on sexual desire and this is not all negative. Some studies indicate women who breastfeed report increased sexual desire and activity compared with when they were not pregnant and that this may be due to increased breast size or increased sensitivity of the breasts (Masters & Johnson, 1996). Some studies report the opposite and say sexual desire is much lower following the birth and this is more likely when women breastfeed (Rowland et al., 2005). Breastfeeding can be associated with painful intercourse in heterosexual relationships, due to a reduced lubrication of the vagina (hormonal changes that accompany breastfeeding) and perineal trauma sustained during the birth (Dahlen & Priddis, 2018). In a study by Avery et al. (2000) most women reported little effect of breastfeeding on their sex lives, with 74.6% of primiparous women saying they were able to combine a sexual relationship with breastfeeding with no problems, though, once they had weaned, 45.3% said breastfeeding interfered with their relationships.

Conclusion

In this chapter we have explored childbirth as a significant event in many women's lives with physical, cultural and psychological changes and challenges. We began with the context women give birth in and that it is a contested space and very medicalized today in many developed countries and in more and more developing countries. We have explored the liminality of childbirth and how this can lead to vulnerability to birth trauma. The physical process of giving birth, including many complex hormonal interactions, can be altered at many points in the process and evidence is mounting that we have gone too far in the way we intervene during childbirth. The next decade will bring a greater understanding of the impact on long-term health, and government and health policy needs to be directed towards humanizing birth and optimizing physiological processes. We have explored sexuality during pregnancy, birth and the postnatal period, and some of the factors that impact on this, including pelvic floor exercises and breastfeeding. Policies that support women to be mothers, including paid maternity leave and breastfeeding-friendly work practices, need to be fought for around the world if we are to see motherhood as a positive choice for women. Barbara Katz Rothman has said, 'Birth is not only about making babies. Birth is about making mothers – strong, competent, capable mothers who trust themselves and know their inner strength' (Katz Rothman, 2019). To achieve this important aim we need to have policy, practice and political alignment to support a social and health care environment that puts the best interests of women who become mothers at its heart.

References

Allen, A. (2007). Experiences of infertility: Liminality and the role of the infertility clinic. *Nursing Inquiry*, *14*(2), 132–139.

Almeida, L. M., Caldas, J., Ayres-de-campos, D., Salcedo-Barrientos, D., & Dias, S. (2013). Maternal healthcare in migrants: A systematic review. *Maternal Child Health*, *17*(8), 1346–1354.

American College of Obstetricians and Gynecologists (ACOG) (2015). ACOG Committee Opinion No. 649: Racial and ethnic disparities in obstetrics and gynecology. *Obstetrics & Gynecology*, *126*(6), e130–e134.

Aslan, G., Aslan, D., Kızılyar, A., Ispahi, C., & Esen, A. (2005). A prospective analysis of sexual functions during pregnancy. *International Journal of Impotence Research*, *17*(2), 154.

Atabay, E., Moreno, G., Nandi, A., Kranz, G., Vincent, I., Assi, T. M., Vaughan Winfrey, E.-M., Earle, A., Raub, A., & Heymann, S. J. (2015). Facilitating working mothers' ability to breastfeed: Global trends in guaranteeing breastfeeding breaks at work, 1995–2014. *Journal of Human Lactation, 31* (1), 81–88.

Australian Government Department of Health (2019). *Australian National Breastfeeding Strategy: 2019 and beyond, consultation report.* Retrieved from https://consultations.health.gov.au/population-health-and-sport-division/breastfeeding.

Avery, M., Duckett, L., & Frantzich, C. (2000). The experience of sexuality during breastfeeding among primiparous women. *Journal of Midwifery & Women's Health, 45*(3), 227–237.

Bartellas, E., Crane, J. M., Daley, M., Bennett, K. A., & Hutchens, D. (2000). Sexuality and sexual activity in pregnancy. *BJOG: An International Journal of Obstetrics & Gynaecology, 107*(8), 964–968.

Buckley, S. (2015). Hormonal physiology of childbearing: Evidence and implications for women, babies, and maternity care. *The Journal of Perinatal Education, 24*(3), 145–153.

Buckley, S. J. (2010). Sexuality in labor and birth: An intimate perspective. In D. Walsh & D. Soo (Eds), *Essential midwifery practice: Intrapartum care* (pp. 213–234). New York, NY: Wiley.

Cardwell, C. R., Stene, L. C., Joner, G., Cinek, O., Svensson, J., Goldacre, M. J., Parslow, R. C., Pozzilli, P., Brigis, G., Stoyanov, D., Urbonaite, B., Sipetić, S., Schober, E., Ionescu-Tirgoviste, C., Devoti, G., de Beaufort, C. E., Buschard, K., & Patterson, C. C. (2008). Caesarean section is associated with an increased risk of childhood-onset type 1 diabetes mellitus: A meta-analysis of observational studies. *Diabetologia, 51*, 726–735.

Clifford, M. (2019, February 21). 'I've run out of time': Terminally ill midwife who battled the HSE says her fight is over. *Irish Examiner.* Retrieved from www.irishexaminer.com/breakingnews/specialreports/ive-run-out-of-time-terminally-ill-midwife-who-battled-the-hse-says-her-fight-is-over-905991.html.

Dahlen, H., Homer, C., Leap, N., & Tracy, S. (2011). Social to surgical: Historic perspectives on perineal care during labour and birth. *Women and Birth, 24*, 105–111.

Dahlen, H., Tracy, S., Tracy, M. B., Bisits, A., Brown, C., & Thornton, C. (2014). Rates of obstetric intervention and associated perinatal mortality and morbidity among low-risk women giving birth in private and public hospitals in NSW (2000–2008): A linked data population-based cohort study. *British Medical Journal Open, 4*, e004551.

Dahlen, H. G., Kennedy, H. P., Anderson, C. M., Bell, A. F., Clark, A., Foureur, M., Ohm, J. E., Shearman, A. M., Taylor, J. Y., Wright, M. L., & Downe, S. (2013). The EPIIC hypothesis: Intrapartum effects on the neonatal epigenome and consequent health outcomes. *Medical Hypothesis, 8*(5), 656–662.

Dahlen, H. G. & Priddis, H. (2018). Perineal care and repair. In S. Pairman, S. Tracy, H. G. Dahlen, & L. Dixon (Eds), *Midwifery preparation for practice* (Vol. 4e, pp. 567–588). Sydney, Australia: Elsevier Australia.

Davis, E. (2010). *Orgasmic birth: Your guide to a safe, satisfying, and pleasurable birth experience.* Emmaus, PA: Rodale Press.

Davis-Floyd, R. (1994). The technocratic body: American childbirth as cultural expression. *Social Science and Medicine, 38*(8), 1125–1140.

Dowling, S. & Pontin, D. (2015). Using liminality to understand mothers' experiences of long-term breastfeeding: 'Betwixt and between', and 'matter out of place'. *Health: An Interdisciplinary Journal for the Social Study of Health, Illness and Medicine, 21*(1), 57–75.

Dykes, F. (2006). The education of health practitioners supporting breastfeeding women: Time for critical reflection. *Maternal and Child Nutrition, 2*, 204–216.

Ehrenreich, B. & English, D. (2010). *Witches, midwives and nurses: A history of women healers.* New York, NY: The Feminist Press.

Elbegway, A. F., Elshamy, F. F., & Hanfy, H. M. (2010). The effect of pelvic floor exercise on sexual function after vaginal delivery. *The Medical Journal of Cairo University, 78*(2), 27–31.

Elmir, R. & Schmied, R. (2016). A meta-ethnographic synthesis of fathers' experiences of complicated births that are potentially traumatic. *Midwifery, 32*, 66–74.

Erol, B., Sanli, O., Korkmaz, D., Seyhan, A., Akman, T., & Kadioglu, A. (2007). A cross-sectional study of female sexual function and dysfunction during pregnancy. *The Journal of Sexual Medicine, 4* (5), 1381–1387.

Ferreira, C. H., Dwyer, P. L., Davidson, M., De Souza, A., Ugarte, J. A., & Frawley, H. C. (2015). Does pelvic floor muscle training improve female sexual function? A systematic review. *International Urogynecology Journal, 26*(12), 1735–1750, doi:10.1007/s00192-015-2749-y.

FIGO (2018). FIGO position paper: How to stop the caesarean section epidemic. *Lancet*, *392*(October 13), 1286–1287.

Forss, A., Tishelman, C., Widmark, C., & Sachs, L. (2004). Women's experiences of cervical cellular changes: An unintentional transition from health to liminality? *Sociology of Health and Illness*, *26*(3), 306–325.

Gałązka, I., Drosdzol-Cop, A., Naworska, B., Czajkowska, M., & Skrzypulec-Plinta, V. (2015). Changes in the sexual function during pregnancy. *The Journal of Sexual Medicine*, *12*(2), 445–454.

Gaskin, I. M. (2002). *Spiritual midwifery*. Cambridge, UK: Summertown.

Gatrell, C. J. (2007). Secrets and lies: Breastfeeding and professional paid work. *Social Science and Medicine*, *65*(2), 393–404.

Gettler, L. T., McDade, T. W., Feranil, A. B., & Kuzawa, W. (2011). Longitudinal evidence that fatherhood decreases testosterone in human males. *The Proceedings of the National Academy of Sciences (PNAS)*, *108*(39), 16194–16199, doi:10.1073/pnas.1105403108.

Global Breastfeeding Collective (2017). *Nurturing the health and wealth of nations: The investment case for breastfeeding*. Geneva, Switzerland: World Health Organization. Retrieved from www.who.int/nutrition/publications/infantfeeding/global-bf-collective-investmentcase.pdf?ua=1.

Golmakani, N., Zare, Z., Khadem, N., Shareh, H., & Shakeri, M. T. (2015). The effect of pelvic floor muscle exercises program on sexual self-efficacy in primiparous women after delivery. *Iranian Journal of Nursing and Midwifery Research*, *20*(3), 347.

Greenfield, B. (2019, February 22). Midwife's arrest shines light on rural America's home-birth 'crisis'. *Yahoo! Lifestyle*. Retrieved from www.yahoo.com/lifestyle/midwifes-arrest-shines-light-rural-americas-home-birth-crisis-200121923.html.

Hairston, A. H. (1996). The debate over twilight sleep: Women influencing their medicine. *Issues in the History of Women's Health*, *5*(5), 489–499.

Hall, H., McLelland, G., Gilmour, C., & Cant, R. (2014). 'It's those first few weeks': Women's views about breastfeeding support in an Australian outer metropolitan region. *Women and Birth*, *27*(4), 259–265.

Handa, V. L., Blomquist, J. L., McDermott, K. C., Friedman, S., & Muñoz, A. (2012). Pelvic floor disorders after childbirth: Effect of episiotomy, perineal laceration, and operative birth. *Obstetrics & Gynecology*, *119*, 233–239.

Hannah, M. E., Hannah, W. J., Hewson, S., Hodnett, E. D., Saigal, S., & Willan, A. R. (2000). Planned caesarean section at term versus planned vaginal birth for breech presentation at term: A randomised controlled multicentred trial. Term Breech Trial Collaborative Group. *Lancet*, *356* (9239), 1375–1383.

Hannah, M. E., Whyte, H., Saigal, S., Hannah, W. J., Hewson, S., & Amankwah, K., Term Breech Trial Collaborative Group (2004). Outcomes of children at 2 years after planned cesarean birth versus planned vaginal birth for breech presentation at term: The international randomized Term Breech Trial. *American Journal of Obstetrics and Gynecology*, *191*(3), 864–871.

Harel, D. (2007). Sexual experiences of women during childbirth (unpublished doctoral dissertation). San Francisco, CA: The Institute for Advanced Study of Human Sexuality.

Hogan, S. (2008). Breasts and the beestings: Re-thinking breastfeeding practices, maternity rituals and maternal attachment in Britain and Ireland. *Journal of International Women's Studies*, *10*(2), 141–160.

Horta, B., Bahl, R., Maritines, J., & Victora, C. G. (2007). *Evidence on the long term effects of breastfeeding*. Geneva, Switzerland: World Health Organization.

Huang, L., Chen, Q., Zhao, Y., Wang, W., Fang, F., & Bao, Y. (2015). Is elective cesarean section associated with a higher risk of asthma? A meta-analysis. *Journal of Asthma*, *52*(1), 16–25.

Hussein, S. A. A. A., Dahlen, H. G., Duff, M., & Schmied, V. (2016). The barriers and facilitators to evidence-based episiotomy practice in Jordan. *Women and Birth*, *29*(4), 321–329.

Hussein, S. S. A. A., Dahlen, H. G., & Schmied, V. (2012). What makes episiotomy rates change? A systematic review of the literature. *International Journal of Childbirth*, *2*(1), 29–39.

Hyde, M. J., Mostyn, A., Modi, N., & Kemp, P. R. (2012). The health implications of birth by caesarean section. *Biological Reviews*, *87*(1), 229–243.

International Labour Organization (ILO) (2019). *International labour standards on maternity protection*. Geneva, Switzerland: Author. Retrieved March 30, 2018 from www.ilo.org/global/standards/subjects-covered-by-international-labour-standards/maternity-protection/lang–en/index.htm.

Jawed-Wessel, S. & Sevick, E. (2017). The impact of pregnancy and childbirth on sexual behaviors: A systematic review. *The Journal of Sex Research*, *54*(4–5), 411–423.

Jones, C., Chan, C., & Farine, D. (2011). Sex in pregnancy. *Canadian Medical Association Journal*, *183*(7), 815–818.

Katz Rothman, B. (2019). Barbara Katz Rothman [website]. Retrieved March 30, 2019 from www.bar barakatzrothman.com.

Keag, O. E., Norman, J. E., & Stock, S. J. (2018). Long-term risks and benefits associated with cesarean delivery for mother, baby, and subsequent pregnancies: Systematic review and meta-analysis. *PLOS Medicine, 15*(1), e1002494.

Kennedy, H. P., Cheyney, M., Dahlen, H. G., Downe, S., Foureur, M., Homer, C. S. E., Jefford, E., McFadden, A., Michel-Schuldt, M., Sandall, J., Soltani, H., Speciale A. M., Stevens, J., Vedam, S., & Renfrew, M. J. (2018). Asking different questions: A call to action for research to improve the quality of care for every woman, every child. *Birth, 63*(5), 516–517.

Kildea, S., Hickey, S., Nelson, C., Currie, J., Carson, A., Reynolds, M., & Tracy, S. (2017). Birthing on country (in our community): A case study of engaging stakeholders and developing a best-practice Indigenous maternity service in an urban setting. *Australian Health Review, 42*(2), 230–238.

Kildea, S., Tracy, S., Sherwood, J., Magick-Dennis, F., & Barclay, L. (2016). Improving maternity services for Indigenous women in Australia: Moving from policy to practice. *The Medical Journal of Australia (MJA), 205*(8), 375–379.

Kitzinger, S. & Simkin, P. (1984). *Episiotomy and the second stage of labour.* (2nd ed.). Seattle, WA: Penny Press Inc.

Leeners, B., Gorres, G., Block, E., & Hengartner, M. P. (2016). Birth experiences in adult women with a history of childhood sexual abuse. *Journal of Psychosomatic Research, 83,* 27–32.

Leite, A. P. L., Campos, A. A. S., Dias, A. R. C., Amed, A. M., De Souza, E., & Camano, L. (2009). Prevalence of sexual dysfunction during pregnancy. *Revista da Associação Médica Brasileira, 55*(5), 563–568.

Locatelli, E. (2017). Images of breastfeeding on instagram: Self-representation, publicness, and privacy management. *Social Media and Society, 3*(2), 1–14.

Lupton, D. & Schmied, V. (2013). Splitting bodies/selves: Women's concepts of embodiment at the moment of birth. *Sociology of Health and Illness, 35*(6), 828–841.

Mahon-Daly, P. & Andrews, G. (2002). Liminality and breastfeeding: Women negotiating space and two bodies. *Health and Place, 8,* 61–76.

Masters, W. & Johnson, V. E. (1996). *Human sexual response.* Boston, MA: Little, Brown and Co.

Mayberry, L. & Daniel, J. (2016). 'Birthgasm'. A literary review of orgasm as an alternative mode of pain relief in childbirth. *Journal of Holistic Nursing, 34*(4), 331–342.

Mecinska, L. (2018). 'Milk Pride': Lactivist online constructions of positive breastfeeding value. *Studies in the Maternal, 10*(1), 9.

Mesch, R. (2009). Housewife or harlot? Sex and the married woman in nineteenth-century France. *Journal of the History of Sexuality, 18*(1), 65–83.

O'Connell, M. A., Leahy-Warren, P., Khashan, A. S., Kenny, L., & O'Neill, S. (2017). Worldwide prevalence of tocophobia in pregnant women: Systematic review and meta-analysis. *Acta Obstetrica et Gynecological Scandinavica, 96*(8), 907–920.

Odent, M. (2014). *Water birth and sexuality.* Glasgow, UK: Clairview Books.

Olsson, A., Lundqvist, M., Faxelid, E., & Nissen, E. (2005). Women's thoughts about sexual life after childbirth: Focus group discussions with women after childbirth. *Scandanavian Journal of Caring Sciences, 19*(4), 381–387.

Oruç, S., Esen, A., Laçin, S., Adigüzel, H., Uyar, Y., & Koyuncu, F. (1999). Sexual behaviour during pregnancy. *Australian and New Zealand Journal of Obstetrics and Gynaecology, 39*(1), 48–50.

Pauls, R. N., Occhino, J. A., & Dryfhout, V. L. (2008). Effects of pregnancy on female sexual function and body image: A prospective study. *The Journal of Sexual Medicine, 5*(8), 1915–1922.

Peters, L. L., Thornton, C., de Jonge, A., Khashan, A., Tracy, M., Downe, S., Feijen-de Jong, E. I., & Dahlen, H. G. (2018). The effect of medical and operative birth interventions on child health outcomes in the first 28 days and up to 5 years of age: A linked data population-based cohort study. *Birth, 45*(4), 347–357.

Polidano, C., Zhu, A., & Bornstein, J. C. (2017). The relation between cesarean birth and child cognitive development. *Scientific Reports, 7*(1), 11483.

Reed, R., Barnes, M., & Rowe, J. (2016). Women's experience of birth: Childbirth as a rite of passage. *International Journal of Childbirth, 6*(1), 46–56.

Renfrew, M., McFadden, A., Bastos, M., Campbell, J., Channon, A. A., Cheung, N. F., Silva, D. R., Downe, S., Kennedy, H. P., Malata, A., McCormick, F., Wick, L., & Declercq, E. (2014). Midwifery and quality care: Findings from a new evidence-informed framework for maternal and newborn care. *Lancet, 384,* 1129–1145.

Ribeiro, M. C., Nakamura, M. U., Torloni, M. R., de Tubino Scanavino, M., do Amaral, M. L. S. A., dos Santos Puga, M. E., & Mattar, R. (2014). Treatments of female sexual dysfunction symptoms during pregnancy: A systematic review of the literature. *Sexual Medicine Reviews*, 2(1), 1–9.

Rosenbaum, T. Y. (2007). Pelvic floor involvement in male and female sexual dysfunction and the role of pelvic floor rehabilitation in treatment: A literature review. *The Journal of Sexual Medicine*, 4(1), 4–13.

Rowland, M., Foxcroft, L., Hopman, W. M., & Patel, R. (2005). Breastfeeding and sexuality immediately post partum. *Canadian Family Physician*, 51(10), 1366–1367.

Sacomori, C., Cardoso, F. L., & Vanderlinde, C. (2010). Pelvic floor muscle strength and body self-perception among Brazilian pregnant women. *Physiotherapy*, 96(4), 337–343.

Sandall, J., Soltani, H., Gates, S., Shennan, A., & Devane, D. (2016). Midwife-led continuity models versus other models of care for childbearing women during pregnancy, birth and early parenting. *Cochrane Database of Systematic Reviews*, 4 (CD004667), doi:10.1002/14651858.CD004667.pub5.

Simpson, M., Schmied, V., Dickson, C., & Dahlen, H. G. (2018). Postnatal post-traumatic stress: An integrative review. *Women and Birth*, 31(5), 367–379.

Sleep, J., Grant, A., Garcia, J., Elbourne, D., Spencer, J., & Chalmers, I. (1984). West Berkshire perineal management trial. *British Medical Journal*, 289, 587–590.

Sobhgol, S. S., Priddis, H., Smith, C. A., & Dahlen, H. G. (2018). The effect of pelvic floor muscle exercise on female sexual function during pregnancy and postpartum: A systematic review. *Sexual Medicine Reviews*, 7(1), 13–28.

Stevens, J., Schmied, V., Burns, E., & Dahlen, H. (2014). Immediate or early skin-to-skin contact after a caesarean section: A review of the literature. *Maternal and Child Nutrition*, 10, 456–473.

Taylor, L. S. (2008). A rites of passage analysis of the families' experience of premature birth. *Journal of Neonatal Nursing*, 14(2), 56–60.

Tew, M. (1990). *Safer childbirth? A critical history of maternity care*. London, UK: Chapman and Hall.

Turner, V. (1969). *The ritual process*. New York, NY: Aldine Transaction.

UNICEF & WHO (2018). *Global breastfeeding scorecard, 2018: Enabling women to breastfeed through better policies and programmes*, Global Breastfeeding Collective. New York, NY, and Geneva: Authors. Retrieved from www.who.int/nutrition/publications/infantfeeding/global-bf-scorecard-2018.pdf?ua=1.

Villarosa, L. (2018, April 11). Why America's black mothers and babies are in a life or death crisis. *The New York Times Magazine*. Retrieved from www.nytimes.com/2018/04/11/magazine/black-mothers-babies-death-maternal-mortality.html.

West, R., Gamble, J., Kelly, J., Milne, T., Duffy, E., & Sidebotham, M. (2016). Culturally capable and culturally safe: Caseload care for Indigenous women by Indigenous midwifery students. *Women and Birth*, 29(6), 524–530.

White, G. (2007). You cope by breaking down in private: Fathers and PTSD following childbirth. *British Journal of Midwifery*, 15, 39–45.

Wilton, T. (2001). Lesbian mothers' experiences of maternity care in the UK. *Midwifery*, 17(3), 203–211.

Wong, P. C. & Kitsantas, P. (2019). A review of maternal mortality and quality of care in the USA. *The Journal of Maternal-Fetal and Neonatal Medicine*. Published online ahead of print, doi: 10.1080/14767058.2019.1571032.

World Health Organization (WHO) (2017). *Protecting, promoting and supporting breastfeeding in facilities providing maternity and newborn services*, World Health Organisation Guideline. Geneva: Author. Retrieved from http://apps.who.int/iris/bitstream/handle/10665/259386/9789241550086-eng.pdf;jsessionid=6E470251709BC8F0CD079EA4EC1F3800?sequence=1.

World Health Organization (WHO) (2018). *WHO recommendations: Intrapartum care for a positive childbirth experience*. Geneva: Author.

Yeniel, A. & Petri, E. (2014). Pregnancy, childbirth, and sexual function: Perceptions and facts. *International Urogynecology Journal*, 25(1), 5–14.

Yıldız, H. (2015). The relation between prepregnancy sexuality and sexual function during pregnancy and the postpartum period: A prospective study. *Journal of Sex & Marital Therapy*, 41(1), 49–59.

23

POSTPARTUM ADJUSTMENT

Psychological aspects

Paula Nicolson

> Becoming a mother has an impact on the life of the woman, each time it occurs, physically, socially, economically and emotionally. The ways in which motherhood affects each woman also crosses over into the lives of her baby, the baby's father, her family and friends. The success of the transition from pregnancy to motherhood has concerned experts and lay people alike. There are distinct rules, written and unwritten, that place the burden for the smooth transition and good mothering firmly upon the individual woman. When she fails to adapt to the role of mothering an infant she is identified as having PND [postnatal depression].
>
> (Nicolson, 2003, *p. 25*)

Nearly two decades have passed since I wrote that account of postpartum adjustment. I suggested then that it demands huge changes to a woman's everyday life, as well as to the lives of those who surround her. Looking back, I wonder how far material conditions have changed for mothers. Superficially it might seem that the current generation of new mothers, particularly women who are privileged, visualize their postpartum adjustment to "normal" life as their absolute right. To illustrate, it was widely reported that on announcing her first pregnancy in January 2018, Jacinda Arden, Prime Minister of New Zealand, declared that after a six-week postpartum break her husband would be the primary baby carer, so that she could continue running the country. She is but one among many women who now return to high-powered occupations within weeks of having given birth. Implicit here is the notion that nothing about a woman's cognitive, emotional, physical, or social world will be unsettled by her having a baby, so that a smooth adjustment to motherhood is simply a matter of a (brief) period of time-out and having effective childcare arrangements in place (Robertson et al., 2004).

So, is motherhood no longer perceived, or even experienced, as disruptive to the flow of everyday life? Or, for those whose lives are less privileged than Arden's, with worries about child care, housing, or money, what might be the consequences of having a baby for their physical and psychological health (Rallis et al., 2014)? There is plenty of evidence from around the globe that motherhood, particularly following the birth of a baby, is interlinked with increased poverty for disadvantaged families, notably single, oppressed, and/or abused mothers in developing countries (Lopez, 2015). The material experience of becoming a mother from pregnancy to the postpartum involves all women in physical and mental discomfort although where poverty, oppression, starvation, lack of medical resources and high levels of infant death intersect, the mother's and baby's health and wellbeing will be greatly at risk. This includes the mother's ability to manage labour, recover from wounds and stitches, and care for the baby's essential needs particularly where there is a lack of clinical support for her physical and emotional pain (Reed et al., 2017).

Disadvantaged families of all types find themselves blamed for their lot – a view that obscures the daily struggles that many poor parents face (O'Campo et al., 2016). This sense that social and health services are not available potentially increases stress for mothers living in poverty, disabled, or single making them vulnerable to mental and physical health problems including diabetes, heart disease, anxiety, and depression (Glosswitch, 2018).

Consequently various factors (i.e., ethnicity, religion, socio-economic, geographic, ability, sexualities, and other identity influences) may conspire to multiply subjugate and disadvantage many women and their families. These potentially overwhelming elements that characterize so many lives do not operate independently but create a system of intersecting oppressions that put many women's mental and physical health at risk (Everson & Ostrach, 2017).

What is postpartum adjustment?

Simply stated, postpartum adjustment refers to the emotional, cultural, psychological, biological, and practical adjustments women face following the birth of a baby. The concept of postpartum adjustment *per se* insinuates that this particular life event is followed by a reinstatement of the new mother's world, either to how it was before the birth, or that she (and her family) will eventually adjust their lives and emotions positively to the change (Fleming et al., 1988). However, for some having a(nother) child can enhance life-prospects, health, and well-being, while for others each birth exacerbates their hardship with dire consequences for the mental and physical health of the woman and her children (Everson & Ostrach, 2017) . This is particularly true when multiple or intersecting oppressions such as poverty, immigrant or minority status, disability, chronic ill health, or social exclusion intersect, as indicated above (Haskins et al., 2016).

Popular magazines, academic articles, blogs, and websites aimed at informing new mothers in Western democratic societies about postpartum adjustment tend to emphasize postpartum *problems*, such as the "baby blues", anxiety, difficulties with breastfeeding, and postnatal depression (Luce et al., 2016). These messages are obliquely embedded in reassurance that feeling anxious, depressed, tired, or lacking in confidence is *normal* because the transition to motherhood is such a profound physical, social, and emotional experience. Which it surely is (Puryear, 2014). Such articles on the whole though avoid issues beyond those directly affected by the arrival of the baby, such as socio-economic matters or longer-term relationship matters (Kendall-Tackett, 2016).

Consequently, thinking about postpartum adjustment presents an interesting paradox. On the one hand, to have the choice of motherhood combined with career for those women fortunate enough to make that decision may be a positive move towards gender equality in both private and public spheres (Ward & Wolf-Wendel, 2016). Whereas domestic abuse, relationship breakdown, physical and mental health concerns, fear for the baby's welfare, and financial worries, which potentially intersect with the transition to motherhood across many societies, act to ensure that some women's lives, even those among the privileged, change irrevocably and negatively, at least for a time, after childbirth (Reck et al., 2012).

Reflecting on this dilemma is not to predict substantive problems for every new mother, whatever her socio-economic or family status, but to note the need to be mindful of evidence collected over many years by feminist and other psychologists and social scientists demonstrating that motherhood often inflicts unexpected changes to a woman's life, which, at the least, require social and emotional work (Seymour-Smith et al., 2017).

In what follows, therefore, I reconsider research on postpartum adjustment, in part illustrated with selected data from two specific studies of the transition to motherhood experienced by three generations of women in the UK and some in the USA. It involved those who gave birth in the 1970s, the 1980s, and towards the end of first decade of the 21st century (Heffernan et al., 2011; Nicolson et al., 2010). The participants had varied socio-economic and cultural backgrounds and provided their own accounts of adjustment of motherhood. The data from the studies is used here in conjunction with other international research to provide insight into women's postpartum adjustment experiences from a psychosocial perspective.

Recovering from pregnancy and birth

Women's reproductive bodies are typically pathologized (Ussher, 1989) such that fluctuating hormones during pregnancy, immediately after birth, and during breastfeeding are positioned within a medicalized discourse as overwhelming women's intellectual and emotional capacities rendering them vulnerable and incapable of managing their emotional and intellectual lives. Feminist psychologists and social scientists more generally (e.g., Oakley, 2016) over the last 40 years, have effectively put forward robust alternatives to this medicalized view with a psychosocial model of postpartum adjustment (Saxbe, 2017).

A psychosocial, feminist understanding of postpartum adjustment reflects the diversity of women's biological, emotional, and social experiences as they interconnect with the health and status of the new baby and the broader historical and political context of each woman's life (McKenzie-Mohr & Lafrance, 2014). Similarly, women's own accounts reflect diversity and ambivalence, and there is some evidence that everyday knowledge(s) and word of mouth have greater influence on a mother's expectations and reported experience than "experts" do (Murphy & Strong, 2018).

Recovering from labour is closely connected to recovery from the emotion of giving birth, although the *pain* of labour and childbirth is central to most women's immediate postpartum experiences. Many women, despite the experts' advice, appear to be unprepared for the strength of the pain that results from childbirth (Jones et al., 2012). Women may therefore feel let down by health professionals who minimize and fail to warn them of the physical trauma and pain during and after birth (Simpson & Catling, 2016). That is the case whether a woman has a vaginal or a caesarean childbirth. Often it is other women who provide the appropriate warnings and support that reinforce resistance to health professionals and might encourage women to opt for a home birth surrounded by friends and family rather than by midwives and obstetricians (Hollander et al., 2017) in contexts where it is possible to do so.

It is worth reflecting on the way in which extreme pain and fear are linked (Junge et al., 2018), so that in some instances unexpected and extreme pain might lead to trauma and thus a poor outcome (Olde et al., 2006). As one participant in our studies, Danni, having her first baby, put it: "I remember my mum saying there was tremendous pain in the beginning – she used to say everybody's different – she said I didn't really want to tell you that the pain is so bad – it would frighten you." It might though have been better for her emotional state if her mother had actually forewarned her. Ali, who had had her first child via caesarean section, was determined to have a natural birth the second time around. However, she too had been unprepared for the level of pain during labour and in the aftermath, which both upset and angered her. Neither was she impressed with the clinical/expert practices she tried to contest. She described the experience:

> I couldn't sleep for pain or the following morning when they examined me the damned stitches had opened up ... I had thought that getting over the [vaginal] delivery would have been faster than getting over the caesarean ... I had this dreadful swelling with the stitches – then the damned thing opened up. ... I couldn't sit down!

Despite the medicalization of contemporary childbirth and apparent acceptance of expert advice on labour, many women, unprepared for the physical shock of having a baby on their postpartum *bodies*, go on to experience a lack of trust in the health care system that influences their experience of mothering in the immediate postpartum period (Sivertsen et al., 2017).

Breastfeeding may also be problematic and painful, and a number of women report having received mixed messages about how to manage this, which were both confusing and frustrating (Moule et al., 2014). Some women are keen to breastfeed, others not so; some find it more difficult than expected, and the quality of advice and support is variable so that much depends upon the woman's own socio-economic, ethnic, and cultural background, all of which impact upon the degree of accession to the predominant advice (Gallegos et al., 2015). Local and family beliefs and taboos and male partners' opinions also impact women's choices (Van Wagenen et al., 2015). Jennifer, who was expecting her second child, explained:

> They [midwives] didn't really put pressure on you ... they give you a leaflet saying: 'Breast is best' ... I felt it was expected of me to breast feed. It's not something I felt great about doing, but it was expected.

Jennifer's ambivalence appeared to be shared across several women from our studies, and in other research, where issues about the dependence of a breastfed baby, lack of sleep, and the difficulties of not having a choice about who does the feeding were raised (Jacob, 2015).

Accepting and resisting the experts

Women do challenge the clinical experts during labour and its aftermath. This resistance to experts became increasingly apparent with the development of interest in psychosocial aspects of the postpartum, motivated by feminist critiques of the medical model of pregnancy, childbirth, and motherhood which championed the value of qualitative and mixed method approaches (e.g., Lafrance & Stoppard, 2006). Consequently, women's own accounts of postpartum adjustment have gradually gained visibility and foregrounded the multiplicity and diversity of experiences that have been absent from medical texts (Taborelli et al., 2016). Some of this work exposed discourses of oppression (Shabot & Korem, 2018), regulation, surveillance, and control by "experts" (Thomas & Lupton, 2015). It also emphasized differences between individual women and groups of women by focussing on subjective experiences rather than pregnancy, childbirth, and early motherhood as a medicalized, homogeneous set of events (Shin & White-Traut, 2007). Thus the experiences of women from different socio-economic and cultural communities, particularly when there are intersecting disadvantages or advantages, is available to inform both academic and popular knowledge(s) (Robinson & Rogers, 2018).

Not only have the confirmation of pregnancy, childbirth, and the postnatal period been traditionally medically driven physiological events, but biomedical discourse has also dominated the self-help literature on pregnancy and childbirth (Van Teijlingen, 2017). This includes advice on antenatal care, labour and birth, diet and lifestyle, all of which serve to limit and control women's behaviour, expectations, and attitudes toward the self. It also influences the public discourse on women's bodies, both during and after pregnancy (Fieril et al., 2017).

Women are now advised what to eat while trying to conceive, while pregnant, and during the postpartum period; recommendations include folic acid, oily fish, fruit, and lean meat (Neiterman & Fox, 2017). The majority of Western women have been convinced that such advice is essential for the health of their baby and their own recovery from labour and childbirth (Fox et al., 2009). Conversely, certain foods are now identified as "taboo" (e.g., soft or blue cheeses, fish that might contain mercury, fats, sugar, nuts, caffeine, alcohol) (van der Pligt et al., 2016). In less developed and/or unstable societies where conflict and general poverty intersect with family disruption, geographical movement, lack of medicine and medical care, the emphasis is upon ensuring adequate nutrition across the transition to motherhood (e.g., Nasreen et al., 2015).

It is clear that there are some potentially harmful effects to the pregnant and postnatal body from particular food and drinks (and cigarettes), yet once again women themselves have been largely peripheral to the evidence gathering (Vincze et al., 2018). It is only relatively recently that equal consideration has been given to the experience and attitudes of the mothers' views on food (see Ussher, 2006), but there is still little indication of how women make choices about implementing professional advice or how the advice influences their everyday postnatal lives (Lucas et al., 2014).

Georgina, pregnant with her second baby, was worried about managing expert nutritional advice during pregnancy and while breastfeeding. She felt both confused and guilty if she were to resist the advice:

> I mean I don't eat soft cheeses, … I'm not sure about shell fish and stuff like that, I have eaten prawns, but … and people have gone 'Oh God' and stuff … you know, cooking your eggs properly, that kind of thing … I feel a bit of a guilt, like if someone sees me drinking a glass of wine.

A significant part of postpartum adjustment involves reactions to others' surveillance alongside a degree of self-surveillance. This happens when women internalize dominant discourses and actively engage with the medicalization of their own pregnancies and postpartum (Malatzky, 2017). This suggests then that postpartum adjustment may be accompanied, almost constantly, by a sense of guilt because few manage the transition to motherhood without breaking some of the experts' rules or transgressing contemporary social norms, which, even though these change over time, challenge women to remain constantly vigilant if they are to be seen as "good (enough)" mothers (Sullivan, 2015).

Despite the worry about managing the effects of medical practices, it was not unusual across the generations for women from our research to respond to their own bodies rather than to accept the dictates of health professionals, especially when there had not been continuity of care from pregnancy through the postpartum (Forster et al., 2016). One such first-time mother resisting pressure from the hospital clinicians responded to her sense of her own postpartum body, bravely and fiercely challenging the tenets of the obstetric team who had classified her in terms of health status rather than as a woman aware of her own health needs. Her blood pressure had been high during pregnancy but her stay in hospital postnatally, demanded by the doctors, became stressful through lack of sleep and the strong desire to go home to her healthy baby who had already been discharged. She said:

> The baby was fine – she was discharged 2 days before me. I knew what it [high blood pressure] was [about] because I hadn't slept ... anxiety and in the end they offered me my own room – I said it wouldn't make any difference anyway 'OK then' they said – 'if anything happens it's not down to us'.

This woman knew that the baby was healthy, and was unconvinced that the hospital team knew much about her specifically. Her resistance suggested a personal strength on her part. It is probable that some of her strong inclination to resist the medical advice and leave the hospital was linked to a desire to build a sense of normality into her new life as a mother, as well as to reinforce a degree of self-awareness about her own body.

Changes, choices, and the psychosocial context

There is little doubt that the context of motherhood has changed over the past 50 years, with greater attention paid by researchers to mothers living in a non-traditional context, such as single, lesbian, disabled, older, adolescent mothers, and mothers from non-Western cultures (Alang & Fomotar, 2015; Collins, 2016; Heffernan et al., 2011). More new mothers in advanced industrial societies return to work, through choice or economic necessity, within weeks of having given birth than they did in the 1970s and 1980s. For instance, in 2017 in England, 4.9 million mothers with dependent children were at work, up from 3.7 million in 1999 (Office for National Statistics, 2017).

Many more unmarried (although not necessarily single) heterosexual and lesbian women have become mothers, often having their first child at a later age than was typical 30 years ago (Golombok et al., 2016). Women from higher socio-economic status groups are less likely than others to live near family or other supportive social networks (Glenn, 2016), which has led to the need for a variety of childcare arrangements (e.g., childminders, nurseries, nannies, or the partner taking the primary responsibilities) (Weiss, 2002). Women from more traditional backgrounds may consider that their family members are too influential and likely to try to interfere with their child care practices (Noriega et al., 2017).

Despite these changes, the common feature across generations is that many girls and women, both heterosexual and lesbian (Hayman & Wilkes, 2017), expect to become mothers, choose to become mothers, and plan *how* to manage their mothering without thoughts of difficulties in postpartum adjustment (Sayil et al., 2007). Furthermore, even though there have been effective challenges to the notion of a maternal instinct driving women towards motherhood (Henderson, 2018), it is possible that the discourse that a woman will "know what to do" as a mother remains present at some level in society, including among women themselves (Lafrance & Stoppard, 2006). Of course, not all mothers consider themselves to be childcare experts, and may experience a sense of failure, guilt, and anxiety for a variety of reasons when facing everyday infant care tasks, which might lead to depression. Further, there are significant groups of women who remain childless by choice (Bień et al., 2017) despite residual social prejudice and pressures (Morison et al., 2016).

Social dynamics change after the birth of a child. This is the case between partners (Clout & Brown, 2016), with friends and family, and with co-workers, above all for mothers whose new baby leaves them at risk of poverty and/or decreased family income

(Blank, 2018). These relationship changes were among the key psychosocial factors for many women's postpartum adjustment in our research. Women find themselves making decisions about day-to-day infant care on their own, when healthcare professionals are no longer paying them attention (Coates et al., 2014) and with less support at home if their partners had returned to work. For example, a woman whose children were born in the 1970s expressed it this way: "Even with [2nd son] being a caesarean, seven days after the operation he [husband] went back to work, and I really just had to get on with it."

Stress and anxiety may also characterize fathers' postnatal experiences (Epifanio et al., 2015). Heightened and unrealistic expectations that intimate partners might have of each other in relation to infant care is a further potential cause of stress and depression (Hoseini et al., 2015). Intimate partner violence and abuse might be exacerbated by the arrival of a baby, possibly fuelled by alcohol or drug intake caused by anxiety (Mumford et al., 2018; Rai, 2017). A further surprise for a new mother, or father if he takes on the primary care role (Locke, 2016), can be the sheer drudgery and loneliness of the daily routine (Bradley, 2016). One woman, who had her first baby in the 1980s, felt especially isolated and exploited while her husband focussed himself on his work, often away from home. But that was: "worse at the weekend because you're stuck – everyone should be at home I think and it's the same damn thing. It's just you and the baby and it really gets you down."

Not everyone felt quite so rejected, but several women in our research experienced that sense of "having to get on with it" on their own and that relationship dynamics were different after the baby had arrived, even if it were not their first child. Loneliness can lead to postnatal depression (Luoma et al., 2015), and it is particularly acute among new mothers who experience social isolation, including migrant women and those who are not integrated into their communities for socio-economic or geo-political reasons (Wittkowski, Patel, & Fox, 2017).

There are both benefits and difficulties for those mothers who return to work (Asai et al., 2015). Benefits include economic and improved mental health prospects, whereas difficulties concern worries about breastfeeding, the overall welfare of the baby, childcare facilities, and exhaustion (Bai et al., 2015). For example, Sophie, who had had her second child, found that the pressure of returning to work provoked anxiety. She considered that her mother's generation had more straightforward postpartum adjustment, because the choices, and therefore the pressures, were not the same – a fact that is acknowledged in other research (Dennis et al., 2016). Sophie said:

> It's harder now [than for her mother] in a lot of ways [being a full-time mother] … it's very physically and emotionally demanding. I've got friends who go to work in the office, and they say that that's actually a rest, compared to the days that they have their toddlers and stuff.

Conversely, there were women we interviewed who had to return to work for financial rather than career reasons. Jerri became depressed because of money worries: "financial worries were a problem! – it was probably something to do something with [the depression]."

The "mother" in contrast to the "other" self

Such a profound experience as becoming a mother, for the first and subsequent times, inevitably causes a woman to re-evaluate herself and her place in her family, friendship groups, and society in general, whatever her background or social status (Taborelli et al., 2016). Ruth, whose older son had started nursery school when she had her second baby, thought hard about the changes in her sense of self and told me that facing these issues prevented a deep sense of despair. She described it as "you're not the one whose important anymore – 'cos your child takes over. You just don't exist anymore – you've got to do things for them before you can even think of yourself!"

Not everyone felt down about the changes in their sense of self, particularly if they were well supported (Çinar & Öztürk, 2014). This is also a characteristic of mothers with disabilities, who often as they adapt to their new roles realize new capacities that impact positively on their self-esteem (Lawler et al., 2015). Several women in our studies reported greater self-confidence once the first few weeks of motherhood had passed. For example, at her third interview (three months postpartum) Nancy, a former health professional who had not yet returned to work, said:

> I've got much more confidence in myself now. I really do feel that. It's just happened. I couldn't say when but his birth and everything gave me strength and I know I came through it without any medical help. And society looks upon me differently. Now I'm a woman. A mother in my own right – no-one is going to tell me what to do any more.

She, along with other women in several international studies, felt transformed into, what they saw as, a valued member of society – in this case by becoming a *woman* (Bleichmar, 2018). Similarly, our participant Janet, who had been depressed for a number of reasons during and shortly after pregnancy, began to feel better as she recognized her mothering as a positive experience. Six months after the birth of her first baby, she reported a positive change to her sense of self:

> I think having the baby has done it ... I think that makes me appear more responsible ... also settling down now. I'm seeing more of a sense of future for myself and the child – or the children. There's a point to it all now.

However, not everyone is able to identify positive changes in their sense of self. Vicki said "I feel a lot older. I don't feel right in certain things I wear and feel like I've got to be a lot more 'respectable'." Vicki stated that she had no clear idea what a mother was supposed to be like, which left her psychologically stranded – somehow knowing that she had changed, and had had to change, but confused as to the nature of the change (Fox & Neiterman, 2015).

It seems that getting back to the "old" self could be run in parallel to being the "new" self and that becoming a mother is experienced as both a "gain" and a "loss" of identities (Javadifar et al., 2016). As Wendy said: "I didn't exactly give work a thought until the Sunday night and when I arrived back it was as if I'd never been away ... it was back to my old self again to be honest." The sense of self, therefore, is discursive. The subjective experience relates to social, biographical, familial, and temporal nuances, with motherhood itself shifting between being a major component and a marginal one. Perhaps being more financially and socially privileged, as is the case for professional women like Wendy, enables a more profound sense of continuity with the old self. Having a sense of a developing ongoing self-hood is a component of privilege, demonstrated by the New Zealand Prime Minister who anticipated continuity of selfhood and prospects after childbirth (Collins, 2016). This stands in stark contrast to women who feel neglected by partner and friends, socially isolated, lonely, and poor, who are simply left to "get on with it," and consequently are at greater risk of anxiety, depression, and post-partum psychosis (Bergink et al., 2016). In recent years, there have been numerous studies of risk factors for postpartum depression, which demonstrate how poverty, disability, intimate partner violence and abuse, and absence of contraception to avoid further pregnancy intersect with the experience of childbirth and new motherhood to further exacerbate psychosocial disadvantage (de Castro et al., 2015).

Living with the changing body

The transition to motherhood involves a degree of pain and exhaustion at each stage (Winson, 2017), although this usually passes relatively quickly. However, the longer, perhaps more gradual, experience of physical change is brought about by and during the pregnancy itself (Berggren et al., 2016). Most women put on excess weight that does not necessarily disappear after birth or on ceasing to breastfeed and may be associated with normal weight gain that occurs with age (Yakusheva et al., 2017). The public discourse of the "thin ideal" continues to influence women's self-surveillance and esteem postpartum (Adegboye et al., 2007).

Not everyone feels pressure to return to their pre-pregnancy weight, but there is a view that mothers are expected to try (Avery et al., 2016). Karen, who had recently had her third baby, made it clear how: "there's pressure to lose weight – definitely but I wouldn't really say there's much to look nice. … yeah there's far too much hype about losing weight definitely." Getting back to "normal" and looking "nice" can be complicated and not necessarily the same thing, and there are different levels of pressure to change or accept changes in the body. There is evidence that challenges about weight gain and loss over the transition to motherhood are closely related to educational level, as well as to relationship and socio-economic status (Rosal et al., 2016).

Elizabeth, just after the birth of her first baby, indicated how she might be influenced by informal norms from her workplace that characterized the "thin ideal" – the public image of a slim/thin woman being both sexy and healthy (Nicolson et al., 2010):

> I wouldn't say I'd be that bothered usually, because I don't pay too much attention to people in magazines anyway, but the only thing I would say I'm a bit bothered about is some people at work, when other people have had babies, have said 'ooh she's not lost her weight has she?'

Generally, for the postnatal women in these studies, exercise appears to be more popular than changing to a lower calorie diet to approach the thin ideal, which may be attributable to the popular discourse of "*fit = healthy*" (McKinley, 2017). Gail identified exercise and sport as means of losing weight, but, more importantly, she acknowledged that her pre-pregnant self, when she was slim and engaged in regular exercise, equated to having a fit and healthy body. Getting back to an exercise regimen would, she believed, go a long way to returning her to her real self. After her first baby she became obsessed with the gym and exercise classes, which exhausted her. On the second occasion she found that: "swimming a couple of times a week and yoga … just kind of gentle stuff … really helped me to be fit. … and in good health as well." This suggests that postpartum adjustment for many women is about adapting to the change of body size, weight and shape, as well as to a different life and relationship dynamics, which might mean different activities and different choices of clothes, which have implications for identity (Fox & Neiterman, 2015; Tiggemann, 2004).

Conclusions

Becoming a mother, in whatever context, has profound physical, socio-economic and emotional implications for every woman. The arrival of a new baby, or an additional child, further impacts on those who surround her, including her partner, her relatives, and her co-workers.

In these respects little may have changed since my reflections at the beginning of this chapter (Nicolson, 2003). What has changed is the increased attention among researchers and clinicians to women from a variety of socio-economic and non-traditional backgrounds. This is because previous research on postpartum adjustment originated in Western countries and focused on women above the poverty line. However, factors that impact on post-partum adjustment, such as lack of health and social care resources, as well as community and family stability, vary to a degree across cultures (see Collins, 2016; de Castro et al., 2015).

In both Western and developing societies food and eating during pregnancy and the postpartum are key issues for researchers and health care practitioners. In the former there is a focus on what not to eat and drink during pregnancy and while breastfeeding. This reflects the relatively recent (e.g., Oakley, 2016) escalation of obstetric technologies with emphasis on the medicalization of childbirth and the postpartum, the health of the baby and mother along with the subsequent need to avoid obesity after birth for the mother and for the infant as she develops. In less developed and/or unstable societies where conflict and general poverty intersect with family disruption, geographical movement, lack of medicine and medical care, the emphasis is upon ensuring adequate nutrition across the transition to motherhood (e.g., Nasreen et al., 2015).

Studies of clinical practice clarify the need to ensure continuity of care across pregnancy, labour and the immediate postpartum, including good quality information for all women on the difficulties that might be faced during labour and while breastfeeding and on effective self-care. However, what this might involve depends very much on culture and beliefs, particularly the social status of women as well as economic stability and familial resources. Although not all women would opt to emulate the New Zealand prime minister, most women aspire to become good enough mothers, with healthy bodies, engaged in positive and supportive relationships, with enough money to avoid poverty and achieve positive mental health.

References

Adegboye, A. A., Linne, Y., & Lourenco, P. (2007). Diet or exercise, or both, for weight reduction in women after childbirth. *Cochrane Database of Systematic Reviews, 3,* 3.

Alang, S. M. & Fomotar, M. (2015). Postpartum depression in an online community of lesbian mothers: Implications for clinical practice. *Journal of Gay & Lesbian Mental Health, 19*(1), 21–39.

Asai, Y., Kambayashi, R., & Yamaguchi, S. (2015). Childcare availability, household structure, and maternal employment. *Journal of the Japanese and International Economies, 38,* 172–192.

Avery, A., Hillier, S., Pallister, C., Barber, J., & Lavin, J. (2016). Factors influencing engagement in post-natal weight management and weight and wellbeing outcomes. *British Journal of Midwifery, 24*(11), 806–812.

Bai, D. L., Fong, D. Y. T., & Tarrant, M. (2015). Factors associated with breastfeeding duration and exclusivity in mothers returning to paid employment postpartum. *Maternal and Child Health Journal, 19* (5), 990–999.

Berggren, E. K., Groh-Wargo, S., Presley, L., Hauguel-de Mouzon, S., & Catalano, P. M. (2016). Maternal fat, but not lean, mass is increased among overweight/obese women with excess gestational weight gain. *American Journal of Obstetrics and Gynecology, 214*(6), 745.e1–745.e5.

Bergink, V., Rasgon, N., & Wisner, K. L. (2016). Postpartum psychosis: Madness, mania, and melancholia in motherhood. *American Journal of Psychiatry, 173*(12), 1179–1188.

Bien, A., Rzonca, E., Iwanowicz-Palus, G., Lecyk, U., & Bojar, I. (2017). The quality of life and satisfaction with life of women who are childless by choice. *Annals of Agricultural and Environmental Medicine, 24*(2), 250–253.

Blank, R. M. (2018). *It takes a nation: A new agenda for fighting poverty,* updated edition. Princeton, NJ: Princeton University Press.

Bleichmar, E. D. (2018). The place of motherhood in primary femininity. In M. Alizade (Ed.), *Motherhood in the twenty-first century* (pp. 73–83). Abingdon, UK: Routledge.

Bradley, H. (2016). *Gender and work*. London, UK: Sage.

Çinar, İ. Ö. & Öztürk, A. (2014). The effect of planned baby care education given to primiparous mothers on maternal attachment and self-confidence levels. *Health Care for Women International, 35*(3), 320–333.

Clout, D. & Brown, R. (2016). Marital relationship and attachment predictors of postpartum stress, anxiety, and depression symptoms. *Journal of Social and Clinical Psychology, 35*(4), 322–341.

Coates, R., Ayers, S., & de Visser, R. (2014). Women's experiences of postnatal distress: A qualitative study. *BMC Pregnancy and Childbirth, 14*(1), 1–14.

Collins, P. H. (2016). Shifting the center: Race, class, and feminist theorizing about motherhood. In E. N. Glen, G. Chang, & L. R. Forcey (Eds), *Mothering* (pp. 45–65). Abingdon, UK: Routledge.

de Castro, F., Place, J. M. S., Billings, D. L., Rivera, L., & Frongillo, E. A. (2015). Risk profiles associated with postnatal depressive symptoms among women in a public sector hospital in Mexico: The role of sociodemographic and psychosocial factors. *Archives of Women's Mental Health, 18*(3), 463–471.

Dennis, C., Falah-Hassani, K., Brown, H., & Vigod, S. (2016). Identifying women at risk for postpartum anxiety: A prospective population-based study. *Acta Psychiatrica Scandinavica, 134*(6), 485–493.

Epifanio, M. S., Genna, V., De Luca, C., Roccella, M., & La Grutta, S. (2015). Paternal and maternal transition to parenthood: The risk of postpartum depression and parenting stress. *Pediatric Reports, 7*(2), 5872.

Everson, C. L. & Ostrach, B. (2017). Pathologized pregnancies and deleterious health outcomes. In B. Ostrach, S. Lerman Ginzburg, & M. Singer (Eds), *Stigma syndemics: New directions in biosocial health* (pp. 61–94). Minneapolis, MN: Lexington Books.

Fieril, D. P., Olsén, P. F., Glantz, D., & Premberg, Å. (2017). Experiences of a lifestyle intervention in obese pregnant women: A qualitative study. *Midwifery, 44*, 1–6.

Fleming, A. S., Ruble, D. N., Flett, G. L., & Shaul, D. L. (1988). Postpartum adjustment in first-time mothers: Relations between mood, maternal attitudes, and mother–infant interactions. *Developmental Psychology, 24*(1), 71–81.

Forster, D. A., McLachlan, H. L., Davey, M., Biro, M. A., Farrell, T., Gold, L., Flood, M., Shafiei, T., & Waldenström, U. (2016). Continuity of care by a primary midwife (caseload midwifery) increases women's satisfaction with antenatal, intrapartum and postpartum care: Results from the COSMOS randomised controlled trial. *BMC Pregnancy and Childbirth, 16*(1), 1–13.

Fox, B. & Neiterman, E. (2015). Embodied motherhood: Women's feelings about their postpartum bodies. *Gender & Society, 29*(5), 670–693.

Fox, R., Nicolson, P., & Heffernan, K. (2009). Pregnancy police? Maternal bodies, surveillance and food. In P. Jackson (Ed.), *Changing families, changing food* (pp. 57–74). New York, NY: Springer.

Gallegos, D., Vicca, N., & Streiner, S. (2015). Breastfeeding beliefs and practices of African women living in Brisbane and Perth, Australia. *Maternal & Child Nutrition, 11*(4), 727–736.

Glenn, E. N. (2016). Social constructions of mothering: A thematic overview. In E. N. Glen, G. Chang, & L. R. Forcey (Eds), *Mothering* (pp. 1–29). Abingdon, UK: Routledge.

Glosswitch (2018, February 21). As we continue to blame single mothers for society's woes, it's no surprise their children are living in poverty. *The Independent*. Retrieved from www.independent.co.uk/voices/single-mothers-parents-research-gingerbread-child-poverty-scapegoating-tories-government-a8221211.html.

Golombok, S., Zadeh, S., Imrie, S., Smith, V., & Freeman, T. (2016). Single mothers by choice: Mother–child relationships and children's psychological adjustment. *Journal of Family Psychology, 30*(4), 409–418.

Haskins, N. H., Ziomek-Daigle, J., Sewell, C., Crumb, L., Appling, B., & Trepal, H. (2016). The intersectionality of African American mothers in counselor education: A phenomenological examination. *Counselor Education and Supervision, 55*(1), 60–75.

Hayman, B. & Wilkes, L. (2017). De novo families: Lesbian motherhood. *Journal of Homosexuality, 64*(5), 577–591.

Heffernan, K., Nicolson, P., & Fox, R. (2011). The next generation of pregnant women: More freedom in the public sphere or just an illusion? *Journal of Gender Studies, 20*, 321–332.

Henderson, S. (2018). *The blurring effect: An exploration of maternal instinct and ambivalence*. (Doctoral Dissertation). Canterbury, UK: University of Kent.

Hollander, M., de Miranda, E., van Dillen, J., de Graaf, I., Vandenbussche, F., & Holten, L. (2017). Women's motivations for choosing a high-risk birth setting against medical advice in the Netherlands: A qualitative analysis. *BMC Pregnancy and Childbirth, 17*(1), 423.

Hoseini, S. S., Panaghi, L., Habibi, M., Davoodi, J., & Monajemi, M. B. (2015). The relation between social support and marital satisfaction & couples' depression after the birth of the first child. *The International Journal of Indian Psychology, 3*(1), 5–14.

Jacob, J. A. (2015). Study reveals gaps in advice to new mothers on infant care. *JAMA: The Journal of the American Medical Association, 314*(12), 1216–1216.

Javadifar, N., Majlesi, F., Nikbakht, A., Nedjat, S., & Montazeri, A. (2016). Journey to motherhood in the first year after child birth. *Journal of Family & Reproductive Health, 10*(3), 146–153.

Jones, L., Othman, M., Dowswell, T., Alfirevic, Z., Gates, S., Newburn, M., Jordan, S., Lavender, T., & Neilson, J. P. (2012). Pain management for women in labour: An overview of systematic reviews. *Cochrane Pregnancy and Childbirth Group*, (3), CD009234.

Junge, C., von Soest, T., Weidner, K., Seidler, A., Eberhard-Gran, M., & Garthus-Niegel, S. (2018). Labor pain in women with and without severe fear of childbirth: A population-based, longitudinal study. *Birth, 45*, 469–477.

Kendall-Tackett, K. A. (2016). *Depression in new mothers: Causes, consequences and treatment alternatives.* Abingdon, UK: Routledge.

Lafrance, M. N. & Stoppard, J. M. (2006). Constructing a non-depressed self: Women's accounts of recovery from depression. *Feminism & Psychology, 16*, 307–325.

Lawler, D., Begley, C., & Lalor, J. (2015). (Re)constructing myself: The process of transition to motherhood for women with a disability. *Journal of Advanced Nursing, 71*(7), 1672–1683.

Locke, A. (2016). Masculinity, subjectivities, and caregiving in the British press: The case of the stay-at-home father. In E. Podnieks (Ed.), *Pops in pop culture* (pp. 195–212). New York, NY: Springer.

Lopez, E. T. (2015). *The lived experience of the transition to motherhood for Mexican American adolescent girls* (Doctoral Dissertation in Nursing). Azusa, CA: Azusa Pacific University.

Lucas, C., Charlton, K. E., & Yeatman, H. (2014). Nutrition advice during pregnancy: Do women receive it and can health professionals provide it? *Maternal and Child Health Journal, 18*(10), 2465–2478.

Luce, A., Cash, M., Hundley, V., Cheyne, H., Van Teijlingen, E., & Angell, C. (2016). "Is it realistic?" the portrayal of pregnancy and childbirth in the media. *BMC Pregnancy and Childbirth, 16*(1), 40. Retrieved from https://bmcpregnancychildbirth.biomedcentral.com/articles/10.1186/s12884-016-0827-x.

Luoma, I., Korhonen, M., Salmelin, R., & Tamminen, T. (2015). Mothers' feelings of loneliness: Prevalence, risk factors and longitudinal associations with depressive symptoms and child adjustment. *European Psychiatry, 30*, 726.

Malatzky, C. A. R. (2017). Australian women's complex engagement with the yummy mummy discourse and the bodily ideals of good motherhood. *Women's Studies International Forum, 62*, 25–33.

McKenzie-Mohr, S. & Lafrance, M. N. (2014). *Women voicing resistance: Discursive and narrative explorations.* Abingdon, UK: Routledge.

McKinley, N. M. (2017). Ideal weight/ideal women: Society constructs the female. In J. Sobal (Ed.), *Weighty issues* (pp. 97–115). Abingdon, UK: Routledge.

Morison, T., Macleod, C., Lynch, I., Mijas, M., & Shivakumar, S. T. (2016). Stigma resistance in online childfree communities: The limitations of choice rhetoric. *Psychology of Women Quarterly, 40*(2), 184–198.

Moule, P., Irvine, R., Subhani, S., Khatri, S., & Cleugh, F. (2014). How good are we at providing breastfeeding advice? *Archives of Disease in Childhood, 99*(Suppl 1), A122–A122.

Mumford, E. A., Liu, W., & Joseph, H. (2018). Postpartum domestic violence in homes with young children: The role of maternal and paternal drinking. *Violence Against Women, 24*(2), 144–162.

Murphy, H. & Strong, J. (2018). Just another ordinary bad birth? A narrative analysis of first-time mothers' traumatic birth experiences. *Health Care for Women International, 39*(6), 619–643.

Nasreen, H. E., Edhborg, M., Petzold, M., Forsell, Y., & Kabir, Z. N. (2015). Incidence and risk factor of postpartum depressive symptoms in women: A population based prospective cohort study in a rural district in Bangladesh. *Journal of Depression and Anxiety, 4*(2), 180.

Neiterman, E. & Fox, B. (2017). Controlling the unruly maternal body: Losing and gaining control over the body during pregnancy and the postpartum period. *Social Science & Medicine, 174*, 142–148.

Nicolson, P. (2003). *Having it all? Choices for today's superwoman.* Chichester, UK: Wiley.

Nicolson, P., Fox, R., & Heffernan, K. (2010). Constructions of pregnant and postnatal embodiment across three generations: Mothers', daughters' and others' experiences of the transition to motherhood. *Journal of Health Psychology, 15*, 575–585.

Noriega, C., López, J., Domínguez, R., & Velasco, C. (2017). Perceptions of grandparents who provide auxiliary care: Value transmission and childrearing practices. *Child & Family Social Work, 22*(3), 1227–1236.

O'Campo, P., Schetter, C. D., Guardino, C. M., Vance, M. R., Hobel, C. J., Ramey, S. L., & Shalowitz, M. U. (2016). Explaining racial and ethnic inequalities in postpartum allostatic load: Results from a multisite study of low to middle income women. *SSM-Population Health, 2*, 850–858.

Oakley, A. (2016). The sociology of childbirth: An autobiographical journey through four decades of research. *Sociology of Health & Illness, 38*(5), 689–705.

Office for National Statistics (2017). *More mothers with young children working full-time.* Newport, UK: Author. Retrieved from www.ons.gov.uk/employmentandlabourmarket/peopleinwork/employmen tandemployeetypes/articles/moremotherswithyoungchildrenworkingfulltime/2017-09-26.

Olde, E., van der Hart, O., Kleber, R., & Van Son, M. (2006). Posttraumatic stress following childbirth: A review. *Clinical Psychology Review, 26*(1), 1–16.

Puryear, L. J. (2014). Postpartum adjustment: What is normal and what is not. In D. L. Barnes (Ed.), *Women's reproductive mental health across the lifespan* (pp. 109–122). New York, NY: Springer.

Rai, G. (2017). *The social context of birth.* Abingdon, UK: Routledge.

Rallis, S., Skouteris, H., McCabe, M., & Milgrom, J. (2014). The transition to motherhood: Towards a broader understanding of perinatal distress. *Women and Birth, 27*(1), 68–71.

Reck, C., Noe, D., Gerstenlauer, J., & Stehle, E. (2012). Effects of postpartum anxiety disorders and depression on maternal self-confidence. *Infant Behavior Development, 35*(2), 264–272.

Reed, R., Sharman, R., & Inglis, C. (2017). Women's descriptions of childbirth trauma relating to care provider actions and interactions. *BMC Pregnancy and Childbirth, 17*(1), 1–10.

Robertson, E., Grace, S., Wallington, T., & Stewart, D. E. (2004). Antenatal risk factors for postpartum depression: A synthesis of recent literature. *General Hospital Psychiatry, 26*(4), 289–295.

Robinson, S. R. & Rogers, K. (2018). "I keep it to myself": A qualitative meta-interpretive synthesis of experiences of postpartum depression among marginalised women. *Health & Social Care in the Community, 27*(3), e23–e36.

Rosal, M. C., Haughton, C. F., Estabrook, B. B., Wang, M. L., Chiriboga, G., Nguyen, O. H. T., Person, S. D., & Lemon, S. C. (2016). Fresh start, a postpartum weight loss intervention for diverse low-income women: Design and methods for a randomized clinical trial. *BMC Public Health, 16*(1), 953.

Saxbe, D. E. (2017). Birth of a new perspective? A call for biopsychosocial research on childbirth. *Current Directions in Psychological Science, 26*(1), 81–86.

Sayil, M., Güre, A., & Uçanok, Z. (2007). First time mothers' anxiety and depressive symptoms across the transition to motherhood: Associations with maternal and environmental characteristics. *Women & Health, 44*(3), 61–77.

Seymour-Smith, M., Cruwys, T., Haslam, S. A., & Brodribb, W. (2017). Loss of group memberships predicts depression in postpartum mothers. *Social Psychiatry and Psychiatric Epidemiology, 52*(2), 201–210.

Shabot, S. C. & Korem, K. (2018). Domesticating bodies: The role of shame in obstetric violence. *Hypatia, 33*(3), 384–401.

Shin, H. & White-Traut, R. (2007). The conceptual structure of transition to motherhood in the neonatal intensive care unit. *Journal of Advanced Nursing, 58*(1), 90–98.

Simpson, M. & Catling, C. (2016). Understanding psychological traumatic birth experiences: A literature review. *Women and Birth, 29*(3), 203–207.

Sivertsen, B., Petrie, K. J., Skogen, J. C., Hysing, M., & Eberhard-Gran, M. (2017). Insomnia before and after childbirth: The risk of developing postpartum pain—A longitudinal population-based study. *European Journal of Obstetrics & Gynecology and Reproductive Biology, 210*, 348–354.

Sullivan, C. (2015). 'Bad mum guilt': The representation of 'work-life balance' in UK women's magazines. *Community, Work & Family, 18*(3), 284–298.

Taborelli, E., Easter, A., Keefe, R., Schmidt, U., Treasure, J., & Micali, N. (2016). Transition to motherhood in women with eating disorders: A qualitative study. *Psychology and Psychotherapy: Theory, Research and Practice, 89*(3), 308–323.

Thomas, G. M. & Lupton, D. (2015). Playing pregnancy: The ludification and gamification of expectant motherhood in smartphone apps. *M/C Journal, 18*(5). Retrieved from http://journal.media-culture.org.au/index.php/mcjournal/article/view/1012.

Tiggemann, M. (2004). Body image across the adult life span: Stability and change. *Body Image, 1*(1), 29–41.

Ussher, J. M. (1989). *The psychology of the female body.* Abingdon, UK: Routledge.

Ussher, J. M. (2006). *Managing the monstrous feminine: Regulating the reproductive body.* Abingdon, UK: Routledge.

van der Pligt, P., Olander, E. K., Ball, K., Crawford, D., Hesketh, K. D., Teychenne, M., & Campbell, K. (2016). Maternal dietary intake and physical activity habits during the postpartum period: Associations with clinician advice in a sample of Australian first time mothers. *BMC Pregnancy and Childbirth, 16*(1), 27. Retrieved from https://bmcpregnancychildbirth.biomedcentral.com/articles/10.1186/s12884-016-0812-4.

Van Teijlingen, E. (2017). The medical and social model of childbirth. *Kontakt, 19*(2), 81–82.

Van Wagenen, S. A., Magnusson, B. M., & Neiger, B. L. (2015). Attitudes toward breastfeeding among an internet panel of US males aged 21–44. *Maternal and Child Health Journal, 19*(9), 2020–2028.

Vincze, L., Rollo, M., Hutchesson, M., Callister, R., & Collins, C. (2018). VITAL change for mums: A feasibility study investigating tailored nutrition and exercise care delivered by video-consultations for women 3–12 months postpartum. *Journal of Human Nutrition and Dietetics, 31*(3), 337–348.

Ward, K. & Wolf-Wendel, L. (2016). Academic motherhood: Mid-career perspectives and the ideal worker norm. *New Directions for Higher Education, 176*(Winter), 11–23.

Weiss, M. J. (2002). Hardiness and social support as predictors of stress in mothers of typical children, children with autism, and children with mental retardation. *Autism, 6*(1), 115–130.

Winson, N. (2017). Transition to motherhood. In G. Rai (Ed.), *The social context of birth* (pp. 159–174). Abingdon, UK: Routledge.

Wittkowski, A., Patel, S., & Fox, J. R. (2017). The experience of postnatal depression in immigrant mothers living in Western countries: A meta-synthesis. *Clinical Psychology & Psychotherapy, 24*(2), 411–427.

Yakusheva, O., Kapinos, K., & Weiss, M. (2017). Maternal weight after childbirth versus aging-related weight changes. *Women's Health Issues, 27*(2), 174–180.

24

UNDERSTANDING PERINATAL MENTAL HEALTH PROBLEMS

Prevalence, risk factors, approaches to prevention, early identification and treatment

Virginia Schmied

It took me a long time to seek support. Too long. I knew something wasn't right but had so many fears about seeking help. I thought my son would be taken away from me, that maybe I was just going crazy or that seeking help would mean I could no longer work as a counsellor again myself. In hindsight it started for me during pregnancy. Our pregnancy was not planned and I was in my early 20s living a carefree life. I can recall moments where I would just leave the house, not tell my partner where I was going and just drive. I did not know where I was driving to, I just drove. On these drives I would have thoughts of how I could take my own life after the baby was born (Hannah's story).

(PANDA, 2019)

Becoming a mother is life changing. Pregnancy and the first year after birth (referred to here as the perinatal period) can be times of excitement and joy for women, their partners, and their families, but many women also encounter unexpected challenges, and, for some, this experience can be very distressing. This is particularly so for women with pre-existing physical or mental health conditions, who enter motherhood with additional needs. The mental health care of women in the perinatal period is a priority internationally (Austin, Highet, & the Expert Working Group, 2017; NICE, 2014). Perinatal mental health problems affect up to 20% of women each year (Schmied et al., 2013), for example, over 800,000 women in the US, over 140,000 women in England and Wales, and over 60,000 women in Australia (Khan, 2015) per year. Perinatal mental health problems impact women themselves, their families and communities, and also the mental, physical, emotional, and psychosocial development of their infants (Glover, O'Donnell, O'Connor, & Fisher, 2018).

In this chapter I examine depression and anxiety experienced by women in the perinatal period. Issues addressed include the symptoms of perinatal depression and anxiety and the prevalence, risk factors, and approaches to early identification, treatment, and prevention of perinatal depression and anxiety in Australia and internationally. The importance of an integrated service system is discussed.

A brief history of perinatal mental illness

In 700 BC Hippocrates wrote about women suffering from emotional difficulties during the postpartum period (O'Hara & Wisner, 2014), and from that point on there have been regular reports of women's postpartum "madness" (Brockington & Kumar, 1982; Marland, 2004). In 1801, Thomas Denman attributed the cause of mental illness to a disturbance beginning in the uterus or the breast and spreading to the brain; he prescribed rest and seclusion, and treatment often required admission of women into a mental asylum (Marland, 2012). Advocates for moral therapy believed that a healthy body in a pleasing environment could heal itself of insanity with the aid of pleasant housing, useful labour, religious instruction, a good diet, plenty of rest, and pleasant activities (Garton, 2009; Mitchinson, 1989).

It was not until the 1850s that the medical profession first recognised postnatal depression (PND) as a disorder. Louis-Victor Marcé (1858) compiled an extensive monograph that surveyed knowledge of psychiatric disorders of women during pregnancy and after childbirth (as cited in Trede, Baldessarini, Viguera, & Bottero, 2009). In it Marcé provided extensive clinical descriptions of syndromes, including 79 case examples, and summarised the theories and treatments of the era (Trede, Baldessarini, Viguera, & Bottero, 2009). Recognising the symptoms of depression, Queen Victoria wrote in a letter to one of her daughters who had just given birth:

> Occasional lowness and tendency to cry you must expect. You of all people will
> be included to this … for it is what every lady suffers with more or less and what
> I during my first two confinements suffered dreadfully with.
>
> *(Break the Silence on Postnatal Illness, n.d.)*

However, women were reluctant to divulge their symptoms, and those who did were often diagnosed as "neurotic". Women who sought help for their symptoms risked being subjected to a variety of harmful and marginalising treatments. During the 1950s electroshock therapy was often the recommended treatment for a "neurotic" woman, or they were prescribed Valium (Jefferies, Duff, & Nicholls, 2018; Ussher, 2011). Women continued to hide their symptoms, and their silence was most likely out of shame that others would think they were neurotic or even insane (Jefferies et al., 2018). In more recent years, several celebrities have discussed their battles with perinatal depression. Through books, blogs, and publicly speaking about their experience, these celebrities have helped to establish that postpartum depression is no longer a "dirty little secret" of which women should be ashamed (Jefferies, Horsfall, & Schmied, 2017).

Perinatal mental illness

Perinatal mental illness refers to psychiatric disorders that are prevalent during pregnancy and for as long as one year after birth. Perinatal disorders that range from mild depression and anxiety to mania or psychosis are all categorised as perinatal mental illness (O'Hara & Wisner, 2014). In addition, disorders that were present before pregnancy, or recurred along with disorders that emerged during pregnancy or in the postpartum period, are also considered perinatal mental illnesses (O'Hara & Wisner, 2014). The focus of this chapter is on depression and anxiety as the two most common mood disorders associated with birth.

Perinatal depression

Perinatal depression disrupts social and physical functioning, and is a precipitating factor for suicide (Humphrey, 2015; Thornton, Schmied, Dennis, Barnett, & Dahlen, 2013). Depression either antenatally or postnatally is often identified symptomatically through a screening measure such as the Edinburgh Postnatal Depression Scale (EPDS) (Cox, Murray, & Chapman, 1993). A score of 13 or greater on the EPDS is generally used for diagnosis, although in some services women with a score of ≥10 will be referred for further evaluation, treatment, or additional support (O'Hara & Wisner, 2014). Following referral, more rigorous assessment occurs in the context of a clinical interview, such as the Structured Clinical Interview (O'Hara & Wisner, 2014). Common symptoms include constant tiredness and lack of energy; having little or no interest in things that bring joy; sleeping too much or not sleeping well at all; losing interest in sex or intimacy; withdrawing from friends and family; feelings of guilt, particularly as a mother; confusion and finding it difficult to focus, concentrate, or remember; feeling constantly sad, low, or crying for no obvious reason; and suicidal ideation (Austin et al., 2017; Dennis, 2014). These symptoms of depression in the perinatal period are the same as those at other times and range from mild to severe (Department of Health, 2018).

Perinatal anxiety disorders

Anxiety during pregnancy or following birth can be a normal but transient reaction to a major life transition. A wide range of anxiety disorders are prevalent in the perinatal period. These include the generalised anxiety, obsessive–compulsive, panic, and social anxiety disorders. In many cases, the severity and effect of anxiety symptoms (e.g., worry, avoidance, obsessions) do not rise to the level of an anxiety disorder diagnosis; nevertheless, they cause at least mild-to-moderate levels of distress and impairment (Dennis, Brown, Falah-Hassani, Marini, & Vigod, 2017). Anxiety is detected with self-report measures such as the Hospital Anxiety and Depression Scale (Zigmond & Snaith, 1983) or the Beck Anxiety Inventory (Steer & Beck, 1997).

Significant anxiety can have debilitating symptoms, including irritability, restlessness, tense muscles, tight chest, and heart palpitations. Women may express these symptoms as feelings of inner turmoil, anger, or agitation; being "wound up" or "not sleeping"; worrying about their baby's development, safety, and well-being; believing something catastrophic will happen; or, in some instances, experiencing panic attacks (Highett, Stevenson, Purtell, & Coo, 2014).

Prevalence of perinatal depression and anxiety

Prevalence rates of perinatal depression reported in low- and middle-income countries (LMIC) are higher than those in high-income countries (HIC) (Woody, Ferrari, Siskind, Whiteford, & Harris, 2017). Globally, the prevalence of antenatal depression is estimated to be between 7% and 20% in HIC, whereas rates of 20% or more have been reported in LMIC (Biaggi, Conroy, Pawlby, & Pariante, 2016; Woody et al., 2017). Biaggi and colleagues (2016) reported that the prevalence of depression is 7.4% during the first trimester of pregnancy, and increases to 12.8% during the second, and 12% during the third trimester.

Prevalence rates of postnatal depression (PND) vary widely, with reports from 5% to 74% in HIC and from 2% to 82% in LMIC (based on self-report) (Norhayati, Hazlina, Asrenee, & Wan Emilin, 2015). For example, Fisher et al. (2012) conducted a systematic review and meta-analysis to establish the mean prevalence of PND in LMIC. They reported the weighted mean prevalence of PND to be 19.8%. When determined by clinical interview, prevalence of PND remains variable but lower, from 0.1% in Finland to 26.3% in India (Norhayati et al., 2015). Prevalence does vary by group; notably in most studies in HIC, women who are migrants have higher rates of PND than non-migrant women. A recent systematic review showed that 20% of migrant women experience PND symptoms in the first year following birth, and this is almost twice as likely as PND in non-migrant women (Falah-Hassani, Shiri, & Dennis, 2016). More recent work in Canada shows that asylum-seeking women had the highest rate of postnatal depression (14.3%), followed by refugee women (11.5%), and non-immigrant women (5.1%) (Dennis, Merry, & Gagnon, 2017).

Rates of perinatal anxiety also vary. Dennis and colleagues (Dennis, Falah-Hassani, & Shiri, 2017) conducted a review of the prevalence of maternal anxiety in the antenatal and postnatal periods. The prevalence of self-reported anxiety symptoms was 18.2% in the first trimester, 19.1% in the second trimester, and 24.6% in the third trimester. The overall prevalence for a clinical diagnosis of any anxiety disorder was 15.2%. The postnatal prevalence of anxiety symptoms overall at 1–24 weeks was 15.0%. The prevalence for any anxiety disorder over the same period was 9.9%. Again rates were higher in LMIC.

Risk and protective factors for perinatal depression and anxiety

Many factors contribute to depression and anxiety during pregnancy and following birth, including stress, hormonal changes, and the decision made by some women or their health professionals to discontinue antidepressant maintenance medications; no single causative factor for perinatal mood disorders has been identified (O'Hara & Wisner, 2014). Around 40% of women who experience symptoms of depression during pregnancy will go on to experience PND if they do not receive treatment (Norhayati et al., 2015). In general, less has been said about factors that protect women from developing perinatal mental health problems. The most commonly reported protective factor is the importance of social support. Social support across all forms (emotional, tangible, affectionate, positive social interaction, and paternal support) has been identified as critical to women's mental well-being and is considered an important protective factor for perinatal depression (Pao, Guintivano, Santos, & Meltzer-Brody, 2019). Other protective demographic factors include having more education; being of the ethnic majority, and having a kind and trustworthy intimate partner (Fisher et al., 2012).

Studies primarily conducted in HIC consistently confirm the following as major risk factors for perinatal mood disorders: previous mental health problems (O'Hara & Wisner, 2014), substance misuse (Devries et al., 2014), and psychosocial variables such as stressful life events, relationship conflict, intimate partner violence, and lack of social support (Woolhouse, Gartland, Hegarty, Donath, & Brown, 2012). Associated risk factors include socio-demographic characteristics such as young age, lower education, unemployment, being a migrant or refugee (Biaggi et al., 2016; O'Hara & Wisner, 2014), idealistic expectations of motherhood, and unsupportive partner and family (Schmied et al., 2013). Women who report unintended pregnancy, or present/past pregnancy complications, or pregnancy loss (Biaggi et al., 2016; O'Hara & Wisner, 2014) are also more likely to experience mood disorders in the perinatal period (see Figure 24.1). Similar risk factors are reported in studies focussed on LMIC (Fisher et al., 2012; James-Hawkins et al., 2019). In addition, PND is also associated in LMIC with having hostile in-laws and, in some settings, giving birth to a daughter (Fisher et al., 2012).

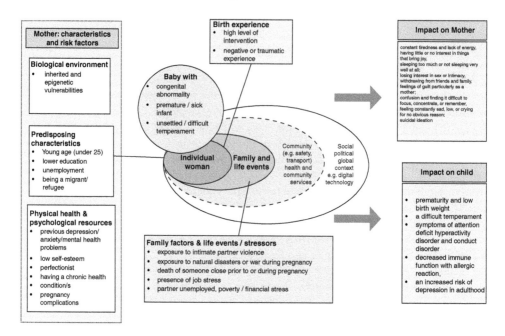

Figure 24.1 Risk factors for perinatal mental health problems (adapted from Schmied et al., 2018).

Commentators have argued that the higher rate of perinatal mental health problems in LMIC is primarily due to the influence of human and economic resources and women's empowerment (James-Hawkins et al., 2019). Empowerment refers to women's access to resources such as financial or economic, education or skills, and social resources such as social support from family or others, and it is crucial to mental health in the perinatal period (James-Hawkins et al., 2019). Recent systematic reviews of risk and protective factors associated with perinatal depression in LMIC underscore the role of limited access to resources, poverty, poor education, and lack of family support (Fisher et al., 2012; James-Hawkins et al., 2019; Schmied, Black, Naidoo, Dahlen, & Liamputtong, 2017). In a systematic review and meta-analysis of PND in the Arab world, James-Hawkins and colleagues (2019) reported that women's empowerment was a critical component of mental health; they reported a negative association between education and depression and a positive association between financial stress and depression among women.

As noted, rates of PND are higher amongst women who are migrants but particularly those who are refugees or asylum seekers. Risk factors for PND amongst immigrant women include a shorter length of residence in the receiving country, lower levels of social support, poorer marital adjustment, and perceived insufficient household income (Falah-Hassani et al., 2016). In a meta-ethnographic study of immigrant women's meanings and experiences of PND (Schmied et al., 2017), four metaphors were identified: "I am alone, worried and angry – this is not me!"; "Making sense of my feelings"; "Dealing with my feelings"; and "What I need to change the way I feel!" Women often attributed "feeling down" to their position as a migrant and a woman living in poor socio-economic circumstances, and they were exhausted keeping up with expected commitments. Many women were resourceful and drew on their personal strengths and family/community resources. All the studies showed that women experienced difficulties in accessing appropriate services (Schmied et al., 2017). This is supported by a recent US-based study of minority women in which differences in social support among various racial and ethnic groups did not appear to explain the increased prevalence of PND. The authors argued that a better explanation for these discrepancies in PND between minority and non-minority groups is the role of immigration and low socioeconomic status (Pao et al., 2019).

Research in the field of psycho-neuro-immunology has revealed that depression is associated with inflammation manifested by increased levels of pro-inflammatory cytokines with physical and psychological stressors increasing inflammation (Kendall-Tackett, 2007). Moreover, inflammation explains why psychosocial, behavioural, and physical risk factors increase the risk of depression. This is true for depression in general and for postpartum depression in particular. Pregnant and postnatal women are especially vulnerable to these effects because their levels of pro-inflammatory cytokines significantly increase during the last trimester of pregnancy – a time when they are also at higher risk for depression (Kendall-Tackett, 2007). Further, common experiences of new motherhood, such as sleep disturbance, postpartum pain, and past or current psychological trauma, are stressors that cause proinflammatory cytokine levels to rise. Breastfeeding has a protective effect on maternal mental health because it attenuates stress and modulates the inflammatory response. However, breastfeeding difficulties, such as nipple pain, can increase the risk of depression (Kendall-Tackett, 2007).

It is very important to understand the complexity of both risk and protective factors. Psychiatric care that focusses solely on symptom reduction, adherence to medication, and attending consultations might not consider the social context that led women to feel humiliated, entrapped, isolated, and thus vulnerable to poor mental health including suicide (Fisher, Chatham, Haseler, Beth, & Thompson, 2012). More consideration needs to be given to the role that social and cultural factors, currently considered "distal" to the individual woman (e.g., communities, health services, national policy context, social media), play in perinatal mental health. In particular, what is the impact of the ideology of the "good mother" (Schmied, Kearney, & The Maternal Anxiety White Paper Group, 2018; see Figure 24.1)? Perinatal depression and anxiety are a social and feminist concern related to the structural issues of access to resources as described above, as well as to the discursive construction of the "good mother" (Mauthner, 2018; Vaswani, Karter, Cosgrove, Peters, & Brodt, 2018). The "good mother" is all-giving, always available, and can knowledgeably meet her child's needs (Pedersen, 2012). Although notions of the "good mother" vary across socio-economic and cultural groups, mothers are acutely aware of being judged by others and are the subject of surveillance by other mothers, medical professionals, and family members (Goodwin & Huppatz, 2010; Liamputtong, 2006). Some women experience motherhood as overwhelming and characterised by guilt, shame, loss, and exhaustion (Armstrong, 2006; Liamputtong, 2006; Schmied et al., 2017; see Figure 24.1). The "good mother" imperative may be particularly felt by mothers living in poverty with little support, mothers from refugee and migrant backgrounds (Liamputtong, 2006; Schmied et al., 2017), those who have other health needs (Parton, Ussher, Natoli, & Perz, 2018), and those with babies who are unwell (Fenwick, Barclay, & Schmied, 2008).

The impact of perinatal depression and anxiety on the fetus and child

Maternal social and emotional distress in the perinatal period can have negative consequences for the child in utero, during infancy, and beyond (Glover et al., 2018). Depression and anxiety in pregnancy are both associated with prematurity and low birth weight (Eastwood, Jalaludin, Kemp, Phung, & Barnett, 2012), as well as deficits in neurological development that result in physical, psychological, language-development, emotional, and behavioural problems (see Figure 24.1). Following birth, depression and anxiety can disrupt a woman's capacity to respond to her infant in an empathic way (Myors, Cleary, Johnson, & Schmied, 2018).

Bowlby (1969) articulated the concept of infant attachment and its importance for child development. Ainsworth and her colleagues identified the importance of maternal sensitivity and proposed that the relationship infants have with their primary caregiver/s has a profound impact throughout life (Ainsworth, Blehar, Waters, & Wall, 1978). Maternal sensitivity is defined as the ability to be aware of and interpret an infant's behavioural cues and respond to the infant in a timely and appropriate manner (Ainsworth et al., 1978). A meta-analysis of research on the effects of PND in mothers during the first three months of the infant's life showed that depressed mothers were less likely to be engaged with their infant, they exhibited less warmth, and played with their infants less than mothers who did not experience PND (Lovejoy, Graczyk, O'Hare, & Neuman, 2000). An infant's risk increases if both parents experience mental health problems that affect their sensitivity to their infant.

Maternal sensitivity to infant cues and behaviours plays a strong role in secure attachment. Research consistently shows that children of depressed mothers have less secure attachments to their mothers, are more fussy, receive lower scores on measures of intellectual and motor development, have more difficult temperaments and react more negatively to stress, show delayed development of self-regulatory strategies, and exhibit poorer academic performance, fewer social competencies, lower levels of self-esteem, and higher levels of behavioural problems – both internalising and externalising problems – than children of non-depressed mothers (Goodman et al., 2011).

Maternal perinatal depression is often linked to unresolved childhood trauma and loss experienced by the mother (Guedeney, Guedeney, Wendland, & Burtchen, 2014). Many women who perceived that they did not receive appropriate love and care as a child have difficulty in providing the love and care their own infant needs, due to few if any positive personal experiences of motherhood (Myors et al., 2018). Thus, a woman's insecure attachment to her own mother can contribute to an insecure attachment with her own infant.

Epigenetics is an emerging field which refers to environmental influences that alter an individual's phenotype (i.e., the expressed characteristics of an individual's genetic code). It is now understood that early caregiving environments have a direct impact on phenotype with resultant positive or negative consequences (Glover et al., 2018). Thus, maternal stress, depression, and anxiety in pregnancy may negatively influence the neurodevelopmental outcomes for the child (O'Hara & Wisner, 2014).

Identifying and assessing women with mental health problems

National and international guidelines indicate that all health care professionals who come into contact with women in the perinatal period should address both mental and physical health (Austin, Colton, Priest, Reilly, & Hadzi-Pavlovic, 2013; NICE, 2014). Australia has led the world in initiating routine antenatal screening for depression. New South Wales (NSW) was the first State to trial routine screening of women using the EPDS for current or potential perinatal mental health problems, and to undertake this in conjunction with a comprehensive psychosocial assessment. This assessment and screening is mandated through maternity and child and family health services (NSW Department of Health, 2009) and is now recommended practice across Australia (Austin et al., 2017), although screening remains limited in the private hospital sector (Kohlhoff, Hickinbotham, Knox, Roach, & Barnett, 2016). International guidelines also increasingly recommend screening for perinatal mood disorders, and the practice is now common in HICs (Austin, 2014; Rahman et al., 2013). Rahman and colleagues (2013) noted, however, that screening and assessment for perinatal mental health disorders is rare in LMICs. The American College of Obstetricians and Gynecologists recommends screening for depression and anxiety symptoms at least once during the perinatal period with a standardised validated tool, and the American Academy of Pediatrics recommends incorporating the EPDS into the one, two, four, and six month visits (Accortt & Wong, 2017). Guidelines from the UK National Institute of Clinical Excellence (NICE) endorse the use of screening tools such as the EPDS:

> Carry out a risk assessment in conjunction with the woman and, if she agrees, her partner, family or carer. Focus on areas that are likely to present possible risk such as self-neglect, self-harm, suicidal thoughts and intent, risks to others (including the baby), smoking, drug or alcohol misuse and domestic violence and abuse.
>
> *(NICE, 2014, p. 846)*

However, routine screening for perinatal depression as well as psychosocial assessment is controversial. Thombs and colleagues (2015) stated that, despite the widespread use of the EPDS, it has not been shown to benefit women in a well-designed and conducted randomised controlled trial, and therefore may lead to misidentification and overtreatment in some women without evidence of benefit. Vaswani and colleagues (2018) similarly critiqued the recommendations by the United States Preventive Services Task Force to screen women for depression during pregnancy and postpartum, and argued that screening is likely to result in over-diagnosis and may increase the number of women prescribed antidepressant medications with unknown safety during pregnancy. Furthermore, limitations of the EPDS have been reported, including ambiguous questions; scoring problems (despite workforce training programs); a high rate of false positives; use of incorrect cut-off scores; and multiple cut-off scores pertaining to gender, culture, timing, and diagnosis (Matthey & Agostini, 2017; Matthey, Della Vedova, & Agostini, 2017). The EPDS was developed as a screening tool, but practice decisions are often made based on an EPDS score alone. Accurate diagnosis is needed to infer the clinical meaning of an EPDS score for individual women. The EPDS and other depression screening tools are available in various languages, but they have not yet been psychometrically tested for the increasing immigrant and refugee populations now living Western countries (Stapleton, Murphy, & Kildea, 2013; Tobin, Dinapoli, & Wood-Gauthier, 2014). Use of the EPDS in culturally diverse populations raises questions regarding routine or indeed mandated perinatal depression screening initiatives.

Lobel and Ibrahim (2018) argued strongly that, to improve the psychological and emotional condition of childbearing women, we must understand and address the factors that contribute to women's emotional responses to the stress of pregnancy, childbirth and postpartum, and determine whether any of these factors are modifiable. Whilst assessment and screening processes in some situations include these social and contextual factors, this does not occur in all settings and women are not necessarily comfortable being asked these sensitive questions by their doctors (Rollans, Schmied, Kemp, & Meade, 2013).

Women's experience of screening and assessment in the perinatal period

Women in HICs report acceptability of screening for perinatal depression in primary care and maternity services (Kingston et al., 2017; Matthey, 2005; Milgrom, Ericksen, Negri, & Gemmill, 2005). However, studies that examined psychosocial assessment in addition to depression screening indicate that women can find questions about their social situation and emotional well-being to be sensitive and confronting, particularly those who are or have previously experienced difficult social and emotional events (e.g., domestic and family violence, sexual assault and abuse) (Rollans et al., 2013). This discomfort may have implications for the way women engage with the maternity services. For example, women may lose trust in service providers if they believe that the intention of the assessment was somehow hidden from them (Bayrampour et al., 2017; Rollans et al., 2013). Nurses have acknowledged that much of the work they do with mothers is hidden "behind the scales" and that the manifest work of weighing the baby is a safe and acceptable way to gain entry to the home (Shepherd, 2011). Rollans et al. (2013) suggested that the extent and nature of questions asked is not adequately explained to women prior to the visits where assessment is conducted. Specifically, women do not expect questions about domestic violence or childhood sexual abuse, with one woman comparing routine domestic violence screening to other mandatory security procedures such as a customs check at the airport. When women and men were asked about their expectations of the health service in pregnancy and after birth, women emphasised that they would want to know in advance the type of sensitive questions they would be asked, and they believed that the questions should only be asked by a trained professional with whom the woman had a relationship (Rowe, Holton, & Fisher, 2012). Men were inclined to be more suspicious of the process and said they would like to know how the information would be used.

Management or treatment of perinatal depression and anxiety

There is a diverse array of approaches to treating perinatal depression and anxiety. The approach will depend on the level of severity of symptoms a woman is experiencing. The first step in treatment always requires a conversation with the woman and her family as appropriate (NICE, 2014). These conversations should include the likely benefits of each treatment, taking into account the severity of the mental health condition; the woman's response to any previous treatment; the possibility of the sudden onset or relapse of symptoms of mental health conditions in pregnancy and the postnatal period; and the risks or harms to the woman and the fetus or baby associated with each treatment option, including risk to mental health and parenting associated with no treatment or stopping or changing a treatment (NICE, 2014).

Pharmacological treatments

Guidelines in HICs (Austin et al., 2017; NICE, 2014) indicate that, for many women with moderate to severe anxiety or depressive disorders, the first-line treatment is medication, with psychological therapies introduced once medication(s) has become effective. UK guidelines indicate that antidepressants in the treatment of depression and anxiety in the general population are effective treatments with a strong evidence base (NICE, 2014). In contrast, in LMICs recommendations prioritise counselling and community interventions (Rahman et al., 2013) with emphasis on training community leaders and local health workers in supporting mothers experiencing depression (Rahman et al., 2012). Evidence for the effectiveness of pharmacological treatments in pregnancy is limited (but not expected to differ from the general population; Austin et al., 2017, p. 51). The important issue is whether the medications are associated with less than optimal birth outcomes or harm to the fetus. Currently there is little indication that the SSRI medications are associated with mortality, major malformations, cardiac malformations, or babies born small for their gestational age, but the quality of evidence is poor. However, the risk of miscarriage is increased with use of these medications in the first 20 weeks of pregnancy (Austin et al., 2017).

A recent systematic review (Prady, Hanlon, Fraser, & Mikocka-Walus, 2018) indicates that there is limited evidence demonstrating detrimental effects of pharmacological treatment on birth weight and child development. Guidelines recommend, however, that careful consideration be given to the use of SSRIs in pregnancy for women with moderate or severe depression or anxiety (Austin et al., 2017, p. 51). But if SSRIs are prescribed, it is important to take into account the woman's past response to treatment and whether she has risk factors for miscarriage (e.g., thyroid dysfunction) or preterm birth (e.g., previous preterm birth, active smoking during pregnancy), and factors that may increase risk of postpartum haemorrhage (Austin et al., 2017).

In contrast, there is strong evidence for use of antidepressants in the postnatal period for women suffering moderate or severe PND. Compared with placebo, treating postnatal depression with an SSRI is associated with good response and remission in a significant proportion of women at 6–8 weeks post-treatment (Molyneaux et al., 2018). Compared with fetal exposure during pregnancy, exposure to medications through breast milk is very low, and there is an even greater need to treat depression postnatally (given its effect on the woman's ability to care for her infant and on mother–infant attachment; Molyneaux et al., 2018). Detailed information regarding medications and breastfeeding, including the degree of transfer of medications into human milk, the effect on mother and infant (if known), the relative risks to the infant (if any), and the adult pharmacokinetics of the medication can be found in Hale (2019).

A recent qualitative review of women's decision making regarding medications during pregnancy showed that women wanted information particularly about longer-term outcomes and to be actively involved in decision-making with decision support. It was important that decisions reflected their beliefs and values, as well as sociocultural expectations. Participants were particularly conscious of the stigma associated not only with having a mental health problem, but also with taking medication during pregnancy (Hippman & Balneaves, 2018).

Given concerns about taking medications during pregnancy and breastfeeding, a number of researchers have examined the efficacy of biological complementary therapies, such as Omega-3 fatty acids. International guidelines indicate that Omega-3 fatty acid supplements do not appear to improve depression symptoms (Miller, Murray, Beckmann, Kent, & Macfarlane, 2013; NICE, 2014). However, there is no evidence of harm to the fetus. Therefore, Omega-3 can be taken, but there is no evidence of benefit (Austin et al., 2017). In contrast, other supplements (e.g., St John's Wort) are not recommended.

Psychological and psychoeducational approaches to treating perinatal depression and anxiety

A range of empirically validated psychological and psycho–educational treatments is available for PND, including cognitive-behavioural counselling with antidepressants. Cognitive-behavioural therapy and non-directive counselling, health-visitor-led non-directive counselling, peer support, and interpersonal psychotherapy have all demonstrated the amenability of postpartum depression to treatment (Dennis, 2014). Psychological and psychoeducational therapies have been commonly used for many years. More recently, there has been an increase in application of diverse complementary therapies such as acupuncture, yoga, and mindfulness-based approaches. At the same time, more emphasis is being placed on trauma-informed care and the use of attachment-based programs where therapists work with both mother and baby.

Cognitive behavioural therapy (CBT) is widely used to treat anxiety and depression, including in pregnancy and the postnatal period. CBT is based on the theory that thoughts, emotions, and behaviours are interconnected and that distorted or negative thinking affects feelings and behaviours and can lead to negative patterns. The focus in CBT is on changing thoughts and behaviours in order to manage problems in a more positive, constructive way (Wadephul, Jones, & Jomeen, 2016). This involves breaking problems down into smaller parts and acquiring coping strategies and skills. The focus is on current issues rather than the past. In pregnancy, these distorted thoughts may relate to pregnancy, labour, and early parenting; addressing these pregnancy-specific negative thoughts may be particularly beneficial (Wadephul et al., 2016).

Psychological approaches such as CBT work by increasing reinforcement and positive appraisal of accomplishments, and offer opportunities to learn through observation and role modelling (Dennis, 2014; Myors et al., 2018). CBT can promote self-reflection and motivation, teach coping strategies, and encourage individuals to anticipate stressful events or experiences and think about them differently (Dennis, 2014).

Interpersonal therapy (IPT) is a time-limited structured form of therapy for psychological distress related to difficulties in interpersonal relationships. IPT focusses on psychological symptoms, relationship conflict, and identifying and strengthening social support (Dennis, 2014). IPT may be a good fit for the perinatal period because parenting transitions entail changes in roles and interpersonal relationships, and thus there is an increased need for social support. There is a wide evidence base for IPT, including its use during the perinatal period (Wadephul et al., 2016). CBT and IPT are also now offered as computer-assisted and internet-based treatments that can provide support to those who do not otherwise have access (e.g., people who live in rural and remote locations) or who prefer anonymity (Dennis, 2014).

Mindfulness-based approaches are becoming increasingly popular and are often used alongside therapies such as CBT. The focus is on cultivating "a mental state of awareness and acceptance of present moment experiences, including one's current sensations, thoughts, bodily states and environment" (Wadephul et al., 2016, p. 2). They use techniques such as progressive muscle relaxation, yoga, and various forms of meditation, and are often taught in groups. Mindfulness-based stress reduction programs have been found to be successful in reducing anxiety and psychological distress, and in improving health outcomes. Mindfulness-based interventions aim to provide strategies for managing negative emotions and stress, and tend to focus on the reduction of anxiety and stress (Wadephul et al., 2016).

Complementary medicines and therapies (CM) are commonly used across the perinatal period and include a diverse range of modalities to promote, treat, and maintain well-being and health. The most common CM are grouped into mind and body practices, such as yoga, chiropractic and osteopathic manipulation, meditation, massage therapy, acupuncture, relaxation techniques (e.g., breathing exercises, guided imagery, progressive muscle relaxation), tai chi, qi gong, healing touch, hypnotherapy, and movement therapies.

Attachment-based parenting programs are based on the relationship between a mother and her infant that evolves during pregnancy. Women who experience high levels of stress have difficulty focussing on their future child and therefore on their relationship, which results in lower levels of maternal–fetal attachment. Intervention that increases the quality of the mother's feelings about her fetus may promote the development of an optimal mother–infant relationship after birth (Maas, Vreeswijk, Braeken, Vingerhoets, & van Bakel, 2014). Attachment-based parent–infant interventions may be helpful as they aim to improve the mother's mood and reduce the impact of antenatal or postnatal depression on the infant

(Guedeney et al., 2014). Two types of attachment-based interventions have been described: interventions that assist the mother to gain insight into the models of attachment that she has formed since she was a child, which may affect her interactions with her infant; and interventions that use video feedback and manualised procedures to assist the mother to identify her infant's cues and thereby better meet her infant's needs (Guedeney et al., 2014).

Efficacy of psychological and psychoeducational approaches for perinatal mood disorders and attachment-based parenting programs

A Cochrane systematic review showed benefits from psychological and psychoeducational interventions. Any psychosocial or psychological intervention, compared with usual postpartum care, was associated with a reduction in the likelihood of depressive symptomatology (Dennis & Hodnett, 2007). A review of psychosocial interventions only for PND (Dennis, 2014) showed that support by a partner or peers, non-directive counselling, home visits by mental health nurses, and collaborative models of care may be beneficial interventions for perinatal depression, especially when PND is linked to a lack of social support.

A recent systematic review (Smith, Shewamene, Galbally, Schmied, & Dahlen, 2019) showed that trials evaluating mindfulness yielded no evidence of reduced perinatal depression, anxiety, stress, or use of medication, although there was a small benefit of reduced relapse of depression during the postnatal period. Smith and colleagues found some evidence that acupuncture reduced the number of women with depression during the antenatal phase, but not in the postnatal period, and it did not reduce the severity of symptoms. Trials evaluating massage yielded evidence of reduced antenatal depression but not anxiety. Bright light therapy was associated with a change in antenatal depression. Relaxation therapy was found to reduce antenatal stress, but there was no evidence of reduced antenatal anxiety. There was no evidence of a benefit from yoga with reducing antenatal anxiety and depression (Smith et al., 2019).

Prevention of perinatal depression and anxiety

The Cochrane systematic review of interventions to prevent PND (Dennis & Dowswell, 2013) showed that women who received a psychosocial or psychological intervention in pregnancy or following birth were significantly less likely than those who received standard care to develop PND. The promising interventions included (1) provision of intensive, individualised postpartum home visits provided by public health nurses or midwives; (2) telephone support provided by lay or peer counsellors for women who had experienced postnatal depression; and IPT. In this meta-analysis, professional- and lay-based interventions were both effective in (3) reducing the risk of developing depressive symptomatology. Successful interventions were characterised by use of screening tools to identify women at risk of PND, individually based interventions, and multiple-contact interventions.

Interventions initiated in the postpartum period that targeted women at risk also significantly reduced the risk of developing depressive symptomatology (Dennis & Dowswell, 2013). However, there is currently no strong evidence to recommend routine antenatal and postnatal classes, postpartum lay-based home visits, early postpartum follow-up, continuity of carer models, in-hospital psychological debriefing, or CBT in the antenatal period to prevent PND (Dennis & Dowswell, 2013).

Group-based interventions to prevent PND are also popular in both antenatal and postnatal maternity and child health settings, and these may be facilitated by either peers or professionals. However, as yet, those provided in the antenatal period do not appear to be effective (Wadephul et al., 2016). Despite the lack of level 1 evidence (systematic reviews of Randomised Controlled Trials [RCT] with meta-analysis) or level 11 evidence (RCT), women reported positive experiences of these interventions (Wadephul et al., 2016). Group-based sessions appear to be a platform through which pregnant women can make important connections with others. Data suggest that women considered "connectivity" particularly important in terms of making friends with other participants.

Barriers to service use. Pregnancy is a time when many women engage with health services and initiate positive lifestyle choices. Research suggests that a number of factors influence women's decisions to uptake services during the perinatal period (Schmied et al., 2016; Smith, Lawrence, Sadler, & Easter, 2019). These include current mental health, symptom awareness, acceptance of postnatal depression, timeliness of care (Schmied et al., 2016), perception of usefulness of service, service quality and responsiveness (Smith et al., 2019; Wadephul et al., 2016), perceived stigma of mental illness and mental health services (Dennis & Chung-Lee, 2006; Foulkes, 2011), reticence to disclose experiences such as abuse (Schmied et al., 2017), the level of trust and quality of the relationship with health professionals (Rollans et al., 2013), and the mother's concern that seeking help is putting her own needs above her infant's needs. Abrams and colleagues (2009) found that women tended to normalise their symptoms of perinatal mood disorders to maintain the image of being a "good mother." Stigma was associated with being labelled a "bad mother," therefore women relied on self-help, including religious or spiritual strategies. A recent review of studies of women's preferences for and motivations to seek treatment for perinatal mental health problems identified that barriers existed at four levels: individual (e.g., stigma, lack of awareness of mental health problem), organisational (e.g., resource inadequacies, service fragmentation), sociocultural (e.g., language/cultural barriers), and structural (e.g., unclear policy) levels (Smith et al., 2019). Given the significant barriers to service use by women experiencing perinatal mental health problems, it is critical that services respond appropriately and sensitively to diverse women's needs.

Policy and health system approaches to prevention and treatment of perinatal depression and anxiety

Women with complex health and social needs can benefit most from services that are part of an integrated system of care with clear care pathways; early identification and intervention programs; and comprehensive management plans to improve their emotional well-being and prevent mental health problems. As many women engage with the healthcare system when they become pregnant, the antenatal period is an ideal time to implement public health policy. Seamless referral pathways require collaboration and integrative care between services. Poor communication and cooperation between services only widens the gap between what is needed and what is available to support women and families experiencing mental ill-health (Myors, Schmied, Johnson, & Cleary, 2013). Women with a history of a serious mental illness need a well-planned, coordinated approach to care that involves case management and the maintenance of support networks (McCauley, Cross, & Kulkarni, 2016).

There is limited literature on women's experiences of collaborative and integrative care for perinatal mental ill-health (Myors et al., 2013). A number of studies, however, have investigated women's experiences of integrated care models for perinatal substance misuse programs (Sword et al., 2013). The positive aspects that women reported from attending these programs are multi-faceted and include decreased stigma; supportive and non-judgmental professionals;

respectful, consistent, and reliable communication; enhanced service engagement; enhanced well-being; decreased substance use/continuation on opioid maintenance treatment; increased social support networks, increased insight, enhanced parenting capacity and maternal–child communication; decreased need for treatment for neonatal abstinence syndrome; increased spontaneous vaginal birth; increased initiation of breastfeeding; and increased housing stability (Myors et al., 2013; Schmied et al., 2015, 2016).

Conclusion

In this chapter, I have addressed perinatal depression and anxiety, two significant mental health problems experienced by around 20% of all pregnant and postpartum women. It is critical that perinatal depression and anxiety are appropriately identified and treated because they have significant ongoing impacts on women, their babies and children as they grow, and on their partners and families. Perinatal depression and anxiety are also associated with difficult and damaging social contexts, such as intimate partner violence and substance misuse. Health professionals, including midwives, child health nurses, and general practitioners, are in key positions to support women at the universal health service level. This is important because experiencing mental health problems still carries significant stigma in some cultures and communities, and many women are reluctant to seek help. It is also important that effective interventions are available and that women have access to appropriate referral pathways and secondary level services.

References

Abrams, L. S., Dornig, K., & Curran, L. (2009). Barriers to service use for postpartum depression symptoms among low-income ethnic minority mothers in the United States. *Qualitative Health Research, 19,* 535–551.

Accortt, E. E. & Wong, M. S. (2017). It is time for routine screening for perinatal mood and anxiety disorders in obstetrics and gynecology settings. *Obstetrical and Gynecological Survey, 72*(9), 553–568.

Ainsworth, M., Blehar, M. C., Waters, E., & Wall, S. (1978). *Patterns of attachment: A psychological study of the strange situation.* Hillsdale, NU: Erlbaum.

Armstrong, J. (2006). Beyond 'juggling' and 'flexibility': Classed and gendered experiences of combining employment and motherhood. *Sociological Research Online, 11*(2), 119–134.

Austin, M. P. (2014). Marcé International Society position on statement psychosocial assessment and depression screening in perinatal women. *Best Practice and Research in Clinical Obstetrics and Gynaecology, 28,* 179–187.

Austin, M. P., Colton, J., Priest, S., Reilly, N., & Hadzi-Pavlovic, D. (2013). The Antenatal Risk Questionnaire (ANRQ): Acceptability and use for psychosocial risk assessment in the maternity setting. *Women and Birth, 26*(1), 17–25.

Austin, M.-P., Highet, N., & the Expert Working Group (2017). *Mental health care in the perinatal period: Australian clinical practice guideline.* Melbourne, Australia: Centre of Perinatal Excellence.

Bayrampour, H., McNeil, D. A., Benzies, K., Salmon, C., Gelb, K., & Tough, S. (2017). A qualitative inquiry on pregnant women's preferences for mental health screening. *BMC Pregnancy and Childbirth, 17*(1), 339, doi:10.1186/s12884-017-1512-4.

Biaggi, A., Conroy, S., Pawlby, S., & Pariante, C. M. (2016). Identifying the women at risk of antenatal anxiety and depression: A systematic review. *Journal of Affective Disorders, 191,* 62–77.

Bowlby, J. (1969). *Attachment and loss v. 3* (Vol. 1). New York, NY: Random House.

Break the Silence on Postnatal Illness (n.d.). Breakthesilence-pni.org [website]. Retrieved from www .breakthesilence-pni.org/about-pni/history.

Brockington, I. F. & Kumar, R. (1982). *Motherhood and mental illness.* London, UK: Academic.

Cox, J., Murray, D., & Chapman, G. (1993). A controlled study of the onset, duration and prevalence of postnatal depression. *The British Journal of Psychiatry, 163,* 27–31.

Dennis, C. L. (2014). Psychosocial interventions for the treatment of perinatal depression. *Best Practice & Research: Clinical Obstetrics and Gynaecology*, *28*(1), 97–111.

Dennis, C. L., Brown, H. K., Falah-Hassani, K., Marini, F. C., & Vigod, S. N. (2017). Identifying women at risk for sustained postpartum anxiety. *Journal of Affective Disorders*, *213*, 131–137.

Dennis, C.-L. & Chung-Lee, L. (2006). Postpartum depression help-seeking barriers and maternal treatment preferences: A qualitative systematic review. *Birth*, *33*(4), 323–331.

Dennis, C. L. & Dowswell, T. (2013). Psychosocial and psychological interventions for preventing postpartum depression. *Cochrane Database of Systematic Reviews (Online)*, *2*, CD001134.,

Dennis, C. L., Falah-Hassani, K., & Shiri, R. (2017). Prevalence of antenatal and postnatal anxiety: Systematic review and meta-analysis. *British Journal of Psychiatry*, *210*(5), 315–323.

Dennis, C. L. & Hodnett, E. D. (2007). Psychosocial and psychological interventions for treating postpartum depression. *Cochrane Database of Systematic Reviews*, *4*, CD006116.

Dennis, C. L., Merry, L., & Gagnon, A. J. (2017). Postpartum depression risk factors among recent refugee, asylum-seeking, non-refugee immigrant, and Canadian-born women: Results from a prospective cohort study. *Social Psychiatry and Psychiatric Epidemiology*, *52*(4), 411–422, doi:10.1007/s00127-017-1353-5.

Department of Health (2018). *Clinical practice guidelines: Pregnancy care*. Canberra, Australia: Australian Government Department of Health.

Devries, K. M., Child, J. C., Bacchus, L. J., Mak, J., Falder, G., Graham, K., Watts, C., & Heise, L. (2014). Intimate partner violence victimization and alcohol consumption in women: A systematic review and meta-analysis. *Addiction*, *109*(3), 379–391.

Eastwood, J. G., Jalaludin, B. B., Kemp, L. A., Phung, H. N., & Barnett, B. E. W. (2012). Relationship of postnatal depressive symptoms to infant temperament, maternal expectations, social support and other potential risk factors: Findings from a large Australian cross-sectional study. *BMC Pregnancy and Childbirth*, *12*, 148.

Falah-Hassani, K., Shiri, R., & Dennis, C. L. (2016). Prevalence and risk factors for comorbid postpartum depressive symptomatology and anxiety. *Journal of Affective Disorders*, *198*, 142–147.

Fenwick, J., Barclay, L., & Schmied, V. (2008). Craving closeness: A grounded theory analysis of women's experiences of mothering in the Special Care Nursery. *Women and Birth*, *21*(2), 71–85.

Fisher, J., Chatham, E., Haseler, S., Beth, M., & Thompson, J. (2012). Uneven implementation of the National Perinatal Depression Initiative: Findings from a survey of Australian women's hospitals. *Australian and New Zealand Journal of Obstetrics and Gynaecology*, *52*(6), 559–564.

Fisher, J., de Mello, M. C., Patel, V., Rahman, A., Tran, T., Holton, S., & Holmesf, W. (2012). Prevalence and determinants of common perinatal mental disorders in women in low-and lower-middle-income countries: A systematic review. *Bulletin of the World Health Organization*, *90*(2), 139–149.

Foulkes, M. (2011). Enablers and barriers to seeking help for a postpartum mood disorder. *JOGNN: Journal of Obstetric, Gynecologic, and Neonatal Nursing*, *40*(4), 450–457.

Garton, S. (2009). Seeking refuge: Why asylum facilities might still be relevant for mental health care services today. *Health History*, *11*(1), 25–45.

Glover, V., O'Donnell, K. J., O'Connor, T. G., & Fisher, J. (2018). Prenatal maternal stress, fetal programming, and mechanisms underlying later psychopathology: A global perspective. *Development and Psychopathology*, *30*(3), 843–854.

Goodman, S. H., Rouse, M. H., Connell, A. M., Broth, M. R., Hall, C. M., & Heyward, D. (2011). Maternal depression and child psychopathology: A meta-analytic review. *Clinical Child and Family Psychology Review*, *14*(1), 1–27.

Goodwin, S. & Huppatz, K. (2010). *The good mother: Contemporary motherhoods in Australia*. Sydney, Australia: Sydney University Press.

Guedeney, A., Guedeney, N., Wendland, J., & Burtchen, N. (2014). Treatment – mother–infant relationship psychotherapy. *Best Practice & Research Clinical Obstetrics & Gynaecology*, *28*(1), 135–145.

Hale, T. (2019). *Medications and mothers milk* (new ed.). New York, NY: Springer Publishing Company.

Highett, N., Stevenson, A., Purtell, C., & Coo, S. (2014). Qualitative insights into women's personal experiences of perinatal depression and anxiety. *Women and Birth*, *27*(3), 179–184.

Hippman, C. & Balneaves, L. G. (2018). Women's decision making about antidepressant use during pregnancy: A narrative review. *Depression and Anxiety*, *35*, 1158–1167.

Humphrey, M. D. (2015). Maternal mortality trends in Australia. *Medical Journal of Australia*, *205*(8), 344–346.

James-Hawkins, L., Shaltout, E., Nur, A. A., Nasrallah, C., Qutteina, Y., Abdul Rahim, H. F., Hennink, M., & Yount, K. M. (2019). Human and economic resources for empowerment and pregnancy-related mental health in the Arab Middle East: A systematic review. *Archives of Women's Mental Health, 22*(1), 1–14.

Jefferies, D., Duff, M., & Nicholls, D. (2018). Understanding the experience of women admitted to a psychiatric hospital in Sydney with psychosis or mania following childbirth after World War II (1945–1955). *International Journal of Mental Health Nursing, 27*(2), 702–711.

Jefferies, D., Horsfall, D., & Schmied, V. (2017). Blurring reality with fiction: Exploring the stories of women, madness, and infanticide. *Women and Birth, 30*(1), e24–e31.

Kendall-Tackett, K. (2007). A new paradigm for depression in new mothers: The central role of inflammation and how breastfeeding and anti-inflammatory treatments protect maternal mental health. *International Breastfeeding Journal, 2*, 6.

Khan, L. (2015). *Falling through the gaps: Perinatal mental health and general practice.* London, UK: Centre for Mental Health.

Kingston, D., Austin, M. P., Van Zanten, S. V., Harvalik, P., Giallo, R., McDonald, S. D., Macqueen, G., Vermeyden, L., Lasiuk, G., Sword, W., & Biringer, A. (2017). Pregnant women's views on the feasibility and acceptability of web-based mental health e-screening versus paper-based screening: A randomized controlled trial. *Journal of Medical Internet Research, 19*(4), e88.

Kohlhoff, J., Hickinbotham, R., Knox, C., Roach, V., & Barnett, B. (2016). Antenatal psychosocial assessment and depression screening in a private hospital. *Australian and New Zealand Journal of Obstetrics and Gynaecology, 56*(2), 173–178.

Liamputtong, P. (2006). Motherhood and "moral career": Discourses of good motherhood among southeast Asian immigrant women in Australia. *Qualitative Sociology, 29*(1), 25–53.

Lobel, M. & Ibrahim, S. (2018). Emotions and mental health during pregnancy and postpartum. *Women's Reproductive Health, 5*(1), 13–19.

Lovejoy, M. C., Graczyk, P. A., O'Hare, E., & Neuman, G. (2000). Maternal depression and parenting behavior: A meta-analytic review. *Clinical Psychology Review, 20*(5), 561–592.

Maas, A. J. B. M., Vreeswijk, C. M. J. M., Braeken, J., Vingerhoets, A. J. J. M., & van Bakel, H. J. A. (2014). Determinants of maternal fetal attachment in women from a community-based sample. *Journal of Reproductive and Infant Psychology, 32*(1), 5–24.

Marland, H. (2004). *Dangerous motherhood: Insanity and childbirth in Victorian Britain.* Basingstoke, UK: Palgrave.

Marland, H. (2012). Under the shadow of maternity: Birth, death and puerperal insanity in Victorian Britain. *History of Psychiatry, 23*(1), 78–90.

Matthey, S. (2005). Assessing for psychosocial morbidity in pregnant women. *Canadian Medical Association Journal, 173*(3), 267–269.

Matthey, S. & Agostini, F. (2017). Using the Edinburgh Postnatal Depression Scale for women and men: Some cautionary thoughts. *Archives of Women's Mental Health, 20*(2), 345–354.

Matthey, S., Della Vedova, A. M., & Agostini, F. (2017). The Edinburgh Postnatal Depression Scale in routine screening: Errors and cautionary advice. *American Journal of Obstetrics and Gynecology, 216*(4), 424.

Mauthner, N. S. (2018). Screening, diagnosing, and medicating depression: Psychiatric methods and the making of mental disorder. *Women's Reproductive Health, 5*(1), 32–36.

McCauley, K. M., Cross, W., & Kulkarni, J. (2016). Mental health: Outcomes of 10 babies of mothers with a history of serious mental illness. *Journal of Psychiatric and Mental Health Nursing, 21*(7), 580–586.

Milgrom, J., Ericksen, J., Negri, L., & Gemmill, A. W. (2005). Screening for postnatal depression in routine primary care: Properties of the Edinburgh Postnatal Depression Scale in an Australian sample. *Australian and New Zealand Journal of Psychiatry, 39*(9), 833–839.

Miller, B. J., Murray, L., Beckmann, M. M., Kent, T., & Macfarlane, B. (2013). Dietary supplements for preventing postnatal depression. *Cochrane Database of Systematic Reviews, 10*, CD009104.

Mitchinson, W. (1989). The Toronto and Gladesville asylums: Humane alternatives for the insane in Canada and Australia? *Bulletin of the History of Medicine, 63*(1), 52–72.

Molyneaux, E., Telesia, L. A., Henshaw, C., Boath, E., Bradley, E., & Howard, L. M. (2018). Antidepressants for preventing postnatal depression. *Cochrane Database of Systematic Reviews, 4*, CD004363.

Myors, K. A., Cleary, M., Johnson, M., & Schmied, V. (2018). 'Modelling a secure-base' for women with complex needs: Attachment-based interventions used by perinatal and infant mental health clinicians. *Issues in Mental Health Nursing, 39*(3), doi:10.1080/01612840.2017.1378784.

Myors, K. A., Schmied, V., Johnson, M., & Cleary, M. (2013). Collaboration and integrated services for perinatal mental health: An integrative review. *Child and Adolescent Mental Health, 18*(1), 1–10.

National Institute for Health and Care Excellence (NICE) (2014). *Antenatal and postnatal mental health: Clinical management and service guidance: Clinical guideline*. London, UK: Author. Retrieved from www .nice.org.uk/guidance/cg192/resources/antenatal-and-postnatal-mental-health-clinical-management-and-service-guidance-pdf-35109869806789.

Norhayati, M. N., Hazlina, N. H., Asrenee, A. R., & Wan Emilin, W. M. A. (2015). Magnitude and risk factors for postpartum symptoms: A literature review. *Journal of Affective Disorders, 175*, 34–52.

NSW Department of Health (2009). *NSW health/families NSW supporting families early package – SAFE START strategic policy*. Sydney, Australia: Author.

O'Hara, M. W. & Wisner, K. L. (2014). Perinatal mental illness: Definition, description and aetiology. *Best Practice & Research Clinical Obstetrics & Gynaecology, 28*(1), 3–12.

Pao, C., Guintivano, J., Santos, H., & Meltzer-Brody, S. (2019). Postpartum depression and social support in a racially and ethnically diverse population of women. *Archives of Women's Mental Health, 22*(1), 105–114.

Parton, C., Ussher, J. M., Natoli, S., & Perz, J. (2018). Being a mother with multiple sclerosis: Negotiating cultural ideals of mother and child. *Feminism and Psychology, 28*(2), 212–230.

Pedersen, D. E. (2012). The good mother, the good father, and the good parent: Gendered definitions of parenting. *Journal of Feminist Family Therapy, 24*(3), 230–246.

Perinatal Anxiety & Depression Australia (PANDA) (2019). *Recovery stories*. North Fitzroy, VIC, Australia: Author. Retrieved from www.panda.org.au/info-support/during-pregnancy/personal-stories-pregnancy.

Prady, S. L., Hanlon, I., Fraser, L. K., & Mikocka-Walus, A. (2018). A systematic review of maternal antidepressant use in pregnancy and short- and long-term offspring's outcomes. *Archives of Women's Mental Health, 21*(2), 127–140.

Rahman, A., Fisher, J., Bower, P., Luchters, S., Tran, T., Yasamy, M., Saxena, S., & Waheed, W. (2013). Interventions for common perinatal mental disorders in women in low- and middle-income countries: A systematic review and meta-analysis. *Bulletin of the World Health Organization, 91*(8), 593–601, doi:10.2471/BLT.12.109819.

Rahman, A., Sikander, S., Malik, A., Ahmed, I., Tomenson, B., & Creed, F. (2012). Effective treatment of perinatal depression for women in debt and lacking financial empowerment in a low-income country. *British Journal of Psychiatry, 201*(6), 451–457.

Rollans, M., Schmied, V., Kemp, L., & Meade, T. (2013). Digging over that old ground: An Australian perspective of women's experience of psychosocial assessment and depression screening in pregnancy and following birth. *BMC Women's Health, 13*(1), 18.

Rowe, H., Holton, S., & Fisher, J. R. W. (2012). Postpartum emotional support: A qualitative study of women's and men's anticipated needs and preferred sources. *Australian Journal of Primary Health, 19*(1), 46–52.

Schmied, V., Black, E., Naidoo, N., Dahlen, H. G., & Liamputtong, P. (2017). Migrant women's experiences, meanings and ways of dealing with postnatal depression: A meta-ethnographic study. *PLoS One, 12*(3), doi:10.1371/journal.pone.0172385.

Schmied, V., Homer, C., Fowler, C., Psaila, K., Barclay, L., Wilson, I., Kemp, L., Fasher, M., & Kruske, S. (2015). Implementing a national approach to universal child and family health services in Australia: Professionals' views of the challenges and opportunities. *Health and Social Care in the Community, 23*(2), 159–170, doi:10.1111/hsc.12129.

Schmied, V., Johnson, M., Naidoo, N., Austin, M. P., Matthey, S., Kemp, L., Mills, A., Meade, T., & ills, Yeo, A. (2013). Maternal mental health in Australia and New Zealand: A review of longitudinal studies. *Women and Birth, 26*(3), 167–178.

Schmied, V., Kearney, E., & The Maternal Anxiety White Paper Group (2018). *Tackling maternal anxiety in the perinatal period: Reconceptualising mothering narratives*. Health and Well-being White Paper Series. Sydney, Australia: Western Sydney University. Retrieved from www.westernsydney.edu.au/__data/assets/pdf_file/0010/1483885/Maternal_Anxiety_White_Papers_FINAL.pdf.

Schmied, V., Langdon, R., Matthey, S., Kemp, L., Austin, M.-P., & Johnson, M. (2016). Antenatal psychosocial risk status and Australian women's use of primary care and specialist mental health services in the year after birth: A prospective study. *BMC Women's Health, 16*(1), 69.

Shepherd, M. L. (2011). Behind the scales: Child and family health nurses taking care of women's emotional wellbeing. *Contemporary Nurse: A Journal for the Australian Nursing Profession, 37*(2), 137–148.

Smith, C. A., Shewamene, Z., Galbally, M., Schmied, V., & Dahlen, H. (2019). The effect of complementary medicines and therapies on maternal anxiety and depression in pregnancy: A systematic review and meta-analysis. *Journal of Affective Disorders, 245*, 428–439, doi:10.1016/j.jad.2018.11.054.

Smith, M., Lawrence, V., Sadler, E., & Easter, A. (2019). Barriers to accessing mental health services for women with perinatal mental illness: Systematic review and meta-synthesis of qualitative studies in the UK. *British Medical Journal Open, 9*(1), e024803, doi:10.1136/bmjopen-2018-024803.

Stapleton, H., Murphy, R., & Kildea, S. (2013). Lost in translation: Staff and interpreters' experiences of the Edinburgh Postnatal Depression Scale with women from refugee backgrounds. *Issues in Mental Health Nursing, 34*, 648–657.

Steer, R. & Beck, A. (1997). Beck anxiety inventory. In C. Zalaquett & R. Wood (Eds), *Evaluating stress: A book of resources* (pp. 23–40). Lanham, MD: Scarecrow Education.

Sword, W., Niccols, A., Yousefi-Nooraie, R., Dobbins, M., Lipman, E., & Smith, P. (2013). Partnerships among Canadian agencies serving women with substance abuse issues and their children. *International Journal of Mental Health and Addiction, 11*(3), 344–357.

Thombs, B. D., Benedetti, A., Kloda, L. A., Levis, B., Riehm, K. E., Azar, M., Cuijpers, P., Gilbody, S., Ioannidis, J. P., McMillan, D., Patten, S. B., Shrier, I., Steele, R. J., Ziegelstein, R. C., Tonelli, M., Mitchell, N., Comeau, L., Schinazi, J., & Vigod, S. (2015). Diagnostic accuracy of the Edinburgh Postnatal Depression Scale (EPDS) for detecting major depression in pregnant and postnatal women: Protocol for a systematic review and individual patient data meta-analyses. *British Medical Journal Open, 5*(10), e009742, doi:10.1136/bmjopen-2015-009742.

Thornton, C., Schmied, V., Dennis, C. L., Barnett, B., & Dahlen, H. G. (2013). Maternal deaths in NSW (2000–2006) from nonmedical causes (suicide and trauma) in the first year following birth. *BioMed Research International, 2013*, ID 623743.

Tobin, C., Dinapoli, P., & Wood-Gauthier, M. (2014). Recognition of risk factors for postpartum depression in refugee and immigrant women: Are current screening practices adequate? *Journal of Immigration and Minority Health, 17*, 1019–1024.

Trede, K., Baldessarini, R., Viguera, A., & Bottero, A. (2009). Treatise on insanity in pregnant, postpartum, and lactating women (1858) by Louis-Victor Marcé: A commentary. *Harvard Review of Psychiatry, 7*(2), 157–165.

Ussher, J. (2011). *The madness of women: Myth and experience.* Abingdon, UK: Routledge.

Vaswani, A., Karter, J. M., Cosgrove, L., Peters, S. M., & Brodt, M. (2018). Depression screening during pregnancy and the postpartum period: Enhancing informed consent practices. *Women's Reproductive Health, 5*(1), 1–12, doi:10.1080/23293691.2018.1429532.

Wadephul, F., Jones, C., & Jomeen, J. (2016). The impact of antenatal psychological group interventions on psychological well-being: A systematic review of the qualitative and quantitative evidence. *Healthcare, 4*(2), 32.

Woody, C. A., Ferrari, A. J., Siskind, D. J., Whiteford, H. A., & Harris, M. G. (2017). A systematic review and meta-regression of the prevalence and incidence of perinatal depression. *Journal of Affective Disorders, 219*, 86–92, doi:10.1016/j.jad.2017.05.003.

Woolhouse, H., Gartland, D., Hegarty, K., Donath, S., & Brown, S. J. (2012). Depressive symptoms and intimate partner violence in the 12 months after childbirth: A prospective pregnancy cohort study. *BJOG: An International Journal of Obstetrics and Gynaecology, 119*(3), 315–323.

Zigmond, A. & Snaith, R. (1983). The hospital anxiety and depression scale. *Acta Psychiatrica Scandinavica, 67*(6), 361–370.

PART V

Sexuality and sexual health

25

WOMEN'S SEXUAL HEALTH AND EMBODIMENT

Niva Piran

Sexual health and embodiment are strongly related. The chapter starts with an examination of the relationship between these two constructs through the lens of the Developmental Theory of Embodiment (DTE; Piran, 2017) and introduces the term *sexual embodiment*. It then continues with an examination of the social conditions that shape both embodiment and sexual health. The same social processes that discipline the experience of embodiment of diverse girls and women and that aim to maintain social structures of power also operate in the sexual domain.

Embodiment and sexual health

> I describe myself as a very sexual person because I was always very much in touch with the sexual feelings that my body had … feeling sexual was a very positive thing. I was curious, so I explored my own body, yeah, there was no shame to it. I have healthy attitudes about sex. I thought, well maybe I am attracted to women and I think that it's more of a continuum … things kind of went on hold when I met [husband] and fell in love with him … I do feel sex was a very good thing for my body. [Jane]
>
> I haven't been sexually active for a while because I can't, and having real issues with intimacy … I just became disgusted having compulsive sex trying to make myself feel better. I went through a very, like, promiscuous phase. I found it very hard to enjoy. I could never, like, orgasm with them … Now with this guy but I'm not gonna let it go down that road. I don't even have to have sex. [Crystal]
>
> *(Piran, 2017, p. 8)*

Both Jane and Crystal participated in a qualitative study with young women, which was one of a series of qualitative and quantitative studies included in a large scale research program on embodiment among girls and women (Piran, 2002, 2016, 2017; Piran & Teall, 2012). Jane and Crystal, both in their early 20s, White, and from a working class background, described very different experiences of embodiment, sexuality, and well-being.

One construct that emerged from girls' and women's narratives on embodiment describes the *quality of embodied lives* (Piran, 2016, 2017; Piran & Teall, 2012). This construct, which is entitled the Experience of Embodiment (EE), includes five dimensions: (a) *Body connection and comfort*; (b) *Agency and functionality* (both physically and through voice); (c) *Experience and expression of desires* (appetite and sexuality); (d) *Attuned self-care* as one engages with the world (physical, emotional, relational, engagement in meaningful pursuits); and (e) *Inhabiting the body as a subjective site* (resisting objectification). Each of the five dimensions ranges from positive to negative; and positive (or negative) experiences on one dimension tend to co-occur with similarly positive (or negative) experiences on other dimensions. Accordingly, EE ranges from positive embodiment (i.e., "positive body connection and comfort, embodied agency and passion, and attuned self-care") to negative embodiment (i.e., "disrupted body connection and discomfort, restricted agency and passion, and self-neglect or harm") (Piran, 2016, p. 47).

Positive, embodied sexuality includes all dimensions of a positive experience of embodiment. As Jane's narrative above indicates, positive experience of sexuality involves *connection to desire*, body comfort and other *positive feelings* in one's body, the experience of *agency in desire*, *attuned self-care* in sexuality (physical, emotional, and *relational*), and immersion in one's experience of sexuality without the interruption of objectification. This description of positive, embodied sexuality aligns with the working definition of the state of sexual health by the World Health Organization (WHO, 2006): "Sexual health requires a *positive* and *respectful* approach to sexuality and *sexual relationships*, as well as the possibility of having *pleasurable* and *safe* sexual experiences, free of coercion, discrimination and violence." The definitions differ in that the WHO description also includes social factors that disrupt sexual health (coercion, discrimination, violence), whereas the Developmental Theory of Embodiment (Piran, 2017) delineates these social conditions separately from the experience of embodied sexuality. As related to the alignment of sexual health and sexual embodiment, the terms are used interchangeably throughout the chapter.

Sexuality, therefore, is one domain of engagement of the body with the physical and social world, where one can experience positive body connection and comfort, embodied agency and passion, and attuned self-care. Further, qualitative and quantitative research suggests that the experience of sexuality relates to the general experience of embodiment. For example, whereas Jane described her general experience of embodiment as "I think of myself as a whole, the mind body all integrated or something like that … I feel comfortable in my own skin and letting go of those prescribed notions of what a girl should look like," Crystal described her experience of embodiment as "I hate my body and I want my body to die, to disintegrate … This body is an obstacle … I feel disconnection … growing up in a woman's body you get the idea that your body is wrong" (Piran, 2017, p. 5). Quantitative research supports the association between sexuality and embodiment; for example, the Experience of Embodiment Scale (Piran & Teall, 2012) is significantly correlated with measures of sexual body esteem, sexual self-efficacy, and sexual assertiveness (Chmielewski, Bowman, & Tolman, 2017; Piran, 2019).

In a recent book on embodiment and the research-based Developmental Theory of Embodiment (Piran, 2017), I described ways in which diverse girls and women are socialized into inequity through the targeting of their bodies, which assures the maintenance of the social status quo. The sexual domain is effective in disenfranchising diverse girls, women, and their bodies. Viewed through the embodiment lens, the lack of sexual health is one expression of inequitable social conditions that bar diverse girls and women from acting in the world with embodied power and agency. Hence, sexual health and social justice are strongly linked.

The Developmental Theory of Embodiment is useful in the examination of women's sexual health and embodiment (Piran, 2017). The DTE includes the relationship between social processes and girls' and women's embodied experiences. According to the DTE, social experiences shape girls' and women's quality of embodied lives via three core pathways: the *physical* domain, the *mental* domain of social discourses and expectations, and the *social power and relational connections* domain. Each of these domains includes protective (and risk) factors: physical freedom (vs corseting), mental freedom (vs corseting), and social power and relational connections (vs disempowerment and disconnection). The embodiment lens therefore provides a way to examine a broad range of social processes that shape sexual health among women.

The physical domain

According to the DTE, physical experiences are powerful in shaping embodiment, in particular: violations to the body territory; opportunities for physical agency and freedom of movement in the public territory; experiences that support and validate bodily desires and encourage attuned, assertive, and joyful responses to them; and the opportunity to practice physical care of the body (Piran, 2017). To focus specifically on sexual embodiment, in this section I explore sexual violations as well as opportunities for physical and sexual agency, connection to sexual desire, and the practice of sexual self-care among women.

Sexual violations, which comprise a major challenge to sexual embodiment, are common among adolescent girls and women. According to a nationally representative sample in the US, about 7.7% of young women reach adulthood having experienced rape for the first time before age 18, a further 6.8% experience rape first between the ages of 18 and 24, and an additional 2.6% of women report first rape at ages 25–34 (Black et al., 2011). Altogether, over 1 in 7 women have experienced rape by age 24 and at least 1 in 6 women have experienced rape across their life span. This challenge is more severe among specific groups of women, such as women of color and members of Indigenous communities in North America (Daniel & Dale, 2013). Research on university campuses reveals that, over a four-year period, the incidence of sexual assault is estimated to be 20–25% (Fisher, Cullen, & Turner, 2000). Women who identify their sexual orientation as lesbian, gay, bisexual, queer, or questioning (LGBTQQ) (Garnets, Herek, & Levy, 1990) or their gender identity as transgender (Grossman & D'Augelli, 2006) face targeted assaults that could include attempts to degrade their sexuality or gender identity. Times of armed conflict, where rape becomes a weapon of war, and forced geographical dislocations severely challenge the safety of women (Hargreaves, 2001; Kirby, 2013).

Beyond rape, other disruptions to respectful ownership of the body within the sexual arena are more common, though never benign. Sexual harassment of girls and women is pervasive. One-third of a sample of about 300 women, who were around 30 years of age and who participated in a work-place sexual harassment study, reported at least one behavioral indicator of harassment, with a higher frequency among non-White women (McLaughlin, Uggen, & Blackstone, 2012; the authors used a dichotomous categorization of race). Similarly, the frequency of everyday stranger harassment in the public domain is high around the world. For example, 36% of a sample of undergraduate women psychology students in the US reported being the victim of unwanted touching or stroking once a month, and 31% reported experiencing catcalls, whistles, or stares every few days or more (Fairchild & Rudman, 2008). High rates of stranger harassment have been reported in other countries, such as Japan ("Japan", 2005) and India (Dhillon & Bakaya, 2014). Research documents that everyday stranger harassment heightens the fear of rape, induces shame, promotes self-objectification, and constricts young women's freedom of movement and use of the public sphere (Dhillon & Bakaya, 2014; Fairchild & Rudman, 2008).

Sexual violence leads to disruption on all five domains of the experience of embodiment. In particular it leads to body dissociation; the association of the body with fear and a host of other negative emotions; vulnerability and restricted embodied agency; disrupted connection to bodily desires; body neglect and engagement in harmful behaviors such as skin cutting or eating disorders; and self-objectification (e.g., van der Kolk, 1996). It is not surprising that sexual violations lead to sexual dysfunction. Analysis of data from the US National and Social Life Survey showed that 32% of young women, ages 18–29, reported a lack of interest in sex, and 26% described an arousal disorder. The survey further indicated that having experienced sexual harassment, been sexually touched before puberty, and been sexually forced by a man were all risk factors for sexual dysfunction across the age spectrum (Laumann, Paik, & Rosen, 1999). It is of note that the Second Australian Study of Health and Relationships found unchanged rates of sexual coercion among women and men compared with a survey conducted 11 years earlier (22% vs 21% among women, and 5% vs 4%, respectively) (de Visser et al., 2014).

A factor that enhances positive embodiment is exposure to experiences that promote physical agency, such as engagement in joyful physical activities and roaming freely in public territories (Piran, 2017). What is generally found for girls is that their agency to act physically in the world is curtailed at puberty, through, for example, differential allocation of resources to girls' and boys' sports, safety concerns, and gender norms (e.g., Piran, 2017; Senne, 2016). The sexual domain, in particular, involves intensive socialization that suppresses physical agency (Gavey, 2005). In a series of qualitative studies (Piran, 2017), girls and women commonly described the expectation that they should wait to be invited to dance by boys or men. While boys' and men's agency in desire was sanctioned, encouraged, and socially rewarded, girls and women were vilified and often received the slut label for engaging sexually, as 16-year-old Ashley, of African-Canadian and working class background described: "There's always the fear of being called a slut. I think it's mostly moderating your own behavior so that you don't get labeled that way" (Piran, 2017, p. 172). It is therefore not surprising that women's narratives indicated challenges to sexual agency: "If I say, 'no', it will be hard on the guy, I would feel bad, like I am a bad person" [Lauren, 19, White, middle class]; "I never got aroused. You had to have a boyfriend and have sex or something like that. It was like a waste of my time" [Beth, mid 20s, White, middle class]; "He wanted and I am, like, what do I have to lose. I don't say no, I just think no" [Sarah, 18–20 age range, White, working class] (Piran, 2017, p. 154).

Sexual assertiveness is relevant to young women's safety and health. Although there is no question that the prevention of sexual violations of women involves social-wide changes (Buchwald, Fletcher, & Roth, 1993), including the critical education of men (Amaro, 1995), addressing women's disrupted agency in the sexual domain has been a component of successful programs aimed at reducing rapes on campus (Senn et al., 2015). For example, the efficacious Enhanced Assess, Acknowledge, Act (Enhanced AAA) Sexual Assault Resistance program addresses, among other components, barriers to resisting unwanted sexual behaviors and verbal coercion by men, practicing physical self-defense, and promoting sexual assertiveness. Agency and assertive communication in the sexual domain are similarly addressed in relation to the negotiation about the use of condoms in sexual contact (Noar, Carlyle, & Cole, 2006); however, women's gender socialization and the context of their lives need to be considered in such programs. *Participatory* approaches to health promotion and the overall goal of addressing the social conditions of diverse women are very important (Amaro, 1995).

The tension between possibilities inherent in embodying sexual agency and the adverse and disempowering social context diverse girls and women encounter daily has stirred disagreements between feminists. The presentation of "embodying agency" versus "embodying culture" as dichotomous options is possibly epitomized by varied responses to the "Slut Walk" activism (e.g., Gavey, 2012; Gill, 2008; Reger, 2015). Reger, for example, discussed the separation and dis-identification between younger and older feminists, as well as the racial divide, whereby, for women of color, the historical trauma of violations is linked to oppression, exploitation, and commodification, and to the construction of *multiple* controlling images, such as the mule, mammy, and Jezebel (Reger, 2015; Simmons, 2011). Another important distinction, made by Bay-Cheng (2015), relates to agency as a psychological construct that reflects "an individual's capacity to exert her will" and a "neoliberal discourse of agency" (p. 280). Further, what may be viewed as agentic action in the public sphere may not be experienced as such by the performing individual (Gavey, 2012). The meaning of sexual agency is therefore multi-layered and can only be understood in relation to varied social contexts.

Research demonstrates the contribution of women's experiences of physical agency to positive embodiment, yet opportunities for physical agency are related to social privilege, and barriers related to gender, age, social class, ethnicity/race, and sexual orientation have been documented (Piran, 2017). It is important that the Enhanced AAA Sexual Assault prevention program (Senn, Gee, & Thake, 2011) includes a sexual education program that follows an emancipatory paradigm focused on dialogical processes about women's sexual desires and alternatives to coitus and learned sexual scripts so as to support women in expressing assertively their own sexual preferences. However, a university campus is a privileged space, and sexual agency cannot be examined without the consideration of the social context within which it is practiced. Indeed, it is within relational spaces for girls and women that the complexity of being sexual agents within an objectifying, sexualizing, unsafe, and inequitable social context can most easily be discussed, interrogated, and critiqued (e.g., Edell, Brown, & Tolman, 2013; Gavey, 2012; Piran, 2017).

Another factor that enhances positive embodiment according to the DTE involves freedom of desire, including experiences that validate desire and encourage attuned, assertive, and joyful responses to bodily desires (Piran, 2017). Such connection to desire enhances positive embodiment, namely positive body connection, physical agency, bodily joy, attuned self-care in the practice of desire, and immersion in the experience of desire (see also Tolman, 2002). In qualitative studies with young women, and retrospective accounts by older women, I have found that women commonly go through challenging journeys towards connecting with their sexual desires and, when engaging sexually with a partner, find it challenging to be attuned to and communicate their own desires, boundaries, and preferences (Piran, 2017). Like other researchers, I have reported multiple challenges to connecting with desire, including the common absence throughout adolescence and early adulthood of validation of experienced female desire and its varied expressions (Fine & McClelland, 2006; Tolman, 2002), the common social vilification of (too much/little or non-heterosexual) female desires (Armstrong, Hamilton, Armstrong, & Seeley, 2014), the social expectation that girls and women be other-attuned and contain male desire (Gavey, 2005), sexual objectification (Murnen & Smolak, 2012), performance expectations in the practice of sexuality (Burns, Futch, & Tolman, 2011), a range of violations (Tolman, 2002), moral and punitive presentations of sexual engagement (Fine & McClelland, 2006), and, overall, adolescent girls' and women's reading of the sexual domain as reflecting social inequity related to gender, age, class, ethnicity/race, and other social variables (e.g., Gavey, 2012).

Opportunity to practice care of the body is a further factor in the physical domain; it contributes to positive embodiment by enhancing body connection, embodied agency, and attuned self-care. Adolescent girls and women experience mounting challenges in the physical care of their bodies (Piran, 2017). One factor that challenges care of the body involves the expectation that adolescent girls and women will override and renounce their own needs in taking care of others (e.g., Ussher & Perz, 2010). This pattern often starts within adolescent girls' nuclear families and continues in young women's heterosexual partnerships, including the inequitable distribution of tasks in the domestic sphere (e.g., Cerrato & Cifre, 2018). Further shaping adolescent girls' and women's challenges to physical self-care is a cultural "abandonment" of women's bodies and physical needs (Piran, 2017; see also Kawachi, Kennedy, Gupta, & Prothrow-Stith, 1999). This pattern is accentuated at puberty. For example, already at menarche, girls confront stigmatization and a lack of resources that can help them manage menstruation. Adolescent girls and women face sexual harassment and sexual violations during dating and in partnership relationships, as noted above, with minimal support (Senn et al., 2015; Tjaden & Thoennes, 2000). Further, their practice of desire is not commonly guided by supportive relational dialogues that invite their own reflections about their sexual preferences, pleasures, boundaries, and assertive communications (Senn et al., 2011). Inequity in the practice of sexuality, in responsibility for unintended pregnancies, and the limited access to abortion also complicates the practice of physical care of the body (Fine & McClelland, 2006). All these challenges are greater for women who are poorer and those whose race/ethnicity, sexual orientation, gender identity, and physical disability expose them to greater discrimination and fewer resources (Fine & McClelland, 2006; Piran, 2017). It is therefore not surprising that challenges to the care of their bodies disrupt women's sexual embodiment.

The domain of social discourses

Examining power, language, and discourse allows for an understanding of constraining molds that women are expected to embody at the intersection of gender, age, ethnicity, social class, and other dimensions of social location. These constraining social discourses maintain the social status quo (Butler, 1996; Weedon, 1987). Collins (2000) referred to such constraining molds as controlling images that work to limit the possibilities of acting in the world, hence making "racism, sexism, poverty, and other forms of social justice appear to be natural, normal and inevitable parts of everyday life" (p. 69). Social discourses that shape diverse women's experiences and ways of inhabiting their bodies also shape their sexual embodiment.

Inhabiting the body as an object of gaze, or self-objectification, involves the internalization of the objectifying gaze so prevalent in patriarchal societies (Fredrickson & Roberts, 1997; McKinley & Hyde, 1996). In addition to the "girl/woman as an object of gaze" discourse present since early childhood in the life of girls, during early puberty a second appearance-related discourse emerges entitled "woman's body as deficient" (Piran, 2017). Inhabiting the body as a deficient object that requires ongoing repair reduces girls' and women's embodied power and agency to act in the world. Studies with young women repeatedly show that self-objectification is associated not only with self-surveillance, body shame, negative self-evaluations (Calogero, 2004; Fredrickson & Roberts, 1997; McKinley & Hyde, 1996), and reduced social agency (Calogero, 2013), but also with depression, disordered eating, and sexual dysfunction (Tiggemann & Williams, 2012).

Inhabiting the body as a deficient object of gaze can affect sexual embodiment adversely by lowering body esteem and hence introducing distress during sexual contact. Studies among mainly heterosexual and White women suggest that self-objectification relates to self-consciousness during sexual contact and to decreased sexual functioning (e.g., Claudat & Warren, 2014; Steer & Tiggemann, 2008), though a similar relationship has been reported among lesbian women in fewer studies (e.g., Peplau et al., 2009). Research also indicates that negative body image and body shame are associated with lower sexual arousability and ability to reach orgasm (Quinn-Nilas, Benson, Milhausen, Buchholz, & Goncalves, 2016; Sanchez & Kiefer, 2007), reduced sexual assertiveness, greater engagement in risky sexual practices (Schooler, Ward, Merriwether, & Caruthers, 2005), and avoidance of bodily exposure during sex (Cash, Maikkula, & Yamamiya, 2004).

Objectification takes place at the intersection of gender with other dimensions of social location. In a chapter on the representation of Black female sexuality, hooks (1997) described the sexualized objectification of the Black body as sexist/racist. In particular, she highlighted the sexist/racist imagery of Black women as hyper-sexed, available, and animalistic, as the colonized representation of their desire. hooks emphasized the importance for Black women to "place erotic recognition, desire, pleasure, and fulfillment at the center of our efforts to create radical black female subjectivity" (p. 128). A qualitative study with African American women similarly validated the sexist/racist presentation of women and its adverse impact on women's embodied experiences (Watson, Robinson, Dispenza, & Nazari, 2012).

In addition to the appearance-related discourses of objectification and deficiency, the DTE describes four other discourses that fall under the comportment-related femininity cluster (Piran, 2017). These comportment-related discourses shape the experience of embodiment and include: "engagement in feminine activities," "woman as submissive/demure," "woman as desired but desire-less," and "patriarchal shaping of relational connections"; of these, the latter three femininity discourses, in particular, shape sexual embodiment.

The "woman as submissive/demure" discourse guides girls and women to act demurely and nice; tells them not to be too dominant, assertive, or needy; and instructs them to subvert their own needs and wishes to those of boys and men (see also Jack, 1991). Research in the sexual domain indeed suggests that this internalized discourse disrupts sexual embodiment and health. In a series of studies, Sanchez and her colleagues (Kiefer & Sanchez, 2007; Sanchez, Kiefer, & Ybarra, 2006) found that gender-role endorsement correlated with more passive behavior for college women. They also found that college women associated sex with submissiveness and that the adoption of a submissive sexual role predicted lower reported arousal and more difficulty becoming aroused. Further, entertainment media shape sexual outcomes by transmitting stereotyped gender-related sexual scripts (Ward, 2003) and decreasing sexual assertiveness, interest, and esteem among women consumers of such media (Aubrey, 2007). An additional aspect of the submissive/demure discourse that can disrupt attunement to sexual desire involves subverting one's own needs and wishes to others, in particular, to boys and men. Satinsky and Jozkowski (2015) found among mainly young heterosexual women that entitlement to pleasure from a partner was related to active consent to oral sex, which they interpreted as comfort with receiving sexual pleasure.

The "woman as desired but desire-less" discourse reflects the dominant sanctioning of male desire and the problem of owning female desire (Piran, 2017). Research (e.g., Gavey, 2005; Piran, 2017) shows that the oppressive layers within which female desire is couched disrupt connection to sexual desire. The slut/prude linguistic labels, which reinforce the "woman as desired but desire-less" discourse, still operate often as a polarizing dichotomy (McLaren, 1995; Piran, 2017), whereby a center location of "sanctioned" desire is precarious and scrutinized, despite a trend towards a greater acceptability of diversity in the expression of desire in terms of sexual orientation (Bay-Cheng, 2015; Hamilton & Armstrong, 2015). However, the stigmatization of women's sexual practices can still instigate social processes of demotion and exclusion, even if sexual events were coercive, as girls and women are also expected to contain and be the gatekeepers of male sexuality (Gavey, 2005; Piran, 2017). Further, adverse sexually linked social processes target, in particular, less privileged members at the intersection of gender with race/ethnicity, social class, physical disability, sexual orientation, and gender identity (e.g., Attwood, 2007; Bay-Cheng, 2015; Piran, 2017). Fear of stigma and blame for sexual violations disrupt women's sexual embodiment and their broader experience of embodiment in the world.

The "patriarchal shaping of relational patterns" discourse reflects an expected pattern of relationships among adolescent girls and women whereby they prioritize sexualized relationships and allegiances with men over relational networks with women, as well as practice competition and policing of other girls and women (Brown, 2003; Piran, 2017). One of the difficult experiences adolescent girls and women experience is the collusion of other girls and women in penalizing them for their sexual activities (Piran, 2017).

A critical stance towards adverse social discourses can be facilitated in relational forums where discourses can be interrogated, named, and their impact on diverse individuals and their social environments examined. Such a cultural critique can mobilize transformations at all levels of the social environment and within individuals. Such dialogues can also repair relational connections interrupted by disruptive social discourses.

Social power and relational connections domain

Adolescent girls' and women's experiences in the physical and social discourses domains are strongly linked to experiences of social power and relational connections with others and with their various communities (Piran, 2017). Women's bodies are viewed as social capital (Bourdieu, 1984), and inhabiting particular bodies determines access to resources and possible exposure to discrimination and harassment. In turn, such prejudicial treatment is informed by ideologies embedded in varied social institutions, including political organizations and associated laws and policies, sites of education and employment, the media, and families. Social power and relational connections at the intersection of gender, age, race/ethnicity, social class, sexual orientation, gender identity, and physical disability can therefore affect embodiment directly through shaping individuals' living conditions, and indirectly through individuals' internalization of inequitable and prejudicial treatment (Piran, 2017). Social justice, feminist, anti-oppressive, and human rights perspectives are therefore all relevant to individuals' experiences of embodiment.

Women's sexual embodiment and sexual health reflect the inextricable connection between societal power structures and individuals' embodied lives (e.g., Amaro, 1995; Fine & McClelland, 2006; Piran, 2017; Tolman, 2002). Level of education and financial standing are examples of contextual factors that impact reproductive health among women. In the US, for example, rates of unintended pregnancies, unprotected sex, and STIs are the highest among those who had not completed high school, were unmarried, of low income, and Black or Hispanic (Amaro, 1995; Finer & Henshaw, 2006).

Another lens through which to examine the relationship between social power and sexual embodiment involves the study of "idealized" visual representations of women. The use of social media by women has enhanced the emphasis on visual representations in shaping social interactions (Cohen, Newton-John, & Slater, 2017; Howard, Heron, MacIntyre,

Myers, & Everhard, 2017). Idealized images of women in the media often reflect the inter-section of disenfranchisement and privilege, presenting women as occupying confined phys-ical spaces and inhabiting altered bodies, while also being hetero-sexualized, clad in brand name clothing, and displaying "White" features (Buchanan, Settles, & Woods, 2019; Piran, 2017). In relation to sexual embodiment, inhabiting idealized bodies denotes access to sought after social and partnership relationships, compelling women in many countries around the world to engage in sometimes risky body-alteration practices to enhance their attractiveness, such as extreme dieting and disordered eating patterns (e.g., Pike & Dunne, 2015), plastic surgeries ("Demand for Cosmetic Surgery Procedures Around the World," 2017), and the application of skin bleachers (e.g., Benn et al., 2016). Idealized images of appearance support body-based harassment and teasing and often target women who are heavier, older, of color, poorer, lesbian, bisexual, queer, questioning, transgender, or who live with physical disabilities (e.g., Buchanan & Ormerod, 2002; Piran, 2017). Body-based harassment affects body image negatively, which, in turn, is associated with increased engagement in potentially risky sexual behaviors (e.g., Gillen, Lefkowitz, & Shearer, 2006).

Conclusion

The understanding of sexual embodiment of girls and women requires the concurrent exploration of their physical experiences; exposure to prevalent social discourses; and experi-ences of social power and relational connections at the place of intersection of gender, age, social class, race/ethnicity, sexual orientation, physical disability, and gender identity. Review of research in these domains suggests multiple disruptions that challenge women's embodied connection to desire, agency in desire, and self-care in the practice of desire. Changes in women's experiences of sexual embodiment require sociocultural transformations informed by social justice, feminist, anti-oppressive, and human rights perspectives. Overall, enhanced sexual embodiment will relate to *embodied equity*. Concurrently, research suggests the value of forming communities of equity and activism, whereby societal structures and ideologies can be interrogated and alternative goals and values can be collectively identified and implemented. Such communities can form locally (schools, universities, workplaces, community centers) or through social media.

References

ABC News (2005, June 10). "Japan tries women-only train cars to stop groping." *ABC News*. Retrieved from http://abcnews.go.com/GMA/International/story?id=803965&CMP=OTC-RSS/feeds0312.

Amaro, H. (1995). Love, sex, and power: Considering women's realities in HIV prevention. *American Psychologist*, 50, 437–447.

Armstrong, E. A., Hamilton, L. T., Armstrong, E. T., & Seeley, J. L. (2014). "Good girls": Gender, social class, and slut discourse on campus. *Social Psychology Quarterly*, 77, 100–122.

Attwood, F. (2007). Sluts and riot grrrls: Female identity and sexual agency. *Journal of Gender Studies*, 16, 233–247.

Aubrey, J. S. (2007). Does television exposure influence college-aged women's sexual self-concept? *Media Psychology*, 10, 157–181.

Bay-Cheng, L. Y. (2015). The agency line: A neoliberal metric for appraising young women's sexuality. *Sex Roles*, 73, 279–291.

Benn, E. K., Alexis, A., Mohamed, N., Wang, Y. H., Khan, I. A., & Liu, B. (2016). Skin bleaching and dermatologic health of African and Afro-Caribbean populations in the US: New directions for meth-odologically rigorous, multidisciplinary, and culturally sensitive research. *Dermatology and Therapy*, 6, 453–459.

Black, M. C., Basile, K. C., Breiding, M. J., Smith, S. G., Walters, M. L., Merrick, M. T., Chen, J., & Stevens, M. R. (2011). *The National Intimate Partner and Sexual Violence Survey (NISVS): 2010 summary report*. Atlanta, GA: National Center for Injury Prevention and Control, Centers for Disease Control and Prevention. Retrieved from www.cdc.gov/violenceprevention/pdf/nisvs_report2010-a.pdf.

Bourdieu, P. (1984). *Distinction: A social critique of the judgment of taste*. Cambridge, MA: Harvard University Press.

Brown, L. M. (2003). *Girlfighting: Betrayal and rejection among girls*. New York, NY: New York University Press.

Buchanan, N. T. & Ormerod, A. J. (2002). Racialized sexual harassment in the lives of African American women. *Women & Therapy*, *25*, 107–124.

Buchanan, N. T., Settles, I. S., & Woods, K. C. (2019). Black women's positive embodiment in the face of race x gender oppression. In T. Tylka & N. Piran (Eds), *Handbook of positive body image and embodiment* (pp. 191–200). New York, NY: Oxford University Press.

Buchwald, E., Fletcher, P. R., & Roth, M. (1993). *Transforming a rape culture*. Minneapolis, MN: Milkweed Editions.

Burns, A., Futch, V. A., & Tolman, D. L. (2011). "It's like doing homework": Academic achievement discourse in adolescent girls' fellatio narratives. *Sexuality Research & Social Policy*, *8*(3), 239–251.

Butler, J. (1996). Imitation and gender insubordination. In A. Garry & M. Pearsall (Eds), *Women, knowledge, and reality: Explorations in feminist philosophy* (2nd ed., pp. 371–387). New York, NY: Routledge Kegan Paul.

Calogero, R. M. (2004). A test of objectification theory: Effect of the male gaze on appearance concerns in college women. *Psychology of Women Quarterly*, *28*, 16–21.

Calogero, R. M. (2013). Objects don't object: Evidence that self-objectification disrupts women's social activism. *Psychological Science*, *24*, 312–318.

Cash, T. F., Maikkula, B. S., & Yamamiya, Y. (2004). Baring the body in the bedroom: Body image, sexual self-schemas, and sexual functioning among college women and men. *Electronic Journal of Human Sexuality*, *7*. Retrieved from www.ejhs.org/volume7/bodyimage.html.

Cerrato, J. & Cifre, E. (2018). Gender inequality in household chores and work–family conflict. *Frontiers in Psychology*, *9*, 1330. Retrieved from www.frontiersin.org/articles/10.3389/fpsyg.2018.01330.

Chmielewski, J., Bowman, C., & Tolman, D. (2017). *Embodiment as intimate justice: Exploring embodiment as a pathway to young women's self esteem*. Unpublished manuscript.

Claudat, K. & Warren, C. S. (2014). Self-objectification, body self-consciousness during sexual activities, and sexual satisfaction in college women. *Body Image*, *11*, 509–515.

Cohen, R., Newton-John, T., & Slater, A. (2017). The relationship between Facebook and Instagram appearance-focused activities and body image concerns in young women. *Body Image*, *23*, 183–187.

Collins, P. H. (2000). *Black feminist thought: Knowledge, consciousness, and the politics of empowerment* (2nd ed.). New York, NY: Routledge.

Daniel, J. H. & Dale, S. K. (2013). Women of color: Violence and trauma. In B. Greene & L. Comas-Diaz (Eds), *Psychological health of women of color* (pp. 133–146). Santa Barbara, CA: Praeger.

de Visser, R. O., Richters, J., Rissel, C., Badcock, P. B., Simpson, J. M., Smith, A. M. A., & Grulich, A. E. (2014). Change and stasis in sexual health and relationships: Comparisons between the first and second Australian studies of health and relationships. *Sexual Health*, *11*(5), 505–509.

Dhillon, M. & Bakaya, S. (2014). Street harassment: A qualitative study of the experience of young women in Delhi. *SAGE Open*, *4*, 1–11.

Edell, D., Brown, L. M., & Tolman, D. (2013). Embodying sexualisation: When theory meets practice in intergenerational feminist activism. *Feminist Theory*, *14*, 275–284.

Fairchild, K. & Rudman, L. A. (2008). Everyday stranger harassment and women's objectification. *Social Justice Research*, *21*, 338–357.

Fine, M. & McClelland, S. (2006). Sexuality education and desire: Still missing after all these years. *Harvard Educational Review*, *76*, 297–338.

Finer, L. B. & Henshaw, S. K. (2006). Disparities in rates of unintended pregnancy in the United States, 1994 and 2001. *Perspectives on Sexual Reproduction Health*, *38*, 90–96.

Fisher, B., Cullen, F., & Turner, M. (2000). *The sexual victimization of college women: Findings from two national-level studies*. Washington, DC: National Institute of Justice and Bureau of Justice Statistics. Retrieved from www.ncjrs.gov/pdffiles1/nij/182369.pdf.

Fredrickson, B. L. & Roberts, T. (1997). Objectification theory: Toward understanding women's lived experiences and mental health risks. *Psychology of Women Quarterly, 21*, 173–206.

Garnets, L., Herek, G. M., & Levy, B. (1990). Violence and victimization of lesbians and gay men: Mental health consequences. *Journal of Interpersonal Violence, 5*, 366–383.

Gavey, N. (2005). *Just sex? The cultural scaffolding of rape.* Abingdon, UK: Routledge.

Gavey, N. (2012). Beyond "empowerment"? Sexuality in a sexist world. *Sex Roles, 66*, 718–724.

Gill, R. (2008). Culture and subjectivity in neoliberal and postfeminist times. *Subjectivity, 25*, 432–445.

Gillen, M. M., Lefkowitz, E. S., & Shearer, C. L. (2006). Does body image play a role in risky sexual behavior and attitudes? *Journal of Youth and Adolescence, 35*, 230–242.

Grossman, A. H. & D'Augelli, A. R. (2006). Transgender youth: Invisible and vulnerable. *Journal of Homosexuality, 51*(1), 111–128.

Hamilton, L. & Armstrong, E. A. (2015). Gendered sexuality in young adulthood: Double binds and flawed options. *Gender & Society, 23*, 589–616.

Hargreaves, S. (2001). Rape as a war crime: Putting policy into practice. *Lancet, 357*, 737.

hooks, b. (1997). Selling hot pussy: Representations of black female sexuality in the cultural marketplace. In K. Conboy, N. Medina, & S. Stanbury (Eds), *Writing on the body: Female embodiment and feminist theory* (pp. 113–128). New York, NY: Columbia University Press.

Howard, L. M., Heron, K. E., MacIntyre, T. I., Myers, T. A., & Everhard, R. S. (2017). Is use of social networking sites associated with young women's body dissatisfaction and disordered eating? A look at Black–White racial differences. *Body Image, 23*, 109–113.

International Society of Aesthetic Plastic Surgery (2017). "Demand for cosmetic surgery procedures around the world continues to skyrocket – USA, Brazil, Japan, Italy and Mexico ranked in the top five countries" [press release]. Hanover, NH: Author. Retrieved from www.isaps.org/wp-content/uploads/2017/10/GlobalStatistics.PressRelease2016-1.pdf.

Jack, D. (1991). *Silencing the self: Women and depression.* Cambridge, MA: Harvard University Press.

Kawachi, I., Kennedy, B. P., Gupta, V., & Prothrow-Stith, D. (1999). Women's status and the health of women and men: A view from the States. *Social Sciences & Medicine, 48*(1), 21–32.

Kiefer, A. K. & Sanchez, D. T. (2007). Scripting sexual passivity: A gender role perspective. *Personal Relationships, 14*, 269–290.

Kirby, P. (2013). How is rape a weapon of war? Feminist international relations, modes of critical explanation and the study of wartime sexual violence. *European Journal of International Relations, 19*, 797–821.

Laumann, E. O., Paik, A., & Rosen, R. C. (1999). Sexual dysfunction in the United States: Prevalence and predictors. *Journal of the American Medical Association, 281*, 537–544.

McKinley, N. M. & Hyde, J. S. (1996). The Objectified Body Consciousness Scale: Development and validation. *Psychology of Women Quarterly, 20*, 181–215.

McLaren, P. (1995). White terror and oppositional agency: Towards a critical multiculturalism. In C. E. Sleeter & P. McLaren (Eds), *Multicultural education, critical pedagogy, and the politics of difference* (pp. 33–70). Albany, NY: State University of New York Press.

McLaughlin, H., Uggen, C., & Blackstone, A. (2012). Sexual harassment, workplace authority, and the paradox of power. *American Sociological Review, 77*, 625–647.

Murnen, S. K. & Smolak, L. (2012). Social considerations related to adolescent girls' sexual empowerment: A response to Lamb and Peterson. *Sex Roles, 66*, 725–735.

Noar, S. M., Carlyle, K., & Cole, C. (2006). Why communication is crucial: Meta-analysis of the relationship between safer sexual communication and condom use. *Journal of Health Communication, 11*, 365–390.

Peplau, L. A., Frederick, D. A., Yee, C., Maisel, N., Lever, J., & Ghavami, N. (2009). Body image satisfaction in heterosexual, gay, and lesbian adults. *Archives of Sexual Behavior, 38*, 713–725.

Pike, K. M. & Dunne, P. (2015). The rise of eating disorders in Asia: A review. *Journal of Eating Disorders, 3*, 33, doi:10.1186/s40337-015-0070-2.

Piran, N. (2002). Embodiment: A mosaic of inquiries in the area of body weight and shape preoccupation. In S. Abbey (Ed.), *Ways of knowing in and through the body: Diverse perspectives on embodiment* (pp. 211–214). Welland, ON: Soleil Publishing.

Piran, N. (2016). Embodied possibilities and disruptions: The emergence of the experience of embodiment construct from qualitative studies with girls and women. *Body Image, 18*, 43–60.

Piran, N. (2017). *Journeys of embodiment at the intersection of body and culture: The developmental theory of embodiment.* San Diego, CA: Elsevier.

Piran, N. (2019). The experience of embodiment construct: Reflecting the quality of embodied lives. In T. Tylka & N. Piran (Eds), *Handbook of positive body image and embodiment* (pp 11–21). New York, NY: Oxford University Press.

Piran, N. & Teall, T. L. (2012). The developmental theory of embodiment. In G. McVey, M. P. Levine, N. Piran, & H. B. Ferguson (Eds), *Preventing eating-related and weight-related disorders: Collaborative research, advocacy, and policy change* (pp. 171–199). Waterloo, ON: Wilfred Laurier Press.

Quinn-Nilas, C., Benson, L., Milhausen, R. R., Buchholz, A. C., & Goncalves, M. (2016). The relationship between body image and domains of sexual functioning among heterosexual, emerging adult women. *Sexual Medicine, 4,* e182–1189.

Reger, J. (2015). The story of a slut walk: Sexuality, race, and generational divisions in contemporary feminist activism. *Journal of Contemporary Ethnography, 44,* 84–112.

Sanchez, D. T. & Kiefer, A. K. (2007). Body concerns in and out of the bedroom: Implications for sexual pleasure and problems. *Archives of Sex Behavior, 36,* 808–820.

Sanchez, D. T., Kiefer, A. K., & Ybarra, O. (2006). Sexual submissiveness in women: Costs for sexual autonomy and arousal. *Personality and Social Psychology Bulletin, 32,* 512–524.

Satinsky, S. & Jozkowski, K. N. (2015). Female sexual subjectivity and verbal consent to receiving oral sex. *Journal of Sex and Marital Therapy, 41,* 413–426.

Schooler, D., Ward, L. M., Merriwether, A., & Caruthers, A. S. (2005). Cycles of shame: Menstrual shame, body shame, and sexual decision-making. *Journal of Sex Research, 42,* 324–334.

Senn, C. Y., Eliasziw, M., Barata, P. C., Thurston, W. E., Newby-Clark, I. R., Radtke, H. L., & Hobden, K. L. (2015). Efficacy of a sexual assault resistance program for university women. *New England Journal of Medicine, 372,* 2326–2335.

Senn, C. Y., Gee, S. S., & Thake, J. (2011). Emancipatory sexuality education and sexual assault resistance: Does the former enhance the latter? *Psychology of Women Quarterly, 35,* 72–91.

Senne, J. (2016). Examination of gender equity and female participation in sport. *Sport Journal, 19,* 1–10.

Simmons, A. S. (2011, August 5). Is the SlutWalk movement relevant for a Black feminist? *Colorlines.* Retrieved from www.colorlines.com/articles/slutwalk-movement-relevant-black-feminist.

Steer, A. & Tiggemann, M. (2008). The role of self-objectification in women's sexual functioning. *Journal of Social and Clinical Psychology, 27,* 205–225.

Tiggemann, M. & Williams, E. (2012). The role of self-objectification in disordered eating, depressed mood, and sexual functioning among women: A comprehensive test of objectification theory. *Psychology of Women Quarterly, 36,* 66–75.

Tjaden, P. & Thoennes, N. (2000, November). *Full report of the prevalence, incidence, and consequences of violence against women.* Washington, DC: U.S. Department of Justice, Office of Justice Programs, National Institute of Justice. Retrieved from www.ncjrs.gov/pdffiles1/nij/183781.pdf.

Tolman, D. L. (2002). *Dilemmas of desire: Teenage girls talk about sexuality.* Cambridge, MA: Harvard University Press.

Ussher, J. & Perz, J. (2010). Gender differences in self-silencing and psychological distress in informal cancer carers. *Psychology of Women Quarterly, 34*(2), 228–242.

van der Kolk, B. A. (1996). The complexity of adaptation to trauma: Self-regulation, stimulus discrimination, and characterological development. In B. A. van der Kolk, A. C. McFarlane, & L. Weisaeth (Eds), *Traumatic stress: The effects of overwhelming experience on mind, body, and society* (pp. 182–213). New York, NY: Guilford Press.

Ward, L. M. (2003). Understanding the role of entertainment media in the sexual socialization of American youth: A review of empirical research. *Developmental Review, 23,* 347–388.

Watson, L. B., Robinson, D., Dispenza, F., & Nazari, N. (2012). African American women's sexual objectification experiences: A qualitative study. *Psychology of Women Quarterly, 36,* 458–475.

Weedon, C. (1987). *Feminist practice & poststructuralist theory.* Oxford, UK: Blackwell.

World Health Organization (WHO) (2006). *Sexual and reproductive health: Defining sexual health .* Geneva, Switzerland: Author. Retrieved from www.who.int/reproductivehealth/topics/sexual_health/sh_defi nitions/en.

26

SEXUAL HEALTH OF ADOLESCENT GIRLS

S. Rachel Skinner, Cristyn Davies, Jennifer Marino, Jessica R. Botfield and Larissa Lewis

For most young people, romantic and sexual relationships are a source of intense interest and activity. In secondary school, the majority of adolescents, sexually active or not, report having had a romantic relationship (Mitchell, Patrick, Heywood, Blackman, & Pitts, 2014). The views and values young people hold about romantic relationships, and the behaviours, values and attitudes they learn in these early relationships, are important for healthy development. Positive relationship experiences in adolescence improve self-esteem and self-concept (Furman & Shaffer, 2003). Within a peer group, they influence status and reinforce shared attitudes, values and interests (Furman & Rose, 2015). They are a primary context for learning about sexuality, including sexual behaviour and orientation (Korchmaros, Ybarra, & Mitchell, 2015). Indeed, large prospective studies show that adolescent romantic relationships are the foundation of healthy young adult romantic relationships (Meier & Allen, 2009).

Adolescence is a time of exploring boundaries and risk-taking is a part of normal adolescent development (Dahl, Allen, Wilbrecht, & Suleiman, 2018). Adolescents pursue new experiences and learn by experimentation in order to achieve adult independence, and they engage deeply with peers to develop adult social competence (Crone, van Duijvenvoorde, & Peper, 2016). However, across the globe, puberty and early adolescence signals a time when gender stereotypical roles and behaviours are strongly reinforced. Family, peers, schools and media are typically responsible for policing these behaviours and expectations (Kagesten et al., 2016). Compared with the relative freedom of childhood, different gendered constraints and expectations are placed on adolescent girls and boys (Blum, Mmari, & Moreau, 2017). Gendered sociocultural constraints can be limiting and potentially detrimental to adolescent girls' wellbeing in particular.

While the majority of adolescents do not experience lasting negative outcomes from taking risks, understanding adolescent risky behaviour is important as it is linked to the leading causes of death and disease burden in adolescents and young adults around the world (which include sexually transmitted infections and complications of adolescent pregnancy and birth) (World Health Organization, 2014). Considering that the morbidity linked to risk-taking in adolescence is entirely preventable and that gains in the health of adolescent populations have been minimal, compared with those seen in childhood and older age, the world has been called to action on adolescent health (Bundy et al., 2018; Patton et al., 2018). Relative inaction is a result of oversight and lack of awareness of the significance of adolescent health to wellbeing across the life course and lack of effective evidence-based interventions (Bundy et al., 2018).

In this chapter, we provide a broad overview of current understandings of adolescent girls' sexual health and behaviour and how these relate to wellbeing across the life course. We discuss the development of gender identity and sexuality as a socially constructed phenomenon. We describe the current status and trends in key indicators of sexual behaviour and wellbeing in adolescence across the globe and discuss key threats to adolescent girls' and young women's sexual health. We highlight the specific challenges that vulnerable young women face, and present evidence for effective population-based and clinical programs that support young women and improve their sexual health. We contextualise our chapter in a health, human rights and social science perspective, reflecting the intersecting contexts in which sexual health and wellbeing of young women is experienced. We argue for the importance of sexual health and wellbeing so that every girl can reach their potential.

Gender identity and sexuality in childhood and adolescence

Gender identity refers to a person's internal self-concept or awareness of gender, which may or may not align with the sex assigned to them at birth, while sex refers to a person's reproductive system and secondary sex characteristics. Until the 1970s, the term 'sex' was commonly used to refer to boys and girls, men and women, and 'sex roles' to refer to the adoption of traditionally feminine and masculine roles and behaviours. Historically, gender has been figured through discourse as a binary (masculinity and femininity) based on perceptions of biological sex (male and female) (Robinson & Jones Díaz, 2016). In more recent times, gender has been understood as socially constructed, fluid and not necessarily aligned with natal sex (Butler, 1990, 2004; Jagose, 1996). However the concept and understanding of gender continues to vary across countries, societies and generations (Lyons, 2009).

Young children generally develop an awareness of gender (including traits and stereotypes) and their own gender identity at around two to three years of age (Davies & Robinson, 2010; Robinson & Davies, 2017). Based on cultural narratives and social practices, children play an active role in constructing gender, most frequently through binary constructions of gender, regulating their own practices according to what they understand as 'appropriate' masculine and feminine cultural scripts and policing the behaviours of peers (Davies & Robinson, 2010; Robinson & Jones Díaz, 2016). Children and young people who transgress gender norms (especially gender diverse and transgender children and young people) generally experience strong disapproval from adults and other children (Davies & Robinson, 2010; Robinson, 2013; Robinson, Bansel, Denson, Ovenden, & Davies, 2014).

Sexual orientation may be conceptualised as comprising three dimensions: identity, attraction and behaviour (Wolff, Wells, Ventura-DiPersia, Renson, & Grov, 2017). Sexual identities are shaped by sociocultural and political values and practices that have changed over time (Robinson & Davies, 2018a, 2018b). In Western cultures, the language used to describe sexual (and gender) identities continues to change, as young people in particular reinscribe or use new discourses to articulate their desires, identities and experiences. Discourses, which operate through language, can be understood as the ways in which a system of statements are used to construct knowledge and meaning (for example, about gender) through power, institutions, social relations and dominant cultural narratives (Foucault, 1972).

It is recognised that gender identity and gender roles, sexual attraction, behaviour and identity are all central to the development of sexuality and sexual identity (Williams, Kang, & Skinner, 2013). Sexual desire, and increased desire for intimacy within relationships during adolescence, means that many young people begin to engage in sexual behaviours during this period of the lifespan (Williams et al., 2013). These experiences also work to shape a sense of who they are as a sexual person.

The study of human sexuality has primarily been constituted through biomedical and psychological discourses that view puberty in adolescence as marking a critical period of sexual development (Foucault, 1978; Robinson & Davies, 2018b). While sexual desire and identity is regarded in biomedical discourses as beginning during adolescence, younger children are also active participants in the development of their sexual subjectivities, desires and relationships (Davies & Robinson, 2010; Renold, 2005; Robinson & Davies, 2018a). The relationship between childhood and sexuality remains a contested space, wherein sexuality is often viewed as 'adult knowledge' and the figure of the child, which has come to represent sexual innocence, is often mobilised to regulate children's and young people's access to information and education about sex and sexuality (Robinson, 2013; Robinson & Davies, 2018b).

Adolescent sexual behaviour and health

Sexual activity includes a spectrum of behaviours and these likely differ by culture, gender and sexual orientation. The most widely studied first sexual experience, particularly in nationally representative surveys, is coitus (vaginal intercourse). Average age of first vaginal intercourse is variable across nations: in low- to middle-income countries, the proportion of girls who have had vaginal intercourse before the age of 15 ranges from 0.3% in Western Asia to 13.4% in sub-Saharan Africa (Santhya & Jejeebhoy, 2015). In Europe, the proportion of 15-year-olds who have had vaginal intercourse averages 24% of boys and 17% of girls (Inchley et al., 2016). In Australia and the United States, respectively, 23% and 36% of year 10 and 50% and 57% of year 12 students have had vaginal intercourse (Kann et al., 2018; Mitchell et al., 2014). In recent decades, adolescent oral sex behaviour has also been studied: it is the most common sexual behaviour among adolescents and first experience occurs before first intercourse for the great majority (Skinner et al., 2015).

Age at first intercourse, across countries, is influenced by social and cultural mores, retention in school, relative socio-economic advantage and, to a lesser extent, the availability of contraception. In most secular high-income nations, the age at first intercourse decreased over the latter half of the 20th century into the 21st, stabilising at around age 16–17. This is the case in Australia and the UK (Lewis et al., 2017; Rissel et al., 2014). In the United States, the same trend was seen until the last decade, when the proportion of all high school students who had had vaginal intercourse *fell* from 48% in 2007 to 40% in 2017 (Centers for Disease Control and Prevention, 2018b). There has been a corresponding increase in age at first vaginal intercourse among younger birth cohorts in the U.S. to 18.1 years in men and 17.8 in women (Finer & Philbin, 2014). Recent data suggests this decrease in sexual activity persists into young adulthood. For example, analyses of the U.S. General Social Survey found that among 20–24 year olds, those born in the 1990s were more than twice as likely to have had no sexual partners since the age of 18 than those born in the 1960s (Twenge, Sherman, & Wells, 2017). The reason for this trend is not yet known: whether related to changing norms and factors specific to the U.S. which other countries may follow, or whether this is simply further stabilisation of a baseline of sexual activity, bringing previous higher rates of adolescent sexual behaviour in the U.S. more in line with the sexual behaviour of adolescents in Western countries elsewhere.

Less is known about low-income nations. In a meta-analysis of timing of first intercourse among unmarried youth in 34 countries in sub-Saharan Africa, the median age was 16 years for women and 17 for men (Amo-Adjei & Tuoyire, 2018), slightly lower than median ages in wealthier nations. In an analysis of demographic and health survey data in 46 countries across Asia, Northern and sub-Saharan Africa, Latin America and the Caribbean, the mean age at first intercourse was noted to have increased over the past 35 years (Bongaarts, Mensch, & Blanc, 2017). In this context, the increase in age at first intercourse was attributed to increasing age at marriage, less child marriage and increasing educational levels of girls. In addition to socio-cultural and political factors, age at first intercourse may also be influenced by individual biological factors such as age of menarche (a late marker of puberty) (Marino et al., 2013).

Whilst earlier age of sexual activity (as compared with the average across a population) in itself is not a health or social concern, it can be a marker for vulnerability to health and social harms. Adolescents who have earlier sexual experiences are more likely to have experienced developmental and social vulnerabilities from early childhood and to have engaged in a range of health risk behaviours (Skinner et al., 2017, 2015). Earlier age of vaginal intercourse has been consistently associated with increased likelihood of multiple partners (recent, lifetime or concurrent), as well as adolescent pregnancy, birth and abortion. Associations with teenage fatherhood and with sexually transmitted infection are not as clear cut (Heywood, Patrick, Smith, & Pitts, 2015).

Having had multiple sexual partners is known to be linked to a general increase in risk of sexually transmitted infection and pregnancy in young people (Kahn & Halpern, 2018). Among Australian secondary school students who had ever had sex, 28% of boys and 20% of girls reported three or more sexual partners with whom they had vaginal intercourse in the previous year (Mitchell et al., 2014). In the U.S., 7.9% of girls and 11.6% of boys reported having had vaginal intercourse with four or more persons over their lives (Kann et al., 2018).

Australian Study on Health and Relationships (ASHR) data show that use of protection at first intercourse has risen steadily in successive birth cohorts. Remarkably, 91% of men and 97% of women in the youngest cohorts used some form of contraception at first intercourse, and 82% of men and 80% of women reported condom use at first vaginal intercourse (Rissel et al., 2014). Condom use drops with subsequent sexual experience as young people transition to regular hormonal contraception: only about half of sexually active girls and two-thirds of boys report using a condom at last intercourse. The proportions who use condoms are slightly higher in Australia and Europe than in the United States. (Inchley et al., 2016; Kann et al., 2018; Mitchell et al., 2014). About 13–14% report not using any method to prevent pregnancy at last intercourse (again slightly higher in the U.S.).

Adolescent pregnancies and births carry significant health and social risks for young mothers and children, and adolescent pregnancies are considered a key indicator of a country's health status. The adolescent (15–19 years) birth rate has decreased in most countries over the past few decades, although the decline has been slower in low- and middle-income countries than in wealthier ones (Santhya & Jejeebhoy, 2015), which is likely a direct result of slower progress in improving educational levels and reducing poverty as much as disparity in resources to enhance sexual and reproductive health. Adolescent pregnancy and birth rates in the U.S. have declined from a peak in 1991 to an all-time low of 22 per 1,000 (Hamilton & Mathews, 2016), although this is still double that of many other Western countries. This decline has been attributed to the general trend to later childbearing and declines seen across the world, decreases in adolescent sexual activity seen in the

U.S., but also to better contraceptive practices, such as use of long acting reversible contraceptives (Kost, Maddow-Zimet, & Arpaia, 2017). Within countries there can be great variation in adolescent births: in Australia, births are relatively high in very remote regions (64.5/1,000), in the poorest areas (24.9/1,000 for those in the lowest quintile versus 2.8/1,000 in the most advantaged quintile) (Australian Institute of Health and Welfare, 2018) and among Indigenous Australians (53.4/1,000) (Australian Bureau of Statistics, 2017).

Declines in adolescent births are in stark contrast to rates of sexually transmitted infections (STIs), which have continued to rise among adolescents and young adults over the same time period (Centers for Disease Control and Prevention, 2018a), indicating a complex interplay of factors. In general, young (versus older) women and girls are more vulnerable to STIs. This is thought to be due to behavioural, epidemiological as well as biological reasons. In the context of established higher prevalence of STI in young people, these infections are also transmitted more efficiently between adolescent partners. As mentioned above, some young people do not use condoms with sexual partners. More importantly though, young people are more likely to have shorter-term relationships and a shorter time interval between relationships (Seiffge-Krenke, 2003). This means that, on average, they have more partners over a similar time frame. STIs are often carried without symptoms, and without treatment, may not clear for several months. Biological reasons such as lower immunity and lack of protection of cervical mucus may also play a role in the epidemiology of STIs in adolescent girls (Kleppa et al., 2015).

STIs such as chlamydia and human papillomavirus are typically most common in adolescent and young adult women and lead to a significant disease burden over the life course. In Australia, notifications of chlamydia genital infections in adolescents and young adults appear to have recently plateaued, after climbing for nearly 20 years (The Kirby Institute, 2018). In some vulnerable populations (such as Indigenous and rural/remote youth), rates remain much higher and other STIs (such as gonorrhea and syphilis) are also of concern (The Kirby Institute, 2018).

The role of online media in adolescent sexual activity

The rise of online media and its popularity amongst young people has been met with moral panic that often accompanies the emergence of new and unfamiliar environments. The ubiquitousness of mobile smart devices means that adolescents' lives and relationships are played out online as much as offline, with experimentation and exploration across both. Many adults are concerned about the effects of young people's exposure to sexual content in social media, which has been shown to be associated with sexual risk behaviour (Lewis, Mooney-Somers, Guy, Watchirs Smith, & Skinner, 2018; Smith et al., 2016). Exposure to explicit sexual content may also influence young people's behavioural and social norms, body image and expectations of sexual activity (Cabecinha et al., 2017).

However, social media platforms like Facebook and Instagram can also provide a forum for young people to receive feedback, practice social skills, interact with peers, and observe others. Furthermore, social media can play an important role in adolescent romantic relationships, not only for relationship initiation and maintenance, but also for a source of relationship models as users watch their friends' relationships unfold (Van Ouytsel, Van Gool, Walrave, Ponnet, & Peeters, 2016). Since adolescents have relatively little romantic experience to draw on and are exposed to many more relationships whilst using social media, it is possible that this pervasiveness as well as the interactivity of social media influences adolescents' views of romantic relationships. It is important we continue to seek to understand the full range of impacts of social media on all aspects of young people's lives.

Gender and sexuality diverse adolescents

Many adolescents can experience marginalisation or 'double discrimination' beyond that experienced by all young people, due to diversity. Gender and sexuality diverse young people are marginalised across all countries and societies. They can experience homo/transphobia in all settings, including school, home and community environments, and this can have a significant impact on their health and wellbeing (Robinson et al., 2014). Due to stigma and homo/transphobia, these young people experience higher levels of mental ill-health than their peers (Davies et al., 2014; McDonald, 2018). While same-sex attraction, gender diversity and intersex status are not themselves pathogenic, they may make young people more vulnerable to negative experiences and discrimination that in turn increases risk for mental ill-health, self-harm and suicide (Davies et al., 2014). They are more likely to be homeless and at greater risk of sexual exploitation, including engaging in survival sex, which can further impact their mental and physical health (McDonald, 2018). They are also at greater risk of contracting sexually transmitted infections and experiencing unintended pregnancies (Ela & Budnick, 2017). The mental health and wellbeing of sexuality and gender diverse young people is intimately related to their sexual health behaviours, including access to sexual and reproductive healthcare information and services (Davies, 2014; Robinson et al., 2014).

Young gender and sexuality diverse people also experience difficulty accessing relevant, accurate and timely sexual health and sexuality education (Robinson et al., 2014; Smith et al., 2014; Steinke, Root-Bowman, Estabrook, Levine, & Kantor, 2017). In the *Growing up Queer* study, when asked about what they were taught as part of sex education at school, very few young people were taught about transgender identities (3.3%) or bisexual identities (7.6%). They were unlikely to be educated about gay and lesbian relationships (11% and 7.8% respectively), or gay and lesbian safe sex (12.9% and 6.1%) (Robinson et al., 2014). These findings are in line with other research in Western countries (Steinke et al., 2017).

Until recently, we have known little about the prevalence of sexuality and gender diversity in youth at the population level, due to lack of recognition of the importance of capturing this data and strong social stigma. In Western countries, where stigma has reduced in recent years, we have seen that young people are more likely than any other age group to identify as gay, lesbian or bisexual: in the UK, this is just over 4% for age group 16–24 (Office for National Statistics, 2017). Among U.S. secondary school students, this figure was just under 4% (with another 4% not sure) (Kann et al., 2018). Including additional items in surveys beyond self-identification – such as attraction and/or behaviour (Geary et al., 2018; Patterson & Jabson, 2018) – substantially increases prevalence and is very important for measuring health outcomes and disparities in sexual minorities (Wolff et al., 2017).

Around 1%–2% of adolescents self-identify as transgender or gender diverse in the few population studies published (Zucker, 2017); higher than in adults at 0.5%. Another difference is that the higher natal male to natal female sex ratio seen among transgender adults (approximately 3:1) is less pronounced in adolescents (Zucker, 2017): the reasons for these differences across generations are as yet unclear. Based on these population prevalence data, only a small proportion of young people who self-identify as gender diverse in the general population will present to clinicians or have clinical diagnoses of gender dysphoria, but there is evidence that both have increased significantly in recent years, possibly related to reductions in stigma (Zucker, 2017).

Sexuality education

Comprehensive sexuality education (CSE) is described as a critical educational component of effective sexual health promotion strategies (see the next section). However, CSE is more than information about sexual health and reproduction education. It is intended to address the knowledge, emotional, physical and social facets of sexuality education. CSE aims to assist in empowering young people to have fulfilling, safe, respectful and productive intimate relationships and sexual futures. It promotes informed decision-making, an ethics of care for the self and others, as well as awareness of sexually transmitted infections (STIs), HIV, unintended pregnancies, gender-based violence (GBV) and inequality (Carmody, 2009; United Nations Educational Scientific and Cultural Organization (UNESCO), 2018).

In dominant health and medical discourses, CSE for young people has most frequently been informed by discourses of risk, while desire and pleasure have not often been addressed. While the call to address pleasure in CSE is not new (Wood, Hirst, Wilson, & Burns-O'Connell, 2019), critical engagement with this concept, without constructing it as an imperative, should be a crucial component of young people's CSE education, contributing to their sexual health literacy and ethical sexual citizenship (Davies & Robinson, 2010).

The design and implementation of a CSE curriculum (or frameworks) in countries is influenced by socio-political and economic climates (Ezer, Jones, Fisher, & Power, 2018; Leahy, O'Flynn, & Wright, 2013). Good partnerships between health and education sectors are critical for effective CSE. The United Nations Population Fund recommend the following nine essential components of evidence-based CSE across both formal and informal sectors: (1) a basis in core universal values of human rights; (2) an integrated focus on gender; (3) thorough and scientifically accurate information; (4) a safe and healthy learning environment; (5) linking to sexual and reproductive health services and other initiatives that address gender, equality, empowerment and access to education, social and economic assets for young people; (6) participatory teaching methods for personalisation of information and strengthened skills in communication, decision-making and critical thinking; (7) strengthening youth advocacy and civic engagement; (8) cultural relevance in tackling human rights violations and gender inequality; and (9) reaching across formal and informal sectors and across age groupings (United Nations Population Fund, 2014). Young people who have access to effective CSE (linked to contraception access) are more likely to engage in safer sex but not increased or earlier sexual activity (Lindberg & Maddow-Zimet, 2012).

In many countries, schools present an ideal opportunity to provide adolescents with access to CSE at a time when they are likely to soon become sexually active. Many parents support accurate, age-appropriate and timely sex education in school settings from early childhood (Robinson, Smith, & Davies, 2017). However, poorly designed and implemented curricula and poorly timed sex education can mean young people need to seek this information online, with varying capacities to obtain accurate, plain language information (Robinson et al., 2014). Keeping in mind age-appropriateness, effective CSE should take a 'sex positive' approach to teaching curricula (having positive attitudes towards sexuality) that is scientifically accurate and non-judgemental (Australian Association for Adolescent Health Ltd, 2018). For effective implementation, CSE requires regular in-school lessons of 'sufficient duration and intensity', integrated within a 'whole school' approach. Teachers should have access to regular evidence-based professional development, and can also be supported to co-teach in partnership with sexual health professionals. Achieving sexual health literacy involves acquiring the sexual health knowledge, attitudes, behavioural intentions, personal skills and self-efficacy so that healthy behaviours are adopted within and beyond education settings (Yu, 2010). Cooperation between young people, families, schools, communities and health services is crucial to ensure the sustainability and ongoing success of CSE.

Effective strategies to support sexual health of adolescent girls

The World Bank's Diseases Control Priorities 3rd Edition (Bundy et al., 2017) present comprehensive evidence for a substantial return on investment when considering resourcing interventions that can (1) support adolescents to achieve their developmental potential, (2) improve their future health, and (3) the health of their children (the so-called triple dividend) (Bundy et al., 2018). Health education and health promotion through schools and the media (including sexual health and human papillomavirus [HPV] vaccination), and youth-friendly health services within and outside schools, are considered 'essential investments' in adolescence (Bundy et al., 2018).

Interventions to reduce sexually transmitted infections (STI), HIV, and unplanned pregnancy in adolescents, and to promote safe sex and sexual health more generally, may be set in schools or communities. School-based interventions range from educational programs (which may promote abstinence, or may teach knowledge, attitudes and skills to inform sexual decision-making) to health clinics in schools. Community interventions include media campaigns to increase knowledge or change norms, family programs to enhance parent–youth communication, STI/HIV testing at youth-friendly venues, positive youth development programs, peer education, primary care programs to assess and address risk, and cash transfer programs (both incentive-based and unconditional). Meta-analysis indicates that, with the exception of abstinence-only programs, most interventions have positive effects on behavioural and biological outcomes (Morales et al., 2018). Interventions most commonly found effective in reducing STI/HIV risk are behaviour change techniques (e.g., condom use skills-training, communication/negotiation skills training, cognitive-behaviour skills training), tailored by age/developmental stage, ethnicity/race and gender, and given in a supportive school environment and targeting immediate social influences (Protogerou & Johnson, 2014). Abstinence-based programs, which have been used widely in the U.S. and in parts of the developing world, show no positive effects on behavioural or biological outcomes (Morales et al., 2018). Technology-based interventions, such as information delivery by computer program, website, email or text message, show promise as an effective addition to the toolbox of interventions (Widman, Nesi, Kamke, Choukas-Bradley, & Stewart, 2018).

Digital health interventions hold particular promise for promoting the sexual health literacy of sexuality and gender diverse youth (Byron et al., 2016). As a result of isolation, stigmatisation and lack of relevant information provided at school, these young people are likely to seek sexual health information online (Steinke et al., 2017). Digital resources should offer diverse and comprehensive sexual health information that links mental and sexual health, and is not only risk focussed but also focusses on the strengths of these communities (Byron et al., 2016; Steinke et al., 2017). An example of a strengths-based mental health help-seeking digital tool in one Australian study is RAD Australia (currently an e-tool prototype), which is a peer-led user-driven online directory to support both LGBTIQ (lesbian, gay, bisexual, transgender, intersex, queer) young people's mental health and wellbeing, and the referral processes of health and community workers (Byron et al., 2016). Ideally these online interventions should complement rather than stand in for regular sexual health education strategies delivered in face-to-face environments, however this group are often ignored in educational interventions. These young people are heterogeneous and have distinct health concerns.

School-based sexual health vaccination programs targeting adolescents have been generally very successful when implemented in a mass program targeting the whole population (Cooper Robbins, Ward, & Skinner, 2011). Most recently we have seen the potential impact of school-based vaccination against a common STI, the human papillomavirus (HPV) (Patel et al., 2018). Australia and other high-income countries, like the UK, Canada and New Zealand, have population-level school-based vaccination of adolescents against HPV. These countries have achieved relatively high coverage, compared with countries using clinic-based programs (e.g., general practitioners), and have demonstrated substantial impacts on infection and HPV-related disease (Patel et al., 2018). The quadrivalent HPV vaccine, used in Australia between 2007–2017,[1] protects against most HPV infections leading to genital warts and at least 70% of infections leading to cervical, ano-genital and head and neck cancers. A nonavalent HPV vaccine is now used, offering additional protection against a further five cancer-causing HPV types, which should translate to protection against over 90% of cervical cancers in women and additional cancers in men.

As a result of over a decade of vaccinating young adolescents against HPV in Australia, genital warts, which was a common presenting complaint to sexual health clinics, is now rarely seen in vaccinated age groups (Patel et al., 2018). Rates of abnormal cervical smears among young women offered the vaccine have declined, as have cervical precancers (Patel et al., 2018). High uptake vaccination combined with high participation in cervical screening using highly sensitive and accurate HPV DNA testing technologies as first line screen, as is current practice in Australia and several other countries, is expected to lead to a marked decline in cervical cancer incidence in the next decade (Velentzis et al., 2019). Indeed, cervical cancer elimination as a public health issue is a tangible goal, as articulated by the World Health Organization (2018).

This example of success in STI prevention and women's sexual and reproductive health is due to the availability of a highly effective technology (the HPV vaccine) in combination with a highly effective public health intervention (school-based vaccination). School-based vaccination programs present many important lessons in how we can overcome stigma around STIs and access barriers to achieve protection of an entire population (Skinner & Cooper Robbins, 2010). Understanding how effective intervention programs work in the adolescent age group is critical in improving their health (Davies et al., 2017; Skinner et al., 2015).

Multi-strategy or multi-level interventions (e.g., comprehensive sex education and condom distribution and/or addressing individual, family and community factors) are considered to be the most effective approaches to promote adolescent sexual and reproductive health overall (Bowring, Wright, Douglass, Gold, & Lim, 2018; Patton et al., 2016). While school-based sexual health education has many merits, alone it is probably not effective in preventing STI/HIV or pregnancy in adolescents (Mason-Jones et al., 2016). However, combining education with contraceptive promotion (including contraceptive distribution) is effective in reducing pregnancy (Oringanje et al., 2009). Although community- and national-level programs are less studied than school-based programs, England's Teenage Pregnancy Strategy took a multicomponent whole-of-government approach to reduce unwanted adolescent parenthood and support teenage parents, with strong outcomes (Skinner & Marino, 2016; Wellings et al., 2016).

Adolescents' access to sexual and reproductive health services

Ensuring accessible health services for adolescents is not only a matter of equity, but also addresses a basic human right. Access to healthcare is essential to achieving sustainable development and to the realisation of optimal health and wellbeing, yet for many adolescents this remains a challenge. This is especially true in countries where adolescents are not permitted or encouraged to seek healthcare on their own behalf, but is seen even in parts of the world where legislation affords adolescents certain healthcare rights. Globally, the right of adolescents to healthcare has been articulated through a universal health coverage framework with accompanying guidelines for the development (World Health Organization, 2012) and implementation (World Health Organization, 2015) of standards for adolescent-friendly health services, including for sexual and reproductive health.

Adolescent girls' sexual and reproductive health is influenced by a range of social, cultural, political, legal, economic and structural factors and inequalities, which increase their barriers to accessing information and services (Svanemyr, Amin, Robles, & Greene, 2015). Their sexual behaviour is sanctioned in societies in a range of ways which can impact on the timely delivery of sexual healthcare. Their unique developmental characteristics may exacerbate feelings of self-consciousness, embarrassment and heightened concerns about confidentiality and privacy, leading to foregone care or unwillingness to disclose sensitive information (Patton et al., 2016). These contextual issues may also be reciprocated in health service provider attitudes, or to be perceived to be by adolescents (Robards et al., 2017).

Romantic relationships can result in distress and are a common reason for help-seeking. For example, among adolescent callers to an Australian national help-line, just under 10% were for concerns about romantic relationships (Price, Hides, Cockshaw, Staneva, & Stoyanov, 2016). Mental health concerns, including self-harm and suicidal ideation linked to their concerns, were frequently identified in this group. Younger adolescents typically report distress linked to relationship formation, while older adolescents experienced distress with relationship break-ups (Price et al., 2016). Attitudes of health service providers regarding adolescent relationship concerns, risk taking and sexual activity; difficulties communicating with adolescents; and concerns about managing parental involvement may restrict provision of optimal care (Kang & Sanci, 2013; Patton et al., 2016).

Structural barriers such as cost and availability of services (for example, location, closeness to transport and opening hours) are also particularly pertinent for adolescents as they may not have independent means of transport, and may face legal or administrative obstacles in accessing care on their own (Robards et al., 2017). Adolescents' relative inexperience in independently accessing healthcare and negotiating health systems, often in combination with lower health literacy, may exacerbate access barriers. Marginalised young people face additional access barriers to those which are common to all young people (Robards, Kang, Usherwood, & Sanci, 2018), as described further below.

Transgender girls can experience unique barriers to healthcare and sometimes challenging decision-making about their reproductive futures (Telfer et al., 2018b). Approaches to the healthcare of transgender and gender diverse girls are different across high-income countries and frequently politicised, which can result in stigma, discrimination and inequities. Many trans girls are unable to access the health services they require to achieve optimal health outcomes to support gender affirmation processes, such as psychosocial support, fertility counselling and preservation, and hormone blockers (gonadotropin-releasing hormone antagonists) to prevent pubertal bodily changes (Chew, Anderson, Williams, May, & Pang, 2018). Hormone blockers do not effect sperm production long-term, but use of oestrogen can cause infertility (RWH, 2014). In settings where fertility counselling and preservation is available, and if it is acceptable to trans girls, they can choose to preserve sperm, ideally before commencing hormone blockers (RWH, 2014). If hormone blocker treatment has commenced, trans girls can cease treatment (but may experience changes associated with male puberty), and after a number of months sperm production can resume (Royal Women's Hospital [RWH], 2014). A testicular biopsy can also be performed, but the results of this in conception of a child are experimental (RWH, 2014). Cost of healthcare services in settings without publicly funded gender clinical services for children and adolescents can operate as a barrier for young people and their families. Globally, in unsupportive settings, trans girls can experience violence, discrimination and limited or no gender-related healthcare. However, in supportive well-resourced healthcare settings, in which gold standard clinical guidelines and standards of care are implemented, trans girls can be empowered to make informed decisions about their sexual and reproductive futures (Telfer, Tollit, Pace, & Pang, 2018b).

Youth-friendly sexual and reproductive health services

Efforts must be made to increase both health service utilisation by and health service provision to adolescents (World Health Organization, 2012). A key approach is ensuring services are 'adolescent-friendly', meaning they are accessible, acceptable, appropriate, equitable and effective (Kang & Sanci, 2013; World Health Organization, 2012). Across all countries and service settings, young people value accessibility of healthcare (including location and affordability), staff attitudes, quality communication, medical competency, guideline-driven care including confidentiality, age-appropriate environments, being involved in decisions about healthcare, and health outcomes (Ambresin, Bennett, Patton, Sanci, & Sawyer, 2013). These aspects of care align with global frameworks on the promotion and provision of quality adolescent-friendly services (World Health Organization, 2012, 2015).

Strategies for increasing adolescent utilisation of services for sexual and reproductive health should include a combination of complementary approaches: welcoming facilities, communication and outreach activities to increase demand for services by adolescents, health workers who are trained and supported to work with adolescents, and community members who are supportive of health service provision to adolescents. Implementing this 'package of interventions' has been found to be successful in many settings, particularly in low- and middle-income countries (Chandra-Mouli, Lane, & Wong, 2015; Patton et al., 2016). To build the confidence and trust of adolescents in using health services, health workers should avoid making assumptions or judgements about young people, use inclusive and appropriate language, and provide assurances of confidentiality (Robinson et al., 2014). Training should include building health workers' confidence and skills in communicating effectively with young people, the consideration of legal issues related to adolescent sexual health, and refresher training on key sexual health issues for young people (Kang & Sanci, 2013; Sanci et al., 2015). To empower adolescents, increase their sense of ownership and ensure relevance and appropriateness of programs and services; adolescents should ideally be involved in the development, implementation and review of services (Braeken & Rondinelli, 2012).

Many gender and sexuality diverse young people frequently do not feel comfortable accessing services for sexual health needs due to experiences with or perceptions of health workers being homo/transphobic or being misinformed about gender and sexuality diversity (Fuzzell, Fedesco, Alexander, Fortenberry, & Shields, 2016; Robinson, 2013). This may include incorrect use of pronouns either in person or in referral/reminder letters; assuming a binary gender, or assuming heterosexual attraction or identity in consultations or on forms. Concerns about homophobia and/or transphobia may be heightened in the presence of mental health issues (Mustanski, Andrews, & Puckett, 2016); homelessness (McDonald,

2018; Snyder et al., 2016); refugee status or Aboriginal and Torres Strait Islander background (Ward et al., 2016); other diverse cultural backgrounds (Wong, Macpherson, Vahabi, & Li, 2017); regional or remote locations (Robards et al., 2017), and/or those with disabilities (McClelland et al., 2012).

In the Australian *Growing up Queer* study, most young people believed it necessary to discuss gender, sexuality or intersex status with health professionals (76%), yet 41% stated they had not engaged in such discussion, and only 46% of young people reported positive experiences if they had (Byron et al., 2016). In this same study, barriers to accessing healthcare reported by gender and sexuality diverse young people included fears of homophobia, transphobia and other discriminations, judgemental responses, gendered assumptions, concerns regarding confidentiality, and difficulties trusting health professionals (Byron et al., 2016). In a study with 51 young people from five countries in Southern Africa,[2] sexuality and gender diverse adolescents were frequently excluded from LGBT-specific sexual health services aimed at adults, while also being excluded from heteronormative sexual and reproductive health services (Müller, Spencer, Meer, & Daskilewicz, 2018). Restrictive legislative frameworks regulating same-sex activity, and/or laws that criminalise same sex behaviour regardless of enforcement, combined with the invisibility of sexual orientation and gender identity in current adolescent sexual and reproductive health policies, marginalise sexual and gender minority young people in Southern Africa. Criminalising minority identities is likely to lead to worse sexual and reproductive health outcomes, and mental health outcomes, for young people (Müller et al., 2018).

Health services can demonstrate inclusivity by visible symbols in countries where non-discrimination is protected by law. This may include: a rainbow symbol visible on the window from the outside of the service; inclusive use of language on service intake forms, websites, administrative systems and in policies; and offering staff professional development and training in the diversity of experiences across the spectrum of gender and sexuality (Byron et al., 2016). In addition, respectful communication, visible user-friendly opening hours and notification of bulk-billing (government subsidised service) can help to create an inclusive environment for young gender and sexuality diverse people (Kang & Sanci, 2013). In recent Australian studies, young people have indicated that they prefer to be asked about their sexuality and/or gender (including preferred pronoun use) by an informed health professional rather than raise this issue themselves (Robinson et al., 2014).

Conclusion

Adolescent sexual development, behaviour and health deserves further attention in the research context globally. We need to embed routine survey data collection on adolescent sexual and gender identities, behaviours, experiences, sexual health knowledge and attitudes, including the role of digital technologies in adolescent sexual health and development, across all countries. We also need to understand better how sexual health and development is linked to other experiences in early life and in adulthood. More in-depth work is required to better understand experiences of vulnerable adolescents, and changes in experience within shifting cultural and environmental contexts over time. A better knowledge of adolescent health and wellbeing pertaining to these key areas will assist in advocating for judicious resourcing of effective intervention programs.

Sexual and reproductive health and universal access to sexual and reproductive health and rights is a global aspiration as per the 2030 Agenda for Sustainable Development. This agenda emphasises reinforced efforts towards ensuring access to sexual and reproductive health and rights for all (United Nations, 2015). To realise this global vision of universal coverage, all young people must have access to quality, comprehensive information, education and health services to support their sexual and reproductive health, regardless of age, gender, marital status, cultural and gender or sexuality diversity. Whilst there is broad recognition of this and significant progress has been made in many parts of the world, adolescents continue to experience inequitable access to sexual and reproductive healthcare.

Notes

1 From 2018, Australia's national HPV vaccination program changed from the quadrivalent HPV vaccine to the 9-valent HPV vaccine.
2 In this study, Southern African countries included: Malawi, Mozambique, Namibia, Zambia, and Zimbabwe.

References

Ambresin, A., Bennett, K., Patton, G. C., Sanci, L. A., & Sawyer, S. M. (2013). Assessment of youth-friendly health care: A systematic review of indicators drawn from young people's perspectives. *Journal of Adolescent Health, 52,* 670–681.

Amo-Adjei, J. & Tuoyire, D. A. (2018). Timing of sexual debut among unmarried youths aged 15–24 years in Sub-Saharan Africa. *Journal of Biosocial Science, 50*(2), 161–177.

Australian Association for Adolescent Health Ltd (2018). *Comprehensive sexuality education in schools: Position paper.* Sydney, Australia: Author.

Australian Bureau of Statistics (2017). *Births, Australia, 2016.* Canberra, Australia: Author.

Australian Institute of Health and Welfare (2018). *Teenage mothers in Australia 2015.* Canberra, Australia: Author.

Blum, R. W., Mmari, K., & Moreau, C. (2017). It begins at 10: How gender expectations shape early adolescence around the world. *Journal of Adolescent Health, 61*(4S), S3–S4.

Bongaarts, J., Mensch, B., & Blanc, A. (2017). Trends in the age at reproductive transitions in the developing world: The role of education. *Population Studies, 71*(2), 139–154.

Bowring, A., Wright, C., Douglass, C., Gold, J., & Lim, M. (2018). Features of successful sexual health promotion programs for young people: Findings from a review of systematic reviews. *Health Promotion Journal of Australia, 29,* 46–57.

Braeken, D. & Rondinelli, I. (2012). Sexual and reproductive health needs of young people: Matching needs with systems. *International Journal of Gynecology and Obstetrics, 119,* S60–S63.

Bundy, D. A. A., de Silva, N., Horton, S., Jamison, D. T., & Patton, G. C. (2017). *Child and adolescent health and development.* Washington, DC: The World Bank.

Bundy, D. A. P., de Silva, N., Horton, S., Patton, G. C., Schultz, L., Jamison, D. T., & Disease Control Priorities-3 Child and Adolescent Health and Development Authors Group (2018). Investment in child and adolescent health and development: Key messages from disease control priorities, 3rd Edition. *Lancet, 391*(10121), 687–699.

Butler, J. (1990). *Gender trouble: Feminism and the subversion of identity.* New York, NY: Routledge.

Butler, J. (2004). *Undoing gender.* New York, NY: Routledge.

Byron, P., Rasmussen, S., Wright Toussaint, D., Lobo, R., Robinson, K. H., & Paradise, B. (2016). *"You learn from each other": LGBTIQ young people's mental health help-seeking and the RAD Australia online directory.* Sydney, Australia: Islandora Repository, Western Sydney University Research Collection. Retrieved from: https://researchdirect.westernsydney.edu.au/islandora/object/uws:38815.

Cabecinha, M., Mercer, C. H., Gravningen, K., Aicken, C., Jones, K. G., Tanton, C., Wellings, K., Sonnenberg, P., & Field, N. (2017). Finding sexual partners online: Prevalence and associations with sexual behaviour, STI diagnoses and other sexual health outcomes in the British population. *Sexually Transmitted Infections, 93*(8), 572–582.

Carmody, M. (2009). *Sex and ethics: Young people and sexual ethics.* Melbourne, Australia: Palgrave Macmillan.

Centers for Disease Control and Prevention (2018a). *Sexually transmitted disease surveillance 2017.* Atlanta, GA: Author. Retrieved from www.cdc.gov/std/stats17/default.htm.

Centers for Disease Control and Prevention (2018b). *Youth risk behavior survey data summary and trends report, 2007–2017.* Atlanta, GA: Author. Retrieved from www.cdc.gov/healthyyouth/data/yrbs/pdf/trendsreport.pdf.

Chandra-Mouli, V., Lane, C., & Wong, S. (2015). What does not work in adolescent sexual and reproductive health: A review of evidence on interventions commonly accepted as best practices. *Global Health: Science and Practice, 3*(3), 333–340.

Chew, D., Anderson, J., Williams, K., May, T., & Pang, K. C. (2018). Hormonal treatment in young people with gender dysphoria: A systematic review. *Pediatrics, 141*(4), pii: e20173742.

Cooper Robbins, C., Ward, K., & Skinner, S. R. (2011). School-based vaccination: A systematic review of process evaluations. *Vaccine, 29*(52), 9588–9599.

Crone, E. A., van Duijvenvoorde, A. C. K., & Peper, J. S. (2016). Annual research review: Neural contributions to risk-taking in adolescence – developmental changes and individual differences. *Journal of Child Psychology and Psychiatry, 57*(3), 353–368.

Dahl, R. E., Allen, N. B., Wilbrecht, L., & Suleiman, A. B. (2018). Importance of investing in adolescence from a developmental science perspective. *Nature, 554,* 441.

Davies, C. (2014). Approaches: Working positively with sexual and gender diversity in schools. In P. Aggleton (Ed.), *Education and sexualities* (Vol. 4, pp. 109–116). Abingdon, UK: Routledge.

Davies, C., Metcalf, A., Robinson, K. H., Bansel, P., Denson, N., & Ovenden, G. (2014). *Intentional self-harm and suicidal behaviour in children. Submission to the Australian Human Rights Commission, National Children's Commissioner.* Sydney, Australia: Australian Human Rights Commission. Retrieved from www.humanrights.gov.au/our-work/childrens-rights/projects/intentional-self-harm-and-suicidal-behaviour-children.

Davies, C. & Robinson, K. (2010). Hatching babies and stork deliveries: Risk and regulation in the construction of children's sexual knowledge. *Contemporary Issues in Early Childhood, 11*(3), 249–263.

Davies, C., Skinner, S. R., Stoney, T., Marshall, H. S., Collins, J., Jones, H., Hutton, H., Parrella, A., Cooper, S., Mcgeechan, K., & Zimet, G. (2017). Is it like one of those infectious kind of things? The importance of educating young people about HPV and HPV vaccination at school. *Sex Education, 17*(3), 256–275.

Ela, E. J. & Budnick, J. (2017). Non-heterosexuality, relationships, and young women's contraceptive behavior. *Demography, 54,* 887–909.

Ezer, P., Jones, T., Fisher, C., & Power, J. (2018). A critical discourse analysis of sexuality education in the Australian curriculum. *Sex Education.* Published online ahead of print: doi:10.1080/14681811.2018.1553709.

Finer, L. B. & Philbin, J. M. (2014). Trends in ages at key reproductive transitions in the United States, 1951–2010. *Women's Health Issues, 24*(3), e271–279.

Foucault, M. (1972). *The archaeology of knowledge and the discourse on language* [translated from the French by A.M. Sheridan Smith]. New York, NY: Pantheon Books.

Foucault, M. (1978). *The history of sexuality: An introduction* (Vol. 1). London, UK: Penguin.

Furman, W. & Rose, A. J. (2015). Friendships, romantic relationships, and peer relationships. In R. M. Lerner & M. E. Lamb (Eds), *Handbook of child psychology and developmental science: Socioemotional processes* (Vol. 3, 7th ed., pp. 1–43). Hoboken, NJ: John Wiley.

Furman, W. & Shaffer, L. (2003). The role of romantic relationships in adolescent development. In P. Florsheim (Ed.), *Adolescent romantic relations and sexual behaviour* (pp. 2–22). Mahwah, NJ: Lawrence Erlbaum Associates.

Fuzzell, L., Fedesco, H. N., Alexander, S. C., Fortenberry, J. D., & Shields, C. G. (2016). "I just think that doctors need to ask more questions": Sexual minority and majority adolescents; experiences talking about sexuality with healthcare providers. *Patient Education and Counseling, 99*(9), 1467–1472.

Geary, R., Tanton, C., Erens, B., Clifton, S., Prah, P., Wellings, K., Mitchell, K. R., Datta, J., Gravningen, K., Fuller, E., Johnson, A. M., Sonnenberg, P., & Mercer, C. (2018). Sexual identity, attraction and behaviour in Britain: The implications of using different dimensions of sexual orientation to estimate the size of sexual minority populations and inform public health interventions. *PLoS One, 13*(1), e0189607.

Hamilton, B. & Mathews, T. (2016). *Continued declines in teen births in the United States, 2015.* Atlanta, GA: Centers for Disease Control and Prevention. Retrieved from www.cdc.gov/nchs/data/databriefs/db259.pdf.

Heywood, W., Patrick, K., Smith, A. M., & Pitts, M. K. (2015). Associations between early first sexual intercourse and later sexual and reproductive outcomes. *Archives of Sexual Behavior, 44*(3), 531–569.

Inchley, J., Currie, D., Young, T., Samdal, O., Torsheim, T., Auguston, L., Mathison, F., Aleman-Diaz, A., Molcho, M., Weber, M., & Barnekow, V. (2016). *Growing up unequal: Gender and socioeconomic differences in young people's health and well-being*. Copenhagen, Denmark: World Health Organization. Retrieved from www.euro.who.int/__data/assets/pdf_file/0003/303438/HSBC-No.7-Growing-up-unequal-Full-Report.pdf.

Jagose, A. (1996). *Queer theory: An introduction*. New York, NY: New York University Press.

Kagesten, A., Gibbs, S., Blum, R. W., Moreau, C., Chandra-Mouli, V., Herbert, A., & Amin, A. (2016). Understanding factors that shape gender attitudes in early adolescence globally: A mixed-methods systematic review. *PLoS One, 11*(6), e0157805.

Kahn, N. F. & Halpern, C. T. (2018). Associations between patterns of sexual initiation, sexual partnering, and sexual health outcomes from adolescence to early adulthood. *Archives of Sexual Behavior, 47*(6), 1791–1810.

Kang, M. & Sanci, L. (2013). Youth friendly practice. In M. Kang, S. R. Skinner, L. Sanci, & S. Sawyer (Eds), *Youth health and adolescent medicine* (pp. 51–56). Melbourne, Australia: IP Communications.

Kann, L., McManus, T., Harris, W. A., Shanklin, S. L., Flint, K. H., Queen, B., Lowry, R., Chyen, D., Whittle, L., Thornton, J., Lim, C., Bradford, D., Yamakawa, Y., Leon, M., Brener, N., & Ethier, K. A. (2018). Youth risk behavior surveillance: United States, 2017. *MMWR Surveillance Summaries, 67*(SS–8), 1–114.

The Kirby Institute (2018). *HIV, viral hepatitis and sexually transmissible infections in Australia: Annual surveillance report 2017*. Kensington, NSW, Australia: Author. Retrieved from https://kirby.unsw.edu.au/sites/default/files/kirby/report/SERP_Annual-Surveillance-Report-2017_compressed.pdf.

Kleppa, E., Holmen, S., Lillebø, K., Kjetland, E., Gundersen, S., Taylor, M., Moodley, P., & Onsrud, M. (2015). Cervical ectopy: Associations with sexually transmitted infections and HIV. A cross-sectional study of high school students in rural South Africa. *Sexually Transmitted Infections, 91*(2), 124–129.

Korchmaros, J. D., Ybarra, M. L., & Mitchell, K. J. (2015). Adolescent online romantic relationship initiation: Differences by sexual and gender identification. *Journal of Adolescence, 40*, 54–64.

Kost, K., Maddow-Zimet, I., & Arpaia, A. (2017). *Pregnancies, births and abortions among adolescents and young women in the United States, 2013: National and state trends by age, race and ethnicity*. New York, NY: The Guttmacher Institute. Retrieved from www.guttmacher.org/report/us-teen-pregnancy-state-trends-2011.

Leahy, D., O'Flynn, G., & Wright, J. (2013). A critical 'critical inquiry' proposition in health and physical education. *Asia-Pacific Journal of Health, Sport and Physical Education, 4*(2), 175–187.

Lewis, L., Mooney-Somers, J. M., Guy, R., Watchirs Smith, L., & Skinner, S. R. (2018). "I see it everywhere …", young Australians unintended exposure to sexual content online. *Sexual Health, 15*(4), 335–341.

Lewis, R., Tanton, C., Mercer, C. H., Mitchell, K. R., Palmer, M., Macdowall, W., & Wellings, K. (2017). Heterosexual practices among young people in Britain: Evidence from three national surveys of sexual attitudes and lifestyles. *Journal of Adolescent Health, 61*(6), 694–702.

Lindberg, L. D. & Maddow-Zimet, I. (2012). Consequences of sex education on teen and young adult sexual behaviors and outcomes. *Journal of Adolescent Health, 51*, 332–338.

Lyons, A. C. (2009). Masculinities, femininities, behaviour and health. *Social and Personality Psychology Compass, 3*(4), 394–412.

Marino, J. L., Skinner, S. R., Doherty, D. A., Rosenthal, S. L., Cooper Robbins, S. C., Cannon, J., & Hickey, M. (2013). Age at menarche and age at first sexual intercourse: A prospective cohort study. *Pediatrics, 132*(6), 1028–1036.

Mason-Jones, A. J., Sinclair, D., Mathews, C., Kagee, A., Hillman, A., & Lombard, C. (2016). School-based interventions for preventing HIV, sexually transmitted infections, and pregnancy in adolescents. *Cochrane Database Systematic Review, 11*, CD006417.

McClelland, A., Flicker, S., Nepveux, D., Nixon, S., Vo, T., Wilson, C., & Proudfoot, D. (2012). Seeking safer sexual spaces: Queer and trans young people labeled with intellectual disabilities and the paradoxical risks of restriction. *Journal of Homosexuality, 59*(6), 808–819.

McDonald, K. (2018). Social support and mental health in LGBTQ adolescents: A review of the literature. *Issues in Mental Health Nursing, 39*(1), 16–29.

Meier, A. & Allen, G. (2009). Romantic relationships from adolescence to young adulthood: Evidence from the national longitudinal study of adolescent health. *The Sociological Quarterly, 50*(2), 308–335.

Mitchell, A., Patrick, K., Heywood, W., Blackman, P., & Pitts, M. (2014). *5th national survey of Australian secondary students and sexual health 2013*. Melbourne, Australia: Australian Research Centre in Sex, Health, and Society, Latrobe University. Retrieved from https://yeah.org.au/wp-content/uploads/2014/10/31631-ARCSHS_NSASSSH_FINAL-A-3.pdf.

Morales, A., Espada, J., Orgiles, M., Escribano, S., Johnson, B., & Lightfoot, M. (2018). Interventions to reduce risk for sexually transmitted infections in adolescents: A meta-analysis of trials, 2008–2016. *PLoS One, 13*(6), e0199421.

Müller, A., Spencer, S., Meer, T., & Daskilewicz, K. (2018). The no-go zone: A qualitative study of access to sexual and reproductive health services for sexual and gender minority adolescents in Southern Africa. *Reproductive Health, 15*(1), 12.

Mustanski, B., Andrews, R., & Puckett, J. A. (2016). The effects of cumulative victimization on mental health among lesbian, gay, bisexual, and transgender adolescents and young adults. *American Journal of Public Health, 106*(3), 527–533.

Office for National Statistics (2017). *Sexual identity, UK: 2016*. Newport, UK: Author. Retrieved from www.ons.gov.uk/peoplepopulationandcommunity/culturalidentity/sexuality/bulletins/sexualidentityuk/2016.

Oringanje, C., Meremikwu, M. M., Eko, H., Esu, E., Meremikwu, A., & Ehiri, J. E. (2009). Interventions for preventing unintended pregnancies among adolescents. *Cochrane Database of Systematic Reviews, 7*(4), CD005215.

Patel, C., Brotherton, J. M., Pillsbury, A., Jayasinghe, S., Donovan, B., Macartney, K., & Marshall, H. (2018). The impact of 10 years of human papillomavirus (HPV) vaccination in Australia: What additional disease burden will a nonavalent vaccine prevent? *Eurosurveillance, 23*(41), 1700737.

Patterson, J. & Jabson, J. (2018). Sexual orientation measurement and chronic disease disparities: National Health and Nutrition Examination Survey, 2009–2014. *Annals of Epidemiology, 28*(2), 72–86.

Patton, G. C., Olsson, C. A., Skirbekk, V., Saffery, R., Wlodek, M. E., Azzopardi, P. S., Stonawski, M., Rasmussen, B., Spry, E., Francis, K., Bhutta, Z. A., Kassebaum, N. J., Mokdad, A. H., Murray, C. J. L., Prentice, A. M., Reavley, N., Sheehan, P., Sweeny, K., Viner, R. M., & Sawyer, S. M. (2018). Adolescence and the next generation. *Nature, 554*(7693), 458–466.

Patton, G. C., Sawyer, S. M., Santelli, J. S., Ross, D. A., Afifi, R., Allen, N. B., Arora, M., Azzopardi, P., Baldwin, W., Bonell, C., Kakuma, R., Kennedy, E., Mahon, J., McGovern, T., Mokdad, A. H., Patel, V., Petroni, S., Reavley, N., Taiwo, K., Waldfogel, J., Wickremarathne, D., Barroso, C., Bhutta, Z., Fatusi, A. O., Mattoo, A., Diers, J., Fang, J., Ferguson, J., Ssewamala, F., & Viner, R. M. (2016). Our future: A *Lancet* commission on adolescent health and wellbeing. *Lancet, 387*, 2423–2478.

Price, M., Hides, L., Cockshaw, W., Staneva, A. A., & Stoyanov, S. R. (2016). Young love: Romantic concerns and associated mental health issues among adolescent help-seekers. *Behavioral Sciences (Basel), 6*(2), pii: E9.

Protogerou, C. & Johnson, B. T. (2014). Success of behavioral HIV-prevention interventions for adolescents: A meta-review. *AIDS Behavior, 18*, 1847–1863.

Renold, E. (2005). *Girls, boys, and junior sexualities: Exploring children's gender and sexual relations in the primary school*. Abingdon, UK: Routledge.

Rissel, C., Heywood, W., de Visser, R. O., Simpson, J. M., Grulich, A. E., Badcock, P. B., Smith, A. M., & Richters, J. (2014). First vaginal intercourse and oral sex among a representative sample of Australian adults: The second Australian study of health and relationships. *Sexual Health, 11*(5), 406–415.

Robards, F., Kang, M., Sanci, L., Steinbeck, K., Jan, S., Hawke, C., & Usherwood, T. (2017). *Access 3: Young people's healthcare journeys, preliminary report*. Sydney, NSW, Australia: The University of Sydney. Retrieved from https://sydney.edu.au/medicine-health/schools/sydney-medical-school/discipline-of-general-practice.html.

Robards, F., Kang, M., Usherwood, T., & Sanci, L. (2018). How marginalized young people access, engage with, and navigate health-care systems in the digital age: Systematic review. *Journal of Adolescent Health, 62*(4), 365–381.

Robinson, K. H. (2013). *Innocence, knowledge and the construction of childhood: The contradictory nature of sexuality and censorship in children's contemporary lives*. Abingdon, UK: Routledge.

Robinson, K. H., Bansel, P., Denson, N., Ovenden, G., & Davies, C. (2014). *Growing up queer: Issues facing young Australians who are gender variant and sexuality diverse.* Bundoora, VIC, Australia: Rainbow Health Victoria, La Trobe University. Retrieved from www.glhv.org.au/sites/default/files/Growin g_Up_Queer2014.pdf.

Robinson, K. H. & Davies, C. (2017). Sexuality education in early childhood. In L. Allen & M. Rasmussen (Eds), *Handbook of sexuality education* (pp. 217–242). London, UK: Palgrave.

Robinson, K. H. & Davies, C. (2018a). A history of constructions of child and youth sexualities, and the construction of the normative citizen subject. In S. Talburt (Ed.), *Youth sexualities: Public feelings and contemporary cultural politics* (Vol. 1, pp. 3–30). Westport, CT: Praeger.

Robinson, K. H. & Davies, C. (2018b). A sociological exploration of childhood sexuality: A discursive analysis of parents' and children's perspectives. In J. G. S. Lamb (Ed.), *The Cambridge handbook of sexual development: Childhood and adolescence* (pp. 54–75). Cambridge, UK: Cambridge University Press.

Robinson, K. H. & Jones Díaz, C. (2016). *Diversity and difference in early childhoods: Implication for theory and practice.* Milton Keynes, UK: Open University Press.

Robinson, K. H., Smith, E., & Davies, C. (2017). Responsibilities, tensions and ways forward: Parents' perspectives on children's sexuality education. *Sex Education, 17*(3), 333–347.

Royal Women's Hospital (2014). *Can I still have children? Information for young people using oestrogen* (2nd ed.). Gender Service, Royal Children's Hospital and the Women's Consumer Health Information team, Melbourne, Australia: Royal Women's Hospital Andrology Unit and Reproductive Services.

Sanci, L. A., Chondros, P., Sawyer, S. M., Pirkis, J., Ozer, E., Hegarty, K., Yang, F., Grabsch, B., Shiell, A., Cahill, H., Ambresin, A. E., Patterson, E., & Patton, G. C. (2015). Responding to young people's health risks in primary care: A cluster randomised trial of training clinicians in screening and motivational interviewing. *PLoS One, 10*(9), e0137581.

Santhya, K. G. & Jejeebhoy, S. J. (2015). Sexual and reproductive health and rights of adolescent girls: Evidence from low- and middle-income countries. *Global Public Health, 10*(2), 189–221.

Seiffge-Krenke, I. (2003). Testing theories of romantic development from adolescence to young adulthood: Evidence of a developmental sequence. *International Journal of Behavioral Development, 27*(6), 519–531.

Skinner, S. R. & Cooper Robbins, S. C. (2010). Voluntary school-based human papillomavirus vaccination: An efficient and acceptable model for achieving high vaccine coverage in adolescents. *Journal of Adolescent Health, 47*(3), 215–218.

Skinner, S. R., Davies, C., Cooper, S., Stoney, T., Marshall, H., Zimet, G., & McGeechan, K. (2015). HPV.edu study protocol: A cluster randomised controlled evaluation of education, decisional support and logistical strategies in school-based Human Papillomavirus (HPV) Vaccination of adolescents. *BMC Public Health, 15*(1), 896.

Skinner, S. R. & Marino, J. L. (2016). England's teenage pregnancy strategy: A hard-won success. *Lancet, 388*(10044), 538–540.

Skinner, S. R., Marino, J. L., Rosenthal, S. L., Cannon, J., Doherty, D. A., & Hickey, M. (2017). Prospective cohort study of childhood behaviour problems and adolescent sexual risk-taking: Gender matters. *Sexual Health, 14*(6), 492–501.

Skinner, S. R., Robinson, M., Smith, M. A., Robbins, S. C., Mattes, E., Cannon, J., Rosenthal, S. L., Marino, J. L., Hickey, M., & Doherty, D. A. (2015). Childhood behavior problems and age at first sexual intercourse: A prospective birth cohort study. *Pediatrics, 135*(2), 255–263.

Smith, E., Jones, T., Ward, R., Dixon, J., Mitchell, A., & Hillier, L. (2014). *From blues to rainbows: Mental health and wellbeing of gender diverse and transgender young people in Australia.* Hawthorn, VIC, Australia: Beyond Blue. Retrieved from www.beyondblue.org.au/docs/default-source/research-project-files/bw0268-from-blues-to-rainbows-report-final-report.pdf?sfvrsn=2.

Smith, L. W., Liu, B., Degenhardt, L., Patton, G., Richters, J., Wand, H., Cross, D., Hocking, J. S., Skinner, S. R., Cooper, S., Lumby, C., Kaldor, J. M., Guy, R., & Lumby, C. (2016). Is sexual content in new media linked to sexual risk behaviour in young people? A systematic review and meta-analysis. *Sexual Health, 13*(6), 501–515, doi:10.1071/SH16037.

Snyder, S. M., Hartinger-Saunders, R., Brezina, T., Beck, E., Wright, E. R., Forge, N., & Bride, B. E. (2016). Homeless youth, strain, and justice system involvement: An application of general strain theory. *Children and Youth Services Review, 62*, 90–96.

Steinke, J., Root-Bowman, M., Estabrook, S., Levine, D. S., & Kantor, L. M. (2017). Meeting the needs of sexual and gender minority youth: Formative research on potential digital health interventions. *Journal of Adolescent Health, 60*(5), 541–548.

Svanemyr, J., Amin, A., Robles, O. J., & Greene, M. E. (2015). Creating an enabling environment for adolescent sexual and reproductive health: A framework and promising approaches. *Journal of Adolescent Health*, *56*, S7–S14.

Telfer, M., Kelly, F., Feldman, D., Stone, G., Robertson, R., & Poulakis, Z. (2018a). Transgender adolescents and legal reform: How improved access to healthcare was achieved through medical, legal and community collaboration. *Journal of Paediatrics and Child Health*, *54*(10), 1096–1099.

Telfer, M. M., Tollit, M. A., Pace, C. C., & Pang, K. C. (2018b). Australian standards of care and treatment guidelines for trans and gender diverse children and adolescents. *Medical Journal of Australia*, *209* (3), 132–136.

Twenge, J. M., Sherman, R. A., & Wells, B. E. (2017). Sexual inactivity during young adulthood is more common among U.S. millennials and iGen: Age, period, and cohort effects on having no sexual partners after age 18. *Archives of Sexual Behavior*, *46*(2), 433–440.

United Nations (2015). *Transforming our world: The 2030 agenda for sustainable development*. New York, NY: Author. Retrieved from https://sustainabledevelopment.un.org/post2015/transformingourworld.

United Nations Educational Scientific and Cultural Organization (UNESCO) (2018). *International technical guidance on sexuality education: An evidence-informed approach*. Geneva, Switzerland: Author.

United Nations Population Fund (2014). *UNFPA operational guidance for comprehensive sexuality education: A focus on human rights and gender*. New York, NY: Author. Retrieved from www.unfpa.org/sites/default/files/pub-pdf/UNFPA_OperationalGuidance_WEB3.pdf.

Van Ouytsel, J., Van Gool, E., Walrave, M., Ponnet, K., & Peeters, E. (2016). Exploring the role of social networking sites within adolescent romantic relationships and dating experiences. *Computers in Human Behavior*, *55*, 76–86.

Velentzis, L. S., Smith, M. A., Simms, K. T., Lew, J. B., Hall, M., Hughes, S., Yuilla, S., Killen, J., Keane, A., Butler, K., Darlington-Brown, J., Hui, H., Brotherton, J. M. L., Skinner, R., Brand, A., Roeske, L., Heley, S., Carter, J., Bateson, D., Frazer, I., Garland, S. M., Guy, R., Hammond, I., Grogan, P., Arbyn, M., Castle, P. E., Saville, M., Armstrong, B. K., & Canfell, K. (2019). Pathways to a cancer-free future: A protocol for modelled evaluations to maximize the future impact of interventions on cervical cancer in Australia. *Gynecologic Oncology*, *152*(1), 465–471.

Ward, J., Wand, H., Bryant, J., Delaney-Thiele, D., Worth, H., Pitts, M., & Kaldor, J. (2016). Prevalence and correlates of a diagnosis of sexually transmitted infection among young Aboriginal and Torres Strait Islander people: A national survey. *Sexually Transmitted Diseases*, *43*(3), 177–184.

Wellings, K., Palmer, M., Geary, R., Gibson, L., Copas, A., Datta, J., Glasier, A., Scott, R. H., Mercer, C. H., Erens, B., Macdowall, W., French, R. S., Jones, K., Johnson, A. M., Tanton, C., & Wilkinson, P. (2016). Changes in conceptions in women younger than 18 years and the circumstances of young mothers in England in 2000–12: An observational study. *Lancet*, *388*, 586–595.

Widman, L., Nesi, J., Kamke, K., Choukas-Bradley, S., & Stewart, J. (2018). Technology-based interventions to reduce sexually transmitted infections and unintended pregnancy among youth. *Journal of Adolescent Health*, *62*, 651–660.

Williams, H., Kang, M., & Skinner, S. R. (2013). Sexual and reproductive health. In R. S. S. M. Kang, L. A. Sanci, & S. M. Sawyer (Eds), *Youth health and adolescent medicine* (pp. 192–214). Melbourne, Australia: IP Communications.

Wolff, M., Wells, B., Ventura-DiPersia, C., Renson, A., & Grov, C. (2017). Measuring sexual orientation: A review and critique of U.S. data collection efforts and implications for health policy. *Journal of Sex Research*, *54*, 4–5.

Wong, J. P., Macpherson, F., Vahabi, M., & Li, A. (2017). Understanding the sexuality and sexual health of Muslim young people in Canada and other Western countries: A scoping review of research literature. *The Canadian Journal of Human Sexuality*, *26*(1), 48–59.

Wood, R., Hirst, J., Wilson, L., & Burns-O'Connell, G. (2019). The pleasure imperative? Reflecting on sexual pleasure's inclusion in sex education and sexual health. *Sex Education*, *19*(1), 1–14.

World Health Organization (WHO) (2012). *Making health services adolescent friendly*. Geneva, Switzerland: Author. Retrieved from www.who.int/maternal_child_adolescent/documents/adolescent_friendly_services/en.

World Health Organization (WHO) (2014). *Health for the world's adolescents. A second chance in the second decade*. Geneva, Switzerland: Author. Retrieved from www.who.int/maternal_child_adolescent/documents/second-decade/en.

World Health Organization (WHO) (2015). *Global standards for quality health services for adolescents.* Geneva, Switzerland: Author. Retrieved from www.who.int/maternal_child_adolescent/documents/global-standards-adolescent-care/en.

World Health Organization (WHO) (2018). *Director-general calls for all countries to take action to help end the suffering caused by cervical cancer.* Geneva, Switzerland: World Health Organization. Retrieved from www.who.int/reproductivehealth/call-to-action-elimination-cervical-cancer/en.

Yu, J. (2010). Sex education beyond school: Implications for practice and research. *Sex Education, 10*(2), 187–199.

Zucker, K. (2017). Epidemiology of gender dysphoria and transgender identity. *Sexual Health, 14*(5), 404–411.

27

OLDER WOMEN AND SEXUAL HEALTH

Social, relational and medical considerations

Camille J. Interligi and Maureen C. McHugh

Older women's sexual health remains a topic of quiet contention and debate globally where evidence of aging women's sexual variability is ceaselessly countered by cultural images of decline, disease, and dysfunction. We define "older women" as postmenopausal women over the age of 60. Though recent research shows that older women around the globe do, in fact, experience sexual desire and remain sexually active into their later years (Hebernick et al., 2010; Lusti-Narasimhan & Beard, 2013; Schick et al., 2010), they are still offered limited and sometimes competing cultural messages concerning their sexuality (McHugh & Interligi, 2015). In contrast to the decline expected of them, older women tend to be satisfied with their sex lives and report moderate-to-high levels of sexual well-being regardless of age-related sexual changes (Field et al., 2013; Mazo & Cardoso, 2011; Santos-Iglesias, Byers, & Moglia, 2016; Wang et al., 2014; Watson, Stelle, & Bell, 2017). Sexually active, unpartnered older women may be considered "exceptions to the norm" and ostracized for their apparent deviance (Montemurro & Siefken, 2014, p. 41), while single older women—like their peers in romantic relationships—report positive attitudes toward aging and sexuality, high sexual satisfaction, and high sexual self-esteem (Fileborn, Thorpe, Hawkes, Minichiello, & Pitt, 2015a).

Despite clear evidence of their varied sexualities, older women are still largely devalued as sexual beings. Declines in sexual attractiveness, desire, and responsiveness are typically viewed as an unavoidable consequence of menopause, which de facto implies declines in sexual behavior and sexual health (McHugh & Interligi, 2015). Yet, older women continue to participate in and enjoy sex. Contrary to stereotypes, research does not solely document decline in older women's sexual response. Studies have demonstrated stability, increases, and other variations in sexual interest and activity during the aging process (McHugh, 2006; McHugh & Interligi, 2015). Between one quarter and one third of women feel more positive about their sexuality and more comfortable in their bodies after menopause (Dillaway, 2005; Koch, Manfield, Thurau, & Carey, 2005). Many older women view sex as important in their relationships, and that importance is a predictor of sustained sexual activity in older adulthood (Ussher, Perz, & Parton, 2015). This holds true for both heterosexual and lesbian women (Ussher et al., 2015). Even in the absence of partnered sex or romantic relationships, older women continue to view themselves as sexual beings (Watson et al., 2017) and engage in solo masturbation (DeLamater & Koepsel, 2015).

However, sexual health includes components beyond sexual activity. The World Health Organization (2006) has defined sexual health as

> a state of physical, emotional, mental and social well-being in relation to sexuality; it is not merely the absence of disease, dysfunction or infirmity. Sexual health requires a positive and respectful approach to sexuality and sexual relationships, as well as the possibility of having pleasurable and safe sexual experiences, free of coercion, discrimination and violence. For sexual health to be attained and maintained, the sexual rights of all persons must be respected, protected and fulfilled.

These sexual rights, as outlined by WHO (2006), include (but are not limited to): (1) "the rights to equality and non-discrimination"; (2) "the rights to information, as well as education"; (3) "the rights to freedom of opinion and expression"; and (4) "the right to an effective remedy for violations of fundamental rights." In this chapter, we ask: Are older women granted these sexual rights? Are they able to achieve sexual health? Do WHO (2006) guidelines forward an inclusive, intersectional, feminist vision of sexual health? And, if not, what "effective remedies" could be used to address these problems? To address these questions, we explore some of the obstacles and options afforded to older women within three arenas of sexual health: the sociopolitical, the relational, and the medical.

The personal is (socio)political

The "achievement" of sexual health is tied to individuals' sexualities, a comprehensive definition of which moves beyond sexual activity and behavior. Research on older women's sexualities has historically adopted a sex-negative approach that perpetuates limited and stereotypical narratives. Common research questions focus on libidinal decline with age, and concerns about (adequate) levels of (hetero)sexual activity, desire, or satisfaction. These markers, which have been deemed *the* defining and important aspects of sexuality, are based on heteronormative and androcentric notions of what "sexuality" is. According to WHO (2006),

> sexuality is experienced and expressed in thoughts, fantasies, desires, beliefs, attitudes, values, behaviours, practices, roles and relationships. While sexuality can include all of these dimensions, not all of them are always experienced or expressed. Sexuality is influenced by the interaction of biological, psychological, social, economic, political, cultural, legal, historical, religious and spiritual factors.

In many cultures, older women's sexualities are informed by sociopolitical systems that perpetuate agism, androcentrism, and heteronormativity. Unfortunately, this reality leaves many older women with rigid, limited, and unfulfilling possibilities for sexual expression, education, and agency.

According to WHO (2006), for individuals to experience sexual health, they must also experience equality and non-discrimination related to their sexual expression. Unfortunately, older women's sexualities are broadly culturally, socially, and systemically policed. Older women face multiple layers of discrimination regarding their sexual lives. As noted by Ussher et al. (2015), "sociocultural discourses shape women's construction of the experience of sex and aging, telling us what is normal and abnormal, which can profoundly impact sexual well being" (p. 451). These discourses include: The *unsexy/asexual* discourse, in which older women are viewed as existing in a state of sexual decline, without interest in/desire for/ability to engage in sexual activity; the *sexy oldie* discourse, in which older adults are expected to remain sexually active in order to be viewed as maintaining vitality and health in the face of aging; the *medicalized* discourse, in which older women's interest in sex is labelled as sexual dysfunction if it is "too low"; the *labor of love/dutiful wife* discourse, in which it is incumbent upon older, heterosexual, married women to attend to and take responsibility for the quality of the sexual relationship; and the *cougar* discourse, in which older, unmarried women are ridiculed for daring to dress provocatively or pursue sex with younger men (Interligi & McHugh, 2017). These discourses are transmitted through spoken and written language (e.g., in informal conversation, in popular media, in formal written communications), and are extremely powerful in shaping the ways in which older women are "allowed" to engage sexually (Interligi & McHugh, 2017). Within these myriad confines and contradictions, older women often find themselves working to achieve a femininity that is "appropriate" for their age, in both appearance and behavior. For example, in an ethnographic study of women in their 50s taking salsa dance classes, participants described becoming increasingly interested in clothes and dressing in clothes that were "feminine" and "fitted" both in and outside of their classes (Milton, 2016). However, these women were also wary of being perceived as libidinous; participants described working hard to ensure that their movement, touch, and body language while dancing was not experienced by their male partners as sexual. The exclusion of older women from sexual participation is further apparent in the construction of physical spaces. Milton (2016) highlighted the ways that social spaces reflect a particular hierarchy of gender, sex, and sexuality (among other variables). Many social spaces that serve the function of partner seeking and embodiment of sexuality (e.g., clubs, bars) are viewed as for—and largely inhabited by—young adults. These spaces may leave older adults feeling "out of place," thus reinforcing the distance between older adulthood and sexuality.

Older women's intersecting identities can qualify, compound, and/or exacerbate the cultural narratives and socially-sanctioned oppressions they face related to sexual expression. Older women of color, LGBTQIA2S+ older women, mentally/physically disabled older women, and working class/poor older women—as well as older women who inhabit other marginalized identities—experience further discrimination regarding their sex lives. For example, older adults who live in care homes due to severe illness or disability face multiple layers of assumptions regarding their sexualities. Research demonstrates that care home workers tend to think of and react to their disabled residents as asexual and that learning to understand and appropriately oversee the expression of these individuals' intimate or sexual needs is experienced by workers as a challenge (Rushbrooke, Murray, & Townsend, 2014). This is related to inherent cultural bias against the perception of disabled persons as sexual beings, as well as larger, systemic oppression of intellectually disabled individuals as evidenced by the facility's policy (or lack thereof). A survey of 175 long-term care facility medical directors demonstrated that only 13% of care homes provided training for staff regarding how to address sexual behavior in the care home, only 20% of care homes had a policy regarding residents' ability to consent to sexual activity, and only 23% had any policy on sexual/intimate behavior (Society for Post-Acute and Long-Term Care Medicine, 2016). Simpson and colleagues (Simpson et al., 2015, p. 243) presented data from a number of studies that highlight the ways older adults in the UK's care homes experience "ageist erotophobia" (i.e., discrimination regarding sexuality based on advanced age). They contended that care home policies and procedures perpetuate a view of older adults' sexuality as limited/nonexistent as a result of physical and mental decline.

Older women with non-heteronormative sexuality identities face the "triple invisibility" of age, gender, and sexual orientation (Phillips & Marks, 2006). Often, older women with "alternative" sexualities are forced into hiding—either as a deliberate act of self-preservation in response to discrimination, or as a byproduct of care home or senior center procedures that presume heterosexuality (e.g., not asking residents about sexual orientation during assessments; Willis et al., 2013).

Older women are also at a disadvantage regarding the necessary "right to information, as well as education" upon which the WHO (2006) definition of sexual health depends. Accurate and inclusive sex education for older women is not widely available, with some older women not having received helpful sexual information at any time in their lives (McHugh & Interligi, 2015). For example, women over 80 may not have received even basic information about sexuality in their youth, and they are unlikely to have learned about orgasm, masturbation, or alternatives to heterosexuality and intercourse.

Until the early 1900s, sex was considered a private matter, unsuitable for public discussion (Huber & Firmin, 2014). Most discussion about sex occurred in the home, if it occurred at all. The content of these conversations was limited to physiology and the morals of sexual behavior. In many cultures, social norms and traditional family values promoted abstinence until marriage. In the early 1900s, the social hygiene movement brought issues of sex and sexuality to social consciousness in the US. Concerned with cleanliness and purity, public health education was a means to transmit information about and prevent STIs, and it promoted marital sex as the most effective prevention method.

Consistent with traditional values, early sex educators were concerned with correcting distorted ideas or information about sex, including the notion that "pleasure might be an acceptable motivation for sex" (Penland, 1981, p. 305). Self-control and sexual restraint were emphasized, and, for women educated within this framework, sex was constructed as solely for procreation. As Ehrlich (2014, p. 145) noted, "there is little room in the abstinence narrative for an authentic expression of female sexual desire." Older women educated in this tradition would have had little access to information about consent, sexual pleasure, and variability in sexual response or desire. Trans, queer, and asexual identities; non-monogamous partnerships; and alternative desires and behaviors were almost certainly excluded from the sex education curricula that was available to today's older women.

Older women have few opportunities to receive education focused on the unique factors that impact their sexuality and often wish for education and resources about sex and aging, especially how to identify and create opportunities for pleasure that are accessible to their changing bodies (Fileborn et al., 2015b). In their interviews with older Australian women, Fileborn and colleagues (2015b) found that a lack of comprehensive and inclusive sex education left older women vulnerable to myths and misinformation regarding sex and aging, and also limited the ways older women think about and/or feel empowered to exact sexual desire. Older adults are generally misinformed about aging processes and often rely on stereotypes to understand the relationships between sex and aging (Minichiello, Plummer, & Loxton, 2004). It is likely that many older women learn about sexuality-related issues from physicians, who tend to view sexuality from a medicalized perspective and focus exclusively on eradicating sexual "problems."

Fortunately, older women's access to sexual health can be fostered through changes to sociopolitical systems of thought, education, and governance. In one (small) step forward, there has been a call in the US for sex education and information to address the increase in STIs among older people. However, this call conceptualizes sex education for elders as parallel to the limited and often negative sex education often offered to adolescents (i.e., focused primarily on the avoidance of risks and negative consequences of sexual activity).

There is currently only one formal sexual health education curriculum in the US (i.e., *Our Whole Lives*) that specifically caters to older adults (Unitarian Universalist Association of Congregations, 2013). Though this program has been operating since 1999, there are no published empirical evaluations of its effectiveness.

Older women's sexual health would also be advanced by changes in cultural discourses of older women's sexuality. The construction of cultural discourse is an ongoing, reciprocal process (Bryant & Schofield, 2007; Butler, 1990). Discourse shapes older women's sexual realities, but older women's actual sexual lives and the ways in which they talk about their experiences shape cultural narratives of what is possible and considered normative (Interligi & McHugh, 2017). As Tolman (2000, p. 70) noted,

> the ways in which we do and do not 'story' sexuality into being are definitive in how we make meaning out of our bodies and relationships, and so the ways in which we do and do not speak about sexuality are crucial.

There is tremendous variability in human sexuality. Women vary enormously in sexual desire, sexual satisfaction, orgasmic experience, and arousability (Kliger & Nedelman, 2005; Leiblum, 1990). Thus, it is harmful to presume that there is a "best" or "right" way for women at any age to experience or enact their sexuality. Many older women have a fulfilling, exciting, and creative life without experiencing any sexual desire or sexual activity. Others report learning to negotiate and express their sensualities in new contexts with advanced age (Milton, 2016).

Our Bodies Ourselves (Boston Women's Health Collective, 2005) has enumerated some of the experiences of women as they age, including: increased sexual desire, changes in sexual preference, feeling removed from sexual practices and urges, finding alternatives to traditional relationships, appreciating a non-sexual sensuality, and recognizing an awakening of old feelings. Such variability and change may be experienced by women of all sexual orientations, preferences, and partnerships (Klinger & Nedelman, 2006). Each woman has the capacity to respond sexually in a variety of ways, and is likely to experience changes in her lifetime related to how she experiences her body, her relationships, and her sexual desire. Sexual fluidity is apparent in many older women's narratives of sexuality across the lifespan. Some women have described their sexualities as wavering between periods of sexual disinterest or celibacy and times of intense desire and frequent sexual activity (Fileborn et al., 2015a). It is our hope that older women both take and make opportunities to share stories —with each other, and with people from other age cohorts—about the richness and variability of their sexualities, including changes across time and partnerships. In doing so, they would promote a cultural shift in which older women can be appreciated as the complex and varied sexual beings that they are.

Older women's sexualities are relational

Cultural narratives of sexuality frequently play out within older women's sexual relationships, which have been shaped by the dominant scripts that they received and enacted across the life course as young, middle-aged, and now older women. In many countries, both historically and currently, it has been considered appropriate for women to be sexually monogamous within a heterosexual, married relationship and to act primarily as pleased, passive, receptors of men's sexual advances (Interligi & McHugh, 2017). However, "the achievement of normal heterosexuality is often hard work" (Cacchioni, 2015, p. 17). Research on women's sexual behavior within the context of long-term relationships frequently demonstrates the "coital imperative"

(McPhillips, Braun, & Gavey, 2001) and privileges a narrow definition of sex that centers on penile–vaginal intercourse (Winterich, 2003). In the US, the UK, and Brazil, older heterosexual women have been shown to assume responsibility for their male partners' sexual satisfaction (Baldissera, Bueno, & Hoga, 2012; Cacchioni, 2015; Nicolson & Burr, 2003; Wood, Mansfield, & Koch, 2007). Older women may continue to engage in penile–vaginal sex even if it is painful due to vaginal dryness (Winterich, 2003) or other age-related physical limitations. In their study of older women and sexuality, Ussher et al. (2015) observed similar patterns of emphasis on male pleasure and coital interactions. They noted that "some heterosexual women may continue to engage in sexual intercourse when they have little desire or pleasure because they or their partners view coital sex as important to the relationship" (p. 454).

The double standard and sexual scripts that privilege men's sexual needs and desire have stifled many women's ability to experience true sexual desire (Cacchioni, 2015). Women learn to "place their sexual desire outside of their own experiences, thereby surrendering their sexual agency" (Wood et al., 2007, p. 196). For some women the choice may be between having non-pleasurable or painful sex, or not having any sex at all. As one woman interviewed by Ussher et al. (2015, p. 455) reported, "Because I don't want to have sexual intercourse, then it has stopped me doing all the other loving things such as hugging, touching, teasing, in case they encourage him to go further." Older women have reported dissatisfaction with the limited variety in their sexual behavior (Woloski-Wruble, Oliel, Leefsma, & Hochner-Celnikier, 2010). This research suggests that, for at least some older women, declines in sexual desire and sexual activity that occur with aging are more a function of relational (and broader societal) issues than of physiological and hormonal aspects of aging.

Further, not all women in long-term relationships experience declines in desire and sexual intimacy. Women in relationships tend to report higher sexual self-esteem, sexual satisfaction, sexual interest, and more positive attitudes toward sexuality and aging than do those who are not in a relationship (Choi, Jang, Lee, & Kim, 2011; DeLamater, 2012; Kontula & Haavio-Mannila, 2009). It is possible that the opportunities for emotional intimacy, support, and sexual expression provided by a romantic partner result in sexual well-being (Minichiello et al., 2004). In committed partnerships, desire, activity, and satisfaction may coexist in a positive feedback loop. Partners in longer-term relationships reported staying passionate, being comfortable asking their partner to meet/attend to their desires, and enjoying a high level of sexual spontaneity (Frederick, Gillepsie, & Garcia, 2016). Furthermore, sexually satisfied older adults report engaging in more foreplay, more oral sex, and more penetrative sex, and they have more orgasms and more variety in sexual activities than those who describe themselves as sexually dissatisfied. "Setting the mood," taking time with non-genital foreplay, and dedicating time and attention to intimacy appear to promote satisfaction and build desire for continued sexual activity.

The sex lives of newly-partnered older women demonstrate an increase in sexual activity. Watson et al. (2017) interviewed a small sample of older women who were in new relationships, and none of them thought aging had negatively impacted their sexuality. In general, the respondents reported renewed sexual desire and enjoyment. Some reported they were experiencing better sex than previously. Some women who had not experienced sexual desire in some time reported that the relationship had reawakened their desire. Several of the women reported enjoyment of sex as a pleasant surprise. Other researchers have similarly reported that new relationships experienced in later life provide more pleasurable and satisfying sex than was experienced earlier (Clarke, 2006; Gott & Hinchliff, 2003).

Some evidence suggests that women in relationships with other women have even more positive experiences concerning sex and aging. Lesbians have been shown to be more open about discussing age-related changes to their bodies and sexualities and less concerned than heterosexual women about being rejected by their partner because of these changes (Winterich, 2003). Ussher et al. (2015) found that older lesbians were more able than older heterosexual women to negotiate diverse behaviors for partnered pleasure and stimulation. For older lesbians, sexual life satisfaction is associated with more positive attitudes toward aging, and a range of affectionate (rather than genitally-focused) behaviors are enjoyed in old age (Averett, Yoon, & Jenkins, 2012).

Older women may find satisfaction in sexual relationships with younger men (Fileborn et al., 2015a). However, those who engage in sex with younger male partners are still frequently subject to ageist assumptions related to biological and social narratives. Taylor et al. (2017) noted that older women may be sought as sexual partners by young men due to assumptions that they do not have STIs, and thus can engage in unprotected sex with minimal risk. The inability to conceive may also make older women more attractive to—and even fetishized by—certain men. However, if an older woman ends a relationship with a younger man, others often perceive the reason to be that she cannot "keep up" with her partner sexually (Fileborn et al., 2015a).

Despite the prevalence of sexist, ageist, and unfulfilling sexual scripts in many (especially Western) cultures, older women often resist these scripts or find ways to (re)negotiate sexuality for their own pleasure and fulfillment. Not all women who experience declines in sexual activity or desire are bothered by this occurrence. For example, many participants in Fileborn et al.'s (2015a) study of single, heterosexual, older Australian women reported being "single by choice" (p. 71), and described a refusal to pursue partnership and (potential) sexual satisfaction over their own independence and goals. These women challenged the societal ideal that they should be in a relationship. Further, many women described a disconnect between the kind of relationship they were interested in (i.e., predicated on mutuality, equality, respect) and the kinds of partnerships they perceived older men to be pursuing (e.g., "the good little wife ... a housekeeper rather than an equal partner") (p. 73). For these women, being single was an overwhelmingly positive and freeing experience. Similarly, many older lesbians experience great satisfaction with the maturity and stability of their relationships even in the absence of sexual activity (Averett et al., 2012). Some women, including those who have never experienced interest in sex, or identify as asexual, may find a sense of ease in the lowered expectations for their level of sexual desire activity in older adulthood.

Older women also report (re)negotiating sex by moving beyond coitus- and genital-focused forms of sexual activity. In the face of bodily changes to due aging, menopause, physical health, and ability status, many older women report making adaptations to their sexual behaviors in order to pursue intimacy and pleasure. For example, in a study of older women with HIV (Taylor et al., 2017), the majority of participants noted that they had adapted to their age and health status by renegotiating sexual boundaries (e.g., preference for different positions during coitus) and making physical accommodations (e.g., to make sex more comfortable). Other older women have described changing the focus of the sexual experience from genital to non-genital activities, such as kissing, cuddling, caressing, and massage (e.g., Santos-Iglesias et al., 2016; Ussher et al., 2015; Winterich, 2003). In the context of relationships, older women continue to defy the heteronormative, coitus-centered sexual scripts that try to define them.

The medicalization of older women's sexualities

Diagnoses and medical conditions, like discourses of sexuality, are socially constructed (Tiefer, 2015). Conceptualizations of women's sexual functioning have been influenced by medical and public discourses since early in the 20th century (Angel, 2010). Historically, women have been criticized for having too much sexual desire (nymphomania) or too little sexual desire (frigidity). Frigidity refers to a variety of women's "sexual failures," including an absence of desire and lack of responsiveness to men's advances (Angel, 2010). However, frigidity has most commonly referred to the failure to experience orgasm through vaginal penetration, and thus women's failure to adhere to gender and sexual roles. Distinctions between vaginal and clitoral orgasms are no longer made, but issues related to women's demonstration of the "correct" levels of desire and appropriate (hetero)sexual response remain of medical concern.

Although no longer referred to as frigidity, questions regarding the adequacy of women's sexuality remain. As previously discussed, postmenopausal women are typically perceived as less sexually active and less interested in sex (Interligi & McHugh, 2017; McHugh & Interligi, 2015). A substantial amount of the research on women's sexuality in midlife and beyond has focused on the role of menopause and has been conducted from a medical or biological perspective, which emphasizes the relationship between hormone levels and declines in women's sexual desire, activity, and satisfaction. Scholars have criticized the medicalized perspective that hormone changes associated with menopause inevitably cause sexual decline and decay (Hinchliff & Gott, 2008; McHugh & Interligi, 2015). This perspective is based on a particular model of human sexual response—a medical or physiological model—and the assumption that sexual desire is heavily influenced by hormones (McHugh & Interligi, 2015; Koch et al., 2005).

Whether related to the hormonal changes of menopause or not, older women's interest in sex may decline with age and may be labeled as a sexual dysfunction if it is "too low" (McHugh & Interligi, 2015). Sexual health can certainly be impacted by physical changes that occur as estrogen levels decline during perimenopause. For example, penetration may become uncomfortable or painful due to reduction in vaginal lubrication (Boston Women's Health Collective, 2005). Likewise, thinning of the vaginal tissue may lead to tears and bleeding during penetration. Vaginal dryness was related to less frequent sexual intercourse and less interest in sex in some research (McCoy, Cutler, & Davidson, 1985). Yet, rather than emphasizing the physiology or hormonal aspects of aging, McCoy and colleagues (McCoy & Davidson, 1985; McCoy et al., 1985) argued for a more multifaceted and integrated approach to study of women's sexuality over the lifespan, as biological, psychological, and social factors all contribute to a woman's sexual health and well-being (Lindau et al., 2007).

As women age, various health conditions may affect their sexual activity (Traen et al., 2017). Women may have less energy and feel less interested in sex due to chronic or acute illnesses. Lack of mobility may limit sexual interactions. Growing facial hair and gaining weight are two aspects of aging that interfered with women's sense of their own attractiveness and desirability and, in turn, have been shown to impact their sexual response and sexual activity (Ussher et al., 2015). However, older women's sexual health may not be as dependent on physical health as older men's. For example, in a study of sexual health of older adults in the UK, chronic health conditions and poor self-rated general health were more associated with decreased sexual activity and functioning for men than for women (Lee, Nazroo, O'Connor, Blake, & Pendleton, 2016). Health problems related to circulation (e.g., heart disease, hypertension) impacted the sexual activities and satisfaction of men, but not women. It is important to note that illness can differentially affect various facets of sexual health. For example, arthritic disease and diabetes attenuated some older women's sexual activity, but did not influence their sexual satisfaction (Lee et al., 2016).

Mental health conditions also affect sexual health and well-being (Traen et al., 2017). Loneliness, depression, and grief are commonly experienced by older women. Symptoms of depression, including fatigue, anhedonia, and sad mood, are not conducive to sexual activity.

Older individuals' mental health concerns may supersede any concerns they have about their sexual well-being. However, individuals diagnosed with depression or grief who also express sexual health concerns must receive careful treatment planning. Pharmaceutical treatments may not be appropriate interventions in this situation as antidepressant drugs may induce sexual dysfunction (Bala, Nguyen, & Hellstrom, 2018), commonly diminish sexual interest and genital sensitivity, and lead to orgasm difficulty in up to 70% of patients (Lorenz, Rullo, & Fabion, 2016). Antipsychotic and neuroleptic medications are also linked to impaired sexual function in women.

The biomedical approach to older women's sexual health is based on the disease concept, in which declines in sexual activity are viewed as pathological (Tiefer, 2001, 2015) and deserving of diagnostic labels such as "female sexual disorder" and "hypoactive sexual desire disorder." In an attempt to reach levels of sexual activity deemed by "experts" as normal, appropriate, or "successful," older women are prescribed medications, treatments, and therapies. Tiefer (2001, 2015) exposed the medicalization of sexuality as an active process, even a strategy, devised by groups whose political and economic interests are served by the medical model.

Underlying the problem of "treating" women's sexual dysfunction is the problem of defining "normal" levels of sexual functioning. For example, feminist scholars have argued that our understanding of women's sexual desire has been based on a androcentric model despite evidence that women's sexual desire is experienced differently (Bancroft, Loftus, & Long, 2003; Basson, 2002; Tiefer, 2001). Tiefer (2001) argued against linear model(s) of sexual response that proceed from desire to arousal to orgasm. Some feminist scholars have proposed alternative models. For many women, desire is experienced consequent to arousal, or desire and arousal are experienced simultaneously. Thus, Basson (2001, 2002) proposed a sexual response model in which sexual desire of women is intimacy based, largely responsive in nature, and less linear than men's sexual desire. Schwartz and Rutter (2000) contended that for heterosexual women, many of whom do not initiate sexual interactions but instead respond to their partner's initiation, the partner's sexual desire is the erotic cue for women's own desire. Women may describe their desire in relation to genital and non-genital physical responses (i.e., arousal) or to cognitive and emotional responses (i.e., desire; Brotto, Heiman, & Tolamn, 2009). That is, women experience sexual desire in multiple ways that differ from a single, linear, and biologically-based way. Further, asexual-spectrum older women, who experience limited to no sexual desire, may be inaccurately diagnosed as dysfunctional in societies that expect "successful" older adults to engage in a prescribed amount of sex (Brotto & Yule, 2017; Yule, Brotto, & Gorzalka, 2017).

Medical, pharmaceutical, and public discussions of female sexual dysfunction (FSD) increased following the successful launch of Viagra. Definitional issues have plagued the FSD literature, despite repeated industry-supported attempts to draw a bright line between healthy sexual function and medical disorder. The search for a pharmaceutical approach to women's sexual functioning continued as the medico-pharmaceutical industry turned its attention to the contemporary version of frigidity: Women with insufficient sexual interest or desire. To diagnose sexual dysfunctions, physicians and others consult the official descriptions of disorders in the *Diagnostic and Statistical Manual of Mental Disorders* (DSM) published by the American Psychiatric Association. The *DSM III* (APA, 1980) and *IV* (APA, 2000) identified women's insufficient desire as hypoactive sexual desire disorder (HSDD), and a prescription medicine, flibanserin, was developed to elevate women's sexual desire to "appropriate" levels. Research demonstrated that flibanserin did not cause substantial improvements in women's sexual pleasure over placebo and resulted in significant side effects. Despite these concerns, some women's groups were rallied into lobbying efforts to encourage the US Food and Drug Administration to approve the drug to "even the score," given that Viagra and other drugs were available to men. Subsequently, in 2015, the FDA approved the use of flibanserin with a warning. Critics (e.g., Tiefer, 2015) decried the approval of a minimally effective drug with serious side effects. Nevertheless, the drug's marketing campaign, designed to cause women to question the adequacy of their sexual interest/desire, is likely to influence older women.

In the *DSM-5* (APA, 2013), the name of the diagnosis concerning sexual desire was changed to sexual interest/arousal disorder (SIAD). SIAD was conceptualized based on the research that accurately reveals women's sexual desire as variable, as responsive, and as a merging of desire and arousal (Laan & Both, 2008). Application of the diagnosis depends on an individual's own identification of low levels of desire as a problem. SIAD is a preferred classification because it differentiates between women who lack desire before the onset of activity (but who are receptive to initiation and/or initiate sexual activity for reasons other than desire) and women who never experience sexual arousal (Brotto, 2010).

Controversy surrounding the diagnosis SIAD has been considerable (Angel, 2013; Balon & Clayton, 2014; Clayton, DeRogatis, Rosen, & Pyke, 2012; Graham, 2016;O' Loughlin, Basson, & Brotto, 2018; Spurgas, 2016), It was criticized as unfairly "raising the bar" for a diagnosis of sexual desire dysfunction in women (Clayton et al., 2012). Based on their research in which 281 women were assessed for both SAID and HSDD, O' Loughlin, Basson, & Brotto (2018) concluded that use of SIAD may prevent healthy individuals with mild (and possibly transient) sexual problems from receiving a diagnosis, although it is sufficiently sensitive to diagnose those with more dysfunction (i.e., more persistent and severe sexual dysfunction). A greater degree of sexual dysfunction in the SIAD group was observed in sexual desire frequency, sexual satisfaction, arousal frequency, reaction to erotic cues, and orgasm achievement. The results suggest that SIAD does raise the bar by effectively distinguishing between mild and moderate-severe symptomatology.

As noted above, women's sexual desire has been conceptualized as "complex," "flexible," "responsive," and "receptive." These descriptors are now incorporated as essential features of female sexuality in the *DSM-5*. Spurgas (2016) disagreed with including lack of responsiveness to a partner's advances as a criterion for diagnosis of women's sexual dysfunction. She was concerned that sexual desire was deleted as a factor in female sexuality and replaced by the more cognitive "interest." These diagnostic and therapeutic shifts influence how women relate to their sexual bodies and those of their partners and have biopolitical, experiential, and psychorelational consequences (Spurgas, 2016). Because of our medicalized cultural milieu, these research and treatment protocols affect all women, not just those who present for treatment (Spurgas, 2016). Thus, the change in the diagnostic label and criteria may result in (positive or negative) transformations in the construction and treatment of women's loss/lack of sexual desire.

Conclusion: a sex-positive future for older women

A sex-positive cultural approach to older women's sexual health would recognize the importance of authenticity, agency, and a broader definition of sex than currently utilized (McHugh & Interligi, 2015). In later life, women might become more authentic in their decision to engage in sexual activity (or not) as they become free from society's expectations of procreation or marital duty. As they age, some women may become more open about their sexual desires and partner attractions, and they might increase their levels of sexual activity. An empowerment perspective on older women's sexuality might emphasize women's right to be sexual (or not) in response to her own sexual desire, and to engage in a range and variety of sexual activities negotiated with her partner(s). Women might feel empowered to advocate for their own sexual rights in personal, relational, and societal arenas.

In this chapter, we have explored the question of the sexual health of older women in relation to the definition endorsed by WHO (2006). Older women's identities as sexual beings persist, even in the face of cultural discourses that label them as declining or diseased, and their sexualities are limitlessly variable. Older women can—and do—engage in sexual activity. Many are satisfied with their levels of sexual activity and desire, regardless of whether that level corresponds to standards of what is considered "normal" or "successful" for women their age. Some older women have learned to make adaptations and accommodations for aging bodies that make sex more pleasurable. These findings appear to hold true for older women regardless of their sexual orientation or nationality. Though older women may experience the "possibility of having pleasurable and safe sexual experiences" required by the WHO (2006) definition of sexual health, they are still subject to many barriers to their free and agentic sexual expression. Older women are not usually provided with the freedom from discrimination that the WHO (2006) definition of sexual health requires. Most older adults have not been provided with adequate, inclusive, sex education, which limits their access to information—another sexual right necessary for sexual health.

We have described the ways in which social, relational, and medical discourses have provided a negative perspective on older women's sexuality and attempted to regulate their sexual expression by promoting narrow narratives that limit women's sexual expression. These discourses implicitly reinforce androcentric and heteronormative mandates on older women's sexualities. Theory, research, and clinical practice related to the sexuality of older women has been critiqued as not consistent with the experiences and narratives of older women. Recent changes in the medical discourse and diagnosis of women's sexual functioning were adopted based on research related to women's sexual desire. These changes may signal a future in which women speak for and about their own sexual desires rather than being evaluated and labelled based on androcentric models of sexual functioning. Yet, discourse does not necessarily define women's sexuality: Through their sexual experiences, women can actively construct or modify their own sexual identities (Bryant & Schofield, 2007). By interpreting these discourses (consciously or unconsciously) and acting in ways that are congruent or incongruent with popular notions of female sexuality, older women can be active agents in shaping social patterns of "normative" sexual behavior (Interligi & McHugh, 2017). Life-long sex education and opportunities for women to speak with one another about sexuality are possible paths to a more positive sexual future for older women. Engaging in these activities can help women to learn validating and accurate information about their bodies and sexuality, to gain tools to critically analyze the dominant discourses that influence their sexuality, to challenge heteronormativity and androcentrism, and to eliminate sexual shame. Through this kind of engagement, the dominant discourses of women's sexuality can be changed, and more positive and diverse discourses can proliferate. We hope that, through these activities, women can imagine, create, and share their own stories of sexuality and further develop a sex positive future for all women, regardless of age.

References

American Psychiatric Association (APA) (1980). *Diagnostic and statistical manual of mental disorders* (3rd ed.). Washington, DC: Author.

American Psychiatric Association (APA) (2000). *Diagnostic and statistical manual of mental disorders* (4th rev. ed.). Washington, DC: Author.

American Psychiatric Association (APA) (2013). *Diagnostic and statistical manual of mental disorders* (5th ed.). Arlington, VA: American Psychiatric Publishing.

Angel, K. (2010). The history of 'female sexual dysfunction' as a mental disorder in the 20th century. *Current Opinions in Psychiatry, 23*, 536–541.

Angel, K. (2013). Commentary on Spurgas's "Interest, arousal, and shifting diagnoses of female sexual dysfunction". *Studies in Gender and Sexuality, 14*, 206–216.

Averett, P., Yoon, I., & Jenkins, C. L. (2012). Older lesbian sexuality: Sexual behavior and the impact of aging. *Journal of Sex Research, 49*, 495–507.

Bala, A., Nguyen, H. M. T., & Hellstrom, W. J. G. (2018). Post-SSRI sexual dysfunction: A literature review. *Sexual Medicine Review, 6*, 29–34.

Baldissera, V. D. A., Bueno, S. M., & Hoga, L. A. K. (2012). Improvement of older women's sexuality through emancipatory education. *Health Care for Women International, 33*, 956–972.

Balon, R. & Clayton, A. (2014). Female sexual interest/arousal disorder: A diagnosis out of thin air. *Archives of Sexual Behavior, 43*, 1227–1229.

Bancroft, J., Loftus, J., & Long, J. S. (2003). Distress about sex: A national survey of women in heterosexual relationships. *Archives of Sexual Behavior, 32*, 193–209.

Basson, R. (2001). Human sex-response cycles. *Journal of Sex and Marital Therapy, 27*, 33–43.

Basson, R. (2002). Rethinking low sexual desire in women. *British Journal of Obstetrics and Gynaecology, 109*, 357–363.

Boston Women's Health Collective (2005). *Our bodies, ourselves.* New York, NY: Touchstone.

Brotto, L. A. (2010). The *DSM* diagnostic criteria for hypoactive sexual desire disorder in women. *Archives of Sexual Behavior, 39*, 221–239.

Brotto, L. A., Heiman, J. R., & Tolamn, D. L. (2009). Narratives of desire in mid-age women with and without arousal difficulties. *Journal of Sex Research, 46*(5), 387–398.

Brotto, L. A. & Yule, M. (2017). Asexuality: Sexual orientation, paraphilia, sexual dysfunction, or none of the above? *Archives of Sexual Behavior, 46*, 619–627.

Bryant, J. & Schofield, T. (2007). Feminine sexual subjectivities: Bodies, agency, and life history. *Sexualities, 10*, 321–340.

Butler, J. (1990). *Gender trouble: Feminism and the subversion of identity.* Abingdon, UK: Routledge.

Cacchioni, T. (2015). *Big pharma, women, and labour of love.* Toronto, Canada: University of Toronto Press.

Choi, K. B., Jang, S. H., Lee, M. Y., & Kim, K. H. (2011). Sexual life and self esteem in married elderly. *Archives of Gerontology and Geriatrics, 53*(1), 17–20.

Clarke, L. H. (2006). Older women and sexuality: Experiences in marital relationships across the life course. *Canadian Journal on Aging, 25*, 129–140.

Clayton, A. H., DeRogatis, L. R., Rosen, R. C., & Pyke, R. (2012). Intended or unintended consequences? The likely implications of raising the bar for sexual dysfunction diagnosis in the proposed DSM-5 revisions: 2. For women with loss of subjective sexual arousal. *Journal of Sexual Medicine, 9*, 2040–2046.

DeLamater, J. (2012). Sexual expression in later life. *Journal of Sex Research, 49*, 125–141.

DeLamater, J. & Koepsel, E. (2015). Relationships and sexual expression in later life: A biopsychosocial perspective. *Sexual and Relationship Therapy, 30*(1), 37–59.

Dillaway, H. E. (2005). (Un)changing menopausal bodies: How women think and act in the face of a reproductive transition and gendered beauty ideals. *Sex Roles, 53*, 1–17.

Ehrlich, J. S. (2014). *Regulating desire: From the virtuous maid to the purity princess.* Albany, NY: State University of New York Press.

Field, N., Mercer, C. H., Sonnenberg, P., Tanton, C., Clifton, S., Mitchell, K. R., & Johnson, A. M. (2013). Associations between health and sexual lifestyles in Britain: Findings from the third national survey of sexual attitudes and lifestyles (Natsal-3). *Lancet, 382*, 1830–1844.

Fileborn, B., Thorpe, R., Hawkes, G., Minichiello, V., & Pitt, M. (2015a). Sex and the older single girl. *Journal of Aging Studies, 33*, 67–75.

Fileborn, B., Thorpe, R., Hawkes, G., Minichiello, V., Pitt, M., & Dune, T. (2015b). Sex, desire and pleasure: Considering the experiences of older Australian women. *Sex and Relationship Therapy, 30*(1), 117–130.

Frederick, D. A., Gillepsie, B. J., & Garcia, J. R. (2016). What keeps passion alive? *Journal of Sex Research*, *54*, 186–201.

Gott, M. & Hinchliff, S. (2003). How important is sex in later life? *Social Science & Medicine, 56*, 1617–1628.

Graham, D. (2016). Reconceptualising women's sexual desire and arousal in DSM-5. *Psychology and Sexuality, 7*(1), 34–47.

Hebernick, D., Reece, M., Schick, V., Sanders, S. A., Dodge, B., & Fortenberry, J. D. (2010). Sexual behavior in the United States: Results from a national probability sample of men and women ages 14–94. *Journal of Sexual Medicine*, 7(Suppl 5), 255–265.

Hinchliff, S. & Gott, M. (2008). Challenging social myths and stereotypes of women and aging: Heterosexual women talk about sex. *Journal of Women & Aging, 20*(1–2), 65–81.

Huber, V. J. & Firmin, M. W. (2014). A history of sex education in the United States since 1900. *International Journal of Educational Reform, 23*(1).

Interligi, C. J. & McHugh, M. C. (2017). Women's sexuality: Victims, objects, or agents? In C. B. Travis & J. White (Eds), *APA handbook of the psychology of women: History, theory, and battlegrounds* (Vol. 1, pp. 297–318). Washington, DC: American Psychological Association.

Kliger, L. & Nedelman, D. (2005, July). Redefining "sexy": Sexual desire and sexual self-esteem in women beyond 50. Paper presented at the New View Conference, Montreal, Canada.

Klinger, L. & Nedelman, D. (2006). *Still sexy after all these years? The 9 unspoken truths about women's desire.* New York, NY: Berkeley Books.

Koch, P. B., Manfield, P. K., Thurau, D., & Carey, M. (2005). "Feeling frumpy": The relationship between body image and sexual response changes in midlife women. *Journal of Sex Research, 42*, 215–222.

Kontula, O. & Haavio-Mannila, E. (2009). The impact of aging on human sexual activity and sexual desire. *Journal of Sex Research, 46*, 45–56.

Laan, E. & Both, S. (2008). What makes women experience desire? *Feminism & Psychology, 18*, 505–514.

Lee, D. M., Nazroo, J., O'Connor, D. B., Blake, M., & Pendleton, N. (2016). Sexual health and well-being among older men and women in England: Findings from the English longitudinal study of ageing. *Archives of Sexual Behavior, 45*, 133–144.

Leiblum, S. R. (1990). Sexuality and the midlife woman. *Psychology of Women Quarterly, 14*, 495–508.

Lindau, S. T., Schumm, L. P., Laumann, E. O., Levinson, W., O'Muircheartaigh, C. A., & Waite, L. J. (2007). A study of sexuality and health among older adults in the United States. *New England Journal of Medicine, 357*, 762–774.

Lorenz, T., Rullo, J., & Fabion, S. (2016). Antidepressant-induced female sexual dysfunction. *Mayo Clinic Proceedings, 91*, 1280–1286.

Lusti-Narasimhan, M. & Beard, J. R. (2013). Sexual health in older women. *Bulletin of the World Health Organization, 91*(9).

Mazo, G. Z. & Cardoso, F. L. (2011). Sexual satisfaction and correlates among elderly Brazilians. *Archives of Gerontology and Geriatrics, 52*, 223–227.

McCoy, N., Cutler, W. B., & Davidson, J. M. (1985). Relationships among sexual behavior, hot flashes, and hormone levels in peri-menopausal women. *Archives of Sexual Behavior, 14*, 381–390.

McCoy, N. L. & Davidson, J. M. (1985). A longitudinal study of the effects of menopause on sexuality. *Maturitas, 7*, 203–210.

McHugh, M. C. (2006). Women at midlife and sex: Desire, dysfunction, diversity. In V. Muhlbauer & J. C. Chrisler (Eds), *Women over 50: Psychological perspectives* (pp. 26–52). New York, NY: Springer.

McHugh, M. C. & Interligi, C. (2015). Sexuality and older women: Desire and desirability. In V. Muhlbauer, J. C. Chrisler, & F. L. Denmark (Eds), *Women & aging: An international, intersectional power perspective* (pp. 89–116). New York, NY: Springer.

McPhillips, K., Braun, V., & Gavey, N. (2001). Defining (hetero)sex: How imperative is the "coital imperative"? *Women's Studies International Forum, 24*, 229–240.

Milton, S. (2016). 'Becoming more of myself': Safe sensuality, salsa, and ageing. *European Journal of Women's Studies, 24*(2), 143–157.

Minichiello, V., Plummer, D., & Loxton, D. (2004). Factors predicting sexual relationships in older people: An Australian study. *Australasian Journal on Ageing, 28*(3), 125–130.

Montemurro, B. & Siefken, J. M. (2014). Cougars on the prowl? New perceptions of older women's sexuality. *Journal of Aging Studies, 28*, 35–43.

Nicolson, P. & Burr, J. (2003). What is 'normal' about women's (hetero)sexual desire and orgasm? A report of an in-depth interview study. *Social Science and Medicine, 57*, 1735–1745.

O'Loughlin, J., Basson, R., & Brotto, L. A. (2018). Women with hypoactive sexual desire disorder versus sexual interest/arousal disorder: An empirical test of raising the bar. *Journal of Sex Research, 55*, 734–746.

Penland, L. R. (1981). Sex education in 1900, 1940, and 1980: A historical sketch. *Journal of School Health, 51*, 305–309.

Phillips, J. & Marks, G. (2006). Coming out, coming in: How do dominant discourses around aged care facilities take into account the identities and needs of ageing lesbians? *Gay and Lesbian Issues and Psychology Review, 2*, 67–77.

Rushbrooke, E., Murray, C., & Townsend, S. (2014). What difficulties are experienced by caregivers in relation to the sexuality of people with intellectual disabilities? *Research in Developmental Disabilities, 35*, 871–886.

Santos-Iglesias, P., Byers, E. S., & Moglia, R. (2016). Sexual well-being of older men and women. *Canadian Journal of Human Sexuality, 25*(2), 86–98.

Schick, V., Herbenick, D., Reece, M., Sanders, S. A., Dodge, B., Middlebstadt, S. E., & Fortenberry, J. D. (2010). Sexual behaviors, condom use, and sexual health of Americans over 50: Implications for sexual health promotion for older adults. *Journal of Sexual Medicine, 7* (Suppl 5), 315–329.

Schwartz, P. & Rutter, V. (2000). *The gender of sexuality.* New York, NY: Rowan & Littlefield.

Simpson, P., Horne, M., Brown, L. J. E., Wilson, C. B., Dickinson, T., & Torkington, K. (2015). Old-(er) care home residents and sexual/intimate citizenship. *Ageing and Society, 37*(2), 1–23.

Society for Post-Acute and Long-Term Care Medicine (2016). Capacity for sexual consent in dementia in long-term care. Columbia, MD: Author. Retrived from https://paltc.org/amda-white-papers-and-resolution-position-statements/capacity-sexual-consent-dementia-long-term-care.

Spurgas, A. K. (2016). Low desire, trauma and femininity in the *DSM-5*: A case for sequelae. *Psychology and Sexuality, 7*, 48–67.

Taylor, T. N., Munoz-Plaza, C. E., Goparaju, L., Martinez, O., Holman, S., Minkoff, H. L., & Wilson, T. E. (2017). "The pleasure is better since I've gotten older": Sexual health, sexuality, and sexual risk behavior among older women living with HIV. *Archives of Sexual Behavior, 46*, 1137–1150.

Tiefer, L. (2001). A new view of women's sexual problems. Why new? Why now? *Journal of Sex Research, 38*, 89–96.

Tiefer, L. (2015). Women's sexual problems: Is there a pill for that? In M. C. McHugh & J. C. Chrisler (Eds), *The wrong prescription for women: How medicine and media create a "need" for treatments, drugs, and surgery* (pp. 147–159). Santa Barbara, CA: Praeger.

Tolman, D. L. (2000). Object lessons: Romance, violation, and female adolescent sexual desire. *Journal of Sex Education and Therapy, 25*(1), 70–79.

Traeen, B., Halt, G. M., Graham, C. A., Enzlin, P., Janssen, E., Kvalem, I. L., Carvalheira, A., & Stulhofer, A. (2017). Sexuality in older adults (65+): An overview of the literature, part 1. Sexual function and its difficulties. *International Journal of Sexual Health, 29*(1), 1–10.

Unitarian Universalist Association of Congregations (2013). Our whole lives: Lifespan sexuality education curricula. Boston, MA: Author. Retrieved from www.uua.org/re/owl/index.shtml, accessed April 2014.

Ussher, J. M., Perz, J., & Parton, C. (2015). Menopause and sexuality: Resisting representations of the abject sexual woman. In M. C. McHugh & J. C. Chrisler (Eds), *The wrong prescription for women: How medicine and media create a "need" for treatments, drugs, and surgery* (pp. 123–146). Santa Barbara, CA: Praeger.

Wang, V., Depp, C. A., Ceglowski, J., Thompson, W. K., Rock, D., & Jeste, D. V. (2014). Sexual health and function in later life: A population-based study of 606 older adults with a partner. *American Journal of Geriatric Psychiatry, 23*, 227–233.

Watson, W. K., Stelle, C., & Bell, N. (2017). Older women in new romantic relationships. *International Journal of Aging and Human Development, 85*(1), 33–43.

Willis, P., Maegusuku-Hewett, T., Raithby, M., Miles, P., Nash, P., Baker, C., & Evans, S. (2013). *Provision of inclusive and anti-discriminatory services to older lesbian, gay, bisexual identifying (LGB) people in residential care environments in Wales.* Swansea, UK: Swansea University. Retrieved from www.swansea.ac.uk/humanandhealthsciences/news-and-events/latest-research/studyoflgbpeopleinresiden tialcarerevealsknowledgegap.php.

Winterich, J. A. (2003). Sex, menopause, and culture: Sexual orientation and the meaning of menopause for women's sex lives. *Gender & Society, 17*, 627–642.

Woloski-Wruble, A., Oliel, Y., Leefsma, M., & Hochner-Celnikier, D. (2010). Sexual activities, sexual and life satisfaction, and successful aging in women. *Journal of Sexual Medicine*, 7, 2401–2410.

Wood, J. M., Mansfield, P. K., & Koch, P. B. (2007). Negotiating sexual agency: Postmenopausal women's meaning and experiences of sexual desire. *Qualitative Health Research*, 17, 189–200.

World Health Organization (WHO) (2006). Defining sexual health. Geneva, Switzerland: Author. Retrieved from www.who.int/reproductivehealth/topics/sexual_health/sh_definitions/en.

Yule, M. A., Brotto, L. A., & Gorzalka, B. B. (2017). Human asexuality: What do we know about the lack of sexual attraction? *Current Sexual Health Reports*, 9(1), 50–56.

28

SEXUALITY AND SEXUAL DYSFUNCTION

Psychological perspectives and interventions

Julia Velten and Sonia Milani

The World Health Organization (WHO, 2006) emphasizes that sexual health includes the ability to have a sex life that is not only safe, but also satisfying. Problems with sexual function are important threats to the sexual health of women across all age groups, ethnicities, and sexual orientations. The most common sexual difficulties are low sexual desire, problems with sexual arousal or orgasm, and genito-pelvic pain related to sexual activity; which occur prevalently among women worldwide (McCabe et al., 2016a).

Little is known about the reasons why some women remain sexually functional despite adverse circumstances (e.g., sexual trauma, relationship discord, chronic stress), whereas others develop one or more sexual dysfunctions at a certain point in their life. We know even less about the time-course of such concerns or why some become serious and distressing chronic dysfunctions, and others vanish into thin air when, for example, a new partnership is entered. It is, however, without question that women's sexual function is influenced not only by biological or medical determinants (e.g., hormone levels), but also by psychological, sociocultural, and partnership-related factors as well.

In this chapter, we start by providing an overview of the most common sexual dysfunctions in women and describe risk and protective factors that can predispose, trigger, or perpetuate sexual concerns. How to adequately diagnose sexual dysfunctions is the focus of the following section. We conclude this chapter by presenting medical and psychological treatments that have been found to be effective in improving women's sexual functioning.

Diagnoses

Overview and recent developments

Women's sexual difficulties include low sexual desire or arousal, pain or discomfort, and problems in reaching orgasm (Rosen et al., 2000). There are three factors that distinguish sexual problems or low levels of sexual functioning from clinically relevant sexual dysfunctions: frequency, duration, and distress. According to the fifth edition of the *Diagnostic and*

Statistical Manual of Mental Disorders (DSM; American Psychiatric Association [APA], 2013), a sexual problem must be present on most of the occasions over a period of six months or more and must lead to clinically significant distress to be classified as a sexual dysfunction. In addition, a sexual dysfunction should only be diagnosed when the symptoms cannot be better explained by a nonsexual mental health issue, are not caused by relationship problems or other stressors, are not the result of substance/medication use, or (almost) exclusively caused by a medical condition (APA, 2013).

Although methods of epidemiological studies conducted to assess the prevalence of sexual dysfunctions vary concerning important factors (e.g., age range of participants), there appears to be reasonable consensus that the prevalence of women who report at least one sexual problem ranges between 40% and 50%, irrespective of age (McCabe et al., 2016a). The most common sexual problem in women is low sexual desire. Studies found that the number of women reporting low levels of desire range from 17% in the United Kingdom, 33% to 35% in the United States, Sweden, and Iran, and up to 55% in Australia (McCabe et al., 2016a). These numbers drop by half if distress is included as a criterion (Brotto, Bitzer, Laan, Leiblum, & Luria, 2010), which means that about half of the women with low desire do not perceive this as problematic, and thus should not be diagnosed with a sexual dysfunction. In the United Kingdom, about 16% of women with sexual problems meet the complete *DSM-5* criteria for sexual dysfunctions, including the three morbidity specifiers, duration, frequency, and distress (Mitchell et al., 2016), suggesting that the high prevalence rates of sexual problems might have to be interpreted with caution. In this study, women who reported at least one same sex partner in the last five years were more likely to experience difficulties with sexual functioning than other women. These findings are, however, in contrast to other studies suggesting higher levels of sexual functioning, especially concerning arousal and orgasm, among lesbian women compared with straight women in steady relationships (Beaber & Werner, 2009; Henderson, Lehavot, & Simoni, 2009).

Low sexual desire and arousal difficulties

The *DSM-5* diagnosis Female Sexual Interest/Arousal Disorder (FSIAD) replaced the two *DSM-IV-TR* diagnoses Hypoactive Sexual Desire Disorder and Female Sexual Arousal Disorder. To receive a FSIAD diagnosis, three out of six criteria of sexual desire and/or arousal must be absent or markedly reduced (i.e., interest in sexual activities, sexual fantasies or thoughts, sexual initiative or receptiveness to partner's initiative, sexual arousal during sexual activity in most sexual encounters, responsive desire to internal or external sexual stimuli, genital or non-genital sensations during sexual activity in most sexual encounters). A sexual desire discrepancy (i.e., a difference in the desire for sexual activities between partners) is not sufficient for a FSIAD diagnosis. Furthermore, whenever a lifelong absent or low desire for sex can be better explained by a woman's self-definition as asexual, she should not receive a FSIAD diagnosis.

Orgasmic dysfunction

Female orgasmic dysfunction is characterized by frequent, long-lasting, and distressing difficulties to reach orgasm or significantly reduced feelings of pleasure during orgasm. Women should only receive this diagnosis when the difficulties occur despite adequate sexual stimulation. Many women require clitoral stimulation in order to reach orgasm; should a woman experience orgasmic difficulties during vaginal intercourse, clinicians should inquire whether adequate clitoral stimulation is provided. Whenever stimulation is not deemed adequate (e.g., no clitoral stimulation, very short or absent foreplay), a diagnosis should not be assigned. The ease with which women experience orgasm shows great variability; estimates suggest that up to 10% of women do not experience orgasm throughout their lifetime (APA, 2013). Thus, clinicians should only use this diagnosis when the absence or delay of orgasms leads to significant personal distress.

Genito-pelvic pain

A Genito-Pelvic Pain/Penetration Disorder (GPPPD) can be diagnosed when at least one of the following four symptoms is experienced over the course of six months and is leading to significant personal distress: problems with intercourse, genito-pelvic pain, fear of this pain or penetration, and increased pelvic-tension during attempted penetration (APA, 2013). GPPPD has replaced the *DSM-IV-TR* diagnoses of Dyspareunia and Vaginismus. Often, women who experience genito-pelvic pain are also diagnosed with medical conditions such as endometriosis, interstitial cystitis, or genital infections (e.g., candidiasis, herpes). In many cases, clinicians cannot reliably assess whether GPPPD or the medical condition is the primary diagnosis. In such instances, a comprehensive treatment strategy—possibly including both pharmacological and non-pharmacological treatments—should be developed to target all relevant symptoms. Pain symptoms associated with GPPPD can be described as burning, stinging, or throbbing, and can be located in different parts of a women's genito-pelvic area (e.g., superficial, vaginal entrance, deep within the pelvis). In some women, symptoms of GPPPD include involuntary-reflexive spasms of the pelvic-floor muscles that surround the vaginal canal. A common genital pain condition in women is Provoked Vestibulodynia. It is characterized by pain at the vulva or the vaginal entrance, which is triggered by touch. Provoked Vestibulodynia is the most frequent cause of dyspareunia (i.e., pain during intercourse) in premenopausal women (Landry, Bergeron, Dupuis, & Desrochers, 2008). Although the time-course of women's genito-pelvic pain has not been thoroughly investigated, some studies suggest that such pain, once present for more than six months, seldom resolves on its own (APA, 2013).

Etiology

Biopsychosocial model

The etiology of women's sexual dysfunctions is multifaceted: Biological, psychological, relationship and social risk, and protective factors interact to influence women's sexual functioning. Many women with sexual dysfunctions might experience several of these risk factors. Others are not affected by risks, while still developing a distressing sexual problem. Some of these factors predispose women to sexual concerns by increasing the likelihood of developing a dysfunction in the future, whereas others trigger a sexual dysfunction more directly (McCabe et al., 2016b). Figure 28.1 shows some of the more common predisposing, triggering, and maintaining factors for women's sexual dysfunctions.

The following sections describe some of the most common risk factors for sexual dysfunctions in more detail.

Biological factors

Sexual dysfunctions are less common among women who describe their physical health as excellent than among women with lower self-perceived health (Richters, Grulich, Visser,

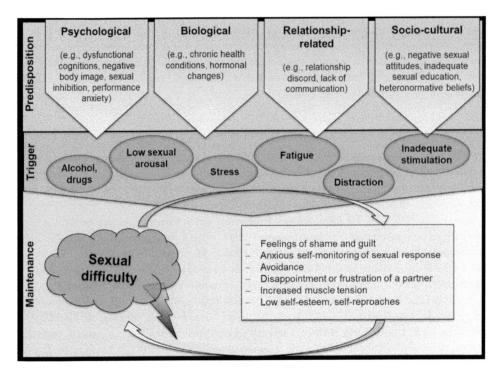

Figure 28.1 Biopsychosocial model of sexual dysfunctions in women. Adapted and translated with permission from Velten, J. (2018). Sexuelle Funktionsstörungen bei Frauen [Sexual dysfunctions in women]. Göttingen, Germany: Hogrefe.

Smith, & Rissel, 2003). Regular physical exercise is related to less frequent problems with orgasm and higher levels of sexual desire (Eplov, Giraldi, Davidsen, Garde, & Kamper-Jørgensen, 2007). Metabolic syndrome and high blood pressure are associated with higher rates of sexual dysfunction in women (Duncan et al., 2001; Martelli et al., 2012). Both hypo- and hyperactivation of pelvic floor muscles can lead to genito-pelvic pain or problems related to arousal and orgasm (Bergeron, Rosen, & Morin, 2011).

Low desire for sex is common among women with serious or life-threatening illnesses (e.g., cancer, cardio-vascular diseases). This is true for acute illnesses, and women with chronic conditions (e.g., thyroid disease, multiple sclerosis, arthritis) are also more likely to experience sexual difficulties (McCabe et al., 2016b). While certain aspects of sexual functioning (e.g., lubrication or reaching orgasm) may be more problematic for women with spinal cord injuries than for able-bodied women, many women with spinal cord injuries report enjoying sexual activities postinjury (Jackson & Wadley, 1999).

Some women who are diagnosed with cancer, in particular gynecological cancer, experience sexual dysfunction that is caused not only by the emotional impact of such a diagnosis, but also by the disease itself and—even more commonly—by treatments that include surgery, radio- and chemotherapy, and/or hormonal therapies (Fobair et al., 2006; Ganz, Rowland, Desmond, Meyerowitz, & Wyatt, 1998).

Menopause is another factor that may lead to sexual problems in women. Reduced ovarian function, which is accompanied by the cessation of menstruation, can lead to a series of physical and mental symptoms including hot flashes, depression, irritability, sleep disturbances, urogenital symptoms, and sexual difficulties (Dennerstein, Dudley, & Burger, 2001). When examining the relationship between menopause and different aspects of female sexual functioning during midlife, a population-based study in Australia reported a significant decrease in women's desire, arousal, orgasm, and frequency of sexual activity, and a significant increase in vaginal dryness (Dennerstein et al., 2001). Similarly, in a European sample of postmenopausal women between the ages of 50 and 60, 35% reported experiencing reduced sex drive, 53% indicated being less interested in sex than before, and they perceived menopause as the leading cause of their reduced sex drive (Nappi & Nijland, 2006). In spite of these high prevalence rates of sexual problems, 71% of women indicated that it was important to them to maintain an active sex life (Nappi & Nijland, 2006). Although sexual responsivity may be adversely affected by both menopause and aging, many women enjoy sexual activities and feel that maintaining a satisfying sex life is important to them beyond midlife and menopause.

Psychological factors

Women who experience sexual dysfunctions differ from women who report no such problems in several psychological characteristics. A meta-analysis shows that the risk of developing a sexual dysfunction for those with *depression* is increased by 50 to 70%, and the risk of depression for those with sexual dysfunctions is increased by 130 to 210% (Atlantis & Sullivan, 2012). Thus, a bidirectional relationship between depressive symptoms and sexual dysfunction is evident.

Early maladaptive schemas have been defined as stable and enduring themes that form in childhood and interfere with adults' ability to meet their basic needs, such as building healthy intimate relationships (Young, Klosko, & Weishaar, 2003). Some women with sexual dysfunctions show stronger endorsements of maladaptive schemas related to feelings of inferiority (e.g., "*I am a failure*") and to feelings of being overly dependent on others (e.g., "*I need other people to help me get by*"; Oliveira & Nobre, 2013). Women might also feel "*inadequate as a woman*" if they are not able to have vaginal intercourse, as shown in a study with heterosexual women with genito-pelvic pain (Ayling & Ussher, 2008).

Women who have a negative attitude toward their body report lower sexual functioning (Woertman & van den Brink, 2012). A negative body image can prevent women from dating or entering a relationship and can lead to self-conscious attempts to conceal their body during sexual activity with a partner. One can easily imagine how self-objectification in the form of preoccupation with (perceived) bodily flaws can negatively affect women's ability to relax and to enjoy potentially pleasurable touch during sex (Steer & Tiggemann, 2008). As feelings of unattractiveness or a perceived lack of femininity negatively affect women who have experienced breast cancer (Ussher, Perz, & Gilbert, 2012) and/or the bodily changes of aging and menopause (Perz & Ussher, 2008), the interaction of biological and psychological factors which influence women's sexual functioning becomes clear.

The psychological consequences of sexual abuse are predictive of sexual problems as an adult (Loeb et al., 2002). While the detrimental effect of sexual abuse on women's psychological and sexual health is well-established, specific associations between traumatic sexual experiences in childhood and certain dysfunctions (e.g., sexual pain disorders) have not been confirmed (Reissing, Binik, Khalif, Cohen, & Amsel, 2003).

Women who have a high level of sexual inhibition—a trait that describes how easily one is distracted during sexual activity or how commonly one experiences the negative impact of sexual worries or performance anxiety on sexual arousal—are at risk for sexual dysfunctions (Bancroft, 1999). For these women, everything has to be "just right" for arousal to occur, and they require a great deal of trust and commitment from a sexual partner in order to "let go" sexually. Similarly, women with low sexual excitation—a trait that describes how easily one is turned on by sexually arousing stimuli (e.g., attractive partner)—are also more likely to experience sexual problems (Bancroft, 1999; Velten, 2017; Velten, Scholten, Graham, & Margraf, 2017). In addition, more general personality traits can also impact women's sexual functioning: Sexual desire is higher in individuals with higher levels of Openness to Experience. Neuroticism is related to higher, and Conscientiousness is related to lower, rates of sexual dysfunction in women (Osborn, Hawton, & Gath, 1988; Velten, Brailovskaia, & Margraf, 2019).

Socio-cultural factors

Socio-cultural factors play a crucial role in determining which sexual behaviors are deemed acceptable and which aspects of women's sexuality are seen as pathological or dysfunctional. *The sexual script perspective*, which is widely used in scientific research on sexuality, posits that sexuality and sexual behavior are social processes (Sakaluk, Todd, Milhausen, & Lachowsky, 2014). Sexual scripts are socially constructed guidelines that, through cognitive schemas, govern appropriate sexual behavior and outline specific roles and interactions (Sakaluk et al., 2014). Parents and major social institutions (e.g., schools, media, governments) promote het-eronormative sexual scripts (Pham, 2016) that prescribe opposite positions for men and women (e.g., the notion that men desire sex, and women are desired but do not themselves desire sex and have weaker sex drives; Masters, Casey, Wells, & Morrison, 2013). These existing scripts, which condemn certain sexual activities for women yet permit the identical actions for men, are problematic because they can serve to obstruct women from expressing their sexual feelings and enjoying sex in many contexts (Baumeister & Twenge, 2002). Cultural norms and expectations that render adolescent girls' sexuality as problematic or danger-ous are still prevalent and may result in turning young women away from the possibilities of empowerment through sexual desire (Tolman, 1994). Culturally speaking, a positive associ-ation has been found between indexes of greater male power and suppression of female sexuality. For instance, in a sample of 186 cultures, Reiss (1986) discovered that the greater the power imbalance in favor of men, the more women's sexuality was suppressed.

Myths about sexuality augment the already existing negative impact that heteronormative scripts have on women's sexual health and well-being. Internalization of unrealistic expect-ations of sex may result in or exacerbate sexual difficulties when these expectations are not met. For example, adherence to the notion that *sexual spontaneity* is necessary for satisfying sex may lead to dissatisfaction or dysfunction. The script of sexual spontaneity asserts that an individual is expected to be aroused instantaneously to facilitate sexual intercourse. Based on this view, women who experience sexual dysfunctions are at a great disadvantage: Low sexual desire disorders violate the expectation that one should desire sexual advances imme-diately, sexual arousal disorders violate the expectation that one should have steady and increasing levels of arousal and vaginal lubrication, orgasmic disorders violate the expectation that one should have an orgasm, and sexual pain disorders may not permit vaginal penetra-tion or make it extremely difficult to enjoy sex (Dune & Shuttleworth, 2009).

Relationship factors

Distress related to sexual difficulties may prevent women from entering a new partnership. In partnered women, it can also cause relationship discord. In women with a steady partner, sexual function and dysfunction are often influenced by their general relationship satisfaction (Dunn, Croft, & Hackett, 2000) as well as their partner's sexual function or dysfunction (Velten & Margraf, 2017). In other words, women who are unhappy in their partnership or whose male or female partners experience sexual difficulties are at risk for sexual dysfunction.

Sexual desire is often highest in the early stages of a relationship and declines afterwards. Among women's reasons for a decline in desire are the institutionalization of the relationship, over-familiarity, and the de-sexualization of roles in these relationships (Sims & Meana, 2010). Another partnership-related factor that can contribute to problems within a sexual relationship is called sexual desire discrepancy. When one sexual partner experiences more desire for sexual activity than the other partner, it can lead to tension within the relationship: The partner with greater desire may get labeled as hypersexual, insatiable, or a sex addict, and the lower desire partner can get blamed as sexually dysfunctional or asexual. While keeping in mind that, of course, both very high and very low desire can be a symptom of a sexual dysfunction, it is more often the case that both partners are simply on two different ends of a continuum between "normal high" and "normal low" sexual desire (Willoughby & Vitas, 2012).

Diagnostic process

Allowing patients to discuss sexual matters, validating and normalizing their concerns, and offering specific suggestions (e.g., to encourage acceptance of normal changes in desire and arousal or to discuss the issue with a partner) can alleviate sexuality-related distress and improve sexual functioning (Annon, 1976). A referral to a sexual health expert is recommended whenever a sexual concern is perceived as severe, long-lasting, and distressing and does not sufficiently respond to these interventions. A thorough gynecological examination is important to identify medical factors that could contribute to a sexual difficulty, and a psychological evaluation of the problem (including predisposing, triggering, and maintaining factors) is necessary to distinguish clinically relevant sexual dysfunctions from short-term, low distress, or sub-clinical sexual problems. As part of this diagnostic process, clinicians trained in sexual health should conduct a comprehensive interview inquiring about all aspects of the sexual response cycle, namely desire, excitement, and orgasm (Kaplan, 1977; Masters & Johnson, 1966) to identify those phases of the sexual response that are perceived as problematic.

Psychometric questionnaires can be helpful to supplement the assessment of women's sexual functioning (Female Sexual Function Index; Rosen et al., 2000), sexual desire (Sexual Interest and Desire Inventory; Clayton et al., 2006), or distress related to sexual concerns (Female Sexual Distress Scale; Derogatis, Rosen, Leiblum, Burnett, & Heiman, 2002). Utilizing such questionnaires can assist clinicians in a multitude of ways (i.e., in their conclusions regarding diagnoses, to identify aspects of women's sexual functioning that are the leading cause for distress, and to individualize treatment approaches). In most cases, clinicians with a background in psychology should encourage patients to also consult a medical expert (e.g., gynecologist), especially when symptoms of genito-pelvic pain are present, to rule out physical causes of the dysfunction.

Medical treatments

Hormonal treatment

Testosterone therapy has been used for decades to treat female sexual dysfunction. This treatment was first introduced in a group of postmenopausal women in the 1950s. Later studies confirmed the beneficial effect of testosterone, namely significant improvement in sexual functioning, not only in postmenopausal women but also in premenopausal women who experience low sexual desire (Khera, 2015). Although there is good evidence regarding the benefit of testosterone treatment, the magnitude of this benefit is small. Despite its common off-label use, long-term safety data on testosterone preparations for women are nonexistent (Wright & O'Connor, 2015).

Oxytocin, a neuropeptide known for its role in parturition and lactation, has attracted interest for its potential impact on sexual arousal and orgasm. One study showed its effectiveness in increasing the intensity of orgasms in couples (Behnia et al., 2014), but a recent review indicates that there is no evidence to support the use of oxytocin for female sexual dysfunction (Worsley, Santoro, Miller, Parish, & Davis, 2016). In addition, the available data also do not support systemic estrogen therapy for the treatment of women's sexual difficulties. Topical vaginal estrogen therapy, however, can improve sexual functioning in postmenopausal women who experience vulvovaginal atrophy (Santoro, Worsley, Miller, Parish, & Davis, 2016).

Flibanserin

Flibanserin, which has pharmacological effects on serotonin and dopamine receptors (Borsini et al., 2002), is the first drug approved by the U.S. Food and Drug Administration for the treatment of female sexual dysfunction (Gellad, Flynn, & Alexander, 2015). While flibanserin was being tested on patients with Major Depressive Disorder, the positive effect of this drug on women's sexual functioning was discovered (Stahl, Sommer, & Allers, 2011). Even though it was ineffective as an antidepressant, it improved sexual functioning in women with depression (Kennedy, 2010). Research suggests that some women with Hypoactive Sexual Desire Disorder can benefit from flibanserin (Katz et al., 2013; Thorp et al., 2012), but the drug has been criticized for its modest effectiveness and an increased risk of hypotension and syncope when used with alcohol (Brotto, 2015).

Other treatments

A review was recently conducted to evaluate the current state of research concerning medical and psychological interventions for vulvodynia (Goldstein et al., 2016). The authors suggested waiting for more empirical evidence before recommending medical treatments such as anti-inflammatory agents, hormonal agents, and anticonvulsant medications. They did *not* recommend lidocaine, topical corticosteroids, or antidepressant medication for the long-term management of vulvodynia, but acknowledged that capsaicin, botulinum toxin, and interferon can be considered second-line avenues in cases where other treatment options (e.g., pelvic-floor muscle therapy, psychological interventions) are not successful. Although the authors agreed that a vestibulectomy, which can include the excision of the mucosa of the entire vulvar vestibule or can be limited to the excision of the mucosa to the posterior vestibule (Tommola, Unkila-Kallio, & Paavonen, 2010), is not recommended as a first line of treatment for Provoked Vestibulodynia, studies suggest that it can be considered once other less invasive treatment options have failed (Goldstein et al., 2016).

Psychological treatments

Most psychological treatments of female sexual dysfunction include couples counseling, behavioral sensate-focus exercises, mindfulness meditation, or a combination of these interventions. Although randomized controlled trials are still scarce, research suggests that psychological therapies—especially cognitive-behavioral and/or mindfulness-based interventions—are effective in treating female sexual dysfunctions (Frühauf, Gerger, Schmidt, Munder, & Barth, 2013). More studies are, however, needed to distinguish which aspects of the commonly used treatment programs are the effective components (Ahn & Wampold, 2001) and whether combinations of psychological and pharmacological treatments improve therapy outcomes (Brotto, 2015).

Psychological and sex education

Psychoeducation combines psychological and educational interventions for the purpose of increasing knowledge and assisting in the development of coping and adaptation skills (Brotto, Basson, & Luria, 2008). Psychoeducational interventions have been found to significantly increase frequency of sexual activity (Capone, Good, Westie, & Jacobson, 1980), reduce fear of intercourse, and improve knowledge about sexuality (Robinson, Faris, & Scott, 1999). Sex education typically focuses on avoiding unintended pregnancy and sexually transmitted infections. Although these two dimensions of sexual health are undoubtedly important, sexual experiences, including women's sexual pleasure, should also be addressed. For example, informing women about physical/genital anatomy, providing information related to different modes of pleasure, and discussing the frequency of women's sexual concerns will not only improve knowledge, but can also lead to greater sexual satisfaction.

Cognitive-behavioral therapy

Cognitive-behavioral therapy (CBT) is the most extensively researched form of psychotherapy for mental health issues (Butler, Chapman, Forman, & Beck, 2006). CBT for sexual dysfunctions in women includes both cognitive and behavioral exercises, which are used comparably for other mental disorders and interventions that aim to target sexual difficulties more specifically.

Using models of sexual response for treatment planning

Use of models of sexual response can be recommended to improve understanding of a woman's sexual interactions, to identify factors that contribute to her sexual difficulty, and to provide a rationale for cognitive or behavioral interventions. Although the linear model of sexual response is useful for diagnostic purposes and for identifying the stages of sexual response that are perceived as dysfunctional, it does not offer insights into the dynamics of specific sexual interactions of a woman and her partner. Basson's circular model of sexual response, however, allows for a detailed analysis of positive and negative aspects of a sexual interaction and is thus a useful tool for deciding which cognitive-behavioral interventions are expected to be effective for a particular sexual difficulty (see Figure 28.2).

Another advantage of this model is the acknowledgment that sexual desire is often not the trigger for sexual interactions in women with sexual dysfunction, especially for those in long-term relationships. According to this view, a woman frequently begins a sexual encounter without any explicit sexual desire, but rather from a place of neutrality. Her reasons for sex can be diverse, such as a wish to feel close to a partner, a desire to please a partner, or a need for stress relief. When she is receptive to sexual stimuli, if the setting and context are pleasing and the woman stays focused and is not

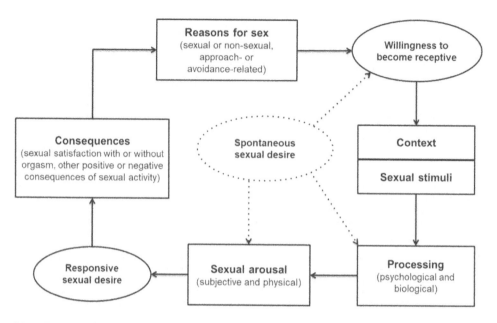

Figure 28.2 Circular sexual response model. Adapted with permission from Basson, R. (2001). Female sexual response: The role of drugs in the management of sexual dysfunction. *Obstetrics & Gynecology, 98,* 350–353.

distracted, her body and mind may respond with some pleasure and beginnings of sexual arousal. Finally, she may have some desire to continue the sexual experience as a result of the enhanced intimacy and/or for the pleasant physical sensations. This alternative model of sexual response clarifies the importance of women's arousal pre-ceding sexual desire (Basson, 2005). Taken together, this model can be used to identify problematic contextual (e.g., lack of privacy or safety, relationship problems), biological (e.g., pain, fatigue, use of certain medications), and psychological (e.g., low mood, negative body image, past negative sexual experiences) factors that may negatively influence women's sexual functioning and thereby facilitate management.

Self-exploration and self-stimulation

Guided masturbation or self-stimulation exercises can be helpful for women with any kind of sexual dysfunction. They are especially useful for women who have few experiences with mastur-bation and have difficulties in identifying what stimuli they find sexually arousing. For women who are not in a committed relationship, these exercises are a key treatment component. By using a hand-held mirror, women can look at their genitals more closely and thereby increase knowledge about their genital anatomy. Women should be encouraged to experiment with dif-ferent kinds of intimate self-touch to learn more about what is pleasurable to them. Knowing what kinds of touch are enjoyable and how sexual arousal can be deliberately triggered is crucial to overcoming not only problems related to a lack of lubrication or problems with orgasm, but also to reducing symptoms of genito-pelvic pain. In cases where a woman has the opportunity and means to purchase sexual aids, clinicians may also discuss whether she is open to experiment-ing with lube, erotic literature, or vibrators to facilitate or enhance her sexual arousal.

Sensate focus exercises

Sensate focus exercises are behavioral interventions that are recommended for couples in which one or both partners experience sexual difficulties (Masters & Johnson, 1970). During the first stages of sensate focus, partners are encouraged to take turns in providing and receiving non-sexual touch. In other words, they limit their caresses to parts of their partner's body that are not considered highly erogenous. Both partners are encouraged to focus on their own sensations, emotions, and thoughts during both active and passive phases and to avoid being guided by a wish to please their partner. In the next stage, partners are allowed to provide sensual touch to the complete body. Still, they should not strive to arouse their partner sexually, but rather experiment with different kinds of touch. In later stages, partners should play with arousal by increasing sexual touch. The main goals of these exercises are to reduce pressure to perform, experience a new kind of intimacy, improve sexual communication, and reveal sexual interaction patterns that may have led to a sexual difficulty. For women with arousal or orgasm difficulties, these interactions might help to focus on one's own sensations of arousal without having to focus on their partner simultaneously. In order to reduce performance anxiety, heterosexual couples should not engage in sexual intercourse during or after these exercises (Carr, 2014).

Cognitive interventions

As outlined above, socialization and cultural factors influence the way women think about sexuality in general and their own personal sexual experiences. Cognitive interventions are effective to modify dysfunctional sexual cognitions and to replace them with more adequate or helpful thoughts. Common thought biases include catastrophizing (e.g., "I worry all the time that the sexual pain will never end"), black-and-white thinking (e.g., "I can never have sex again"), or personalization (e.g., "It is all my fault that my partner is sexually dissatisfied"). As most of these thoughts are rather automatic and not completely conscious, keeping thought records can help women to be more aware of these thoughts, to be able to distinguish these thoughts from facts, and to be able to see how they impact their mood as well as their sexual relationships. A thought diary can also be used to consider alternative thoughts that may result in a more positive emotional state and more functional behavior patterns (e.g., approaching sexual situations with a more helpful attitude; Fenn & Byrne, 2013). Clients might complete a seven-column thought diary (Greenberger & Padesky, 1995), which involves detailing the situation; mood; negative automatic thoughts related to sexuality; evidence for and against each thought; the development of an alternative, more adequate, or functional response; and a rerating of mood that would be associated with this alternative thought. Identifying cognitive errors, examining evidence for and against sexuality-related thoughts, listing rational alternatives, and other techniques related to cognitive restructuring can help women to evaluate their sexual difficulties or their sex life in a more favorable light (Fenn & Byrne, 2013).

Mindfulness-based treatments

Mindfulness, an ancient Eastern practice, is a present-moment, nonjudgmental awareness of one's feelings, physical sensations, and thoughts. Kabat-Zinn introduced this phenomenon into Western mental health services in the late 1970s (Kabat-Zinn, 1982). Mindfulness exercises have since been integrated with interventions for a broad range of mental health issues (e.g., depression, chronic pain). Mindfulness-based treatments for sexual dysfunctions in women have become increasingly popular over the last decade (Brotto, Chivers, Millman, & Albert, 2016). This is not surprising as recent studies have shown that such treatments are effective in improving women's sexual pain, reducing sexuality-related distress in women who are recovering from gynecological cancer, and increasing sexual desire and arousal in women with FSIAD (Brotto, Basson, Smith, Driscoll, & Sadownik, 2014; Brotto & Heiman, 2007; Paterson, Handy, & Brotto, 2016).

The mechanisms, however, by which mindfulness improves women's sexual concerns remain unclear (Arora & Brotto, 2017). It has been suggested that mindfulness improves women's sexual functioning by reducing spectatoring (i.e., the process of watching oneself during sexual activity from a third-person perspective), decreasing distraction by nonsexual thoughts, increasing acceptance and nonjudgment with respect to a sexual experience, and/or directly influencing the different levels of women's sexual arousal response (Paterson, Handy, & Brotto, 2016; Velten, Margraf, Chivers, & Brotto, 2018). Exercises that are commonly used in sex therapy include mindfulness during a regular activity (e.g., eating, walking, engaging in conversation), body-scans, and breathing exercises. These are supplemented by more sexuality-related practices that guide women to focus on sensations on different parts of the body, including the genitals. Treatments include in-session mindfulness practices as well as daily at-home exercises. Women are also encouraged to set long-term goals for a personal mindfulness practice.

Conclusion

Millions of women worldwide struggle with sexual difficulties such as low desire, arousal problems, or genito-pelvic pain (McCabe et al., 2016a). When these problems are experienced frequently and persistently, and are the cause of significant personal distress, a sexual dysfunction may be present. As problems with sexual functioning are still a taboo topic, mental health professionals are encouraged to inquire whether a woman experiences any sexuality-related concerns, rather than waiting for a patient or client to take the first step. For most sexual dysfunctions, psycho-social interventions are the treatment of choice. Consultation of medical experts is, however, recommended to rule out physical causes of sexual difficulties. In many cases, educating women about their sexual response; explaining the relationships between mood, stress, and sexual arousal; and introducing some behavioral exercises can help to alleviate symptoms. Cognitive-behavioral exercises as well as mindfulness-based therapies are promising treatments for many women with sexual dysfunctions. With the advancement of technology, there is a major shift towards utilizing Internet-based platforms. More specifically, researchers are focusing on developing online resources (i.e., web- and phone-based apps) that can provide educational information as part of self-help interventions, with the goal of reaching and helping women who live in rural areas and/or do not have access to other resources. Improving access to effective treatments for sexual dysfunctions across all age groups, ethnicities, and sexual orientations is needed to improve the women's sexual health around the globe.

References

Ahn, H. & Wampold, B. E. (2001). Where oh where are the specific ingredients? A meta-analysis of component studies in counseling and psychotherapy. *Journal of Counseling Psychology, 48,* 251–257.

American Psychiatric Association (APA) (2013). *Diagnostic and statistical manual of mental disorders* (5th ed.). Washington, DC: Author.

Annon, J. S. (1976). The PLISSIT model: A proposed conceptual scheme for the behavioral treatment of sexual problems. *Journal of Sex Education and Therapy, 2,* 1–15.

Arora, N. & Brotto, L. A. (2017). How does paying attention improve sexual functioning in women? A review of mechanisms. *Sexual Medicine Review, 5*, 266–274.

Atlantis, E. & Sullivan, T. (2012). Bidirectional association between depression and sexual dysfunction: A systematic review and meta-analysis. *Journal of Sexual Medicine, 9*, 1497–1507.

Ayling, K. & Ussher, J. M. (2008). "If sex hurts, am I still a woman?" The subjective experience of vulvodynia in hetero-sexual women. *Archives of Sexual Behavior, 37*, 294–304.

Bancroft, J. (1999). Central inhibition of sexual response in the male: A theoretical perspective. *Neuroscience & Biobehavioral Reviews, 23*, 763–784.

Basson, R. (2001). Female sexual response: The role of drugs in the management of sexual dysfunction. *Obstetrics & Gynecology, 98*, 350–353.

Basson, R. (2005). Women's sexual dysfunction: Revised and expanded definitions. *Canadian Medical Association Journal, 172*, 1327–1333.

Baumeister, R. F. & Twenge, J. M. (2002). Cultural suppression of female sexuality. *Review of General Psychology, 6*, 166–203.

Beaber, T. E. & Werner, P. D. (2009). The relationship between anxiety and sexual functioning in lesbians and heterosexual women. *Journal of Homosexuality, 56*, 639–654.

Behnia, B., Heinrichs, M., Bergmann, W., Jung, S., Germann, J., Schedlowski, M., Hartmann, U., & Kruger, T. H. C. (2014). Differential effects of intranasal oxytocin on sexual experiences and partner interactions in couples. *Hormones and Behavior, 65*, 308–318.

Bergeron, S., Rosen, N. O., & Morin, M. (2011). Genital pain in women: Beyond interference with intercourse. *Pain, 152*, 1223–1225.

Borsini, F., Evans, K., Jason, K., Rohde, F., Alexander, B., & Pollentier, S. (2002). Pharmacology of flibanserin. *CNS Drug Reviews, 8*, 117–142.

Brotto, L. A. (2015). Flibanserin. *Archives of Sexual Behavior, 44*, 2103–2105.

Brotto, L. A., Basson, R., & Luria, M. (2008). A mindfulness-based group psychoeducational intervention targeting sexual arousal disorder in women. *Journal of Sexual Medicine, 5*, 1646–1659.

Brotto, L. A., Basson, R., Smith, K. B., Driscoll, M., & Sadownik, L. (2014). Mindfulness-based group therapy for women with provoked vestibulodynia. *Mindfulness, 6*, 1–16.

Brotto, L. A., Bitzer, J., Laan, E., Leiblum, S., & Luria, M. (2010). Women's sexual desire and arousal disorders. *Journal of Sexual Medicine, 7*, 586–614.

Brotto, L. A., Chivers, M. L., Millman, R. D., & Albert, A. (2016). Mindfulness-based sex therapy improves genital-subjective arousal concordance in women with sexual desire/arousal difficulties. *Archives of Sexual Behavior, 45*, 1907–1921.

Brotto, L. A. & Heiman, J. R. (2007). Mindfulness in sex therapy: Applications for women with sexual difficulties following gynecologic cancer. *Sexual and Relationship Therapy, 22*, 3–11.

Butler, A. C., Chapman, J. E., Forman, E. M., & Beck, A. T. (2006). The empirical status of cognitive-behavioral therapy: A review of meta-analyses. *Clinical Psychology Review, 26*, 17–31.

Capone, M., Good, R. S., Westie, K. S., & Jacobson, A. F. (1980). Psychosocial rehabilitation of gynecologic oncology patients. *Archives of Physical Medicine and Rehabilitation, 61*, 128–132.

Carr, A. (2014). The evidence base for couple therapy, family therapy and systemic interventions for adult-focused problems. *Journal of Family Therapy, 36*, 158–194.

Clayton, A. H., Segraves, R. T., Leiblum, S., Basson, R., Pyke, R., Cotton, D., Lewis-D'Agostino, D., Evans, K. R., Sills, T. L., & Wunderlich, G. R. (2006). Reliability and validity of the Sexual Interest and Desire Inventory–Female (SIDI-F), a scale designed to measure severity of female hypoactive sexual desire disorder. *Journal of Sex & Marital Therapy, 32*, 115–135.

Dennerstein, L., Dudley, E., & Burger, H. (2001). Are changes in sexual functioning during midlife due to aging or menopause? *Fertility and Sterility, 76*, 456–460, doi:10.1016/S0015-0282(01)01978-0.

Derogatis, L. R., Rosen, R. C., Leiblum, S., Burnett, A., & Heiman, J. (2002). The Female Sexual Distress Scale (FSDS): Initial validation of a standardized scale for assessment of sexually related personal distress in women. *Journal of Sex & Marital Therapy, 28*, 317–330.

Duncan, L. E., Lewis, C., Smith, C. E., Jenkins, P., Nichols, M., & Pearson, T. A. (2001). Sex, drugs, and hypertension: A methodological approach for studying a sensitive subject. *International Journal of Impotence Research, 13*, 31–40.

Dune, T. M. & Shuttleworth, R. P. (2009). "It's just supposed to happen": The myth of sexual spontaneity and the sexually marginalized. *Sexuality and Disability, 27*, 97–108.

Dunn, K. M., Croft, P. R., & Hackett, G. I. (2000). Satisfaction in the sex life of a general population sample. *Journal of Sex & Marital Therapy, 26*, 141–151.

Eplov, L., Giraldi, A., Davidsen, M., Garde, K., & Kamper-Jørgensen, F. (2007). Sexual desire in a nationally representative Danish population. *Journal of Sexual Medicine, 4*, 47–56.

Fenn, K. & Byrne, M. (2013). The key principles of cognitive behavioural therapy. *InnovAiT: Education and Inspiration for General Practice, 6*, 579–585.

Fobair, P., Stewart, S. L., Chang, S., D'Onofrio, C., Banks, P. J., & Bloom, J. R. (2006). Body image and sexual problems in young women with breast cancer. *Psycho-Oncology, 15*, 579–594.

Frühauf, S., Gerger, H., Schmidt, H. M., Munder, T., & Barth, J. (2013). Efficacy of psychological interventions for sexual dysfunction: A systematic review and meta-analysis. *Archives of Sexual Behavior, 42*, 915–933.

Ganz, P. A., Rowland, J. H., Desmond, K., Meyerowitz, B. E., & Wyatt, G. E. (1998). Life after breast cancer: Understanding women's health-related quality of life and sexual functioning. *Journal of Clinical Oncology, 16*, 501–514.

Gellad, W. F., Flynn, K. E., & Alexander, G. (2015). Evaluation of flibanserin: Science and advocacy at the FDA. *Journal of the American Medical Association, 314*, 869–870.

Goldstein, A. T., Pukall, C. F., Brown, C., Bergeron, S., Stein, A., & Kellogg-Spadt, S. (2016). Vulvodynia: Assessment and treatment. *Journal of Sexual Medicine, 13*, 572–590.

Greenberger, D. & Padesky, C. A. (1995). *Mind over mood: A cognitive therapy treatment manual for clients.* New York: Guilford.

Henderson, A. W., Lehavot, K., & Simoni, J. M. (2009). Ecological models of sexual satisfaction among lesbian/bisexual and heterosexual women. *Archives of Sexual Behavior, 38*, 50–65.

Jackson, A. B. & Wadley, V. (1999). A multicenter study of women's self-reported reproductive health after spinal cord injury. *Archives of Physical Medicine and Rehabilitation, 80*(11), 1420–1428.

Kabat-Zinn, J. (1982). An outpatient program in behavioral medicine for chronic pain patients based on the practice of mindfulness meditation: Theoretical considerations and preliminary results. *General Hospital Psychiatry, 4*, 33–47.

Kaplan, H. S. (1977). Hypoactive sexual desire. *Journal of Sex & Marital Therapy, 3*, 3–9.

Katz, M., DeRogatis, L. R., Ackerman, R., Hedges, P., Lesko, L., Garcia, M., & Sand, M. (2013). Efficacy of flibanserin in women with hypoactive sexual desire disorder: Results from the BEGONIA trial. *Journal of Sexual Medicine, 10*, 1807–1815.

Kennedy, S. (2010). Flibanserin: Initial evidence of efficacy on sexual dysfunction, in patients with major depressive disorder. *Journal of Sexual Medicine, 7*, 3449–3459.

Khera, M. (2015). Testosterone therapy for female sexual dysfunction. *Sexual Medicine Reviews, 3*, 137–144.

Landry, T., Bergeron, S., Dupuis, M. J., & Desrochers, G. (2008). The treatment of provoked vestibulodynia: A critical review. *Clinical Journal of Pain, 24*, 155–171.

Loeb, T. B., Rivkin, I., Williams, J. K., Wyatt, G. E., Carmona, J. V., & Chin, D. (2002). Child sexual abuse: Associations with the sexual functioning of adolescents and adults. *Annual Review of Sex Research, 13*, 307–345.

Martelli, V., Valisella, S., Moscatiello, S., Matteucci, C., Lantadilla, C., Costantino, A., Pelusi, G., Marchesini, G., & Meriggiola, M. C. (2012). Prevalence of sexual dysfunction among postmenopausal women with and without metabolic syndrome. *Journal of Sexual Medicine, 9*, 434–441.

Masters, N. T., Casey, E., Wells, E. A., & Morrison, D. M. (2013). Sexual scripts among young heterosexually active men and women: Continuity and change. *Journal of Sex Research, 50*, 409–420.

Masters, W. H. & Johnson, V. E. (1966). *Human sexual response.* Boston, MA: Little, Brown, and Company.

Masters, W. H. & Johnson, V. E. (1970). *Human sexual inadequacy.* Boston, MA: Little, Brown, and Company.

McCabe, M. P., Sharlip, I. D., Lewis, R., Atalla, E., Balon, R., Fisher, A. D., Laumann, E., Lee, S. W., & Segraves, R. T. (2016a). Incidence and prevalence of sexual dysfunction in women and men: A consensus statement from the fourth international consultation on sexual medicine 2015. *Journal of Sexual Medicine, 13*, 144–152.

McCabe, M. P., Sharlip, I. D., Lewis, R., Atalla, E., Balon, R., Fisher, A. D., Laumann, E., Lee, S. W., & Segraves, R. T. (2016b). Risk factors for sexual dysfunction among women and men: A consensus statement from the fourth international consultation on sexual medicine 2015. *Journal of Sexual Medicine, 13*, 153–167.

Mitchell, K. R., Jones, K. G., Wellings, K., Johnson, A. M., Graham, C. A., Datta, J., Copas, A. J., Bancroft, J., Sonnenberg, P., Macdowall, W., Field, N., & Mercer, C. H. (2016). Estimating the prevalence of sexual function problems: The impact of morbidity criteria. *Journal of Sex Research, 53*, 955–967.

Nappi, R. E. & Nijland, E. A. (2006). Women's perception of sexuality around the menopause: Outcomes of a European telephone survey. *European Journal of Obstetrics & Gynecology and Reproductive Biology*, *137*, 10–16.

Oliveira, C. & Nobre, P. J. (2013). The role of trait-affect, depression, and anxiety in women with sexual dysfunction: A pilot study. *Journal of Sex & Marital Therapy*, *39*, 436–452.

Osborn, M., Hawton, K., & Gath, D. (1988). Sexual dysfunction among middle aged women in the community. *British Medical Journal*, *296*, 959–962.

Paterson, L. Q. P., Handy, A. B., & Brotto, L. A. (2016). A pilot study of eight-session mindfulness-based cognitive therapy adapted for women's sexual interest/arousal disorder. *Journal of Sex Research*, *54*, 850–861.

Perz, J. & Ussher, J. M. (2008). "The horror of this living decay": Women's negotiation and resistance of medical discourses around menopause and midlife. *Women's Studies International Forum*, *31*, 293–299.

Pham, J. M. (2016). The limits of heteronormative sexual scripting: College student development of individual sexual scripts and descriptions of lesbian sexual behavior. *Frontiers in Sociology*, *1*, 1–10.

Reiss, I. L. (1986). *Journey into sexuality: An exploratory voyage*. Upper Saddle River, NJ: Prentice Hall.

Reissing, E. D., Binik, Y. M., Khalif, S., Cohen, D., & Amsel, R. (2003). Etiological correlates of vaginismus: Sexual and physical abuse, sexual knowledge, sexual self-schema, and relationship adjustment. *Journal of Sex & Marital Therapy*, *29*, 47–59.

Richters, J., Grulich, A. E., Visser, R. O., Smith, A., & Rissel, C. E. (2003). Sex in Australia: Autoerotic, esoteric and other sexual practices engaged in by a representative sample of adults. *Australian and New Zealand Journal of Public Health*, *27*, 180–190.

Robinson, J. W., Faris, P. D., & Scott, C. B. (1999). Psychoeducational group increases vaginal dilation for younger women and reduces sexual fears for women of all ages with gynecological carcinoma treated with radiotherapy. *International Journal of Radiation Oncology Biology Physics*, *44*, 497–506.

Rosen, R. C., Brown, J., Heiman, S., Leiblum, C., Meston, R., Shabsigh, D., Ferguson, R., & D'Agostino, R. (2000). The Female Sexual Function Index (FSFI): A multidimensional self-report instrument for the assessment of female sexual function. *Journal of Sex & Marital Therapy*, *26*, 191–208.

Sakaluk, J. K., Todd, L. M., Milhausen, R., & Lachowsky, N. J. (2014). Dominant heterosexual sexual scripts in emerging adulthood: Conceptualization and measurement. *Journal of Sex Research*, *51*, 516–531.

Santoro, N., Worsley, R., Miller, K. K., Parish, S. J., & Davis, S. R. (2016). Role of estrogens and estrogen-like compounds in female sexual function and dysfunction. *Journal of Sexual Medicine*, *13*, 305–316.

Sims, K. E. & Meana, M. (2010). Why did passion wane? A qualitative study of married women's attributions for declines in sexual desire. *Journal of Sex & Marital Therapy*, *36*, 360–380.

Stahl, S. M., Sommer, B., & Allers, K. A. (2011). Multifunctional pharmacology of flibanserin: Possible mechanism of therapeutic action in hypoactive sexual desire disorder. *Journal of Sexual Medicine*, *8*, 15–27.

Steer, A. & Tiggemann, M. (2008). The role of self-objectification in women's sexual functioning. *Journal of Social and Clinical Psychology*, *27*, 205–225.

Thorp, J., Simon, J., Dattani, D., Taylor, L., Kimura, T., Garcia, Jr, M., Lesko, L., & Pyke, R. (2012). Treatment of hypoactive sexual desire disorder in premenopausal women: Efficacy of flibanserin in the daisy study. *Journal of Sexual Medicine*, *9*, 793–804.

Tolman, D. L. (1994). Doing desire: Adolescent girls' struggle for/with sexuality. *Gender & Society*, *8*, 324–342.

Tommola, P., Unkila-Kallio, L., & Paavonen, J. (2010). Surgical treatment of vulvar vestibulitis: A review. *Acta Obstetricia Et Gynecologica Scandinavica*, *89*, 1385–1395.

Ussher, J. M., Perz, J. & Gilbert, E. (2012). Changes to sexual wellbeing and intimacy after breast cancer. *Cancer Nursing*, *35*(6), 456–465.

Velten, J. (2017). The dual control model of sexual response: Relevance of sexual excitation and sexual inhibition for sexual function. *Current Sexual Health Reports*, *9*, 90–97.

Velten, J. (2018). *Sexuelle Funktionsstörungen bei Frauen*. Göttingen: Hogrefe.

Velten, J., Brailovskaia, J., & Margraf, J. (2019). Exploring the impact of personal and partner traits on sexuality: Sexual excitation, sexual inhibition, and big five predict sexual function in couples. *Journal of Sex Research*, *56*, 287–299.

Velten, J. & Margraf, J. (2017). Satisfaction guaranteed? How actor, partner, and relationship factors impact sexual satisfaction within partnerships. *PLoS One*, *12*, e0172855.

Velten, J., Margraf, J., Chivers, M. L., & Brotto, L. A. (2018). Effects of a mindfulness task on women's sexual response. *Journal of Sex Research*, *55*, 747–757.

Velten, J., Scholten, S., Graham, C. A., & Margraf, J. (2017). Sexual excitation and sexual inhibition as predictors of sexual function in women: A cross sectional and longitudinal study. *Journal of Sex & Marital Therapy*, *43*, 95–109.

Willoughby, B. J. & Vitas, J. (2012). Sexual desire discrepancy: The effect of individual differences in desired and actual sexual frequency on dating couples. *Archives of Sexual Behavior*, *41*, 477–486.

Woertman, L. & van den Brink, F. (2012). Body image and female sexual functioning and behavior: A review. *Journal of Sex Research*, *49*, 184–211.

World Health Organization (WHO) (2006). *Defining sexual health*. Geneva, Switzerland: Author. Retrieved 29 July 2019, from www.who.int/reproductivehealth/topics/sexual_health/sh_definitions/en.

Worsley, R., Santoro, N., Miller, K. K., Parish, S. J., & Davis, S. R. (2016). Hormones and female sexual dysfunction: Beyond estrogens and androgens-findings from the fourth international consultation on sexual medicine. *Journal of Sexual Medicine*, *13*, 283–290.

Wright, J. J. & O'Connor, K. M. (2015). Female sexual dysfunction. *Medical Clinics of North America*, *99*, 607–628.

Young, J. E., Klosko, J. S., & Weishaar, M. E. (2003). *Schema therapy: A practitioner's guide*. New York: Guilford.

29

SEXUALITY AND SEXUAL DYSFUNCTIONS

Critical analyses

Peggy J. Kleinplatz, Lianne A. Rosen, Maxime Charest and Alyson K. Spurgas

The topic of this chapter is ostensibly women's sexuality and its problems or dysfunctions. However, in order to provide a critical analysis of this subject, we are first required to consider queries such as: What are sex and sexuality? How are we to conceptualize sexual problems? How are we to diagnose women's sexual problems? What gets defined as problematic for women and by whom? Although sexology, sex therapy, and sexual medicine all give lip-service to the notion of a "biopsychosocial" model of women's sexuality, the role of biological factors tends to be emphasized while the psychosocial factors tend to be underestimated (cf., American Psychiatric Association [APA], 2013, as described by McCarthy & McDonald, 2009). Similarly, although diagnoses of sexual problems are to be based on distress and dysfunction, the role of women's distress has been de-contextualized and minimized while "objective" indicators increasingly have been emphasized (Nathan, 2010; Ussher, 1993).

The current system of diagnosis and treatment of women's sexual problems is largely a product of Western cultural norms and values about sexuality, though these models tend to be presented as value-neutral and free from bias. In this chapter, we contextualize and critique the three major diagnostic categories of sexual dysfunctions specific to women, as defined by the fifth edition of the *Diagnostic and Statistical Manual of Mental Disorders* (*DSM-5*; APA, 2013): Female Orgasmic Disorder, Genito-Pelvic Pain/Penetration Disorder (GPPPD), and Female Sexual Interest/Arousal Disorder (FSIAD).

Contextualizing theories of women's sexualities

The sex-related diagnoses contained in the *DSM-5* (APA, 2013) must be situated in socio-historical context. "Sexual dysfunctions" have been defined such that they refer primarily to first-world problems. The majority of girls and women on Earth have more fundamental sexual problems to contend with than do most individuals in Western countries. Sexologists are more than aware that over 200,000,000 women have been subjected to female genital mutilation (WHO, 2018). However, most of us are not aware of other problems equally or more pervasive than FGM, which prevent women in developing countries from even the most basic sexual health. Here are a few examples: In Western societies, we assume that women who fail to lubricate have a problem. In much of Africa and the Middle East, vaginas are supposed to be dry to make for a tighter fit for the husband (Levin, 2005; Mbikusita-Lewanika, Stephen, & Thomas, 2009). As such, women are instructed to engage in "salt-packing" of their vaginas, or a liberal application of astringents to their vaginal mucosa, so as to create the aesthetic of dried-out vaginal tissues. This cross-cultural juxtaposition highlights the social construction of the female body.

Another common problem is the direct result of lack of the most basic health care for women in childbirth. Prolonged, arduous labour without the support of a midwife too often results in the development of vaginal-rectal fistulas. The resulting incontinence and accompanying stigma result in women being forced to withdraw permanently to their homes, never able to go out in public; even the thought of further sexual activity can be abhorrent for them and often their husbands (Heller & Hannig, 2017). Paradoxically, the United States, home to the highest rates of medical interventions – again, generally without midwives – is also the site of the highest rate of maternal and fetal mortality in the Western world (Studnicki & Fisher, 2018). Not surprisingly, the highest rate of Caesarean sections in the world is in the US as well (American College of Obstetricians and Gynecologists, 2014). In some instances, women request the procedure to preserve attractively youthful vaginal tone and the appearance of the genitals. Whereas it is commonplace for pelvic floor physiotherapists and sex therapists to deal with the sequelae of potentially unnecessary episiotomies and subsequent scarring, the preventative sex education necessary for women the world over and their caregivers is sadly lacking.

Assumptions about what counts as "normal," "objective" genital sexual response eclipse subjective experience and pleasure. These assumptions are so ingrained in sexuality theory and research that many do not even realize that these are indeed assumptions. For example, women's and men's sexualities are not as divergent as they are often claimed to be. Studies have demonstrated that there is more within-sex variation in sexuality than there is between-sex variation (Conley et al., 2011; Petersen & Hyde, 2010). However, these assumptions are injected into much of the research at the outset and the accompanying diagnostic nosologies. Accordingly, these unexplored assumptions have become the tenuous foundations upon which the field of modern sexology rests. They are the product of more than a century of purportedly objective medical, psychological, and scientific inquiry into what counts as "normal" sexuality and its deviations.

The modern study of sexual dysfunctions and sex therapy began in the U.S. in the 1950s, when Masters and Johnson set out to liberate human sexuality from the domains of theology, philosophy, and psychoanalysis. They stated that sexual response is a bodily function, as "natural" as "respiratory, bowel, and bladder functions" (Masters & Johnson, 1986, p. 2). Their studies led to the development of Masters and Johnson's (1966) model of the Human Sexual Response Cycle (HSRC), which consists of four stages in both women and men: excitement, plateau, orgasm, and resolution.

Their model has been criticized for concerns about generalizability and the limitations of the data beyond the physiological (e.g., Irvine, 2005; Reiss, 1990; Schnarch, 1991; Tiefer, 1996; Zilbergeld & Ellison, 1980). The unintended consequences of this line of research were to limit the understanding of human sexuality and its problems to that which could be examined via physiological measures, thereby obscuring the lived experience of human phenomena. Notwithstanding these criticisms, the HSRC model became the basis for defining "normal" sexual response and clinical diagnosis and treatment, beginning with diagnoses such as anorgasmia and vaginismus in the *DSM-III* (APA, 1980).

In the 1980s, low desire was added to the diagnostic nomenclature (APA, 1980). In the 1990s, the disorder was named as the presumably "atheoretical" Hypoactive Sexual Desire Disorder (HSDD). HSDD later came to be diagnosed more frequently in women than in men, and eventually came to be understood, at least in the popular sphere, as women's most common and pressing sexual difficulty.

As indicated by the editors of the *DSM-III* (APA, 1980), new editions were to be empirically based, and therefore the earlier diagnoses (APA, 1952, 1968) of nymphomania and satyriasis were removed because they were gender-biased. It was presumably no coincidence that in the aftermath of the "sexual revolution," suddenly too much sex could no longer be pathologized, whereas low desire was newly deemed pathological. A complete review of the changes in the nosology of female sexual dysfunctions in the *DSM* from 1952 to 2013 is beyond the scope of this chapter. (For a more complete discussion of nosology, see Angel, 2012; Kleinplatz, 2018.)

The medicalization of female sexuality

Because the initial academic and clinical discourse in sexology rested on tenuous footing, it was not surprising to see even the existing structures collapse upon the introduction of medical and pharmacologic solutions to sexual problems. Sexual difficulties were suddenly reconstituted as problems in sexual health to be treated by specialists in sexual medicine. Any hope for trans-disciplinary sharing of knowledge, challenging of one another's assumptions, conceptualizations of the goals of treatment, and general contextualizing of women's health care needs and aspirations has been lost. (For a fuller exposition of these changes over time, see Kleinplatz, 2003, 2012, 2018.)

Upon its introduction in 1998, the initially impressive sales of Viagra created a market for pharmaceutical companies to produce an equivalent drug for women (Hartley, 2006; Loe, 2004). The problem for those in research and development was in specifying what disorder ought to be targeted. The industry created the new nomenclature of "Female Sexual Dysfunction" (FSD). This term – note the singular form – began to appear regularly in the media. It was unclear to researchers and clinicians what "disorder" FSD might be. It appeared to be an amalgam of any and all previous female sexual dysfunctions with an emphasis on women's low desire or HSDD, but FSD was never defined. In other words, the goal was to develop treatments for whatever might sell best by creating an increasingly oblique diagnostic catch-all (Moynihan, 2003; Potts, 2008; Tiefer, 2001, 2006). The race was on to create new treatments for FSD (as documented in the film *Orgasm Inc.* by Canner, 2009).

Pfizer investigators began to study whether or not Viagra might have sales potential for women. After six years of gathering data, Pfizer concluded that women are more "complicated" than men (as cited in Harris, 2004). Women were said to require more wooing in order to engage them sexually. Ironically, Viagra works identically, physiologically and pharmacologically, on the erectile tissues of the genitalia regardless of biological sex. However, in a society that defines "sex" as heterosexual intercourse, an erect penis is a more salient sign to initiate sex than is an engorged clitoris. As a result, Pfizer announced it would cease its research on the use of Viagra in women. This opened up the field for new conceptualizations of what could possibly be wrong with women's sexual functioning by the pharmaceutical industry and in the research literature.

What has been continuous is that women's sexual dysfunctions have been treated piecemeal, as if each of the dysfunctions were independent and discrete entities, rather than noticing how, for example, lack of appropriate stimulation might lead to low arousal, which might lead to lack of orgasm, which might lead to pain on intercourse, and eventually to both lowered desire for sex (diagnosed as FSIAD) and bodily aversion to penetration (diagnosed as GPPPD). In the interim, what has been lost is a focus on women's pleasure. Each of these diagnoses and their history will be discussed below.

Female orgasmic disorder

Controversies surrounding female orgasm have gone in and out of fashion. The first two editions of the *DSM* (APA, 1952, 1968) listed women's "frigidity" without specifying what this might comprise. Implicit in mid-20th-century Western society was the notion that women should be sexually responsive to their husbands' desires, and ideally, this should culminate in orgasm during heterosexual intercourse. Thus, during the first three decades of the *DSM*, arousal, orgasm, and desire were conflated. The 1950s notion that women *should* have orgasms during intercourse was reversed when Masters and Johnson reported that women have no nerve endings for touch in the inner two-thirds of their vaginas, thereby making orgasm via thrusting alone a physical impossibility. During the 1970s and 1980s, feminist sex therapists such as Lonnie Barbach (2000) and Betty Dodson (1987) encouraged women to discover orgasm in whatever ways they might find pleasurable. Barbach (1980) even suggested that the term "anorgasmia" is a misnomer: There is no such thing as a woman incapable of orgasm – only one who has not experienced orgasm, yet. Thus, she favored the term "pre-orgasmic." Thereafter, women who presented in therapy complaining of difficulties with orgasm were provided with psychoeducational counselling that emphasized the role of the clitoris in female sexual pleasure rather than "treatment" as such. The various editions of the *DSM* from the 1980s to the present have indicated that it is for the clinician to determine whether or not the woman has received adequate and sufficient stimulation to reach orgasm. Notwithstanding the clinical leeway, during the 1980s there was renewed controversy about whether women should be having "vaginal" versus "clitoral" orgasms. The best-selling book, *The G Spot* (Ladas, Whipple, & Perry, 1983/2004), had been misconstrued so as to suggest, again, that "mature" women should, in fact, be having orgasms during intercourse. This struck its authors as ironic. They had sought to liberate women from being told what the right kind of orgasm ought to be. Instead, their work was subverted by the popular press, which continued to debate how women should "achieve" orgasm (Tavris, 1992). The controversy lingers, fueled by mainstream media and pornographic depictions of women reaching climaxes effortlessly upon penetration. Some researchers continue to suggest that there is a hierarchy of women's orgasms with the alleged "vaginal" orgasm as the ideal (Brody & Costa, 2008, 2017), while others condemn this notion strongly (e.g., Brotto, 2017; Therrien & Brotto, 2016). In clinical practice, we are now more, rather than less, likely to encounter young women who feel defective by virtue of their inability to reach orgasm during coital "sex" than we were 25 years ago.

A cursory cross-cultural analysis betrays the biological reductionism and Western-centric notions present in the diagnostic manuals. For example, the 42.2% prevalence rate of Female Orgasmic Disorder in Southeast Asia, as cited by the *DSM-5*, clearly demonstrates a worldwide lack of adequate access to appropriate/sex-positive sex education rather than incredibly widespread psychological disorders. The underlying assumption is that if a woman cannot experience orgasm, there is something wrong with her rather than with the culture in which she was brought up, teaching her to hide, curb, disregard, or deny her own pleasure and desire. It must be noted that in most societies across the globe, women are socialized to put their partners' sexual desire and pleasure first. Our argument here is not about Southeast Asian women in particular, but about the problems that accompany a lack of sex education, sex-positivity, and female empowerment all over the world.

A review of the state of the field regarding GPPPD

The pain and tension that cause muscular contraction at the vaginal opening has long been acknowledged as an obstacle to intercourse. Sex therapy and sexual medicine have been less interested in the causes of dyspareunia (pain) and vaginismus (muscular contraction) than in removing obstacles to intercourse. Sometimes the focus is not even on the woman's capacity to engage in intercourse but on childbearing. In the 1980s with the rise of assistive reproductive technologies, the infertility literature advised against providing infertility treatment to women with vaginismus in case the closed vagina represented an unconscious desire to avoid pregnancy. By the 1990s, with the rise of sexual medicine, women's feelings seemed to become less relevant. New technologies emerged that allowed physicians to bypass the symptoms without necessarily addressing the cause (e.g., the relaxation of the vaginal muscles through dilators and, later, Botox). For example, treatment of survivors of child sexual abuse who had difficulty with intercourse aimed to "help" women open and close their pelvic floor muscles, with no regard for why their muscles were tight and painful in the first place; thus, the underlying trauma was circumvented and designated irrelevant (Kleinplatz, 1998). Such treatment reinforced the coital imperative. The very real pain that women experience during sexual and other contact has been decontextualized, thereby minimizing the suffering of the women attached to the genitals (Ayling & Ussher, 2008).

For decades, studies have indicated that the majority of women with what was previously termed vaginismus are orgasmic through oral and manual partnered stimulation (Hawton & Catalan, 1990; Leiblum, Pervin, & Campbell, 1989). What is our responsibility as a society and as health care providers in supporting women who may or may not actually choose to engage in intercourse if they are already enjoying their sex lives as they are?

When Binik (2009a, 2009b) suggested collapsing dyspareunia and vaginismus into GPPPD, his intention was to ensure that women would receive comprehensive clinical care rather than only diagnoses of psychopathology. In addition, he wondered why women with genital pain were considered to have psychopathology, whereas patients suffering from other physical problems that cause pain are not similarly diagnosed (Binik, 2005; Binik, Meana, Berkley, & Khalifé, 1999). For instance, athletes who are distressed by tennis elbow are not diagnosed with psychopathology and are instead referred to both a health/sports psychologist *and* a rheumatologist. However, women who reported genital pain were receiving comparatively fragmented care. In addition, for women diagnosed with GPPPD, the role of pressure from the partner and/or family to engage in intercourse and to conceive are rarely assessed, let alone taken into consideration.

The current standard of care for GPPPD is considered to be interdisciplinary treatment by pain specialists, psychotherapists, sex and/or marital therapists, gynecologists, and pelvic floor physiotherapists (Bergeron et al., 2002). However, patients are increasingly being referred from the primary care physician directly to the physical therapist for dilator therapy rather than to a mental health professional who is better trained to deal with the person or relationship (Rosenbaum, 2018). Please note that the literature is conspicuously lacking any case material on queer and lesbian women, who may not be subject to the heteronormative coital imperative, but may experience sexual difficulties or concerns.

Even more strikingly, the treatment of GPPPD introduced by cosmetic surgeon Peter Pacik (2010) of injecting Botox into the woman's vaginal and pelvic floor muscles to prevent her from opening and closing her vaginal muscles is increasingly becoming a viable treatment option (Moga et al., 2018). The heteronormative and reproductive focus of these treatments is clear and has very real consequences for women's agency, empowerment, and ability to make choices about their own sexual and reproductive health.

"Treatment" of women's genitals – no disorder required

Pacik's intervention paved the way for other cosmetic surgeons and cosmetic dermatologists to offer stand-alone treatment for "problems" that may or may not exist. Over the last 30 years, the increasing access to online pornography and its particular aesthetics have created the belief that women's genitals need alterations. Pubic hair is to be removed, labia minimized and denuded, vulvas and anuses bleached, and labia even stained cosmetically in different shades of pink (in an apparent effort to be sensitive to the diversity of women's bodies in a "multicultural" vein). Cosmetic genital surgery is not limited to the vulva; this new and highly lucrative field has introduced such procedures as O-shots and platelet-rich plasma (PRP) injections, intended to plump the clitoris and/or the anterior wall of the vagina to facilitate orgasms during intercourse (Runels, Melnick, Debourbon, & Roy, 2014), as well as laser treatment of the vaginal mucosa (Gaspar, Addamo, & Brandi, 2011). Ironically, whereas some interventions are designed to force tensed vaginas open, these latter interventions are designed to tighten other, presumably looser, vaginas in procedures referred to as "vaginal rejuvenation," "vaginal revirginization," and so forth. Thus, although it is never articulated, there is purportedly some standard for exactly how pliable and resilient vaginal tissue "ought" to be. Although it is not clear which sexual dysfunctions these medical interventions are designed to treat, disease mongering continues to proliferate (Moynihan & Mintzes, 2010; Tiefer, 2001, 2006).

Female sexual arousal and desire problems

Perhaps the most controversial and convoluted vicissitudes within the female sexual dysfunction diagnoses of the *DSM* are those related to arousal and desire. As indicated above, the first two editions of the *DSM* listed the amorphous "frigidity." There was no distinction between arousal and desire. Arousal and desire disorders were introduced formally in the *DSM-III* (APA, 1980), paralleling diagnoses of erectile dysfunction and inhibited sexual desire in men. These new gender-neutral diagnoses (i.e., low arousal and low desire) remained in the *DSM*'s classifications until 2013.

With the advent of the *DSM-5*, the working group on sexual and gender identity disorders maintained the existing nosology for men. However, in the case of women, arousal and desire were collapsed. The rationale for collapsing these diagnoses in women was introduced by Graham (2010) and Brotto (2010). They suggested that low arousal and desire are discrete phenomena in men, whereas in women they were often mingled. Some of this thinking reflects the work of Basson (2000, 2001), who suggested that women were different from men in terms of desire. Specifically, Basson indicated that whereas men tend to experience spontaneous and initiatory desire, women were more likely to have responsive desire. This was a provocative line of reasoning. When women are conceived of as more "receptive" or "responsive" than men, women may come to see themselves this way. This internalization may affect women's own sense of sexual agency and desire (or lack thereof) (see Spurgas, 2013a, 2013b, 2016a, 2016b for a discussion of the evolution of the FSIAD diagnosis).

From a diagnostic perspective, the working group on the sexual and gender identity disorders of the *DSM-5* (Brotto, 2010; Graham, 2010) argued that many women present for sex therapy without distinguishing whether their infrequent sex is based in arousal difficulties or low desire. It is normally incumbent upon the clinician to conduct the differential diagnosis, even when symptoms seem amorphous. It is the clinician's responsibility, rather than the patient's, to tease out the distinction between what a woman wants and what she finds arousing, even if these distinctions seem nebulous to a woman who finds sex undesirable (Kleinplatz, 2011).

As discussed above, profits from Viagra created an incentive for pharmaceutical companies to create a market for "female sexual dysfunction." Following the "failure" of Viagra for women, Proctor and Gamble suggested that the "problem" was not genital but rather hormonal, and therefore attempted to introduce a testosterone patch for women. Their Intrinsa patch was rejected by the U.S. Food and Drug Administration and by Health Canada. The U.K. allowed the introduction of the Intrinsa patch, but its marked lack of sales led to its withdrawal shortly thereafter. Clinical trials were then initiated for a variety of other pharmaceutical products that did not reach the FDA approval process in the U.S. ("Melanotan"/PT-141, "Lybrido," "Lybridos," "Libigel").

The discourse that followed these attempts suggested that if women's desire was not situated in or driven by the genitals, nor the hormones, then it must be in the brain. In 2010, Boehringer-Ingelheim developed flibanserin, a drug designed to affect the 5-HT receptors in the brain. (Note: Despite the pervasiveness of low desire in men, their needs have been all but ignored. No one has even tried to develop a drug for low desire for men; Maurice, 2007.) The exclusion criteria cited by Boehringer-Ingelheim were extraordinary, including marital problems, being on any drug whatsoever over the previous six months (including contraceptives), family problems, depression, anxiety, lactation, menstrual disorders, menopause, and more (for a complete list, see US FDA, 2015). The drug was rejected by the FDA in 2010 and 2013. Sprout Pharmaceuticals, the pharmaceutical company that later obtained the rights to flibanserin, created a clever new marketing strategy, "Even the Score" (2014), which co-opted feminist discourse. Sue Goldstein (2009, p. 302), an administrator who oversaw clinical trials for flibanserin, wrote: "Would anyone deny a man the right to an erection? ... When is it really my turn?" In 2015, for the third time, the FDA's advisory committee concluded that flibanserin still had not been proven to be effective, efficacious, or safe. However, in an unusual turn of events, the FDA board, notwithstanding the recommendations of its own advisory committee, overturned the conclusions and approved flibanserin, now sold under brand name Addyi. A subsequent meta-analysis (Jaspers et al., 2016) found it was not even as (in)effective as promised – an increase of 0.5 satisfying sexual events per month – by its manufacturers.

The conceptualization of women's sexual desire

The social construction of women's sexual desire must be considered in understanding what comes to be diagnosed and treated as FSIAD. Feminist psychologists, such as Deborah Tolman (1994, 2002), Michelle Fine (1988), Breanne Fahs, and Sara McClelland (Fahs & McClelland, 2016; McClelland, 2014), have undertaken qualitative studies of young women's sexualities, in particular, to uncover the social pressures these women experience to be sexual in specific ways. According to Tolman (2002), many young women feel a simultaneous push and pull – to be both sexual in ways that service men, but also to protect themselves or engage in "gatekeeping," as sex is framed as dangerous. This alludes to what Fine (1988, p. 29) called the "missing discourse of desire" for women. For social psychologists like Fine and Tolman, women's agency – and, thus, the possibility of them pursuing sex for the sake of their own pleasure – is what is missing from sex education, from media representations, and often from women's own narratives. Young women in particular are encouraged not to understand themselves as sexual beings, unless in the service of male satisfaction. There is a widespread notion that women should be responsive to men's desires yet that they should also be hypervigilant and protect themselves from sex (specifically sex with men). Some feminist scholars have also explored the role of social factors (e.g., gender roles, safety, fear, social stigma, trauma) that women must consider when seeking their own sexual pleasure (e.g., Irvine, 2005; Spurgas, 2016a, 2016b). Women are figuratively put between "a rock and a hard place" when it comes to sex.

Recent innovations

The entire enterprise of the scientific focus on female sexual psychopathology has been questioned over the course of the last 20 years. In 2001, the Working Group for the New View of Women's Sexual Problems (Alperstein et al., 2001) aimed to provide an alternative to the diagnostic nosologies of the *DSM* and *ICD*. The attempt was to create an alternative classification system that incorporated the intrapsychic, interpersonal, psychosocial, and organic causes of women's sexual problems. The resulting document describes the origins of women's sexual problems rather than merely outlining a nosology based on "symptoms." However, this work continued to focus on sexual problems, rather than the entire range of sexualities and sexual experiences, from the problematic to the "normal" to the optimal.

In the same way that pharmaceutical treatments such as Addyi reflect gender-biased ideas about female sexuality, other clinical interventions may also endorse gendered conceptualizations of female sexuality. One such example is Mindfulness-Based Sex Therapy (MBST; Brotto, 2018; Brotto, Basson, Carlson, & Zhu, 2013) for treatment of GPPPD and FSIAD. The goal of mindfulness interventions in sex therapy is for women to attend to their bodily sensations non-judgmentally, in order to increase their subjective experience of arousal. It is interesting that this protocol for low desire has been targeted primarily at women rather than also at men or couples (at the time of this writing, only one published study has described using MBST with men with situational erectile dysfunction – see Bossio et al., 2018). Regardless, mindfulness continues to be promoted within the realm of third-wave cognitive-behavioural therapies as a way to help female patients attend to the present moment, despite negative thoughts and feelings that may arise during sex. While this approach has suggested positive outcomes for some women, an inappropriate application of these techniques may instead teach women to disregard relevant thoughts and feelings regarding their lives and relationships (Barker, 2013). In other words, the concern here is that new clinical interventions may unintentionally reify traditional, heteronormative goals without questioning the broader social context in which women's "dysfunctions" are situated (Spurgas, 2013a, 2013b, 2016a). Women have increasingly become the identified patients, that is, the targets of treatment in cases of sexual desire discrepancy; this is a reversal of Masters and Johnson's initial formulation in which the couple/system was to be the focus of sex therapy (Charest & Kleinplatz, 2018).

Weiner and Avery-Clark (2017) recently reintroduced Masters and Johnson's much-maligned and misunderstood approach for women and men – sensate focus exercises. They believed it was time to describe the exercises more accurately and effectively to a new generation of sex therapists and their patients. More than Masters and Johnson, Weiner and Avery-Clark emphasized sensuality and pleasure for both men and women, across sexual orientations.

Feminist Gina Ogden (2008, 2018) developed an approach which integrated mental, physical, emotional, and spiritual dimensions in sex therapy. Her 4D Wheel model supported and advocated for individuals and couples who sought holistic orientations towards healing. Her innovative use of group therapy promoted personal and interpersonal development with no need to pathologize sexual difficulties.

An alternative to the focus on women's sexual problems has been proposed by the Optimal Sexual Research Team of the University of Ottawa (Kleinplatz et al., 2009; Ménard et al., 2015). The focus has been on shifting conceptions of sexuality from a system of categories to a continuum of sexual experience. Here, the focus is not on diagnosing and treating pathology but on enhancing the ordinary and troubled sex lives of women and men. For example, in dealing with individuals with low or no desire or low or no sexual frequency, there is no attempt to situate the problem in the individual. Rather, the goal is to facilitate hopes and aspirations for fulfilling erotic intimacy and helping couples – women and men, heterosexual and LGBTQ – to experience sex that is worth wanting. Preliminary data suggest that the clinical endeavours resulting from this approach are successful (Kleinplatz et al., 2018).

Conclusion

Where do we go from here? Who are "we," who even have the luxury to pose such a question? So many of the problems we have described throughout this chapter could be averted with comprehensive sex education for women, men, children, and health care providers, who might truly – rather than merely ideally and fancifully – work together to improve sexual health and sexual satisfaction. Women's agency in determining their own sexual health care and their sexual wishes must be promoted. To put it succinctly, women's voices are often absent from narratives of "female sexual dysfunction" and its "treatment." By broadening perspectives to include intersectional voices in research, teaching, and clinical practice, we can hope to create a future that we cannot yet even foresee.

References

Alperstein, L., Ellison, C., Fishman, J. R., Hall, M., Handwerker, L., Hartley, H., Kaschak, E., Kleinplatz, P., Loe, M., Mamo, L., Tavris, C., & Tiefer, L. (2001). A new view of women's sexual problems. *Women & Therapy, 24*, 1–8.

American College of Obstetricians and Gynecologists and Society for Maternal-Fetal Medicine. (2014). Safe prevention of the primary cesarean delivery. Obstetric Care Consensus, March (1). Retrieved September 24, 2015, from www.acog.org/Resources-And-Publications/Obstetric-Care-Consensus-Series/Safe-Prevention-of-the-Primary-Cesarean-Delivery.

American Psychiatric Association (1952). *Diagnostic and statistical manual of mental disorders*. Washington, DC: Author.

American Psychiatric Association (1968). *Diagnostic and statistical manual of mental disorders* (2nd ed.). Washington, DC: Author.

American Psychiatric Association (1980). *Diagnostic and statistical manual of mental disorders* (3rd ed.). Washington, DC: Author.

American Psychiatric Association (2013). *Diagnostic and statistical manual of mental disorders* (5th ed.). Washington, DC: Author.

Angel, K. (2012). Contested psychiatric ontology and feminist critique: "Female sexual dysfunction" and the *DSM. History of the Human Sciences, 25*(4), 3–24.

Ayling, K. & Ussher, J. M. (2008). If sex hurts, am I still a woman? The subjective experience of vulvodynia in hetero-sexual women. *Archives of Sexual Behaviour, 37*, 294–304.

Barbach, L. (1980). *Women discover orgasm*. New York, NY: Free Press.

Barbach, L. (2000). *For yourself: The fulfillment of female sexuality.* New York, NY: Signet Books.

Barker, M. (2013). Reflections: Towards a mindful sexual and relationship therapy. *Sexual and Relationship Therapy, 28,* 147–153.

Basson, R. (2000). The female sexual response: A different model. *Journal of Sex & Marital Therapy, 26,* 51–65.

Basson, R. (2001). Using a different model for female sexual response to address women's problematic low sexual desire. *Journal of Sex & Marital Therapy, 27,* 395–403.

Bergeron, S., Brown, C., Lord, M.-J., Oala, A. M., Binik, Y. M., & Khalife, S. (2002). Physical therapy for vulvar vestibulitis syndrome: A retrospective study. *Journal of Sex & Marital Therapy, 28,* 183–192.

Binik, Y. M. (2005). Should dyspareunia be retained as a sexual dysfunction in DSM-V? A painful classification decision. *Archives of Sexual Behavior, 34,* 11–22.

Binik, Y. M. (2009a). The *DSM* diagnostic criteria for dyspareunia. *Archives of Sexual Behavior, 39,* 292–303.

Binik, Y. M. (2009b). The *DSM* diagnostic criteria for vaginismus. *Archives of Sexual Behavior, 39,* 278–291.

Binik, Y. M., Meana, M., Berkley, K., & Khalifé, S. (1999). The sexual pain disorders: Is the pain sexual or is the sex painful? *Annual Review of Sex Research, 10,* 210–235.

Bossio, J. A., Basson, R., Driscoll, M., Correia, S., & Brotto, L. A. (2018). Mindfulness-based group therapy for men with situational erectile dysfunction: A mixed-methods feasibility analysis and pilot study. *Journal of Sexual Medicine, 15,* 1478–1490.

Brody, S. & Costa, R. M. (2008). Vaginal orgasm is associated with less use of immature psychological defense mechanisms. *The Journal of Sexual Medicine, 5,* 1167–1176.

Brody, S. & Costa, R. M. (2017). Vaginal orgasm is associated with indices of women's better psychological, intimate relationship, and psychophysiological function. *The Canadian Journal of Human Sexuality, 26,* 3–4.

Brotto, L. A. (2010). The *DSM* diagnostic criteria for hypoactive sexual desire disorder in women. *Archives of Sexual Behavior, 39,* 221–239.

Brotto, L. A. (2017). Vaginal versus clitoral? Or, vaginal and clitoral? A reply to Brody and Costa. *The Canadian Journal of Human Sexuality, 26,* 5–6.

Brotto, L. A. (2018). *Better sex through mindfulness.* Vancouver, BC: Greystone Books.

Brotto, L. A., Basson, R., Carlson, M., & Zhu, C. (2013). Impact of an integrated mindfulness and cognitive behavioural treatment for provoked vestibulodynia (IMPROVED): A qualitative study. *Sexual and Relationship Therapy, 28,* 3–19, doi:10.1080/14681994.2012.686661.

Canner, L. (2009). *Orgasm Inc.* [film]. West Groton, MA: Astrea Media.

Charest, M. & Kleinplatz, P. J. (2018). A review of recent innovations in the treatment of low sexual desire. *Current Sexual Health Reports, 10,* 281–286.

Conley, T. D., Moors, A. C., Matsick, J. L., Ziegler, A., & Valentine, B. A. (2011). Women, men, and the bedroom: Methodological and conceptual insights that narrow, reframe, and eliminate gender differences in sexuality. *Current Directions in Psychological Science, 20,* 296–300.

Dodson, B. (1987). *Sex for one: Joy of self-loving.* New York, NY: Crown.

Fahs, B. & McClelland, S. (2016). When sex and power collide: An argument for critical sexuality studies. *The Journal of Sex Research, 53,* 392–416.

Fine, M. (1988). Sexuality, schooling, and adolescent females: The missing discourse of desire. *Harvard Educational Review, 58,* 29–53.

Gaspar, A., Addamo, G., & Brandi, H. (2011). Vaginal fractional CO_2 laser: A minimally invasive option for vaginal rejuvenation. *The American Journal of Cosmetic Surgery, 28,* 156–162.

Goldstein, S. W. (2009). My turn … finally. *Journal of Sexual Medicine, 6,* 301–302.

Graham, C. A. (2010). The *DSM* diagnostic criteria for female sexual arousal disorder. *Archives of Sexual Behavior, 39,* 240–255.

Harris, G. (2004, February 28). Pfizer gives up testing Viagra on women. *New York Times,* p. C1.

Hartley, H. (2006). The 'pinking' of Viagra culture. *Sexualities, 9,* 363–378.

Hawton, K. & Catalan, J. (1990). Sex therapy for vaginismus: Characteristics of couples and treatment outcome. *Sexual and Marital Therapy, 5,* 39–48.

Heller, A. & Hannig, A. (2017). Unsettling the fistula narrative: Cultural pathology, biomedical redemption, and inequities of health access in Niger and Ethiopia. *Anthropology & Medicine, 24,* 81–95.

Irvine, J. M. (2005). *Disorders of desire: Sex and gender in modern American sexology.* Philadelphia, PA: Temple University Press.

Jaspers, L., Feys, F., Bramer, W. M., Franco, O. H., Leusink, P., & Laan, E. T. (2016). Efficacy and safety of flibanserin for the treatment of hypoactive sexual desire disorder in women: A systematic review and meta-analysis. *Journal of the American Medical Association Internal Medicine, 176*, 453–462.

Kleinplatz, P. J. (1998). Sex therapy for vaginismus: A review, critique, and humanistic alternative. *Journal of Humanistic Psychology, 38*, 51–81.

Kleinplatz, P. J. (2003). What's new in sex therapy: From stagnation to fragmentation. *Sex and Relationship Therapy, 18*, 95–106.

Kleinplatz, P. J. (2011). Arousal and desire problems: Conceptual, research, and clinical considerations or the more things change the more they stay the same. *Sex and Relationship Therapy, 26*, 3–15.

Kleinplatz, P. J. (2012). Advancing sex therapy or is that the best you can do? In P. J. Kleinplatz (Ed.), *New directions in sex therapy: Innovations and alternatives* (2nd ed., pp. xix–xxxvi). New York, NY: Routledge.

Kleinplatz, P. J. (2018). History of the treatment of female sexual dysfunction(s). *Annual Review of Clinical Psychology, 14*, 29–54.

Kleinplatz, P. J., Ménard, A. D., Paquet, M.-P., Paradis, N., Campbell, M., Zuccarini, D., & Mehak, L. (2009). The components of optimal sexuality: A portrait of "great sex". *Canadian Journal of Human Sexuality, 18*, 1–13.

Kleinplatz, P. J., Paradis, N., Charest, M., Lawless, S., Neufeld, M., Neufeld, R., Pratt, D., Ménard, A. D., Buduru, B., & Rosen, L. (2018). From sexual desire discrepancies to desirable sex: Creating the optimal connection. *Journal of Sex & Marital Therapy, 44*, 438–449.

Ladas, A. K., Whipple, B., & Perry, J. D. (1983/2004). *The G spot*. New York, NY: Holt.

Leiblum, S. R., Pervin, L. A., & Campbell, E. H. (1989). The treatment of vaginismus: Success and failure. In S. R. Leiblum & R. C. Rosen (Eds), *Principles and practice of sex therapy: Update for the 1990s* (pp. 113–138). New York, NY: Guilford.

Levin, R. J. (2005). Wet and dry sex: The impact of cultural influence in modifying vaginal function. *Sex and Relationship Therapy, 20*, 465–474.

Loe, M. (2004). *The rise of Viagra: How the little blue pill changed sex in America*. New York, NY: New York University Press.

Masters, W. H. & Johnson, V. E. (1966). *Human sexual response*. Boston, MA: Little, Brown.

Masters, W. H. & Johnson, V. E. (1986). *Sex therapy on its twenty-fifth anniversary: Why it survives*. St. Louis, MO: Masters and Johnson Institute.

Maurice, W. (2007). Sexual desire disorders in men. In S. R. Leiblum (Ed.), *Principles and practice of sex therapy* (4th ed., pp. 181–211). New York, NY: Guilford.

Mbikusita-Lewanika, M., Stephen, H., & Thomas, J. (2009). The prevalence and the use of 'dry sex' traditional medicines, among Zambian women, and the profile of the users. *Psychology, Health & Medicine, 14*, 227–238.

McCarthy, B. & McDonald, O. D. (2009). Psychobiosocial versus biomedical models of treatment: Semantics or substance. *Sexual and Relationship Therapy, 24*, 30–37.

McClelland, S. (2014). "What do you mean when you say that you are sexually satisfied?" A mixed methods study. *Feminism & Psychology, 24*, 74–96.

Ménard, A. D., Kleinplatz, P. J., Rosen, L., Lawless, S., Paradis, N., Campbell, M., & Huber, J. D. (2015). Individual and relational contributors to optimal sexual experiences in older men and women. *Sexual and Relationship Therapy, 30*, 78–93.

Moga, M., Dimienescu, O., Bălan, A., Scârneciu, I., Barabaş, B., & Pleş, L. (2018). Therapeutic approaches of botulinum toxin in gynecology. *Toxins, 10*, E169.

Moynihan, R. (2003). The making of a disease: Female sexual dysfunction. *British Medical Journal, 326*, 45–47.

Moynihan, R. & Mintzes, B. (2010). *Sex, lies and pharmaceuticals: How drug companies plan to profit from female sexual dysfunction*. Vancouver, BC: Greystone Books.

Nathan, S. (2010). When do we say a woman's sexuality is dysfunctional? In S. Levine, C. Reisen, & S. Althof (Eds), *Handbook of clinical sexuality for mental health professionals* (pp. 95–110). New York, NY: Brunner-Routledge.

Ogden, G. (2008). *The return of desire: A guide to rediscovering your sexual passion*. Boston, MA: Trumpeter.

Ogden, G. (2018). *Expanding the practice of sex therapy: The neuro update edition – An integrative model for exploring desire and intimacy* (2nd ed.). New York, NY: Routledge.

Pacik, P. T. (2010). *When sex seems impossible: Stories of vaginismus and how you can achieve intimacy*. Manchester, NH: Odyne Publishing.

Petersen, J. L. & Hyde, J. S. (2010). A meta-analytic review of research on gender differences in sexuality, 1993–2007. *Psychological Bulletin, 136,* 21–38.

Potts, A. (2008). The female sexual dysfunction debate: Different 'problems', new drugs – More pressures? In P. Moss & K. Teghtsoonian (Eds), *Contesting illness: Processes and practices* (pp. 259–280). Toronto, ON: Toronto University Press.

Reiss, I. L. (1990). *An end to shame: Shaping our next sexual revolution.* New York, NY: Prometheus Books.

Rosenbaum, T. Y. (2018). Limits of pelvic floor physical therapy in the treatment of GPPD. *Current Sexual Health Reports, 10*(2), 35–37.

Runels, C., Melnick, H., Debourbon, E., & Roy, L. (2014). A pilot study of the effect of localized injections of autologous platelet rich plasma (PRP) for the treatment of female sexual dysfunction. *Journal of Women's Health Care, 3,* 4.

Schnarch, D. (1991). *Constructing the sexual crucible: An integration of sexual and marital therapy.* New York, NY: Norton.

Spurgas, A. K. (2013a). Interest, arousal, and shifting diagnoses of female sexual dysfunction, or: How women learn about desire. *Studies in Gender and Sexuality, 14,* 187–205.

Spurgas, A. K. (2013b). Gendered populations and trauma beyond Oedipus: Reply to Angel's commentary. *Studies in Gender and Sexuality, 14,* 217–223.

Spurgas, A. K. (2016a). Low desire, trauma, and femininity in the *DSM-5*: A case for sequelae. *Psychology & Sexuality, 7,* 48–67.

Spurgas, A. K. (2016b, March 9). Solving desire. *New Inquiry.* Retrieved from http://thenewinquiry.com/essays/solving-desire.

Studnicki, J. & Fisher, J. W. (2018). Recent increases in the U.S. maternal mortality rate: Disentangling trends from measurement issues. *Obstetrics & Gynecology, 131,* 932–934.

Tavris, C. (1992). *The mismeasure of woman.* New York, NY: Touchstone.

Therrien, S. & Brotto, L. A. (2016). A critical examination of the relationship between vaginal orgasm consistency and measures of psychological and sexual functioning and sexual concordance in women with sexual dysfunction. *The Canadian Journal of Human Sexuality, 25,* 109–118.

Tiefer, L. (1996). The medicalization of sexuality: Conceptual, normative, and professional issues. *Annual Review of Sex Research, VII,* 252–282.

Tiefer, L. (2001). The selling of "female sexual dysfunction". *Journal of Sex & Marital Therapy, 27,* 625–628.

Tiefer, L. (2006). Female sexual dysfunction: A case study of disease mongering and activist resistance. *PLoS Medicine, 3*(4), e178.

Tolman, D. L. (1994). Doing desire: Adolescent girls' struggles for/with sexuality. *Gender & Society, 8,* 324–342.

Tolman, D. L. (2002). *Dilemmas of desire: Teenage girls talk about sexuality.* Cambridge, MA: Harvard University Press.

U.S. Food and Drug Administration (2015). *FDA briefing document: Joint meeting of the Bone, Reproductive and Urologic Drugs Advisory Committee (BRUDAC) and the Drug Safety and Risk Management (DSaRM) Advisory Committee (NDA 022526).* Silver Spring, MD: Author.

Ussher, J. M. (1993). The construction of female sexual problems: Regulating sex, regulating woman. In J. M. Ussher & C. D. Baker (Eds), *Psychological perspectives on sexual problems: New directions in theory and practice* (pp. 10–40). New York, NY: Routledge.

Weiner, L. & Avery-Clark, C. (2017). *Sensate focus in sex therapy: The illustrated manual.* New York, NY: Routledge.

World Health Organization (WHO) (2018). *WHO marks the international day of zero tolerance for female genital mutilation.* Geneva, Switzerland: Author. Retrieved from www.who.int/reproductivehealth/topics/fgm/en.

Zilbergeld, B. & Ellison, C. R. (1980). Desire discrepancies and arousal problems in sex therapy. In S. R. Leiblum & L. A. Pervin (Eds), *Principles and practice of sex therapy* (pp. 65–101). New York, NY: Guilford.

30

HIV, STIS, RISK TAKING AND SEXUAL HEALTH

Jennifer Power

Human sexual health is increasingly understood in social terms. The World Health Organization (WHO, 2015) defined sexual health as a complete state of physical, emotional, mental, and social well-being in relation to sexuality. This means that good sexual health is measured not just by absence of disease, but through a person's capacity to pursue a safe and pleasurable sexual life that contributes to their overall well-being. This definition aligns with an increasing body of international research that shows that the incidence of sexually transmitted infections (STIs) and human immunodeficiency virus (HIV) among women is strongly associated with structural, social, and cultural factors. Women who are most vulnerable to HIV or STIs are those who have less agency over their sexuality and sexual relationships or more limited access to education and clinical care. In this way, sexual health is a product of the social environment and the day-to-day realities of women's lives. This chapter provides an overview of STI and HIV rates among women across the world, drawing attention to the relationship between social and structural factors – including poverty, gender-based inequality, and violence – and women's vulnerability to poor sexual health outcomes.

Epidemiological trends in HIV and STIs

STIs

Estimating global prevalence of STIs is complicated due to lack of standardised reporting systems between countries and limited capacity for reporting in many low-income regions (Ortayli, Ringheim, Collins, & Sladden, 2014). Nonetheless, recent efforts by the WHO, and other international bodies, to enhance consistency in STI surveillance means that some data are available to track general patterns in STI transmission globally (Newman et al., 2015; World Health Organization, 2016).

There is evidence that global incidence of four major curable STIs is increasing: *chlamydia trachomatis* (chlamydia), *neisseria gonorrhoeae* (gonorrhoea), syphilis, and *trichomanisasis vaginalis* (trichomaniasis). Data indicate that new infections of these STIs increased by nearly 50% between 1995 and 2008 (Ortayli et al., 2014). The vast burden of disease associated with these STIs is in low- and middle-income countries, particularly in the African and Western

455

Pacific regions (Newman et al., 2015). If left untreated, these STIs can lead to a range of serious complications for women and their children, including pelvic inflammatory disease (PID), infertility, ectopic pregnancy, foetal death, and congenital infections in infants (Newman et al., 2015)

These STIs are curable with antibiotic medication, but many women do not receive adequate treatment due to lack of testing or follow up post-diagnosis. There may be several reasons for this. Infections such as gonorrhoea and chlamydia are often asymptomatic, and many women do not seek testing unless they experience symptoms or discomfort. For some women, even those experiencing symptoms, concerns about privacy, self-consciousness, embarrassment, or cost may make them reluctant to seek testing (Denison, Bromhead, Grainger, Dennison, & Jutel, 2017). Even when women do present for testing, they may not follow through with treatment if it requires further clinic visits or multi-dose treatment regimens (World Health Organization, 2013). However, in many resource-poor areas, the biggest barrier to STI testing is lack of facilities. Clinical and laboratory infrastructure to test for STIs is expensive and requires specifically trained staff, who are often not available in low-income settings. Where testing capacity is limited, clinics often rely on syndromic management of STIs, whereby patients presenting with symptoms receive treatment. However, this misses asymptomatic cases and leads to a high proportion of complications and adverse health outcomes (Ortayli et al., 2014; World Health Organization, 2013).

Non-curable viral STIs, other than HIV, also affect large numbers of women across the world, and may lead to serious health complications. Human papillomavirus (HPV) is the most common STI globally; over 290 million women are estimated to be infected worldwide at any one time (World Health Organization, 2016). HPV is the leading cause of cervical cancer, one of the most common cancers among women – particularly women in low- and middle-income countries where routine screening for cervical cancer is limited (World Health Organization, 2013). Vaccines are available to protect against strains of HPV that lead to the majority of cervical cancers, although these are not universally available in many low-income settings (LaMontagne et al, 2017). In 2014, high-income countries accounted for 70% of women who had received the HPV vaccine worldwide (Bruni et al., 2016). Nevertheless, there is a continued global effort to increase HPV vaccination (World Health Organization, 2017b), and there is evidence that this will be effective in reducing rates of cervical cancer, particularly among young women (Brotherton, Zuber, & Bloem, 2016).

Herpes simplex virus (HSV-2) is a common STI characterised by periodic appearance of genital ulcers in many people who are infected, although it may be asymptomatic. In 2012, it was estimated that, globally, 14.8% of women aged 15–49 were infected with HSV-2 (Looker et al., 2015). HSV-2 is a lifelong infection. Although the virus in itself does not necessarily cause serious health problems for adult women, there is a risk, albeit small, of neonatal transmission, which can lead to severe morbidity in infants. In addition, HSV-2 infection has been shown to significantly increase susceptibility to HIV infection (Looker et al., 2017).

HIV

In many high-income countries, such as Australia and the USA, HIV disproportionately affects men who have sex with men, and so rates among women are comparatively low (Centers for Disease Control, 2017a; Kirby Institute, 2017). However, across the globe, the majority of people living with HIV are women. In 2018, UNAIDS reported that 18.8 million women and girls were living with HIV, more than half of the estimated 36.7 million HIV+ people. Low-income countries have significantly higher rates of HIV infection than high-income countries; sub-Saharan Africa bears the largest burden, accounting for 64% of new HIV infections in 2016 (UNAIDS, 2017). Despite effective antiretroviral treatment for HIV, inadequate access to it in many regions means AIDS-related illnesses are the leading cause of death among girls and women aged 15–49 (UNAIDS, 2018). Estimates by UNAIDS suggest that, in 2015, approximately 46% of people living with HIV across the world had access to antiretroviral treatment (UN Women, 2017).

Vulnerable or marginalised sub-populations

Key international bodies, such as UNAIDS, recognise particular groups of women as highly vulnerable at-risk populations for HIV or STIs. This includes female sex workers, transgender people, young women, and pregnant women (Gall et al., 2017; UNAIDS, 2018). In addition to this, particular sub-groups of women, including sexual and gender minority women and older women, may be more vulnerable to poor sexual health outcomes due to exclusion from sexual health education, information, or clinical care (Marrazzo, 2013; Minichiello, Hawkes, & Pitts, 2011).

Adolescent and young women

Every year, there are close to 870,000 new HIV infections among women and girls globally, and young women are twice as likely as young men to acquire HIV (Harrison, Colvin, Kuo, Swartz, & Lurie, 2015; UNAIDS, 2018; UN Women, 2017). This is particularly pronounced in certain regions. For example, across eastern and southern Africa, young women (aged 15–24) are up to five times more likely than men of the same age to be infected with HIV (Fleischman & Peck, 2015).

HIV is less common among young women in high-income countries. However, in recent years, rates of STIs, particularly chlamydia and gonorrhoea, have increased among women aged 15–24 in many high-income countries (Centers for Disease Control, 2016; Kirby Institute, 2017; Public Health England, 2017). Data on STI diagnoses in low- and middle-income countries are harder to access (Dellar, Dlamini, & Karim, 2015), but there is evidence that STI rates are high among young women in these countries, following a similar pattern to HIV (Torrone et al., 2018).

Pregnant women

Pregnancy poses particular sexual health problems for women due to the risk of negative consequences for infants. Of major concern are the risks of congenital syphilis or mother-to-child transmission of HIV (Taylor et al., 2018). In 2012, approximately 900,000 pregnant women were infected with syphilis, which resulted in approximately 350,000 estimated adverse pregnancy outcomes, including 200,000 stillbirths or neonatal deaths (World Health Organization, 2017a). Although rates are still high, there has been a significant reduction in congenital syphilis diagnoses since the initiation of a global campaign to encourage systematic screening of pregnant women and their partners (Wijesooriya et al., 2016).

It is estimated that mother-to-child transmission of HIV is the cause of 90% of HIV infections in children worldwide. Appropriately administered antiretroviral treatment can prevent HIV transmission from a mother to her child, but many women in low-income countries do not have access to this HIV treatment (World Health Organization, 2007). In 2015, approximately 77% of pregnant women, globally, had access to antiretroviral treatment (UN Women, 2017).

Female sex workers

In some high-income countries, such as Australia, the incidence of HIV and other STIs among sex workers is very low due to sustained and successful efforts within the industry to normalise condom use – efforts that are often supported by laws that decriminalise or regulate the sex industry (Boily & Shannon, 2017; Lee, Binger, Hocking, & Fairley, 2005). However, globally, the rate of HIV among female sex workers is significantly higher than among other women, particularly in low-income settings (Shannon et al., 2015). A recent review by the World Bank showed that overall HIV prevalence among female sex workers was 11.8%, which is up to 13.5 times the prevalence rate in the general population of woman aged 15–49 years (Kerrigan, et al., 2013).

Female sex workers are at heightened risk of HIV due to poor working conditions and economic insecurity, which makes them vulnerable to high levels of violence, sexual assault, and pressure to have unprotected sex (Decker et al., 2015; Dunkle & Decker, 2013; World Health Organization, 2015). Modelling undertaken by Shannon and colleagues (2015) estimated that decriminalisation of sex work could reduce the incidence of HIV transmission among sex workers by 33–46% over the next decade. This would be achieved by a combination of reduced violence against sex workers and improvements in safe work environments (Shannon et al., 2015).

Transgender people

Transgender women may include male-to-female transgender people, people who identify as transfeminine, or people who were assigned the male sex at birth but identify as gender-diverse or gender-non-binary. Recent international research indicates that transgender women are disproportionately affected by HIV and other STIs; one study showed an HIV prevalence rate among transgender women of 19.1% (Baral et al., 2013; Reisner & Murchison, 2016). The high rate of HIV among transgender women may relate to several factors, including having sex with gay or bisexual men, high levels of harmful substance use, a high likelihood of experiencing sexual or physical violence, and high numbers of transgender women working in the sex industry (Poteat, German, & Kerrigan, 2013; World Health Organization, 2015).

Transgender men may include female-to-male transgender people, people who identify as transmasculine, or people who were assigned the female sex at birth but identify as gender-diverse or gender-non-binary. It would be more appropriate to consider the needs of transgender men in a review of men's sexual health. However, the sexual and reproductive health needs of transgender men (which may include the need for cervical screening or reproductive health services) are generally aligned with women's health and excluded from men's health research and practice. There is very little research on the sexual health needs of transgender men, including rates of HIV or STIs (Stephenson et al., 2017). However, transgender men who have sex with other men may be vulnerable to HIV or STIs due to a high rate of these infections among gay and bisexual men and/or because basic HIV or STI prevention services are inappropriate for transgender men (Scheim et al., 2016).

Women who have sex with women

Women who have sex with women (WSW), which may include lesbian and bisexual women as well as women who identify primarily as heterosexual but who have sex with women, are often perceived to be at low risk for STIs or HIV (Marrazzo, 2013). However, there is evidence that the lifetime rate of STIs among WSW is equivalent to that of heterosexual women. This may be, in part, because many WSW – even those who identify as exclusively lesbian – have also had (or continue to have) sex with men. For some WSW, this involves sexual play with gay or bisexual men, among whom there are higher rates of both HIV and STIs (Koh, Gómez, Shade, & Rowley, 2005; Marrazzo, 2013).

The perception that WSW are at lower risk for STIs or HIV means many WSW do not seek sexual health testing, assume women's sexual health information is irrelevant for their needs, and do not engage in safe-sex practices (Marrazzo et al., 2015; Mullinax, Schick, Rosenberg, Herbenick, & Reece, 2016; Power, McNair, & Carr, 2009). Sexual health services are also often not inclusive of WSW, and many healthcare providers have limited understanding of the sexual behaviours, or the sexual health risks and needs, of WSW (McNair, 2005).

Older women

In contemporary life, where people are living longer, many women are sexually active well into their older years (Herbenick et al., 2010; Schick et al., 2010). A large survey of adults aged over 50 living in the USA, for example, showed that up to 30% of women and men remained regularly sexually active into their 80s (Schick et al., 2010), and many older people seek new sexual partners following the end of a long-term relationship through death or divorce (Fileborn et al., 2015). There is only limited available information on STI rates among older women, but data from some high-income countries shows an increase in STI diagnoses within this population group in recent years (Minichiello et al., 2011; Poynten, Grulich, & Templeton, 2013). However, older women are often excluded from policy, public dialogue, or education about sexual health due to assumptions that older people are not (or should not be) sexually active and/or the interlinking of sexual and reproductive health in education or clinical care, thereby excluding women beyond childbearing age (Cooper & Crockett, 2015; Fileborn et al., 2015; Minichiello et al., 2011).

Understanding risk and vulnerability in women's sexual health

The likelihood that someone will become infected with an STI or HIV is often conceptualised in terms of risk. In some cases, this 'risk' is associated with being part of a population group that is at higher risk of certain illnesses due to a high incidence within that population. Gay and bisexual men, for example, are considered to be at elevated risk of HIV due to a high prevalence of HIV within their sexual networks (Beyrer et al., 2016). HIV or STI risk is also associated with certain behaviours. Commonly identified 'risky behaviours' are unsafe sex (e.g., sex without a condom, sex with multiple partners, sex without other forms of protection against STIs or HIV), high levels of substance use, or sex while intoxicated (Rosenstock, Strecher, & Becker, 1994). These concepts are not mutually exclusive. Often, 'risk groups' are identified due to a higher incidence of particular behaviours within that group. Young people, for example, are often considered to be at high risk for STIs due to a perceived tendency for young people to be less risk averse, along with high rates of STIs among heterosexual youth (Leclerc-Madlala, 2002).

The concept of 'risk' groups and behaviours can be useful to target or design sexual health interventions or HIV/STI prevention resources. However, conceptualising risk in these terms obscures the social context in which people make decisions or take actions – or broader structural factors that may determine or limit their choices. This can lead to stigma or blame of people identified as 'at risk' (Frohlich & Potvin, 2008). Human behaviour (e.g., desires, decisions, actions) occurs within a social framework that is shaped by cultural norms and values as well as structural conditions, including economic and political circumstances (Auerbach, Parkhurst, & Cáceres, 2011). For instance, a woman may 'choose' not to use a condom for sex, but this choice is shaped by multiple factors, including her own or her partner's desires, social norms regarding condom use, accessibility and affordability of condoms, her capacity to negotiate or insist upon condom use with her partner, and/or her ability to refuse sex with her partner. All these dynamics are situated within much broader structures of gender and power, which shape the expectations of women and men in their sexual relationships and restrict the capacity of many women to assert their sexual health needs (Dunkle & Decker, 2013; Haberland, 2015).

In contemporary HIV/STI research and policy, 'risk' is increasingly conceived of in terms of vulnerable populations. This term refers to populations whose situation or social context makes them vulnerable to HIV or STIs due to inequality, prejudice, or marginalisation, or due to limits placed them by social, economic, or cultural conditions (Frohlich & Potvin, 2008; Greenall, Kunii, Thomson, Bangert, & Nathan, 2017; Link & Phelan, 2010; Semenza, 2010). Economic and social conditions affect people's vulnerability to HIV or STIs by limiting accessing to information, education, or clinical care (Kim & Watts, 2005). On a global level, poverty is a major driver of HIV because it creates conditions that heighten people's vulnerability to HIV. This might include lack of education, limited access to clinical care or treatment, and few prevention services (Auerbach et al., 2011).

In both low- and high-income countries, epidemiological trends for STIs and HIV reveal patterns of social inequality, prejudice, and marginalisation (Auerbach et al., 2011). Within high-income countries, for example, racial or ethnic minority people are often disproportionately affected by HIV and STIs. In the US, the 2016 rate of gonorrhoea infection among African American women was 8.6 times higher than among White women. Similarly, the rate of chlamydia was 5.1 times higher, and syphilis 4.7 times higher, among African American women (Centers for Disease Control, 2017b). In Australia, the rate of new HIV cases among Indigenous women is significantly higher than among non-Indigenous Australian-born women (Kirby Institute, 2017). The rates of chlamydia, gonorrhoea, and syphilis are also significantly higher among Aboriginal Australians (Kirby Institute, 2017).

For women, vulnerability to HIV or STIs is often an outcome of multiple social inequalities – including socio-economic status, race, ethnicity, and sexuality – each of which intersects with gender. For example, in low-income settings where there is not universal education for children, it usually women and girls who are undereducated. This is because expectations about a woman's social role as a wife and mother means that girls' education is often less valued than boys' education. Lack of education, strict adherence to traditional gender roles, and limited employment opportunities mean that many women will never be financially independent from their husbands (Türmen, 2003). This restricts some women's capacity to protect themselves from HIV or STIs by removing their choice to refuse sex, leave a violent relationship, or seek clinical care (Auerbach et al., 2011; Dunkle & Decker, 2013).

Gender-inequality, and gender-based socials norms, also shape women's interactions with male sexual partners in ways that can increase their vulnerability to HIV or STIs. Traditional gender norms suggest that women should be both passive and sexually available, whereas masculine norms place high value on male heterosexual power and the presentation of mas-culinity as strong and assertive (Connell, 2005; Dunkle & Decker, 2013; Türmen, 2003; Wingood & DiClemente, 2000). The implicit imbalance of power embedded in these gender norms has been challenged through feminist action over the past 50 years. However, this model is still enacted in many women's sexual encounters with men. For some women gender norms can be a barrier to asserting their needs or desires in sexual interactions or insisting on safe sex; the norms also perpetuate cultures of violence against women (Dunkle & Decker, 2013).

Gender-based violence

The relationship between gender-based inequality and sexual health outcomes is starkly evi-dent in the increasing body of international research that shows an association between women's experience of gender-based violence (or intimate-partner violence) and HIV or STI infection (Li et al., 2014).

There may be multiple reasons why a woman who is experiencing – or who has previ-ously experienced – violence may be more vulnerable to HIV or other STIs. There is evi-dence from around the world that men who exhibit violent or aggressive forms of masculinity, or who are violent toward female partners, are more likely than other men to have been diagnosed with an STI or HIV at some point in their life (Decker et al., 2009; Raj et al., 2006). Violent men are also more likely to engage in riskier sex, including mul-tiple sexual partners, sex while highly intoxicated, or sex with female sex workers (which is associated with higher levels of HIV risk in many settings) (Dunkle & Decker, 2013; Dunkle et al., 2006; Raj et al., 2006; Schulkind, Mbonye, Watts, & Seeley, 2016). The experience of intimate partner violence may also negatively affect a woman's self-confidence and increase her level of psychological distress, which in turn can reduce her capacity to be assertive within a sexual encounter or relationship. This loss of confidence can have an impact on a woman's life for many years after her first experience of violence (Pettifor, Measham, Rees, & Padian, 2004; Schwartz et al., 2014; Wingood & DiClemente, 1998). Women who have experienced violence are more likely to engage in risky substance use, sex while intoxicated, unprotected sex, and sex work. They are also at heightened risk of experiencing further violence (Decker et al., 2014; Schulkind et al., 2016).

Responding to gender-based inequality in HIV/STI prevention and sexual health education

Biomedical interventions

Recent technological advances mean that there are now a range of biomedical approaches to preventing HIV and STIs (Padian et al., 2011). Where available, vaccination is a highly effective means of reducing STI rates. HPV vaccination programs have led to a significant reduction in HPV in settings where there has been wide-scale roll out of the vaccine (Brotherton et al., 2016). Along with this, widespread testing and treatment programs have the potential to increase early diagnosis of HIV or STIs in order to expedite uptake of treat-ment and prevent onward infection (Ortayli et al., 2014). Novel approaches to HIV/STI testing, such as home-testing kits and point-of-care testing (which provides results within the clinical session), are creating new opportunities to expand and increase testing (Taylor, Frasure-Williams, Burnett, & Park, 2016; Toskin, Blondeel, Peeling, Deal, & Kiarie, 2017).

For HIV, pre-exposure prophylaxis (PrEP) provides the possibility for a significant reduction in new HIV infection rates in coming years (Padian et al., 2011). PrEP is antiretroviral medication taken orally by HIV-negative people to prevent HIV infection. Studies to date show that PrEP is highly effective in reducing HIV transmission among women and men given proper adherence to the treatment regimen (Flash, Dale, & Krakower, 2017).

It is beyond the scope of this chapter to present a detailed analysis of the impact of PrEP or other biomedical HIV or STI prevention options on women's sexual health. But it is worth noting that the potential benefit of new prevention technologies (e.g., PrEP) is that they enable women to have control over HIV prevention rather than relying on negotiation of safe sex with male sexual partners (Padian et al., 2011). Although there are major economic and logistic barriers to the global supply of PrEP, it has the potential to reduce the risk of HIV transmission among some groups of women, such as sex workers (Bekker et al., 2015; Beyrer et al., 2015).

Economic incentives and support

Programs that address the structural drivers of HIV and STI transmission, including poverty and gender-based inequality, have become more common in recent years. Many of these programs take the form of microfinance, which are small loans to assist women to begin a business or invest in education, or direct cash payments to incentivise behavioural change by paying cash to people who engage in HIV/STI testing or who remain HIV/STI-free. Some programs offer a combination of both approaches, such as payment to assist with school fees alongside cash payments for HIV or pregnancy testing (Pettifor, MacPhail, Nguyen, & Rosenberg, 2012).

The complex relationships between poverty, economic independence, gender, and sexual health make it difficult to evaluate the impact of microfinance programs on HIV or STI rates. But some studies do indicate that microfinance programs can reduce factors associated with increased vulnerability to HIV or STIs, including intimate partner violence (Auerbach et al., 2011; Kennedy, Fonner, O'Reilly, & Sweat, 2014; Seeley, 2015). Microfinance programs have also been shown to increase use of contraception among women and to reduce household poverty in the longer term (Krishnan et al., 2008). Programs that provide direct cash payments to young people who remain HIV or STI free over a period of time have been effective in achieving behavioural change some settings (De Walque et al., 2012; Kohler & Thornton, 2012; Padian et al., 2011). However, it is not known how well this strategy would be replicable, including in higher-income areas (Pettifor et al., 2012).

Comprehensive sexuality education

Sexuality education supports STI and HIV prevention by informing women about their prevention options and improving their understanding of sex, bodies, and relationships. When it is done well, comprehensive sexuality education empowers women to protect their sexual and reproductive health in ways that best suit their needs (Ponzetti, 2015). Studies on comprehensive sexuality education show that this form of education is effective in increasing HIV/STI prevention behaviours among young people and is therefore an important component of overall prevention efforts (Chin et al., 2012; Fonner, Armstrong, Kennedy, O'Reilly, & Sweat, 2014). Contemporary approaches to sexuality education include a focus on gender and power within the curriculum. This may include explicit discussion of gender norms, gender equality, and gender and power, and/or encouragement of self-reflection and personal consideration of how gender and power shape participants' lives (Haberland, 2015).

A recent review of sexuality education programs from a range of countries showed that programs that included a gender/power component were more likely than those that did not to achieve a decrease in at least one sexual health outcome indicator (i.e., pregnancy, childbearing, STI infection) (Haberland, 2015).

Conclusion

This chapter has focused on STIs and HIV, with an emphasis on transmission rates and approaches to HIV and STI prevention. This is an important aspect of women's sexual health. However, sexual health is not only the absence of disease. Women's sexual health is also about the capacity for women to pursue satisfying sexual relationships and intimacy without fear of discrimination, violence, or coercion (Lottes, 2013). In an ideal world, people's sexuality and sexual relationships would support their overall well-being. However, this is often not the case, and there are multiple structural, social, and cultural factors that may make women vulnerable to poorer sexual health and higher rates of HIV or STIs. Health systems inevitably play a key role in supporting women's sexual health, but action to improve sexual health outcomes must also involve broader civil society, including policy and the legal and educational systems (Aggleton, de Wit, Myers, & Du Mont, 2014).

References

Aggleton, P., de Wit, J., Myers, T., & Du Mont, J. (2014). New outcomes for sexual health promotion. *Health Education Research, 29*(4), 547–553.

Auerbach, J. D., Parkhurst, J. O., & Cáceres, C. F. (2011). Addressing social drivers of HIV/AIDS for the long-term response: Conceptual and methodological considerations. *Global Public Health, 6*(sup3), S293–S309.

Baral, S. D., Poteat, T., Strömdahl, S., Wirtz, A. L., Guadamuz, T. E., & Beyrer, C. (2013). Worldwide burden of HIV in transgender women: A systematic review and meta-analysis. *The Lancet Infectious Diseases, 13*(3), 214–222.

Bekker, L.-G., Johnson, L., Cowan, F., Overs, C., Besada, D., Hillier, S., & Cates, W. (2015). Combination HIV prevention for female sex workers: What is the evidence?. *The Lancet, 385* (9962), 72–87.

Beyrer, C., Baral, S. D., Collins, C., Richardson, E. T., Sullivan, P. S., Sanchez, J., Trapence, G., Katabira, E., Kazatchkine, M., Ryan, O., Wirtz, A. L., & Mayer, K. H. (2016). The global response to HIV in men who have sex with men. *The Lancet, 388*(10040), 198–206.

Beyrer, C., Crago, A.-L., Bekker, L.-G., Butler, J., Shannon, K., Kerrigan, D., Decker, M. R., Baral, S. D., Poteat, T., Wirtz, A. L., Weir, B. W., Barré-Sinoussi, F., Kazatchkine, M., Sidibé, M., Dehne, K. L., Boily, M. C., & Strathdee, S. A. (2015). An action agenda for HIV and sex workers. *The Lancet, 385*(9964), 287–301.

Boily, M.-C. & Shannon, K. (2017). Criminal law, sex work, HIV: Need for multi-level research. *The Lancet HIV, 4*(3), 98–99.

Brotherton, J. M., Zuber, P. L., & Bloem, P. J. (2016). Primary prevention of HPV through vaccination: Update on the current global status. *Current Obstetrics and Gynecology Reports, 5*(3), 210–224.

Bruni, L., Diaz, M., Barrionuevo-Rosas, L., Herrero, R., Bray, F., Bosch, F. X., de Sanjosé, S., & Castellsagué, X. (2016). Global estimates of human papillomavirus vaccination coverage by region and income level: A pooled analysis. *The Lancet Global Health, 4*(7), e453–e463.

Centers for Disease Control (2016). *2016 Sexually transmitted diseases surveillance.* Atlanta, GA: Author. Retrieved from www.cdc.gov/std/stats16/toc.htm.

Centers for Disease Control (2017a). *HIV among women.* Atlanta, GA: Author. Retrieved from www .cdc.gov/hiv/group/gender/women/index.html.

Centers for Disease Control (2017b). *STDs in racial and ethnic minorities.* Atlanta, GA: Author. Retrieved from www.cdc.gov/std/stats16/minorities.htm.

Chin, H. B., Sipe, T. A., Elder, R., Mercer, S. L., Chattopadhyay, S. K., Jacob, V., Wethington, H. R., Kirby, D., Elliston, D. B., Griffith, M. Chuke, S. O., Briss, S. C., Ericksen, I., Galbraith, J. S.,

Herbst, J. H., Johnson, R. L., Kraft, J. M., Noar, S. M., Romero, L. M., Santelli, J.; Community Preventive Services Task Force (2012). The effectiveness of group-based comprehensive risk-reduction and abstinence education interventions to prevent or reduce the risk of adolescent pregnancy, human immunodeficiency virus, and sexually transmitted infections: Two systematic reviews for the guide to community preventive services. *American Journal of Preventive Medicine*, *42*(3), 272–294.

Connell, R. (2005). *Masculinities* (2nd ed.). Berkely, CA: University of California Press.

Cooper, B. & Crockett, C. (2015). Gender-based violence and HIV across the life course: Adopting a sexual rights framework to include older women. *Reproductive Health Matters*, *23*(46), 56–61.

De Walque, D., Dow, W. H., Nathan, R., Abdul, R., Abilahi, F., Gong, E., Isdahl, Z., Jamison, J., Jullu, B., Krishnan, S., Majura, A., Miguel, E., Moncada, J., Mtenga, S., Mwanyangala, M. A., Packel, L., Schachter, J., Shirima, K., & Medlin, C. A. (2012). Incentivising safe sex: A randomised trial of conditional cash transfers for HIV and sexually transmitted infection prevention in rural Tanzania. *British Medical Journal Open*, *2*(1), e000747.

Decker, M. R., Crago, A.-L., Chu, S. K., Sherman, S. G., Seshu, M. S., Buthelezi, K., Dhaliwal, M., & Beyrer, C. (2015). Human rights violations against sex workers: Burden and effect on HIV. *The Lancet*, *385*(9963), 186–199.

Decker, M. R., Miller, E., McCauley, H. L., Tancredi, D. J., Anderson, H., Levenson, R. R., & Silverman, J. G. (2014). Recent partner violence and sexual and drug-related STI/HIV risk among adolescent and young adult women attending family planning clinics. *Sexually Transmitted Infections*, *90* (2), 145–149.

Decker, M. R., Seage, 3rd, G., Hemenway, D., Gupta, J., Raj, A., & Silverman, J. G. (2009). Intimate partner violence perpetration, standard and gendered STI/HIV risk behaviour, and STI/HIV diagnosis among a clinic-based sample of men. *Sexually Transmitted Infections*, *85*(7), 555–560.

Dellar, R. C., Dlamini, S., & Karim, Q. A. (2015). Adolescent girls and young women: Key populations for HIV epidemic control. *Journal of the International AIDS Society*, *18*(S1), 64–70.

Denison, H. J., Bromhead, C., Grainger, R., Dennison, E. M., & Jutel, A. (2017). Barriers to sexually transmitted infection testing in New Zealand: A qualitative study. *Australian and New Zealand Journal of Public Health*, *41*(4), 432–437.

Dunkle, K. L. & Decker, M. R. (2013). Gender-based violence and HIV: Reviewing the evidence for links and causal pathways in the general population and high-risk groups. *American Journal of Reproductive Immunology*, *69*(s1), 20–26.

Dunkle, K. L., Jewkes, R. K., Nduna, M., Levin, J., Jama, N., Khuzwayo, N., Koss, M. P., & Duvvury, N. (2006). Perpetration of partner violence and HIV risk behaviour among young men in the rural Eastern Cape, South Africa. *AIDS*, *20*(16), 2107–2114.

Fileborn, B., Thorpe, R., Hawkes, G., Minichiello, V., Pitts, M., & Dune, T. (2015). Sex, desire and pleasure: Considering the experiences of older Australian women. *Sexual and Relationship Therapy*, *30* (1), 117–130.

Flash, C. A., Dale, S. D., & Krakower, D. S. (2017). Pre-exposure prophylaxis for HIV prevention in women: Current perspectives. *International Journal of Women's Health*, *9*, 391–401.

Fleischman, J. & Peck, K. (2015). *Addressing HIV risk in adolescent girls and young women.* Washington, DC: Center for Strategic & International Studies (CSIS).

Fonner, V. A., Armstrong, K. S., Kennedy, C. E., O'Reilly, K. R., & Sweat, M. D. (2014). School based sex education and HIV prevention in low-and middle-income countries: A systematic review and meta-analysis. *PloS One*, *9*(3), e89692.

Frohlich, K. L. & Potvin, L. (2008). Transcending the known in public health practice: The inequality paradox: The population approach and vulnerable populations. *American Journal of Public Health*, *98*(2), 216–221.

Gall, J., Sabin, K., Frescura, L., Sabin, M. L., Erkkola, T., & Toskin, I. (2017). Global trends of monitoring and data collection on the HIV response among key populations since the 2001 UN declaration of commitment on HIV/AIDS. *AIDS and Behavior*, *21*(1), 34–43.

Greenall, M., Kunii, O., Thomson, K., Bangert, R., & Nathan, O. (2017). Reaching vulnerable populations: Lessons from the global fund to fight AIDS, tuberculosis and malaria. *Bulletin of the World Health Organization*, *95*(2), 159–161.

Haberland, N. A. (2015). The case for addressing gender and power in sexuality and HIV education: A comprehensive review of evaluation studies. *International Perspectives on Sexual and Reproductive Health*, *41*(1), 31–42.

Harrison, A., Colvin, C. J., Kuo, C., Swartz, A., & Lurie, M. (2015). Sustained high HIV incidence in young women in Southern Africa: Social, behavioral, and structural factors and emerging intervention approaches. *Current HIV/AIDS Reports, 12*(2), 207–215.

Herbenick, D., Reece, M., Schick, V., Sanders, S. A., Dodge, B., & Fortenberry, J. D. (2010). Sexual behavior in the United States: Results from a national probability sample of men and women ages 14–94. *Journal of Sexual Medicine, 7*(s5), 255–265.

Kennedy, C. E., Fonner, V. A., O'Reilly, K. R., & Sweat, M. D. (2014). A systematic review of income generation interventions, including microfinance and vocational skills training, for HIV prevention. *AIDS Care, 26*(6), 659–673.

Kerrigan, D., Wirtz, A., Baral, S., Decker, M., Murray, L., Poteat, P., Pretorius, C., Sherman, S., Sweat, M., Semini, I., N'Jie, N., Stanciole, A., Butler, J., Osornprasop, O., Oelrichs, R., & Beyrer, C. (2013). *The global HIV epidemics among sex workers.* Washington, DC: World Bank.

Kim, J. C. & Watts, C. H. (2005). Gaining a foothold: Tackling poverty, gender inequality, and HIV in Africa. *British Medical Journal, 331*(7519), 769–772.

Kirby Institute (2017). *Annual Surveillance Report on HIV, viral hepatitis and STIs in Australia 2017.* Sydney, Australia: Kirby Institute.

Koh, S. A., Gómez, A. C., Shade, A. S., & Rowley, A. E. (2005). Sexual risk factors among self-identified lesbians, bisexual women, and heterosexual women accessing primary care settings. *Sexually Transmitted Diseases, 32*(9), 563–569.

Kohler, H.-P. & Thornton, R. L. (2012). Conditional cash transfers and HIV/AIDS prevention: Unconditionally promising? *The World Bank Economic Review, 26*(2), 165–190.

Krishnan, S., Dunbar, M. S., Minnis, A. M., Medlin, C. A., Gerdts, C. E., & Padian, N. S. (2008). Poverty, gender inequities, and women's risk of human immunodeficiency virus/AIDS. *Annals of the New York Academy of Sciences, 1136*(1), 101–110.

LaMontagne, D. S., Bloem, P. J., Brotherton, J. M., Gallagher, K. E., Badiane, O. & Ndiaye, C. (2017). Progress in HPV vaccination in low- and lower-middle-income countries. *International Journal of Gynecology & Obstetrics, 138*, 7–14.

Leclerc-Madlala, S. (2002). Youth, HIV/AIDS and the importance of sexual culture and context. *Social Dynamics, 28*(1), 20–41.

Lee, D., Binger, A., Hocking, J., & Fairley, C. (2005). The incidence of sexually transmitted infections among frequently screened sex workers in a decriminalised and regulated system in Melbourne. *Sexually Transmitted Infections, 81*(5), 434–436.

Li, Y., Marshall, C. M., Rees, H. C., Nunez, A., Ezeanolue, E. E., & Ehiri, J. E. (2014). Intimate partner violence and HIV infection among women: A systematic review and meta-analysis. *Journal of the International AIDS Society, 17*(1), ID 18845.

Link, B. G. & Phelan, J. (2010). Social conditions as fundamental causes of health inequalities. In C. Bird, P. Conrad, A. Fremont, & S. Timmermans (Eds), *Handbook of medical sociology* (Vol. 6, pp. 3–16). Nashville, TN: Vanderbilt University Press.

Looker, K. J., Elmes, J. A., Gottlieb, S. L., Schiffer, J. T., Vickerman, P., Turner, K. M., & Boily, M.-C. (2017). Effect of HSV-2 infection on subsequent HIV acquisition: An updated systematic review and meta-analysis. *The Lancet Infectious Diseases, 17*(12), 1303–1316.

Looker, K. J., Magaret, A. S., Turner, K. M., Vickerman, P., Gottlieb, S. L., & Newman, L. M. (2015). Global estimates of prevalent and incident herpes simplex virus type 2 infections in 2012. *PloS One, 10* (1), e114989.

Lottes, I. (2013). Sexual rights: Meanings, controversies, and sexual health promotion. *Journal of Sex Research, 50*(3–4), 367–391.

Marrazzo, J. M. (2013). Enhancing women's sexual health: Prevention measures in diverse populations of women. In S. Aral, K. Fenton, & J. Lipshutz (Eds), *The new public health and STD/HIV prevention: Personal, public and health systems approaches* (pp. 197–219). New York, NY: Springer.

Marrazzo, J. M., Ramjee, G., Richardson, B. A., Gomez, K., Mgodi, N., Nair, G., Palanee, T., Nakabiito, C., van der Straten, A., Noguchi, L., Hendrix, C. W., Dai, J. Y., Ganesh, S., Mkhize, B., Taljaard, M., Parikh, U. M., Piper, J., Mâsse, B., Grossman, C., Rooney, J., Schwartz, J. L., Watts, H., Marzinke, M. A., Hillier, S. L., McGowan, I. M., & Z. M. Chirenje (2015). Tenofovir-based preexposure prophylaxis for HIV infection among African women. *New England Journal of Medicine, 372*(6), 509–518.

McNair, R. (2005). Risks and prevention of sexually transmissible infections among women who have sex with women. *Sexual Health, 2*(4), 209–217.

Minichiello, V., Hawkes, G., & Pitts, M. (2011). HIV, sexually transmitted infections, and sexuality in later life. *Current Infectious Disease Reports, 13*(2), 182–187.

Mullinax, M., Schick, V., Rosenberg, J., Herbenick, D., & Reece, M. (2016). Screening for sexually transmitted infections (STIs) among a heterogeneous group of WSW(M). *International Journal of Sexual Health, 28*(1), 9–15.

Newman, L., Rowley, J., Vander Hoorn, S., Wijesooriya, N. S., Unemo, M., Low, N., Stevens, G., Gottlieb, S., Kiarie, J., & Temmerman, M. (2015). Global estimates of the prevalence and incidence of four curable sexually transmitted infections in 2012 based on systematic review and global reporting. *PloS One, 10*(12), e0143304.

Ortayli, N., Ringheim, K., Collins, L., & Sladden, T. (2014). Sexually transmitted infections: Progress and challenges since the 1994 International Conference on Population and Development (ICPD). *Contraception, 90*(6), S22–S31.

Padian, N. S., McCoy, S. I., Karim, S. S. A., Hasen, N., Kim, J., Bartos, M., Katabira, E., Bertozzi, S. M., Schwartländer, B., & Cohen, M. S. (2011). HIV prevention transformed: The new prevention research agenda. *The Lancet, 378*(9787), 269–278.

Pettifor, A., MacPhail, C., Nguyen, N., & Rosenberg, M. (2012). Can money prevent the spread of HIV? A review of cash payments for HIV prevention. *AIDS and Behavior, 16*(7), 1729–1738.

Pettifor, A. E., Measham, D. M., Rees, H. V., & Padian, N. S. (2004). Sexual power and HIV risk, South Africa. *Emerging Infectious Diseases, 10*(11), 1996.

Ponzetti, Jr, J. J. (2015). Sexuality education: Yesterday, today, and tomorrow. In J. J. Ponzetti, Jr (Ed.), *Evidence-based approaches to sexuality education: A global perspective* (pp. 1–14). New York, NY: Routledge.

Poteat, T., German, D., & Kerrigan, D. (2013). Managing uncertainty: A grounded theory of stigma in transgender health care encounters. *Social Science & Medicine, 84*, 22–29.

Power, J., McNair, R., & Carr, S. (2009). Absent sexual scripts: Lesbian and bisexual women's knowledge, attitudes and action regarding safer sex and sexual health information. *Culture, Health & Sexuality, 11*(1), 67–81.

Poynten, I. M., Grulich, A. E., & Templeton, D. J. (2013). Sexually transmitted infections in older populations. *Current Opinion in Infectious Diseases, 26*(1), 80–85.

Public Health England (2017). *Sexually transmitted infections and chlamydia screening in England, 2016.* London, UK: Public Health England.

Raj, A., Santana, M. C., La Marche, A., Amaro, H., Cranston, K., & Silverman, J. G. (2006). Perpetration of intimate partner violence associated with sexual risk behaviors among young adult men. *American Journal of Public Health, 96*(10), 1873–1878.

Reisner, S. L. & Murchison, G. R. (2016). A global research synthesis of HIV and STI biobehavioural risks in female-to-male transgender adults. *Global Public Health, 11*(7–8), 866–887.

Rosenstock, I. M., Strecher, V. J., & Becker, M. H. (1994). The health belief model and HIV risk behavior change. In R. J. DiClemente & J. Peterson (Eds), *Preventing AIDS* (pp. 5–24). Boston, MA: Springer.

Scheim, A. I., Santos, G.-M., Arreola, S., Makofane, K., Do, T. D., Hebert, P., Thomann, M., & Ayala, G. (2016). Inequities in access to HIV prevention services for transgender men: Results of a global survey of men who have sex with men. *Journal of the International AIDS Society, 19*(S2: 20779), 1–7.

Schick, V., Herbenick, D., Reece, M., Sanders, S. A., Dodge, B., Middlestadt, S. E., & Fortenberry, J. D. (2010). Sexual behaviors, condom use, and sexual health of Americans over 50: Implications for sexual health promotion for older adults. *The Journal of Sexual Medicine, 7*(s5), 315–329.

Schulkind, J., Mbonye, M., Watts, C., & Seeley, J. (2016). The social context of gender-based violence, alcohol use and HIV risk among women involved in high-risk sexual behaviour and their intimate partners in Kampala, Uganda. *Culture, Health & Sexuality, 18*(7), 770–784.

Schwartz, R. M., Weber, K. M., Schechter, G. E., Connors, N. C., Gousse, Y., Young, M. A., & Cohen, M. H. (2014). Psychosocial correlates of gender-based violence among HIV-infected and HIV-uninfected women in three US cities. *AIDS Patient Care and STDs, 28*(5), 260–267.

Seeley, J. (2015). Microfinance and HIV prevention. *Review of African Political Economy, 42*(145), 488–496.

Semenza, J. (2010). Strategies to intervene on social determinants of infectious diseases. *Eurosurveillance, 15*(27), 19611.

Shannon, K., Strathdee, S. A., Goldenberg, S. M., Duff, P., Mwangi, P., Rusakova, M., Reza-Paul, S., Lau, J., Deering, K., Pickles, M. R., Boily, M. C., & Pickles, M. R. (2015). Global epidemiology of HIV among female sex workers: Influence of structural determinants. *The Lancet, 385*(9962), 55–71.

Stephenson, R., Riley, E., Rogers, E., Suarez, N., Metheny, N., Senda, J., Saylor, K. M., & Bauermeister, J. A. (2017). The sexual health of transgender men: A scoping review. *The Journal of Sex Research, 54*(4–5), 424–445.

Taylor, M., Gliddon, H., Nurse-Findlay, S., Laverty, M., Broutet, N., Pyne-Mercier, L., & Liljestrand, J. (2018). Revisiting strategies to eliminate mother-to-child transmission of syphilis. *The Lancet Global Health, 6*(1), e26–e28.

Taylor, M. M., Frasure-Williams, J., Burnett, P., & Park, I. U. (2016). Interventions to improve sexually transmitted disease screening in clinic-based settings. *Sexually Transmitted Diseases, 43*(2S), S28–S41.

Torrone, E. A., Morrison, C. S., Chen, P.-L., Kwok, C., Francis, S. C., Hayes, R. J., Looker, K. J., McCormack, S., McGrath, N., van de Wijgert, J. H. H. M., Watson-Jones, D., Low, N., Gottlieb, S. L., STIMA Working Group, & van de Wijgert, J. H. (2018). Prevalence of sexually transmitted infections and bacterial vaginosis among women in sub-Saharan Africa: An individual participant data meta-analysis of 18 HIV prevention studies. *PLoS Medicine, 15*(2), e1002511.

Toskin, I., Blondeel, K., Peeling, R. W., Deal, C., & Kiarie, J. (2017). Advancing point of care diagnostics for the control and prevention of STIs: The way forward. *Sexually Transmitted Infections, 93*(S4), S81–S88.

Türmen, T. (2003). Gender and HIV/aids. *International Journal of Gynecology & Obstetrics, 82*(3), 411–418.

UN Women (2017). *Facts and figures: HIV and AIDS.* New York, NY: Author. Retrieved March 8, 2018, from www.unwomen.org/en/what-we-do/hiv-and-aids/facts-and-figures#notes.

UNAIDS (2017). *UNAIDS data 2017.* Geneva, Switzerland: Author. Retrieved from www.unaids.org /en/resources/documents/2017/2017_data_book.

UNAIDS (2018). *Women and girls and HIV.* Geneva, Switzerland: Author . Retrieved from www .unaids.org/en/resources/documents/2018/women_girls_hiv.

Wijesooriya, N. S., Rochat, R. W., Kamb, M. L., Turlapati, P., Temmerman, M., Broutet, N., & Newman, L. M. (2016). Global burden of maternal and congenital syphilis in 2008 and 2012: A health systems modelling study. *The Lancet Global Health, 4*(8), e525–e533.

Wingood, G. M. & DiClemente, R. J. (1998). Rape among African American women: Sexual, psychological, and social correlates predisposing survivors to risk of STD/HIV. *Journal of Women's Health, 7* (1), 77–84.

Wingood, G. M. & DiClemente, R. J. (2000). Application of the theory of gender and power to examine HIV-related exposures, risk factors, and effective interventions for women. *Health Education & Behavior, 27*(5), 539–565.

World Health Organization (WHO) (2007). *Guidance on global scale-up of the prevention of mother to child transmission of HIV.* Geneva, Switzerland: Author . Retrieved from www.unfpa.org/publications/guid ance-global-scale-prevention-mother-child-transmission-hiv.

World Health Organization (WHO) (2013). *Sexually Transmitted Infections (STIs): The importance of a renewed commitment to STI prevention and control in achieving global sexual and reproductive health.* Geneva, Switzerland: Author . Retrieved from http://apps.who.int/iris/handle/10665/75838.

World Health Organization (WHO) (2015). *Sexual health, human rights and the law* (9241564989). Geneva, Switzerland: Author . Retrieved from www.who.int/reproductivehealth/publications/sex ual_health/sexual-health-human-rights-law/en.

World Health Organization (WHO) (2016). *Report on global sexually transmitted infection surveillance 2015.* Geneva, Switzerland: Author . Retrieved from www.who.int/reproductivehealth/publications/rtis/ stis-surveillance-2015/en.

World Health Organization (WHO) (2017a). *Global guidance on criteria and processes for validation: Elimination of mother-to-child transmission of HIV and syphilis* (9241513276). Geneva, Switzerland: Author . Retrieved from www.who.int/reproductivehealth/publications/emtct-hiv-syphilis/en.

World Health Organization (WHO) (2017b). *Human pappilomavirus vaccines: WHO position paper.* Geneva, Switzerland: Author . Retrieved from www.who.int/immunization/policy/position_papers/ hpv/en.

31

IMPACTS OF SEXUAL VIOLENCE ON WOMEN'S SEXUAL HEALTH

Kyja Noack-Lundberg

Sexual violence is a widespread health issue that has broad impacts on women's lives. On a daily basis, many women live with the threat of sexual violence and fears for their safety that can limit their mobility and access to spaces. As sexual violence more often takes place in domestic spaces with known offenders, many women's most intimate and domestic lives are marked by the threat of sexual violence. A significant proportion of women have experienced childhood or adult sexual abuse or assault. For example, a meta-analysis of child sexual abuse prevalence rates showed that 18% of girls had experienced sexual abuse (Stoltenborgh et al., 2011). The World Health Organization (2013) found that 7.2% of women over the age of 15 had experienced non-partner sexual violence. In the United States, 21.3% of women had experienced rape or attempted rape as an adult or a child, and 43.6% had been subject to contact sexual violence (Smith et al., 2018). Although estimates of sexual violence vary, high prevalence rates point to sexual violence as a major public health problem globally.

Discourse about rape, and social justifications or explanations of rape including "rape myths," often individualizes sexual violence and locates fault with the individual victim, who could have monitored her actions more carefully to prevent rape; the perpetrator is often portrayed as a deviant monster, or a man whose normal masculine sexuality is not easily controlled. However, it can be argued that women around the world live in cultures that support, if not facilitate, sexual violence. Gavey (2005, p. 2), for example, argued that "normative forms of heterosexuality work as forms of cultural scaffolding" for rape. In other words, there is a whole social infrastructure and discourse that supports forced sex, such as prevalent cultural ideas of women's inherent passivity and men's unstoppable sexual agency and right to women's bodies (Gavey, 2005).

In many women's lives experiences of violence are cumulative and may be interlinked. For example, sexual assault can occur as part of intimate partner violence, and women who experience child sexual abuse are more likely to be involved in interpersonally violent relationships as adults (Alexander, 2009). Sexual violence often co-occurs with physical violence and with emotional, verbal, or psychological abuse. Therefore, it is not solely the global epidemic of sexual violence that needs to be addressed, but also the sociocultural climate in which it becomes acceptable to belittle, degrade, and victimize women; to ignore women's rights to self-determination over their bodies; and to deny their agency and ownership over their own lives.

Definitions of sexual violence

There is considerable debate amongst feminists and sexual violence researchers about how to define sexual violence in general, and rape and sexual assault in particular (Healicon, 2016; Reitan, 2001). Gavey (2005), for example, discusses events that women may not label as rape, but may have included being pressured, rough sex, unwanted sex, and sex that women felt unable to refuse. These incidents may not necessarily be considered rape or meet legal definitions. However, women's understandings of sex are shaped by discourses about hetero-sexual sex, which include sexual scripts of how men and women should act, including men's sexuality as unstoppable and women as passive (Hollway, 1989). Some feminists have argued that the definition of sexual violence should include staring or inappropriate touching and take into consideration that such acts occur in an environment, or "rape culture," that facilitates, allows, or appears to accept sexual assault (O'Neal, 2017). The effects on health of living in a rape culture may be cumulative and ongoing, as women are raised in societies in which they experience persistent threat of assault and ongoing pressure to acquiesce to men's sexual demands (Gavey, 2005).

This is reflected in the #metoo movement that was originated by the activist Tarana Burke in 2006, but only gained worldwide currency after its recent uptake by Hollywood celebrities, who encouraged women who had experienced harassment or sexual assault to tweet "If you've been sexually harassed or assaulted write 'me too' as a reply to this tweet." Rodino-Colocino (2018, p. 97) claimed that activists, including Burke, seek to not only garner empathy for individual suffering, but "also to become an agent for exposing systems of oppression and privilege of which sexual harassment and assault are cause and effect." This intersectional approach focuses on "power and privilege," including White supremacy and patriarchy, as systems that facilitate sexual violence (Rodino-Colocino, 2018, p. 97).

It is important to maintain clear definitions of rape and sexual assault as separate from harassment and other forms of violence, however it is also necessary to acknowledge the environmental and social factors that support rape and sexual assault. Although some of these factors have changed over time (e.g., disbelief of survivors), criminal justice systems in which defendants are rarely prosecuted, rape myths, rape supportive attitudes, and limited ideas of what constitutes "real rape" render some forms of sexual violence (e.g., rape within marriage) as legitimate sexual activity in the eyes of many people (Gavey, 2005).

Direct effects of sexual violence on women's sexual and reproductive health

Impacts of sexual violence in conflict zones

In recent decades, attention has been drawn to wartime rape. Scholars became particularly interested in theorizing this issue after the war in Bosnia and Herzegovina (1992–1995), which involved widespread and brutal sexual violence (Henry, Ward, & Hirshberg, 2004). However, historical records demonstrate that sexual violence during conflict has taken place since ancient Greece (Schott, 2011). The United Nations defines conflict-related sexual violence as "rape, sexual slavery, forced prostitution, forced pregnancy, forced abortion, enforced sterilization, forced marriage and any other form of sexual violence of comparable gravity perpetrated against women, men, girls or boys that is directly or indirectly linked to a conflict" (Office of the Special Representative of the Secretary-General on Sexual Violence in Conflict, 2018, p. 3). Sexual violence is currently prevalent in conflict situations around the world. It may be employed by state or non-state actors, including military groups, paramilitary groups, and terrorist organizations. Victims may be targeted due to their membership of an ethnic minority group, or on the basis of gender or sexual orientation (Office of the Special Representative of the Secretary-General on Sexual Violence in Conflict, 2018). There is some disagreement on the conditions that underpin wartime sexual violence. Key criminological and sociological explanations of conflict-related sexual violence include a breakdown in social norms, rape as a form of ethnic expansion through impregnation, the inherent hyper-sexuality of military environments, rape as a reward for combat, and gang rape as a form of masculine bonding and way of signalling masculinity to other men (Henry et al., 2004).

A qualitative literature review undertaken by Farr (2009) showed that what has been termed "extreme war rape" (e.g., group rapes, rape with mutilation and objects) was common in the 27 civil war contexts she analyzed. These included conflicts in South and Central America, Europe, South Asia, Central Asia, South East Asia, and Africa. Given that tens or hundreds of thousands of women have been raped in many of these conflicts (Crawford, 2013), rape with severe violence during war is a global issue, and millions of women worldwide are living with the after-effects of rape during war. Here I take the Democratic Republic of the Congo as a case study, given the relative recency of that civil war (which ended officially in 2003) and the ongoing extreme sexual violence that is occurring as part of conflicts between rebel military groups in the eastern region of the country.

It has been argued that loyalties to one's military unit, and secondarily to one's nation or ethnic group, may override ethical concerns in conflict situations (Connor, 2010). Civilian social norms must be broken down or overridden for those in the military to be able to kill others, and recruits are therefore inculcated with military values. Connor (2010) argued that loyalty to one's military peers may lead to "malfeasance" or unethical acts, such as violence, in some situations. This can be seen as similar to processes that occur in civilian group rape, which is often committed by young men. In Franklin's (2004) study of group rape among New York high school students, group rape worked "to increase group solidarity and cohesion through cooperative enterprise," and, in group contexts, individuals were more likely to participate in behaviour that did not fit with their personal values (2004, p. 26).

Conflict-related sexual violence can cause specific effects on women's health, such as injuries, STIs, and pregnancy. Much of the research on traumatic genital injuries has been conducted in the Kivu Region in the eastern Democratic Republic of Congo, as that region has some of the world's highest recorded sexual violence prevalence, due to military conflict between rival armies who control the region's mines and lucrative mineral trade (Mukwege & Nangini, 2009). According to Longombe, Claude, and Ruminjo (2008), genital injuries such as vaginal tears are often reported in Western countries, however sexual violence that results in fistula have not been recorded there. This may be due to a lack of recent studies on sexual violence during conflict situations in these areas.

Research by Dossa, Zunzunegui, Hatem, and Fraser (2014) in the Democratic Republic of Congo compared health outcomes of women who had experienced sexual violence in conflict and non-conflict situations. The researchers were unable to establish a direct causal link between conflict-related violence and fistula, but they found that there was an increased odds ratio (11.1%) of fistula in women who experienced sexual violence in a conflict context. Longombe et al. (2008) cited statistics from Doctors on Call, who reported 702 cases of sexual violence-related fistula in a three-year, two-month period from April 2003 to June 2006. In Longombe's case studies in the eastern Democratic Republic of the Congo, many of the women had been gang-raped, taken into sexual slavery, or raped during pregnancy; the latter often experienced obstructed labour.

Onsrud, Sjøveian, Luhiriri, and Mukwege (2008) found that 0.8% of fistula were directly attributable to sexual violence, after excluding women who had experienced issues such as urinary incontinence prior to rape (although sexual violence may have exacerbated these injuries). Some in this group of women were raped at a very young age, were gang-raped, or raped with objects. The prevalence of severe traumatic genital injury resulting in fistula is disputed. Onsrud claims that this may be either because it is a very uncommon issue, or that insufficient research has been conducted to determine its prevalence (Onsrud et al., 2008).

In Panzi Hospital in South Kivu province, 71% of women who attended hospital for sexual violence in 2006 had experienced gang rape, and 4.9% had experienced sexual slavery (Bartels et al., 2010); 27% of the perpetrators were in the military. Denis Mukwege, a Nobel Peace Prize winner and doctor at Panzi Hospital, coined the term "rape with extreme violence" to account for the kinds of violence the hospital staff has witnessed and its sequelae. Mukwege and Nangini (2009) wrote that they frequently saw gang rapes, which have a higher risk of injury, mutilation, torture, and deliberate infection with STIs. In their study of 7,519 sexual violence survivors who received treatment between 1999 and 2006, 72% of the victims were also tortured, and 12.4% were raped with objects.

Other African studies show an association between sexual violence and incontinence, which Dossa et al. (2014) claimed is often used as a proxy for fistula. In one study of fistula in hospitals in Africa, the vast majority of cases were found to be related to obstetric complications, however 4% was caused by sexual violence (Dossa et al., 2014). There was also much higher prevalence of chronic pelvic pain, "absence of desire for sexual intercourse," and "absence of desire for children" (Dossa et al., 2014, p. 10) among women who had experienced conflict-related sexual violence. A group of women in the Democratic Republic of the Congo who were raped while pregnant experienced interuterine fetal death, gave birth prematurely, and/or experienced iatrogenic fistula caused by evacuation procedures (Onsrud et al., 2008). In Addis Ababa, Ethiopia, 71 young women were treated for fistula or tears that resulted from sexual intercourse when attending the Addis Ababa Fistula hospital for total fecal incontinence (Muleta & Williams, 1999); most of these injuries occurred in marital relationships (Onsrud et al., 2008). However, it must be noted that other women in conflict situations may also experience marital violence, as the two kinds of violence are not mutually exclusive.

In addition to physical health symptoms, conflict-related sexual violence has strong impacts on psychological and societal welfare. In one study, young single women were more likely to experience gang-rape or sexual slavery, both of which were more likely to result in pregnancy (Bartels et al., 2010). The stigma of being a single parent means that marriage and career options become extremely limited, and the stigma of having experienced sexual assault also limits women's chances of marriage (Bartels et al., 2010). Women who experience fistula may face isolation or abandonment by their husbands or communities. In the Dossa et al. (2014) study of young women in Goma, in the Democratic Republic of the Congo, 16% of those who had fistula were deserted by their husbands. Chronic pelvic pain was also associated with relationship and mood issues (Dossa et al., 2014). As the sexual assault took place in a war zone, it was often also complicated by loss of loved ones, grieving, property loss, and housing and income insecurity (Dossa, Zunzunegui, Hatem, & Fraser, 2015).

Impacts of sexual violence in non-conflict zones

Direct effects of sexual violence in non-conflict situations can include vaginal bleeding, genital pain, urinary tract infections, sexually transmitted infection, and pregnancy (Krug, Dahlberg, Mercy, Zwi, & Lozano, 2002). Injuries are relatively common among women who have experienced rape, although different studies have shown different prevalence rates. Vaginal and anal tears and ecchymoses (a type of bruise resulting from damaged blood vessels) are common injuries (Slaughter, Brown, Crowley, & Peck, 1997). Traumatic genital injury rates range from 68% of victims in a US study (Slaughter et al., 1997), to 32% in a Danish study (Hilden, Schei, & Sidenius, 2005), to 22% in an Australian study (Zilkens et al., 2017). In their review of the literature on acute injuries caused by sexual assault, Resnick, Acierno, and Kilpatrick (1997) found that previous studies of hospital emergency rooms (ER) indicate that over 50% of victims showed signs of vaginal and perineal trauma, and 15% had significant tearing. The authors claimed that rape does not generally cause severe physical injuries, yet women may also seek medical attention for cuts, knife wounds, strangulation, or other physical impacts of sexual violence.

Although some studies (Bartoi & Kinder, 1998) indicate differences in psychological variables but not in sexual functioning, Campbell, Lichty, Sturza, and Raja (2006) found that gynecological symptoms (e.g., dysmenorrhea, menorrhagia) and sexual dysfunction were sometimes the result of sexual assault. There was an association between gynecological symptoms and sexual assault history, as participants who reported a gynecological symptom were 66% more likely than those who reported none to have experienced sexual assault. Certain assault characteristics were also associated with gynecological symptoms. Women who had experienced more than one assault or a "highly distressing" assault were more likely to have chronic pelvic pain. Campbell et al. (2006) also found that women with more forced penetrations and more severe penetrations reported more symptoms.

Women who had experienced assaults were more likely to use the health system at a 1.5 to 4 times greater frequency (Campbell, Sefl, & Ahrens, 2003) and to report more ongoing health problems and worse physical health (Campbell et al., 2006). Although there have been concerns that women who had experienced sexual violence might neglect healthcare, Lang et al. (2003) found that they were actually more likely to undertake pap smear tests and breast self-examinations. Having experienced sexual assault was found to be associated with higher levels of anxiety around health and greater "somatization" of symptoms (Stein et al., 2004). These factors also statistically predicted a higher level of healthcare visits (Stein et al., 2004). Seeking healthcare may result in "secondary victimization" if healthcare providers do not understand the relationship between sexual violence and physical health effects; this may lead to feelings of self-blame and guilt, which may negatively affect victims' recovery, both physically and mentally (Campbell et al., 2003).

Women who experience premenstrual syndrome (PMS) report higher rates of sexual abuse than the broader population (Golding, Taylor, Menard, & King, 2000). In their study, Golding et al. found that 95% of women attending a clinic for treatment of premenstrual symptoms had experienced "attempted or completed sexual abuse" (Golding et al., 2000, p. 74). Campbell et al. (2006) cautioned that attention should be focused on both direct injuries and indirect pathways to ill health.

Indirect effects related to sexual violence

Issues in the perinatal period

Some women who have experienced sexual violence may find procedures during pre-natal care or childbirth intrusive or re-traumatizing (Reeves, 2015). This has led to recommendations that healthcare services should identify women who have experienced sexual violence through screening practices (Geller & Stasko, 2017; Muzik et al., 2016) or provide trauma-informed care and less intrusive practices to everyone, on the assumption that many women will have experienced sexual violence (Geller & Stasko, 2017). Collaboration, choice, and empowerment form some of the principles of trauma-informed care (Sperlich et al., 2017), which help victims to establish a sense of safety and control. In one study, most women said that they would prefer screening for sexual assault; only 3.5% disagreed (Reeves, 2015).

Kendall-Tackett (2007) found that many women who had experienced child sexual abuse or intimate partner violence developed post-partum depression or PTSD, which led to negative physical and mental health outcomes, including inflammation responses. These findings need to be seen in the context of reports that 17–65% of women who have experienced sexual violence develop PTSD (Campbell, Dworkin, & Cabral, 2009). In turn, women with depression or PTSD also experience an increased risk of childbirth, pregnancy, and neonatal complications (Kendall-Tackett, 2007). Breastfeeding may also be affected by prior experiences of sexual violence. Although more women with histories of sexual violence expressed a wish to breastfeed, decreased cortisol issues could cause a delay in the onset of milk supply after birth for these women, which may result in the women ceasing to breastfeed (Kendall-Tackett, 2007).

Breastfeeding women may also experience uncomfortable sensations, given that breasts are viewed as sexual as well as maternal (Jansson, Velez, & Butz, 2017). For some women who had experienced child sexual abuse, touching and suckling triggered memories of child sexual abuse, and this resulted in dissociative symptoms such as detachment from the experience of breastfeeding for many women (Elfgen, Hagenbuch, Görres, Block, & Leeners, 2017). Barriers to continued breastfeeding included feelings of panic and agitation, concerns about becoming an abuse perpetrator, and difficulty in trusting healthcare practitioners (Elfgen et al., 2017).

Women who have been sexually assaulted are particularly at risk of experiencing mental health issues in the perinatal period. In one study, women who had experienced sexual trauma faced a greater risk (2.81 times higher) of developing postnatal depression (Geller & Stasko, 2017). Women who had experienced child sexual assault also developed perinatal depression at particularly high rates (Geller & Stasko, 2017). Mental health issues may also affect bonding and attachment with children and by implication have an impact on the mother–child relationship and thus the mental health of the next generation (Kendall-Tackett, 2007; Sperlich et al., 2017).

Women with PTSD have greater levels of high-risk health behaviours and adverse health outcomes during pregnancy. For example, women who have experienced sexual assault are more likely to use alcohol, tobacco, and other drugs (Lang et al., 2003). A literature review showed associations between PTSD and both low birth weight and decreased gestational length (Geller & Stasko, 2017). The review included women with PTSD caused by events other than sexual abuse, but made it clear that sexual abuse is a particularly distressing form of interpersonal trauma, which may lead to PTSD. Complications such as "ectopic pregnancy, spontaneous abortion, hyperemesis, preterm contractions, and excessive fetal growth" as well as "preterm birth and pre-eclampsia" (Geller & Stasko, 2017, p. 918) were more common among women with PTSD. There is also a risk of intergenerational transmission of trauma and neuro-endocrine dysfunction (Geller & Stasko, 2017).

Perinatal care often involves invasive procedures over which women may have little control. These include "vaginal examinations, delivery procedures, [and] breastfeeding support" (Sperlich & Seng, 2015, p. 75). Medical practitioners and policy makers have been undertaking studies and developing guidelines for trauma-informed care across a range of healthcare settings (Reeves, 2015). Such interventions can involve adjustments to procedures to make them less invasive, such as allowing participants to remove less clothing or remain fully-clothed during medical procedures. A study of a modified surgical gown showed that it helped women who had experienced child sexual abuse to feel more comfortable during gynecological examinations (Smith & Smith, 2000). Other components of trauma-informed perinatal care include explaining each procedure carefully beforehand, asking for consent, and giving patients control over their environment (Reeves, 2015).

The South Australian Government's Department of Health and Ageing (2018) provides an example of best practice policies related to sexual violence and the perinatal period. Documents address the effects of child sexual abuse on pregnant women, such as remembering abuse during this time or being triggered or re-traumatized during childbirth and examinations. These guidelines describe how to identify women who have experienced child abuse in ante-natal visits and intrapartum care, how healthcare practitioners can support women who have experienced child sexual abuse, and advice on bonding and breastfeeding that address specific concerns of women who have experienced child sexual abuse.

Revictimization, polyvictimization, and intergenerational transmission of trauma

Many women have experienced cumulative violence, including sexual, physical, and emotional or psychological violence, throughout their lifetimes, which may result in ongoing physical, psychological, relational, and self-care problems. Women who experience sexual abuse as children are far more likely to have relationships involving intimate partner violence as adults (which may itself involve sexual assault) (Alexander, 2009) and are also at risk of experiencing revictimization as adults (Banyard, Williams, & Siegel, 2001). The health effects of repeated sexual and physical violence over many years are difficult to disentangle, and both may cause mental health problems such as PTSD. Most children who are victims of childhood violence experience more than one kind of violence (Blom, Högberg, Olofsson, & Danielsson, 2016; Turner, Finkelhor, & Ormrod, 2006). It is therefore important, when considering sexual violence and its impacts on women's sexual and reproductive health, to understand that its aetiology may be complex and multi-factorial, rather than resulting from one incident or one type of violence.

Some women are at greater risk of experiencing multiple forms of trauma across their lifetimes. Campbell and her colleagues have conducted research focused on sexual violence experienced by women in the US military, which they have identified as a "high-risk" group (Campbell, Greeson, Bybee, & Raja, 2008). Many participants in their research were Black women from lower socioeconomic backgrounds, who had often experienced sexual or intimate partner violence or childhood abuse prior to entering the military, and then went to work in an environment with high levels of sexual harassment and assault (Campbell et al., 2008). They have called for more research to be undertaken on experiences of sexual assault disproportionately affecting minority groups, such as Black (Campbell et al., 2008), indigenous (Taylor & Putt, 2007), and transgender (Stotzer, 2009) women. It is therefore important to take an intersectional approach to understanding differences in experiences of sexual violence and to undertake research studies focused on the groups most likely to experience severe or ongoing victimization. This will help to better address the specific healthcare and coping needs of women who may have experienced cumulative trauma and polyvictimization.

Women who have previously experienced sexual assault, whether as a child or an adult, face a high likelihood of revictimization; around two-thirds of women experience further assaults (Classen, Palesh, & Aggarwal, 2005). Women who experienced child sexual abuse are also more likely to experience intimate partner violence as adults. There are multiple explanations to account for revictimization. These include disordered attachment; affect dys-regulation including dissociation, cognitive attributions, and threat perception; and the role of coping mechanisms such as drug and alcohol use (Alexander, 2009; Chu, Deprince, & Mauss, 2013; Classen et al., 2005; Kwako, Noll, Putnam, & Trickett, 2010). Given that there are many competing theories about how revictimization takes place, it can be argued that pathways to revictimization may be complex. It is also important that explanations for revictimization take into account the development of coping strategies such as dissociation that may have emerged in response to situations of severe violence, but may no longer be effective mechanisms (Hulette, Kaehler, & Freyd, 2011). I argue that, when this is not acknowledged, it individualizes the issue, locating the problem inherently within women who have experienced trauma. It is important to avoid pathologizing strategies that devel-oped in situations of extreme stress and may have worked to keep women safe at the time.

Although one might expect a clear relationship between previously having experienced sexual violence and re-experiencing sexual violence, forms of violence are interrelated; as discussed above, experiences of other kinds of violence, such as physical abuse, predict sexual violence later in life. Violence can have an additive effect whereby having experi-enced multiple types of trauma is related to risk of revictimization (Classen et al., 2005; Lippus, Laanpere, Part, Ringmets, & Karro, 2018). Women who have experienced child sexual abuse and witnessed intimate partner violence as children are more likely than other women to experience abusive relationships as adults (Alexander, 2009). Further, youth who experienced multiple forms of violence as children also have an early age of first sexual intercourse, and those who had experienced both physical and sexual violence had an increased risk of adolescent pregnancy (Blom et al., 2016). Sexual dysfunction, depression, health issues, stress, and symptom severity are associated with the number of types of vio-lence experienced (Lippus et al., 2018); women with histories of physical and sexual intim-ate partner violence have low self-rated health and report more symptoms (Bonomi, Anderson, Rivara, & Thompson, 2007).

Impaired attachment is one mechanism through which revictimization may occur and intergenerational trauma is passed down. Kwako et al. (2010, p. 407) referred to this process as "intergenerational transmission of the risks." They argued that flexible protective strategies are necessary to protect oneself against danger, but that women who have experienced childhood sexual abuse tend to use "rigid" protective strategies. Children whose mothers had experienced child sexual abuse demonstrated what the authors termed "extreme" attach-ment strategies. These included inhibited attachment, which resulted in children becoming overly independent and inhibiting their affect, and coercive strategies, including exaggerated negative affect. These strategies were termed extreme as they went beyond behaviours nor-mally used either to gain attention or protect themselves, and were different than those used by children with normative attachment (either secure or anxious) (Kwako et al., 2010).

In her research on the links between adult and child sexual abuse and victimization by mul-tiple intimate partners, Alexander (2009) found that women who had experienced intimate partner violence from multiple partners did not necessarily have unresolved attachment. Unre-solved attachment is the adult equivalent of the fourth attachment category of disorganized or disoriented attachment in children, and is related to unresolved loss or trauma (Alexander, 2009). However, although she found no relationship between neglect and multiple partner victimization, there was an association between parent–child role reversal and multiple partner victimization. Ninety percent of women in the study who had unresolved attachment had experienced multiple intimate partner victimization. This lends support to the idea that dis-ordered attachment is a factor that may cause women to be vulnerable to revictimization.

The biopsychoimmunological model

The biopsychoimmunologic model was originated by Woods et al. (2005), who focused on intimate partner violence, which can include, but is not limited to, sexual violence. First, a stress response occurs in reaction to the violence. Both the sympathetic nervous system and the hypothalamic–pituitary–adrenal axis are activated. The HPA axis releases cortico-trophin releasing hormone (CRH), which causes adrenocorticotropin releasing hormone (ACTH) to be discharged. This in turn causes the release of cortisol. Under normal condi-tions, this process would cease once the threat had abated; however ongoing or chronic stress can interrupt this process and result in abnormal release of cortisol. Both PTSD and depression may influence or be influenced by this process, as those with PTSD tend to have lower basal cortisol levels and those with depression have higher basal cortisol levels (Woods et al., 2005).

The biopsychoimmunologic model may account for chronic pain and increased health problems among women who have experienced sexual violence. Increased cortisol has been linked to chronic stress and immune system dysfunction (Lippus et al., 2018), although there is limited understanding of these processes. Bonomi et al. (2007) also linked chronic stress caused by sexual intimate partner violence to a range of physical outcomes, including abdominal pain, loss of appetite, headaches, back pain, fainting, and seizures. They linked isolation to psychological impacts such as fear and guilt and blaming oneself, and argued that the stress caused by isolation is associated with smoking, substance use, chronic pain, and cardiovascular issues (Bonomi et al., 2007). Campbell et al. (2008) also linked their findings to the biopsychoimmunological model, as they found that different kinds of assault were linked to different pain responses. Chronic violence such as IPV was more strongly linked to pelvic pain, for example, which could be explained by the "stress-immune functioning hypothesis" (Campbell et al., 2008, p. 411).

Changes in reactions to stressors can impair immune responses, and this is theorized to drive the chronic pain that many sexual violence survivors experience. Inflammation gener-ally occurs in relation to a threat or infection. Inflammation is part of the immune system response to threat: "[it] is a physiological process meant to alert the immune system of pathogen presence, tissue injury or other aggression" (Xu & Larbi, 2018, p. 98). T-lympho-cytes are deployed as part of the body's immune response. These kill infected cells. There are two main types of T-cells: Th1 and Th2. Both release proteins called cytokines that tell surrounding cells how to act. One type of cytokine produced by Th1 cells is interferon-γ. A change in Th1 cells results in immune suppression, which can lead to an increase in infec-tions and allergies, whereas a change in Th2 cells can result in autoimmune conditions, skin conditions, miscarriage, chronic inflammation, and chronic pain (Woods et al., 2005).

Woods et al. (2005) studied 97 women who had experienced intimate partner violence (IPV), one half of whom had experienced sexual violence. They had hypothesized that women who had experienced IPV would have higher levels of proinflammatory cytokine IFN-γ in comparison with women who had not, and their findings showed that levels were significantly higher in women who reported partner abuse. Women with PTSD were also found to have higher levels of proinflammatory cytokine IFN-γ than women without PTSD. The authors argued that this response is mediated by PTSD; the mental health effects drive the changes in cortisol, leading to inflammatory processes. The IPV also preceded PTSD, which demonstrates that PTSD could be the mediating factor between IPV and chronic health conditions. Although not measured in the Woods et al. (2005) study, lower cortisol levels in women with PTSD may be associated with an increase in prostaglandin release, which causes pain.

Earlier studies, such as that undertaken by Altemus, Cloitre, and Dhabhar (2003), show similar results, including different immune responses among women with and without PTSD, as well as delayed type (Type IV) hypersensitivity, which is related to Th1 cell mediation of immune response. In the Woods et al. (2005) framework, a delayed type hypersensitivity reaction is part of an autoimmune/inflammatory response caused by Th1 cell shift.

Influence of experiencing sexual violence on intimacy and sexual relationships

Although, anecdotally, avoidance of sexual intimacy is seen as a natural consequence of sexual violence, not all studies have shown support for this premise. Van Berlo and Ensink's (2000) review of the impact of sexual assault on sexual functioning showed that in older studies (from the 1980s) women who had been sexually assaulted reported decreased sexual satisfaction in some but not all sexual activities; activities such as hugging and stroking were not found to be affected. Across studies, some, but not all, women who had experienced sexual assault reported lower interest or less sexual pleasure or more fear. The characteristics of the assault (e.g., age of abuse, known or unknown perpetrator) impacted impairments in sexual functioning in different ways.

Multiple studies have shown that physiological responses are not impaired, whereas psychological responses are (Bartoi & Kinder, 1998; Becker, Skinner, Abel, & Treacy, 1982). Bartoi and Kinder (1998) found that the differences between women who had and had not experienced sexual assault were in the psychological variables of "sexual dissatisfaction" and "nonsensuality." A more recent study corroborates these findings, showing that women who had experienced sexual assault differed from women who had not only in the dimensions of "avoidance" and "nonsensuality" (Sanjuan, Langenbucher, & Labouvie, 2009). However, another study showed that, after controlling for other variables, PTSD best explained sexual problems (Letourneau, Resnick, Kilpatrick, Saunders, & Best, 1996).

Sexual intimacy and sexual relationships may trigger intrusive PTSD symptoms (Dimauro, Renshaw, & Blais, 2018). According to Tran, Dunckel, and Teng (2015), who studied survivors of sexual trauma in the military, "they are likely to experience intrusive or disturbing sexual thoughts and images, as sexual activity is a direct reminder of the sexual assault" (Tran et al., 2015, p. 849). They may also experience flashbacks or memories of the assault. Women with PTSD from sexual assault may experience anger, guilt, and or disgust when they are touched by their partners, and sex may be undertaken as a duty to partners (Healicon, 2016).

Feelings of powerlessness associated with having experienced sexual assault impacted women's abilities to negotiate contraception. Although contraception negotiation is often framed in terms of women's assertiveness or agency, negotiations of contraception take place within a cultural context that serves to facilitate men's sexual desires and delimit women's agency. Therefore, condom use needs to be viewed not solely as an indicator of individual women's willingness to value herself and practice safer sex behaviours, but also as affected by contextual and environmental factors such as cultural norms. Some male partners may prefer sex without condoms and use coercive or manipulative tactics, even where condom usage has been discussed and negotiated prior to or during sexual encounters.

Research has shown that some women who have experienced sexual violence engage in higher-risk sexual behaviours after the assault (Jina & Thomas, 2012). However, findings in this area have been inconsistent, as studies have shown that women engaged in less sexual behaviour overall after a sexual assault (Campbell, Sefl, & Ahrens, 2004). In the Resnick et al. (1997) review of health outcomes for women who had experienced sexual assault, higher rates of smoking, drinking, drug use, eating disorders, and sexually transmitted infections were found. Drawing on a learning theory model, Resnick et al. hypothesized that negative health outcomes may be mediated by depression, PTSD, panic, and their effects on functioning. In turn, panic may be triggered by cues and stimuli related to the assault that result in an automatic fear response. According to this theory, as women with PTSD avoid traumatic stimuli, the cues continue to trigger a response if the victim is not exposed to them in order to minimize their effects.

Conclusion

The effects of sexual violence on women's sexual and reproductive health are manifold and affect multiple areas of life and functioning. I have focused on sexual and reproductive health, rather than on mental health. However, a history of sexual violence can influence mental health through a greater likelihood of a diagnosis of PTSD, anxiety, or depression. Mental health issues and chronic stress can influence immune pathways and result in increases in inflammation (Campbell et al., 2006; Woods et al., 2005). It is well-documented that women who have experienced sexual assault suffer from a wide variety of medical conditions and have higher involvement in the healthcare system (Campbell et al., 2003).

Although some women may experience single incidents of sexual violence, it is clear that there are certain at-risk groups for whom sexual violence is part of a broader picture of repeated or ongoing violence. Violence in these women's lives is cumulative and may be interlinked. It is therefore important for healthcare practitioners, researchers, and policy-makers to take a broader, more holistic view of the effects of violence on women's lives, and to be aware that some women may be more vulnerable to sexual violence. Disaggregating data, and determining who is at risk and why, may go some way to explaining conflicting findings in this area.

Further interventions may be needed to ensure that women who have experienced sexual assault are able to access and be comfortable with medical care. Screening may ensure that patients are able to access modified procedures and that practitioners are aware of the potential cause of discomfort or distress, particularly when they are performing invasive procedures. In practice, both trauma-specific interventions, such as alterations to practices where possible, and trauma-informed care, which maintains an awareness that trauma is prevalent in the broader population and that many women have experienced sexual assault, may be necessary to ensure that healthcare is experienced as comfortable rather than disempowering or re-traumatizing.

References

Alexander, P. C. (2009). Childhood trauma, attachment, and abuse by multiple partners. *Psychological Trauma: Theory, Research, Practice, and Policy, 1*(1), 78–88.

Altemus, M., Cloitre, M., & Dhabhar, F. S. (2003). Enhanced cellular immune response in women with PTSD related to childhood abuse. *American Journal of Psychiatry, 160*(9), 1705.

Banyard, V. L., Williams, L. M., & Siegel, J. A. (2001). The long-term mental health consequences of child sexual abuse: An exploratory study of the impact of multiple traumas in a sample of women. *Journal of Traumatic Stress, 14*(4), 697–715.

Bartels, S. A., Scott, J. A., Mukwege, D., Lipton, R. I., Vanrooyen, M. J., & Leaning, J. (2010). Patterns of sexual violence in Eastern Democratic Republic of Congo: Reports from survivors presenting to Panzi Hospital in 2006. *Conflict and Health, 4*(1), 1–10.

Bartoi, M. G. & Kinder, B. N. (1998). Effects of child and adult sexual abuse on adult sexuality. *Journal of Sex & Marital Therapy, 24*(2), 75–90.

Becker, J. V., Skinner, L. J., Abel, G. G., & Treacy, E. C. (1982). Incidence and types of sexual dysfunctions in rape and incest victims. *Journal of Sex & Marital Therapy, 8*(1), 65–74.

Blom, H., Högberg, U., Olofsson, N., & Danielsson, I. (2016). Multiple violence victimisation associated with sexual ill health and sexual risk behaviours in Swedish youth. *The European Journal of Contraception & Reproductive Health Care, 21*(1), 49–56.

Bonomi, A. E., Anderson, M. L., Rivara, F. P., & Thompson, R. S. (2007). Health outcomes in women with physical and sexual intimate partner violence exposure. *Journal of Women's Health, 16*(7), 987–997.

Campbell, R., Dworkin, E., & Cabral, G. (2009). An ecological model of the impact of sexual assault on women's mental health. *Trauma, Violence, & Abuse, 10*(3), 225–246.

Campbell, R., Greeson, M. R., Bybee, D., & Raja, S. (2008). The co-occurrence of childhood sexual abuse, adult sexual assault, intimate partner violence, and sexual harassment: A mediational model of posttraumatic stress disorder and physical health outcomes. *Journal of Consulting and Clinical Psychology, 76*(2), 194.

Campbell, R., Lichty, L. F., Sturza, M., & Raja, S. (2006). Gynecological health impact of sexual assault. *Research in Nursing & Health, 29*(5), 399–413.

Campbell, R., Sefl, T., & Ahrens, C. E. (2003). The physical health consequences of rape: Assessing survivors' somatic symptoms in a racially diverse population. *Women's Studies Quarterly, 31*(1/2), 90–104.

Campbell, R., Sefl, T., & Ahrens, C. E. (2004). The impact of rape on women's sexual health risk behaviors. *Health Psychology, 23*(1), 67–74.

Chu, A. T., Deprince, A. P., & Mauss, I. B. (2013). Exploring revictimization risk in a community sample of sexual assault survivors. *Journal of Trauma & Dissociation, 15*(3), 319–331.

Classen, C. C., Palesh, O. G., & Aggarwal, R. (2005). Sexual revictimization: A review of the empirical literature. *Trauma, Violence, & Abuse, 6*(2), 103–129.

Connor, J. M. (2010). Military loyalty: A functional vice? *Criminal Justice Ethics, 29*(3), 278–290.

Crawford, K. F. (2013). From spoils to weapons: Framing wartime sexual violence. *Gender & Development, 21*(3), 505–517.

Department for Health and Ageing, G. o. S. A. (2018). *South Australian perinatal practice guideline sexual abuse in childhood – pregnancy care considerations.* Adelaide, South Australia: Department for Health and Ageing, Government of South Australia.

Dimauro, J., Renshaw, K. D., & Blais, R. K. (2018). Sexual vs. non-sexual trauma, sexual satisfaction and function, and mental health in female veterans. *Journal of Trauma & Dissociation, 19*(4), 403–416.

Dossa, N. I., Zunzunegui, M. V., Hatem, M., & Fraser, W. (2014). Fistula and other adverse reproductive health outcomes among women victims of conflict-related sexual violence: A population-based cross-sectional study. *Birth, 41*(1), 5–13.

Dossa, N. I., Zunzunegui, M. V., Hatem, M., & Fraser, W. D. (2015). Mental health disorders among women victims of conflict-related sexual violence in the Democratic Republic of Congo. *Journal of Interpersonal Violence, 30*(13), 2199–2220.

Elfgen, C., Hagenbuch, N., Görres, G., Block, E., & Leeners, B. (2017). Breastfeeding in women having experienced childhood sexual abuse. *Journal of Human Lactation, 33*(1), 119–127.

Farr, K. (2009). Extreme war rape in today's civil-war-torn states: A contextual and comparative analysis. *Gender Issues, 26*(1), 1–41.

Franklin, K. (2004). Enacting masculinity: Antigay violence and group rape as participatory theater. *Sexuality Research and Social Policy, 1*(2), 25–40.

Gavey, N. (2005). *Just sex? The cultural scaffolding of rape.* Abingdon, UK: Routledge.

Geller, P. A. & Stasko, E. C. (2017). Effect of previous posttraumatic stress in the perinatal period. *Journal of Obstetric, Gynecologic & Neonatal Nursing, 46*(6), 912–922.

Golding, J., Taylor, D. L., Menard, L., & King, M. (2000). Prevalence of sexual abuse history in a sample of women seeking treatment for premenstrual syndrome. *Journal of Psychosomatic Obstetrics & Gynecology, 21*(2), 69–80.

Healicon, A. A. (2016). *The politics of sexual violence: Rape, identity and feminism.* New York, NY: Palgrave Pivot.

Henry, N., Ward, T., & Hirshberg, M. (2004). A multifactorial model of wartime rape. *Aggression and Violent Behavior, 9*(5), 535–562.

Hilden, M., Schei, B., & Sidenius, K. (2005). Genitoanal injury in adult female victims of sexual assault. *Forensic Science International, 154*(2), 200–205.

Hollway, W. (1989). *Subjectivity and method in psychology: Gender, meaning and science.* London, UK: Sage.

Hulette, A., Kaehler, L., & Freyd, J. (2011). Intergenerational associations between trauma and dissociation. *Journal of Family Violence, 26*(3), 217–225.

Jansson, L. M., Velez, M. L., & Butz, A. M. (2017). The effect of sexual abuse and prenatal substance use on successful breastfeeding. *Journal of Obstetric, Gynecologic & Neonatal Nursing, 46*(3), 480–484.

Jina, R. & Thomas, L. S. (2012). Health consequences of sexual violence against women. *Best Practice & Research Clinical Obstetrics & Gynaecology, 27*(1), 15–26.

Kendall-Tackett, K. A. (2007). Violence against women and the perinatal period: The impact of lifetime violence and abuse on pregnancy, postpartum, and breastfeeding. *Trauma, Violence, & Abuse, 8*(3), 344–353.

Krug, E. G., Dahlberg, L. L., Mercy, J. A., Zwi, A. B., & Lozano, R. (2002). *World report on violence and health.* Geneva, Switzerland: World Health Organization.

Kwako, L. E., Noll, J. G., Putnam, F. W., & Trickett, P. K. (2010). Childhood sexual abuse and attachment: An intergenerational perspective. *Clinical Child Psychology and Psychiatry, 15*(3), 407–422.

Lang, A. J., Rodgers, C. S., Laffaye, C., Satz, L. E., Dresselhaus, T. R., & Stein, M. B. (2003). Sexual trauma, posttraumatic stress disorder, and health behavior. *Behavioral Medicine, 28*(4), 150–158.

Letourneau, E. J., Resnick, H. S., Kilpatrick, D. G., Saunders, B. E., & Best, C. L. (1996). Comorbidity of sexual problems and posttraumatic stress disorder in female crime victims. *Behavior Therapy, 27*(3), 321–336.

Lippus, H., Laanpere, M., Part, K., Ringmets, I., & Karro, H. (2018). Polyvictimization and the associations between poor self-perceived health, dissatisfaction with life, and sexual dysfunction among women in Estonia. *Journal of Interpersonal Violence,* doi: 10.1177/0886260518780412 [epub ahead of print].

Longombe, A. O., Claude, K. M., & Ruminjo, J. (2008). Fistula and traumatic genital injury from sexual violence in a conflict setting in Eastern Congo: Case studies. *Reproductive Health Matters, 16*(31), 132–141.

Mukwege, D. & Nangini, C. (2009). Rape with extreme violence: The new pathology in South Kivu, Democratic Republic of Congo. *PLoS Medicine, 6*(12), e1000204.

Muleta, M. & Williams, G. (1999). Postcoital injuries treated at the Addis Ababa Fistula Hospital, 1991–97. *Lancet, 354*(9195), 2051–2052.

Muzik, M., McGinnis, E. W., Bocknek, E., Morelen, D., Rosenblum, K. L., Liberzon, I., Seng, J., & Abelson, J. L. (2016). PTSD symptoms across pregnancy and early postpartum among women with lifetime PTSD diagnosis. *Depression and Anxiety, 33*(7), 584–591.

O'Neal, E. N. (2017). "Victim is not credible": The influence of rape culture on police perceptions of sexual assault complainants. *Justice Quarterly, 36*(1), 1–34.

Office of the Special Representative of the Secretary-General on Sexual Violence in Conflict (2018). *Report of the secretary-general on conflict-related sexual violence.* Geneva, Switzerland: United Nations.

Onsrud, M., Sjøveian, S., Luhiriri, R., & Mukwege, D. (2008). Sexual violence-related fistulas in the Democratic Republic of Congo. *International Journal of Gynecology & Obstetrics, 103*(3), 265–269.

Reeves, E. (2015). A synthesis of the literature on trauma-informed care. *Issues in Mental Health Nursing, 36*(9), 698–709.

Reitan, E. (2001). Rape as an essentially contested concept. *Hypatia, 16*(2), 43–66.

Resnick, H. S., Acierno, R., & Kilpatrick, D. G. (1997). Health impact of interpersonal violence 2: Medical and mental health outcomes. *Behavioral Medicine, 23*(2), 65–78.

Rodino-Colocino, M. (2018). Me too, #MeToo: Countering cruelty with empathy. *Communication and Critical/Cultural Studies, 15*(1), 96–100.

Sanjuan, P. M., Langenbucher, J. W., & Labouvie, E. (2009). The role of sexual assault and sexual dysfunction in alcohol/other drug use disorders. *Alcoholism Treatment Quarterly, 27*(2), 150–163.

Schott, R. M. (2011). War rape, natality and genocide. *Journal of Genocide Research, 13*(1–2), 5–21.

Slaughter, L., Brown, C. R. V., Crowley, S., & Peck, R. (1997). Patterns of genital injury in female sexual assault victims. *American Journal of Obstetrics and Gynecology, 176*(3), 609–616.

Smith, M. S. & Smith, M. T. (2000). A stimulus control intervention in the gynecological exam with sexual abuse survivors. *Women & Health, 30*(2), 39–51.

Smith, S. G., Zhang, X., Basile, K. C., Merrick, M. T., Wang, J., Kresnow, M.-J., & Chen, J. (2018). *National intimate partner and sexual violence survey: 2015 data brief – updated release.* Atlanta, GA: Centers for Disease Control and Prevention.

Sperlich, M. & Seng, J. (2015). What does trauma informed perinatal care look like? In J. Seng (Ed.), *Trauma informed care in the perinatal period* (pp. 72–82). Edinburgh: Dunedin Academic Press.

Sperlich, M., Seng, J., Rowe, H., Fisher, J., Cuthbert, C., & Taylor, J. (2017). A cycles-breaking framework to disrupt intergenerational patterns of maltreatment and vulnerability during the childbearing year. *Journal of Obstetric, Gynecologic & Neonatal Nursing, 46*(3), 378–389.

Stein, M. B., Lang, A. J., Laffaye, C., Satz, L. E., Lenox, R. J., & Dresselhaus, T. R. (2004). Relationship of sexual assault history to somatic symptoms and health anxiety in women. *General Hospital Psychiatry, 26*(3), 178–183.

Stoltenborgh, M., van Ijzendoorn, M. H., Euser, E. M., & Bakermans-Kranenburg, M. J. (2011). A global perspective on child sexual abuse: Meta-analysis of prevalence around the world. *Child Maltreatment, 16*(2), 79–101.

Stotzer, R. L. (2009). Violence against transgender people: A review of United States data. *Aggression and Violent Behavior, 14*(3), 170–179.

Taylor, N. & Putt, J. (2007). *Adult sexual violence in Indigenous and culturally and linguistically diverse communities in Australia.* Trends and issues in crime and criminal justice (Vol. 345). Canberra, Australia: Australian Institute of Criminology.

Tran, J., Dunckel, G., & Teng, E. (2015). Sexual dysfunction in veterans with post-traumatic stress disorder. *The Journal of Sexual Medicine, 12*(4), 847–855.

Turner, H. A., Finkelhor, D., & Ormrod, R. (2006). The effect of lifetime victimization on the mental health of children and adolescents. *Social Science & Medicine, 62*(1), 13–27.

Van Berlo, W. & Ensink, B. (2000). Problems with sexuality after sexual assault. *Annual Review of Sex Research, 11*, 235–257.

Woods, A. B., Page, G. G., O'Campo, P., Pugh, L. C., Ford, D., & Campbell, J. C. (2005). The mediation effect of posttraumatic stress disorder symptoms on the relationship of intimate partner violence and IFN-Ⓧ levels. *American Journal of Community Psychology, 36*(1–2), 159–175.

World Health Organization (WHO) (2013). *Global and regional estimates of violence against women: Prevalence and health effects of intimate partner violence and non-partner sexual violence.* Geneva, Switzerland: World Health Organization.

Xu, W. & Larbi, A. (2018). Immunity and inflammation: From Jekyll to Hyde. *Experimental Gerontology, 107*, 98–101.

Zilkens, R. R., Smith, D. A., Phillips, M. A., Mukhtar, S. A., Semmens, J. B., & Kelly, M. C. (2017). Genital and anal injuries: A cross-sectional Australian study of 1266 women alleging recent sexual assault. *Forensic Science International, 275*, 195–202.

32

FEMINIST PERSPECTIVES ON CHILD SEXUAL ABUSE

Sam Warner

Child sexual abuse can have life-long impacts on women's sexual and reproductive health. It is a body-directed crime that shapes girls' relationship with, and their experiences of, themselves and their bodies thereafter. It directly undermines girls' and women's control over their own bodies, and this lack of control intersects with and may be reinforced by the socioeconomic, cultural, and political environments in which they live. How sexually victimized girls and women experience their embodied gender is, therefore, both intensely personalized as well as being culturally and socially shaped and sedimented. Child sexual abuse is a global problem that has multiple local iterations intersected by competing priorities and ideologies. In order to make sense of this, I start by elaborating an inclusive knowledge base about child sexual abuse and utilize a feminist framework to unfold developments in theory and practice. I explicate some of the psychosocial mechanisms through which sexually abused girls and women are controlled, and consider the predominant ways in which they are impacted by, and cope with, such experiences. Finally, I demonstrate how feminism's attention to power inequalities informs work with sexually abused girls and women.

Making and maintaining an inclusive knowledge base

Identifying the best available research evidence about child sexual abuse is a complex practice. The scientific method is presumed to be value-free, yet prevailing social values are implicated in and serve to constrain the evidence base (Warner & Spandler, 2012). As such, *evidence-based practice* is often limited because how we determine what is important remains hidden and unexplored. For example, it has long been accepted as 'true' that women who have experienced child sexual abuse are more likely than their non-abused peers to have a diagnosis of mental illness and personality disorder (e.g., Spataro, Mullen, Burgess, & Wells, 2004). However, when diagnosis is both the starting point and end result of research, the medicalization of psychosocial difficulties cannot be challenged.

There is a richer, less conventional seam of analysis in grey literature (New York Academy of Medicine, 2019). Grey literature is produced outside of traditional academic publishing and dissemination methods, and is a form of *practice-based evidence* (see Warner & Spandler, 2012), which is inclusive of research, papers, government documents, evaluations, and reviews. The grey literature, being outside of the Academy, may be more able to reflect critically and rapidly on current concerns and issues. Both the scientific and grey literature shapes and is shaped by popular media, which is produced by journalists on-line and in newspapers and magazines. Newspaper reports tend to reflect dominant cultural beliefs about child sexual abuse (Davies, O'Leary, & Read, 2015) although, sometimes, journalists have been advocates for social change, such as the treatment of sexually exploited girls (e.g., Bindel, 2017).

Underlying and informing all forms of the above literature are the autobiographical accounts shared by survivors orally and in blogs, books, and poetry. It is these personal stories and accounts, the *experience-based evidence*, that provides deep understanding about child sexual abuse and fuels social change. Yet survivors, as all-knowing subjects, are also social subjects whose ability to speak and to be heard is always socially mediated (Althusser, 1971). This gives rise to the need for a further form of intersecting knowledge, which can be termed *theory-based* and/or *values-based evidence*. This last form of knowledge invites reflective specificity about the various issues that shape where we speak from; what we speak about; and to which theory and/or values-based 'communities of knowledge' (Ramazanoglu & Holland, 1999) we feel ourselves to be most accountable.

I write from my multiple experiences: as a survivor of sexual violence, a community activist, an academic, and a clinical psychologist with over 30 years' experience in the field of child sexual abuse. The politics I draw on are feminist. I am aware that feminism covers a vast terrain and that any overarching approach (such as feminism or psychology) fails when its ability to 'speak the truth' is unquestioningly assumed (Warner, 2009). Thus, I use post-structuralism (Foucault, 1978; Warner, 2016a) to guard against the automatic acceptance of any grand narrative or ideology by maintaining a space for critical reflexivity. I maintain an awareness of how language constructs intersecting identities and is implicated in practices of marginalization (see Butler, 1990; Crenshaw, 1993). This approach enables me to think through the social systems that keep all intersecting oppressions in place, termed the kyriarchy by Fiorenza (2001). This chapter thus draws on the range of knowledges outlined above and it has an explicit, socially-situated feminist agenda.

Recognizing child sexual abuse

A herstory

There is no worldwide consensus on what constitutes childhood and therefore the legal age of consent to sex. What constitutes child sexual abuse is also contested, and our understandings of it have changed throughout history. For example, Freedman (2013; see also Bindell, 2013) detailed the changes in British law, which provided the basis for many North American laws, for the term 'rape' (from the Latin *raptus* or *rapere*), which originally referred to the nonsexual crime of violent theft. In the 12th century a distinction was made between abduction and rape, with the latter defined as forced sexual intercourse. As girls and women were not understood to be fully human under the law, they could not be offended against. Rather, in the 15th century, it was the father or husband of a rape victim who pressed criminal charges because the legal definition of rape only applied to the theft of a woman's virtue: either a daughter's virginity or a married woman's honour.

The foundations for a more 'woman-centred' understanding of sexual abuse parallels women's fight to be recognized as fully human. Feminist campaigners in the UK raised concerns about the sexual abuse and exploitation of girls and young women, which culminated in 1925 in the Government's publication of the forward-looking *Report of the Departmental*

Committee on Sexual Offences Against Young Persons (British Government, 1925). The Second World War, however, brought changing priorities. Concerns about sexually victimized girls were replaced with moral panics about promiscuous young women or 'good time girls' (Bingham, Delap, Jackson, & Settle, 2016). A period of relative stability and prosperity after the Second World War in most developed countries heralded the growth of liberation movements in the 1960s and the inception of second-wave feminism. This brought significant opportunities for reinvigorating concerns about child sexual abuse. Through 'consciousness-raising' groups, women theorized their everyday experiences of oppression and began to speak about, and organize against, sexual and physical abuse by men. This led to the establishment of the first rape crisis centres and domestic violence refuges in these countries in the 1970s, followed by women-only specialist child sexual abuse services thereafter (e.g., Taboo, a service for women and girl survivors of child sexual abuse, Manchester, UK).

Meanwhile, the general public was struggling to accept the increasingly visible concern about child sexual abuse. This was evident in people's refusal to believe in organized abuse, such as the so-called satanic sexual abuse of children in the 1980s (Campbell, 1988) and the 'memory wars' of the 1990s (Crews, 1995). Feminist believers (e.g., Bass & Davies, 1988) were pitted against sexual abuse deniers (see Loftus, 1993), who argued that, because some therapists implanted *false* memories of child abuse in (their mainly female) clients' minds, most or all *recovered* memories of child sexual abuse were untrue. This was, and is, not the case.

The third wave of feminism (the politics of deconstruction: 1990s–2000s) arose out of the need to make sense of women's intersections and differences. This phase heralded a 'turn to language' (see Warner, 2016a, for an overview) and was particularly influenced by academic theorizing. Perhaps the biggest shift in thinking was, and continues to be, in the implicit, but increasingly widespread use of social constructionism in recognizing that abuser grooming strategies shape how child sexual abuse is structured, how victimization is maintained, and how its effects are experienced (e.g., Warner, 2000, 2009). Grooming refers to the various processes that abusers use to build emotional bonds with, and control over, a child for the purposes of sexual abuse and which engender the child's trust, dependence and powerlessness.

Current concerns

Most contemporary definitions of child sexual abuse cover issues of sex, power, consent, and age. For example, the World Health Organization (WHO, 2006) stated that child sexual abuse is inclusive of any sexual activity with a child who does not fully understand, is not developmentally ready for, or is unable to give informed consent to the activity; and/or a sexual activity with a child that violates the laws and social mores of a society. Sexual abuse is understood to be perpetrated by adults and children who are, because of their age or developmental stage, in a position of power, trust, or responsibility over the victim; the aim of the activity is to gratify or satisfy the needs of the abuser. Definitions of sexual abuse have recently been expanded from contact abuse (being physically present with/touching the child during abuse) to include non-contact abuse, which covers all non-touching activities, such as grooming, on-line abuse and sexually exploiting a child for money, power or status (see National Society for the Prevention of Cruelty to Children/NSPCC, 2019).

Sex crimes are often not reported because of enduring fear and stigma. UNICEF (2017a) reported that, in some countries, as few as 1% of adolescent girls who have experienced forced sex reached out for professional help. This is especially the case for children in cultures where family honour is placed above the safety and well-being of children; where reporting sexual violence can lead to ostracism, further violence or even death (Radford, Allnock, & Hynes, 2018); and where rigid and unequal gender power relations are embedded and support discriminatory social, cultural and economic norms (Simon-Butler & McSherry, 2019). Men overwhelmingly predominate as perpetrators (see United Nations/UN, 2019a) because men's privilege, superiority and entitlement to sex are deeply entrenched in many cultures.

Marginalizing language is also often used to describe victims of child sexual abuse (Greijer & Doek, 2016). In the UK, for example, this is evident over the recent history of responses to sexually exploited girls. For much of the 20th century, such girls were depicted as prostitutes, rather than as victims, as in this *Independent* newspaper headline: 'Prostitute dies of drug overdose – at 13' (Kossoff, 1999). In 1998, the British charity Barnardo's published *Whose Daughter Next? Children Abused Through Prostitution* (Van Meeuwen, Sara Swann, McNeish, & Edwards, 1998), in which they argued that child prostitution *is* child abuse. Yet, children's power and control continued to be over-emphasized, perhaps through the misappropriation of a children's rights discourse. A series of reports on child sexual exploitation scandals in the UK demonstrated that abused children were repeatedly dismissed for having made 'poor choices' and had 'problematic lifestyles' (Topping, 2015). It is only recently that sexual *exploitation* has reframed work with such girls. This is a result of sustained efforts to remediate previous failures and of organizing partners around the world to address the plight of child victims of sexual exploitation, human trafficking, and modern slavery. Yet as Greijer and Doek (2016, p.1) argued:

> Even where the same terms are used, there is quite often disagreement concerning their actual meaning. This has created significant challenges for policy development and programming, development of legislation, and data collection, leading to flawed responses and limited and ineffective methods of measuring impact or setting targets. In the context of international/cross-border child sexual exploitation and abuse, these difficulties are magnified.

Although children of every age are susceptible to sexual violence, adolescence is a period of pronounced vulnerability, especially for girls (Radford et al., 2018). Domestic abuse also impacts young women at higher rates than other age groups. For example, the British Crime Survey (Office for National Statistics, 2018) showed that young women were the group most likely to suffer abuse from a partner. The most consistent risk factor, then, for sexual abuse is gender.

Impact of child sexual abuse

Physical and mental health effects

Child sexual abuse can be deeply traumatic and can lead to immediate and long-term physical health problems and life-long mental health and social difficulties. The physical body has a great capacity for recovery, which means that, in most cases, there is no conclusive physical evidence of sexual abuse. However, sometimes there may be life-changing injuries, other health impacts and even death (Christie, 2018; Irish, Kobayashi, & Delahanty, 2010; Mills, Majeed-Ariss, & White, 2018; Nelson, 2016; Simon-Butler & McSherry, 2019), particularly in the context of conflict/war situations (UN, 2019b).

Physical ill-health difficulties concurrent to sexual abuse can also result from unwanted pregnancies and repeated, sometimes forced abortions; continually disrupted sleep (and adult insomnia); leaving abusive homes to live on the streets; declining or avoiding preventative health checks (avoidance that may continue throughout adulthood); and self-harm (including self-injury, disordered eating, and misuse of alcohol and drugs) (Nelson, 2016). Further, sometimes life-long, negative physical effects can result from gynecological trauma and sexually transmitted infections. This can lead to increased complications during childbirth and higher rates of associated gynecological problems including chronic pelvic pain, urinary tract infections and pain during intercourse (see WHO, 2012). Because sex may be painful and/or trigger stress responses such as dissociation this can negatively impact women's sexual desire, arousal, and ability to orgasm (American College of Obstetrics and Gynecology, 2017). Additionally, as a result of lowered self-worth, women who have experienced childhood sexual abuse may be more likely to engage in risky sex and/or may be at increased risk of further victimization (Spicer, 2018). Furthermore, sexual violence does not automatically stop at 18 years old (López et al., 2017): women and girls may be targeted and groomed because of their existing vulnerabilities rather than their (younger) age (Spicer, 2018).

Tactics, grooming and coercive control

Emotional trauma often persists longer than the physical effects of abuse because the grooming or training tactics used to control children are internalized by the child and, once internalized, are difficult to resist or unload (Warner, 2009). This can leave victims feeling betrayed, scared, powerless, ashamed, depressed, despairing, unable and/or not knowing whom to trust, confused, conflicted (e.g., feeling both love and fear), angry, hopeless and sometimes suicidal (Warner, 2000).

If sexual abuse occurs when children are very young, it may also impact on women's later sense of their sex/gender identity. This is because, in early childhood, identity is experienced as inherently changeable, whereas, after about seven years old, identity feels more constant and stable (Kohlberg, 1966). Early sexual abuse can therefore feel very much part of identity development. Furthermore, talk about child sexual abuse can too often be used to invalidate survivors' positive sexual and gender experiences, particularly when those experiences are associated with marginalized identities such as LGBTQ+ (Walding, 2016).

The negative effects of sexual abuse may be further intensified through other criminal, financial, and/or care-giving social exploitation, and through social exclusion in terms of intersecting identity and community marginalizations (e.g., women from refugee or traveller communities) (e.g., UNICEF, 2017b). There may be additional family abuse and neglect. All this can increase the risk of further trauma associated with family separation as a result of coming into care, psychiatric hospital, and/or prison. Women's sense of relationship may be so damaged that this can result in later having their own children removed (Mothers living apart from their children, 2014) and/or women avoiding services for fear of having their children removed (Warner, 2009).

Grooming occurs in all sexual abuse contexts. This is in terms of cultures, societies and contexts that legitimate male entitlement and control. Physical force tends to predominate in conflict situations. However, similar processes of individual and group control and grooming are present in most other contexts in which girls are sexually abused, including the family, their community, with peers, in intimate partner relationships and on-line. The recognition that grooming is endemic to sexual abuse has led some countries to place new crimes on record. For example, 'sexual communication with a child' (whether on-line or off-line) is a criminal offence in the UK (Ministry of Justice, 2017), Australia (Australian Institute of Criminology, 2008) and the USA (US Legal, 2019).

Increased recognition of grooming has led some countries to extend their powers to deprive of their liberties girls and women who are judged, as a result of having been groomed, to lack the mental capacity to make informed choices about their behaviour (Spicer, 2018). The aim of restricting liberty in secure and semi-secure placements is to provide the space in which victims might be 'deprogrammed'. However, in the absence of wider interventions with abusers and the families, intimate partners and communities to which girls and women return, such specialist placements have limited effect.

Coping and surviving

The ways in which girls and women cope with the impact of child sexual abuse are influenced by their ability to access protective relationships, their age, their learning ability and intersecting forms of social marginalization. However, during the moments of abuse, there are methods that most children use to avoid focussing on the emotional terror and physical harm. These include denial (which is difficult to sustain when abuse is repetitive), distraction (which is intensely effortful), and dissociation (which can feel effortless and uncontrollable) (see Warner, 2000). Because emotional terror does not stop when the physical act of abuse ends, these coping strategies can generalize and persist into adulthood. And, although they may be emotionally necessary, they can be problematic.

People are less socially aware when they are distracted and/or dissociated, and this can increase their vulnerability. When abuse has been severe, enduring and ubiquitous, dissociation can sometimes lead to different aspects of the child and the child's memories being reconstructed as separate voices, visions or different parts of the self within the same abused person (Longden, 2017). Dissociative coping strategies, coupled with active attempts not to notice, think and talk about abuse (augmented by distraction), can result in patchy and fragmented memories of abuse thereafter. It is rare for children to be completely successful in repressing *all* traumatic memories (American Psychological Association, 2019). This is why the idea that completely lost memories of abuse can be recovered in therapy was challenged (Loftus, 1993).

Abuse survivors are commonly plagued by their traumatic memories, and this can result in post-traumatic stress effects. These include intrusive and reoccurring thoughts and flashbacks, night terrors, reduced concentration, high anxiety, panic attacks, hyperarousal, avoidance of trauma triggers, hypervigilance and reduced trust in others (Christie, 2018). Dementia can further exacerbate stress responses to memories of childhood sexual abuse as the separation between past and present breaks down (Martinez-Clavera, James, Bowditch, & Kuruvilla, 2017). Survivors across the lifespan may come to rely on externalized forms of distraction and dissociation to help them cope with their hyper-emotional arousal and, conversely, hypo-emotional arousal or numbness.

Specific strategies include self-injury (which is more likely to occur when the body has already been invalidated through experiences such as abuse), alcohol and drugs (often also promoted by abusers as an additional means of control), and food (restricting intake, over-eating and/or purging). Self-harm, in all these forms, is associated with reoccurring themes of powerlessness, exclusion and identity stigmatization, and hence child sexual abuse (Warner & Shaw, 2016).

Coping strategies such as these can add additional layers of marginalization, as girls and women may be pejoratively described as self-harmers, addicts or anorexics, and/or fat-shamed when judged to be overweight. Embedded distraction and dissociation may also attract labels such as ADHD, schizophrenia and personality disorder (see Warner, 2009). Whilst some women and girls find relief in receiving a psychiatric label because it serves to validate their distress, for many others it adds to their feelings of self-loathing and low self-esteem (Shaw & Shaw, 2007). In addition, it can be argued that the medicalization of socially located mental distress can lead to a false hope that there is a chemical cure for the after-effects of sexual abuse. At best, like self-harm, psychiatric drugs can help to suppress feelings and thoughts or, conversely, to increase alertness and energy. This can help girls and women cope with overwhelming feelings, numbness, and/or visons, voices and flashbacks (Moncrieff, 2013). It should be noted that prescription drugs work in the same way as street drugs. Both can be toxic and both can be used to control victims and to supress girls' and women's rightful anger at, and ability to resist, abuse. What is needed is a more socially aware understanding of the tactics and effects of child sexual abuse and the strategies girls and women use to cope with these.

Working with the impact of child sexual abuse

Therapy and assessment

Feminist therapy aims to empower clients by supporting them to challenge the tactics of abuse that impact how girls and women view themselves. A key aspect of this approach is in the deliberate use of language to subvert normalized notions of girls' and women's passivity by validating clients' strength as survivors and refusing the idea that they are only and forever victims (e.g., Brown, 1994). Further, feminist therapy often encourages clients to reassert their power by becoming activists on the issues that brought them to therapy and/or to find support and common cause by joining survivor-activist groups. At an individual level, girls and women can be enabled to work out how their sense of self has been constrained through abusive relationships and how this can impact their sexual and reproductive health and decision making (McCloskey, 2016). Hence, girls' and women's unresolved abuse-trauma is addressed through talking about the context to abuse, rather than maintaining a retraumatizing focus on the physical acts of abuse (which is more relevant in criminal investigations). Abuse-effects are understood to relate to the particular (psychological, social and physical) tactics of control utilized by the abuser, within their specific cultural context. This type of approach informs specialist sexual exploitation services that explicitly aim to help girls reframe their understandings about themselves and their relationships by, for example, addressing how grooming works (Warner, 2019). Schema therapy can also help women to learn how to change schemas associated with negative experiences such as abuse (Young & Klosko, 1993).

A feminist understanding of interactional power encourages professionals to consider how professional relationships can mirror earlier grooming/relationship experiences and to ward against this (Warner, 2009). Clients should not be positioned as passive recipients of expert knowledge, as this reinforces victimhood. Conversely, professionals who deny their experience and expertise in understanding child sexual abuse act like abusers who trick and manipulate. As such, it is important that professionals are explicit about the frameworks they use to make sense of sexual abuse, rather than presenting perspective as truth (Warner, 2009). This kind of approach can inform therapy and court assessments. Court reports that deliberately contextualize knowledge provide a form of theory/values-based evidence or what has also been termed 'social framework evidence' (e.g., Raitt & Zeedyk, 2000). This, then, is about making all knowledge forms and claims visible and open to exploration and elaboration.

There are multiple ways relationship meanings can be explored, including in respect of the past, present and/or hopes for the future; in dreams; and/or the voices, visions, dissociation and dissociated parts victims sometimes experience. All of these symbolic spaces can be used to make sense of how power is transacted, used and resisted, and how abuser-realities are maintained post-abuse and shaped through subsequent experiences. This type of approach requires dissociative phenomena to be accepted as meaningful, not simply a symptom of psychiatric disorder. For example, voices and visions, or different dissociated parts of the self, can become stronger and more compelling at times of stress (Longden, 2017). Women can be encouraged not to take voices literally (e.g., the imperative to hurt oneself or others), but rather to explore what this might symbolize for them. Even negative voices, or negative parts of the self, can act as 'early warning systems' that enable unconscious or uncomfortable thoughts and feelings to be spoken aloud and addressed (Warner, 2009). The aim should not be to provide a fixed or authoritative reading of women's visions, voices and sometimes unusual beliefs, but to help them find meaning in them rather than fear them and to recognize that they may be trauma-based, but they are also indicative of the capacity and strength to survive.

The meanings of self-harm also need exploring so that girls and women are enabled to achieve a greater sense of control over their self-harm. Approaches that do not take harm-stopping as their primary aim are referred to as harm-minimization or harm-reduction approaches. As Pembroke, 2006, p. 166) argued, 'harm-minimisation is about accepting the need to self-harm as a valid method of survival until survival is possible by other means'. Personal meanings of self-harm are not static, but can change and be mediated by triggers and amplifications in the present, such as key dates associated with sexual abuse or further experiences of being controlled (Warner & Shaw, 2017). This is why restricting opportunities to self-harm can paradoxically increase risk. For example, at times of heightened suicidality, direct physical methods are often used to restrict girls' and woman's access to methods of self-harm and their opportunities to use them. Anything that may be used to cause harm to the body (e.g., CDs, knives, tablets, belts) may be removed. Conversely, the person may be encouraged or even forced to take increased medication (e.g., when detained under Mental Health Acts). Such measures may be necessary to keep the girl or woman alive, but they have very many negative consequences, such as re-invoking feelings of being controlled, hurt, violated, scared and angry (Warner & Shaw, 2017).

Psychological methods that are designed to stop suicide may be experienced more positively. Such methods are designed to build *pause* between the desire to end life and the suicidal act. In the short term, 'psychological barriers' can help. This may simply involve saying, 'Can we talk first?' Over the longer term, services can develop *advance agreements* with service users that can help professionals identify when the person is starting to become hopeless, what triggers are around, and what helps and hinders in such circumstances. In this way girls and women can be enabled to take their thinking into their most out-of-control moments. Sometimes girls and women feel so out of control of their coping strategies that they themselves seek out harm-cessation services, such as Alcohol and Narcotics Anonymous (e.g., alcoholics-anonymous.org.uk). Girls' and women's choices should be understood in context and, as far as possible, be supported; service-controlled harm-stopping approaches should be proportionate and time limited (Warner & Shaw, 2017; Warner & Spandler, 2012).

Girls and women may, then, be traumatized not just by their experiences of sexual abuse, but by service responses to them. This has led to a rediscovered interest in providing trauma-informed care. Current approaches are largely informed by Felitti et al. (1998), whose research shows that adverse childhood experiences (known as ACEs) can have long-term negative effects and that biological and neurological mechanisms are impacted by trauma (Christie, 2018). The idea that abuse-trauma only becomes 'real' when given the gloss of a neuro-makeover is problematic. Abused girls and women do not come to therapy to 'get their neurons firing', but to feel safe, find hope, make better relationships and recover. Additionally, ACEs can be misunderstood as providing a predictive diagnosis. This type of understanding can serve to underestimate women's capacities for survival, adaptation and change. Perhaps the key benefit of trauma-informed services is that there is a presumption of the need to ask 'what has happened to you?' rather than simply to diagnose mental disorder. However, when psychiatric diagnosis remains the key to accessing treatment services, then trauma concerns remain tokenistic: services may be trauma-informed, but they are not trauma-led.

Support, investigation and prosecution

Different service approaches can, therefore, act to re-traumatize women. Re-traumatization is also engendered when support is not integrated and survivors must navigate multiple services, repeating their statement to each agency they encounter (UK Children's Commissioner, 2017). The need to provide seamless services for girls and women underpins the development of dedicated Sexual Assault Referral Centres (SARCs) in the UK and other countries. The aim of SARCs is to provide an integrated service regarding support and the criminal justice system. This work is supported by independent sexual violence advisers (ISVAs), who help victims to gain access to other services and provide support through the criminal justice system if required, including supporting the person through the trial. This model has been extended to include children and family safe houses, following the Icelandic Barnahus model (see UK Children's Commissioner, 2017), which provide sexually abused children and their families with safe houses in which they can stay whilst accessing medical, investigative and emotional support under the same one roof. At the same time, police forces in the UK are being more creative in pursuing sex offenders. For example, some UK police forces now follow a policy of 'interference and disruption' in the wider activities of child sexual exploiters, leafletting hotels and taxi firms, and encouraging community responsibility (Spicer, 2018). Additionally, Royal Commissions on institutionalized child sexual abuse in Australia and the UK (Child Abuse Royal Commission, 2019; Independent Inquiry Child Sexual Abuse, 2019), which have exposed abuse in churches, schools and other community contexts, has once again focussed public attention on the institutionally located vulnerability of many children, but has also increased opportunities for institutional abuse survivors to speak out and be believed.

Conclusion

Child sexual abuse is an embedded social practice that can have devastating effects on girls' and women's sexual and reproductive health, mental health and well-being, and socio-economic potential. It is a gender-based crime, a violation of human rights, and a crime against humanity. There are intersections across countries in sexual exploitation, modern slavery, trafficking, sex tourism, and the growing impact of the internet in facilitating sexual abuse on an industrial scale. This is why if *all* victims of sexual abuse are to be helped, then it is crucial to develop treaties, laws, policies, and frameworks for support and investigation at international, national, and local levels (Warner, 2016b). Work on child sexual abuse is ever-evolving as new forms of knowledge-action come to prevail. A commitment to prevention should inform all work on child sexual abuse and, as generations of feminists and others have argued, a sexually violent world should not be accepted as inevitable.

Like Shaw (2012), I do not believe in silence. It is crucial to continue to voice concerns about child sexual abuse and to reflect on how language impacts our ability to recognize and resist abuse. This approach has been adopted by fourth-wave feminists, who have returned to an embodied identity-based feminism, to use the internet to 'call-out' and raise concerns about sexual violence. Whether on-line or off-line, in terms of professional practices or in community spaces, in peace or in conflict situations, we all need to challenge child sexual abuse and to keep fighting for a better, fairer, more inclusive world. Only then will human wrongs be transformed into human rights.

References

Althusser, L. (1971). *Lenin and philosophy and other essays*. London, UK: New Left Books.

American College of Obstetrics and Gynecology (ACOG) (2017). *Committee opinion number 498: Adult manifestations of child sexual abuse*. Washington, DC: Author. Retrieved from www.acog.org/Clinical-Guidance-and-Publications/Committee-Opinions/Committee-on-Health-Care-for-Underserved-Women/Adult-Manifestations-of-Childhood-Sexual-Abuse.

American Psychological Association (2019). *Memories of childhood abuse*. Washington, DC: Author. Retrieved from www.apa.org/topics/trauma/memories.

Australian Institute of Criminology (2008). *Online child grooming laws*. High tech crime brief No. 17. Canberra, Australia: Author. Retrieved from https://aic.gov.au/publications/htcb/htcb017.

Bass, E. & Davies, L. (1988). *The courage to heal: A guide for women survivors of child sexual abuse*. London, UK: Cedar.

Bindel, J. (2017, May 16). I wrote the first ever piece about the grooming gangs in northern English towns in 2006, but the media didn't want to know. *Independent*. Retrieved from www.independent.co.uk/voices/three-girls-drama-child-sexual-exploitation-rochdale-blackpool-pimping-a7739006.html.

Bindell, J. (2013, August 13). Rape: A burning injustice. *Guardian*. Retrieved from www.theguardian.com%2flifeandstyle%2f2013%2faug%2f13%2frape-defined-sexual-crime-history&type=article&internalpagecode=1949815.

Bingham, A., Delap, L., Jackson, L., & Settle, L. (2016). Historical child sexual abuse in England and Wales: The role of historians. *History of Education*, *45*(4), 411–429, doi:10.1080/0046760X.2016.1177122.

British Government (1925). Report of the departmental committee on sexual offences against young persons, Command Paper (fourth series, 1918–56), 2561, 67.

Brown, L. S. (1994). *Subversive dialogues: Theory in feminist therapy*. New York, NY: Basic Books.

Butler, J. (1990). *Gender trouble: Feminism and the subversion of identity*. London, UK: Routledge.

Campbell, B. (1988). *Unofficial secrets: Child sexual abuse, the Cleveland case*. London, UK: Virago Press Ltd.

Children's Commissioner (2017). *Barnahus: Improving the response to child sexual abuse in England*. London, UK: Author.

Christie, C. (2018, May). *A trauma-informed health and care approach for responding to child sexual abuse and exploitation current knowledge report*. London, UK: Crown copyright. Retrieved from https://assets.publishing.service.gov.uk/government/uploads/system/uploads/attachment_data/file/712725/trauma-informed-health-and-care-approach-report.pdf.

Crenshaw, K. (1993). Mapping the margins: Intersectionality, identity politics and violence against women of color. *Stanford Law Review*, *43*, 1241–1299.

Crews, F. (1995). *The memory wars: Freud's legacy in dispute*. New York, NY: The New York Review of Books.

Davies, E., O'Leary, E., & Read, J. (2015). Child abuse in England and Wales 2003–2013: Newspaper reporting versus reality. *Journalism*, *18*(6), 754–771, doi:10.1136/emermed-2015-205285.

Felitti, V. J., Anda, R. F., Nordenberg, D., Williamson, D. F., Spitz, A. M., Edwards, V., Koss. P., & Marks, J. S. (1998). Relationship of childhood abuse and household dysfunction to many of the leading causes of death in adults. *American Journal of Preventive Medicine, 14*(4), 245–258.

Fiorenza, E. S. (2001). *Wisdom ways: Introducing feminist biblical interpretation.* New York, NY: Orbis.

Foucault, M. (1978). *The history of sexuality, volume one: An introduction.* Harmondsworth, UK: Penguin.

Freedman, E. B. (2013). *Redefining rape: Sexual violence in the era of suffrage and segregation.* Cambridge, MA: Harvard University Press.

Greijer, S. & Doek, J. (2016, January 28). *Terminology guidelines for the protection of children from sexual exploitation and sexual abuse.* Bangkok, Thailand: ECPAT International & ECPAT Luxembourg. Retrieved from www.icmec.org/wp-content/uploads/2016/10/Terminology-guidelines_EN.pdf.

Independent Inquiry Child Sexual Abuse (2019). London, UK: Author. Retrieved from www .iicsa.org.uk.

Irish, L., Kobayashi, I., & Delahanty, D. L. (2010). Long-term physical health consequences of childhood sexual abuse: A meta-analytic review. *Journal of Pediatric Psychology, 35*(5), 450–461, doi:10.1093/ jpepsy/jsp118.

Kohlberg, L. A. (1966). A cognitive-developmental analysis of children's sex role concepts and attitudes. In E. Maccoby (Ed.), *The development of sex differences* (pp. 82–173). Stanford, CA: Stanford University Press.

Kossoff, J. (1999, February 7). Prostitute dies of drug overdose –at 13. *Independent.* Retrieved from www .independent.co.uk/news/prostitute-dies-of-overdose-at-13-1069223.html.

Loftus, E. F. (1993). The reality of repressed memories. *American Psychologist, 48,* 518–537.

Longden, E. (2017). Listening to the voices people hear: Auditory hallucinations beyond a diagnostic framework. *Journal of Humanistic Psychology, 57*(6), 573.

López, S., Faro, C., Lopetegui, L., Pujol-Ribera, E., Monteagudo, M., Avecilla-Palau, A., Martínez, C., Cobo, J., & Fernández, M.-I. (2017). Child and adolescent sexual abuse in women seeking help for sexual and reproductive mental health problems: Prevalence, characteristics, and disclosure. *Journal of Child Sexual Abuse, 26*(3), 246–269, doi:10.1080/10538712.2017.1288186.

Martinez-Clavera, C., James, S., Bowditch, E., & Kuruvilla, T. (2017). Delayed-onset post-traumatic stress disorder symptoms in dementia. *Progress in Neurology and Psychiatry, 21*(3), 26–31.

McCloskey, L. A. (2016). The effects of gender-based violence on women's unwanted pregnancy and abortion. *The Yale Journal of Biology and Medicine, 89*(2), 153–159.

Mills, H., Majeed-Ariss, R., & White, C. (2018). *Prevalence of anal injuries in clients attending Saint Mary's sexual assault referral centre following an allegation of anal penetration.* Manchester, UK: St. Mary's Sexual Assault Referral Centre's 16th Annual Conference, doi:10.13140/RG.2.2.19302.32321.

Ministry of Justice (2017). Sexual communication with a child: Implementation of section 67 of the Serious Crime Act 2015. London, UK: Author. Retrieved from https://assets.publishing.service.gov.uk /government/uploads/system/uploads/attachment_data/file/604931/circular-commencement-s67- serious-crime-act-2015.pdf.

Moncrieff, J. (2013). *The bitterest pills: The troubling story of antipsychotic drugs.* Basingstoke, UK: Palgrave Macmillan.

Mothers living apart from their children (2014). *In our hearts: Stories and wisdom of mothers living apart from their children.* Kirklees and Calderdale, UK: WomensCentre.

National Society for the Prevention of Cruelty to Children (NSPCC) (2019). *Sexual abuse: What is sexual abuse.* London, UK: NSPCC [website]. Retrieved from www.nspcc.org.uk/preventing-abuse/child- abuse-and-neglect/child-sexual-abuse.

Nelson, S. (2016). *Tackling child sexual abuse: Radical approaches to prevention, protection and support.* Bristol, UK: Policy Press.

New York Academy of Medicine (2019). *Grey literature report.* New York, NY: Author. Retrieved from www.greylit.org.

Office for National Statistics (ONS) (2018, November 22). *Domestic abuse: Findings from the crime survey for England and Wales: Year ending March 2018.* London, UK: Author. Retrieved from www.ons.gov.uk /peoplepopulationandcommunity/crimeandjustice/articles/domesticabusefindingsfromthecrimesurvey forenglandandwales/yearendingmarch2018#toc.

Pembroke, L. R. (2006). Harm minimisation: Limiting the damage of self-injury. In H. Spandler & S. Warner (Eds), *Beyond fear and control: Working with young people who self-harm* (pp. 163–171). Ross-on -Wye, UK: PCCS Books.

Radford, L., Allnock, D., & Hynes, P. (2018, August 31). *Preventing and responding to child sexual abuse and exploitation: Evidence review*. New York, NY: UNICEF. Retrieved from www.unicef.org/protection/files/Evidence_Review_SEA_(Radford_et_al)(final).pdf.

Raitt, F. E. & Zeedyk, S. (2000). *The implicit relation of psychology and the law: Women and syndrome evidence*. London, UK: Routledge.

Ramazanoglu, C. & Holland, J. (1999). Tripping over experience: Some problems in feminist epistemology. *Discourse: Studies in the Cultural Politics of Education, 20*(3), 381–392.

Royal Commission into Institutional Responses to Child Sexual Abuse (2019). Royal Commission into Institutional Responses to Child Sexual Abuse. Retrieved from www.childabuseroyalcommission.gov.au.

Shaw, C. (2012). I do not believe in silence. *Head on*. Henley, UK: Bloodaxe Books.

Shaw, C. & Shaw, T. (2007). A dialogue of hope and survival. In H. Spandler & S. Warner (Eds), *Beyond fear and control: Working with young people who self-harm* (pp. 25–36). Ross-on-Wye, UK: PCCS Books.

Simon-Butler, A. & McSherry, B. (2019). *Defining sexual and gender-based violence in the refugee context: IRiS working paper series*, 28. Birmingham, UK: The University of Birmingham/Institute for Research into Superdiversity. Retrieved from www.birmingham.ac.uk/Documents/college-social-sciences/social-policy/iris/2019/iris-working-papers-28-2019.pdf.

Spataro, J., Mullen, P. E., Burgess, P. M., & Wells, D. L. (2004). Impact of child sexual abuse on mental health: Prospective study in males and females. *British Journal of Psychiatry, 184*(5), 416–421, doi:10.1192/bjp.184.5.416.

Spicer, D. (2018, March). *Joint serious case review concerning sexual exploitation of children and adults with needs for care and support in Newcastle-upon-Tyne*. Newcastle-upon-Tyne, UK: Newcastle Safeguarding Children Board and Newcastle Safeguarding Adults Board. Retrieved from www.newcastle.gov.uk/sites/default/files/wwwfileroot/final_jscr_report_160218_pw.pdf.

Topping, A. (2015, January 6). End use of outdated term 'child prostitution', says MP. *Guardian*. Retrieved from www.theguardian.com/society/2015/jan/06/child-prostitution-term-outdated-mp-ann-coffey.

United Nations (UN) (2019a). *Preventing sexual exploitation and abuse*. New York, NY: Author. Retrieved from www.un.org/preventing-sexual-exploitation-and-abuse/content/prevention.

United Nations (UN) (2019b, March 29). *Conflict related sexual violence: Report of the United Nations Secretary-General*. New York, NY: Author. Retrieved from www.un.org/sexualviolenceinconflict/wp-content/uploads/2019/04/report/s-2019-280/Annual-report-2018.pdf.

United Nations Children's Fund (UNICEF) (2017a). *A familiar face: Violence in the lives of children and adolescents*. New York, NY: Author. Retrieved from www.unicef.org/publications/files/Violence_in_the_lives_of_children_and_adolescents.pdf.

United Nations Children's Fund (UNICEF) (2017b, February). *A deadly journey for children the central Mediterranean migration route*. New York, NY: Author. Retrieved from www.unicef.org/publications/index_94905.html.

US Legal, Inc. (2019). *Child grooming law and legal definition*. Definitions.uslegal.com. USLegal, Inc. [website]. Retrieved from https://definitions.uslegal.com/c/child-grooming.

Van Meeuwen, A., Sara Swann, S., McNeish, D., & Edwards, S. S. M. (1998). *Whose daughter next? Children abused through prostitution*. London, UK: Barnardos.

Walding, J. (2016). *Our stories: Lizzie's story of experiencing abuse*. Manchester, UK: LGBT Foundation.

Warner, S. (2000). *Understanding child sexual abuse: Making the tactics visible*. Gloucester, UK: Handsell Publishing.

Warner, S. (2009). Understanding the effects of child sexual abuse: Feminist revolutions in theory, research and practice. London, UK: Routledge.

Warner, S. (2016a). Structuralism, feminist approaches and feminist critique. In N. Naples, R. C. Hoogland, M. Wickramasinghe, & W. C. A. Wong (Eds), *The Wiley Blackwell encyclopedia of gender and sexuality studies* (doi: 10.1002/9781118663219.wbegss642). London, UK: Wiley-Blackwells.

Warner, S. (2016b). Child sexual abuse and trauma. In N. Naples, R. C. Hoogland, M. Wickramasinghe, & W. C. A. Wong (Eds), *The Wiley Blackwell encyclopedia of gender and sexuality studies* (doi: 10.1002/9781118663219.wbegss454). London, UK: Wiley-Blackwells.

Warner, S. (2019). *Child sexual exploitation placements: Clinical service statement of purpose [unpublished]*. London, UK: Cambian Group.

Warner, S. & Shaw, C. (2016). Working with looked after children who self-harm: Understanding coping, communication and suicide. In J. Guisharde-Pine, G. Coleman-Oluwabusola, & S. McCall (Eds.), *Supporting the mental health needs of children in care: Evidence for practice* (pp. 40–52). London, UK: Jessica Kingsley Publishers.

Warner, S. & Shaw, C. (2017). Working with looked after children who self-harm: understanding coping, communication and suicide. *Annual Review of Critical Psychology, 13*, 1–12.

Warner, S. & Spandler, H. (2012). New strategies for practice based evidence: A focus on self–harm. *Journal of Qualitative Research in Psychology, 9*(1), 13–26.

World Health Organization (WHO) (2006). *Preventing child maltreatment: A guide to taking action and generating evidence*. Geneva, Switzerland: Author. Retrieved from https://apps.who.int/iris/bitstream/handle/10665/43499/9241594365_eng.pdf;sequence=1.

World Health Organization (WHO) (2012). *Understanding and addressing violence against women: Health consequences*. Geneva, Switzerland: WHO Publications. Retrieved from https://apps.who.int/iris/bitstream/handle/10665/77431/WHO_RHR_12.43_eng.pdf;sequence=1.

Young, J. E. & Klosko, J. S. (1993). *Reinventing your life: The breakthrough program to end negative behavior and feel great again*. New York, NY: Plume.

33

FEMALE GENITAL MUTILATION AND GENITAL SURGERIES

Hilary Burrage

'The practise of FGM is struggling to remain relevant', reported the lawyer Christine Nan-jala-Ndenga (2016), 'and as a result it keeps on changing every single day'. Ms. Nanjala-Ndenga is well placed to make this observation, given her experience in Kenya as a lead officer in the female genital mutilation (FGM) prosecution unit in the Office of the Director of Public Prosecutions. Like many others around the world, she started her career with little idea that the eradication of FGM would become the focus of her work, but also like many others, her commitment to ending this cruel, entrenched, human rights abuse has become compelling.

Despite valiant efforts there is little evidence of significant reduction of rates of FGM globally. Estimates suggest that around 200 million women and girls alive today have under-gone some form of 'cutting', and around three million more experience FGM every year. FGM occurs everywhere across the globe. In both the USA (Milken Institute School of Public Health, 2017) and Europe (Access to European Law (Eur-LEX), 2013) half a million girls and women are thought to have experienced, or to be at serious risk of, mutilation. FGM is found in parts of Asia and South America as well as in the usually acknowledged nations of Africa and the Middle East (Burrage, 2015; World Health Organisation, 2018). In some countries local programmes to stop FGM have been successful, as rates have dropped significantly (Koski & Heymann, 2017), but overall the numbers of girls and young women who experience FGM continue to rise (UNICEF, 2016).

The stark truth is that in the 21st century we continue to face an epidemic of both child and gendered abuse, of which FGM is one of the most prevalent and appalling elem-ents. FGM stretches back millennia. It is a vestige of authoritarian patriarchy (Makama, 2013), as are many other forms of harmful traditional practice (HTPs) (International Planned Parenthood Federation, 2013). In many traditional communities FGM is an unquestionable imperative; as Nanjala-Ndenga (2016) said above, it morphs to suit local conditions and evade detection. Formal notions of individual human rights and child pro-tection have little or no impact in often-isolated communities that have conducted busi-ness unchanged for hundreds of years. Traditions define groups and can be absolute, and absolute authoritarianism is just as true for some tight-knit communities (usually diaspora groups) in Western countries as it is for various heritage-defined groups in the 'develop-ing' nations (de Vos, 2013).

In this chapter I explore how female genital mutilation fits in the context of a world where almost all informed opinion now perceives it as a harmful tradition to be consigned to history as soon as possible, yet it continues to have powerful sway in many places around the globe.

What is female genital mutilation?

Female genital mutilation comprises cutting or otherwise harming female genitalia (sexual organs) in the absence of medical necessity. It has no positive outcomes except, in practicing communities, as a marker of virtue, 'purity', marriageability or group identity. It may cause significant long-term physical and/or psychological damage to women, or even result in death. For example, it has been suggested that in parts of Somalia where there are no anti-biotics as many as 1 in 3 girls who undergo FGM die of the practice (Nordqvist, 2017). Many countries have now made FGM formally illegal, whether by explicit legislation or, as in the case of France, in the context of the prohibition of bodily harm (Burrage, 2015).

The World Health Organization (2007a) defined four main types of FGM:

1 *Clitoridectomy* – damage to, or removal of, some part of the clitoris, the female erectile sex organ. Contrary to common belief, total removal of the clitoris is effectively impossible, as only the small front 'button' is visible, but the entire organ extends backwards in a wishbone shape around the vagina (O'Connell, Sanjeevan, & Hutson, 2005). Similarly, sometimes 'only' the prepuce (visible skin fold) is removed in a 'minimal' practice – which some communities insist is not FGM at all – known as sunna, khafz, or khafna (Abrol, 2018). But realistically 'minimal' removal is almost impossible, given the very modest skills of most operators and the likely erratic physical movements of the victim (Horowitz & Jackson, 1997).

2 *Excision* – partial removal by whatever means (even sharp objects such as nails, stones or snail shells) of the clitoris and of the labia minora, plus sometimes also of the labia majora.

3 *Infibulation* – securing the outer labia (e.g., with pins, thorns, thread) (Rashid & Rashid, 2007), usually after excision, to leave only a small hole for urine, menstrual blood, and other body fluids. The hole may not align with internal anatomy, thereby causing enduring blockages, infection and pain; it is often sealed by tying the legs together until the wound heals to whatever extent it can.

4 *Other* – piercing, scraping, burning, pricking, labia pulling, or otherwise damaging the female genitalia. This category has given rise to much heated debate because it includes and overlaps with Western-style piercing, to which little attention has been paid by enforcement authorities. The debate about whether adult female genital cosmetic surgery (FCGS) constitutes FGM remains in some minds unresolved (Magon & Alinsod, 2017) but, as discussed below, in general legal advice has been to proceed very cautiously.

Not everyone however is convinced that the formal categorisation of types of FGM are needed. As Dr. Morissanda Kouyate (2016), Director of the Inter-African Committee on Harmful Traditional Practices (which focusses especially on FGM), said (Kouyate, 2016), all types of 'cutting' are mutilation (Burrage, 2013).

The history of FGM goes back as far as ancient Egypt, when first princesses and later also female slaves were infibulated to ensure that they became pregnant only when their husbands or owners wanted this to happen. FGM has also been associated in various societies across history with notions of coming of age, purity and sexuality (though never named as such), as well as notions of dominance/subjugation. FGM also increases (or simply makes possible) the economic 'value' that can be secured when a daughter is sold in marriage (Burrage, 2015).

FGM is practiced in groups that link it to various formal religions including Islamic, Christian, animist, and other communities (Drum, 2017). It has as its rationale everything from the belief that the clitoris is a lethal organ, which, if left unattended, will grow enormously and kill any man or new-born whom it touches, or that a girl will not be female, or cannot be an adult, unless it is removed, or that hygiene and child-birth are improved by clitoridectomy (New Zealand FGM Education Programme, 2019). Mackie (1996) referred to these terrifying claims that no-one dare test as 'belief traps' (p. 101). Whilst such beliefs are more common in Islamic communities, there is no validated reference in Islamic scripture to a requirement for FGM (Asmani & Abdi, 2008).

What are the outcomes of FGM for girls and women?

The consequences for every aspect of the woman's life may be very serious. The specifics of the damage are reported in many professional publications (World Health Organization, 2018) and summarised below. It is self-evident that the harm of FGM produces many clinical challenges.

Impacts on physical and psychological health

In the immediate term, FGM is often imposed by brute force, often without pain relief and in (frequently extremely) unsterile conditions, sometimes with crude utensils used to cut numbers of girls at one time. Inevitably severe pain, shock and the risk of infection, tetanus or even death (Norwegian Institute of Public Health, 2014) are amongst the consequences of this assault. The harm inflicted may be amplified if girls struggle as FGM is undertaken. In the long term, FGM may result in chronic infection, anaemia, anal and/or urinary incontinence, chronic pain, cheloids and scarring (fibrosis) (Hearst & Molnar, 2013) caused by FGM wounds, haematocolpos (internal accumulation of menstrual blood), hepatitis, genital hypersensitivity and/or tissue rotation (e.g., birth passage adheres to the pelvis, with significant risks to both mother and child) (Reisel & Creighton, 2015). Recto-vaginal/obstetric fistulae, in which tearing results in permanent leakage of urine and/or faeces via the FGM orifice, is a devastating outcome of giving birth for some women, especially when labour is extended due to the young age of the mother or other FGM-related obstruction of the birth canal (Vaughan, 2017).

Sexual problems that result from FGM may include pain (dyspareunia) or other issues with sexual intercourse (including lack of desire/arousal) (Biglu, Farnam, Abotalebi, Biglu, & Ghavami, 2016), vaginal dryness, greater risk of HIV (due to unhealed wounds), morbidity due to anal intercourse, and both primary infertility (due to damage to reproductive organs) and secondary infertility (due to lack of access for intercourse). FGM can also impact on sexual relationships; broken marriages may occur if husbands resort to 'uncut' prostitutes, or if the woman cannot respond sexually and her husband finds solace elsewhere (Ismail et al., 2017). Fistulae may result in social ostracism for the woman. In recent years some surgeons have developed techniques to reconstruct the clitoris, in the hope that this may enhance the enjoyment of sex. As discussed below, much work to evaluate these complex issues remains to be done (Sigurjonsson & Jordal, 2018), but there are some reports of successful outcomes (Abdulcadir, Rodriguez, Petignat, & Say, 2015).

The nature of imposition of FGM – often unanticipated by the victim and imposed forcefully by people she has trusted to care for her – can trigger anger, anxiety/fear, flash-backs, depression, emotional insecurity and distance, hyper-vigilance and sleep disorders (Daughters of Eve, n.d.). Vulnerability, low self-esteem, lack of trust and problems with relationships may occur, as may phobias, stigma, a sense of helplessness and post-traumatic stress disorder (PTSD) (Behrendt & Moritz, 2005). Individual therapy may offer valuable support to women familiar with Western psychological treatments, if not for others in trad-itional settings, but wider questions concerning the impacts, generation after generation, of FGM on the mental health of whole communities of women remain to be addressed (Glover, Liebling, Barrett, & Goodman, 2017).

Asylum seekers with or at risk of FGM are often poorly served (University of Oxford Refugee Study Centre, 2015), and women from the diaspora are unlikely to mention FGM when they first encounter the asylum gatekeepers. Thereafter, if such women share their concerns (perhaps fears for their daughters' safety), they may be disbelieved, or officials may claim that FGM is not a hazard in the region of origin. Distress, deportation and enforced exposure to risk is the not infrequent outcome (Burrage, 2014b).

Obstetric impacts for mother and child

Female genital mutilation has adverse impact on obstetric outcomes – perhaps one or two additional maternal deaths per 100 women (World Health Organization, 2006). It requires specific care throughout pregnancy (Balogun, Hirayama, Wariki, Koyanagi, & Mori, 2013). Pelvic examination (including non-pregnant health checks) may be difficult or impossible prior to de-infibulation, and there is increased need for episiotomy and caesarean delivery (where these services are available) (Rodriguez, Seuc, Say, & Hindin, 2016). The second stage of labour may be extended and result in haemorrhage and risk of torn uterus, perineal damage and sepsis. Repeated pregnancies after pregnancy loss may occur, with a higher risk overall of premature maternal death and high infant mortality (World Health Organization, 2006); all the impacts are tragedies for surviving family members.

Given the obstructions of the birth canal that FGM can cause, the likelihoods of stillbirth, neonatal distress or mortality, and need for resuscitation, are increased by FGM. One report showed that over 20% of perinatal deaths in infants born to women with FGM can be attributed to the FGM (Eke & Nkanginieme, 2006). Failure to thrive and serious long-term incapacity are also significant risks for the child, as is post-partum or later death of the mother, which places the infant at subsequent high risk (Atrash, 2011).

There is still, however, much to learn about the obstetric impact of FGM. One large-scale study in African countries by WHO demonstrated that FGM does have adverse obstetric out-comes (Rymer, 2006), but further investigation showed that, in a Western metropolitan con-text, this disadvantage can be mitigated (Varol et al., 2016). Other researchers have explored the particular context of migrant women who frequently encounter negative attitudes when accessing the maternity services in their host countries (Scamell & Ghumman, 2019). Also studied have been the perspectives of both those with FGM who seek healthcare and those who provide that care in high-income countries (Evans et al., 2017).

Socio-economic outcomes

Negative socio-economic impacts of FGM occur at all levels, from the individual girl or woman, to the family and community, and ultimately to the nation state itself (Burrage,

2016b; Mpinga et al., 2016). There is much still to learn about such impacts, but there is little doubt that the chronic physical and mental ill-health that results from FGM can put a life-strain on women's social and economic functioning. Equally, girls who fail to undergo FGM may be deemed unmarriageable, unable to attain adult status, and thereby not permitted to own land or other resources, and girls who do have FGM may receive little further education (another hindrance to social outcomes). Further, child 'brides', perhaps as young as ten years old, are told they are now 'women' with the personal autonomy in some areas that goes with that status – and which inevitably a child cannot handle well. Women who are unable to 'enjoy' sex with their husbands or who are incontinent or have fistulae may be discarded and destitute (Ernest, Howard-Merill, Norman, & Otoo-Otortey, 2014). Women with chronic anaemia or other ill-health find it difficult to support and care for their families. They may even in desperation turn to prostitution – a tragic irony given that FGM is believed by some to stop promiscuity.

When mothers are incapacitated (or dead) their children are at severe risk, which also impacts at every social level. At the national level, entirely avoidable premature morbidity and mortality is a heavy burden on any country's resources, legislature and socio-political infrastructure.

Medicalisation of FGM: how clinicians have become 'cutters'

Not all clinicians see FGM as an act of harm. In some countries, such as Egypt, Kenya and parts of southeast Asia, medicalised FGM is increasingly the norm, performed by clinicians who maintain they remove risks associated with a traditional practitioner or see opportunities to amplify their income (Doucet, Pallitto, & Groleau, 2017). Neonatal services may include regular maternal and infant care alongside procedures such as ear-piercing, vaccination and genital mutilation (Watch Indonesia, 2014).

The World Health Organization (2010) and others are clear that the medicalisation of FGM is a matter of very serious concern. Whilst medicalised FGM is generally conducted with asepsis and anaesthetics, it also provides an aura of normality and acceptability to this harmful practice – evident in the symbolic 'just a prick or tiny cut' idea promoted by some US physicians (Kimani & Shell-Duncan, 2018). This medicalised normalisation is strongly resisted by most EndFGM activists, who say it may be interpreted by FGM traditionalists as validation of the notion that FGM is necessary or even beneficial (Serour, 2013). Thus, weighty legal questions and ethical issues apart, the widely held consensus is that medicalisation is now perhaps the greatest obstacle to FGM eradication (Batha, 2017).

The condemnation of the medicalisation of FGM is not a straightforward matter. Whilst it is obvious that any unnecessary 'surgery' is unacceptable, the issue becomes complicated when modern Western clinical procedures, such as female cosmetic genital surgery (FGCS) and intersex gender reassignment, particularly in infants and children, are considered. The accusation can be made that there is a double standard (Northern Ireland Human Rights Commission, 2016): FGM done by minority ethnic people is 'wrong', but FGCS provided by White clinicians – or, in any circumstance, male circumcision – is acceptable (Shahvisi & Earp, 2018).

Female genital cosmetic surgery

Female genital cosmetic surgery is a clinical field that has grown considerably in the Western world and beyond over the past few decades (Braun & Tiefer, 2010; Desai & Dixit, 2018).

It is often referred to in public discussion as procedures intended to achieve a 'designer vagina', an indication of the lack of public understanding of the anatomy of the female genital organs (Telfer, 2018). The more accurate terms include labiaplasty (NHS, 2016), vaginoplasty (or 'vaginal rejuvenation') (WebMD, 2017), hymenoplasty (Diane, 2016) and vulvoplasty (Zelmanovich, 2017). As the documents cited here demonstrate, such surgeries are most commonly conducted within the for-profit sector of clinical practice with the concomitant marketing language. Some health provision services, such as the British National Health Service (NHS), may provide these procedures without cost (approximately 2,000 procedures were conducted in the UK in 2011), however there is resistance to the use of public money for the large majority of women who desire cosmetic surgery (Roberts, 2011).

Another form of genital aesthetic is piercing (BMEZINE.com, 2007), which is done as a purely cosmetic procedure and/or in the belief that it will heighten sexual sensation. The procedure, usually carried out by non-clinical operators in commercial premises, is formally categorised as Type 4 FGM (World Health Organisation, 2007a) and, as such, is included in FGM data sets, such as the UK records of FGM (The National Archives, 2017). However, it has been argued that, whilst FGCS has parallels with FGM, piercings do not permanently excise bodily tissue, and they can be reversed simply by the person concerned removing the piercing object (Nelius et al., 2012). In this vein, practitioners in Scotland have recently been given the all-clear to conduct piercing, having previously been prohibited from such practices, following WHO designation of piercing as FGM (*The Times*, 2018).

Why do women request FGCS?

The evidence so far suggests that women and girls who request FGCS do so for reasons such as poorly informed, non-diverse ideas about bodily 'perfection' and how other women's genitals appear; perceived physical discomfort and/or embarrassment because of clothing or sports activity; pressures from advertising and marketing; the trend, especially in younger women, toward removal of pudendal hair (with subsequent exposure of genitals); and, in women and girls from some communities, the necessity for an 'intact' hymen before marriage (Sharp, Mattiske, & Vale, 2016; Tiefer, 2008). Women and girls expect FGCS to make them more confident or comfortable or happier and perhaps also to enhance their sex lives (RCOG, 2013). Whilst online pornography and digitally manipulated images have been associated with increased dissatisfaction with the genitals, feminist critics have argued that the medical profession authenticates the idea that female genitalia can routinely be 'improved' by cosmetic surgery (Braun & Tiefer, 2010; Keil, 2010).

As the BritSPAG statement (Mayo Clinic, n.d.) makes clear, however, there is scant evidence to support the expectation that FGCS will resolve women's concerns, and the experience itself may be harmful or unpleasant. There are reports of bleeding, infection, wound dehiscence and scarring, as well as the risk of decreased genital sensitivity and other hazards (Liao & Creighton, 2011). There is at present no substantive research that provides clarity about these possibilities; no stringent longitudinal studies have been undertaken, at least in part because much of this surgery is conducted in private clinics away from the scrutiny of large or state institutions. Indeed, FGCS is a generally unregulated field with little in the way of accredited post-qualifying training (see, for example, the RACGP letter to the Chair of the Medical Board of Australia (2015)), in which private medicine is delivered by clinicians with a substantial financial interest to patients who are anxious about their bodies and how they present to others.

The relevant medical colleges of several nations, especially but not only in the global North (Reingold, 2017), have recommended that FGCS should not be undertaken and that under no circumstance should it be offered unless medically essential to girls under 18 (Medical Board of Australia, 2017). Guidance emphasises the importance of psychological and psychiatric assessments where appropriate; surgery should never be the first option and consent to surgery should never be obtained on first consultation. In addition, a UK legal report suggests that a second opinion should be sought, if possible from the patient's GP, before any surgery is undertaken (Mills & Reeve, 2016). Clinicians are strongly advised by professional bodies (RACGP, 2015) always to keep full written records of consultations, including medical details and signed consents (of which patients should also have a copy); these may be needed in any possible future legal situation. Doctors must listen carefully to the explanations patients give of their concerns. They must also consider wider health and sexual matters, offer respectful general and gynaecological examination, and (if there is no evidence of disease) reassure and emphasise that the variation in female genital morphology is normal and that the female genital organs change considerably over a lifetime.

However, it could be said that clinicians, in agreeing to perform FGCS, are endorsing social structures that construe women and girls to be objects rather than individuals in their own right. These cosmetic procedures are aligned with ideas regarding 'sexuality as technical performance' (Barbara et al., 2017) and with traditional notions of 'purity', which also impact perceptions of the female body (Ussher et al., 2017). Indeed, some commentators have suggested that, whilst most current medical models about FGCS underpin assumptions about the 'need' for private clinical services, doctors should reflect on how their actions reinforce wider and unquestioned assumptions about women that are embedded in social-political-cultural beliefs and structures (Lippman, 1999). In condoning FGCS clinicians position themselves as cultural guardians, reflect masculine aspirations and fears (Liao & Creighton, 2011), and undermine gender equality (Tiefer, 2008).

Genital surgery for intersex neonates

Genital surgeries may also be conducted, without consent, in instances where a child is born without clearly sex-defined genitalia or reproductive organs, referred to as 'intersex' (Viau-Colindres, Axelrad, & Karaviti, 2017). The most pressing clinical question is the extent to which the child's genitalia and internal organs are able to support normal physiological functions such as excretion. For parents, however, the discovery that their new-born has no immediately identifiable 'gender' is understandably confusing and upsetting (Oliveira Mde, de Paiva-e-Silva, Guerra-Junior, & Maciel-Guerra, 2015). A case has often been made for surgical intervention at a very early stage, so that children grow up with clearly defined notions of their gender (Kleeman, 2016).

The serious drawback of this determination is that, when children are older, they may not feel comfortable in the gender assigned to them, thus genital surgery on such children is considered a violation of their human rights (Carpenter, 2018). Likewise, the clinical assumption, based on inadequate evidence, that there should be physical and psychological congruence is no longer always accepted (Kipnis & Diamond, n.d.). As personal testimony has sometimes made clear (Zieselman, 2017), physical attributes, whether surgically imposed or original, do not inevitably attune as children develop with psychological gender preferences (NHS, 2018).

More nuanced legal and protocol considerations, beyond physiological function, are needed in relation to surgical intervention for infant and paediatric intersex patients (Davis, 2015). Further, as Markosyan and Ahmed (2017) observed, assignments are influenced by temporal, social and geographical variations. In some countries, such as Australia, Bangladesh, Germany, India, New Zealand, Nepal and Pakistan, the sex of the child can be registered as undetermined – a move increasingly adopted around the globe, along with calls not to require registration of sex at all (Markosyan & Ahmed, 2017). It is worth noting that some traditional (non-Western) communities have also acknowledged non-binary gender status. For example, the TwoSpirit people, Fa'afafine and Hijra all include 'third' gender individuals (American Psychological Association, 2015).

Resistance or withdrawal of support is growing to the 'treatments' that have been developed to begin anatomical sex transition in childhood (American Academy of Pediatrics, 2007). Unless there is a clinically justifiable requirement beyond the parents' simple preference for surgery, the view is often now that irreversible treatments should not be imposed before the child is genuinely able to make the choice, convincingly, in person (Carpenter, 2018).

Caring for women and girls with FGM

Globally FGM, like modern-day inessential genital surgeries, is increasingly seen as a matter of human rights and reproductive justice (Braun, 2012). This rights perspective on FGM is reflected in the United Nations Sustainable Development Goal 5 (Wendoh, 2018), which aims to 'achieve gender equality and empower all women and girls' (United Nations, n.d.).

In order to achieve this, in some parts of the world the emphasis is on low-technology approaches and education of communities. Significant here are developments such as the Barefoot Grannies (Burrage, 2016a) and Grandmother Project initiatives (Associated Press, 2019), where older women in a community – sometimes themselves former 'cutters' – receive training in basic health care and why FGM must not be done. These women then take the message to others in their community. In developing countries, safe houses have been established for girls who run away to avoid FGM, where long-term education and later possible reconciliation with parents is offered (Tremblay & Carson, 2016). One practical initiative in African communities is some form of alternative rite of passage (ARP) (Cook, 2018) in which, with the community's consent, girls (and sometimes boys) are taught how their bodies function and are encouraged to continue their education. The programme concludes with a ceremony during which everyone in the community accords the girls adult status without the imposition of FGM. ARPs offer increasing scope for success, particularly if introduced alongside education and at the optimal point of readiness for intervention (Brown, Beecham, & Barrett, 2013).

The World Health Organization (2016) has issued guidance on clinical practice in the care of women and girls with FGM, as have national health bodies in countries such as Australia (Jordan, Neophytou, & James, 2014) and the UK (Royal College of General Practitioners, 2016). Increasingly, instruction is available for clinicians and other carers on-line (AHAFoundation, 2019; Forensic Healthcare Online, 2018; World Health Organization, 2019) in the development of interventions and support to address specific damage following FGM. Likewise, specific instruction is available for those who provide obstetric care, sometimes via a 'pathway' such as that prescribed by the UK NHS (Royal College of Obstetricians and Gynaecologists, 2015).

The most common medical intervention is deinfibulation, which can be conducted by suitably trained midwives and doctors as well as specialist gynaecologists and obstetricians (FGM National Clinical Group, n.d.). Deinfibulation may be done at any time if the woman wishes to achieve a degree of reversal of the more serious forms of FGM, and it can be necessary for safe childbirth. More complex procedures intended to reconstruct or 'restore' clitoral response have also been developed (Abdulcadir, et al., 2015; Thabet & Thabet, 2003). Surgery is not necessarily the first or best option; sometimes simply learning that she has a 'hidden' clitoris is enough to reassure a woman who has presented for help (Surugue, 2017). For other women, some forms of surgical intervention can provide pain relief, enable pleasurable sexual sensation, and induce a feeling of 'wholeness' or improved self-image (Manero & Labanca, 2018). However, there is always a need in referrals for multi-disciplinary support – physical, psychological and social – and often therapy across a range of agencies and specialisations is required.

Guidance on good clinical practice continues to be marred by omissions in areas of considerable importance. For example, in the UK, there has only recently been advice for general medical practitioners on how to deal with FGM (Royal College of General Practitioners, 2016). If the clinician has not thought through her or his response to unanticipated disclosure, that may be the last time the patient ever tries to discuss her mutilation, the problems arising from it, or other aspects of gendered violence (VAWG) she may be experiencing (Department of Health, 2016). This silence may have severe consequences both for the woman and for her children, particularly because the risk of intimate partner violence may be higher in cases where the woman has undergone FGM (Peltzer & Pengpid, 2014; UN Women, 2017). Many of the observations above point to the criticality of awareness by the whole health and social care team – including school nurses, social workers, teachers, law enforcement officers and professionals in formal clinical settings. In the UK and some other countries attempts are being made to bring these various roles into an integrated whole via versions of the 'multi-agency' approach (HM Government, 2016), but on-the-ground realities may not always reflect that policy position.

Nor has legal action in some developed nations so far achieved much success. There have been several successful prosecutions in France (Bouchoucha, 2016; Burrage, 2012) but, as of early 2019, just one with that outcome in the UK (Marsh, 2019) and one in Australia, later overturned (Lawrence, 2018). Until an articulated clinical and legal paradigm for dealing with FGM is developed, with genuine formal, identified and top-level leadership, we cannot address the problem adequately (Burrage, 2015).

The vocabularies of FGM and 'circumcision'

Given the harm FGM can inflict, the terms used to discuss FGM have particular significance. There is a trend (e.g., in parts of the USA) to ignore the advice of WHO and UNFPA (World Health Organisation, 2006) and instead consistently to refer to FGM as female genital 'cutting' or 'circumcision' (FGC) (New York State Department of Health, 2016). Levin (2010) referred to this position as Anthr/Apology, the claim that people must not 'judge' the action and its consequences, but rather record it solely in the contexts of the understandings of those directly involved – hence the use of softer terms such as 'cutting' (Cassman, 2008). This may help those close to the tradition to feel comfortable, but euphemisms in formal settings risk lessening the gravity of the tradition in wider community and professional perceptions (28 Too Many, n.d.). FGM is not a serendipitous ill-health condition to be borne bravely; it is patriarchy incarnate (Burrage, 2016c), a violent affront to human rights and reproductive justice, an intended criminal act inflicted in the interests of powerful people, usually on minors, who by default cannot consent. Nonetheless, there are occasions when alternatives to the term 'mutilation' may be appropriate, particularly in discussion with those women and girls who have undergone FGM, or with other people who live in communities where it is done, in order to aid communication between local people and visiting health or education workers.

The term 'circumcision' brings to some minds a suggestion that, as male circumcision (more accurately, male genital mutilation, MGM) is deemed – in error – to do no harm, then FGM is also harmless. Boy babies can die as a result of circumcision, even in developed nations (e.g., the USA) (Earp, Allareddy, Allareddy, & Rotta, 2018), and in parts of the developing world hundreds of adolescent boys are killed by the procedure every year (World Health Organization, 2007b). There is an emerging opinion in some parts of the EndFGM community that neither FGM or MGM will cease entirely until the other does (Burrage, 2018a).

Conclusion

Female genital mutilation is at epidemic levels (UNICEF, 2016), but to see FGM as a single issue is to miss a fundamental truth: FGM is 'only' one aspect of patriarchy incarnate, the imposition of some men's will and economic interests (regardless of the genders of the implementing actors) on the bodies of women and girls. FGM is closely associated with domestic violence (Peltzer & Pengpid, 2014) and other harmful traditional practices, includ-ing bride price and child 'marriage', various forms of slavery and trafficking, breast 'ironing', and other assaults and human rights abuses (Women's Rights – Ethiopia, 2013).

For these reasons (sub-)national programmes to eradicate FGM need to be bolstered by international and global messages and cooperation. The contributions from the United Nations (2014), World Health Organization (2016, 2018), UNFPA (2018), the EU (EndFGM European Network, n.d.) and others are essential to setting this harmful tradition firmly within the human and reproductive rights contexts they promote. Work on the ground must be supported, whether with girls and women directly, with community and faith leaders (mostly men, plus powerful female cutters who agree to abandon the knife), or in the context of a broader approach, for instance training young indigenous journalists to challenge and expose FGM in traditionally practising locations (Global Media Campaign to End FGM, n.d.) – a strategy particularly effective in engaging powerful politicians with the influence to steer facilities and allocate funds.

FGM eradication programmes operate in many parts of the world and take various forms (UNICEF, 2016; World Health Organization, 2010). The elements of eradication to be addressed within communities constitute the '4Es': Engagement, Education, Enforcement, and Economics (or, indeed, the 'Many Es' – including also Empathy, Empowerment, and Epidemics) (Burrage, 2018b) all of them within the remit of public health. Simple prohib-ition (enforcement) is rarely effective; the practice may then just be hidden (Dubuis, 2016).

FGM is deeply embedded in the beliefs and practices of long-established communities, both in the developing world and in the Western diaspora. It is not, however, a 'cultural matter'; it is a tradition, and as such can, with due care (Burrage, 2017), be stopped without necessarily contesting deeply embedded community identities. Eradicating female genital muti-lation and other harmful traditional practices is a journey in which everyone has something to contribute but no one can travel far without co-campaigners and workers. The analysis is complex, as it moves across many disciplines from anthropology and socio-economics, via politics and policy to enforcement, education, and psychology. But often the first point of contact regarding FGM is medical. Clinicians and public health practitioners have an especially important part to play in FGM eradication.

References

28 Too Many (n.d.). *Terminology and FGM*. London, UK: Author. Retrieved from www.28toomany.org/thematic/terminology-and-fgm.

Abdulcadir, J., Rodriguez, M. I., Petignat, P., & Say, L. (2015). Clitoral reconstruction after female genital mutilation/cutting: Case studies. *The Journal of Sexual Medicine, 12*(1), 274–281.

Abrol, S. (2018, February 6). Yes, female genital mutilation happens in India; here's everything you need to know. We bring you the why, how and why-not of female genital mutilation in India. *India Today*. Retrieved from www.indiatoday.in/lifestyle/people/story/female-genital-mutilation-india-clitoris-pleasure-muslim-bohra-community-1162510-2018-02-06.

Access to European Law (Eur-LEX) (2013). *Towards the elimination of female genital mutilation*. Eur-LEX [database]. Retrieved from https://eur-lex.europa.eu/legal-content/EN/TXT/?uri=COM:2013:0833:FIN.

AHAFoundation (2019). *A training curriculum for professionals likely to encounter victims of genital mutilation/cutting*. New York, NY: Author. Retrieved from www.theahafoundation.org/online-training/female-genital-mutilationcutting-fgmc-training-for-professionals-working-with-victims-and-communities.

American Academy of Pediatrics (2007). AAP Publications Retired or Reaffirmed, October 2006. *Pediatrics, 119*(2), 405.

American Psychological Association (APA) (2015). *Non-binary gender identities, APA factsheet*, APA division 4, society for the psychology of sexual orientation and gender diversity. Washington, DC: Author. Retrieved from www.apadivisions.org/division-44/resources/advocacy/non-binary-facts.pdf.

Asmani, I. L. & Abdi, M. S. (2008). *Delinking female genital mutilation/cutting from Islam*. New York, NY: United Nations Population Fund. Retrieved from www.unfpa.org/sites/default/files/pub-pdf/Delinking%20FGM%20from%20Islam%20final%20report.pdf.

Associated Press (2019, February 6). Grandmothers fight to banish female genital mutilation, *New York Post*. Retrieved from https://nypost.com/2019/02/06/grandmothers-fight-to-banish-female-genital-mutilation.

Atrash, H. K. (2011). Parents' death and its implications for child survival. *Revista Brasileira De Crescimento E Desenvolvimento Humano, 21*(3), 759–770.

Balogun, O. O., Hirayama, F., Wariki, W. M. V., Koyanagi, A., & Mori, R. (2013). Interventions for improving outcomes for pregnant women who have experienced genital cutting. *Cochrane Database of Systematic Reviews, 2*, CD009872.

Barbara, G., Facchin, F., Buggio, L., Alberico, D., Frattaruolo, M. P., & Kustermann, A. (2017). Vaginal rejuvenation: Current perspectives. *International Journal of Women's Health, 9*, 513–519.

Batha, E. (2017). Why 'medicalization' of FGM is a serious threat to women. New York, NY: *Global Citizen*. Retrieved from www.globalcitizen.org/en/content/medicalization-fgm-serious-threat.

Behrendt, A. & Moritz, S. (2005). Posttraumatic stress disorder and memory problems after female genital mutilation. *American Journal of Psychiatry, 162*(5), 1000–1002.

Biglu, M. H., Farnam, A., Abotalebi, P., Biglu, S., & Ghavami, M. (2016). Effect of female genital mutilation/cutting on sexual functions. *Sexual and Reproductive Healthcare, 10*, 3–8.

BMEZINE.com (2007). Category: Female genital piercings. BMEZINE.com [website]. Retrieved from https://wiki.bme.com/index.php?title=Category:Female_Genital_Piercings.

Bouchoucha, L. (2016, March 7). In France, FGM is reason to fear homelands, seek Asylum. *We News*. Retrieved from https://womensenews.org/2016/03/in-france-fgm-is-reason-to-fear-homelands-seek-asylum.

Braun, V. (2012). Female genital cutting around the globe: A matter of reproductive justice? In J. C. Chrisler (Ed.), *Reproductive justice: A global concern* (pp. 29–55). Santa Barbara, CA: Praeger.

Braun, V. & Tiefer, L. (2010). The 'designer vagina' and the pathologisation of female genital diversity: Interventions for change. *Radical Psychology, 8*(1), 11–18.

Brown, K., Beecham, D., & Barrett, H. (2013). The applicability of behaviour change in intervention programmes targeted at ending female genital mutilation in the EU: Integrating social cognitive and community level approaches. *Obstetrics and Gynecology International, 2013*, 1–12.

Burrage, H. (2012). *The UK can learn from France on female genital mutilation prosecutions.* Hilaryburrage.com [website]. Retrieved from https://hilaryburrage.com/2012/11/28/the-uk-can-learn-from-france-on-fgm-prosecutions.

Burrage, H. (2013). *Feminist statement on female genital mutilation.* Retrieved from https://statementonfgm.com.

Burrage, H. (2014, April 25). How can Britain deport a child at risk of FGM? Theresa May must think again. *Guardian.* Retrieved from www.theguardian.com/commentisfree/2014/apr/25/britain-deport-child-at-risk-fgm-theresa-may-nigeria.

Burrage, H. (2015). *Eradicating female genital mutilation.* Abingdon, UK: Routledge.

Burrage, H. (2016a). *Female mutilation: The truth behind the horrifying global practice of female genital mutilation.* Sydney, Australia: New Holland Press.

Burrage, H. (2016b) *The 4 'E's Of FGM eradication – My paper on the economics of FGM, at the UN Geneva IAC meeting.* Hilaryburrage.com [website]. Retrieved from https://hilaryburrage.com/2016/05/12/the-4-es-of-fgm-eradication-my-paper-on-economics-at-the-un-geneva-iac-meeting.

Burrage, H. (2016c) *Patriarchy incarnate: The horrifying practice of female genital mutilation.* Hilaryburrage.com [website]. Retrieved from https://hilaryburrage.com/2016/03/05/patriarchy-incarnate-the-horrifying-practice-of-female-genital-mutilation.

Burrage, H. (2017). *Thinking about ethics in tackling Female Genital Mutilation (FGM).* Hilaryburrage.com [website]. Retrieved from https://hilaryburrage.com/2017/05/19/thinking-about-ethics-in-tackling-fgm.

Burrage, H. (2018a). *#EndFGM campaigners and intactivists against male circumcision (MGM) have many concerns in common.* Hilaryburrage.com [website]. Retrieved from https://hilaryburrage.com/2018/11/11/endfgm-and-intactivists-against-male-circumcision-mgm-have-many-concerns-in-common.

Burrage, H. (2018b). *The many 'E's of FGM eradication – And why they all lead via 'economics' and 'epidemics' to public health.* Hilaryburrage.com [website]. Retrieved from https://hilaryburrage.com/2018/04/24/the-many-es-of-fgm-eradication-and-why-they-all-lead-via-economics-and-epidemics-to-public-health.

Carpenter, M. (2018). Intersex variations, human rights, and the international classification of diseases. *Health & Human Rights: An International Journal, 20*(2), 205–214.

Cassman, R. (2008). Fighting to make the cut: Female genital cutting studied within the context of cultural relativism. *Journal of Human Rights, 6*(1), 1–15.

Cook, S. (2018). *Do alternative rites of passage (ARP) work?* London, UK: 28 Too Many. Retrieved from www.28toomany.org/blog/2018/mar/7/do-alternative-rites-of-passage-arp-approaches-work.

Daughters of Eve (n.d.). *Living with FGM.* Retrieved from www.dofeve.org/living-with-fgm.html.

Davis, G. (2015). *Contesting intersex: The dubious diagnosis.* New York, NY: NYU Press.

de Vos, P. (2013). Do members of traditional communities have any democratic rights? *Constitutionally Speaking* [website]. Retrieved from https://constitutionallyspeaking.co.za/do-members-of-traditional-communities-have-any-democratic-rights.

Department of Health (2016). *Female genital mutilation: Risk and safeguarding guidance for professionals.* London, UK: Author. Retrieved from https://assets.publishing.service.gov.uk/government/uploads/system/uploads/attachment_data/file/525390/FGM_safeguarding_report_A.pdf.

Desai, S. A. & Dixit, V. V. (2018). Audit of female genital aesthetic surgery: Changing trends in India. *Journal of Obstetrics and Gynaecology of India, 68*(3), 214–220.

Diane (2016). *What is hymenoplasty?* Woodstock and Canton, GA: Cherokee Women's Health Specialists. Retrieved from https://cherokeewomenshealth.com/2016/08/what-is-hymenoplasty.

Doucet, M.-H., Pallitto, C., & Groleau, D. (2017). Understanding the motivations of health-care providers in performing female genital mutilation: An integrative review of the literature. *Reproductive Health, 14*(1), 46.

Drum, K. (2017, February 6). Female genital mutilation is not a uniquely Muslim problem. *Mother Jones.* Retrieved from www.motherjones.com/kevin-drum/2016/02/female-genital-mutilation-not-uniquely-muslim-problem.

Dubuis, A. (2016, December 12). Kenyan clan elders are profiting off female genital mutilation. *Huffington Post.* Retrieved from https://www.huffpost.com/entry/kenyan-clan-elders-are-profiting-off-female-genital-mutilation_n_584ec02ee4b0bd9c3dfd8816.

Earp, B. D., Allareddy, V., Allareddy, V., & Rotta, A. T. (2018). Factors associated with early deaths following neonatal male circumcision in the United States, 2001 to 2010. *Clinical Pediatrics, 57*(13), 1532–1540.

Eke, N. & Nkanginieme, K. (2006). Female genital mutilation and obstetric outcome. *Lancet, 367*, 1799.

EndFGM European Network (n.d.). *EU Policy Framework*. Brussels, Belgium: Author. Retrieved from www.endfgm.eu/resources/eu-framework.

Ernest, D., Howard-Merill, L., Norman, K., & Otoo-Otortey, N. (2014). *'Do not hide yourselves, you are not cursed': A PEER study of obstetric fistula.* Mpwapwa, Dodoma, Tanzania. London, UK: Forward UK. Retrieved from https://forwarduk.org.uk/wp-content/uploads/2014/12/Do-not-hide-yourself_PEER-Study.pdf.

Evans, C., Tweheyo, R., McGarry, J., Eldridge, J., McCormick, C., Nkoyo, V., & Higginbottom, G. M. A. (2017). What are the experiences of seeking, receiving and providing FGM-related healthcare? Perspectives of health professionals and women/girls who have undergone FGM: Protocol for a systematic review of qualitative evidence. *British Medical Journal Open, 7*(12), e018170.

FGM National Clinical Group (n.d.). *FGM treatment: What is deinfibulation?* London, UK: Author. Retrieved from www.fgmnationalgroup.org/fgm_treatment.htm.

Forensic Healthcare Online (2018). *Clinical guide: Female genital mutilation/ cutting.* Forensic Healthcare Online [website]. Retrieved from www.forensichealth.com/clinical-guides/female-genital-mutilation.

Global Media Campaign to End FGM (n.d.). London, UK: Author. Retrieved from www.facebook.com/gmcendfgm.

Glover, J., Liebling, H., Barrett, H., & Goodman, S. (2017). The psychological and social impact of female genital mutilation. *Journal of International Studies, 10*(2), 219–238.

HM Government (2016). *Multi-agency statutory guidance on female genital mutilation.* London, UK: Author.

Hearst, A. A. & Molnar, A. M. (2013). Female genital cutting: An evidence-based approach to clinical management for the primary care physician. *Mayo Clinic Proceedings, 88*(6), 618–629.

Horowitz, C. R. & Jackson, J. C. (1997). Female 'circumcision': African women confront American medicine. *Journal of General Internal Medicine, 12*(8), 491–499.

International Planned Parenthood Federation (2013). *Harmful traditional practices affecting women and girls.* London, UK: Author.Retrieved from www.ippf.org/sites/default/files/harmful_traditional_practices.pdf.

Ismail, S. A., Abbas, A. M., Habib, D., Morsy, H., Saleh, M. A., & Bahloul, M. (2017). Effect of female genital mutilation/cutting; types I and II on sexual function: Case-controlled study. *Reproductive Health, 14*(1), 108.

Jordan, L., Neophytou, K., & James, C. (2014). *Improving the health care of women and girls affected by female genital mutilation/cutting: A national approach to service coordination.* Melbourne, Australia: Family Planning Victoria.

Keil, A. & Greenhalgh, S. (2010). Genital anxiety and the quest for the perfect vulva: A feminist analysis of female genital cosmetic surgery [unpublished manuscript]. University of California Irvine, California, USA.

Kimani, S. & Shell-Duncan, B. (2018). Medicalized female genital mutilation/cutting: Contentious practices and persistent debates. *Current Sexual Health Reports, 10*(1), 25–34.

Kipnis, K. & Diamond, M. (n.d.). *Pediatric ethics and the surgical assignment of sex.* London, UK: The UK Intersex Association.

Kleeman, J. (2016, July 2). 'We don't know if your baby's a boy or a girl': Growing up intersex. *Guardian.* Retrieved from www.theguardian.com/world/2016/jul/02/male-and-female-what-is-it-like-to-be-intersex.

Koski, A. & Heymann, J. (2017). Thirty-year trends in the prevalence and severity of female genital mutilation: A comparison of 22 countries. *British Medical Journal Global Health, 2*(4), e000467.

Kouyate, M. (2016). Preface. In H. Burrage (Ed.), *Female mutilation: The truth behind the horrifying global practice of female genital mutilation* (pp. 6–7). Sydney, Australia: New Holland Publishers.

Lawrence, E. (2018, August 12). Genital mutilation convictions overturned after new evidence showing victims remain intact. *ABC News.* Retrieved from www.abc.net.au/news/2018-08-11/genital-mutilation-convictions-overturned/10108106.

Levin, T. (2010). 'Highly valued by both sexes': Activists, anthr/apologists and FGM. *Journal on Female Genital Mutilation and Other Harmful Traditional Practices, 3*(1), 52–61.

Liao, L.-M. & Creighton, S. M. (2011). Female genital cosmetic surgery: A new dilemma for GPs. *The British Journal of General Practice: The Journal of the Royal College of General Practitioners, 61*(582), 7–8.

Lippman, A. (1999). Choice as a risk to women's health. *Health, Risk & Society, 1*(3), 281–291.

Mackie, G. (1996). Ending footbinding and infibulation: A convention account. *American Sociological Review, 61*(6), 999–1017.

Magon, N. & Alinsod, R. (2017). Female cosmetic genital surgery: Delivering what women want. *Journal of Obstetrics and Gynaecology of India, 67*(1), 15–19.

Makama, G. A. (2013). Patriarchy and gender inequality in Nigeria: The way forward. *European Scientific Journal, 19*(7), 115–144.

Manero, I. & Labanca, T. (2018). Clitoral reconstruction using a vaginal graft after female genital mutilation. *Obstetrics and Gynecology International, 131*(4), 701–706.

Markosyan, R. & Ahmed, S. F. (2017). Sex assignment in conditions affecting sex development. *Journal of Clinical Research in Pediatric Endocrinology, 9*(Suppl 2), 106–112.

Marsh, S. (2019, March 8). Mother jailed for 11 years in first British FGM conviction. *Guardian*. Retrieved from www.theguardian.com/society/2019/mar/08/mother-of-three-year-old-is-first-in-uk-to-be-convicted-of-fgm.

Mayo Clinic (n.d.). Body dysmorphic disorder. Rochester, MN: Author. Retrieved from www.mayoclinic.org/diseases-conditions/body-dysmorphic-disorder/symptoms-causes/syc-20353938.

Medical Board of Australia (2017). Guidelines for registered medical practitioners who perform cosmetic medical and surgical procedures. Melbourne, VIC, Australia: Author. Retrieved from www.medicalboard.gov.au/Codes-Guidelines-Policies/Cosmetic-medical-and-surgical-procedures-guidelines.aspx.

Milken Institute School of Public Health (2017). Female genital mutilation/cutting: Half a million girls & women in the United States at risk. Washington, DC: The George Washington University. Retrieved from https://publichealth.gwu.edu/content/female-genital-mutilationcutting-half-million-girls-women-united-states-risk.

Mills and Reeve (2016). *The Female Genital Mutilation Act: An update*. London, UK: Author. Retrieved from www.mills-reeve.com/insights/publications/the-female-genital-mutilation-act-an-update.

Mpinga, E. K., Macias, A., Hasselgard-Rowe, J., Kandala, N.-B., Félicien, T. K., Verloo, H., Bukonda, N. K., & Chastonay, P. (2016). Female genital mutilation: A systematic review of research on its economic and social impacts across four decades. *Global Health Action, 9*, 31489.

Nanjala-Ndenga, C. (2016). Sub-Saharan and Southern Africa. In H. Burrage (Ed.), *Female mutilation: The truth behind the horrifying global practice of female genital mutilation* (p. 46). Sydney, Australia: New Holland Publishers.

National Health Service (NHS) (2016). *Your guide to cosmetic procedures: Labiaplasty (vulval surgery)*. London, UK: Author. Retrieved from www.nhs.uk/conditions/cosmetic-treatments/labiaplasty.

National Health Service (NHS) (2018). *Think your child may be trans or non-binary? Healthy body*. London, UK: Author. Retrieved from www.nhs.uk/live-well/healthy-body/think-your-child-might-be-trans-or-non-binary.

Nelius, T., Armstrong, M. L., Angel, E., Hogan, L., Young, C., & Rinard, K. (2012). A relationship between female genital piercings and genital mutilation? *BJOG: An International Journal of Obstetrics and Gynaecology, 119*(7), 895–896.

New York State Department of Health (2016). *Female genital mutilation/female circumcision reference card for health care providers. Communication Guidelines and Physician Obligations*. Albany, NY: Author. Retrieved from www.health.ny.gov/community/adults/women/female_circumcision/providers.htm.

New Zealand FGM Education Programme (2019). *Beliefs and issues. Female genital mutilation information for health and child protection professionals*. Auckland, New Zealand: Author. Retrieved from http://fgm.co.nz/beliefs-and-issues.

Nordqvist, C. (2017, May 15). What is female genital mutilation? *Medical News Today*. Retrieved from www.medicalnewstoday.com/articles/241726.php.

Northern Ireland Human Rights Commission (2016). *Female genital mutilation in the United Kingdom*. Belfast, Northern Ireland: Author. Retrieved from www.nihrc.org/uploads/publications/FGMinUK-15.08.2016.pdf.

Norwegian Institute of Public Health (2014). *Immediate health consequences of female genital mutilation/cutting (FGM/C)*. Oslo, Norway: Author. Retrieved from www.fhi.no/en/publ/2014/immediate-health-consequences-of-female-genital-mutilationcutting-fgmc-.

O'Connell, H. E., Sanjeevan, K. V., & Hutson, J. M. (2005). Anatomy of the clitoris. *Journal of Urology, 174*(4 Pt 1), 1189–1195.

Oliveira Mde, S., de Paiva-E-Silva, R. B., Guerra-Junior, G., & Maciel-Guerra, A. T. (2015). Parents' experiences of having a baby with ambiguous genitalia. *Journal of Pediatric Endocrinology & Metabolism: JPEM, 28*(7–8), 833–838.

Peltzer, K. & Pengpid, S. (2014). Female genital mutilation and intimate partner violence in the Ivory Coast. *BMC Women's Health, 14*, 13.

Rashid, M. & Rashid, M. H. (2007). Obstetric management of women with female genital mutilation. *The Obstetrician & Gynaecologist, 9*, 95–101.

Reingold, R. (2017). *The differential treatment of FGCS and FGM/C: A legal double standard?* Washington, DC: O'Neill Institute, Georgetown University. Retrieved from http://oneill.law.georgetown.edu/the-differential-treatment-of-fgcs-fgmc-a-legal-double-standard.

Reisel, D. & Creighton, S. M. (2015). Long term health consequences of Female Genital Mutilation (FGM). *Maturitas, 80*(1), 48–51.

Roberts, M. (2011, August 24). Designer vagina NHS operations unwarranted. *BBC Health News.* Retrieved from www.bbc.com/news/health-14627659.

Rodriguez, M. I., Seuc, A., Say, L., & Hindin, M. J. (2016). Episiotomy and obstetric outcomes among women living with type 3 female genital mutilation: A secondary analysis. *Reproductive Health, 13*(1), 131.

Royal Australian College of General Practitioners (RACGP) (2015). *Female genital cosmetic surgery: A resource for general practitioners and other health professionals.* Melbourne, Australia: Author.

Royal College of General Practitioners (RCGP) (2016). Female genital mutilation. Retrieved from www.rcgp.org.uk/policy/rcgp-policy-areas/female-genital-mutilation.aspx

Royal College of Obstetricians and Gynaecologists (RCOG) (2013). *Ethical opinion paper: Ethical considerations in relation to female genital cosmetic surgery.* London, UK: Author.

Royal College of Obstetricians and Gynaecologists (RCOG) (2015). *Female genital mutilation and its management, Green-top Guideline No. 53.* London, UK: Author.

Rymer, J. (2006). Female genital mutilation. *The Lancet, 368*(9535), 579.

Scamell, M. & Ghumman, A. (2019). The experience of maternity care for migrant women living with female genital mutilation: A qualitative synthesis. *Birth, 46*(1), 15–23.

Serour, G. I. (2013). Medicalization of female genital mutilation/cutting. *African Journal of Urology, 19*, 145–149.

Shahvisi, A. & Earp, B. (2018). The law and ethics of female genital cutting. In S. Creighton & L.-M. Liao (Eds), *Female genital cosmetic surgery: Interdisciplinary analysis and solution* (pp. 52–64). Cambridge, UK: Cambridge University Press.

Sharp, G., Mattiske, J., & Vale, K. I. (2016). Motivations, expectations, and experiences of labiaplasty: A qualitative study. *Aesthetic Surgery Journal, 36*(8), 920–928.

Sigurjonsson, H. & Jordal, M. (2018). Addressing Female Genital Mutilation/Cutting (FGM/C) in the era of clitoral reconstruction: Plastic surgery. *Current Sexual Health Reports, 10*(2), 50–56.

Surugue, L. (2017, February 7). Meet the surgeon who made the fight against FGM his life-long battle: Hearing women's voices. *International Business Times.* Retrieved from www.ibtimes.co.uk/meet-surgeon-who-made-fight-against-fgm-his-life-long-battle-1602246.

Telfer, N. (2018). Vaginas 101. *HelloClue* [website]. Retrieved from https://helloclue.com/articles/cycle-a-z/vaginas-101.

Thabet, S. M. A. & Thabet, A. S. M. A. (2003). Defective sexuality and female circumcision: The cause and the possible management. *Journal of Obstetrics and Gynaecology Research, 29*(1), 12–19.

The National Archives (2017). *FGM enhanced dataset – Frequently asked questions.* Richmond, UK: Author. Retrieved from https://webarchive.nationalarchives.gov.uk/20180328130852tf_/http://content.digital.nhs.uk/media/22977/Frequently-Asked-Questions-updated-16-11-2016/pdf/Frequently_Asked_Questions_updated_16-11-2016.pdf.

The Times (2018, April 12). Intimate piercings win legal all-clear after FGM muddle. *The Times.* Retrieved from www.thetimes.co.uk/article/intimate-piercings-win-legal-all-clear-after-fgm-muddle-x679b6275.

Tiefer, L. (2008). Female genital cosmetic surgery: Freakish or inevitable? Analysis from medical marketing, bioethics, and feminist theory. *Feminism & Psychology, 18*(4), 466–479.

Tremblay, S. & Carson, M. (2016, February 6). End FGM Guardian global media campaign: Online mapping tool gives FGM runaways a path to help. *Guardian.* Retrieved from www.theguardian.com/society/2017/feb/06/online-mapping-tool-gives-fgm-runaways-a-path-to-help.

United Nations Children's Fund (UNICEF) (2016). *New statistical report on female genital mutilation shows harmful practice is a global concern.* New York, NY: Author.

United Nations (n.d.). *Sustainable development goals 5: Gender equality.* New York, NY: Author. Retrieved from www.un.org/sustainabledevelopment/gender-equality.

United Nations Population Fund (UNFPA) (2018). *Female genital mutilation: Overview/news on female genital mutilation.* New York, NY: Author. Retrieved from www.unfpa.org/female-genital-mutilation.

University of Oxford Refugee Study Centre (2015). *Forced migration review mini-feature: FGM and asylum in Europe. Forced Migration Review.* Oxford, UK: Author.

UN Women (2017). *Female genital mutilation/cutting and violence against women and girls: Strengthening the policy linkages between different forms of violence.* New York, NY: Author.

Ussher, J. M., Perz, J., Metusela, C., Hawkey, A. J., Morrow, M., Narchal, R., & Estoesta, J. (2017). Negotiating discourses of shame, secrecy, and silence: Migrant and refugee women's experiences of sexual embodiment. *Archives of Sexual Behavior, 46*(7), 1901–1921.

Varol, N., Dawson, A., Turkmani, S., Hall, J. J., Nanayakkara, S., Jenkins, G., Homer, C. S., & McGeechan, K. (2016). Obstetric outcomes for women with female genital mutilation at an Australian hospital, 2006–2012: A descriptive study. *BMC Pregnancy and Childbirth, 16*(1), 328.

Vaughan, J. (2017). *Obstetric fistula: A silent death for millions of women and girls.* London, UK: Thomson Reuters Foundation. Retrieved from http://news.trust.org/item/20170523104025-9ctkl.

Viau-Colindres, J., Axelrad, M., & Karaviti, L. P. (2017). Bringing back the term 'Intersex'. *Pediatrics, 140*(5), e20170505.

Watch Indonesia (2014). Additional submission to the United Nations committee on the rights of the child 66th session. In Medicalization of FGM in Indonesia. Berlin, Germany: Author. Retrieved from https://tbinternet.ohchr.org/Treaties/CRC/Shared%20Documents/IDN/INT_CRC_NGO_IDN_16628_E.pdf.

WebMD (2017). What is vaginoplasty and labiaplasty? *WebMD* [website]. Retrieved from www.webmd.com/women/qa/what-is-vaginoplasty-and-labiaplasty.

Wendoh, S. (2018). *Female genital mutilation (FGM) is a human rights violation.* London, UK: International Planned Parenthood Federation. Retrieved from www.ippf.org/blogs/female-genital-mutilation-fgm-human-rights-violation.

Women's Rights – Ethiopia (2013). *Combating female genital mutilation and other harmful traditional practices.* Brussels, Belgium: European Union External Action. Retrieved from www.eeas.europa.eu/archives/delegations/ethiopia/documents/eidhr/eidhr_ethiopia_2013.pdf.

World Health Organization (WHO) (2006). Female genital mutilation: New knowledge spurs optimism. *Progress newsletter 72.* Geneva, Switzerland: Author. Retrieved from www.who.int/reproductivehealth/publications/fgm/newsletter72/en.

World Health Organization (WHO) (2007a). *Classification of female genital mutilation.* Geneva, Switzerland: Author. Retrieved from www.who.int/reproductivehealth/topics/fgm/overview/en.

World Health Organization (WHO) (2007b). *Male circumcision: Global trends and determinants of prevalence, safety and acceptability.* Geneva, Switzerland: . Author Retrieved from http://apps.who.int/iris/bitstream/handle/10665/43749/9789241596169_eng.pdf;jsessionid=BFFA8FAEB03A4FE6EF0E8689A150C7B9?sequence=1.

World Health Organization (WHO) (2010). *Global strategy to stop health-care providers from performing female genital mutilation.* Geneva, Switzerland: Author. Retrieved from www.who.int/reproductivehealth/publications/fgm/rhr_10_9/en.

World Health Organization (WHO) (2018). *Female genital mutilation.* Geneva, Switzerland: Author. Retrieved from www.who.int/reproductivehealth/topics/fgm/prevalence/en.

World Health Organization (WHO) (2019). *Sexual and reproductive health: High-quality health care for girls and women living with FGM: WHO launches new clinical handbook.* Geneva, Switzerland: Author. Retrieved from www.who.int/reproductivehealth/health-care-girls-women-living-with-FGM/en.

World Health Organization (WHO) (2006). *New study shows female genital mutilation exposes women and babies to significant risk at childbirth.* Geneva, Switzerland: Author. Retrieved from www.who.int/mediacentre/news/releases/2006/pr30/en/

World Health Organization (WHO) (2016). *Guidelines on the management of health complications from female genital mutilation.* Geneva, Switzerland: Author. Retrieved from www.who.int/reproductivehealth/topics/fgm/management-health-complications-fgm/en.

World Health Organization (WHO) (2018). Health risks of female genital mutilation (FGM). Geneva, Switzerland: Author. Retrieved from www.who.int/reproductivehealth/topics/fgm/health_conse quences_fgm/en.

Zelmanovich, A. (2017). *Vulvoplasty*. New York, NY: Manhattan Women's Health & Wellness. Retrieved from www.obgynecologistnyc.com/procedures/vulvoplasty.

Zieselman, K. M. (2017, August 10). I was an intersex child who had surgery. Don't put other kids through this. *USA Today*. Retrieved from https://eu.usatoday.com/story/opinion/2017/08/09/inter sex-children-no-surgery-without-consent-zieselman-column/539853001.

PART VI

Marginalized women's health

34

SHAME, SILENCE AND SECRECY

Migrant and refugee women's sexual and reproductive health and embodiment

Alexandra Hawkey

In this chapter we utilise a life-course approach to explore migrant and refugee women's sexual and reproductive health. We focus on how women negotiate discourses (i.e., the different ways of representing the world, meanings, or statements that shape a specific version of events (Burr, 2015)) and practices in relation to their sexual and reproductive health when transitioning from countries where cultural beliefs, norms, and practices may differ from the Western, high-income contexts (e.g., Australia, Canada, the U.S., the U.K.) to which they relocate. We draw on a range of sources, including previously published research and interviews we have conducted with migrant and refugee women in relation to sexual and reproductive health.

Understanding migrant and refugee women's constructions and experiences of sexual and reproductive health is important for a number of reasons. Migrant and refugee women are less likely than native-born populations to access and utilise sexual and reproductive health-care services (Botfield, Newman, & Zwi, 2016; Rade, Crawford, Lobo, Gray, & Brown, 2018). This is problematic as accessing appropriate sexual and reproductive health services is also associated with positive mental health outcomes, greater quality of life, and higher sexual well-being (Aggleton & Campbell, 2000; WHO, 2009). It provides an opportunity for women to obtain adequate information for informed decision-making and is associated with good sexual and reproductive health outcomes (Benson, Maldari, Williams, & Hanifi, 2010). Those women who do not access services are less likely to know about, and participate in, preventative health strategies, such as cervical cancer screening, human papillomavirus (HPV) vaccination, sexually transmitted infection (STI) testing, and contraception use (Salad, Verdonk, de Boer, & Abma, 2015; Watts, Liamputtong, & Carolan, 2014). This places women at increased risk of cervical cancer (Allotey, Manderson, Baho, & Demian, 2004) and unintended pregnancy (Rademakers, Mouthaan, & de Neef, 2005), which has implications for women's health and psychosocial well-being (Kirkman, Rowe, Hardiman, & Rosenthal, 2011; Tsui, McDonald-Mosley, & Burke, 2010).

Psychologists, social scientists, and feminist researchers are increasingly seeking to capture women's embodied constructions and experiences of sexual and reproductive health. This involves a close examination into "the experience of living in, perceiving, and experiencing the world from the very specific location of our bodies" (Tolman, Bowman, & Fahs, 2014, p. 706). Everything we know and do is mediated through the body (Chrisler & Johnston-Robledo, 2018). Yet, the human body is a fluid and permeable barrier between ourselves and the outside world (Fahs & Swank, 2015, p. 149), as our corporeality, or "bodiliness," influences our relations with other people (Csordas, 2011, p. 137). How we experience our bodies, and our bodily sensations, is culturally and socially determined, and subject to dominant discourses, practices, and bodily disciplines (Csordas, 2002). However, often embodiment studies focus on White, Western, middle-class, heterosexual, able-bodied women; constructions and experiences of sexual and reproductive health amongst minority women, including migrant or refugee women, are less widely known.

Understanding migrant and refugee women's embodied sexual and reproductive knowledge is of particular importance. Migration has the potential to introduce women to new and competing discourses about aspects of their sexual and reproductive health (Dean, Mitchell, Stewart, & Debattista, 2017; Salad et al., 2015), while at the same time changing the social, cultural, and political context in which their embodiment is lived (Spitzer, 2009). Given that migrant and refugee women migrate from various cultural contexts, practice different religions, and have different pathways to migration, it is important that an intersectional perspective be drawn on to understand women's sexual and reproductive health, embodiment, and subjective experiences (Grzanka, 2018; Hankivsky et al., 2010). Such a perspective strives to understand "what is created and experienced at the intersection of two or more axes" (Hankivsky et al., 2010, p. 3) and demands analyses that do not focus on gender alone, but contextualise women in their diverse sociocultural settings by simultaneously taking into account other forms of social difference such as race, culture, religion, class, and ability (Varcoe, Hankivsky, & Morrow, 2007).

A life-course approach acknowledges that sexual and reproductive health is important at all stages of life and that women may have differing challenges at each of these phases. We begin this chapter by considering the ways in which menarche and menstruation are experienced by migrant and refugee women, and build on this by considering the ways in which migrant and refugee women experience and construct their sexuality as young women and as adults. We then unpick the cultural, religious, and gendered factors that shape the acceptability of cervical cancer screening and contraception use for fertility control. We conclude by providing an overview of migrant and refugee women's constructions and experiences of menopause. To illustrate our arguments, we draw on the findings from a recent study (Ussher et al., 2017) in which we examined the sexual and reproductive health of newly arrived migrant and refugee women, from a range of cultural backgrounds, who migrated to Australia or Canada.

Bleeding bodies and borders: menarche and menstruation

Menarche, a woman's first menstruation, is the beginning of the reproductive lifecycle, and is considered an important milestone in sexual development (Lee, 1994). It is intimately linked to fertility, sexual health, a women's sense of belonging, and gender identity (Brantelid, Nilvér, & Alehagen, 2014; Teitelman, 2004). There have been a number of studies where menarche and menstrual experiences of women are considered and compared across cultural settings (Sommer, Ackatia-Armah, Connolly, & Smiles, 2015; Uskul, 2004), yet research on migrant and refugee women's constructions and experiences is limited. What is known is that menarche is discursively positioned as a marker of adulthood and reproductive maturity across many sociocultural contexts (Chang, Hayter, & Wu, 2010), as has been found amongst migrant and refugee women (Hawkey, Ussher, Perz, & Metusela, 2017; Im

& Meleis, 2000). For example, across cultural groups, participants in our study described menarche as a time when "you start bleeding and you become a woman" and reported that, in their home countries, "it's associated with marriage … you're going to get married and you are going to have babies" (Hawkey et al., 2017, p. 1477).

Preparedness for menarche plays an important role in how it is experienced; girls who receive menstrual education prior to menarche report more positive experiences of this transition (Marván, Morales, & Cortés-Iniestra, 2006). However, many migrant and refugee women come from cultural contexts where menstruation is not discussed prior to menarche because of shame and the taboo nature of talking about topics related to sexuality and the reproductive body (Hawkey et al., 2017). This results in girls and young women receiving little or no pre-menarcheal education in their countries of origin, and consequently, many experienced menarche as shocking, shameful, and scary and associate menstrual blood with excrement, injury, and guilt (Hawkey et al., 2017; Im & Meleis, 2000). It also means that women have limited knowledge about the function of menstruation in relation to reproduction; for example, participants in our study stated that they did not know this connection until "we grew up aged 20 years, that's when I know this makes this" (Hawkey et al., 2017, p. 1481). These findings reiterate the importance of adequate menstrual education prior to menarche (Costos, Ackerman, & Paradis, 2002), particularly given that negative constructions of menstrual blood lead women to feel humiliated and unclean, and might result in women developing ongoing associations between menstruation and contamination (Lee, 2009).

Migration has been found to shape the way in which girls and women learn about menstruation, not always for the better. For example, in a study by Mendlinger and Cwikel (2005), Ethiopian women who migrated to Israel said that menstrual talk became more taboo once they had migrated. This was said to occur as women lost opportunities to gain embodied knowledge, such as observing their mothers address menstruation in their daily lives. Women disclosed that they found it difficult to provide a substitute for this type of learning following migration. In contrast, as a consequence of having received little or no menstrual education themselves, other migrant and refugee women resisted menstrual silencing by disclosing that they wanted to be more open about menstruation with their daughters given they "don't want them to be shocked, like I was" (Hawkey et al., 2017, p. 1481). However, despite this, some migrant and refugee women have disclosed being shy, embarrassed, or unsure about when to talk to their daughters about menstruation, which suggests that some migrant and refugee mothers need information and support to facilitate their daughters' menarcheal transition (Hawkey et al., 2017).

The virginity imperative: premarital sex as taboo

Across sociocultural settings and epochs, constructions of normative sexuality vary and influence women's subjective experiences of sexual identity and sexual practices (Weeks, 2014). Past research with recent migrant and refugee women has shown that traditional cultural and religious views towards premarital sexuality and virginity continue to be upheld following migration; premarital sex is often positioned as "not permissible at all" and "a sin and … a major mistake" (Hawkey, Ussher, & Perz, 2017, p. 6; Wray, Ussher, & Perz, 2014). In addition to remaining virginal until marriage, women have described the expectation that they will maintain ignorance of all things of a sexual nature, including the avoidance of conversations about sex, which they positioned as "bad" or "shameful," and social segregation from men (Hawkey et al., 2017; Ussher et al., 2012).

Transgression of the virginity imperative has been found to put women at risk of severe consequences, such as family exclusion, a loss of reputation, stigmatisation, and violence; participants in our study said that "nobody will respect her in society" and that "people start saying, 'she is a used woman, so I am not going to marry her'" (Hawkey et al., 2017, p. 7). Following migration, negotiating cultural differences regarding virginity has been described as difficult by some young Muslim women living in Australia, given they must balance meanings and expression of sexuality according to Islam, the Muslim culture of their community, and the Australian culture (Meldrum, Liamputtong, & Wollersheim, 2014). Other migrant women living in Australia and Canada have given accounts that suggest resistance to the virginity imperative and stated that this expectation is not fair to women, particularly given that men's behaviour and sexual practices prior to marriage are not under such scrutiny (Hawkey et al., 2017).

Meanings of virginity among migrant and refugee women have been reported in both an abstract manner (e.g., as representing purity, cleanliness, and honour) and as the material presence of a vaginal hymen (Hawkey et al., 2017). However, the focus on the hymen as "proof" of virginity puts pressure on women to bleed following first coitus, which leaves women vulnerable to anxiety, violence, depression, and family ostracism if bleeding does not occur (Cinthio, 2015; Hawkey et al., 2017). For example, one Afghan participant in our study said, "I'm very worried. I know I should bleed, but … when the girls talk about this issue, I get kind of nerve-wracking in my body … this sort of thing is a big part of my life" (Hawkey et al., 2017, p. 1123). In European countries which host migrant communities, healthcare professionals are increasingly being asked questions regarding virginity, including requests to perform hymen reconstructions or to provide virginity certificates to culturally diverse young women, many of whom are from migrant or refugee backgrounds (Essén, Blomkvist, Helström, & Johnsdotter, 2010; Tschudin et al., 2013). Such requests go against official health policy, and healthcare professionals have described being in an ethical dilemma; if they do not carry out such procedures, they are concerned the young woman involved would be subject to honour-related violence (Juth, Tännsjö, Hansson, & Lynöe, 2013). This situation suggests a need to integrate education about virginity into sexual health information for new migrant and refugee women and men, their families, and community leaders (Hawkey et al., 2017). This education should challenge the construction of the hymen as a tangible structure that can verify virginity, as has been done in a European context (Magnusson, 2009).

Given that premarital virginity remains important across a number of cultural contexts, young or unmarried women may be prohibited from accessing appropriate sexual health services, as being seen at a clinic could jeopardise their personal or family's reputation (Beck, Majumdar, Estcourt, & Petrak, 2005; Rogers & Earnest, 2015). They may also avoid contraception use as they fear their parents may discover that they are sexually active (Watts et al., 2014). Similarly, in culturally diverse communities that promote premarital virginity, preventative measures (e.g., HPV vaccination) may be seen as inappropriate or not necessary for young and unmarried women, as chastity in itself is seen as protection against disease (Forster et al., 2017; Salad et al., 2015). Vaccination may also be avoided as parents believe it may result in daughters engaging in promiscuous behaviours due to the protection it offers (Mupandawana & Cross, 2016). In some communities, parents may be reluctant to talk about sexual health with their children (Botfield, Zwi, Rutherford, & Newman, 2018; Dean et al., 2017), or may discourage their daughters from receiving sexual health education, as it is thought to encourage premarital sexual behaviour (Ussher et al., 2012). These findings indicate that ethnic minority migrant and refugee women may be vulnerable to negative sexual health outcomes, due to poor use of sexual health services, lack of knowledge, and social stigma associated with the discussion of sexuality (Hawkey et al., 2017; Wray et al., 2014).

Marital sexual duty: silencing sexual desire and pain

Although premarital sex is often prohibited for migrant and refugee women, marital sex has been reported to be an imperative and described as a "duty" and "the meaning of marriage" within religious and cultural discourse (Ussher et al., 2012, 2017, p. 1911). For example, amongst some Iranian migrant women, sexual obedience is considered a religious duty that is symbolic of idealised Muslim femininity and an indicator of modesty or self-respect (Khoei, Whelan, & Cohen, 2008). A number of migrant and refugee women have also disclosed having experienced sexual discomfort or pain but have felt unable to communicate it to their partners (Ussher et al., 2012). For example, a participant in our study stated, "I feel pain in my vagina ... I can't talk to my husband or complain ... In my culture its shame to talk about this pain, it is considered a normal [part] of having sex" (Ussher et al., 2017, p. 1912). Migrant and refugee women have also said that they have limited knowledge of solutions to address sexual pain and are reluctant to seek medical attention (Hawkey, Ussher, & Perz, 2018b). These experiences are not confined to migrant and refugee women, as a significant proportion of women in the general population have also stated that they did not seek help from a healthcare professional for sexual pain (Berman et al., 2003). Addressing pain during sex is important as a rights-based issue (i.e., women are entitled to pain-free sex), but is also important in relation to women's sexual subjectivity, as sexual pain is often associated with shame, distress, and feelings of inadequacy as a woman (Ayling & Ussher, 2008).

Some migrant and refugee women have also told us that idealised femininity requires women to supress their own sexual desires, and women have only rarely given accounts of expression of their own sexual desire (Hawkey et al., 2018b). Some migrant women's accounts suggest the internalisation of a critical male gaze (Fredrickson & Roberts, 1997) in explaining their inability to disclose their desire for sex, as a husband "would think about it as inappropriate [to initiate sex], therefore it is better to stay silent" (Hawkey et al., 2018b). Adoption of gendered sexual scripts, wherein women are positioned as passive and receptive to the needs of men, has implications for sexual health, including negative impacts on women's sexual arousal (Sanchez, Kiefer, & Ybarra, 2006), decreased sexual-risk knowledge (Curtin et al, 2011), and sexual coercion, which is strongly associated with women's experiences of unintended pregnancy (Rowe et al., 2016).

In contrast to these findings, Connor et al. (2016) found that Muslim Somali migrant women generally had the right to refuse unwanted sexual encounters, particularly those which are religiously prohibited (e.g., oral or anal sex) and that within Islam married women have the right to seek sexual satisfaction from their husbands. Similar findings were reported amongst Muslim women in our study who positioned sexual pleasure as a religious right as it "says it in the Koran" (Hawkey et al., 2018b). Migration to Western contexts has been found to challenge traditional patriarchal norms of sexuality; it has resulted, for example, in Iranian women demanding sexual satisfaction for themselves (Ahmadi, 2003) and migrant and refugee women's increased ability to refuse unwanted sex (Hawkey et al., 2018b). These findings suggest that exposure to different sexual ideologies and a discourse of sexual rights may facilitate women's ability to negotiate sexual agency.

Negotiating contraception use for fertility control

In a number of industrialised Western countries, migrant and refugee women are less likely than native-born women to use any form of contraception (Omland, Ruths, & Diaz, 2014; Wiebe, 2013). They are also more likely than native-born women to report using less effective methods of contraception, such as condoms, withdrawal, and the rhythm method (Family Planning NSW, 2013; Richters et al., 2016). Mazza et al. (2012) found that women in Australia who spoke a language other than English were 50% less likely than women in English-speaking households to have had contraceptive consultations with a general practitioner. This is similar to findings in the Netherlands, where migrant and refugee women had significantly fewer general practitioner consultations where contraception was discussed or prescribed than was the case for native-born women (Raben & van Den Muijsenbergh, 2018). Within some communities, such as Sri Lankan migrants in Australia, women (and men) are less likely to have heard of more effective means of contraception, and are more likely to disclose having difficulty in accessing helpful contraception advice, than are Australian-born women and men (Ellawela et al., 2017). Research in a number of European countries which host migrant and refugee women also shows higher rates of abortion in migrant than in native-born women (Goosen, Uitenbroek, Wijsen, & Stronks, 2009; Rodriguez-Alvarez, Borrell, González-Rábago, Martín, & Lanborena, 2016) or a higher prevalence of repeat abortions; this finding has also been reflected amongst migrant women in Canada (Fisher et al., 2005).

Qualitative research with migrant and refugee women has shown that women often arrive in their host countries with limited knowledge about contraception and the reproductive body (Hawkey, Ussher, & Perz, 2018a; Watts et al., 2014). For instance, women in our study stated that they "don't know anything" and have "zero awareness" or "no idea" about contraception (Hawkey et al., 2018a). One reason migrant women believe contributes to their lack of sexual and reproductive health knowledge is that talking about sex is viewed as sinful or inappropriate, and thus is avoided in the family context (Quelopana & Alcalde, 2014). Similarly, young African migrant mothers living in Australia have reported that their parents are often not knowledgeable about contraception, retain strong cultural beliefs about its use, and are not comfortable discussing it with their daughters, thereby greatly impeding their ability to provide informed guidance and support (Rogers & Earnest, 2014; Watts, McMichael, & Liamputtong, 2015). Traditional cultural values may also mean that parents deny that their children are sexually active outside of wedlock, and believe that knowledge of contraception would lead to the initiation of sexual relationships (Rogers & Earnest, 2014; Watts et al., 2015). Migrant and refugee women have also reported a lack of cultural competency and ineffective communication with healthcare professionals when they have attended health services for family planning advice (Degni, Koivusilta, & Ojanlatva, 2006; Rogers & Earnest, 2014), which further limits their opportunities to learn about effective contraceptive methods.

Some migrant and refugee women are aware of contraception options, but this does not mean they are always utilised (Hawkey et al., 2018a; Watts et al., 2014). Fear about contraception's side effects and efficacy and negative experiences of use shape women's willingness to use hormonal methods of fertility control (Kolak, Jensen, & Johansson, 2017; Rogers & Earnest, 2014). For example, even when young women are having unprotected sex and risk pregnancy, contraception may be avoided as it is feared to result in infertility (Watts et al., 2014). For women from cultures with a strong motherhood imperative, this is a major deterrent to its use; participants in our study have stated that, "we didn't want to use contraceptives because through my friends I knew it can mess up conceiving" (Hawkey et al., 2018a). Other fears and misconceptions associated with contraception use include weight gain, irregular menstrual cycles, cancer, and the irreversibility of specific contraception methods (Hawkey et al., 2018a; Watts et al., 2014). Such fears contribute to avoiding advice in relation to effective or continuous use of contraception, which leads to unintended pregnancies (Watts et al., 2014).

Gender dynamics also influence the acceptability of contraception use amongst women in migrant and refugee communities (Kolak et al., 2017; Rogers & Earnest, 2014). Healthcare professionals have observed that, even when migrant and refugee women are knowledgeable about their contraceptive options, their husbands do not always consent to its use (Kolak et al., 2017; Mengesha, Perz, Dune, & Ussher, 2017). Migrant women have also described experiences of forced sex, pregnancy coercion, and control over the use of contraception, which severely restricts women's reproductive autonomy (Quelopana & Alcalde, 2014). The use of contraception by women in some migrant communities has also been positioned as problematic because it is associated with promiscuity (Drummond, Mizan, & Wright, 2008; Watts et al., 2014). For example, West African migrant women in Australia have reported that, if their partner suggests using a condom, this may indicate that he is suspicious about her past sexual behaviour (Drummond et al., 2008). Similarly, young African Australian mothers fear that men in their sexual relationships will see contraceptive use as evidence of sexual experience or of the intention to cheat on them with other men (Watts et al., 2015).

Religion also shapes the acceptability of contraception use for fertility control in a number of migrant and refugee communities (Degni et al., 2006; Rogers & Earnest, 2014). Some migrant and refugee women have stated that, under Islam, women are not permitted to control their family size (Allotey et al., 2004; Hawkey et al., 2018a); contraception is associated with "killing" and "punishment" from God if they were to use it (Degni et al., 2006, p. 195). Young Latinas living in the U.S., who are predominantly Catholic, have described being influenced by their family's religious beliefs, where birth control is prohibited, stigmatised, and looked down upon (Gilliam, Warden, & Tapia, 2004). Although religion is an important factor in contraception decision-making within a portion of the general population in resettlement countries such as Australia, past research suggests that, in some migrant communities, it is more likely to influence fertility and contraceptive choices than it is among native-born Australians (Ellawela et al., 2017).

It is important to note, however, that not all migrant and refugee women experience restrictions to contraception use or describe negative experiences in relation to contraception use for fertility control. Some migrant and refugee women have reported positive impacts of contraception use on their health, particularly in relation to childbirth spacing and the management of heavy menstrual flow (Hawkey et al., 2018a; Rogers & Earnest, 2014). Others have described its acceptability and use to postpone pregnancies, as women wanted to continue their education (Degni et al., 2006). Women from migrant and refugee communities have also reported that migration to countries such as the U.S. and Australia has facilitated access to information and methods of contraception unavailable in their home countries, which made them feel more empowered about their reproductive choices (Hawkey et al., 2018a; Quelopana & Alcalde, 2014). It is important that healthcare professionals recognise migrant and refugee women's different constructions and experiences of contraception and provide individualised sexual and reproductive care that avoids stereotypical constructions often attached to specific cultural or religious groups (Srikanthan & Reid, 2008).

Cervical cancer screening amongst migrant and refugee women

Women from migrant and refugee backgrounds are less likely to take part in cervical cancer screening, and they have higher rates of cancer than native-born women (Aminisani, Armstrong, & Canfell, 2012; Downs, Smith, Scarinci, Flowers, & Parham, 2008). Barriers to screening include women's perception of their risk of cervical cancer (Brown, Wilson, Boothe, & Harris, 2011), as well as limited understanding of cancer and screening (Abdullahi, Copping, Kessel, Luck, & Bonell, 2009). For instance, some women in our study said that the reason they did not get screened was "lack of knowledge … we don't know what it is … how much is that important for us" and that they "don't know anything about them, it's very shocking" (Ussher et al., 2017, p. 1913). Other reasons for non-engagement with screening amongst migrant women include embarrassment, fear of or misconceptions about screening (Gany, Herrera, Avallone, & Changrani, 2006), fatalistic beliefs that undermine prevention (Ghebre et al., 2015), and mistrust related to healthcare engagement (Ussher et al., 2012). This suggests that, to improve screening rates, community-based strategies aimed at increasing women's health literacy, allaying women's fears about screening, and incorporating women's various belief systems into explanation and communications for cervical screening is critical (Cullerton et al., 2016).

Migration and menopause: changing cultural boundaries

The symbolic meanings attached to the menopause may change drastically as a result of migration and modernisation (Hall, Callister, Berry, & Matsumura, 2007), which makes it an important topic in migrant and refugee women's health. For example, Macedonian migrant women living in Australia stated that they had neither heard of, or experienced symptoms of, menopause prior migration (Strezova et al., 2017). Further, women from the Indian sub-continent who had migrated to the U.K. reported vasomotor and psychological symptoms similar to those of White women living in the U.K., in contrast to women from the same cultural background who had remained in India and who reported low levels of symptomatology (Hunter, Gupta, Papitsch-Clark, & Sturdee, 2009). This suggests that acculturation may affect the construction and experience of menopause for migrant and refugee women (Sommer et al., 1999).

Migrant women may need to negotiate contradictory meanings of menopause in their country of origin and their host country (Ussher, Hawkey, & Perz, 2019), as part of making sense of novel or modified notions of embodiment (Spitzer, 2009). In a study of Korean women who had migrated to the United States, menopause was reported to be an ambivalent experience, associated with the end of womanhood due to failing fertility, but also an unspoken experience, due to cultural taboos against talking about menstruation and sexuality (Im & Meleis, 2000). Similar findings of silencing were reported by migrant and refugee women in Australia and Canada, where menopause was described by Sudanese women as "Sin Al Ya-iss," which translates to "age of despair" (Ussher et al., 2019). Among Italian migrant women in Australia, "cambiamento di vita" (the change of life) is constructed and experienced as a time of vulnerability, as the positive roles that they had expected to take on as older women in Italy remain unrealised in Australia and led to menopause being positioned as "a time of sorrow for a life left behind" (Richters, 1997).

However, migrant and refugee women do challenge negative constructions or experiences of menopause; they resist the positioning of the menopausal woman as abject, and menopause as a deficiency disease. For example, some participants in our study said that "after menopause life starts" and that it is "the beginning of the second stage," which is a "natural" transition that they were "curious" about (Ussher et al., 2019). Women in our study also positioned the cessation of menstruation associated with menopause as a positive experience and associated the absence of fertility with a reduction in worries about the need to use effective means of contraception. Other women, such as Chilean migrants in Canada, have reported that menopause is insignificant compared with the trials of immigration and exile; although they adopted the biomedical discourse familiar from their home country, they resisted biomedical intervention in the form of hormone therapy, and many saw menopause as a time of self-reflection, or a new beginning (Spitzer, 2009). Macedonian women living in Australia report that although talk of sexuality for young women is taboo within their cultural contexts, some found the experience of menopause liberating, as they had a new-found "freedom of speech" that came with getting older (Strezova et al., 2017, p. 311).

Resistance to negative discourse about menopause has been associated with reproductive health education and more open communication about menopausal changes experienced by women following migration (Ussher et al., 2019). However, a number of studies that explore migrant and refugee women's experiences of menopause have found that women often have inadequate knowledge in relation to changes to the reproductive body in later life; with women stating that they had received little or no information, even following migration (Strezova et al., 2017; Ussher et al., 2019). Given that education and reproductive health information can facilitate affirming aspects of menopause for migrant and refugee women and ease the severity of symptoms experienced by women (Rotem, Kushnir, Levine, & Ehrenfeld, 2005), it is important that migrant and refugee women have access to culturally tailored menopause information and education. When providing education about menopause, health care professionals and community workers should also assess cultural beliefs and knowledge, and demonstrate respect for those beliefs, as well as assess women's desire for further information and intervention options (Hall et al., 2007).

Conclusion

We have highlighted the ways in which religious beliefs and cultural traditions intersect to regulate migrant and refugee women and their sexual and reproductive bodies. This begins at puberty, where a discourse of shame, secrecy, and silence often prohibits women from learning about their reproductive bodies at menarche. It continues through adulthood, and serves to inhibit young women from exploring themselves as sexual beings (at least prior to marriage) and shapes the ways in which they can express themselves sexually. It also strongly influences women's autonomy in contraception choices and informs women's embodiment at menopause. However, migrant and refugee women are not simply positioned within existing discourses; they re-position themselves, variably adopting, resisting, negotiating, and tailoring discourses and practices associated with sexual and reproductive health in order to achieve a desired sexual subjectivity and acquire a degree of sexual agency (Day, Johnson, Milnes, & Rickett, 2010, p. 238). Thus, migrant and refugee women are not voiceless victims, rather they are active agents working to determine and engage in their own sexual and reproductive rights.

It is important not to position the West as a utopia for women's sexual and reproductive health and rights. As stated by Hélie (2012), women's "bodily rights, sexual conduct and gender expression are regulated in all societies" (p. 1). For instance, young Western women's sexuality continues to be regulated through the persistence of the sexual double standard and the "threat" of a negative sexual reputation (Farvid, Braun, & Rowney, 2017).

Women are now also "expected" to experience sexual pleasure and desire, and they are pathologised if they experience an absence of desire (Tiefer, 2003). Cultural scripts in the West also dictate that women are required to provide their (male) partners with sexual access to their bodies (Fahs, 2011), such that women often describe narratives of obligatory or coerced sex (Gavey, 2005). These findings demonstrate that regulation of women's sexual and reproductive health is not limited to migrant and refugee populations, but occurs across cultural contexts within different rubrics of sociocultural discourses, many of which can have serious consequences for the health and well-being of women.

What we have highlighted in this chapter is that migrant and refugee women in particular are at risk of experiencing unmet sexual and reproductive health needs and negative health outcomes due to sociocultural norms that contribute to the potential for inadequate knowledge and low uptake of sexual health services. This shows the need for healthcare providers, in consultation with communities and community leaders, to develop culturally appropriate and spiritually significant sexual health promotion initiatives (Heard, Auvaa, & Pickering, 2015), to draw on approaches that are tailored for specific cultures (Beiser, 2005), and to ensure that services are accessible to all migrant and refugee women at resettlement, irrespective of their sociocultural background or category of migration (McMichael & Gifford, 2009).

Sexual and reproductive health information needs to be provided in a range of modalities to meet women's diverse needs (Ussher et al., 2017). The focus should be not only on health education and increasing women's knowledge, but also on understanding the sociocultural constraints that may impede knowledge and behaviour (Aggleton & Campbell, 2000). Migrant and refugee women and their sexual and reproductive health needs should be treated holistically, with a focus on the whole person within her sociocultural context (Maleku & Aguirre, 2014).

References

Abdullahi, A., Copping, J., Kessel, A., Luck, M., & Bonell, C. (2009). Cervical screening: Perceptions and barriers to uptake among Somali women in Camden. *Public Health*, *123*(10), 680–685.

Aggleton, P. & Campbell, C. (2000). Working with young people: Towards an agenda for sexual health. *Sexual and Relationship Therapy*, *15*(3), 283–296.

Ahmadi, N. (2003). Migration challenges views on sexuality. *Ethnic and Racial Studies*, *26*, 684–706.

Allotey, P., Manderson, L., Baho, S., & Demian, L. (2004). Reproductive health for resettling refugee and migrant women. *Health Issues*, *78*, 12–17.

Aminisani, N., Armstrong, B. K., & Canfell, K. (2012). Cervical cancer screening in Middle Eastern and Asian migrants to Australia: A record linkage study. *Cancer Epidemiology*, *36*(6), e394–e400.

Ayling, K. & Ussher, J. M. (2008). "If sex hurts, am I still a woman?" The subjective experience of vulvodynia in hetero-sexual women. *Archives of Sexual Behavior*, *37*(2), 294–304.

Beck, A., Majumdar, A., Estcourt, C., & Petrak, J. (2005). "We don't really have cause to discuss these things, they don't affect us": A collaborative model for developing culturally appropriate sexual health services with the Bangladeshi community of Tower Hamlets. *Sexually Transmitted Infections*, *81*(2), 158–162.

Beiser, M. (2005). The health of immigrants and refugees in Canada. *Canadian Journal of Public Health*, *96*, S30–S44.

Benson, J., Maldari, T., Williams, J., & Hanifi, H. (2010). The impact of culture and ethnicity on women's perceived role in society and their attendant health beliefs. *InnovAiT*, *3*(6), 358–365.

Berman, L., Berman, J., Felder, S., Pollets, D., Chhabra, S., Miles, M., & Powell, J. A. (2003). Seeking help for sexual function complaints: What gynecologists need to know about the female patient's experience. *Fertility and Sterility*, *79*(3), 572–576.

Botfield, J. R., Newman, C. E., & Zwi, A. B. (2016). Young people from culturally diverse backgrounds and their use of services for sexual and reproductive health needs: A structured scoping review. *Sexual Health*, *13*(1), 1–9.

Botfield, J. R., Zwi, A. B., Rutherford, A., & Newman, C. E. (2018). Learning about sex and relation-ships among migrant and refugee young people in Sydney, Australia: "I never got the talk about the birds and the bees". *Sex Education, 18*(6), 1–16.

Brantelid, I. E., Nilvér, H., & Alehagen, S. (2014). Menstruation during a lifespan: A qualitative study of women's experiences. *Health Care for Women International, 35*(6), 600–616.

Brown, D. R., Wilson, R. M., Boothe, M. A. S., & Harris, C. E. S. (2011). Cervical cancer screening among ethnically diverse Black women: Knowledge, attitudes, beliefs, and practices. *Journal of the National Medical Association, 103*(8), 719–728.

Burr, V. (2015). *Social constructionism.* New York, NY: Routledge.

Chang, Y. T., Hayter, M., & Wu, S. C. (2010). A systematic review and meta-ethnography of the quali-tative literature: Experiences of the menarche. *Journal of Clinical Nursing, 19*, 447–460.

Chrisler, J. C. & Johnston-Robledo, I. (2018). *Woman's embodied self: Feminist perspectives on identity and image.* Washington, DC: American Psychological Association.

Cinthio, H. (2015). "You go home and tell that to my dad!" Conflicting claims and understandings on hymen and virginity. *Sexuality & Culture, 19*(1), 172–189.

Connor, J. J., Hunt, S., Finsaas, M., Ciesinski, A., Ahmed, A., & Robinson, B. B. E. (2016). Sexual health care, sexual behaviors and functioning, and female genital cutting: Perspectives from Somali women living in the United States. *The Journal of Sex Research, 53*(3), 346–359.

Costos, D., Ackerman, R., & Paradis, L. (2002). Recollections of menarche: Communication between mothers and daughters regarding menstruation. *Sex Roles, 46*(1), 49–59.

Csordas, T. (2002). *Body/meaning/healing.* Basingstoke, UK: Palgrave.

Csordas, T. (2011). Cultural phenomenology: Embodiment: Agency, sexual difference, and illness. In F. E. Mascia-Lees (Ed.), *A companion to the anthropology of the body and embodiment* (pp. 137–156). Chichester, UK: WileyBlackwell.

Cullerton, K., Gallegos, D., Ashley, E., Do, H., Voloschenko, A., Fleming, M., Ramsey, R., & Gould, T. (2016). Cancer screening education: Can it change knowledge and attitudes among cultur-ally and linguistically diverse communities in Queensland, Australia?. *Health Promotion Journal of Austra-lia, 27*(2), 140–147.

Curtin, N., Ward, L. M., Merriwether, A., & Caruthers, A. (2011). Feminity ideology and sexual health in young women: A focus on sexual knowledge, embodiment, and agency. *International Journal of Sexual Health, 23*(1), 48–62.

Day, K., Johnson, S., Milnes, K., & Rickett, B. (2010). Exploring women's agency and resistance in health-related contexts: Contributors' introduction. *Feminism & Psychology, 20*(2), 238–241.

Dean, J., Mitchell, M., Stewart, D., & Debattista, J. (2017). Intergenerational variation in sexual health attitudes and beliefs among Sudanese refugee communities in Australia. *Culture, Health & Sexuality, 19* (1), 17–31.

Degni, F., Koivusilta, L., & Ojanlatva, A. (2006). Attitudes towards and perceptions about contraceptive use among married refugee women of Somali descent living in Finland. *The European Journal of Contra-ception & Reproductive Health Care, 11*(3), 190–196.

Downs, L. S., Smith, J. S., Scarinci, I., Flowers, L., & Parham, G. (2008). The disparity of cervical cancer in diverse populations. *Gynecologic Oncology, 109*(2, Supplement), S22–S30.

Drummond, P. D., Mizan, A., & Wright, B. (2008). HIV/AIDS knowledge and attitudes among West African immigrant women in Western Australia. *Sexual Health, 5*(3), 251–259.

Ellawela, Y., Nilaweera, I., Holton, S., Rowe, H., Kirkman, M., Jordan, L., McNamee, K., Bayly, C., McBain, J., Sinnott, V., & Fisher, J. (2017). Contraceptive use and contraceptive health care needs among Sri Lankan migrants living in Australia: Findings from the Understanding Fertility Management in Contemporary Australia survey. *Sexual & Reproductive Healthcare, 12*, 70–75.

Essén, B., Blomkvist, A., Helström, L., & Johnsdotter, S. (2010). The experience and responses of Swedish health professionals to patients requesting virginity restoration (hymen repair). *Reproductive Health Matters, 18*(35), 38–46.

Fahs, B. (2011). *Performing sex: The making and unmaking of women's erotic lives.* Albany, NY: State Univer-sity of New York Press.

Fahs, B. & Swank, E. (2015). Unpacking sexual embodiment and embodied resistance. In J. DeLamater & R. F. Plante (Eds), *Handbook of the sociology of sexualities* (pp. 149–167). Cham, Switzerland: Springer.

Family Planning NSW (2013). *Reproductive and sexual health in Australia.* Ashfield, Sydney: Author. Retrieved from http://familyplanningallianceaustralia.org.au/wp-content/uploads/2015/09/rshi naust_book_webedition_1.pdf.

Farvid, P., Braun, V., & Rowney, C. (2017). "No girl wants to be called a slut!": Women, heterosexual casual sex and the sexual double standard. *Journal of Gender Studies, 26*(5), 544–560.

Fisher, W. A., Singh, S. S., Shuper, P. A., Carey, M., Otchet, F., MacLean-Brine, D., Dal Bello, D., & Gunter, J. (2005). Characteristics of women undergoing repeat induced abortion. *Canadian Medical Association Journal, 172*(5), 637–641.

Forster, A. S., Rockliffe, L., Marlow, L. A. V., Bedford, H., McBride, E., & Waller, J. (2017). Exploring human papillomavirus vaccination refusal among ethnic minorities in England: A comparative qualitative study. *Psycho-Oncology, 26*(9), 1278–1284.

Fredrickson, B. L. & Roberts, T.-A. (1997). Objectification theory: Toward understanding women's lived experiences and mental health risks. *Psychology of Women Quarterly, 21*(2), 173–206.

Gany, F. M., Herrera, A. P., Avallone, M., & Changrani, J. (2006). Attitudes, knowledge, and health-seeking behaviors of five immigrant minority communities in the prevention and screening of cancer: A focus group approach. *Ethnicity & Health, 11*(1), 19–39.

Gavey, N. (2005). *Just sex? The cultural scaffolding of rape.* New York, NY: Routledge.

Ghebre, R. G., Sewali, B., Osman, S., Adawe, A., Nguyen, H. T., Okuyemi, K. S., & Joseph, A. (2015). Cervical cancer: Barriers to screening in the Somali community in Minnesota. *Journal of Immigrant and Minority Health, 17*(3), 722–728.

Gilliam, M. L., Warden, M. M., & Tapia, B. (2004). Young latinas recall contraceptive use before and after pregnancy: A focus group study. *Journal of Pediatric and Adolescent Gynecology, 17*(4), 279–287.

Goosen, S., Uitenbroek, D., Wijsen, C., & Stronks, K. (2009). Induced abortions and teenage births among asylum seekers in the Netherlands: Analysis of national surveillance data. *Journal of Epidemiology and Community Health, 63*, 528–533.

Grzanka, P. (2018). *Intersectionality: A foundations and frontiers reader.* Abingdon, UK: Routledge.

Hall, L., Callister, L. C., Berry, J. A., & Matsumura, G. (2007). Meanings of menopause: Cultural influences on perception and management of menopause. *Journal of Holistic Nursing, 25*(2), 106–118.

Hankivsky, O., Reid, C., Cormier, R., Varcoe, C., Clark, N., Benoit, C., & Brotman, S. (2010). Exploring the promises of intersectionality for advancing women's health research. *International Journal for Equity in Health, 9*(1), 5.

Hawkey, A. J., Ussher, J. M., & Perz, J. (2017). Regulation and resistance: Negotiation of premarital sexuality in the context of migrant and refugee women. *The Journal of Sex Research, 55*(9), 1–18.

Hawkey, A. J., Ussher, J. M., & Perz, J. (2018a). "If you don't have a baby, you can't be in our culture": Migrant and refugee women's experiences and constructions of fertility and fertility control. *Women's Reproductive Health, 5*, 2.

Hawkey, A. J., Ussher, J. M., & Perz, J. (2018b). Negotiating sexual agency in marriage: The experience of migrant and refugee women. *Healthcare for Women International,* forthcoming.

Hawkey, A. J., Ussher, J. M., Perz, J., & Metusela, C. (2017). Experiences and constructions of menarche and menstruation among migrant and refugee women. *Qualitative Health Research, 27*(10), 1473–1490.

Heard, E., Auvaa, L., & Pickering, C. (2015). Love bugs: Promoting sexual health among young people in Samoa. *Health Promotion Journal of Australia, 26*(1), 30–32.

Hélie, A. (2012). Policing gender, sexuality and "Muslimness". In A. Hélie & H. Hoodfar (Eds), *Sexuality in Muslim contexts: Restrictions and resistance* (pp. 1–14). London, UK: Zed Books.

Hunter, M. S., Gupta, P., Papitsch-Clark, A., & Sturdee, D. W. (2009). Mid-aged health in women from the Indian subcontinent (MAHWIS): A further quantitative and qualitative investigation of experience of menopause in UK Asian women, compared to UK Caucasian women and women living in Delhi. *Climacteric, 12*(1), 26–37.

Im, E.-O. & Meleis, A. I. (2000). Meanings of menopause to Korean immigrant women. *Western Journal of Nursing Research, 22*(1), 84–102.

Juth, N., Tännsjö, T., Hansson, S.-O., & Lynöe, N. (2013). Honour-related threats and human rights: A qualitative study of Swedish healthcare providers' attitudes towards young women requesting a virginity certificate or hymen reconstruction. *The European Journal of Contraception & Reproductive Health Care, 18*(6), 451–459.

Khoei, E. M., Whelan, A., & Cohen, J. (2008). Sharing beliefs: What sexuality means to Muslim Iranian women living in Australia. *Culture, Health & Sexuality, 10*(3), 237–248.

Kirkman, M., Rowe, H., Hardiman, A., & Rosenthal, D. (2011). Abortion is a difficult solution to a problem: A discursive analysis of interviews with women considering or undergoing abortion in Australia. *Women's Studies International Forum, 34*(2), 121–129.

Kolak, M., Jensen, C., & Johansson, M. (2017). Midwives' experiences of providing contraception coun-selling to immigrant women. *Sexual & Reproductive Healthcare*, *12*, 100–106.

Lee, J. (1994). Menarche and the (hetero)sexualization of the female body. *Gender & Society*, *8*(3), 343–362.

Lee, J. (2009). Bodies at menarche: Stories of shame, concealment, and sexual maturation. *Sex Roles*, *60* (9–10), 615–627.

Magnusson, A. K. (2009). *Vaginal corona: Myths surrounding virginity: Your questions answered*. Stockholm, Sweden: Riksförbundet för Sexuell Upplysning (the Swedish Association for Sexuality Education). Retrieved from www.rfsu.se/globalassets/pdf/vaginal-corona-english.pdf.

Maleku, A. & Aguirre, R. T. P. (2014). Culturally competent health care from the immigrant lens: A qualitative interpretive meta-synthesis (QIMS). *Social Work in Public Health*, *29*(6), 561–580.

Marván, M., Morales, C., & Cortés-Iniestra, S. (2006). Emotional reactions to menarche among Mexican women of different generations. *Sex Roles*, *54*(5), 323–330.

Mazza, D., Harrison, C., Taft, A., Brijnath, B., Britt, H., Hobbs, M., Stewart, K., & Hussainy, S. (2012). Current contraceptive management in Australian general practice: An analysis of BEACH data. *The Medical Journal of Australia*, *197*(2), 110.

McMichael, C. & Gifford, S. (2009). "It is good to know now … before it's too late": Promoting sexual health literacy amongst resettled young people with refugee backgrounds. *Sexuality & Culture*, *13*(4), 218–236.

Meldrum, R., Liamputtong, P., & Wollersheim, D. (2014). Caught between two worlds: Sexuality and young Muslim women in Melbourne, Australia. *Sexuality & Culture*, *18*(1), 166–179.

Mendlinger, S. & Cwikel, J. (2005). Learning about menstruation: Knowledge aquisition and cultural diversity. *International Journal of Diversity in Organisations, Communities & Nations*, *5*(3), 53–62.

Mengesha, Z., Perz, J., Dune, T., & Ussher, J. (2017). Refugee and migrant women's engagement with sexual and reproductive health care in Australia: A socio-ecological analysis of health care professional perspectives. *PLoS One*, *12*(7), e0181421.

Mupandawana, E. T. & Cross, R. (2016). Attitudes towards human papillomavirus vaccination among African parents in a city in the north of England: A qualitative study. *Reproductive Health*, *13*(1), 97.

Omland, G., Ruths, S., & Diaz, E. (2014). Use of hormonal contraceptives among immigrant and native women in Norway: Data from the Norwegian prescription database. *BJOG: An International Journal of Obstetrics and Gynaecology*, *121*(10), 1221–1228.

Quelopana, A. & Alcalde, C. (2014). Exploring knowledge, belief and experiences in sexual and reproductive health in immigrant Hispanic women. *Journal of Immigrant and Minority Health*, *16*(5), 1001–1006.

Raben, L. A. D. & van Den Muijsenbergh, M. E. T. C. (2018). Inequity in contraceptive care between refugees and other migrant women? A retrospective study in Dutch general practice. *Family Practice*, *35*, 468–474.

Rade, D., Crawford, G., Lobo, R., Gray, C., & Brown, G. (2018). Sexual health help-seeking behavior among migrants from Sub-Saharan Africa and South East Asia living in high income countries: A systematic review. *International Journal of Environmental Research and Public Health*, *15*(7), 1311.

Rademakers, J., Mouthaan, I., & de Neef, M. (2005). Diversity in sexual health: Problems and dilemmas. *The European Journal of Contraception & Reproductive Health Care*, *10*(4), 207–211.

Richters, J. (1997). Menopause in different cultures. *Journal of Psychosomatic Obstetrics & Gynecology*, *18*(2), 73–80.

Richters, J., Fitzadam, S., Yeung, A., Caruana, T., Rissel, C., Simpson, J. M., & de Visser, R. O. (2016). Contraceptive practices among women: The second Australian study of health and relationships. *Contraception*, *94*(5), 548–555.

Rodriguez-Alvarez, E., Borrell, L. N., González-Rábago, Y., Martín, U., & Lanborena, N. (2016). Induced abortion in a Southern European region: Examining inequalities between native and immigrant women. *International Journal of Public Health*, *61*(7), 829–836.

Rogers, C. & Earnest, J. (2014). A cross-generational study of contraception and reproductive health among Sudanese and Eritrean women in Brisbane, Australia. *Health Care for Women International*, *35*(3), 334–356.

Rogers, C. & Earnest, J. (2015). Sexual and reproductive health communication among Sudanese and Eritrean women: An exploratory study from Brisbane, Australia. *Culture, Health & Sexuality*, *17*(2), 223–236.

Rotem, M., Kushnir, T., Levine, R., & Ehrenfeld, M. (2005). A psycho-educational program for improving women's attitudes and coping with menopause symptoms. *Journal of Obstetric, Gynecologic, & Neonatal Nursing, 34*(2), 233–240.

Rowe, J., Holton, S., Kirkman, M., Bayly, C., Jordan, L., MacNamee, K., & Fisher, J. (2016). Prevalence and distribution of unintended pregnancy: The Understanding Fertility Management in Australia National Survey. *Australia and New Zealand Journal of Public Health, 40*(2), 104–109.

Salad, J., Verdonk, P., de Boer, F., & Abma, T. A. (2015). "A Somali girl is Muslim and does not have premarital sex. Is vaccination really necessary?" A qualitative study into the perceptions of Somali women in the Netherlands about the prevention of cervical cancer. *International Journal for Equity in Health, 14*(1), 1–13.

Sanchez, D. T., Kiefer, A. K., & Ybarra, O. (2006). Sexual submissiveness in women: Costs for sexual autonomy and arousal. *Personality and Social Psychology Bulletin, 32*, 512–524.

Sommer, B., Avis, N., Meyer, P., Ory, M., Madden, T., Kagawa-Singer, M., Mouton, C., Rasor, N. O., & Adler, S. (1999). Attitudes toward menopause and aging across ethnic/racial groups. *Psychosomatic Medicine, 61*(6), 868–875.

Sommer, M., Ackatia-Armah, N., Connolly, S., & Smiles, D. (2015). A comparison of the menstruation and education experiences of girls in Tanzania, Ghana, Cambodia and Ethiopia. *Compare: A Journal of Comparative and International Education, 45*(4), 589–609.

Spitzer, D. L. (2009). Crossing cultural and bodily boundaries of migration and menopause. In L. Hernandez & S. Krajewski (Eds), *Crossing cultural boundaries: Taboo, bodies and identities* (pp. 148–158). Newcastle upon Tyne: Cambridge Scholars Publishing.

Srikanthan, A. & Reid, R. L. (2008). Religious and cultural influences on contraception. *Journal of Obstetrics and Gynaecology Canada, 30*(2), 129–137.

Strezova, A., O'Neill, S., O'Callaghan, C., Perry, A., Liu, J., & Eden, J. (2017). Cultural issues in menopause: An exploratory qualitative study of Macedonian women in Australia. *Menopause, 24* (3), 308–315.

Teitelman, A. M. (2004). Adolescent girls' perspectives of family interactions related to menarche and sexual health. *Qualitative Health Research, 14*(9), 1292–1308.

Tiefer, L. (2003). Female Sexual Dysfunction (FSD): Witnessing social construction in action 1. *Sexualities, Evolution & Gender, 5*(1), 33–36.

Tolman, D., Bowman, C. P., & Fahs, B. (2014). Sexuality and embodiment. In D. L. Tolman, L. M. Diamond, J. Bauermeister, W. H. George, J. Pfaus, & M. Ward (Eds), *Handbook of sexuality and psychology* (Vol. 1, pp. 759–804). Washington, DC: American Psychological Association Books.

Tschudin, S., Schuster, S., Dumont Dos Santos, D., Huang, D., Bitzer, J., & Leeners, B. (2013). Restoration of virginity: Women's demand and health care providers' response in Switzerland. *Journal of Sexual Medicine, 10*(9), 2334–2342.

Tsui, A. O., McDonald-Mosley, R., & Burke, A. E. (2010). Family planning and the burden of unintended pregnancies. *Epidemiologic Reviews, 32*(1), 152–174, doi:10.1093/epirev/mxq012.

Uskul, A. K. (2004). Women's menarche stories from a multicultural sample. *Social Science & Medicine, 59* (4), 667–679.

Ussher, J. M., Hawkey, A., & Perz, J. (2019). "Age of despair", or "When Life starts": Migrant and refugee women negotiate constructions of menopause. *Culture, Health & Sexuality, 21*(7), 741–756.

Ussher, J. M., Perz, J., Metusela, C., Hawkey, A. J., Morrow, M., Narchal, R., & Estoesta, J. (2017). Negotiating discourses of shame, secrecy, and silence: Migrant and refugee women's experiences of sexual embodiment. *Archives of Sexual Behavior, 46*(7), 1901–1921.

Ussher, J. M., Rhyder-Obid, M., Perz, J., Rae, M., Wong, T. W. K., & Newman, P. (2012). Purity, privacy and procreation: Constructions and experiences of sexual and reproductive health in Assyrian and Karen women living in Australia. *Sexuality & Culture, 16*(4), 467–485.

Varcoe, C., Hankivsky, O., & Morrow, M. (2007). Introduction: Beyond gender matters. In M. Morrow, O. Hankivsky, & C. Varcoe (Eds), *Women's health in Canada: Critical perspectives on theory and policy* (pp. 3–30). Toronto, Canada: University of Toronto Press.

Watts, M. C. N. C., Liamputtong, P., & Carolan, M. (2014). Contraception knowledge and attitudes: Truths and myths among African Australian teenage mothers in Greater Melbourne, Australia. *Journal of Clinical Nursing, 23*(15–16), 2131–2141.

Watts, M. C. N. C., McMichael, C., & Liamputtong, P. (2015). Factors influencing contraception awareness and use: The experiences of young African Australian mothers. *Journal of Refugee Studies, 28* (3), 368–387.

Weeks, J. (2014). *Sex, politics and society: The regulations of sexuality since 1800.* New York, NY: Routledge.

World Health Organization (WHO) (2009). *Mental health aspects of women's reproductive health: A global review of the literature.* Geneva, Switzerland: Author. Retrieved from www.who.int/reproductive health/publications/general/9789241563567/en.

Wiebe, E. (2013). Contraceptive practices and attitudes among immigrant and nonimmigrant women in Canada. *Canadian Family Physician, 59*(10), e451–e455.

Wray, A., Ussher, J. M., & Perz, J. (2014). Constructions and experiences of sexual health among young, heterosexual, unmarried Muslim women immigrants in Australia. *Culture, Health & Sexuality, 16*(1), 76–89.

35

REPRODUCTIVE HEALTH DISPARITIES AMONG WOMEN EXPERIENCING HOMELESSNESS

Courtney Cronley and Shamsun Nahar

Control over one's body and reproductive health are fundamental human rights (World Health Organization, 2018b), yet women at risk of, or currently experiencing, homelessness are frequently denied this right. In fact, one of the main forces that pushes women into homelessness is reproductive health issues such as unintended pregnancy and sexual trauma (Reeve, 2018), and homelessness itself can lead to a host of negative reproductive health outcomes (Cronley, Hohn, & Nahar, 2018). Women's reproductive health requires specialized care related to pregnancy, birth, menopause, and sexual trauma; however, homeless women are often staying in environments that are ill equipped to provide this level of care (e.g., the street, a friend's couch, a shelter, a hotel). As such, homelessness presents a unique and acute health risk in regard to deleterious reproductive health behaviors and outcomes (Committee on Health Care for Women, 2013; Esen, 2017). Thus, the more we understand the association between reproductive health risks and homelessness, the more we can reduce reproductive health disparities among women in situations of homelessness and precarious housing. In this chapter, we explore the inter-relationship between homelessness and reproductive health among women globally, starting with definitions of homelessness, the scope of the problem, empirical associations with reproductive health issues, and concluding with a theoretical explanation and recommendations for mitigating the risks that homelessness poses to women's reproductive health.

Definitions of homelessness

Definitions of *homelessness* differ, often based on technicalities, policy, and funding decisions in various countries, but the United Nations Office of Human Rights (UNOHR) (2018) offered a synthesized, three-dimensional, overarching definition: Homelessness is (1) the absence of a home "both in terms of physical structure and its social aspects"; (2) "a form of systemic discrimination and social exclusion, whereby the 'homeless' become a social group subject to stigmatization"; and (3) an experience of individuals who are "resilient in the struggle for survival and dignity and potential agents of change as rights holders" (p. 1). Inherent in the UNOHR's definition is the recognition that adequate housing is a basic human right and that housing is not merely shelter but also validation of an individual's inclusion in broader society. Among women, the term "homeless" encompasses single parents with dependent children fleeing intimate partner violence, unaccompanied young women living on the street, women with partners living in emergency shelters, and older adult women staying in permanent supportive housing.

Scope of the problem

Quantifying the prevalence of homeless women worldwide is a challenging endeavor due to differences in methodologies, definitions and terminology, and when homeless counts are conducted; thus, prevalence varies widely across countries. Women account for approximately 41% of homeless people in Australia (Australian Bureau of Statistics, 2016), 40% in the United States (Henry, Watt, Rosenthal, & Shivji, 2016), 38% in Sweden (National Board of Health and Welfare, 2011), and 27.3% in Canada (Gaetz, Dej, Richter, & Redman, 2016); women accounted for 14% of people sleeping unsheltered on the street in England in 2017 (Homeless Link, 2017), and just 3% in the City of Nagoya, Japan, in 2003 (Ministry of Health, Labour, and Welfare, 2003).

In general, homeless prevalence rates for women are difficult to obtain in African, South American, and southeast Asian countries, and homelessness may appear differently in developing than in more Westernized countries. For example, urban homeless people often live in slums in developing nations; slums are characterized by challenging living conditions, poverty, housing of poor structural integrity, overcrowding, and poor access to water, sanitation and other facilities (WHO, 2018a). Homeless women in developing nations are severely disadvantaged because of social, cultural, and economic obstacles to access to education, social services, and property (Sikich, 2008). Sexual and reproductive health risks, such as high rates of unwanted pregnancies, sexually transmitted infections (STIs), and poor maternal and child health outcomes, are common among slum women due to lack of access to services and information, modern means of contraception, and skilled attendants at birth (Mberu, Mumah, Kabiru, & Brinton, 2014).

In addition, researchers have reported increasing concern about the rising prevalence of family homelessness within countries such as England (Houston, Reuschke, Sabater, Maynard, & Stewart, 2014) and Australia (Johnson, Scutella, Tseng, & Wood, 2015); in the US, homeless families are disproportionately headed by women (Gewirtz, DeGarmo, Lee, Morrell, & August, 2015; HUD, 2016), and many live with other family or friends (Hallett, 2012; U.S. Interagency Council on Homelessness, 2014), thereby avoiding traditional services and not appearing in official homelessness counts. In sum, prevalence data most likely underestimate the extent of the problem, which may lead to low public awareness and under-allocation of funding to reduce women's risks for homelessness and help women currently homeless to secure permanent housing.

Empirical associations between homelessness and reproductive health conditions

Menstruation and homelessness

Although menstruation is a basic, biological reproductive process, it becomes a physical challenge for homeless women due to lack of access to sanitary menstrual products and cultural and religious stigma surrounding menstruation (WHO, 2018c). Homeless women experience unique health injustices that result from lack of access to menstrual hygiene resources and private facilities in which to change and dispose of sanitary products (Parrillo & Edward Feller, 2017). In the US, tampons and pads are some of the least donated items to homeless shelters, and thus, many homeless women resort to using paper towels, napkins, socks, or no menstrual products at all (Meadows-Fernandez, 2017). Moreover, negative and misguided information about menstruation promotes shame, isolation, and gender discrimination around the world. In Kenya, Nepal, Malawi, India, and Iran, low-income women face additional challenges to care for their health during menstruation (Scaramella & Fagan, 2016). Due to lack of safe and affordable hygiene products, women turn to dirty cloths, foliage, scraps, mattress stuffing, and mud to care for their flow in Kenya, which often leads to infection and disease. Sometimes religiosity also promotes menstrual stigma. Lack of education and poor menstrual management contribute to consideration of menstruation as a dirty, disgraceful, and shameful act rather than a natural biological process (McNamara, 2017; Scaramella & Fagan, 2016; WHO, 2018c).

Unintended pregnancy

There appears to be a significant association between pregnancy and homelessness (Crawford, Trotter, Hartshorn, & Whitbeck, 2011; Winetrobe et al., 2013), and data from the US show that, among homeless women aged 15–44, 50–60% were pregnant in 2009 compared with about 10% of their housed peers (Halcon & Lifson, 2004). Women experiencing homelessness often report unintended pregnancies. In London, England, for example, nearly 24% of homeless women's pregnancies were unplanned in 2015 (Hogg, Haynes, Baradon, & Cuthbert, 2015).

The data indicate that the elevated risk for unintended pregnancy may be due, in part, to the desperation some women face while living on the street such that they are forced to engage in survival sex in order to procure basic needs such as food and clothing (Cronley, Cimino, Hohn, Davis, & Madden, 2016) or in exchange for drugs (Duff, Deering, Gibson, Tyndall, & Shannon, 2011; Walls & Bell, 2011). Survival sex undoubtedly entails multiple sexual partners (Halcon & Lifson, 2004) and inconsistent contraception use. Unintended pregnancy may prolong homelessness by delaying a woman's ability to secure employment and giving rise to new economic obstacles to employment, such as paying for childcare. Not all pregnancies are unintended, however; some homeless women may actually try to become pregnant in order to gain access to shelters and housing or due to a strong desire to have a family and experience motherhood (Cronley et al., 2018; Killion, 1995), often in contrast to their own disrupted childhoods.

Pregnancy complications

Not surprisingly, many homeless women who become pregnant report difficult pregnancies (Scappaticci & Blay, 2009) and are ill prepared for childbirth (Cronley et al., 2018; Esen, 2017). Women experiencing homelessness report higher rates of pregnancy terminations, both spontaneous (i.e., miscarriages) and planned (i.e., abortions), while homeless than do their non-homeless peers (Begun, 2015; Ensign, 2000). For some homeless women, pregnancy terminations can be particularly high-risk in that they have reported ending unintended pregnancies through self-induced (Ensign, 2000) or forced (Cronley et al., 2018) abortions. This may be due, in part, to significant obstacles to healthy prenatal behaviors, such as maintaining optimal dietary intake and accessing adequate prenatal care (Moore,

2014; Richards, Merrill, & Baksh, 2011). Research indicates that the stress and negative emotions related to homelessness influence women's feelings about their pregnancies, perhaps leading to reduced intentionality to engage in positive health behaviors (Kennedy, Grewal, Roberts, Steinauer, & Dehlendorf, 2014; Moore, 2014).

Ake and colleagues (2018) found that women who were pregnant while homeless lacked access to education (e.g., Lamaze classes) to promote healthy perinatal behaviors. Issues such as costs and logistics such as clinic locations (Bloom, Canning, & Sevilla, 2004) and transportation (Ake et al., 2018) constitute additional barriers to adequate perinatal health care. Moreover, some women report choosing not to utilize perinatal care due to perceived stigma from health care providers (Gelberg, Browner, Lejano, & Arangua, 2004; Milligan et al., 2002). They are sensitive to issues of discrimination based on their social class and living conditions, and to negative judgments based on their health behaviors such as inconsistent or lack of contraception use (Kennedy et al., 2014) or multiple sexual partners (Halcon & Lifson, 2004). Ironically, one study showed that pregnancy was a deterrent to staying at a shelter due to the perceived health risk posed by the shelter environment (Ha, Narendorf, Santa Maria, & Bezette-Flores, 2015). The reluctance to stay in a shelter could lead to under-engagement in services such as case management and referrals designed to facilitate health care access. Some homeless individuals report an inability to prioritize health due to competing demands (Koh & O'Connell, 2016), and shelter-related obstacles that impede access to reproductive health care services and the use of contraception may further diminish women's perceptions of autonomy over their decisions and life outcomes. Furthermore, pre-existing conditions such as STIs (Haley, Roy, Leclerc, Boudreau, & Boivin, 2004; Thompson, Bender, Lewis, & Watkins, 2008), mental illness (Crawford et al., 2011; Scappaticci & Blay, 2009), and substance abuse (Hathazi, Lankenau, Sanders, & Bloom, 2009; Scappaticci & Blay, 2009) may affect women's health during pregnancy and the health of their babies.

Pregnancy outcomes

It is not surprising, given the prenatal risks, that pregnancy outcomes for homeless women are worse than those of their consistently housed peers (Cutts et al., 2015; Merrill, Richards, & Sloan, 2011; Richards et al., 2011). When women lack permanent housing, they experience psycho-emotional stress, depression, and anxiety, which heighten their risk for adverse reproductive health and child outcomes, such as shorter gestation, lower fetal neurodevelopment, and persistent mental health problems among children (Crawford et al., 2011; Schetter & Tanner, 2012). Multiple studies have identified homelessness as an independent risk factor for low birth weight (Committee on Health Care for Underserved Women, 2013; Cutts et al., 2015; Merrill et al., 2011), and severity of homelessness has been associated with more adverse birth outcomes (Stein, Lu, & Gelberg, 2000). Factors such as untreated mental illness and addictions may impede women's abilities to maintain health care or place some women at high risk of postpartum depression. Moreover, babies whose mothers were using drugs while pregnant are often born with drug-dependence (Tolia et al., 2015).

New mothers who are homeless may also find it difficult to engage in proactive postnatal behaviors. For example, a national survey in the US showed that women experiencing homelessness during pregnancy were less likely to breastfeed or did so for a shorter duration than their non-homeless peers (Richards et al., 2011), and sustained lack of health care access among homeless families exacerbates infants' health conditions and may lead to long-term and permanent health problems (Koh & O'Connell, 2016). Finally, some data indicate that the intersection of minority status with homelessness intensifies reproductive health dis-parities; US studies show that Black and Latina women who are homeless while pregnant have worse pregnancy experiences and outcomes (e.g., low birth weight child, preterm labor, vaginal bleeding, nausea, kidney/bladder infections) than their White peers (Commit-tee on Health Care for Underserved Women, 2013; Cutts et al., 2015; Merrill et al., 2011).

Reproductive cancers

Homeless women have higher rates of reproductive and breast cancers than housed women do (Gawron et al., 2017), and data from some studies show that they are at elevated risk for cervical cancer (Asgary et al., 2016; Wittenberg et al., 2015). These risks are due in part to lower rates of cancer screening (Chau et al., 2002; Teruya et al., 2010; Weinreb, Goldberg, & Lessard, 2002). Women may find it particularly difficult to access and/or prioritize pre-ventative health care, such as cancer screenings, when they are facing significant logistical and economic obstacles and are preoccupied with trying to meet their daily needs, such as food, clothing, and shelter (Koh & O'Connell, 2016). Treatment for cervical and other reproductive cancers is of particular concern for women because, when left untreated, they nearly always lead to infertility (Levine, Kelvin, Quinn, & Gracia, 2015).

Reproductive health traumas

Reproductive health-related trauma is disturbingly common among homeless women, including forced abortions, rape and sexual assault, and survival sex (Cronley et al., 2018; Goodman, Fels, & Glenn, 2006). Results from a prevalence study in the US showed that nearly every woman living on the street (92%) had experienced severe physical and/or sexual violence at some point in her life (Browne & Bassuk, 1997); a sample of homeless individuals in five US cities indicated that women were at greater risk than men of rape and prolonged suffering from violence (Meinbresse et al., 2014). Sexual assault increases the risk of unprotected sex, and thus elevates women's risks for HIV/AIDs and STIs, as well as mental health outcomes such as post-traumatic stress disorder and substance abuse (Coker et al., 2002; Jordan, Campbell, & Follingstad, 2010). Sexual trauma is also associated with an increased risk of death from homicide (Campbell, 2002). Moreover, sexual assault increases homeless women's risk for unintended pregnancy and/or birth control sabotage, as well as for spontaneous miscarriage (Campbell, 2002; Johri et al., 2011). Women who are victims of sexual violence during pregnancy are more likely to develop postnatal depression (Luder-mir, Lewis, Valongueiro, de Araújo, & Araya, 2010) and pregnancy-related physical symp-toms (Lukasse, Henriksen, Vangen, & Schei, 2012). In addition, the WHO (2013) reported that sexual violence also appears to increase the risk for poor infant outcomes, such as low birth weight, premature birth, growth restriction in utero, and/or small for gestational age.

Overcoming barriers

Despite the reproductive health challenges that homeless women face within the context of structural barriers and, for minority homeless women, multiplicative risks based on race, class, gender, or religion, research suggests that these women are resourceful and engage in a variety of coping strategies to mitigate the negative effects of their circumstances (Cron-ley et al., 2018; Little, Gorman, Dzendoletas, & Moravac, 2007; Moore, 2014; Ruttan, Laboucane-Benson, & Munro, 2012). In fact, becoming pregnant can motivate women to try to get off the street (Killion, 1995; Ruttan et al., 2012) and may incentivize them to cease substance use and seek family reunification (Keys, 2007). For example, one study showed that homeless women who were pregnant reported pregnancy as a reason to persist in the face of previously insurmountable bureaucratic obstacles to obtain permanent housing (Ha et al., 2015).

Health interventions can also help women to overcome challenges and access care sooner. Wood and Watts (2005) recommended training midwives in models of trauma-informed care with high-risk patients such as women who are homeless while pregnant. These health care providers may be more attuned to the issues that complicate homeless women's access to and utilization of health care, including perceptions of stigma, histories of sexual trauma, and limited economic resources. Furthermore, practitioners seeking to improve women's reproductive health outcomes can reduce more practical logistical barriers to care such as transportation by providing bus or train passes or by bringing health care to the streets and shelters.

Some communities have begun utilizing peer navigators to help homeless individuals to access health care (e.g., Bishop, Edwards, & Nadkarni, 2009; Corrigan et al., 2017; Sarango, de Groot, Hirschi, Umeh, & Rajabium, 2017). The peer navigator model borrows from patient navigator models, which were designed to help reduce health disparities in situations such as cancer care for under-served populations (Gabram et al., 2008; Natale-Pereira, Enard, Nevarez, & Jones, 2011). Peer navigators assist clients in accessing health care, as well as advocating for clients and potentially mitigating real and perceived stigma that under-served populations face in health care settings. Given that women in several studies reported (Gelberg et al., 2004; Milligan et al., 2002) eschewing health care while pregnant and homeless due to stigma, peer navigators may be a particularly promising innovation for improving reproductive health outcomes this population. Moreover, minority women in most countries are at increased risk for both homelessness and poor health outcomes, so peer navigators would be able to help women overcome the exponential stigma and disparate care associated with their multiplicative positions of disadvantage.

Social determinants of health and risks to reproductive health among homeless women

The theory of social determinants of health (SDH; Marmot, Friel, Bell, Houweling, & Taylor, 2009) helps to explain how homelessness is associated with poor reproductive health outcomes among women. According to SDH, past and current life circumstances at individual, local, and national levels interact to shape people's health outcomes and contribute to disparities. These may include one's gender, race, education, and employment status, as well as factors of the built environment such as neighborhood safety and proximity to health care, and state-level laws and regulations that ensure basic standards of living and provide funding for social welfare programs (Marmot et al., 2009).

Health, access to quality health care, and homelessness are all correlated with poverty, social systems, and minority status. According to the theory of SDH, states with better social welfare programs tend to show more equitable distribution of wealth and fewer health disparities (Marmot et al., 2009). One of the key social welfare programs is housing. At its core, homelessness is a structural issue of inadequate housing supply and lack of state intervention to mitigate this shortage; individuals who have lower income, particularly women and minority status populations, are at disproportionate risk for housing disadvantage due to social exclusion and social and structural conditions, such as lower educational attainment

(Cronley et al., 2018; Hurlbut, Robbins, & Hoke, 2011), lower-paying jobs, and insufficient social welfare programs (UNOHR, 2018).

These disparities among women draw attention to the issue of intersectionality (Cho, Crenshaw, & McCall, 2013; Crenshaw, 1989) within SDH and the idea that some individuals inhabit a position of multiplicative risks due to combinations of gender, race, and income status. Moreover, these same factors are also risks for poor reproductive health outcomes (Marmot, Allen, Bell, Bloomer, & Goldblatt, 2012). For example, minority race, at least within the US, appears to correlate with a higher risk of homelessness (Henry, Watt, Rosenthal, & Shivji, 2017). Thus, when a minority woman experiences homelessness, finding herself at the intersection of poverty and an inadequate housing safety net in conjunction with gender-based health disparities, she may be at disparately high risk for poor reproductive health outcomes.

Researchers who study the association between homelessness and reproductive health tend to emphasize women's individual behaviors during episodes of homelessness and housing instability and devote less attention to structural factors. In fact, the intersection of housing policies, housing discrimination, employment policies, and social welfare policies may be equally, if not more, critical to women's long-term reproductive health and housing security than individual behaviors. Prevention and intervention efforts aimed at policy- and state-level targets, in combination with individually focused interventions, may produce the greatest reduction in reproductive health disparities among women who are homeless and precariously housed. Such efforts include increasing housing affordability and supply, expanding health and social welfare benefits, providing access to care, expanding high-quality education and employment opportunities for women, and offering services such as subsidized childcare and transportation, which homeless women report as critical ancillary services to exiting homelessness (Denton & Walters, 1999; Lantz et al., 1998; Viner et al., 2012).

Summary

The association between pregnancy, particularly unintended pregnancy, and homelessness underscores the incontrovertible importance of providing women with equitable access to reliable and safe contraception, both as a means of promoting upward economic mobility and preventing health disparities, prolonged poverty, and homelessness. Given that many homeless women have reported having felt forced to engage in risky sexual behaviors, it is critical that communities and service providers expand access to reproductive and sexual health care and contraception within homeless environments. Harm-reduction strategies such as contraception education may empower women to engage in proactive sexual and reproductive health behaviors and thus prevent and minimize negative reproductive health outcomes such as unintended pregnancy, STIs, and diseases such as cervical cancer, which place women at extremely high risk for infertility.

Moreover, policy changes must be attuned to how the intersection of gender, race, and class plays a role in social exclusion, risks for housing insecurity and homelessness, unintended pregnancy, and poor reproductive and sexual health outcomes. Expanding the supply of affordable, quality housing may enable women who become homeless while pregnant to access permanent housing more rapidly and help promote proactive reproductive health behaviors. Providing attendant social welfare benefits (e.g., subsidized childcare and transportation, income support) is critical to helping mothers trying to leave homelessness. Particularly in capitalist, free-market economic systems with limited labor regulations, these ancillary benefits support a woman's independence when she may be working a low-wage job and lacking adequate social support. Finally, systems must be attuned to how women of minority status in situations of homelessness may be at heightened risk for poor reproductive health outcomes; thus, any potential solutions must address racial, ethnic, and religious barriers to housing and healthcare, in addition to those that exist due to gender inequities. Ultimately, the global empirical evidence shows that housing insecurity creates substantial reproductive health vulnerabilities and that minority women and their children are at highest risk for the negative outcomes. In order to uphold the WHO's (2018b) definition of reproductive health as a fundamental human right for all women, housing must become part of the public health approach to reducing reproductive health disparities among homeless women.

References

Ake, T., Diehr, S., Ruffalo, L., Farias, E., Fitzgerald, A., Good, S. D., Howard, L. B., Kostelyna, S. P., & Meurer, L. N. (2018). Needs assessment for creating a patient-centered, community-engaged health program for homeless pregnant women. *Journal of Patient-Centered Research and Reviews, 5*(1), 36–44.

Asgary, R., Alcabes, A., Feldman, R., Garland, V., Naderi, R., Ogedegbe, G., & Sckell, B. (2016). Cervical cancer screening among homeless women of New York City shelters. *Maternal and Child Health Journal, 20*(6), 1143–1150.

Australian Bureau of Statistics (2016). *Census of population and housing, Estimating homelessness 2016.* Canberra, Australia: Author. Retrieved from www.abs.gov.au/ausstats/abs@.nsf/mf/2049.0.

Begun, S. (2015). The paradox of homeless youth pregnancy: A review of challenges and opportunities. *Social Work in Health Care, 54*(5), 444–460.

Bishop, S. E., Edwards, J. M., & Nadkarni, M. (2009). Charlottesville health access: A locality-based model of health care navigation for the homeless. *Journal of Health Care for the Poor and Underserved, 20,* 958–963.

Bloom, D. E., Canning, D., & Sevilla, J. (2004). The effect of health on economic growth: A production function approach. *World Development, 32*(1), 1–13.

Browne, A. & Bassuk, S. S. (1997). Intimate violence in the lives of homeless and poor housed women: Prevalence and patterns in an ethnically diverse sample. *American Journal of Orthopsychiatry, 67*(2), 261.

Campbell, J. C. (2002). Health consequences of intimate partner violence. *Lancet, 359*(9314), 1331–1336.

Chau, S., Chin, M., Chang, J., Luecha, A., Cheng, E., Schlesinger, J., Rao, V., Huang, D., Maxwell, A. E., Usatine, R., Bastani, R., & Gelberg, L. (2002). Cancer risk behaviors and screening rates among homeless adults in Los Angeles County. *Cancer Epidemiology and Prevention Biomarkers, 11*(5), 431–438.

Cho, S., Crenshaw, K. M., & McCall, L. (2013). Toward a field of intersectionality studies: Theory, applications, and praxis. *Signs, 38*(4), 785–810.

Coker, A. L., Davis, K. E., Arias, I., Desai, S., Sanderson, M., Brandt, H. M., & Smith, P. H. (2002). Physical and mental health effects of intimate partner violence for men and women. *American Journal of Preventive Medicine, 23*(4), 260–268.

Committee on Health Care for Underserved Women (2013). *Health care for homeless women.* Washington, DC: American College of Obstetricians and Gynecologists. Retrieved from www.acog.org/-/media/Committee-Opinions/Committee-on-Health-Care-for-Underserved-Women/co576.pdf?dmc=1&ts=20170812T1108043268.

Corrigan, P. W., Pickett, S., Schmidt, A., Stellon, E., Hantke, E., Kraus, D., & Dubke, R. (2017). Peer navigators to promote engagement of homeless African Americans with serious mental illness in primary care. *Psychiatry Research, 255,* 101–103.

Crawford, D. M., Trotter, E. C., Hartshorn, K. J. S., & Whitbeck, L. B. (2011). Pregnancy and mental health of young homeless women. *American Journal of Orthopsychiatry, 81*(2), 173–183.

Crenshaw, K. (1989). Demarginalizing the intersection of race and sex: A Black feminist critique of antidiscrimination doctrine, feminist theory, and antiracist politics. *University of Chicago Legal Forum, 140,* 139–167.

Cronley, C., Cimino, A. N., Hohn, K., Davis, J., & Madden, E. (2016). Entering prostitution in adolescence: History of youth homelessness predicts earlier entry. *Journal of Aggression, Maltreatment & Trauma, 25*(9), 893–908.

Cronley, C., Hohn, K., & Nahar, S. (2018). Reproductive health rights and survival: The voices of mothers experiencing homelessness. *Women & Health, 58*(3), 320–333.

Cutts, D. B., Coleman, S., Black, M. M., Chilton, M. M., Cook, J. T., de Cuba, S. E., Heeren, T. C., Meyers, A., Sandel, M., Casey, P. H., & Frank, D. A. (2015). Homelessness during pregnancy: A unique, time-dependent risk factor of birth outcomes. *Maternal and Child Health Journal, 19*(6), 1276–1283.

Denton, M. & Walters, V. (1999). Gender differences in structural and behavioral determinants of health: An analysis of the social production of health. *Social Science & Medicine, 48*(9), 1221–1235.

Duff, P., Deering, K., Gibson, K., Tyndall, M., & Shannon, K. (2011). Homelessness among a cohort of women in street-based sex work: The need for safer environment interventions. *BMC Public Health, 11*(1), 643.

Ensign, J. (2000). Reproductive health of homeless adolescent women in Seattle, Washington, USA Josephine. *Women & Health, 31*(2–3), 117–131.

Esen, U. I. (2017). The homeless pregnant woman. *The Journal of Maternal-Fetal & Neonatal Medicine, 30*(17), 2115–2118.

Gabram, S. G., Lund, M. J. B., Gardner, J., Hatchett, N., Bumpers, H. L., Okoli, J., Rizzo, M., Johnson, B. J., Kirkpatrick, G. B., & Brawley, O. W. (2008). Effects of an outreach and internal navigation program on breast cancer diagnosis in an urban cancer center with a large African-American population. *Cancer, 113*(3), 602–607.

Gaetz, S., Dej, E., Richter, T., & Redman, M. (2016). *The state of homelessness in Canada 2016.* Toronto, ON: The Canadian Observatory on Homelessness/Homeless Hub. Retrieved from http://homelesshub.ca/sites/default/files/SOHC16_final_20Oct2016.pdf.

Gawron, L. M., Redd, A., Suo, Y., Pettey, W., Turok, D. K., & Gundlapalli, A. V. (2017). Long-acting reversible contraception among homeless women veterans with chronic health conditions: A retrospective cohort study. *Medical Care, 55*(5), S111–S120.

Gelberg, L., Browner, C. H., Lejano, E., & Arangua, L. (2004). Access to women's health care: A qualitative study of barriers perceived by homeless women. *Women & Health, 40*(2), 87–100.

Gewirtz, A. H., DeGarmo, D. S., Lee, S., Morrell, N., & August, G. (2015). Two-year outcomes of the early risers prevention trial with formerly homeless families residing in supportive housing. *Journal of Family Psychology, 29*, 242–252.

Goodman, L., Fels, K., & Glenn, C. (2006). *No safe place: Sexual assault in the lives of homeless women.* Harrisburg, PA: National Online Resource Center on Violence Against Women. Retrieved from https://vawnet.org/sites/default/files/materials/files/2016-09/AR_SAHomelessness.pdf.

Ha, Y., Narendorf, S. C., Santa Maria, D., & Bezette-Flores, N. (2015). Barriers and facilitators to shelter utilization among homeless young adults. *Evaluation and Program Planning, 53*, 25–33.

Halcon, L. L. & Lifson, A. R. (2004). Prevalence and predictors of sexual risks among homeless young women. *Journal of Young Women and Adolescence, 33*, 71–80.

Haley, N., Roy, E., Leclerc, P., Boudreau, J. F., & Boivin, J. F. 2004. Characteristics of adolescent street youth with a history of pregnancy. *Journal of Pediatric Adolescent Gynecology, 17*, 313–320.

Hallett, R. E. (2012). *Educational experiences of hidden homeless teenagers: Living doubled-up.* New York, NY: Routledge.

Hathazi, D., Lankenau, S. E., Sanders, B., & Bloom, J. J. (2009). Pregnancy and sexual health among homeless young injection drug users. *Journal of Adolescence, 32*(2), 339–355.

Henry, M., Watt, R., Rosenthal, L., & Shivji, A. (2016). *The 2016 Annual Homeless Assessment Report (AHAR) to Congress.* Washington, DC: The U.S. Department of Housing and Urban Development. Retrieved from: www.hudexchange.info/resources/documents/2016-AHAR-Part-1.pdf.

Henry, M., Watt, R., Rosenthal, L., & Shivji, A. (2017). *The 2017 Annual Homeless Assessment Report (AHAR) to Congress.* Washington, DC: The U.S. Department of Housing and Urban Development. Retrieved from: www.hudexchange.info/resources/documents/2017-AHAR-Part-1.pdf.

Hogg, S., Haynes, A., Baradon, T., & Cuthbert, C. (2015). *All babies count: Spotlight on homelessness.* London, UK: NSPCC. Retrieved from www.nspcc.org.uk/globalassets/documents/research-reports/all-babies-count-unstable-start.pdf.

Houston, D. S., Reuschke, D., Sabater, A., Maynard, K., & Stewart, N. (2014). *Gaps in the housing safety net*. St Andrews, UK: St Andrews Centre for Housing Research. Retrieved from https://research-repository.st-andrews.ac.uk/bitstream/handle/10023/6223/gaps_chr.pdf?sequence=1&isAllowed=y.

Hurlbut, J. M., Robbins, L. K., & Hoke, M. M. (2011). Correlations between spirituality and health-promoting behaviors among sheltered homeless women. *Journal of Community Health Nursing, 28*(2), 81–91.

Johnson, G., Scutella, R., Tseng, Y., & Wood, G. (2015). *Entries and exits from homelessness: A dynamic analysis of the relationship between structural conditions and individual characteristics*, AHURI Final Report No. 248. Melbourne, Australia: Australian Housing and Urban Research Institute. Retrieved from https://researchbank.rmit.edu.au/view/rmit:33299/n2006055386.pdf.

Johri, M., Morales, R. E., Boivin, J. F., Samayoa, B. E., Hoch, J. S., Grazioso, C. F., Barrios Matta, I. J., Sommen, C., Baide Diaz, E. L., Fong, H. R., & Arathoon, E. G. (2011). Increased risk of miscarriage among women experiencing physical or sexual intimate partner violence during pregnancy in Guatemala City, Guatemala: Cross-sectional study. *BMC Pregnancy and Childbirth, 11*(1), 49.

Jordan, C. E., Campbell, R., & Follingstad, D. (2010). Violence and women's mental health: The impact of physical, sexual, and psychological aggression. *Annual Review of Clinical Psychology, 6*, 607–628.

Kennedy, S., Grewal, M. M., Roberts, E. M., Steinauer, J., & Dehlendorf, C. (2014). A qualitative study of pregnancy intention and the use of contraception among homeless women with children. *Journal of Health Care for the Poor and Underserved, 25*(2), 757–770.

Keys, D. (2007). Complex lives: Young motherhood, homelessness, and partner relationships. *Journal of the Association for Research on Mothering, 9*(1), 101–110. Retrieved from https://jarm.journals.yorku.ca/index.php/jarm/article/viewFile/5139/4335.

Killion, C. M. (1995). Special health care needs of homeless pregnant women. *Advances in Nursing Science, 18*(2), 44–56.

Koh, H. W. & O'Connell, J. J. (2016). Improving health care for homeless people. *Journal of the American Medical Association, 316*(24), 2536–2587.

Lantz, P. M., House, J. S., Lepkowski, J. M., Williams, D. R., Mero, R. P., & Chen, J. (1998). Socio-economic factors, health behaviors, and mortality: Results from a nationally representative prospective study of US adults. *Journal of the American Medical Association, 279*(21), 1703–1708.

Levine, J. M., Kelvin, J. F., Quinn, G. P., & Gracia, C. R. (2015). Infertility in reproductive-age female cancer survivors. *Cancer, 121*(10), 1532–1539.

Link, H. (2017). *Support for single homeless people in England*. London, UK: Homeless Link. Retrieved from www.homeless.org.uk/sites/default/files/siteattachments/Annual%20Review%202017_0.pdf.

Little, M., Gorman, A., Dzendoletas, D., & Moravac, C. (2007). Caring for the most vulnerable: A collaborative approach to supporting pregnancy homeless youth. *Nursing for Women's Health, 11*(5), 458–466.

Ludemir, A. B., Lewis, G., Valongueiro, S. A., de Araújo, T. V. B., & Araya, R. (2010). Violence against women by their intimate partner during pregnancy and postnatal depression: A prospective cohort study. *Lancet, 376*(9744), 903–910.

Lukasse, M., Henriksen, L., Vangen, S., & Schei, B. (2012). Sexual violence and pregnancy-related physical symptoms. *BMC Pregnancy and Childbirth, 12*(1), 83.

Marmot, M., Allen, J., Bell, R., Bloomer, E., & Goldblatt, P. (2012). WHO European review of social determinants of health and the health divide. *Lancet, 380*(9846), 1011–1029.

Marmot, M., Friel, S., Bell, R., Houweling, T. A. J., & Taylor, S. (2009). Closing the gap in a generation: Health equity through action on the social determinants of health. *Child Care, Health, and Development, 35*(2), 285.

Mberu, B., Mumah, J., Kabiru, C., & Brinton, J. (2014). Bringing sexual and reproductive health in the urban contexts to the forefront of the development agenda: The case for prioritizing the urban poor. *Maternal and Child Health Journal, 18*(7), 1572–1577.

McNamara, B. (2017, December 20). How periods perpetuate homelessness. *Teen Vogue*. Retrieved from www.teenvogue.com/story/homelessness-and-periods.

Meadows-Fernandez, R. (2017, July 27). Getting your period can be a pain. Getting it while homeless is even worse. *YES!* Retrieved from www.yesmagazine.org/people-power/getting-your-period-can-be-a-pain-getting-it-while-homeless-is-even-worse-20170727.

Meinbresse, M., Brinkley-Rubinstein, L., Grassette, A., Benson, J., Hamilton, R., Malott, M., & Jenkins, D. (2014). Exploring the experiences of violence among individuals who are homeless using a consumer-led approach. *Violence and Victims, 29*(1), 122–136.

Merrill, R. M., Richards, R., & Sloan, A. (2011). Prenatal maternal stress and physical abuse among homeless women and infant health outcomes in the United States. *Epidemiology Research International, 2011,* 1–10.

Milligan, R., Wingrove, B. K., Richards, L., Rodan, M., Monroe-Lord, L., Jackson, V., Hatcher, B., Harris, C., Henderson, C., & Johnson, A. A. (2002). Perceptions about prenatal care: Views of urban vulnerable groups. *BMC Public Health, 2*(1), 1–9.

Ministry of Health, Labour, and Welfare (2003). *For people, for life, for the future.* Tokyo, Japan: Author. Retrieved from www.mhlw.go.jp/english.

Moore, R. (2014). Coping with homelessness: An expectant mother's homeless pathway. *Housing, Care and Support, 17*(3), 142–150.

Natale-Pereira, A., Enard, K., Nevarez, L., & Jones, L. (2011). The role of patient navigators in eliminating health disparities. *Cancer, 117,* S3543–S3552.

National Board of Health and Welfare (2011). *Homelessness in Sweden 2011.* Stockholm, Sweden: Author. Retrieved from www.socialstyrelsen.se/publikationer2012/homelessnessinsweden2011.

Parrillo, A. & Edward Feller, M. D. (2017). Menstrual hygiene plight of homeless women, a public health disgrace. *Rhode Island Medical Journal, 100*(12), 14–15.

Reeve, K. (2018). Women and homelessness: Putting gender back on the agenda. *People, Place & Policy Online, 11*(3), 165–174. Retrieved from https://extra.shu.ac.uk/ppp-online/wp-content/uploads/2018/01/women-homelessness-putting-gender-on-the-agenda.pdf.

Richards, R., Merrill, R. M., & Baksh, L. (2011). Health behaviors and infant health outcomes in homeless pregnant women in the United States. *Pediatrics, 128*(3), 438–446.

Ruttan, L., Laboucane-Benson, P., & Munro, B. (2012). Does a baby help young women transition out of homelessness? Motivation, coping, and parenting. *Journal of Family Social Work, 15*(1), 34–49.

Sarango, M., de Groot, A., Hirschi, M., Umeh, C. A., & Rajabium, S. (2017). The role of patient navigators in building a medical home for multiply diagnosed HIV-positive homeless populations. *Journal of Public Health Management and Practice, 23*(3), 276–282.

Scappaticci, A. L. S. & Blay, S. L. (2009). Homeless teen mothers: Social and psychological aspects. *Journal of Public Health, 17*(1), 19.

Scaramella, N. & Fagan, J. M. (2016). *It's a part of life. Period.* New Brunswick, NJ: Rutgers, The State University of New Jersey. Retrieved from https://rucore.libraries.rutgers.edu/rutgers-lib/51726.

Schetter, C. D. & Tanner, L. (2012). Anxiety, depression and stress in pregnancy: Implications for mothers, children, research, and practice. *Current Opinion in Psychiatry, 25*(2), 141.

Sikich, K. W. (2008). Global female homelessness: A multi-faceted problem. *Gender Issues, 25*(3), 147–156.

Stein, J. A., Lu, M. C., & Gelberg, L. (2000). Severity of homelessness and adverse birth outcomes. *Health Psychology, 19*(6), 524–534.

Teruya, C., Longshore, D., Andersen, R. M., Arangua, L., Nyamathi, A., Leake, B., & Gelberg, L. (2010). Health and health care disparities among homeless women. *Women & Health, 50*(8), 719–736.

Thompson, S. J., Bender, K. A., Lewis, C. M., & Watkins, R. (2008). Runaway and pregnant: Risk factors associated with pregnancy in a national sample of runaway/homeless female adolescents. *Journal of Adolescent Health, 43*(2), 125–132.

Tolia, V. N., Patrick, S. W., Bennett, M. M., Murthy, K., Sousa, J., Smith, B., Clark, R. H., & Spitzer, R. (2015). Increasing incidence of the neonatal abstinence syndrome in U.S. neonatal ICUs. *New England Journal of Medicine, 372,* 2118–2126.

United Nations Office of Human Rights (2018). Homelessness and human rights. New York, NY: Author. Retrieved from www.ohchr.org/_layouts/15/WopiFrame.aspx?sourcedoc=/Documents/Issues/Housing/HomelessSummary_en.pdf&action=default&DefaultItemOpen=1.

U.S. Department of Housing and Urban Department (HUD) (2016). *The 2016 Annual Homeless Assessment Report (AHAR) to Congress.* Washington, DC: Author. Retrieved from www.hudexchange.info/resources/documents/2016-AHAR-Part-1.pdf.

U.S. Interagency Council on Homelessness (2014). *Fiscal year 2014 performance and accountability report.* Washington, DC: Author. Retrieved from www.usich.gov/resources/uploads/asset_library/FIN_FY_2014_USICH_PAR_Final.pdf.

Viner, R. M., Ozer, E. M., Denny, S., Marmot, M., Resnick, M., Fatusi, A., & Currie, C. (2012). Adolescence and the social determinants of health. *Lancet, 379*(9826), 1641–1652.

Walls, N. E. & Bell, S. (2011). Correlates of engaging in survival sex among homeless youth and young adults. *Journal of Sex Research, 48*(5), 423–436.

Weinreb, L., Goldberg, R., & Lessard, D. (2002). Pap smear testing among homeless and very low-income housed mothers. *Journal of Health Care for the Poor and Underserved, 13*(2), 141–150, doi:10.1353/hpu.2010.0528.

Winetrobe, H., Rhoades, H., Barman-Adhikari, A., Cederbaum, J., Rice, E., & Milburn, N. (2013). Pregnancy attitudes, contraceptive service utilization, and other factors associated with Los Angeles homeless youths' use of effective contraception and withdrawal. *Journal of Pediatric and Adolescent Gynecology, 26*(6), 314–322.

Wittenberg, E., Bharel, M., Saada, A., Santiago, E., Bridges, J. F. P., & Weinreb, L. (2015). Measuring the preferences of homeless women for cervical cancer screening interventions: development of a best-worst scaling survey. *Patient, 8*(5), 455–467.

Wood, T. & Watts, K. (2005). Challenges of caring for homeless pregnant women–1. *British Journal of Midwifery, 13*(3), 138–140, doi:10.12968/bjom.2005.13.3.17631.

World Health Organization (WHO) (2013). *Global and regional estimates of violence against women: Prevalence and health effects of intimate partner violence and non-partner sexual violence.* Geneva, Switzerland: Author. Retrieved from http://apps.who.int/iris/bitstream/handle/10665/85239/9789241564625_eng.pdf; jsessionid=2EE639ABC247A1376EC201A123C958DD?sequence=1.

World Health Organization (WHO) (2018a). *Health and sustainable development.* Geneva, Switzerland: Author. Retrieved from www.who.int/sustainable-development/cities/health-risks/slums/en.

World Health Organization (WHO) (2018b). *Reproductive health.* Geneva, Switzerland: Author. Retrieved from www.wpro.who.int/topics/reproductive_health/en.

World Health Organization (WHO) (2018c). *World Health Organization stigmatization of menstruation.* Geneva, Switzerland: Author. Retrieved from http://modelun.com/cjmunc/wp-content/uploads/sites/14/2018/05/WHO-Stigmatization-of-Menstruation-1.pdf.

36

REPRODUCTIVE JUSTICE AND CULTURALLY SAFE APPROACHES TO SEXUAL AND REPRODUCTIVE HEALTH FOR INDIGENOUS WOMEN AND GIRLS

Pat Dudgeon and Abigail Bray

We recognize the impacts and tragedies that have occurred because of environmental violence, but we also celebrate our victories, strength, resilience and resistance. We commit to continue our struggles and fulfill our responsibilities to our children and the generations still to come. We commit to continue revitalizing our traditional ways of life, languages, and cultures, and to implement solutions in our own communities based on our traditional knowledge, practices and ways of knowing. We commit to reclaim our wellness and power as Indigenous women and Peoples and reaffirm that our children have a right to be born healthy and to live in a clean environment. To heal our Peoples and Mother Earth, we must continue to heal ourselves, tell our stories, build our unity, defend out rights and be who we are.

(*The 3rd International Indigenous Women's Environmental and Reproductive Health Symposium, 2018*)

In this chapter we take a de-colonising, strengths-based approach to the subject of Indigenous women's and girls' sexual and reproductive health. Indigenous strengths-based approaches are asset-based; focussed on resilience, protective factors, and capacity building; culturally safe; engaged with social and cultural determinants; and governed by Indigenous research methodologies and concepts of well-being (Fogarty, Lovell, Langenberg, & Heron, 2018). The importance of strengths-based, culturally safe, comprehensive primary health care has long been recognised by Indigenous communities, is enshrined in the United Nations Declaration of the Rights of Indigenous Peoples, and is an emerging best practice across many neo-colonial states (Brascoupe & Walters, 2009; Ramsden, 1990; Taylor & Guerin, 2010). However, there is limited research on how Indigenous health sciences can inform a culturally safe, strengths-based approach to Indigenous women's and girls' sexual and reproductive health (Bell, Aggelton, Ward, & Maher, 2017).

Here we describe an innovative Aboriginal and Torres Strait Islander model for strengthening the sexual and reproductive health of Aboriginal and Torres Strait Islander women and girls. Composed of seven inter-related Indigenous domains of well-being—Country, spirituality, culture, community, family and kinship, mind and emotions, and body—Social and Emotional Wellbeing (SEWB) is widely recognised as a culturally appropriate Indigenous health model within Australia (Dudgeon, Bray, D'Costa, & Walker, 2017). This holistic model of health was refined by Gee, Dudgeon, Schultz, Hart, and Kelly (2014) after substantial community consultations, was further developed by Dudgeon and Walker (2015), and informs important state and federal health policies and strategies such as the *National Strategic Framework for Aboriginal and Torres Strait Islander Peoples' Mental Health and Social and Emotional Wellbeing 2017–2023*.

Before we explore this Indigenous model it is necessary to provide some context. In what follows we present an overview of dominant findings about Indigenous women's and girls' sexual and reproductive health with a concentration on population health data from the neocolonial states of Australia, New Zealand, and North America. We then describe some of the major Indigenous health models that have emerged from the global resurgence of Indigenous self-determination in primary health care. The Aboriginal and Torres Strait Islander model of SEWB is then explored, with a focus on how each of the seven domains contribute to the strengthening of women's and girls' sexual and reproductive health.

Indigenous women's reproductive oppression

International Indigenous women's groups have become increasingly vocal about the importance of achieving *reproductive justice* through self-determination. Self-determination has long been recognised as the solution to overcoming the stark health disparities between Indigenous and non-Indigenous people and vital in combating the destructive impacts of the main social determinant of this disparity, namely *colonisation* (International Symposium on the Social Determinants of Indigenous Health, 2007), however the relationship between reproductive justice and self-determination is a relatively new focus. The concept of reproductive justice comes out of research and activism conducted by women of colour committed to expanding culturally safe access to comprehensive primary health care and ending reproductive oppression (Ross & Solinger, 2018). Reproductive oppression is intersectional and mobilised by shifting forces of racism, sexism, and classism that control and exploit women's and girls' bodies, sexuality, labour, and reproduction. The reproductive oppression of Indigenous women is now well documented both in Australia (Behrendt, 2001; Sykes, 1977/1975); Watson, 2009) and internationally (Stannard, 1992), with groups such as *SisterSong*, a women's health lobby led by Native American and other women of colour, campaigning for reproductive justice. The reproductive oppression of Indigenous women and girls includes rape, the forced removal of children from their families, involuntary sterilisation, coerced abortions, lack of access to culturally appropriate health care and education (including prenatal care for pregnant women), and the exclusion of Indigenous women's traditional health systems and culture. There is an emerging movement against the colonial contamination of Indigenous waterways, land, and air; the concept of *environmental reproductive justice* (Hoover, 2018) is being increasingly used by Indigenous women. The impact of reproductive oppression is complex, cross-generational, and entrenched, and it can be understood as an underlying driver of the health gap between Indigenous and non-Indigenous women and girls across the world.

First Nations, Inuit, and Metis women in Canada suffer higher maternal mortality and more coercive sterilisation, gestational diabetes, smoking during pregnancy, STIs, and reproductive cancers than other Canadian women do (Halseth, 2013). Native American women have less access to safe antenatal care, maternity hospitals, and family planning (Gurr, 2012), and endure the trauma of sterilisation (Torpy, 2000). In New Zealand/Aotearoa, Maori women and girls suffer higher levels of STIs (Tipene & Green, 2017), have less access to antenatal care, birth more premature babies, smoke more often during pregnancy, have greater maternal and neonatal mortality, and higher levels of fatal cervical and breast cancer than other women in New Zealand (Parton, 2015). In Australia, Indigenous women experience higher rates of maternal sepsis, gestational diabetes, and perinatal morbidity; give birth to more low weight babies; experience more maternal smoking and STIs (Bell et al., 2017; Lowell, Kildea, Liddle, Cox, & Paterson, 2015), and have higher mortality rates from reproductive cancers (Tapia, Garvey, McEntee, Rickard, & Brennan, 2017) than other Australian women do.

Indigenous women and girls across the world are also subjected to chronic levels of traumatising and fatal sexual violence. For example, the plight of First Nations missing and murdered women and girls in Canada and sexual violence against Native American women is an internationally recognised crisis (Legal Strategy Coalition on Violence Against Indigenous Women, 2018). The ongoing trauma of colonisation (cross-generational and historical trauma) also results in significant numbers of pregnant Indigenous women with mental health challenges (Mah et al., 2017).

Indigenous women, especially those who live in rural and remote areas, often do not have access to culturally safe, comprehensive, primary health care services; one consequence is that girls and women are not adequately screened for cancers that impact their sexual and reproductive health (Hutchinson, Tobin, Muirhead, & Robinson, 2018). There is a consensus across the literature that access to culturally informed and culturally safe health services is vital to the strengthening of Indigenous women's and girls' sexual and reproductive health (Hutchinson et al., 2018). This access is upheld by Article 24 (1) in the United Nations Declaration of the Rights of Indigenous Peoples:

> Indigenous people have the right to their traditional medicine and to maintain their health practices, including the conservation of their vital medicinal plants, animals and minerals. Indigenous people also have the right to access, without any discrimination, to all social and health services.
>
> *(UNDRIP, 2007)*

Self-determination, cultural safety, and Indigenous health models

There is substantial evidence that Indigenous self-determination restores health and wellbeing (Chandler & Lalonde, 1998; King, Smith, & Gracey, 2009; Oster, Grier, Lightning, Mayan, & Toth, 2014). Indigenous control over the governance of communities, and in particular control over comprehensive primary health care services, is emerging as a strong solution to the health gap between Indigenous and non-Indigenous women and girls. A clear reason is that Indigenous women are best placed to provide culturally safe (i.e., knowledgeable and non-racist) services to Indigenous women and girls. Long histories of severe institutionalised racism and sexism within the colonial health care sector have led many Indigenous women to an understandable reluctance to experience further punitive contact (Bradley, Dunn, Lowell, & Nagel, 2015; Dietsch, Shackleton, Davies, McLeod, & Alston, 2010). In this context, Indigenous controlled health care practices that support cultural safety can be understood to be forms of counter-colonial resistance and ways of fighting for Indigenous women's reproductive justice. In Australia and other colonised countries, Indigenous women's and girls' well-being has benefited from Indigenous con-trolled comprehensive primary health care services (Howell, Auger, Gomes, Brown, & Leion, 2016; Lowell et al., 2015). Central to the global project of Indigenous healing through self-determination is the restoration of Indigenous health systems.

Culturally safe Indigenous healing systems are being used by communities to de-colonise health discourses and practices across the world. Some examples of the emerging Indigenous health discourses are the Cree model of Being Alive Well or *miyupimaasisiiun* (Adelson, 2000); the Maori models of well-being, *Te Whetu* The Star (Mark & Lyons, 2010), *Whare Tapa Maori* The Four-Sided House (Durie, 2001), and *Te Wheke* The Octopus (Pere, 1995); the Matsigenka of the Amazon jungle's model (Izquierdo, 2005); and Native American well-being models founded on traditional Medicine Wheel teachings (Canales, 2004; Rountree & Smith, 2016). For Indigenous people, health is a holistic concept that "encompasses everything important in a person's life, including land, environment, physical body, community, relationships, and law" (Burns, Maling, & Thomson, 2010, p. 1). Indigenous sexual and reproductive well-being is hol-istic and relational, collective and ecocentric. Land is central to Indigenous well-being and is emerging as a topic of research in the determinants of health literature (de Leeuw, 2018).

Aboriginal and Torres Strait Islander-led holistic de-colonising approaches that support the empowerment of women and their families and communities have existed since at least the 1970s, when the self-determination movement successfully mobilised for Aboriginal Community Controlled Health Organisations (Foley, 1991). As we write this in 2018, there are roughly 150 such organisations across Australia. Similar processes have occurred in other Indigenous cultures across the world. One result of the Indigenous self-determination move-ment in Australia has been the development of nine guiding principles of Aboriginal and Torres Strait Islander Social and Emotional Wellbeing. In brief, the 1989 National Aborigi-nal Health Strategy identified nine engagement principles, which were developed by the landmark *Ways Forward* (Swan & Raphael, 1995) and also contained in the *National Strategic Framework for Aboriginal and Torres Strait Islander Peoples Mental Health and Social and Emotional Wellbeing 2004–2009*. These nine principles inform a central text in the field, *Working Together: Aboriginal and Torres Strait Islander Mental Health and Wellbeing: Principles and Practice* (Dudgeon, Milroy, & Walker, 2014). The revised 2017–2023 national SEWB Framework promotes these principles, which are underpinned by a recognition that self-determination in the health sector is the solution to overcoming the complex burdens of colonisation (Dudgeon, Bray, D'Costa, & Walker, 2017). These nine guiding principles embody a holistic and whole-of-life view of health held by Aboriginal and Torres Strait Islander people and emphasise that SEWB is a strengths-based understanding of health.

Aboriginal and Torres Strait Islander women's and girls' social and emotional well-being

It is the right of Aboriginal and Torres Strait Islander women to determine what their health system will look like. Aboriginal and Torres Strait Islander women and their organisations must have a pivotal role in consulting, designing, developing, implementing and evaluating health services for Aboriginal and Torres Strait Islander women.

(Fredericks, Adams, Angus, & the Australian Women's Health Network Talking Circle, 2011, p. 25)

The social and emotional well-being of Aboriginal and Torres Strait Islander women and girls is acknowledged to be an under-researched area; for example, the minimal amount of research into motherhood has tended to be epidemiological and child-outcome-focussed (Ussher, Parton, & Perz, 2016). Moreover, "initiatives in which Indigenous approaches and the role of culture are integrated into women-centered, trauma-informed approaches are scarce", and "[p]rograms generally tend to focus on only one or two elements of women's wellbeing and few have explicitly and/or effectively embraced the intersection of culture, gender and trauma to support recovery" (Wyndow, Walker, & Reibel, 2018, p. 6). Furthermore, as Bell et al. (2017) concluded in their review of young Indigenous women's sexual health in Australia, there is a lack of acknowledgement of the strengthening power of women's culture in peer-reviewed articles in the area. They identified a "major gap in understanding how indigenous cultural values and practices support, rather than inhibit, young people's sexual health and promote, rather than constrain, practices of harm reduction" (Bell et al., 2017, p. 14). Action is also urgently needed to improve the dire conditions of Indigenous women's everyday life.

As *The Birthing on Country Position Statement* (CATSINaM, 2016), which addresses strengthening sexual and reproductive well-being, puts it, women's health disadvantage is:

> underpinned by the inequity across all of the 'Social Determinants of Health' (SDH) such as, poor housing, insecure employment, lower educational outcomes and access to health care, including care during pregnancy. Alongside the SDH, there are many other factors, which influence an Aboriginal and/or Torres Strait Islander women's engagement with, and early presentation for, care in pregnancy. Specifically, those include the availability of culturally safe services, institutional racism in our health services, the frequency (or absence) of local services.
>
> *(p. 1)*

These SDH are recognised in the numerous Indigenous health policies that promote SEWB, and are an integral part of SEWB, which recognises the influence of social and historical determinants. This is depicted below in Figure 36.1, adapted from Gee et al. (2014).

In what follows, each strengths-based domain of SEWB is discussed in terms of Indigenous women's sexual and reproductive well-being. This is not meant to be prescriptive. How might sexual and reproductive health be strengthened by connections to the seven domains of SEWB?

Connection to Country

Indigenous women are the traditional custodians of the land and waterways of Australia. Relationship to Country is vital to their strength and to the ecocentric concept of subjectivity that underpins Indigenous ontology. Country is often respected as female, as mother, or as the Noongar people call her, "'Boodjar' or 'nourishing terrain', a nurturing, creative, fertile place" (Wooltorton, Collard, & Horwitz, 2017, p. 1). There is robust evidence that links connection to Country to improved SEWB (Biddle, 2011; Biddle & Swee, 2012; Burgess, Berry, Gunthorpe, & Baille, 2008; Burgess et al., 2009). Indigenous health programs for girls and women take pregnant women onto Country, to get exercise, learn about healthy bush tucker, and visit culturally important places with other women and girls (Lowell et al., 2015).

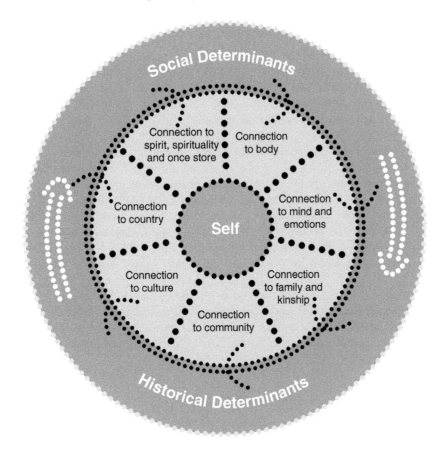

Figure 36.1 Social and emotional well-being framework depicting the interplay of social and historical
  determinants.

Source: https://www.pmc.gov.au/sites/default/files/publications/mhsewb-framework_0.pdf

Connection to Country is important for caring for sacred women's sites, where women's
business can occur, and central to initiation ceremonies that celebrate transitions in sexual
and reproductive well-being. Country is a place where one can be nourished, strengthened,
replenished, and seek guidance. Within classical Indigenous culture, great importance was
placed on where women gave birth, and in recent years there has been strong movement to
reclaim the power of this SEWB practice, termed Birthing on Country (Kildea et al., 2018).
Giving birth is an important rite of passage. "Many Aboriginal women living in rural and
remote areas want the opportunity, in low risk situations, to be able to birth 'on Country'
with the knowledge and support of their Elders" (Dudgeon & Walker, 2011, p. 116). Culturally and spiritually, this birthing is linked to strengthening and protecting infants and
mothers, and barriers to being able to do so are argued to lead to a "weakened spirit in
baby and higher rates of infant mortality" (Dudgeon & Walker, 2011, p. 116; see also Wardaguga & Kildea, 2004), as well as the breakdown of the protective qualities of culture and
subsequent disharmony in communities. The right to birth on Country is supported by
SNAICC: National Voice for Our Children, a powerful, community-controlled organisation
dedicated to protecting children, young people, and families and strengthening self-
determination through cultural identity (SNAICC, 2018).

Connection to spirituality

Spirituality is recognised across the literature to be an important source of well-being (Grieves, 2009; Yap & Yu, 2016; Ypinazar, Margolis, Haswell-Elkins, & Tsey, 2007). There are strong links to spirituality and well-being across the literature, and many concepts of Indigenous well-being are anchored in spirituality. For example, the Yawuru people speak of *mabu liyan* "a continuity and connection between the mind, body, spirit, culture and land" (Yap & Yu, 2016, p. 28).

Indigenous spirituality is a sophisticated ecocentric philosophy and a law that maps relationships and obligations, which are passed down in stories and ceremonies, and it is a complex knowledge system that includes women's understandings of sexual and reproductive well-being from a holistic perspective. Traditional women healers, for example, draw on spiritual knowledge, and classical midwives are also often healers, counsellors, and Elders. For example, the powerful Ngaanyatjarra Pitjantjatjara Yankunytjatjara Women's Council Aboriginal Corporation support traditional Ngangkari women healers who strengthen the sexual and reproductive health of women and girls across central Australia (Dudgeon & Bray, 2018).

Strengthening women's sexual and reproductive well-being through the SEWB domain of spirituality means, among other things, providing access to traditional women healers and midwives and to sacred women's birthing places and the stories they carry, as well as access to the cultural knowledge systems that support women's strength and power (Bell, 1982; Bell & Ditton, 1980).

Connection to culture

The Congress of Aboriginal and Torres Strait Islander Nurses and Midwives' *Birthing on Country Position Statement* (CATSINaM, 2016) asserts that culture "underpins" Indigenous health priorities "including that mothers and babies get the best possible care and support for a good start to life" (CATSINaM, 2016, p. 1). Culture is also central to the successful Strong Women, Strong Babies, Strong Culture Program, which recognises "culture and cultural renewal as the wellspring of health" (Lowell et al., 2015, p. 2). The Program has been supporting women and girls in the Northern Territory since 1993 and runs "culture camps for young girls and women" (Lowell et al., 2015, p. 3) to strengthen their cultural identity. The success of this Program depends on the continuation of community control and self-determination.

Prior to colonisation women had a powerful, respected, and central place in society and enjoyed freedom, security, rights to land, and equality with men; they were a vital part of the governance of communities and active participants in cultural activities and the development and continuation of Indigenous knowledge systems in Australia. Indigenous "women were 'bosses for themselves', a self-perception that was manifest in their economic, social, familial, spiritual and ritual roles" (Dudgeon & Walker, 2011, p. 98). As Elders, and women of High Degree, women had considerable power, were integral to the handing on of knowledge and Lore to younger generations and enabling important transitions from childhood and adolescence to adulthood, and had sovereign rights as custodians of Country. Indigenous culture was highly structured; there were numerous laws in place to regulate sexual relations and birth, and women were honoured. As Elder George Gaymarrangi Pasco put it: "[i]n our cultural Lore, it says we need to protect our women because she represents the earth. Women are very special in this world and our customs and Lore says that we must protect them" (People Culture Environment, 2014, p. 46).

Indigenous women's sexual and reproductive health is shaped by the Dreaming, sacred laws passed down across thousands of years through story, ritual, and art, which, for example, honour pregnancy as a sacred experience when a spirit child came into being. The health of pregnant women was very important: There were various rules about what could and could not be eaten, and the whole community cared for her (Dudgeon & Walker, 2011). The reproductive stages of a woman's life were marked by initiations, and when a girl entered womanhood she was instructed in secret women's business, rituals, songs, knowledge, and Lore about marriage by grandmothers and female Elders. "An Aboriginal woman gained status after the birth of a child, becoming equal to other women of the camp and enjoying certain freedoms and privileges" (Dudgeon & Walker, 2011, p. 100). There was strong solidarity between women that centred around a collective nourishing of the sexual and reproductive health of other women.

Strengthening women's sexual and reproductive well-being through the domain of culture includes providing access to culturally safe services, including women treating other women and woman-only services (Dudgeon et al., 2014); celebrating the transition into womanhood to deepen a connection to culture; participating in secret women's business; respecting cultural ways of caring for self when pregnant; birthing ceremonies and celebration of motherhood as a higher status and a form of power and respect. Strengths-based women's empowerment camps such as those organised by the Kanyirninpa Jukurrpa Puntura-ya Ninti Program and Martu Rangers can be understood within this context. In 2017 the Martu Rangers focussed on the theme of the Jakulyukulyu (Seven Sisters) Dreaming Story "to keep the story strong and to pass on elders' knowledge and culture to younger women" (Country Needs People, 2018, p. 87). A number of cultural laws related to women's sexuality are part of this narrative.

Connection to family and kinship

Various studies have shown that connecting to kinship networks improves the maternal health of Indigenous women (e.g., Dietsche et al., 2011). Women's sexual and reproductive health is culturally supported by other women in the family and kinship network. Older women, not just mothers, teach girls about sexual and reproductive health when they are of age, and the transition from childhood to adolescence is about learning how to build up knowledge and power as a woman and mother.

> The relationship between grandmothers, mothers, and daughters was particularly important; grandmothers had a special relationship with, and responsibilities to, their grandchildren to assist them in the transition to adulthood and motherhood. *Grandmothers' laws* refer to the authority of senior women when men and women held sovereignty over the land and Aboriginal women shared equal rights and responsibilities with men to provide a safe and healthy environment for women and children.
>
> *(Watson, 2008, as cited in Dudgeon & Walker, 2011, p. 99)*

Sexual and reproductive well-being is also strengthened by cultural knowledge of kinship rules, support and guidance from other women, and a sense of pride in Indigenous identity. The destruction of these protective relationships, for example through the forced removal of girls from their mothers across generations, is a well-known source of complex trauma, as the 1997 *Bringing Them Home: Report of the National Inquiry into the Separation of Aboriginal and Torres Strait Islander Children from Their Families* documented (Australia & Wilkie, 1997).

Secure and appropriate long-term housing, food security, the material conditions to support thriving families, and access to non-discriminatory health care, welfare services, education, and employment, in effect *self-determination* over the material conditions of everyday life, would support the sexual and reproductive well-being of women and girls in the SEWB domain of the family.

Connection to community

As *The Birthing on Country Position Statement* (CATSINaM, 2016) asserts, access to community-controlled health services that support women and girls strengthens sexual and reproductive well-being. Among the benefits of such culturally safe services are access to cancer screening and the early detection and treatment of breast cancer (Tapia et al., 2017). Sharing experiences with other women in the community, especially with clients who are service users, has also been identified as a protective factor (Jennings, Bond, & Hill, 2018). Studies have shown that pregnant women who were supported by woman Elders in the community had stronger neonatal and postnatal health (Andersson & Ledogar, 2008). Within Aboriginal and Torres Strait Islander communities "[a] female Elder had the power and responsibility to hand on knowledge, traditions, customs, rights, and myths that underlay and sanctioned the social and political life of the group" (Dudgeon & Walker, 2011, p. 99). Access to Indigenous midwives who are embedded in the community has been identified as a protective factor for childbearing women and their families (Kelly et al., 2014). Family and community involvement in the control of maternity services has been identified as a recommendation to improve the well-being of women (Parker, McKinnon, & Kruske, 2014). The support of senior women in the community is one of the key reasons the Strong Women, Strong Babies, Strong Culture Program is successful.

Connection to mind and emotions

The discipline of Indigenous psychology has provided evidence that Indigenous self-determination over how Indigenous people's mental and emotional health is strengthened is a best-practice approach (Chandler & Lalonde, 2004). Healing the complex forms of trauma (i.e., historical trauma, cross-generational trauma, intergenerational trauma) that are the result of the Australian genocide through culturally safe healing programs designed by and for women would strengthen women's and girls' well-being (Dudgeon et al., 2014; Wyndow et al., 2018). Within Australia, The Healing Foundation is a national Indigenous-controlled organisation dedicated to healing the survivors of the Stolen Generations (i.e., those impacted by the forced removal of children from families). As they state: "healing programs for women have included the use of traditional healing methods and bush medicines, and cultural renewal activities such as dance, song, craft and rituals". They support Coota Girls Aboriginal Corporation, survivors of the Cootamundra Domestic Training Home for Aboriginal Girls, and women's leadership in the domain of healing. There is evidence that connecting to culture and Country restores emotional and mental health (Biddle & Swee, 2012).

Connection to body

Addressing poverty, and the associated ill-health and psychological stress poverty produces across generations, is urgent. The invading culture often targeted Indigenous women's access to food by poisoning their supplies or fencing them off from land where they gathered food. Indigenous women and girls living in rural and remote areas experience food shortages, which impact on their health. Appropriate and safe housing is an important foundation for physical well-being along with secure access to nutritious food. Far too many Indigenous women and girls do not have access to these basic human rights despite the vast wealth of Australia.

Strengthening women's sexual and reproductive well-being through the domain of the body, and from an Indigenous standpoint, also involves access to culturally safe health services and holistic Indigenous health systems. The Indigenous Martu women rangers, for example, teach knowledge of edible plants: "each plant has its own songs, places, stories and laws, and has special techniques, tools, knowledge and skills to prepare them" (Country Needs People: Protecting Nature, Transforming Lives, 2018, p. 88). Bush medicine is used in the Strong Women, Strong Baby, Strong Culture Program to treat women.

Conclusion

Culturally safe care for Indigenous women's sexual and reproductive well-being that is founded on holistic Indigenous knowledge systems and designed and delivered by Indigenous people is of central importance to closing the gap between Indigenous and non-Indigenous people's health and to ensuring that future generations flourish. We have suggested an Indigenous model for thinking through a strength-based understanding of sexual and reproductive well-being through the domains of SEWB: Country, culture, spirituality, family and kinship, community, mind and emotions, and body. Many of the suggestions here are related to the social determinate of the sexual and reproductive health of Indigenous women and girls, of which colonisation is the over-arching determinant. For reproductive justice to be achieved, self-determination and decolonisation is needed across all sectors that impact on well-being. We hope that this model will open up a decolonised space for thinking through the sexual and reproductive well-being of women and girls from an Indigenous standpoint. The re-emergence of women-led eco-centric Indigenous health movements dedicated to strengthening sexual and reproductive well-being represents an urgently needed cultural re-birth of women's knowledge systems across the Earth.

References

Adelson, N. (2000). *"Being alive well": Health and the politics of Cree well-being.* Toronto, Canada: University of Toronto Press.

Andersson, N. & Ledogar, R. L. (2008). The CEIT aboriginal youth resilience study: 14 years of capacity building and methods development in Canada. *Pimatisiwin, 6*(2), 65–88.

Australia & Wilkie, M. (1997). *Bringing them home: Report of the national inquiry into the separation of Aboriginal and Torres Strait Islander children from their families.* Sydney, Australia: Human Rights and Equal Opportunity Commission.

Behrendt, L. (2001). Genocide: The distance between law and life. *Aboriginal History, 25,* 132–147.

Bell, D. (1982). Women's changing role in health maintenance in a central Aboriginal community. In J. Reid (Ed.), *Body, land and spirit: Health and healing in Aboriginal society* (pp. 197–224). St. Lucia, Australia: University of Queensland Press.

Bell, D. & Ditton, P. (1980). *Law: The old and new: Aboriginal women in central Australia speak out.* Canberra, Australia: Central Australian Aboriginal Legal Aid Service, Aboriginal History.

Bell, S., Aggelton, P., Ward, J., & Maher, L. (2017). Sexual agency, risk, and vulnerability: A scoping review of young Indigenous Australians' sexual health. *Journal of Youth Studies, 20,* 1208–1224.

Biddle, N. (2011). *Physical and mental health. Measures of Indigenous wellbeing and their determinants across the life course* [CAEPR lecture series, lecture 3]. Canberra, Australia: Centre for Aboriginal Economic Policy Research, Australian National University. Retrieved from http://caepr.anu.edu.au/sites/default/files/page/2011/01/Lecture03Paper.pdf.

Biddle, N. & Swee, H. (2012). The relationship between wellbeing and Indigenous land, language, and culture in Australia. *Australian Geographer, 43*(3), 215–232.

Bradley, P., Dunn, S., Lowell, A., & Nagel, T. (2015). Acute mental health service delivery to Indigenous women: What is known? *International Journal of Mental Health Nursing, 24*, 471–477.

Brascoupe, S. & Walters, C. (2009). Cultural safety: Exploring the applicability of the concept of cultural safety to Aboriginal health and community wellness. *Journal of Aboriginal Health, 5*(2), 6–41.

Burgess, C. P., Berry, H. L., Gunthorpe, W., & Baille, R. S. (2008). Development and preliminary validation of the 'Caring for Country' questionnaire: Measurement of an Indigenous Australian health determinant. *International Journal for Equity in Health, 7*(10), 1.

Burgess, C. P., Johnston, F. H., Berry, H. L., McDonnell, J., Yibarbuk, D., Gunabarra, C., & Baille, R. S. (2009). Healthy country, healthy people: The relationship between Indigenous health status and caring for country. *Medical Journal of Australia, 190*(10), 567–572.

Burns, J., Maling, C. M., & Thomson, N. (2010). *Summary of Indigenous women's health.* Perth, Australia: Australian Indigenous HealthInfoNet.

Canales, M. K. (2004). Taking care of self: Healthcare decision making of American Indian women. *Health Care for Women International, 25*, 411–435.

Chandler, M. J. & Lalonde, C. (1998). Cultural continuity as a hedge against suicide in Canada's First Nations. *Transcultural Psychiatry, 35*(2), 191–219.

Chandler, M. J. & Lalonde, C. E. (2004). Transferring whose knowledge? Exchanging whose best practices? On knowing about Indigenous knowledge and Aboriginal suicide. *Aboriginal Policy Research Consortium International (APRCi)* [Paper 144]. Retrieved from http://ir.lib.uwo.ca/aprci/144.

Congress of Aboriginal and Torres Strait Islander Nurses and Midwives (CATSINaM) (2016). *The birthing on country position statement.* Majura Park, ACT, Australia: Author. Retrieved from www.catsinam.org.au/static/uploads/files/birthing-on-country-position-statement-endorsed-march-2016-wfaxpyhvmxrw.pdf.

Country Needs People: Protecting Nature, Transforming Lives (2018). *Strong women on country: The success of women caring for country as Indigenous ranges and on Indigenous protected areas.* Canberra, Australia: Author. Retrieved from countryneedspeople.org.au.

de Leeuw, S. (2018). Activating place: Geography as a determinant of Indigenous people's health and well-being. In M. Greenwood, S. de Leeuw, & N. M. Lindsay (Eds), *Determinants of Indigenous people's health: Beyond the social* (pp. 187–203). Toronto, Canada: Canadian Scholars.

Dietsch, E., Shackleton, P., Davies, C., McLeod, M., & Alston, M. (2010). 'You can drop dead': Midwives bullying women. *Women and Birth, 23*, 53–59.

Dietsche, E., Martin, T., Shackelton, P., Davies, C., McLeod, M., & Alston, M. (2011). Australian Aboriginal kinship: A means to enhance maternal well-being. *Women and Birth, 24*(2), 58–64.

Dudgeon, D., Milroy, H., & Walker, R. (2014). *Working together: Aboriginal and Torres Strait Islander mental health and wellbeing principles and practices.* Canberra, Australia: Commonwealth Government.

Dudgeon, P. & Bray, A. (2018). Indigenous healing practices in Australia. *Women & Therapy, 41*, 97–113.

Dudgeon, P., Bray, A., D'Costa, B., & Walker, R. (2017). Decolonising psychology: Validating social and emotional wellbeing. *Australian Psychologist, 52*, 316–325.

Dudgeon, P. & Walker, R. (2011). The health, social and emotional wellbeing of Aboriginal women. In R. Thackrah & K. Scott (Eds), *Indigenous Australian health and culture: An introduction for health professionals* (pp. 96–126). Sydney, Australia: Pearson Education.

Dudgeon, P. & Walker, R. (2015). Decolonizing Australian psychology: Discourses, strategies, and practice. *Journal of Social and Political Psychology, 3*(1), 276–297.

Durie, M. (2001). *Mauri Ora: The dynamic of Maori health.* Auckland, New Zealand: Oxford University Press.

Fogarty, W., Lovell, M., Langenberg, J., & Heron, M.-J. (2018). *Deficit discourse and strengths-based approaches: Changing the narrative of Aboriginal and Torres Strait Islander health and wellbeing.* Carlton, Australia: Lowitja Institute.

Foley, G. (1991). *Redfern Aboriginal medical service 1971–1991: Twenty years of community service*. Redfern, NSW, Australia: Aboriginal Medical Service Cooperative Ltd. Retrieved from http://vuir.vu.edu.au/27033/1/Redfern%20Aboriginal%20Medical%20Service%201971-1991.pdf.

Fredericks, B., Adams, K., Angus, S., & the Australian Women's Health Network Taking Circle (2011). *National Aboriginal and Torres Strait Islander women's health strategy*. Melbourne, Australia: Australian Women's Health Network. Retrieved from https://eprints.qut.edu.au/32256/1/FINAL_National_Aboriginal_and_Torres_Strait_Islander_Women%27s_Strategy_May_2010.pdf.

Gee, G., Dudgeon, P., Schultz, C., Hart, A., & Kelly, K. (2014). Aboriginal and Torres Strait Islander social and emotional wellbeing. In P. Dudgeon, H. Milroy, & R. Walker (Eds), *Working together: Aboriginal and Torres Strait Islander mental health and wellbeing principles and practice* (2nd ed., pp. 55–68). Canberra, Australia: Department of the Prime Minister and Cabinet.

Grieves, V. (2009). *Aboriginal spirituality: Aboriginal philosophy, the basis of Aboriginal social and emotional wellbeing* [Discussion paper no. 9]. Darwin, NT, Australia: Cooperative Research Centre for Aboriginal Health. Retrieved from www.lowitja.org.au/sites/default/files/docs/DP9-Aboriginal-Spirituality.pdf.

Gurr, B. (2012). The failures and possibilities of a human rights approach to secure Native American women's reproductive justice. *Societies Without Borders*, 7(1), 1–28.

Halseth, R. (2013). *Aboriginal Women in Canada: Gender, socio-economic determinants of health, and initiatives to close the wellness-gap*. Prince George, Canada: National Collaborating Centre for Aboriginal Health.

Hoover, E. (2018). Environmental reproductive justice: Intersections in an American Indian community impacted by environmental contamination. *Environmental Sociology*, 4(1), 8–21.

Howell, T., Auger, M., Gomes, T., Brown, F. L., & Leion, A. Y. (2016). Sharing our wisdom: A holistic Aboriginal health initiative. *International Journal of Indigenous Health*, 11, 1.

Hutchinson, P., Tobin, P., Muirhead, A., & Robinson, N. (2018). Closing the gaps in cancer screening with First Nations, Inuit, and Metis populations: A narrative literature review. *Journal of Indigenous Wellbeing*, 3(1), 3–17.

International Symposium on the Social Determinants of Indigenous Health (2007). *Social determinants and Indigenous health: The international experience and its policy implications*. Adelaide, Australia: Commission on Social Determinants of Health. Retrieved from www.who.int/social_determinants/resources/indigenous_health_adelaide_report_07.pdf.

Izquierdo, C. (2005). When 'health' is not enough: Societal, individual and biomedical assessments of wellbeing among the Matsigenka of the Peruvian Amazon. *Social Science and Medicine*, 61, 767–783.

Jennings, W., Bond, C., & Hill, P. S. (2018). The power of talk and power in talk: A systematic review of Indigenous narratives of culturally safe healthcare communication. *Australian Journal of Primary Health*, 24, 109–115.

Kelly, J., West, R., Gamble, J., Sidebotham, M., Carson, V., & Duffy, E. (2014). 'She knows how we feel': Australian Aboriginal and Torres Strait Islander childbearing women's experience of Continuity of Care with an Australian Aboriginal and Torres Strait Islander midwife student. *Women and Birth*, 27, 157–162.

Kildea, S., Hickey, S., Neson, C., Currie, J., Carson, A., Reynolds, M., Wilson, K., Kruske, S., Passey, M., Roe, Y., West, R., Clifford, A., Kosiak, M., Watego, S., & Traey, S. (2018). Birthing on country (in our community): A case study of engaging stakeholders and developing a best-practice Indigenous maternity service in an urban setting. *Australian Health Review*, 42(2), 230–238.

King, M., Smith, A., & Gracey, M. (2009). Indigenous health part 2: The underlying causes of the health gap. *Lancet*, 374, 76–85.

Legal Strategy Coalition on Violence against Indigenous Women (2018). *Ongoing systemic inequalities and violence against Indigenous women in Canada* [LCS Discussion Paper]. Ottawa, ON, Canada: Amnesty International Canada. Retrieved from www.amnesty.ca/sites/amnesty/files/LSC%20Discussion%20Paper%20to%20Special%20Rapporteur%20-%20Final.pdf.

Lowell, A., Kildea, S., Liddle, M., Cox, B., & Paterson, B. (2015). Supporting Aboriginal knowledge and practice in health care: Lessons from a qualitative evaluation of the strong women, strong babies, strong culture program. *BMC Pregnancy and Childbirth*, 15, 19.

Mah, B., Weatherall, L., Burrows, J., Blackwell, C. C., Gwynn, J., Wadhwa, P., Lumbers, E. R., Smith, R., & Rae, K. M. (2017). Post-traumatic stress disorder symptoms in pregnant Australian Indigenous women residing in rural and remote New South Wales: A cross-sectional descriptive study. *Australian and New Zealand Journal of Obstetrics and Gynaecology*, 57, 520–525.

Mark, G. T. & Lyons, A. C. (2010). Maori healers' view on wellbeing; the importance of mind, body, spirit, family and land. *Social Science and Medicine, 70*, 1756–1764.

National Voice for Our Children (SNAICC) (2018). Retrieved from www.snaicc.org.au.

Oster, R. T., Grier, A., Lightning, R., Mayan, M. J., & Toth, E. L. (2014). Cultural continuity, traditional Indigenous language, and diabetes in Alberta First nations: A mixed methods study. *International Journal of Equity in Health, 13*, 92.

Parker, S., McKinnon, L., & Kruske, S. (2014). 'Choice, culture and confidence': Key findings from the 2012 having a baby in Queensland Aboriginal and Torres Strait Islander survey. *BMC Health Service Research, 14*, 196.

Parton, B. M. (2015). *Maori women, health care, and contemporary realities: A critical reflection.* [Doctoral dissertation], Massey University, Wellington, New Zealand. Retrieved from https://mro.massey.ac.nz/bitstream/handle/10179/7213/02_whole.pdf?sequence=2&isAllowed=y.

People Culture Environment (2014). *The Elder's report into preventing indigenous self-harm & youth suicide.* Melbourne, Australia: Author. Retrieved from www.cultureislife.org/bepartofthehealing/EldersReport.pdf.

Pere, R. (1995). *Te wheke: A celebration of infinite wisdom.* Gisborne, New Zealand: Ao Ako.

Ramsden, I. M. (1990). *Whakaruruhau: Cultural safety in nursing education in Aotearoa: A report for Maori health and nursing.* Wellington, New Zealand: Ministry of Education New Zealand.

Ross, L. & Solinger, R. (2018). *Reproductive justice: An introduction.* Berkeley, CA: University of California Press.

Rountree, J. & Smith, A. (2016). Strength-based well-being indicators for Indigenous children and families: A literature review of Indigenous communities' identified well-being indicators. *American Indian and Alaska Native Mental Health Research, 23*, 206–220.

Stannard, D. E. (1992). *American holocaust: The conquest of the new world.* New York, NY: Oxford University Press.

Swan, P. & Raphael, B. (1995). *'Ways forward': National consultancy report on Aboriginal and Torres Strait Islander mental health.* Canberra, Australia: AGPS.

Sykes, B. (1977/1975). The other half: Women in Australian society. In J. Mercer (Ed.), *Black women in Australia* (pp. 313–321). Melbourne, Australia: Penguin.

Tapia, K., Garvey, G., McEntee, M., Rickard, M., & Brennan, P. (2017). Breast cancer in Australian Indigenous women: Incidence, mortality, and risk factors. *Asia Pacific Journal of Cancer Prevention, 18*, 873–884.

Taylor, M. & Guerin, P. (2010). *Health care and Indigenous Australians: Cultural safety in practice* (2nd ed.). South Yarra, Australia: Palgrave Macmillan.

The 3rd International Indigenous Women's Environmental and Reproductive Health Symposium (2018). The 3rd Declaration for Health, Life and Defense of Our Lands, Rights and Future Generations. *Indigenous Policy Journal, 29*, 1. Retrieved from: www.indigenouspolicy.org/index.php/ipj/article/view/559/548.

Tipene, J. & Green, A. (2017). *He Pukenga Korero: Rangatahi and sexually transmitted infections in the Waikato: A Report submitted to the health research council of New Zealand.* Auckland, New Zealand: Te Whāriki Takapou. Retrieved from https://tewhariki.org.nz/assets/He-Pukenga-Korero-Final-Report-31-Aug-2017.pdf.

Torpy, S. (2000). Native American women and coerced sterilization: On the trail of tears in the 1970s. *American Indian Culture and Research Journal, 24*(2), 1–22.

United Nations (2007). *United Nations Declaration on the Rights of Indigenous People.* New York, NY: United Nations. Retrieved June, 2010, from www.un.org/esa/socdev/unpfii/documents/DRIPS_en.pdf.

Ussher, J., Parton, C., & Perz, J. (2016). Constructions and experience of motherhood in the context of an early intervention for Aboriginal mothers and their children: Mother and healthcare workers perspectives. *BMC Public Health, 16*, 620.

Wardaguga, M. & Kildea, S. (2004). Senior Aboriginal health worker tells medical conferences: It's time to listen! *Aboriginal and Islander Health Worker Journal, 28*(6), 10–11.

Watson, I. (2008). Aboriginal women's law and lives: How might we keep growing the law? In D. Rigney, E. Johnston, & M. Hinton (Eds), *Indigenous Australians and the law* (2nd ed., pp. 15–30). London, UK: Routledge-Cavendish.

Watson, I. (2009). Sovereign spaces, caring for country and the homeless position of Aboriginal people. *South Atlantic Quarterly, 108*(1), 27–51.

Wooltorton, S., Collard, L., & Horwitz, P. (2017). The land still speaks: Ni, Katitj! *PAN: Philosophy, Activism, Nature, 13,* 57–67.

Wyndow, P., Walker, R., & Reibel, T. (2018). A novel approach to transforming smoking cessation practice for pregnant Aboriginal women and girls living in the Pilbara. *Healthcare, 6,* 1.

Yap, M. & Yu, E. (2016). *Community wellbeing from the ground up: A Yawuru example* [Research report no. 3/16]. Perth, Australia: Bankwest Curtin Economics Centre.

Ypinazar, V. A., Margolis, S. A., Haswell-Elkins, M., & Tsey, K. (2007). Indigenous Australians' understandings regarding mental health and disorders. *Australian and New Zealand Journal of Psychiatry, 41,* 467–478.

37

REPRODUCTIVE HEALTH OF WOMEN IN LOW- AND MIDDLE-INCOME COUNTRIES

Kirsten I. Black and Miriam O'Connor

For reproductive-aged women and girls in low- and middle-income countries (LMICs), poor sexual and reproductive health outcomes contribute to one third of the total global burden of disease, and violence and unsafe sex continue to be major risk factors for death and disability (Temmerman, Khosla, Laski, Mathews, & Say, 2015a; World Health Organization, 2014b). The global health agenda recognises this burden, and the United Nations Sustainable Development Goals highlight the need to address issues of sexual and reproductive health (SRH) under 2 of the 17 goals that focus on sexual and reproductive rights and access to SRH services. The shift from an agenda focussed on population control and family planning programs to one that addresses the overall reproductive health needs of women and men, as well as the importance of social and economic policy measures designed to empower women and to strengthen their rights, was first raised at the International Conference on Population and Development in Cairo in 1994 (The International Bank for Reconstruction and Development/The World Bank, 2007). However, in the years since the conference, much of the global reproductive health attention shifted to HIV infection and AIDS, and, between 1995 and 2009, funding for family planning fell globally from 55% to 7% of all SRH funding (Cleland et al., 2006). Subsequently further ground was lost through US government policies that resulted in the defunding of many contraception services. In the last 5–10 years there has been a re-emergence of recognition of the central importance of SRH and how it is inextricably linked to an individual's physical, mental, environmental, and economic well-being. This chapter provides an overview of the ongoing challenges to improving the reproductive lives of women and their families and considers some interventions and service models that have been tried in various low- and middle-income settings.

Epidemiology of reproductive health issues in low- and middle-income countries

The definition of SRH used by the World Health Organization encompasses the concept that people should be able to have responsible, fulfilling, and safe sex lives and the capability to have children if, and when, they choose to do so. Implicit in this is the notion that women and men will be able to access "safe, effective, affordable and acceptable methods of fertility regulation" along with access to health services that provide safe care for women during pregnancy and childbirth to optimise the chance of a healthy infant. Currently, in many countries, universal SRH is limited by poverty, gender inequality, cultural and religious influences, geographical location, and health system barriers. The burden of sexual and reproductive ill health falls disproportionately on those in low-income countries (Gross National Income [GNI] per capita of $1,005 or less in 2017–2018; e.g., the Solomon Islands), lower-middle income countries (LMIC; GNI between $1,006 and $3,955; e.g., Indonesia), and some upper middle-income countries (GNI per capita between $3,956 and $12,235; e.g., Samoa) (World Bank, 2018). In addition, it is important to be aware that, even though the national purse appears to have fattened (on paper) for several LMICs, many of the national health plans, particularly in contexts such as the Pacific Islands, have not augmented funding to SRH (Countdown to 2030 collaboration, 2018; Government of Papua New Guinea, 2017; World Health Organization, 2017).

Sexual and reproductive health is now recognised as a core concern of global development. The ability to plan and space the number of children strengthens most other efforts to improve human life, including in the realms of education, gender equality, health, economic development, and the environment. However, the Millennium Development Goals (MDG) were late to recognise the importance of SRH and, when launched in 1990, targets that referenced contraception and sexual health were initially absent. It was not until 2007 that the MDG 3 adopted "universal access to sexual and reproductive health" as one of the goals. Unfortunately, significant ground was lost during those 17 years between 1995 and 2009 when less than one quarter of the estimated US$ 3.2 billion needed per year was spent on family planning. Contraceptive prevalence increased only 9% from 55% in 1990 to 64% in 2015 (United Nations Department of Economic and Socia Affairs Population Division, 2015). Towards the end of the MGD period, of all the interventions across the reproductive lifespan, one of the lowest success rates was in the area of contraceptive needs: only 57% of women reported access to modern methods of contraception (Countdown to 2030 Collaboration, 2018; World Health Organization, 2014a).

In other aspects of reproductive health, significant progress has been made, albeit with ongoing notable inequities. The global Maternal Mortality Ratio (MMR) is *estimated* (given that in many countries data collection is not robust) to have fallen by 45% worldwide between 1990 and 2013 from 380 to 210 per 100,000 live births, but this fell short of the two-thirds reduction target (United Nations, 2015). The greatest progress was seen in southern Asia, where the MMR declined by 64% during this time period. Nevertheless, most of the maternal deaths in 2013 occurred in low- and middle-income countries where the maternal mortality ratio was around 14 times higher than in high-income countries.

By 2014 more than 71% of births were assisted by "skilled health personnel" globally, a rise from 59% in 1990. There were, however, large differences between urban and rural areas. In developing regions, only 56% of births in rural areas were attended by skilled health personnel compared with 87% in urban areas. There was also an increase in the proportion of women attending four or more antenatal visits; this was particularly marked in northern Africa where there was an increase from 50% in 1990 to 89% in 2014 (United Nations, 2015). Figure 37.1 shows the 2017 median national coverage of interventions in reproductive, maternal, and child health and again illustrates that the demand for family planning performed poorly against other interventions (Countdown to 2030 Collaboration, 2018).

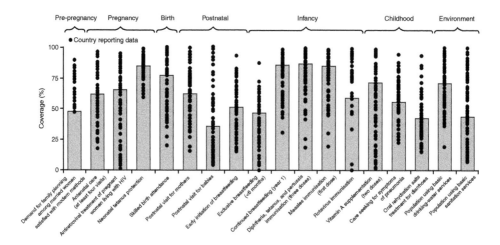

Figure 37.1 Major gaps in intervention countries remain (Countdown to 2030 Collaboration, 2018).

The Sustainable Development Goals (SDGs) have recognised the importance of SRH in both goal 3 and goal 5. Goal 3.7 is "by 2030, to ensure universal access to sexual and reproductive health-care services" and goal 5.6 is "to ensure universal access to sexual and reproductive health and reproductive rights" (United Nations, 2016). To clarify the areas of priority for the SDGs the Copenhagen Consensus brought together experts from the United Nations, non-governmental organisations, and universities along with teams of economists to examine evidence about the most effective targets for the post-2015 development agenda. The group looked at a range of issues that would potentially benefit development, including climate change, education, infant mortality, and maternal health, and prioritised them in terms of "value for money". SRH, in particular universal access to contraception, ranked third of 22 interventions, behind reducing world trade restrictions and free regional Asia Pacific trade as the most cost-effective intervention (Kohler & Behrman, 2014). For every dollar spent on contraception, it is estimated that $120 will be recouped in health, education, and other costs.

Universal access to contraception increases the likelihood that a greater proportion of pregnancies are intended; it is one of the most effective interventions for development, and its measurement and monitoring is critical. Individual countries' Demographic and Health Surveys measure current use of contraception amongst women who are married or in a union. Women who are pregnant are asked whether or not they had wanted to get pregnant at that time and whether the pregnancy was wanted later or not wanted at all (The DHS Program, 2018). These latter questions are prone to recall bias as notions of pregnancy intendedness have been found to change as a pregnancy progresses. Responses are also affected by gender relations and religious and sociocultural factors that may restrict women's freedom to make choices about use of contraception and pregnancy planning. For example, in a report that examined the case for investing in family planning in the Solomon Islands, there was a large gap between reported rate of mistimed and unwanted pregnancies (58%) and reported unmet need (34.4%) for contraception, which suggests that the needs of populations may not be well articulated (Kennedy et al., 2013).

Social, gender, and cultural norms and religious influences on SRH

The degree to which women and girls are able to exert any control over the various aspects of their SRH lives (e.g., the ability to negotiate the marriage partner of their choice, the timing of sex, the conditions under which sex takes place, the use of contraceptives, family size and spacing) plays a critical role in determining their vulnerability to infections, unintended pregnancies, and, in many instances, gender-based violence. This varies between and within countries, but is affected, inter alia, by perceived cultural and social norms and by religious teachings and practices. Where the status of women is poor, and human rights issues are low on the local/national agenda, these factors have a stronger influence on SRH morbidity and mortality. This is especially so where women's participation in education (at least to secondary level) remains low (Ugwu & de Kok, 2015).

In Papua New Guinea, for example, there are more than 830 living languages and separate cultures within a country of over eight million people. This environment makes service provision complex, especially given the additional topographical and demographic challenges whereby 87% live in rural and remote areas and only 53% are estimated to be literate (National Statistical Office, 2009). "Bride price"[1] remains common, but very early marriage is declining. However, in several sub-Saharan African countries, especially in circumstances of family poverty, early (usually arranged) marriage and child-bearing remains prevalent. Women have little reproductive autonomy, and many who are forced into early marriage bear children during adolescence, which places them at higher risk of a range of adverse perinatal outcomes (Muleta, 2006).

In many LMIC settings women's access to services may be impossible without support from their male partners/relatives. Barriers to that access can be cultural, financial, geographical (e.g., distance, topographical, transport, roads, law and order issues), opportunity costs (e.g., arranging for someone else to manage her family and community duties), legal, and/or religious (World Health Organization, 2012). In Ghana, for example, whether or not a woman accesses a skilled birth attendant depends to a large extent on the values and opinions of husbands, mothers-in-law, traditional birth attendants, and other family and community members rather than on the woman's own desires (Ganle et al., 2015). Without the agreement that is locally required, she may not be supported to seek care (the opportunity costs related to her daily "duties") or be able to access the necessary funds (even a cheap bus fare) (Oshi, Oshi, Alobu, & Ukwaja, 2016). Where family planning and contraceptive programs are offered, it is often seen as a women's issue, so men are not included in any aspect of the program, to the point that they then refuse women's participation in positive choices because of their own ignorance and uncertainty regarding contraceptive methods. Health programmers must take some responsibility for this because, although avenues to include men in family planning programs are part of any effective design these days, men have been largely kept out (yet also blamed) for not supporting their partners' choices (Croce-Galis, Salazar, & Lundgren, 2014; Hardee, Croce-Galis, & Gay, 2017). Health service providers may not accede to requests for modern contraceptives (especially permanent methods such as sterilisation) without written evidence of a partner's consent, even if a national policy dictates otherwise. The health workers themselves carry their own values, attitudes, and beliefs (especially in relation to adolescent girls or single women attempting to get the services they need) that can negatively impact access to care, and, where service management is lacking or poor performance by staff goes unremarked and unmanaged, women suffer. Workers tend to reflect prevailing societal and cultural norms (Holmes & Goldstein, 2012; Tilburt, 2010).

Prevailing religious teachings and beliefs often negatively influence access to services and SRH outcomes (UNFPA, 2016). In many countries there is a legal prohibition against health workers supplying single women and girls with contraception, against LGBTIQ clients, and against termination of pregnancy, as these are based on religious beliefs and teachings. Religious facilities frequently provide pre-service training for lower levels of health workers in LMICs, and many have taken the opportunity to alter the curricula according to their religion's teachings. Religious beliefs and teachings may also influence clients' acceptance of poor outcomes (e.g., God's will, fate) and, in so doing, decrease development of demand for improved services. Religion can also hold significant sway in the development of national health policy and its implementation.

Beyond the LMICs' sphere of influence over their own programs and services, the cultural and religious beliefs of the international development partner communities can negatively influence SRH outcomes. The *Mexico City Policy* (Cincotta & Crane, 2001), sometimes referred to by critics as the "global gag rule", is a United States government policy that blocks U.S. federal funding for non-governmental organisations that provide abortion counselling and referrals or advocate to decriminalise abortion or expand abortion services. The denial of funding applies to all SRH services that these organisations provide, not just to abortion.

SRH health service competence

There can be no health without an appropriate health workforce. Many LMICs continue to face challenges due to worker shortages, skill mix imbalance, maldistribution of resources, a work environment challenged by poor physical conditions and lack of basic equipment, and a weak knowledge and skills base (Chen et al., 2004; World Health Organization, 2006). The SRH workforce has received particular attention with a special emphasis on bringing quality midwifery services closer to the community (Berer, 2006). WHO and the Global Health Workforce Network have established a *Global Strategy on Human Resources for Health*, but the challenges of training staff, retaining them, and ensuring their professional development and recognition are immense (Fourth Global Forum on Human Resources for Health, 2017). Training of SRH staff is difficult because of the low baseline education of the health care professionals and the lack of context-specific curriculum and educators. Retaining staff with positions and conditions that are attractive for graduates, and maintaining staff skills, providing opportunities for ongoing professional development, and formalising registration and regulation procedures remain significant barriers to a high functioning SRH workforce.

Gendered issues (especially in countries where women's status is low in comparison with men's) are important in so far as the providers of SRH services are usually female, often have lower levels of knowledge and skills (e.g., in PNG where the majority of health care providers are Community Health Workers[2] and nurses), and, in many instances, do not have the training required to provide optimal care (e.g., obstetric emergencies, post-abortion care, provision of quality family planning services). Too often, health workers who have graduated from their pre-service training get little or no in-service training. For example, in PNG, a study of the delivery of essential and emergency obstetric care in-service training to primary health care workers in rural and remote facilities showed that over 50% of the participant primary health care workers had been offered no in-service courses at all in any health issues since they had graduated, in some cases 25 years ago (O'Connor M. 2018, Personal Communication).

A key issue that many governments have failed to recognise whilst planning their workforce is that the population growth rate far outstrips the human resource planning and implementation to provide enough skilled workers to provide for their citizens' health needs (Global Health Workforce Alliance, 2013). This is further sabotaged by the "brain drain" to more prosperous countries due to insufficient opportunities for professional advancement locally, political and social conflict, and their concerns for their families' safety (Frenk et al., 2010). Further, health services will be effective only in so far as the staff can be satisfactorily deployed and retained. This means adequate remuneration (and incentives), housing, supportive performance management and an enabling environment in which to apply their skills, career pathways, regular in-service opportunities, and appropriate regulation and re-registration.

Effective strategies to improve SRH in low- and middle-income country settings

Researchers and policy makers understand the epidemiology and know what interventions decrease both mortality and morbidity across a range of SRH problems in women and girls (Gülmezoglu et al., 2016; Ronsmans & Graham, 2006; Temmerman, Khosla, Laski, Mathews, & Say, 2015b). The challenges confronting many LMICs are moving from a solely *curative* approach to a *health promotion/preventative* approach and providing services for marginalised groups (Frieden, 2014).

Within the field of SRH, the majority of morbidity and mortality relates to pregnancy and childbirth. This is because 15% of women have a complication during pregnancy, childbirth, or the post-natal period, and 1.4% have a life-threatening emergency (the majority of which cannot be predicted and require emergency care without which 50% will die) (Dubourg et al., 2002; World Health Organization, 2006). The two most cost-effective strategies for reducing maternal mortality are family planning and quality contraceptive choices *plus* labour, childbirth, and post-natal care supervised by a skilled health care worker, with access to Emergency Obstetric Care (EmOC), if required.

Family planning

Numerous economic modelling exercises have demonstrated that enabling access to family planning is one of the most cost-effective development interventions that has a wide range of benefits for society (Kohler & Behrman, 2014). Studies of several countries in the Pacific have been undertaken. For example, in 2012 a study indicated that one in nine reproductive-aged women in the Solomon Islands who were married or in a union wanted to avoid pregnancy but were not using any contraceptive method (Kennedy et al., 2013). The authors reported that, if all family planning needs were met by 2025, there would be a 12% reduction in the number of maternal deaths and a 20% reduction in infant deaths each year. For each $1 spent on unmet needs for contraception by 2020, $9–16 would be saved in health and education expenditure, which would make other development goals more attainable (Kennedy et al., 2013). In Africa each year 211,000 women die from complications of abortion, miscarriage, or childbirth, but if all women received the contraceptive care they *desired*, the number of deaths would be reduced by 52,000 (Guttmacher Institute, 2017).

If women can control their fertility they can stay in education longer and have increased participation in the workforce to the economic benefit of their families and communities. Data from 170 countries between 1970 and 2009 show that, for every single additional year of education a woman of reproductive age has, there was a corresponding decrease in child mortality of 9.5% (Gakidou, Cowling, Lozano, & Murray, 2010). Women's workforce participation in the Asia-Pacific region continues to be low, costing the region more than $89 billion each year (United Nations Economic and Social Commission for Asia and the Pacific, 2018). A World Bank analysis illustrates that, if women's economic activity were on par with men's, economic growth in many Asia-Pacific countries could increase by as much as 18% (The World Bank, 2012).

Lower pregnancy rates and adequate spacing between pregnancies results in improvement in children's health. Children born less than two years apart are twice as likely to die in the first year of life as are those born three or more years apart (Fotso, Cleland, Mberu, Mutua, & Elungata, 2013). Short inter-pregnancy intervals (from the birth of one baby to the conception of the next) are associated with a range of adverse perinatal outcomes including increased rates of growth restriction, premature birth, and stillbirth (Conde-Agudelo, Belizan, Norton, & Rosas-Bermudez, 2005) and also interfere with breastfeeding, a proven and cost-effective way to improve child nutrition and resistance to infectious disease (Ball & Bennett, 2001).

Despite this myriad of benefits, the unmet need for contraception in many regions of the world remains high. This leads to unintended pregnancies and abortion, which in low- and middle-income countries is too often illegal and unsafe, and thus contributes to 8% of global maternal mortality (Say et al., 2014).

Antenatal care and skilled birth attendance

The workforce caring for pregnant women has been particularly scrutinised because the MDG's fifth target to improve maternal health was not met: only nine countries decreased their MMR by 75%, 26 countries made no progress, and 12 countries increased Maternal Mortality Ratios (United Nations, 2015; World Health Organization, 2015, 2017). Facility-based childbirth with skilled birth attendants increased (United Nations, 2015), but there is concern that countries have focussed too much on the *numbers* and that phrases such as "skilled birth attendant" and "emergency obstetric care" have masked poor *quality* care to the point that some consider it unethical to encourage women to give birth in places with poor capability, or where no actual care is received, or where that care is not guided by nationally agreed protocols (Campbell et al., 2016). Millions of women have received care that is delayed, inadequate, unnecessary, harmful, or no care at all due to the dual issues of poor quality and/or inaccessible care. Respectful Maternity Care[3] is, rightly, gaining an increasing prominence, and clients' experience and feedback is increasingly considered in monitoring and evaluation, as well as in research (Miller et al., 2016). Research has shown that women who experience mistreatment report that they are less likely to return for future confinements (Mannava, Durrant, Fisher, Chersich, & Luchters, 2015).

The *Lancet*'s Midwifery Series (Renfrew et al., 2014b) identified that the lowest cost option for care with the best outcomes is midwives as care providers with access to emergency services (Renfrew et al., 2014b). The countries that have been most successful in tackling MDG 5 have done so by bringing quality context-specific midwifery graduates closer to the people (Renfrew et al., 2014b). However, use of evidence to design and implement appropriate strategies to improve maternal health in LMIC settings remains a challenge related to the issues regarding service quality as previously discussed, including the number and competence of the health care providers, inadequate supervision of staff, environmental limitations including infrastructure problems (e.g., no water or electricity), and supply chain failures for medicines and equipment. There is a clear need to improve the quality of locally contextualised clinical practice guidelines, their formulation and dissemination, and to increase regular audit and research to enable services to examine how well the recommended interventions are *actually* provided (e.g., frequency of active management of the third stage of labour).

Engaging men and boys

It has been increasingly acknowledged that sustainable development cannot be achieved without addressing the issue of gender parity (Sweetman, 2002; United Nations, 2015). The SDG for gender equality (Goal 5) recognises that a multifaceted process is required by nations to address the spectrum of gender-related issues including gender-based violence, equality of employment opportunities for women, and sexual and reproductive health and rights; this includes legislative changes that support women's empowerment and their access to economic resources and technology. Gender issues are also reflected in other SGDs related to health improvement and poverty alleviation.

Strategies to address the impacts of gender inequity have previously focussed largely on empowering women, but many groups working on gender equity have recognised that change is best achieved if both men and women are engaged in examining their cultural practices and social norms (WorldFish, 2018). One example in South America is the *Instituto Promundo*, which researches practical strategies for engaging men in gender equality, particularly in the areas of SRH and gender-based violence (Promundo and UNFPA, 2016). In South Africa, the *Sonke Gender Justice Network* works with young women and men to enhance their knowledge and skills regarding gender equality and to educate them about sexual and reproductive health and rights and the prevention of HIV and gender-based violence (Sonke Gender Justice, 2016).

Factors that have limited men's and boys' involvement in SRH to date include prevailing views of masculinities, "old" stereotypes that "SRH is women's business", that SRH means "maternal and child health", myths and misunderstandings, unfavourable social and cultural climates, limited or no specific training for health providers in relation to men's SRH service requirements, primary health centre programs not geared to meet men's needs, and limited contraceptive options for men (The Alan Guttmacher Institute, 2003). Globally, men are poor users of health facilities and too often have limited or inaccurate information, but if they feel welcome and are offered the knowledge base from which to make good decisions for themselves, their partners, their families, and their communities, they may do so (Edström, Hassink, Shahrokh, & Stern, 2015). They need their own safe places to access accurate information and men-friendly services (Greene et al., 2006; IPPF & UNFPA, 2017). Armed with accurate information, they will be better placed to engage in discussion and good decision-making with their partner/s and community. If they are left out, the underlying root causes of gender inequality and poor SRH and gender-based violence may remain unaddressed.

SRH and the youth cohort

The present generation of 10–24-year-olds is the largest in history at 1.8 billion (25% of the global population), and 90% of them live in LIMCs (Sawyer et al., 2012). Until recently, they have been overlooked in global health and other social policies, and thus have had fewer health gains than other age groups.

Young people live in an increasingly threatening world and SRH challenges, along with undernutrition and infectious diseases, disproportionately affect those in sub-Saharan Africa, southeast Asia, and Oceania, yet they remain largely invisible to health systems as health information systems collect very little age-aggregated data and even more limited morbidity data. Most ill health is not captured in mortality data, and reported mortality rates probably underestimate adolescents, as published data are overwhelmingly focussed on the <5-year age group. However, we do know that adolescent mothers face higher risk of complications in pregnancy and their babies have increased rates of adverse outcomes (World Health Organization, 2018). Yet there are limited SRH services targeted to this age group, and multiple cultural, religious, and legal obstacles to be overcome in planning and implementing appropriate adolescent-friendly services (Patton et al., 2016).

One of the main barriers to service provision is that adolescent pregnancy remains stigmatised in many countries, and punitive responses (including blaming young women for promiscuity) exclude them from education. LMICs need partnerships to develop relevant youth SRH policy, legislation, National Youth Forums, models of care that are youth-friendly, health worker curricula and education (especially in relation to Respectful Maternity Care for this group), as well as a focus on collecting morbidity and mortality data for this age group (Patton et al., 2016; Starrs et al., 2018). SRH issues under consideration should include menstrual hygiene options and support to stay in school whilst menstruating; contraception; safer sex; pregnancy, childbirth, and post-natal care that is supportive and non-judgemental, with an emphasis on deferring a subsequent pregnancy until a time of their own choosing; the importance of staying in school; protection from violence and sex trafficking; and care and support if they are exploited/attacked.

Conclusion

Access to reproductive health services is fundamental to healthcare and is recognised by the United Nations Human Rights Council (UNHRC) as a pressing human rights issue. Restriction of access to safe family planning violates women's rights to health, life, education, dignity, and vital information. However, there are numerous challenges to meeting the world's SRH needs, including social, religious, and cultural barriers along with gender-power relations. Even though most countries have endorsed the Declaration for Human Rights and the Convention on the Elimination of all Forms of Discrimination Against Women (CEDAW), specific marginalised groups (adolescents, refugees, women with HIV, sex workers, women with a disability) will always suffer more in relation to these cultural, social, and religious beliefs. With improved health and nutrition, young people are reaching sexual maturity and sexual debut earlier, but many LMICs are not well prepared for their SRH needs, and few countries currently offer services that are accessible to these young, usually unmarried populations. Health workforce issues are critical in many settings, and greater support for training, adequate remuneration, and continuing professional development are required if human resources are to grow. Any SRH program, if it is to have an impact, must create an enabling environment that acknowledges local cultural and social norms, consults with community leaders, and works with partner organisations and researchers to deliver clinical and public health practice that is evidence-based and appropriate.

Notes

1 In PNG traditional society, the groom's family pay what is known as a "bride price" to his partner's family and the value of this might depend on the political value of the new relationship joining the

families together, her education, her health and good looks, and her proven ability to produce children for him. In some tribal cultures this leads to a perception of "ownership" of the woman by her husband and his family. To some degree exposure to a Western consumer culture is changing the tradition. Large amounts of cash and goods can be exchanged, and women increasingly feel as though they are a commodity to be bartered.

2 PNG CHWs are part of the formal health system; they have had at least two years full-time training in Primary Health Care, as distinct from Village Health Volunteers.

3 www.who.int/woman_child_accountability/ierg/reports/2012_01S_Respectful_Maternity_Care_Charter_The_Universal_Rights_of_Childbearing_Women.pdf.

References

Ball, T. M. & Bennett, D. M. (2001). The economic impact of breastfeeding. *Pediatric Clinics of North America, 48*(1), 253–262.

Berer, M. (2006). Human resources: An impersonal term for the people providing health care. *Reproductive Health Matters, 14*(27), 6–11.

Campbell, O. M. R., Calvert, C., Testa, A., Strehlow, M., Benova, L., Keyes, E., Donnay, F., Macleod, D., Gabrysch, S., Rong, L., Ronsmans, C., Sadruddin, S., Koblinsky, M., & Bailey, P. (2016). The scale, scope, coverage, and capability of childbirth care. *The Lancet, 388*(10056), 2193–2208.

Chen, L., Evans, T., Anand, S., Boufford, J. I., Brown, H., Chowdhury, M., Cueto, M., Dare, L., Dussault, G., Elzinga, G., Fee, E., Habte, D., Hanvoravongchai, P., Jacobs, M., Kurowski, C., Michael, S., Pablos-Mendez, A., Sewankambo, N., Solimano, G., Stilwell, B., de Waal, A., & Wibulpolprasert, S. (2004). Human resources for health: Overcoming the crisis. *The Lancet, 364* (9449), 1984–1990.

Cincotta, R. P. & Crane, B. B. (2001). The Mexico city policy and U.S. family planning assistance. *Science, 294*(5542), 525–526.

Cleland, J., Bernstein, S., Ezeh, A., Faundes, A., Glasier, A., & Innis, J. (2006). Family planning: The unfinished agenda. *The Lancet, 368*(9549), 1810–1827.

Conde-Agudelo, A., Belizan, J. M., Norton, M. H., & Rosas-Bermudez, A. (2005). Effect of the interpregnancy interval on perinatal outcomes in Latin America. *Obstetrics & Gynecology, 106*(2), 359–366.

Countdown to 2030 collaboration (2018). Countdown to 2030: Tracking progress towards universal coverage for reproductive, maternal, newborn, and child health. *The Lancet, 391*(10129), 1538–1548.

Croce-Galis, M., Salazar, E., & Lundgren, R. (2014). *Male engagement in family planning: Reducing unmet need for family planning by addressing gender norm.* Washington, DC: Institute for Reproductive Health.

Dubourg, D., De Brouwere, V., Van Lerberghe, W., Richard, F., Litt, V., & Derveeuw, M. D. (2002). *Final report.* Belgium: Unmet Need Obstetrics Network.

Edström, J., Hassink, A., Shahrokh, T., & Stern, E. (2015). *Engendering men a collaborative review of evidence on men and boys in social change and gender equality: EMERGE evidence review.* Washington, DC: Promundo-US, Sonke Gender Justice and the Institute of Development Studies.

Fotso, J. C., Cleland, J., Mberu, B., Mutua, M., & Elungata, P. (2013). Birth spacing and child mortality: An analysis of prospective data from the Nairobi urban health and demographic surveillance system. *Journal of Biosocial Science, 45*(6), 779–798.

Fourth Global Forum on Human Resources for Health (2017). *Dublin declaration on human resources for health: Building the health workforce of the future.* Paper presented at the Human Resouces for Health conference, Dublin, Ireland.

Frenk, J., Chen, L., Bhutta, Z. A., Cohen, J., Crisp, N., Evans, T., Fineberg, H., Garcia, P., Ke, Y., Kelley, P., Kistnasamy, B., Meleis, A., Naylor, D., Pablos-Mendez, A., Reddy, S., Scrimshaw, S., Sepulveda, J., Serwadda, D., & Zurayk, H. (2010). Health professionals for a new century: Transforming education to strengthen health systems in an interdependent world. *The Lancet, 376*(9756), 1923–1958.

Frieden, T. R. (2014). Six components necessary for effective public health program implementation. *American Journal of Public Health, 104*(1), 17–22.

Gakidou, E., Cowling, K., Lozano, R., & Murray, C. J. (2010). Increased educational attainment and its effect on child mortality in 175 countries between 1970 and 2009: A systematic analysis. *The Lancet, 376*(9745), 959–974.

Ganle, J. K., Obeng, B., Segbefia, A. Y., Mwinyuri, V., Yeboah, J. Y., & Baatiema, L. (2015). How intra-familial decision-making affects women's access to, and use of maternal healthcare services in Ghana: A qualitative study. *BMC Pregnancy and Childbirth, 15*, 173.

Global Health Workforce Alliance (2013). *A universal truth: No health without a workforce. Third global forum on human resources for health report.* Geneva, Switzerland: World Health Organization.

Government of Papua New Guinea (2017). *Papua New Guinea 2017 national budget.* Port Moreseby, Papua New Guinea: Author.

Greene, M. E., Mehta, M., Pulerwitz, P., Wulf, D., Bankole, A., & Singh, S. (2006). *Involving men in reproductive health: Contributions to development.* Geneva, Switzerland: Un Millenium Project.

Gülmezoglu, A. M., Lawrie, T. A., Hezelgrave, N., Oladapo, O. T., Souza, J., Gielen, M., Lawn, J. E., Bahl, R., Althabe, F., Colaci, D., & Hofmeyr, G. (2016). Interventions to reduce maternal and new-born morbidity and mortality. In R. E. Black, R. Laxminarayan, M. Temmerman, & N. Walker (Eds), *Reproductive, maternal, newborn, and child health: Disease control priorities* (Third Edition, Vol. 2, pp. 115–136). Washington, DC: The International Bank for Reconstruction and Development/The World Bank.

Guttmacher Institute (2017). *ADDING IT UP: Investing in contraception and maternal and newborn health in Africa.* New York, NY: Guttmacher Institute.

Han, N., Wright, S. T., O'Connor, C. C., Hoy, J., Ponnampalavanar, S., Grotowski, M., Zhao, H. X., Kamarulzaman, A., Ellis, D., & Bloch, M. (2015). HIV and aging: Insights from the Asia Pacific HIV Observational Database (APHOD). *HIV Medicine, 16*, 152–160.

Hardee, K., Croce-Galis, M., & Gay, J. (2017). Are men well served by family planning programs? *Reproductive Health, 14*(1), 14.

Holmes, W. & Goldstein, M. (2012). *Being treated like a human being: Attitudes and behaviours of reproductive and maternal health workers.* Melbourne, Australia: Burnet Institute.

IPPF & UNFPA (2017). *Global sexual and reproductive health service package for men and adolescent boys.* London, UK and New York, NY: IPPF & UNFPA.

Kennedy, E. C., Mackesy-Buckley, S., Subramaniam, S., Demmke, A., Latu, R., Robertson, A. S., Tiban, K., Tokon, A., & Luchters, S. (2013). The case for investing in family planning in the Pacific: Costs and benefits of reducing unmet need for contraception in Vanuatu and the Solomon Islands. *Reproductive Health, 10*, 30.

Kohler, H. P. & Behrman, J. R. (2014). *Benefits and costs of the population and demography targets for the post-2015 development agenda: Post-2015 consensus.* Copenhagen, Denmark: Copenhagen Consensus Center.

Mannava, P., Durrant, K., Fisher, J., Chersich, M., & Luchters, S. (2015). Attitudes and behaviours of maternal health care providers in interactions with clients: A systematic review. *Globalization and Health, 11*, 36.

Miller, S., Abalos, E., Chamillard, M., Ciapponi, A., Colaci, D., Comande, D., Diaz, V., Geller, S., Hanson, C., Langer, A., Manuelli, V., Millar, K., Morhason-Bello, I., Castro, C. P., Pileggi, V. N., Robinson, N., Skaer, M., Souza, J. P., Vogel, J. P., & Althabe, F. (2016). Beyond too little, too late and too much, too soon: A pathway towards evidence-based, respectful maternity care worldwide. *The Lancet, 388*(10056), 2176–2192.

Muleta, M. (2006). Obstetric fistula in developing countries: A review article. *Journal of Obstetrics and Gynaecology Canada, 28*(11), 962–966.

National Statistical Office (2009). *PNG demographic and health survey 2006. National report.* Port Moresby, Papua New Guinea: National Statistical Office.

Oshi, D. C., Oshi, S. N., Alobu, I. N., & Ukwaja, K. (2016). Gender-related factors influencing women's health seeking for tuberculosis care in Ebonyi State, Nigeria. *Journal of Biosocial Science, 48*(1), 37–50.

Patton, G. C., Sawyer, S. M., Santelli, J. S., Ross, D. A., Afifi, R., Allen, N. B., Arora, M., Azzopardi, P., Baldwin, W., Bonell, C., Kakuma, R., Kennedy, E., Mahon, J., McGovern, T., Mokdad, A. H., Patel, V., Petroni, S., Reavley. N., Taiwo, K., Waldfogel, J., Wickremarathne, D., Barroso, C., Bhutta, Z., Fatusi, A. O., Mattoo, A., Diers, J., Fang, J., Ferguson, J., Ssewamala, F., & Viner, R. M. (2016). Our future: A Lancet commission on adolescent health and wellbeing. *The Lancet, 387*(10036), 2423–2478.

Promundo and UNFPA (2016). *Strengthening CSO-government partnerships to scale up approaches engaging men and boys for gender equality and SRHR: A tool for action.* Washington, DC: PromundoUS and New York City, NY: UNFPA.

Renfrew, M. J., Homer, C., Downe, S., & Mcfadden, A. (2014a). Midwifery. An executive summary for the Lancet's series. *The Lancet, 384*, 2–8.

Renfrew, M. J., McFadden, A., Bastos, M. H., Campbell, J., Channon, A. A., Cheung, N. F., Silva, D. R., Downe, S., Kennedy, H. P., Malata, A., McCormick, F., Wick, L., & Declercq, E. (2014b). Midwifery and quality care: Findings from a new evidence-informed framework for maternal and newborn care. *The Lancet, 384*(9948), 1129–1145.

Ronsmans, C. & Graham, W. J. (2006). Maternal mortality: Who, when, where, and why. *The Lancet, 368*(9542), 1189–1200.

Sawyer, S. M., Afifi, R. A., Bearinger, L. H., Blakemore, S. J., Dick, B., Ezeh, A. C., & Patton, G. C. (2012). Adolescence: a foundation for future health. *Lancet, 379*(9826), 1630–1640.

Say, L., Chou, D., Gemmill, A., Tuncalp, O., Moller, A. B., Daniels, J., Gülmezoglu, A. M., Temmerman, M., & Alkema, L. (2014). Global causes of maternal death: A WHO systematic analysis. *Lancet Global Health, 2*(6), e323–333.

Sonke Gender Justice (2016). *Annual report March 2015–February 2016 celebrating 10 years of advancing gender justice.* Cape Town, South Africa: Sonke Gender Justice.

Starrs, A. M., Ezeh, A. C., Barker, G., Basu, A., Bertrand, J. T., Blum, R., Coll-Seck, A. M., Grover, A., Laski, L., Roa, M., Sathar, Z. A., Say, L., Serour, G. I., Singh, S., Stenberg, K., Temmerman, M., Biddlecom, A., Popinchalk, A., Summers, C., & Ashford, L. S. (2018). Accelerate progress – sexual and reproductive health and rights for all: Report of the Guttmacher-Lancet Commission. *The Lancet, 391*(10140), 2642–2692.

Sweetman, C. (Ed.) (2002). *Gender, development and poverty.* Oxford, UK: Oxfam.

Temmerman, M., Khosla, R., Laski, L., Mathews, Z., & Say, L. (2015a). Women's health priorities and interventions. *BMJ: British Medical Journal, 351*, doi.org.ezproxy.uws.edu.au/10.1136/bmj.h4147.

Temmerman, M., Khosla, R., Laski, L., Mathews, Z., & Say, L. (2015b). Women's health priorities and interventions. *BMJ: British Medical Journal, 351*, h4147.

The Alan Guttmacher Institute (2003). *In their own right: Addressing the sexual and reproductive health needs of men worldwide.* New York, NY: The Alan Guttmacher Institute.

The DHS Program (2018). *Model women's questionnaire.* Rockville, MD: Author. Retrieved 14/04/2018, from https://dhsprogram.com/pubs/pdf/DHSQ7/DHS7-Womans-QRE-EN-07Jun2017-DHSQ7.pdf.

The International Bank for Reconstruction and Development/The World Bank (2007). *The global family planning revolution. Three decades of population policies and programs.* Washington, DC: Author.

The World Bank (2012). *Towards gender equality in east Asia and the Pacific: A companion to the world development report – conferenece edition.* Washington, DC: Author.

The World Bank (2018). World Bank Country and Lending Groups. Washington, DC: Author. Retrieved 14/04/2018, from https://datahelpdesk.worldbank.org/knowledgebase/articles/906519-world-bank-country-and-lending-groups.

Tilburt, J. (2010). The role of worldviews in health disparities education. *Journal of General Internal Medicine, 25*(Suppl 2), 178–181.

Ugwu, N. U. & de Kok, B. (2015). Socio-cultural factors, gender roles and religious ideologies contributing to Caesarian-section refusal in Nigeria. *Reproductive Health, 12*(1), 70.

United Nations (2015). *The Millenium development goals report.* New York, NY: Author.

United Nations (2016). Sustainable development goals. New York, NY: Author. Retrieved 22/10/2018, from www.undp.org/content/undp/en/home/sustainable-development-goals.

United Nations Department of Economic and Socia Affairs Population Division (2015). *Trends in contraceptive use worldwide.* New York, NY: United Nations.

United Nations Economic and Social Commission for Asia and the Pacific (ESCAP) (2018). *Empowering women is the smart approach to sustainable development.* Bangkok, Thailand: Author. Retrieved 21/04/2018, from www.unescap.org/op-ed/empowering-women-smart-approach-sustainable-development.

United Nations Population Fund (UNFPA) (2016). *Religion, women's health and rights: Points of contention and paths of opportunities.* New York, NY: Author.

World Health Organization (2006). *World health report 2006.* Geneva, Switzerland: Author.

World Health Organization (2012). *Addressing the challenges of women's health in Africa: Report of the commission on women's health in the African region.* Brazzaville, Republic of Congo: WHO Regional Office for Africa.

World Health Organization (2014a). *Contraception fact sheet.* Geneva, Switzerland: Author. Retrieved 22/10/2018, from www.who.int/en/news-room/fact-sheets/detail/family-planning-contraception.

World Health Organization (2014b). *Global health estimates 2000–2012.* Geneva, Switzerland: Author.

World Health Organization (2015). *Trends in maternal mortality: 1990 to 2015: Estimates by WHO, UNICEF, UNFPA, World Bank Group and the United Nations Population Division.* Geneva, Switzerland: Author.

World Health Organization (2017). *World health statistics 2017: Monitoring health for the SDGs, sustainable development goals.* Geneva, Switzerland: Author.

World Health Organization (2018). *Adolescent pregnancy.* Geneva, Switzerland: Author. Retrieved 29/10/2018, from www.who.int/news-room/fact-sheets/detail/adolescent-pregnancy.

WorldFish (2018). *Gender strategy brief: A gender transformative approach to research in development in aquatic agricultural systems.* Penang, Malaysia: Author. Retrieved 20/06/2018, from www.worldfishcenter.org/content/gender-strategy-brief-gender-transformative-approach-research-development-aquatic.

38

EXPERIENCES OF REPRODUCTIVE AND SEXUAL HEALTH AND HEALTH CARE AMONG WOMEN WITH DISABILITIES

Heather Dillaway, Brianna Marzolf, Heather Fritz, Wassim Tarraf and Catherine Lysack

Approximately 15% of the global population, or close to one billion people, have disabilities, nearly 200 million of which limit physical functioning (WHO, 2011). Rates of disability are also currently higher internationally among women than men (Emmett & Alant, 2006; Kiani, 2009; WHO, 2011). Kiani (2009) reported that the gender difference is because women live longer than men and because there is gender bias in the allocation of resources and access to health services in many parts of the world (see also Emmett & Alant, 2006). Disability rates among women are even higher in low-income countries, where 22.1% of women have a disability, as compared with 14.4% in higher-income countries (WHO, 2011).

Access to good health has been declared a human right by the World Health Organization (WHO), yet there are many barriers for marginalized populations such as women with disabilities (WHO, 2017). Rates of disability among women have increased in recent years (WHO, 2011, 2013). Securing good reproductive and sexual health is critical for their well-being since they are more likely than women without disabilities to report poor reproductive and sexual outcomes (especially perinatal outcomes) (Signore, 2016). In this chapter we discuss basic barriers to good health and, more specifically, to good reproductive and sexual health and health care for women with physical disabilities. We then focus on the case of women with spinal cord injuries to provide readers with a more nuanced understanding of the experiences of one group of women with disabilities. Throughout this chapter we hone in on women's experiences within the U.S., but urge others to extend this important discussion to broader contexts.

A feminist disability perspective emphasizes how both *gender* and *disability* are essential in shaping the thoughts and experiences of women with disabilities (Deegan & Brooks, 1985; Gill, 1994; Morris, 2001; Naples, Mauldin, & Dillaway, 2019; Wendell, 1996). Following this perspective, we argue that gendered meanings and experiences are filtered through the context of having a disability as much as through gendered social contexts. Merleau-Ponty (1962, p. 206) wrote that the "lived body" is a location of meaning and identity as well as a material entity: "We are in the world through our body, and … we perceive that world within our body." Turner (2001, p. 253) argued that we must look at the "governmentality" or production of bodies within society (i.e., the social rules, constraints, and barriers put forth for how we should define and engage in bodily experience), and Thomas (1999) reminded us to pay attention to the embodied experience of impairment while also paying attention to the sociocultural barriers associated with impairment. Likewise, the International Classification of Functioning Disability and Health (ICF) purposely defined disability as not just an "attribute of the individual" but, rather, a state that results from the interaction between person and environment (Tarraf, Mahmoudi, Dillaway, & Gonzalez, 2016). Impairment is not a fixed property of a person but, rather, a social-relational entity, which means that how one lives with a physical impairment is more telling about what an impairment truly is for a person than is any material reality of the body.

Barriers to good health and health care among people with disabilities

It is well documented that significant physical, political and social barriers limit access to health and social services as well as job and educational opportunities among people with disabilities (WHO, 2011). As such, individuals with disabilities have lower educational achievement, lower labor force participation, and greater risk of poverty relative to those without disabilities. Overall, they also receive substandard health care, have lower levels of basic or preventive health services utilization, report higher dissatisfaction with health care providers, and have poorer health outcomes (McColl, 2002; Pharr & Chino, 2013; WHO, 2011).

Historically, research about barriers to quality health care for individuals with disabilities has focused on barriers in the external physical environment (e.g., lack of suitable infrastructure) that limit access to health care (Dillaway & Lysack, 2014a). Various health care technologies and diagnostic tools (e.g., mammography machines) and the internal design of health care facilities also pose barriers to physically impaired bodies, and complicate care provision during diagnostic appointments (Dillaway & Lysack, 2014a). Geographic limitations for certain health services, and the lack of access to affordable and reliable transportation often compound the problem (Kiani, 2009; WHO, 2011).

Though public policy can address some of these issues, the political will for large scale action is often insufficient, and change is commonly hindered by vague policy guidelines and inadequate funding for implementation of policy. Still, attempts to establish policy indicate growing awareness of the problems of accessibility and the need to address them. Internationally, the United Nations' 2006 Convention on the Rights of Persons with Disabilities (CRPD) identified several structural barriers to good health and recommended both "national and international action" to remedy these barriers (WHO, 2011, p. 7). In the U.S., the implementation of the Americans with Disabilities Act (ADA) lessened some, but not all physical barriers. For example, public access to buildings and transportation has improved, but less has been done within health care settings (Dillaway & Lysack, 2015; McColl, 2002; Pharr & Chino, 2013).

Limited knowledge about policy (e.g., ADA) or exposure to patients with disabilities among providers indirectly shape attitudes, influence compliance with rules, and can reinforce existing barriers and lower care quality (Dillaway & Lysack, 2014a, 2015; Kiani, 2009; Symons, Morley, McGuigan, & Akl, 2014; WHO, 2011). Despite worldwide calls to revamp medical curricula to increase awareness and enhance training, medical providers continue to lack training in the unique needs of people with disabilities or how to manage care for those with diagnosed disabilities (WHO, 2011). Medical students, residents, and even practicing physicians often demonstrate deficiencies in working knowledge of disability, and patients with disabilities often report the need to educate their physicians about the basic elements of their disability (Dillaway & Lysack, 2015; Symons et al., 2014).

Reproductive and sexual health and health care among women with disabilities

Many reproductive events and processes are experienced differently by women with disabilities, such as menstruation, fertility, prenatal care and pregnancy, contraception, and reproductive health screenings (McColl, 2002; Signore, 2016). Reasons for unique experiences vary but can include: difficulties with menstrual hygiene management (Dillaway, Cross, Lysack, & Schwartz, 2013); societal biases about whether women with disabilities can handle, or are "fit" for, motherhood (Dillaway & Lysack, 2014b; Frederick, 2017; Signore, 2016); skepticism about prenatal testing (Signore, 2016); unique complications in labor and delivery (Signore, 2016; WHO, 2009); doctors' lack of recognition of the need for STD and STI testing or cancer screenings (Signore, 2016); and lack of attention to their contraceptive needs (Kaplan, 2006; McCarthy, 2009; McColl, 2002; Welner, 1999). Among the biggest reproductive health challenges facing women with disabilities are the inadequate provision of primary and preventative gynecological health care (McColl, 2002), the lack of access to family planning services (WHO, 2009, p. 10), and the overreliance on specialists for basic care (Frederick, 2017). These challenges are driven by the lack of availability of suitable resources and infrastructure (Signore, 2016; Symons et al., 2014), and compounded by limited know-how and physicians' and other providers' (e.g., midwives) discomfort in interacting with and caring for disabled bodies (see also Dillaway & Lysack, 2014a, 2014b).

It is important to note that, although there are some unique risks posed by impairments at times (Signore, 2016; WHO, 2009, 2011), most variations in reproductive experiences are caused by the social-relational interactions between women with disabilities and their environments (Dillaway & Lysack, 2014a; Frederick, 2017; Turner, 2001; WHO, 2009). Furthermore, most of the existing knowledge about the reproductive and sexual experiences of women with disabilities is derived from research on women with physical disabilities (Signore, 2016; WHO, 2011). We know less about the experiences of women with intellectual, developmental and sensory disabilities.

The literature on the reproductive experiences of women with disabilities also largely ignores how experiences of sexuality and intimacy are part of, and also influence, reproductive experiences (Fritz, Dillaway, & Lysack, 2015; McCarthy, 2009). The reproductive and sexual health experiences of women with disabilities are intertwined, as they are for all women. For instance, decisions about engaging in sexual activity may coincide with decisions about family planning. Research on intimacy among women with disabilities focuses on sexual functioning and the impairment-related conditions that can affect sexual activity, such as urinary and bowel incontinence, rather than on women's actual involvement in intimate relationships, expectations for intimacy, reproductive decision-making, or sexual identities (Fritz et al., 2015). Much more research is needed on how reproductive and sexual health decisions and experiences intersect and overlap across the life span before we can understand women's reproductive and sexual health holistically.

Sexual health and wellness includes having a positive sexual identity, adequate information about one's sexuality, positive and productive relationships, the ability to manage barriers to sexual health or intimacy, and the ability to achieve optimal physical sexual functioning (Signore, 2016). Some barriers to sexual activity may result from impairments themselves but, as with other dimensions of reproductive health, most aspects of sexual health are determined by factors in the social or physical environment (Fritz et al., 2015; Signore, 2016). For example, according to data from the World Health Survey, women and girls with disabilities often lack access to sex education, including information on safe sex, STIs, and healthy relationships (Kiani, 2009; WHO, 2009, 2011); this is a global problem.

Negative attitudes

Sociocultural contexts can infringe upon women's ability to achieve good reproductive and sexual health and access quality health care. According to Signore (2016, p. 94), worldwide, women with disabilities confront what she deemed "stubborn attitudinal barriers." They often experience stigma, insensitivity, and discrimination within interactions with families, peers, and health care providers, and the result may be substandard, abridged, or incomplete health care that leads to poor reproductive and sexual health (Frederick, 2017; Fritz et al., 2015; Kiani, 2009; McCarthy, 2009; Pharr & Chino, 2013; WHO, 2009). Women with disabilities must also confront their "double disadvantage" of being women *and* disabled (Deegan & Brooks, 1985) and facing prejudice and discrimination because of both social locations. For instance, disabled women are stereotyped as "asexual," "celibate," "non-reproductive," or "infertile," and not mothers (Becker, Stuifbergen, & Tinkle, 1997; Nosek, 2000; Welner, 1999; Wendell, 1996), because sexual beings and mothers are assumed to be able-bodied, whereas disabled bodies are assumed to be broken, childlike and incapable of "normal" reproductive and sexual activities (e.g., Frederick, 2017). Frederick (2017, p. 76) argued that cultural ideologies dictate a "normalcy project" that "prizes" a typical (non-disabled) maternal body and "sees 'abnormality' [as] an unwelcome drain on society." In other words, cultural ideologies about motherhood call for women to be "perfectly normal reproducers" (Frederick, 2017, p. 76).

These cultural prejudices have serious consequences for the health of women with disabilities, as they affect how families, peers, health care providers, and even women themselves see their reproductive and sexual trajectories (Frederick, 2017). For example, although some women with disabilities do have family support for their reproductive decisions, others receive negative reactions from family members after they share news of pregnancies (Signore, 2016). Some women may not even be allowed to establish intimate relationships (WHO, 2009). Health professionals may also react adversely when women with disabilities come to them for prenatal care (Frederick, 2017; Prunty, Sharpe, Butow, & Fulcher, 2008). In fact, in countries where care is coordinated by local community health workers (e.g., midwives), women with disabilities are sometimes turned away from prenatal care and told that "they should not be pregnant, or scolded because they have decided to have a child" (Maxwell, Belser, & David, 2007, as cited in WHO, 2009, p. 10).

As a result of these attitudes, women with disabilities can feel "degendered" in health care settings, "perceiving their roles as women, lovers, spouses, or mothers as unrecognizable or ignored by clinicians" (Signore, 2016, p. 94). Health care providers' perceptions (and misperceptions) and their disability-specific knowledge and training (or lack thereof) comprise the social context within which reproductive and sexual health care takes place (Dillaway & Lysack, 2014a; Frederick, 2017; Signore, 2016). Because health care providers' training has not covered the reproductive and sexual health of women with disabilities, and because the cultural assumption is that women with disabilities are "risky" mothers (Frederick, 2017), providers may concentrate on the impairment itself when a woman comes in for care, rather than treating the woman for the reason she arrives in the setting (Signore,

2016). Thinking about the actual human encounters that take place during these situations is critical in order to understand what shapes the accessibility and availability of good reproductive and sexual health and health care for women with disabilities.

A concrete example: women with spinal cord injuries

To truly understand the experiences of women with physical disabilities and the barriers such women face as they attempt to lead their reproductive and sexual lives or access health care, we examine research on one group of women with a very specific type of physical disability: spinal cord injuries (SCI). Traumatic SCI refers to a sudden injury that causes paralysis and loss of sensation. Some persons lose the ability to use their legs and lower body (paraplegia), whereas others lose this ability from the neck down (tetraplegia or quadriplegia). Complete or partial motor paralysis necessitates wheelchair use and lifelong coping with a range of serious medical complications (Jensen, Kuehn, Amtmann, & Cardenas, 2007). Thus, survivors of SCI must deal with the physical effects of their impairment while also struggling with the social-relational barriers created by an ableist society that defines their bodies as "abnormal" (Hughes & Patterson, 1997).

Based on 2012 world population estimates, 250,000 to 500,000 people suffer a SCI every year (WHO, 2013). In 2015, approximately 288,000 people were currently living with SCI in the U.S., and almost 18,000 new injuries occur each year (NSCISC, 2018). The average age at injury in the U.S. has moved from 29 years in the 1970s to 42 years in 2015; this increase can also be seen internationally (National Spinal Cord Injury Statistics Center (NSCISC), 2018; WHO, 2013). Both in the U.S. and abroad, motor vehicle crashes are the most common cause of SCI (38–40% of all injuries depending on the reporting country), followed by falls (14–36%), acts of violence (including war-related injuries and intimate partner violence) (11–14%), and sports accidents (8%) (NSCISC, 2018; WHO, 2013). Historically, about 90% of SCIs have been traumatic in nature, but non-traumatic SCIs are also growing in number internationally, due to work-related accidents, attempted suicides, tuberculosis, and other chronic diseases (WHO, 2013). Unfortunately, persons with SCI are more disadvantaged and more dissatisfied than the able-bodied population on many quality of life indicators including employment, financial well-being, family life, psychological adjustment, and a range of personal health outcomes, (Hammell, 2007). Women with SCI face poorer quality of life outcomes than men overall (Hammell, 2007; Nosek, 2000).

The focus on women's issues after SCI is a relatively new phenomenon, in part because men are the majority of SCI patients worldwide (approximately 70%) (Rutberg, Friden, & Karlsson, 2008). More women and older adults are suffering SCI in recent years (WHO, 2013). However, we know little about women's everyday experiences post-injury, and even less about their everyday reproductive and sexual health experiences after SCI, even though there is more research on women with SCI than on women with other disabilities overall. Questions remain about how women with SCI make decisions about reproductive and sexual health within a context of limited medical knowledge and negative attitudes towards women with disabilities.

Unique experiences?

Endocrinologists, physiologists, neuroscientists and rehabilitation scholars in a variety of countries confirm that a temporary period of amenorrhea is probable immediately after SCI (Bughi, Shaw, Mahmood, Atkins, & Szlachcic, 2008; DeForge et al., 2005; Estores & Sipski, 2004; Rutberg et al., 2008). Research findings are mixed about how likely, or how long, this period of amenorrhea might be, or how it affects women's fertility, although most of these studies suggest that menstrual cycles resume for most women after about 12–24 months (DeForge et al., 2005). Signore (2016) reported that women with higher-level injuries (at or above the sixth thoracic vertebra) can also experience blood pressure elevations (called autonomic dysreflexia), and these elevations may coincide with dysmenorrhea. These complications are well documented but we have little understanding of how women with SCI manage menstruation or deal with unique complications on a regular basis.

Further, there is some evidence that women with SCI face higher risks in pregnancy and childbirth because of their higher risk of diabetes and high blood pressure (Nosek, Howland, Rintala, Young, & Chanpong, 2001; Signore, 2016); thus, some impairment-related contexts may shape prenatal experience. The rates of forceps use, vacuum extraction, and caesarean section are also higher than for able-bodied women, but data are anecdotal and incomplete (WHO, 2009). It is unclear why these interventions are utilized more often with disabled women, but the reasons may be related to doctors' lack of knowledge about how to deal with pregnant or birthing bodies that are disabled (Signore, 2016; WHO, 2009). DeForge et al. (2005, p. 700) documented a general "paucity of literature regarding SCI, female fertility, and pregnancy-related complications."

Studies of women's sexual and reproductive health after SCI are often written in response to myths about the "non-reproductive" and "asexual" nature of women with disabilities (Dillaway & Lysack, 2014b). For instance, much of the existing literature has simply argued that women *can* still become pregnant after SCI (Dillaway & Lysack, 2014b). Other research seems to have been generated purposely to inform health care providers about special screening and treatment issues that arise from the effects of physical impairment (e.g., bladder management, labor management, osteoporosis, cardiac problems, lack of sexual feeling) or the risks of particular birth control methods (DeForge et al., 2005; Estores & Sipski, 2004; Welner, 1999). That research reinforces the definition of women with SCI as different and "abnormal," and stands in contrast to research that documents the normality of women with SCI (Dillaway & Lysack, 2014b; Signore, 2016). Thus, a tension exists in this small body of literature: do women with SCI have "normal" or "abnormal" reproductive and sexual health experiences? By focusing on difference alone, we may forget that women with SCI live full reproductive and sexual lives that are affected, but not completely determined, by physical impairments alone.

Learning from interviews with women with SCI

We can understand the everyday reproductive and sexual health experiences of women with SCI more clearly when we listen to individual women's voices. In this section we highlight examples of how women in our own research have talked about reproductive and sexual experiences to indicate the complexities of disability, reproductive health and sexuality across the life span. Specifically, we draw on data from 20 in-depth qualitative interviews with women with SCI in a Midwestern city in the U.S. to highlight their everyday experiences of menstruation, fertility, pregnancy, childbirth, and sexual relationships (see Dillaway et al. (2013) for a detailed description of our methods).

Menstruation

Following disability-related amenorrhea, one-third of the women in our study reported additional hassles with menstruation because of their impairment, and almost one-half reported using birth control methods and/or reproductive surgery to lessen or stop menstruation because of these hassles (Dillaway et al., 2013). For example, one of our interviewees, Kendra, discussed the "extra clean-up work" that had to be done because she could not feel when she needed to change a pad, or move from her bed to a wheelchair and then a toilet easily (p. 114). Rachel described trying to use tampons while dealing with her shaky legs and how she resorted to wearing gloves in order to decrease the amount of clean-up she had to do after insertion. Nina felt lucky that she had had a hysterectomy before her SCI because she had avoided post-injury menstrual hassles completely.

Even though one-half of the women in our sample reported feeling positive about resuming menstruation after injury, the impact of the SCI on women's menstrual management resulted in mixed feelings. On the one hand, to be similar to other, able-bodied women or to their pre-injury self was a positive thing, as women who menstruate regularly are assumed to be "normal" and healthy (Dillaway et al., 2013). On the other hand, managing the logistical hassles associated with menstruation, especially in cases of quadriplegia, can be hard for women with SCI (Dillaway et al., 2013). One of our interviewees, Kelsey, explained: "I liked it the first year [after SCI] because I didn't have [a regular menstrual cycle] after the trauma. That was really nice but not for the right reason." She was somewhat disappointed to menstruate again because she had to deal with the hassle of managing periods, but knew it was "natural" (Dillaway et al., 2013, p. 114).

Pregnancy and childbirth

As other researchers have found (AACE, 2006; Welner, 1999), the majority of women in our study were told by doctors that they could still get pregnant. Yet, although doctors reminded them of their "normal" status, they also warned them about the risks of using contraception or becoming pregnant in light of their impairments (Dillaway & Lysack, 2014b). For instance, Terry was told by one doctor, "If you take birth control you will die" (Dillaway & Lysack, 2014b, p. 142). The doctor wanted to make sure that Terry knew that she could not use hormone-based birth control (e.g., the pill) because of the risk of blood clots. Damita explained how a doctor discouraged her from getting pregnant right after injury: "If you're going to engage in [sex] you need to protect yourself" (p. 142). Both Terry and Damita had difficulty interpreting their doctors' declarations and assessing the real risks at hand because the doctors did not explain why they made these statements. The result was that both women felt unsure about what they could and could not do post-injury.

Signore (2016) also documented doctors' concerns about pregnancy and labor, including women's inability to feel labor pains and their risk for autonomic dysreflexia (elevated blood pressure). Stacie, a participant in our study, described how her lack of sensation affected her interactions with hospital staff and her ability to push during labor:

> [B]efore the baby came, [hospital staff members] were asking me, "Did your water break"? [And I said,] "How would I know, 'cause I'm always incontinent!" … [And w]hen the baby was coming, when it got close to coming out, I began to have [autonomic] dysreflexia. Yeah, I couldn't push anymore.

There are higher rates of caesarean section among women with physical disabilities like SCI because of doctors' attempts to control perceived risks and eliminate possible complications in labor and delivery (Signore, 2016; WHO, 2009). Without full understanding of how fertility, pregnancy and childbirth will manifest in women with disabilities, doctors label all pregnancies among women with SCI as "high risk" (Frederick, 2017; Signore, 2016). Caesarean sections, of course, have their own risks and complications.

Just thinking about fertility was complicated for women in our study, especially because they were unsure about what the risks of pregnancy really were in the face of their impairment. Some women in our study (Dillaway & Lysack, 2014b) decided they would rather forgo having children post-injury than deal with the uncertain risks to their personal health. Kelsey, for instance, told us how she did not expect to have children post-injury. She and her husband were intimate "because the 'apparatus' [body parts, her quotations] that I have are fully functional," but "we have talked about it and we don't want any children. I'm afraid if there are side effects that could complicate my spinal cord injury. I'm afraid of the complications." Terry's concerns paralleled Kelsey's. Terry had two children before injury, and she and her husband thought about having a third after her SCI: "It's scarier [post-injury] than it was before [injury]. ... [W]e didn't know what risk it was going to put on me and so it was better to go without having another child."

Thus, even though many women in our study became mothers post-injury, reproductive options and choices sometimes came with qualifications and constraints because of impairment-related concerns. Doctors relayed information about potential complications due to SCI but did not always explain the risk for these complications, which induced uncertainty, and sometimes fear, among our interviewees. The women in our study also documented others' negative attitudes toward mothers with disabilities, as others assumed that they were "asexual" or "unable" to mother well. The most negative attitudes came from unsupportive medical staff or lay individuals who challenged their legitimacy as mothers. As Damita explained,

> I think the hardest thing that I've had to come to grips with is that people look at me as an asexual being ... [F]or example, you and I could be walking down the street and my kid is with me and they'll probably think that my kid is your kid. You know, 'cause they think, "How could she have sex?" ... I think sometimes we're viewed as half-people, not whole individuals. Or, as children. You know, as if we're not capable of doing things.
>
> *(Dillaway & Lysack, 2014b, p. 146)*

It is important to note, however, that almost one-third of our sample bore children post-injury, and many women made choices post-injury about menstrual management, birth control, sexual relationships, hysterectomies, and other reproductive procedures. Thus, attitudinal barriers did not always prevent them from making a variety of reproductive and sexual decisions post-injury. Nonetheless, some of our interviewees never had children, and this may be because they were discouraged from opting into certain reproductive experiences after injury. Others were finished with childbearing before injury and did not feel the direct impact of disability on fertility (Dillaway & Lysack, 2014b). For instance, Justine was injured later in life when her children were in high school and college. Although she was still navigating an intimate relationship and raising children, she was not concerned about whether she would be able to bear additional children (Fritz et al., 2015).

Sexuality and sexual relationships post-injury

The sexual health consequences of SCI can be substantial, especially because the majority of SCIs happen during early adulthood when women may be anticipating active reproductive and sexual lives (Fritz et al., 2015). Positive sexual experiences after SCI increase quality of life after injury (Fritz et al., 2015). The interaction between disability and sexuality is particularly important for women with SCI because women are more likely than their male counterparts with SCI to engage in partnered sexual activity after injury (McCabe & Taleporos, 2003).

Research also suggests that heterosexual women with SCI identify regaining sexual function as a higher priority than men do, perhaps because women worry about whether their husbands will leave them if intimacy is affected (Fritz et al., 2015; Kiani, 2009). A WHO (2013) report on SCI indicated that relationship dissolution and divorce are common in the early years after injury. This was the case for at least one of the women in our sample.

Nonetheless, there is a dearth of research on women's sexuality after SCI. We still know very little about how sexuality or sexual intimacy is defined by women with SCI, how women with physical disabilities defined positive sexual experiences, the ways in which they decide whether to engage in sexual activity after injury, and how they obtain information about sexual functioning after injury. Moreover, because women with SCI are seen as asexual and non-reproductive, doctors' assumptions may be that women with SCI do not need comprehensive information about intimacy and sexual activity (Signore, 2016; WHO, 2013). Compared with non-disabled women, women with physical disabilities report delayed sexual activity and limited access to intimate relationships (Nosek et al., 2001; Signore, 2016). Women with disabilities may also not be seen as "suitable" partners, if cultural attitudes degender them and define them as seemingly "unfit" to be mothers and/or caregivers (Becker et al., 1997; Gill, 1994; Signore, 2016; Welner, 1999).

Women in our study wanted more education about sexual intimacy after SCI, yet they did not receive it from their rehabilitation team initially, or from other doctors in the longer term (Fritz et al., 2015). Our interviewees suggested that providers may feel uncomfortable talking about sexuality, especially about broaching the topic with women who did not bring it up themselves. Women themselves may feel shame and anxiety about broaching the topic with professionals (Signore, 2016). Our findings suggest that good sexual health is important to women and that providers, family members, partners, and peers must think about the life stage of the woman who is disabled, her relationship status and expectations, and her desires for the future (e.g., marriage, family planning, healthy aging) when trying to support women's pursuits of good reproductive and sexual health (Fritz et al., 2015). For example, a 20-year-old woman with SCI may be interested in initiating sexual activity for the first time and may be wondering about basic sexual functioning or whether she might be able to have children someday, whereas a woman with SCI in her 40s might be wondering whether she can maintain an established intimate relationship and how to have good sexual health at midlife.

Women in our study also highlighted their varied definitions of sexual intimacy after injury, and indicated that sex education and doctor–patient conversation should refer to those different meanings. Existing research has often focused on women's sexuality within heteronormative contexts, such as attempts to have penetrative sexual intercourse (Fritz et al., 2015; Rembis, 2010; Tarasoff, 2016). However, our findings suggest that women with SCI may desire different kinds of sexual activity, especially within the context of changing and aging bodies. For instance, Damita said,

> At this point in my life, it isn't just the, you know, the [sex]. It's also an emotional thing. It's a common response for women with spinal cord injury. It's just wanting to be intimate, you know, holding hands, being held, it's that kind of thing. I think that's where I am at this point. It's not just the act itself.
>
> *(Fritz et al., 2015, p. 5).*

Idell affirmed Damita's perspective; she stated that women with SCI "want to be … affectionate [and have] romance" (Fritz et al., 2015, p. 5). Expanding the notion of what it means to be "intimate" or "close" was important to many of the women in our study. On the other hand, when penetrative sexual intercourse was important, it was typically associated with starting (or expanding) a family. Just over half of our participants had not borne children before injury, and others did not feel "done" having children upon injury (Fritz et al., 2015). Therefore, sex education for women with SCI should take into account women's reproductive life stage and relationship status because sexual activity may have different purposes at different times.

Conclusion

As outlined in WHO (2009, p. 31), women with disabilities have the right to achieve the "highest attainable standard of health," but, as evidenced in this chapter, currently this right is not guaranteed for all. Ensuring this right means providing accessible health care services that are gender- and disability-sensitive, so that all women with disabilities can secure good reproductive and sexual health and health care. Protecting this right also means acknowledging the normalcy of women with disabilities, in that women with disabilities desire to, and do, lead reproductive and sexual lives, just like other women.

In order to secure good reproductive and sexual health as a basic right, women with disabilities need several additional and broad guarantees: (1) greater provision and accessibility of health care services, so that all women with disabilities can experience good reproductive and sexual health regardless of their social locations; (2) better education and training of medical providers, so that women with disabilities can seek health care from providers who understand both their unique needs and their normalcy as compared with women without disabilities; (3) increased cultural understanding of the reproductive and sexual expectations and experiences of women with disabilities, including the recognition that women with disabilities are sexual, are fertile, are mothers, and are making reproductive and sexual decisions on a daily basis; and (4) further research on the reproductive and sexual experiences of women with different types of impairments, so that we know just as much about women with intellectual, developmental, or sensory disabilities as we do about women with certain types of physical disabilities. Women with disabilities residing in different regions of the world need to be consulted on how to better assure good reproductive and sexual health because providers and policy makers can learn from listening to women's voices. Using all means possible and with the above guarantees in mind, we must continue to update our understandings of both the effects of impairment itself and the social-relational contexts within which women and their impairments exist, so that we can better understand, and remove, the barriers that women with disabilities face as they attempt to achieve good reproductive and sexual health and health care.

References

American Association of Clinical Endocrinologists (AACE) (2006). *Women who have experienced temporary amenorrhea at the time of spinal cord injury may still achieve pregnancy.* Jacksonville, FL. Retrieved January 31, 2012 from www.newswise.com/articles/women-who-have-experienced-temporary-amenorrhea-at-time-of-spinal-cord-injury-may-still-achieve-pregnancy.

Becker, H., Stuifbergen, A., & Tinkle, M. (1997). Reproductive health care experiences of women with physical disabilities: A qualitative study. *Archives of Physical Medicine and Rehabilitation, 78,* S26–S33.

Bughi, S., Shaw, S., Mahmood, G., Atkins, R., & Szlachcic, Y. (2008). Amenorrhea, pregnancy, and pregnancy outcomes in women following spinal cord injury: A retrospective cross-sectional study. *Endocrine Practice, 14,* 437–441.

Deegan, M. J. & Brooks, N. A. (Eds) (1985). *Women and disability: The double handicap.* New Brunswick, NJ: Transaction Books.

DeForge, D., Blackmer, J., Garrity, C., Yazdi, F., Cronin, V., Barrowman, N., Fang, M., Mamaladze, V., Zhang, L., Sampson, M., & Moher, D. (2005). Fertility following spinal cord injury: A systematic review. *Spinal Cord, 43,* 693–703.

Dillaway, H., Cross, K., Lysack, C., & Schwartz, J. (2013). Normal and natural, or burdensome and terrible? Women with spinal cord injuries discuss ambivalence about menstruation. *Sex Roles, 68,* 107–120.

Dillaway, H. & Lysack, C. (2014a). Encounters with inaccessibility: The contexts women with spinal cord injury face when seeking gynecological health care. In B. Altman & S. Barnartt (Eds), *Research in social science and disability* (Vol. 8, pp. 233–259). Bingley, UK: Emerald Group.

Dillaway, H. & Lysack, C. (2014b). "My doctor told me I can still have children but …": Contradictions in women's reproductive health experiences after spinal cord injury. In M. Nash (Ed.), *Reframing reproduction* (pp. 135–149). London, UK: Palgrave Mcmillan.

Dillaway, H. & Lysack, C. (2015). "Most of them are amateurs": Women with spinal cord injury experience the lack of education and training among medical providers while seeking gynecological care. *Disability Studies Quarterly, 35*(3). Retrieved from http://dsq-sds.org/article/view/4934.

Emmett, T. & Alant, E. (2006). Women and disability: Exploring the interface of multiple disadvantage. *Development Southern Africa, 23*(4), 445–460.

Estores, I. M. & Sipski, M. L. (2004). Women's issues after SCI. *Topics in Spinal Cord Injury Rehabilitation, 10*(2), 107–125.

Frederick, A. (2017). Risky mothers and the normalcy project: Women with disabilities negotiate scientific motherhood. *Gender & Society, 31*(1), 74–95.

Fritz, H., Dillaway, H., & Lysack, C. (2015). "Don't think paralysis takes away your womanhood": Sexual intimacy after SCI. *American Journal of Occupational Therapy, 69*(1), 1–10.

Gill, C. J. (1994). When is a woman not a woman? *Sexuality and Disability, 12,* 117–119.

Hammell, K. W. (2007). Quality of life after spinal cord injury: A meta-synthesis of qualitative findings. *Spinal Cord, 45,* 124–139.

Hughes, B. & Patterson, K. (1997). The social model of disability and the disappearing body: Towards a sociology of impairment. *Disability & Society, 12*(3), 325–340.

Jensen, M., Kuehn, D., Amtmann, D., & Cardenas, D. (2007). Symptom burden in persons with spinal cord injury. *Archives of Physical Medicine and Rehabilitation, 88,* 638–645.

Kaplan, C. (2006). Special issues in contraception: Caring for women with disabilities. *Journal of Midwifery & Women's Health, 51,* 450–456.

Kiani, S. (2009). Women with disabilities in the North West province of Cameroon: Resilient and deserving of greater attention. *Disability & Society, 24*(4), 517–531.

Maxwell, J., Belser, J. W., & David, D. (2007). *A health handbook for women with disabilities.* Berkley, CA: Hesperian Foundation.

McCabe, M. P. & Taleporos, G. (2003). Sexual esteem, sexual satisfaction, and sexual behavior among people with physical disability. *Archives of Sexual Behavior, 32,* 359–369.

McCarthy, M. (2009). "I have the jab so I can't be blamed for getting pregnant": Contraception and women with learning disabilities. *Women's Studies International Forum, 32,* 198–208.

McColl, M. (2002). A house of cards: Women, aging and spinal cord injury. *Spinal Cord, 40,* 371–373.

Merleau-Ponty, M. (1962). *Phenomenology of perception.* Abingdon, UK: Routledge.

Morris, J. (2001). Impairment and disability: Constructing an ethics of care that promotes human rights. *Hypatia, 16*(4), 1–16.

Naples, N., Mauldin, L., & Dillaway, H. (2019). Gender, disability, and intersectionality. *Gender & Society, 33*(1), 5–18.

National Spinal Cord Injury Statistics Center (NSCISC) (2018). *Facts and figures at a glance.* Birmingham, AL: Author. Retrieved from www.nscisc.uab.edu/Public/Facts%20and%20Figures%20-%202018.pdf.

Nosek, M. (2000). Overcoming the odds: The health of women with physical disabilities in the United States. *Archives of Physical Medicine and Rehabilitation, 81,* 135–138.

Nosek, M. A., Howland, C., Rintala, D. H., Young, M. E., & Chanpong, G. F. (2001). National study of women with physical disabilities: Final report. *Sexuality and Disability, 19*(1), 5–39.

Pharr, J. & Chino, M. (2013). Predicting barriers to primary care for patients with disabilities: A mixed methods study of practice administrators. *Disability and Health Journal, 6,* 116–123.

Prunty, M., Sharpe, L., Butow, P., & Fulcher, G. (2008, June). The motherhood choice: Themes arising in the decision-making process for women with multiple sclerosis. *Multiple Sclerosis, 14,* 701–704.

Rembis, M. A. (2010). Beyond the binary: Rethinking the social model of disabled sexuality. *Sexuality and Disability, 28*(1), 51–60, doi:10.1007/s11195-009-9133-0.

Rutberg, L., Friden, B., & Karlsson, A. K. (2008). Amenorrhea in newly spinal cord injured women: An effect of hyperprolactinaemia? *Spinal Cord, 46,* 189–191.

Signore, C. (2016). Reproductive and sexual health for women with disabilities. In S. E. Miles-Cohen & C. Signore (Eds), *Eliminating inequities for women with disabilities: An agenda for health and wellness* (pp. 93–114). Washington, DC: American Psychological Association.

Symons, A., Morley, C., McGuigan, D., & Akl, E. (2014). A curriculum on care for people with disabilities: Effects on medical student self-reported attitudes and comfort level. *Disability and Health Journal, 7,* 88–95.

Tarasoff, L. A. (2016). "We exist": The health and well-being of sexual minority women and trans people with disabilities. In S. E. Miles-Cohen & C. Signore (Eds), *Eliminating inequities for women with disabilities: An agenda for health and wellness* (pp. 179–208). Washington, DC: American Psychological Association.

Tarraf, W., Mahmoudi, E., Dillaway, H., & Gonzalez, H. (2016). Health spending among working-age immigrants with disabilities compared to those born in the US. *Disability and Health Journal, 9,* 479–490.

Thomas, C. (1999). *Female forms: Experiencing and understanding disability.* Buckingham, UK: Open University Press.

Turner, B. S. (2001). Disability and the sociology of the body. In G. L. Albreacht, K. D. Seelman, & M. Bury (Eds), *Handbook of disability studies* (pp. 252–264). Thousand Oaks, CA: Sage.

Welner, S. (1999). Contraceptive choices for women with disabilities. *Sexuality and Disability, 17,* 209–214.

Wendell, S. (1996). *The rejected body: Feminist philosophical reflections on disability.* New York, NY: Routledge.

World Health Organization (WHO) (2009). *WHO/UNFPA guidance note: Promoting sexual and reproductive health for women with disabilities.* Geneva, Switzerland: Author. Retrieved from file:///C:/Users/Admin/Documents/WHO-UNFPA%20guidance%20note%20on%20promoting%20sexual%20and%20reproductive%20health%20for%20women%20with%20disabilities%202009.pdf.

World Health Organization (WHO) (2011). *Summary: World report on disability.* Geneva, Switzerland: Author. Retrieved from www.who.int/disabilities/world_report/2011/report/en.

World Health Organization (WHO) (2013). *International perspectives on spinal cord injury.* Geneva, Switzerland: Author. Retrieved from www.who.int/disabilities/policies/spinal_cord_injury/en.

World Health Organization (WHO) (2017, December 29). *Fact sheet: Human rights and health.* Geneva, Switzerland: Author. Retrieved from www.who.int/news-room/fact-sheets/detail/human-rights-and-health.

39

WOMEN WITH INTELLECTUAL AND DEVELOPMENTAL IMPAIRMENTS

Differences not deficits

Jan Burns

This chapter describes the current landscape with regard to the sexual and reproductive rights of women with intellectual impairments through early, middle, and later life. Sexual and reproductive health inequalities for women with disabilities have existed for decades (Burns, 1993). Despite medical and psychological advances, this inequality has sustained and the gap potentially widened; as the array of opportunities for women with intellectual impairments has increased, the resources and support to access these opportunities has not kept pace. Women with intellectual impairments, by the very nature of their impairments, often lack the voice and opportunity to advocate for their rights, including their sexual and reproductive rights. This leads not just to impoverished lives in terms of sexual and reproductive health, but can ultimately result in life or death. For example, research has shown that people with intellectual disabilities die on average 20 years younger, of more avoidable causes than those without such disabilities (O'Leary, Cooper, Hughes-McCormack, 2018). This includes poor gynaecological and obstetrical care, which leads to increased morbidity for both women and their offspring (Brown, Cobigo, Lunsky, & Vigod, 2016). Such shocking health inequality would usually spark governmental enquiries, public campaigns, and reparatory health initiatives. However, this has not been the case for this population of women. In this chapter, I explore these inequalities within sexual and reproductive health in depth; their causation, and why this inequality continues, despite having been acknowledged for decades.

Part of the issue is that health inequalities in this population are under-researched, which is even more evident in the case of sexual and reproductive health care. In comparison with other areas of women's health, due to the nature of intellectual impairments and the power position of these women, their voice is largely missing, and much of the available research is from the perspective of practitioners, families, and paid carers (Krahn, Hammond, & Turner, 2006). Given that people with intellectual impairments constitute at least 2% of the world's population, and the population of people with autism is growing, this represents a large number of women. In countries less well-resourced in terms of health care, where stigma towards disabled populations occurs and cultural attitudes towards women are oppressive, this discrimination is likely to be even greater (United Nations Population Fund, 2018a). Unfortunately, for women who are not only intellectually impaired, but also belong to other marginalised groups, intersectionality further exaggerates such discrimination. (Dean, Tolhurst, Khanna, & Jehan, 2017). Intersectionality includes both the intersection of vulnerable identities such as the occurrence of multiple health conditions, which are common in this group of women, but also the intersection of disability and other marginalised identities. This includes the known negative interactional effects of the intersection of race, ethnicity, class, sexuality and sexual identity. Such intersectionality for disabled women makes them some of the most economically, politically, and socio-emotionally vulnerable groups in any society (WHO, 2017).

Definitions and terminology

The terminology of intellectual impairment and developmental disability includes both people with intellectual disabilities and people with autism. Whilst these two conditions have a high rate of co-morbidity, they are separate conditions with their own unique characteristics, which, when they intersect, have a cumulative impact in terms of increased limitations and prevalence of health conditions. Hence, it is important to consider both populations under the remit of this chapter as they are often served by the same agencies and combined within research populations.

Intellectual impairment is the terminology now used by the World Health Organization International Classification of Diseases (ICD 11) to describe people who have limitations, usually congenital or through early trauma, to their intellectual capacities (WHO, 2017). This affects their developmental trajectory and presents greater challenges in everyday life, but also places them at economic, social, psychological, educational, and environmental risk of reduced opportunities and adverse life events. Various terms have been used over time and in different nations, most commonly 'intellectual disabilities', 'mental retardation', and 'learning disabilities'.

Autism is a developmental condition that includes impairments in two specific domains; difficulties in interaction and social communication, and restricted interests and repetitive behaviours (ICD 11). Other commonly associated characteristics include unusual sensory sensitivities. Researchers have estimated that 20–30% of people with intellectual impairments also have autism (Dunn, Rydzewska, MacIntyre, Rintoul, & Cooper, 2019). Whilst there is a demonstrated difference in the prevalence rates of autism between men and women, with a ratio of around 3:1, this is now decreasing. Previously, assessment instruments have been primarily developed on the male phenotype, however autistic characteristics in women may be evidenced differently than in men and so may be underdiagnosed using these instruments (Tierney, Burns, & Kilbey, 2016). As a result of this new understanding more girls and young women with autism are now being diagnosed, and those who have been misdiagnosed are now being diagnosed later in life.

Early development and adolescence

Understanding one's body and the changes it undergoes during puberty, and how this relates to sex, sexuality, and reproduction through appropriate sex education, is a fundamental need

(UNESCO, 2018). However, there is continuing evidence that sex and reproductive health education for young people with intellectual impairments is either absent or of poor quality (Stein, Kohut, & Dillenburger, 2018).

Given the risks of sexual abuse faced by young women with intellectual impairments, this is a grave omission. Evidence suggests that individuals with intellectual impairments experience much higher rates than non-disabled individuals of forced sexual interactions. The reported incidence in children ranges from 15% to 52% (Wissink, van Vugt, Moonen, Stams, & Hendriks, 2015). For example, in a New Zealand study Briggs (2006) interviewed 161 children with intellectual impairments and found rates of sexual abuse at 32% across the genders. The author related this to the high incidence of lack of knowledge about sex, as 17% of her sample did not know if adults were allowed to have sex with children. Given that this was a self-report study and there was confusion about what behaviours constituted an offence, the actual prevalence of sexual abuse was likely to have been even greater.

Rates of sexual abuse in adults are reported to be higher than in children. One study showed a prevalence of 83% (Johnson & Sigler, 2000). However, a recent Spanish study highlighted some of the problems of obtaining robust data in this area by demonstrating variance across self-report and reports by professionals (Gil-Llario, Morell-Mengual, & Díaz-Rodríguez, 2019). In their study of 360 adults with intellectual impairments, aged 18–55, 50% of whom were women, self-reported sexual abuse was reported by 6.1% of the sample, however professionals reported the prevalence as 28.6%. For the women themselves, having always being in a position of low power and status, feeding a desire for acceptance and inclusion, and possibly being excluded from opportunities to know and be able to assert their sexual rights, it is not surprising that self-report of abuse is lower than might be expected.

Whilst it is imperative that women at risk of predatory sexual abuse are not blamed for the abuse perpetrated upon them, a foundation of safeguarding is required to ensure that they are able to protect themselves as much as possible. However, the link between poor sex and relationship education and risk is rarely remarked upon. Indeed, in a recent study that compared the perceived need for sex education between parents of children with and without disabilities, Stein et al. (2018) found that the parents of children with intellectual impairments were less likely to believe their children will have consensual or non-consensual sex before age 18 than were parents of children without impairments. However, they did believe their impaired children should be educated, but by their parents with help from professionals.

Undeniably, protection versus freedom is a difficult balance to draw, but what can occur is that the defence of protecting the 'individual rights and freedoms' of the individual is actually used to mask passivity, denial, and a lack of intervention to protect and safeguard the woman. Likewise, protection can also be used as an excuse to restrict unnecessarily the individual rights and freedoms, usually for the convenience of others. This complexity was a recent topic of discussion in the UK in the case of a young woman headlined in newspapers as 'Autistic woman pimped out in care scandal'. A judge had given permission for her to make her own choices about sexual partners, on the basis that her carers were said to have believed that high-risk sexual encounters with strangers might, as reported in the press, help her to 'learn from her mistakes' (www.thetimes.co.uk/article/autistic-woman-pimped-out-in-care-scandal-665b6xpl9). This ruling was subsequently overturned in the High Court by another judge. The court records reveal that this highly complex case has been ongoing for five years, involving many professionals and requiring a delicate and changing balance between the autonomy and protection of the young woman.

Service responses to supporting girls and young women with intellectual impairments

As our understanding advances in these areas, such cases are likely to get more complex, and these require sophisticated, multidisciplinary, and dynamic responses. To facilitate this, services systems must be robust and flexible enough to respond in more refined ways. Much of the current literature relates to nations that have established educational, welfare, and health systems, and, whilst high levels of vulnerability and need are becoming recognised, this situation is much worse in nations without this infrastructure and in cultures where the equality of girls and women, let alone children and young people with disabilities, is not accepted. The United Nations Populations Fund (UNPFA, 2018b) published a report on gender-based violence and sexual and reproductive rights for young people with disabilities and concluded:

> Young persons with disabilities, especially young women and girls with disabilities, are more vulnerable to violence than are their peers without disabilities. They face different forms of violence, including physical, sexual, psychological, and emotional abuse; bullying, coercion, institutionalisation, trafficking, and forced sterilisation; and beliefs and practices not conducive to human rights such as child marriage and female genital mutilation.
>
> *(p.17)*

Young persons with disabilities, especially young women and girls with disabilities, are often denied access to justice and response services for survivors of sexual violence and GBV (p. 17). www.unfpa.org/sites/default/files/pub-pdf/Final_Global_Study_English_3_Oct.pdf

The report refers to research carried out in Africa, which documented that all of the 1,000 young people sampled in a study reported physical abuse, and the girls reported extensive sexual abuse in addition to increased rates of physical abuse (UNPFA, 2018a, p. 26). Particularly important for girls with intellectual impairments was the denial of their legal capacity and advocacy services, which eliminated their ability to testify and made them additionally targeted and vulnerable, adding to the detrimental psychological consequences of not being heard (UNFPA, 2018b, p. 38).

Identified in the United Nations Convention of Rights of Persons with Disabilities is the right to access inclusive education, and this includes sex and reproductive health education (United Nation, 2006). Not only does sex and relationship education need to be of good quality, but it needs to recognise some of the differences associated with this group of girls and young women, not only in terms of making the material accessible to accommodate cognitive differences, but also related to some marked embodied differences. For example, research has continued to show that girls with intellectual impairments tend to start their menstrual cycles earlier than average (Walsh, Heller, Schupf, & Van Schrojenstein Lantman-de Valk, 2001). Hence, an important adaptation in terms of education is to ensure that girls with intellectual impairments receive education about menarche at an earlier age than usual.

Whilst appropriate sex education may be missing, that which is provided may be of poor quality. There has been movement to an acceptance that sexual behaviour is an individual right, but within sex education it still tends to be problematised, and the content aimed at managing risk and ultimately ensuring pregnancy does not occur. Behind this can be both a moralistic discourse, in terms of making value judgements about who should and who should not procreate and under what circumstances, but also an active way of avoiding involvement in complex decision-making, risk management, and, at worst, uncovering abuse by services and staff members. 'Surprise' pregnancies in the field of intellectual impairments have historically been the most obvious way abuse has surfaced, and, whilst services may not always be able to stop such offences, reliance on the systematic curtailment of reproduction by the routine use of female contraception as a risk management procedure is inappropriate. Another approach to manage unplanned pregnancies is forced involuntary sterilisation of girls and women with disabilities, described by UNFPA (2018b, p. 45) as still 'widespread'. Rather than 'protecting', which is often the discursive narrative used to promote sterilisation, this practice increases vulnerability to abuse by allowing the perpetrators to avoid detection.

As the disability rights movement has had more influence, sex education has become more positive in some countries and better resources produced (e.g., The Arc–Autism Now, n.d.; Teaching Sexual Health Canada, n.d.; Allen, 2003; Asagba, Burns, & Doswell, 2019). However, due to a lack of access to appropriate opportunities, young women with intellectual impairments often have to resort to informal education. Their social networks tend to be more restricted, with fewer friends, some of whom may be in similar situations to themselves (Lippold & Burns, 2009). They thus may be more reliant on representations of sex and relationships through popular culture and social media, and, as a result, may have unrealistic ideas about what is 'normal', which is compounded by their more restricted actual life experiences (Wilkinson, Theodore, & Raczka, 2015). Use of the Internet does provide a possible gateway into accessing useful information, but without education on the dangers of the Internet, this presents its own risks. Health education online may be inaccurate and unbalanced, and the user must be equipped with the skill of knowing where to look in the first place, and then be able to evaluate the information appropriately (Asagba et al., 2019).

Gender dysphoria and autism

A more recently noted association is the relationship between gender dysphoria and autism, which is reflected in the changing patterns of referral rates to gender dysphoria (GD) clinics. Research across a number of countries, including the UK, Netherlands, US, and Australia, has shown a dramatic increase in the rates of referrals to GD clinics of children and young people with Autism Spectrum Disorder (ASD) (Glidden, Bouman, Jones, & Arcelus, 2016). For example, in a review of the existing research, Van Der Miesen et al. (2016) suggested that approximately 20% of referrals identified co-occurring GD and ASD and that presentation was atypical, with more cisgender girls than boys who have a diagnosis of ASD coming forward for potential gender reassignment.

Causality theories accounting for this co-occurrence fall into three main areas. First, biological factors associated with the 'extreme male brain' hypothesis promoted by Baron-Cohen (2002) suggest that there are sex differences related to the capacity to empathise and systemise and that people with autism show highly masculine tendencies with developed systemisation skills and more limited empathy skills. Hence, girls with autism may want to transition as they feel more affinity with masculinity (Pasterski, Gilligan, & Curtis, 2014). The second theory relates to social factors associated with the communication differences associated with ASD. People with ASD tend to communicate differently, which can be challenging and socially isolating (Ehrensaft, 2016). Research suggests that girls with autism find communication with boys more straightforward as it is less nuanced and sophisticated than the complex interactions between girls and their social networks. This greater affinity with boys is then interpreted by the ASD girls as 'being like a boy' (Cooper, Smith, & Russell, 2018). The third explanation relates to the diagnostic characteristic of 'restricted, repetitive patterns of behaviour and interests', often called 'special interests'. Here it is suggested that transitioning becomes a 'special interest' and that the person with ASD becomes 'stuck' on this issue (Lemaire, Thomazeau, & Bonnet-Brilhault, 2014). This explanation is weak as it does not account for the gender difference, and transitioning gender is unlike other types of special interests people with ASD tend to focus upon. However, the thinking styles and emotional differences often associated with ASD are likely to play a part in this phenomenon, alongside other suggested causal factors, including psychodynamic, hormonal, and multi-dimensional explanations (e.g., Robinow, 2009).

Gender dysphoria and its association with ASD is a burgeoning field of enquiry within the ever-expanding deconstruction of a static and binary approach to gender identity. The purpose of mentioning this here is twofold. First, to illustrate the need for sex education to adapt to the specific needs of this population, such as trans issues in young women with autism. Second, to demonstrate that traditionally there has been a lag in the research behind mainstream concerns about sexuality and identity (Burns & Davies, 2011).

Adulthood: sex, reproduction, and living healthy lives

As women with intellectual impairments enter adulthood they share many of the same concerns as women without disabilities, such as having enjoyable and fulfilling sexual relationships, leading healthy lives, and contemplating motherhood. However, their actual experience has tended to be very different from their expectations. Earlier work in this area suggested that women with intellectual impairments experienced sex as largely negative, heteronormative, practised in contexts of coercion, and often used as a 'trade-off' to gain the status of a desired woman (Burns, 1993). More recent research sadly does not paint a more positive picture. On the whole, women with intellectual impairment do not see sex as a pleasurable activity (Bernert & Ogletree, 2013), and 'repeated victimisation' is a common experience (Eastgate, Van Driel, Lennox, & Scheermeyer, 2011, p. 229). Sex still seems to be used as a trading option in taking up the societally valued role of a normal, desirable, heterosexual woman, in contrast to a single, undesired, de-sexed, disabled person (McCarthy, 2014).

Whilst the right to equal access to relationships, reproduction, and parenthood as a basic human right has attained a greater recognition (e.g., article 23, Convention on the Rights for Persons with Disabilities; UN, 2006), participants in recent studies in this area have recounted examples of how their sexuality was managed or restricted by partners, staff, services, and families. For example, Hollomotz (2011) recounted one woman's experience of when she wished to use a vibrator and had to ask staff, who then signed it in and out of a locked medication cabinet. Other women recounted restrictions that led to subversive behaviour, such as secretly having sex, which then became seen as 'problem behaviours' and the women concerned consequently being positioned in a 'permanent state of adolescence' (Hollomotz, 2011, p. 68). This control of the sexual and reproductive lives of women with intellectual impairments is an even greater problem in non-Western contexts where the marginalised and disempowered position of the woman intersects with cultural restraints and traditions. An extreme example of this is described in the UNPFA (2018b) report:

> Many women with disabilities suffer from extreme poverty and will use transactional sex for survival. A female board member of a national cross-disability organisation of persons with disabilities in Maputo explained, 'If she is hungry, she will have sex with a man for a meal. There is no question about condoms. Not if she needs to eat'.
>
> *(p. 39)*

When it comes to reproduction, Earle (2001) summarised the situation as 'Disabled people are expected to neither reproduce nor be reproduced' (p. 435). Sterilisation has had a long and sad history concerning women with intellectual impairments (Sifris, 2016). Whilst enforced sterilisation for eugenic purposes has now largely ceased, sterilisation and long-acting contraception are still practiced as a method of controlling the reproductive bodies of women with intellectual impairments. In their fascinating history of the international sterilisation of women with intellectual impairments, which focussed on a review of multiple case histories, Tilley, Walmsley, Earle, and Atkinson (2016) put forward three rationales used for the continuation of control of these women's reproductive rights. The first was 'a permanent solution to potential pregnancy' (p. 29). The discourse behind this is that repeated unplanned pregnancies will result in a 'burden of care' and this will fall on other members of the family, who are already caring for the woman herself. This will impact the resources of the family to care for themselves, the woman with intellectual impairments, and the offspring, placing them in a downward cycle of deprivation. However, as Tilley et al. (2016) pointed out, many of the women in these studies were not in consensual sexual relationships, and had few options in terms of sex education and support in managing these issues. Hence, sterilisation might be seen as an easy prophylactic solution in a toxic context of high rates of sexual abuse and poor safeguarding.

Ironically, protection from the consequences of sexual abuse was cited as the second rationale for these medical interventions. Tilley et al. (2016) suggested that 'giving contraception to women because they are at risk of sexual abuse is in itself abusive, and points to a lack of regard for their well-being' (p. 31). Using contraception in this way can be seen as a way of aiding and abetting continued sexual abuse. The third rationale relates to the management of menstruation and its associated symptoms (Tilley et al., 2016). This rationale includes concerns about the practical management of menstruation and the potential distress caused by the monthly cycle. The use of long-acting contraception, and in some cases hysterectomy, for this reason has tended to focus on women with more severe intellectual disabilities, who may have the capacity to demonstrate distress associated with menstruation, but not the capacity to engage in decisions about preventative interventions (McCarthy, 2009). This is an under-researched area, with only one known study so far of the experience of menstruation and premenstrual distress (Kyrkou, 2005). The results suggest that women with intellectual impairments, and particularly those with Down Syndrome and ASD, 'appeared to have a higher rate of period pain than women in the general population, but the presence of pain more often had to be deduced from behavioural changes' (p. 770). Decisions about management of menstruation are commonly made for women with intellectual impairments in the context of 'best interest', but it should be noted that managing medication or a one-off medical procedure may be much more attractive to carers than continuously managing menstruation for a severely impaired woman. Hence, the convenience of support structures versus the autonomy of the woman can be a balancing act.

Whilst there may be genuine and consensual reasons for choosing medical interventions to prevent pregnancy, Tilley et al. (2016) rightly pointed out that the involvement of the woman herself and the power she holds in the decision-making process is pivotal. National and international human rights declarations, mental capacity, and consent legislation, including the UN Convention on the Rights of Persons with Disabilities (UN, 2006), are increasingly being used in courts of law by advocates on behalf of women without the capacity to make more woman-centred decisions in this respect.

Pregnancy and women with intellectual impairments

When a woman with intellectual impairments becomes pregnant, instead of her status being seen as a person who needs extra care, the evidence suggests that her pregnancy status is more likely to lead to negligent care. Homeyard, Montgomery, Chinn, and Patelarou (2016) carried out a systematic review of antenatal care and concluded that women with intellectual impairments often experienced disempowering practices by professionals, a lack of autonomy, and little accessible information or targeted support. This sometimes resulted in a lack of engagement with services, due to missed appointments and missing information that the women were unable to supply, which in turn caused increased risk and negative attitudes from the service personnel and perpetuated the 'unsuitable mother stereotype' (p. 55). Midwives involved in women's care reported a lack of knowledge about the needs of women with intellectual impairments and little guidance about how to adapt their practices. In a wider review of gynaecological care, Abells, Kirkham, and Ornstein (2016) noted that some women with intellectual impairments may not engage with services until quite late in the pregnancy, leading to unwanted pregnancies and higher health risks. Delayed access to services was attributed to educational inadequacies, the potential disapproval of those around them, and fears about the possible loss of custody of their baby.

The extent and profile of higher health risks that women with intellectual impairments face for both themselves and their babies has been demonstrated by two large cohort studies. The extensive work by Brown and colleagues in Canada and Mitra and colleagues in the US provides some rich insights within an area generally deficient of good quality research. Brown et al. (2016) looked at the social and health characteristics of mothers with intellectual impairments who gave birth in one fiscal year in Ontario, found 450 live births to this population, and reported that the general fertility rate (live births in a year) was approximately one half (20.3 per 1,000) that of the general female population (43.4 per 1,000). Whilst the age specific fertility rate was similar to those without impairments for younger women, the gap increased significantly for older women with intellectual impairments, which suggests that the reduction in fertility occurs more rapidly for women with intellectual impairments. The results show that women with intellectual impairments who did conceive also faced multiple social and health disparities, including being poorer and younger first-time parents, with higher rates of obesity, epilepsy, mental health issues, and medication usage.

Brown et al. (2016) also looked at the health outcomes of 3,932 childbirths by mothers with intellectual impairments. In terms of maternal outcomes, the women with intellectual impairments had a higher prevalence of pre-eclampsia and venous thromboembolism. The outcomes for the children included increased risk of preterm birth, being small for the gestational age, perinatal mortality (the majority were still births), and perinatal morbidity including respiratory distress syndrome, haemorrhage, and seizures. In a similar large study in the US, Mitra, Parish, Clements, Cui, and Diop (2015) compared childbirths in women with intellectual impairments against the general population of women and found similar outcomes. Thirty-two percent of the mothers with intellectual impairments did not disclose the father's name on the birth certificate compared with 8.3% of the general population. Childbirths by women with intellectual impairments were likely to be preterm, low weight, and by caesarean section, and there was increased risk of perinatal mortality. Both research teams concluded that there is a need to address modifiable risk factors and to enhance monitoring peri-natally. They also acknowledged both the lack of research in this area and inadequacies in support resources. Despite research that clearly identifies the well-evidenced link with intergenerational disadvantage, services seem poorly equipped to support this highly vulner-able group. As Brown et al. (2016) summarised, these women are likely to 'have intensive pregnancy support needs and should be included in perinatal strategies aimed at vulnerable population groups' (p. 14).

Brown and colleagues followed up their cohort of mothers with intellectual impairments to explore their experiences postpartum, particularly in the areas of postpartum contracep-tion and repeat pregnancy. Women with intellectual impairments were statistically more likely than non-disabled women to be in receipt of non-barrier and injectable contraception (Brown, Kirkham, Lunsky, Cobigo, & Vigod, 2018a). Rapid repeat pregnancy (RRP; i.e., a live birth within 12 months of a previous birth) was also higher in this group, which is associated with adverse perinatal outcomes (Brown, Ray, Liu, Lunsky, & Vigod, 2018b). However, this risk was reduced after health, social, and support factors were taken into account, which demonstrates that RRP is not a characteristic of having intellectual impair-ments, but a result of what happens to women who have these disabilities and are placed in seriously disadvantaged and marginalised social positions. This is despite the label 'intellectual impairments' acknowledging that such women have a compromised ability to manage adverse circumstances. Whilst the majority of these studies did not look at the consequences of intersecting identities, it is likely that Black, lesbian, and migrant women with ID may be even further disadvantaged.

Day-to-day health care management

It is not only in managing reproduction that sexual and reproductive health disadvantages occur for women with intellectual impairment, but also in day-to-day health management. For example, general practitioners (GPs) in the UK reported believing that women with intellectual impairments would not have sex and thus did not need cervical screening (Havercamp & Scott, 2015). A New Zealand study replicated these findings, and also showed that the women themselves were frequently ill-informed about the need for such screening, the procedures involved, and how they may access such services, which resulted in a lower demand for regular health checks or avoidant behaviour (Conder et al., 2019).

These studies and previous work suggest that systemic changes need to occur to improve the routine health care of women with intellectual impairments. This includes funding annual health checks for this group of women, especially given the likelihood of co-morbid conditions and the possibility of the woman falling through established health care systems. Since 2009 in the UK, everybody over 14 with intellectual impairments and registered with a GP is invited for an annual health check (NHS, 2017). Whilst uptake has been gradual, there is some evidence that this has impacted positively on the health of people with intellectual impairments (Carey et al., 2017). Similar schemes have been established in other countries, including Canada, Australia, the Netherlands, and New Zealand. However, despite the implementation of such policies and governmental incentives, uptake varies regionally and remains below the optimal standards, which suggests that other systemic changes need to occur (Durbin et al., 2016).

Improving training for primary care staff and those involved in health promotion has also been a focus of change and evaluation. Research has indicted that health promotion for women with intellectual impairments tends not to be included in professional health training and is often seen as a post-qualification option, which results in lack of understanding and de-prioritisation (Salvador-Carulla, 2015). Change in this area has tended to be led by char-ities associated with intellectual impairments and also by cancer or health-promotion organisations. For example, the Canadian Breast Cancer Network provided an excellent report that includes specific guidance on staff training, roles, and procedural adaptations (Rajan et al., 2013). The Norah Fry Research Centre (2016) has published a very helpful strategy and toolkit aimed at improving the uptake of five types of health screening, including breast and cervical. The UK Royal College of Practitioners has produced a step-by-step toolkit aimed at educating general practitioners about how to carry out an annual health assessment of people with ID and what to look for (Royal College of General Practitioners, 2017). This includes how to organise the check, what it should include (e.g., menstrual issues, but not contraception), mental health and behavioural issues, syndrome-specific issues (including early menopause for women with Down Syndrome, average age 44), the legislative framework, and additional resources.

Managing day-to-day health issues is reliant on being informed about the issues, however much health promotional material is not accessible to this population and in recent years efforts have been focussed on redressing this omission. Charities, health care providers, and health promotion agencies have developed excellent resources in response. A good example from the UK is the charity Jo's Cervical Cancer Trust, which has produced an excellent web-based resource including a video of a smear test, accessible information about what a smear test is, why and how it is done, and a help line (www.jostrust.org.uk/about-cervical-cancer/cervical-screening/cervical-screening-learning-disability). Another good example is the *Beyond Words* series of paperback books, also available as e-books, which provide pictorial guides to a variety of health issues including health screening, breast care, managing cancer, and hospital procedures (https://booksbeyondwords.co.uk). These are in the format of a simple story and accompanying pictures that take a person through the issue in chronological order of how the health issue might be noticed, what action to take, how the matter might be discussed and with whom, and what might be some of the outcomes.

Sexual and reproductive care in older life

Many of the problems identified earlier in this chapter continue to cause sexual and reproductive health inequalities for women with intellectual impairments later in life. However, there is an even greater paucity of research at this stage of women's lives, especially regarding the menopause and chronic conditions such as osteoporosis (WHO, 2000). Risks of sexual abuse continue, and, due to exclusion from the workforce, poverty may be an ongoing risk with implications for ability to manage health risks and psychological welfare (Walsh, Heller, & Schupf, 2001).

The research that has been carried out on the menopause in women with intellectual impairments has primarily been small-scale qualitative studies focused on the women's understanding and experience of this developmental transition and the understanding of their carers (e.g., McCarthy, 2002a, 2002b; Willis, 2010). The findings commonly point to the familiar issues of the necessity of better health resources tailored to the needs of these women and more relevant health education training for staff. One issue that needs further research is the suggestion in some literature that menopause may occur earlier in women with intellectual impairments, especially in the case of women with Down Syndrome (Nelson Goff et al., 2013). This is linked to earlier menarche in women with Down Syndrome and in later life to an increased prevalence of dementia, associated with the accelerated aging hypothesis (Esbensen, 2010).

As concerns about reproduction diminish post-menopause, caregivers' concerns about the reproductive health of women with intellectual impairments also diminish, and women may not be offered or able to access interventions that could be beneficial. For example, although the research literature is very limited, there is evidence that hormone therapy is less commonly offered to menopausal women with intellectual impairments (Ward, 2002). This decision may entirely be in the hands of the practitioners or carers, as the women may be considered not to have the capacity to make informed decisions where complex advantages and disadvantages need weighing up and consent for treatment is required, so they are simply not presented with the option (McCarthy, 2002b). The consequences of this lack of attention to age-related health conditions in women with intellectual impairment are serious and wide-ranging. In their review of the health surveillance of older adults with intellectual and developmental disabilities, Ouell-ette-Kuntz, Martin, and McKenzie (2015) pointed out not just the personal cost to the individual in terms of quality of life, but also the costs to the health and social care system in terms of increased home care and potential institutionalisation.

Summary and conclusions

A theme that runs through this chapter is that the disability is most commonly fore-grounded as the individual woman's primary identity. Only after this might their gender be considered and, as a consequence of this disability-centric view, health issues associated with gender may either not receive the attention needed (health screening; menstruation; reproduction; menopause) or may receive discriminatory attention (contraceptive methods; perinatal care). Whilst the sexual and reproductive health care needs of women with intellectual impairments have been increasingly recognised, accessible resources made available, and standards set, services and providers have been slow to respond and are dependent upon economic vitality, cultural acceptance of gender equality and women-focussed services.

It is clear that the low social worth given to women with intellectual impairments contributes to this ongoing inequality, alongside the limited opportunities they have to get their voices heard and the restricted experience they may have in self-advocacy. For change to occur, McCarthy (2014) pointed to four important founding principles: (1) accessible information, (2) time to make decisions, (3) support from significant others, and (4) freedom from coercion. Although they are simple in conception, the principles are harder to implement, but do provide a helpful starting point. However, perhaps a fifth should be added: collaboration. 'Nothing about us without us' is a slogan that had its origins in European politics and was later adopted by the Disability Rights Movement with the rise of self-advocacy in the 1990s (Charlton, 2000), and it is central to intersectional and feminist perspectives both in health care and research. As such the phrase still sets out a very relevant principle for the current context. For true change to occur there must be a coalition of disability groups, health care providers, and policy makers. Disability must be moved away from a medical discourse to a discourse of difference that allows assumptions about differential standards of health care to be questioned and the expectation of fulfilled, healthy, gendered lives to become an assumed human right for all.

References

Abells, D., Kirkham, Y., & Ornstein, M. (2016). Review of gynecologic and reproductive care for women with developmental disabilities. *Current Opinion in Obstetrics and Gynecology, 28*, 350–358.

Allen, D. (2003). *Gay, lesbian, bisexual, and transgender people with developmental disabilities and mental retardation: Stories of the rainbow support group*. Abingdon, UK: Routledge.

The Arc – Autism Now [website] (n.d.). Washington, DC: Author. Retrieved from https://autism now.org/about-us/;https://autismnow.org/about-us.

Asagba, K., Burns, J., & Doswell, S. (2019). *Sex and relationships education for young people and adults with intellectual disabilities.* Brighton, UK: Pavilion.

Baron-Cohen, S. (2002). The extreme male brain theory of autism. *Trends in Cognitive Sciences, 6,* 248–254.

Bernert, D. J. & Ogletree, R. J. (2013). Women with intellectual disabilities talk about their perceptions of sex. *Journal on Intellectual Disability Research, 57,* 240–249.

Briggs, F. (2006). Safety issues in the lives of children with learning disabilities. *Social Policy Journal of New Zealand, 29,* 43–59.

Brown, H. K., Cobigo, V., Lunsky, Y., & Vigod, S. N. (2016). Maternal and offspring outcomes in women with intellectual and developmental disabilities: A population-based cohort study. *BJOG: An International Journal of Obstetrics and Gynaecology, 124,* 757–765.

Brown, H. K., Kirkham, Y. A., Lunsky, Y., Cobigo, V., & Vigod, S. N. (2018a). Contraceptive provision to postpartum women with intellectual and developmental disabilities: A population-based cohort study. *Perspectives on Sexual and Reproductive Health, 50,* 93–99.

Brown, H. K., Ray, J. G., Liu, N., Lunsky, Y., & Vigod, S. N. (2018b). Rapid repeat pregnancy among women with intellectual and developmental disabilities: A population-based cohort study. *Canadian Medical Association Journal, 190,* 949–E956.

Burns, J. (1993). Invisible women: Women who have learning disabilities. *The Psychologist, 6,* 102–110.

Burns, J. & Davies, D. (2011). Same-sex relationships and women with intellectual disabilities. *Journal of Applied Research in Intellectual Disabilities, 24*(4), 351–360.

Carey, I. M., Hosking, F. J., Harris, T., DeWilde, S., Beighton, C., Shah, S. M., & Cook, D. G. (2017). Do health checks for adults with intellectual disability reduce emergency hospital admissions? Evaluation of a natural experiment. *Journal of Epidemiology and Community Health, 71,* 52–58.

Charlton, J. (2000). *Nothing about us without us: Disability oppression and empowerment.* San Francisco, CA: University of California Press.

Conder, J., Mirfin-Veitch, B., Payne, D., Channon, A., & Richardson, G. (2019) Increasing the participation of women with intellectual disabilities in women's health screening: A role for disability support services. *Research and Practice in Intellectual and Developmental Disabilities, 6*(1), 86–96.

Cooper, K., Smith, L. G. E., & Russell, A. J. (2018). Gender identity in autism: Sex differences in social affiliation with gender groups. *Journal of Autism Developmental Disorders, 48,* 3995–4006.

Dean, L., Tolhurst, R. J., Khanna, R., & Jehan, K. (2017). 'You're disabled, why did you have sex in the first place?' An intersectional analysis of experiences of disabled women with regard to their sexual and reproductive health and rights in Gujarat State, India. *Global Health Action,* Jan.–Dec.;*10*(sup2), 1290316.

Dunn, K., Rydzewska, E., MacIntyre, C., Rintoul, J., & Cooper, S.-A. (2019). The prevalence and general health status of people with intellectual disabilities and autism co-occurring together: A total population study. *Journal of Intellectual Disability Research, 63,* 277–285.

Durbin, J., Selick, A., Casson, I., Green, L., Spassiani, N., Perry, A., & Lunsky, Y. (2016). Evaluating the implementation of health checks for adults with intellectual and developmental disabilities in primary care: The importance of organizational context. *Intellectual and Developmental Disabilities, 54,* 136–150.

Earle, S. (2001). Disability, facilitated sex and the role of the nurse. *Journal of Advanced Nursing, 36,* 433–440.

Eastgate, G., Van Driel, M. L., Lennox, N. G., & Scheermeyer, E. (2011). Women with intellectual disabilities: A study of sexuality, sexual abuse and protection skills. *Australian Family Physician, 40,* 226–230.

Ehrensaft, D. (2016). *The gender creative child: Pathways for nurturing and supporting children who live outside gender boxes.* New York, NY: The Experiment.

Esbensen, A. J. (2010). Health conditions associated with aging and end of life of adults with Down syndrome. *International Review of Research in Mental Retardation, 39,* 107–126.

Glidden, D., Bouman, W., Jones, B., & Arcelus, J. (2016). Gender Dysphoria and Autism spectrum disorder: A systematic review of the literature. *Sexual Medicine Reviews, 4*(1), 3–14.

Gil-Llario, M. D., Morell-Mengual, V., Díaz-Rodríguez, I., & Ballester-Arnal, R. (2019). Prevalence and sequelae of self-reported and other-reported sexual abuse in adults with intellectual disability. *Journal of Intellectual Disability Research, 63,* 138–148.

Havercamp, S. & Scott, H. (2015). National health surveillance of adults with disabilities, adults with intellectual and developmental disabilities, and adults with no disabilities. *Disability and Health Journal, 8*, 165–172.

Hollomotz, A. (2011). *Learning difficulties and sexual vulnerability: A social approach*. London, UK: Kingsley.

Homeyard, C., Montgomery, E., Chinn, D., & Patelarou, E. (2016). Current evidence on antenatal care provision for women with intellectual disabilities: A systematic review. *Midwifery, 32*, 45–57.

Johnson, I. M. & Sigler, R. T. (2000). Forced sexual intercourse among intimates. *Journal of Family Violence, 15*, 95–108.

Krahn, G. L., Hammond, L., & Turner, A. (2006). A cascade of disparities: Health and health care access for people with intellectual disabilities. *Mental Retardation and Developmental Disabilities Research Review, 12*, 70–82.

Kyrkou, M. (2005). Health issues and quality of life in women with intellectual disability. *Journal of Intellectual Disability Research, 49*, 770–772.

Lemaire, M., Thomazeau, B., & Bonnet-Brilhault, F. (2014). Gender identity disorder and autism spectrum disorder in a 23-year-old female. *Archives of Sexual Behaviour, 43*, 395–398.

Lippold, T. & Burns, J. (2009). Social support and intellectual disabilities: A comparison between social networks of adults with intellectual disability and those with physical disability. *Journal of Intellectual Disability Research, 53*, 463–473.

McCarthy, M. (2002a). Going through the menopause: Perceptions and experiences of women with learning disability. *Journal of Intellectual & Developmental Disability, 27*, 281–295.

McCarthy, M. (2002b). Responses of GPs, paid carers and mothers to women with learning disabilities as they go through the menopause. *Tizard Learning Disability Review, 7*, 4–12.

McCarthy M. (2009). 'I have the jab so I can't be blamed for getting pregnant': contraception and women with learning disabilities. *Women's Studies International Forum, 32*, 198–208.

McCarthy M. (2014). Women with intellectual disability: their sexual lives in the 21st century. *Journal of Intellectual and Developmental Disability, 39*, 124–131.

Mitra, M., Parish, S. L., Clements, K. M., Cui, X., & Diop, H. (2015). Pregnancy outcomes among women with intellectual and developmental disabilities. *American Journal of Preventative Medicine, 48*, 300–308.

National Health Service (NHS) (2017). *A summary and overview of the learning disability annual health check electronic clinical template*. London, UK: Author. Retrieved from www.england.nhs.uk/wp-content/uploads/2017/05/nat-elec-health-check-ld-clinical-template.pdf.

Nelson Goff, B. S., Springer, N., Foote, L. C., Frantz, C., Peak, M., Tracy, C., Veh, T., Bentley, G. E., & Cross, K. A. (2013). Receiving the initial Down syndrome diagnosis: A comparison of prenatal and postnatal parent group experiences. *Journal of Intellectual and Developmental Disability, 51*(6), 446–457.

Norah Fry Research Centre & National Development Team for Inclusion (2016). *Improving the uptake of screening services by people with learning disabilities across the South West Peninsula*. Bath, UK: National Development Team for Inclusion. Retrieved from www.ndti.org.uk/uploads/files/Screening_Services_Strategy_Toolkit_final.pdf.

O'Leary, L., Cooper, S.-A., & Hughes-McCormack, L. (2018). Early death and causes of death of people with intellectual disabilities: A systematic review. *Journal of Applied Research in Intellectual Disabilities, 31*, 325–342.

Ouellette-Kuntz, E., Martin, L., & McKenzie, K. (2015). A review of health surveillance in older adults with intellectual and developmental disabilities. In C. Hatton & E. Emerson (Eds), *International review of research in developmental disabilities* (Vol. 48, pp. 151–194). Cambridge, MA: Academic Press.

Pasterski, V., Gilligan, L., & Curtis, R. (2014). Traits of autism spectrum disorders in adults with gender dysphoria. *Archives of Sexual Behaviour, 43*, 387–393.

Rajan, S., Foreman, J., Wallis, M. G., Caldas, C., & Britton, P. (2013). Multidisciplinary decisions in breast cancer: does the patient receive what the team has recommended? *British Journal of Cancer, 108*, 2442–2447.

Robinow, O. (2009). Paraphilia and transgenderism: A connection with Asperger's Disorder? *Sexual and Relationship Therapy, 24*, 143–151.

Royal College of General Practitioners (2017). *Health checks for people with learning disabilities toolkit*. Author.Retrieved from: www.rcgp.org.uk/clinical-and-research/resources/toolkits/health-check-toolkit.aspx.

Salvador-Carulla, L., Martínez-Leal, R., Heyler, C., Alvarez-Galvez, J., Veenstra, M. Y., García-Ibáñez, J., Carpenter, S., Bertelli, M., Munir, K., Torr, J., & Van Schrojenstein Lantman-de

Valk, H. M. J. (2015). Training on intellectual disability in health sciences: The European perspective. *International Journal of Developmental Disabilities*, *61*, 20–31.

Sifris, R. (2016). The involuntary sterilisation of marginalised women: Power, discrimination, and intersectionality. *Griffith Law Review*, *25*, 45–70.

Stein, S., Kohut, T., & Dillenburger, K. (2018). The importance of sexuality education for children with and without intellectual disabilities: What parents think. *Sexuality and Disability*, *36*, 141–148.

Teaching Sexual Health Canada [website] (n.d.). Retrieved from http://teachers.teachingsexualhealth. ca/lesson-plans/differing-abilities.

Tierney, S., Burns, J., & Kilbey, E. (2016). Looking behind the mask: Social coping strategies of girls on the autistic spectrum. *Research in Autism Spectrum Disorder*, *23*, 73–83.

Tilley, L., Walmsley, J., Earle, S., & Atkinson, D. (2016). International perspectives on the sterilization of women with intellectual disabilities. In S. Earle, C. Komoaromy, & L. Layne, (Eds), *Understanding reproductive loss: Perspectives on life, death and fertility* (pp. 23–36). Abingdon, UK: Routledge.

United Nations Educational, Scientific and Cultural Organization (UNESCO) (2018). *International technical guidance on sexuality education: An evidence-informed approach*. Paris, France: Author.

United Nations (UN) (2006). *Convention on the Rights of Persons with Disabilities (CRPD)*. Geneva, Switzerland: Author.

United Nations Population Fund (UNPFA) (2018a). *Women and young persons with disabilities guidelines for providing rights-based and gender-responsive services to address gender-based violence and sexual and reproductive health and rights for women and young persons with disabilities*. Geneva, Switzerland: Author. Available from www.unfpa.org/featured-publication/women-and-young-persons-disabilities.

United Nations Populations Fund (UNPFA) (2018b). *Young persons with disabilitiesglobal study on ending gender-based violence and realizing sexual and reproductive health and rights*. Geneva, Switzerland: Author. Retrieved from www.unfpa.org/publications/young-persons-disabilities.

Van Der Miesen, A., Hurley, H., & de Vries, A. (2016). Gender dysphoria and autism spectrum disorder: A narrative review. *International Review of Psychiatry*, *28*(1), 70–80.

Walsh, P. N., Heller, T., Schupf, N., & Van Schrojenstein Lantman-de Valk, H. (2001). Healthy ageing – Adults with intellectual disabilities: Women's health and related issues. *Journal of Applied Research in Intellectual Disabilities*, *14*, 195–217.

Ward, L. (2002). Women with learning disabilities and the menopause. *Tizard Learning Disability Review*, *7* 13–16.

Wilkinson, V. J., Theodore, K., & Raczka, R. (2015). 'As normal as possible': Sexual identity development in people with intellectual disabilities transitioning to adulthood. *Sexuality and Disability*, *33*, 93–105.

Willis, D. S., Wishart, J. G., & Muir, W. J. (2010). Carer knowledge and experiences with menopause in women with intellectual disabilities. *Journal of Policy and Practice in Intellectual Disabilities*, *7*, 42–48.

Wissink, I., van Vugt, E., Moonen, X., Stams, G. J., & Hendriks, J. (2015). Sexual abuse involving children with an intellectual disability (ID): A narrative review. *Research in Developmental Disabilities*, *36* (2015), 20–35.

World Health Organization (WHO) (2000). *Ageing and intellectual disabilities - improving longevity and promoting healthy ageing: Summative report*. Geneva, Switzerland: Author.

World Health Organization (WHO) (2017). *ICD-11*. Geneva, Switzerland: Author. Available from https://icd.who.int.

40

LESBIAN, BISEXUAL, QUEER AND TRANSGENDER WOMEN'S SEXUAL AND REPRODUCTIVE HEALTH

Ruth P. McNair

The sexual and reproductive health behaviours of lesbian,[1] bisexual,[2] and queer[3] (LBQ) women can be revolutionary and diverse. For over a century, LBQ women have dared to challenge orthodoxy, and they continue to do so. Emerging trends are a microcosm of the widespread movement of sexuality and gender diversity that is apparent in multiple areas of life. These include relationships, parenting, sexual adventurism, multiple identities, and intersections that challenge normative values and embrace alternative viewpoints. In many ways the sexual and reproductive health of LBQ women is flourishing. However, any counter cultural movement has its challenges, often resulting from individual or collective experiences of marginalisation and discrimination. Healthcare providers must keep pace with these changes to ensure they can provide the best possible care. Understanding differences between identity and expression, changes in terminologies, new and emerging social groups, and the impacts of discrimination are all essential knowledge. LBQ women deserve our attention as a specific sub-group with health inequalities and health needs.

In this chapter, I first explore sexual and gender identities and how these intersect with sexual and gender expression. This provides the background to understanding intimate relationships and experiences of reproduction and family creation. I then discuss sexual health and sexually transmitted infections (STIs), and finally suggest targeted health promotion strategies. Gender and sexual identities are interwoven in the lives of many LBQ women, so I will discuss transgender[4] and gender diversity[5] as well as sexual diversity. I will not cover people with intersex variations, although I acknowledge that some LBQ women and transgender people have intersex variations. Sexual and gender identity acronyms in this field are ever-expanding. I use LBQ when discussing issues specific to women, LBQT when the topic includes transgender and gender diverse (TGD) people, and LGBTQ when gay and bisexual men are also included.

Diverse sexual and gender identities and expressions

Parks (1999) described lesbian sexual identity as "an achieved, not ascribed, status" (Parks, 1999, p. 347). Unlike heterosexuality, which is largely assumed, LBQ women must identify their own desires and reality as same-sex attracted and then "come out" to others. Psychologists have described the developmental process of attaining minority sexual identities since the early work of Vivienne Cass (1979), who described six stages of "homosexual" identity formation: identity confusion, comparison, tolerance, acceptance, pride, and synthesis. Claiming a minority sexual identity has been framed as an act of empowerment in the face of moral arguments against homosexuality (Swigonski, 1995). More recently, the role of families of origin has been identified as crucial to the mental health and resilience of LBQ young people. For example, in one recent US study of 843 LBQ women aged 18–25, up to 41% had experienced rejection from their families after coming out, and this affected self-esteem and community connection for many (Zimmerman, Darnell, Rhew, Lee, & Kaysen, 2015). Conversely, family support builds resilience, self-esteem, and well-being (Legate, Ryan, & Weinstein, 2012).

Women and men experience their sexual identity and expression differently. For example, population-based studies consistently show that more women than men identify as bisexual (Richters et al., 2014), and women have more fluid sexual desires than men (Ussher, 2017). Cass (2006) has eloquently argued that "human behaviour, especially behaviour as richly faceted as sexual orientation, cannot be explained in simple, single-causation and reductionist terms" (p. 33). Both genetic and environmental factors influence same-sex behaviours, but women are more heavily influenced by social, and men by genetic, factors (Långström, Rahman, Carlström, & Lichtenstein, 2010). It may be that sociocultural attitudes and beliefs in Western societies enable women to express their sexuality more freely and to be less constrained by internalised stigma than men are; thus, women can express diverse sexual behaviours without the need for identity labelling (e.g., lesbian, bisexual).

Bisexuality has been a contested sexual identity, marginalised and even "erased" in decades of research as merely a phase or transitional identity (Monro, Hines, & Osborne, 2017). However, bisexuality is an identity in its own right, and bisexual people can feel ostracised both from heterosexual and lesbian and gay communities (Hayfield, Clarke, & Halliwell, 2014). They face accusations of confusion, immaturity, untrustworthiness, and promiscuity. These experiences influence the physical and mental health of bisexual people. So, although all LBQ women have higher risk than heterosexuals of mental health issues related to experiences of discrimination and violence, bisexual women are even more disadvantaged (Ross et al., 2016). However, researchers have started to identify positive aspects of bisexuality, including freedom of sexual expression and acceptance of diversity (Rostosky, Riggle, Pascale-Hague, & McCants, 2010). Reframing bisexuality as a secure sexual identity for some and a sexual expression for others may begin to overcome the stigma and inequalities that arise. Further, there is an increasing array of non-binary sexual identities including pansexuality and queer that emphasise the fluid nature of sexuality (Callis, 2014).

Gender identity and sexual identity also intersect in interesting and diverse ways. Historically, some lesbian or bisexually identified women expressed their gender as either femme or butch. This binary gender dichotomy was perhaps a reflection of heterosexual gender stereotypes applied to same-sex relationships. Butch lesbians were described as "gender atypical", and tended to engage in more risky behaviours, such as substance use and smoking, related possibly to higher levels of stress as well as methods to express their gender (Rosario, Schrimshaw, & Hunter, 2008, p. 1002). The butch–femme conceptualisation persists in some circles, but it has largely been replaced by more fluid understandings of gender. New terms being used globally reflect these changes, including gender queer, gender diverse, gender non-binary, gender flexible, omnigender, and gender expansive (Dowshen et al., 2016). From a health perspective, gender diversity can be associated with poorer mental health and lower help seeking, due in part to experiences of marginalisation (McNair &

Bush, 2016). However, in supportive social contexts, such as schools with affirming policies and practices, gender diverse people can thrive (Jones et al., 2015).

Intimate relationships in the context of sexual and gender diversity

Relationships that have traditionally been labelled simply as "same-sex" must now be conceptualised differently (Better & Simula, 2015). They might involve two cisgender[6] lesbians or a bisexual and a lesbian woman, but might instead involve two gender-diverse people, or a trans man and a lesbian-identified woman, or be polyamorous. I term these poly-gender rather than same-sex relationships. These emerging relationships can challenge the identities of the individuals within those relationships. For example, how does a lesbian identify when her female partner comes out as a trans man or as gender non-binary? Which communities will the couple find most affirming and comfortable? Poly-gender relationships may be for life, they may be for experimentation, or for affirmation of a particular sexual identity, or they may be for fun. Again, no assumptions or stereotypes can be applied.

Initiation of poly-gender relationships for young people can require both opportunity and willingness to transgress the hetero-normative assumptions that surround them. Lesbian desire may be invisible and seen as dangerous by some young women (Ussher & Mooney-Somers, 2000). However, it can also be innovative and enlightening. Negotiating relationships for transgender and gender diverse (TGD) people can be even more complex. A study of 160 Australian TGD people described relationship barriers including anxiety about possible rejection, discrimination from partners, and a lack of self-acceptance (Riggs, von Doussa, & Power, 2015). At the other end of the age spectrum, intimate poly-gender relationships can be a rare safe space for people to express authentic sexual identities (Barrett, Whyte, Lyons, Crameri, & Comfort, 2015). This can become difficult as the couple ages, due to fears of having to expose their relationship in the aged-care system. They might find themselves becoming a care-giver in the relationship rather than seeking external help, which can create unnecessary stress to both individuals. They might also experience even more isolation after a partner dies, particularly if their relationship was hidden and therefore their grief is unrecognised.

While most countries have not legislated for poly-gender relationship recognition, legal recognition of same-sex relationships has advanced through the democratic world since the first registered partnerships in Denmark in 1989 and the first same-sex marriage legislation in the Netherlands in 2001. The health of same-sex couples in jurisdictions with legal recognition is better than in those without, as it reduces structural stigma and improves social and legal belonging (Wight, LeBlanc, & Badgett, 2012). Conversely, many countries still do not have same-sex marriage, and in many of these, homosexuality is illegal. This adversely effects health; for example, in US communities without legal safeguards, LGB people had a shorter life expectancy than heterosexual people by 12 years (95% C.I.: 4–20 years), due to suicide, violence, or cardiovascular diseases (Hatzenbuehler et al., 2014). In addition, we must understand that marriage is not desired by all same-sex couples and remains inaccessible to people who are polyamorous or in gender-diverse partnerships. Analysis of media reporting about the UK 2004 civil union legislation suggests that the "seismic change" of same-sex relationship recognition is framed in a heteronormative world that does not recognise non-monogamy, nor more radical types of partnerships (Jowett & Peel, 2010).

Intimate partner violence (IPV) in same-sex and poly-gender relationships is likely to be at least as prevalent as amongst heterosexual couples, and some data suggest it is higher. For example, in the US National Violence Against Women Survey (n=14,182), all types of IPV were, on average, twice as likely amongst the lesbian and bisexual women as amongst the heterosexual women (Messinger, 2011). Emotional or psychological abuse can also be higher than physical abuse between lesbian couples. Correlates with IPV for same-sex couples include a family history of violence, past IPV, fusion (where the couple have few social outlets as individuals), and alcohol intake (Badenes-Ribera, Bonilla-Campos, Frias-Navarro, Pons-Salvador, & Monterde, 2016). Emerging work indicates that transgender and gender-diverse individuals may be more likely than cisgender LGB people to have experienced IPV (Langenderfer-Magruder, Whitfield, Walls, Kattari, & Ramos, 2016). The field is complicated by assumptions that gender-based power imbalances underpin much IPV, which does not translate well to female same-sex and poly-gender relationships. This is likely to result in under-reporting of IPV both in clinical settings and in research.

Access to appropriate and supportive services for both victims and perpetrators of IPV is limited and problematic in relation to same-sex and poly-gender relationships. Services tend to be gendered, and staff lack cultural training in diverse relationships (Campo & Tayton, 2015). Fear of discriminatory responses can prevent individuals from seeking support (Ard & Makadon, 2011) and reporting violence. For example, in an Australian study of 813 LGBQT people, 55% had experienced IPV but only 15% had reported this to police (LGBTIQ Domestic Violence Interagency, 2014). Lesbian and trans women were less likely than gay men or bisexual people to report, and gender diverse people were least likely to report. Barriers to reporting included fear of police, concerns about not being believed or being outed, and fear of retaliation by the partner. Other barriers to accessing help include community assumptions that IPV does not exist in same-sex or poly-gender relationships. People are also reluctant to disclose for fear of further pathologising their relationships. Therefore, to provide appropriate support for people experiencing IPV, service providers must actively inquire in an environment that is affirming of LBQT identities and knowledgeable of LGBTQ-specific support needs.

Family formation including reproduction

Lesbians, bisexuals, and gay men have always been involved in parenting, either through previous heterosexual relationships, or through individual negotiations with friends. However, the so-called lesbian baby boom (or the "gayby boom" (Weeks, Heaphy, & Donovan, 2001) of the 1980s was the start of a rapid increase in parenting desire. From this period, lesbians, usually as couples, have created family through conceiving with sperm donors, often in defiance of family objections and legal threats. Legislative reforms in family and reproductive law followed these social changes and actively engaged human rights principles, including that the rights of the child should be fulfilled regardless of the sexual orientation of the parents (Tobin & McNair, 2009). Conservative rhetoric persists in equal marriage debates; it typically emphasises that marriage is primarily for procreation and that children should be raised by two biological parents. However, outcomes for children in same-sex-parented families are generally positive (Dempsey, 2013). Social attitudes have rapidly shifted as same-sex-parented families have become increasingly visible and their children have grown into well-adjusted and vocal adults.

More recent trends include families with more than two parents (e.g., a lesbian couple and their donor dads) and parenting through adoption, fostering, and surrogacy (particularly for gay and bisexual men) (Crouch, Waters, McNair, Power, & Davis, 2014). The literature continues to describe this diversity, although it has been critiqued for the persistent gaps in relation to race, ethnicity, and social class (Goldberg & Gartrell, 2014). The increasing access to assisted reproductive technologies has enabled re-imagining of the links between the biological and the social parent. For example, some lesbian couples have had the egg from one woman fertilised through IVF with donor sperm, and then the embryo carried by the other woman. Ethicists argue over the ethical and social risks and benefits of these arrangements, but they ultimately agree that the psychosocial benefits for the family and children outweigh the counter arguments (Pennings, 2016). In particular, lesbian parents have been found to have a range of strengths over heterosexual parents, including more egalitarian couple and parenting relationships and more child-focussed, higher quality parent–child interactions (Power et al., 2010).

Outcomes for children in same-sex-parented families are also generally positive. One of the largest studies to date involving 315 same-sex-attracted parents (including 80% lesbian/ bisexual women and 18% gay/bisexual men) and 500 children compared various child health and wellbeing outcomes against population norms (Crouch et al., 2014). Most outcomes were equivalent to the general population, and general behaviour, general health and family cohesion were better for the study children. The one disadvantage for some of these families was stigma related to the sexual orientation of the parents. For the 67% of parents that reported experiencing sexuality-related stigma at least once, family cohesion was lower, child mental health was worse, and child emotional symptoms were higher than population norms, however most of the young people viewed their families as normal and sought out supportive community and peers (Crouch, Waters, McNair, & Power, 2014).

Young TGD people are now grappling with the complexities of forming families in their affirmed identities, as a significant minority are interested in becoming parents (Riggs et al., 2015). Thomas Beattie is something of a celebrity in the US after having become pregnant and given birth to three children as a trans man (Riggs et al., 2015). He accomplished this by stopping his testosterone, which allowed his body to ovulate again and to conceive. However, the medical evidence is slim at this stage regarding the proportion of people who can ovulate after having taken testosterone. Cisgender women coupled with trans men have been described as challenging parenting norms in important ways (Pfeffer, 2012), yet there is little awareness of the specific needs of trans men during pregnancy care (Light, Obedin-Maliver, Sevelius, & Kerns, 2014). Fertility preservation for pubertal children who are embarking on gender affirmation is a vital conversation but fraught at this age when their parenting aspirations in the distant future are the last thing they may want to consider. Innovations include collecting and freezing sperm via testicular biopsy or freezing ovarian sections before commencing puberty-blocking treatments, however it is not clear whether these immature tissues could produce fertile gametes in the future (Faure et al., 2016). Best practice in adults is currently to recommend sperm freezing prior to initiation of oestrogen in trans women (Hembree et al., 2017). For trans men, freezing of eggs is a much more complex and expensive IVF procedure that is not appealing to most in the context of gender dysphoria.[7] This is an emerging area that requires open and frank conversation with TGD people, some of whom desire family formation.

Pregnancy prevention for LBQ women and TGD people is a related issue. Young LBQ women are at higher risk than their heterosexual peers for unintended pregnancy (Saewyc, Bearinger, Blum, & Resnick, 1999). The US National Survey of Family Growth collected data about pregnancies in women aged 18 to 44 from 2006 to 2013 (n = 25,403) (Hartnett, Lindley, & Walsemann, 2017). LBQ women had higher odds of unintended pregnancy (odds ratio 1.26), associated with a higher number of male partners, compared with heterosexual women. The US National Longitudinal Study of Adolescent to Adult Health (n = 5,972) identified that the bisexual women were more likely (odds ratio 1.70) and the lesbian women were less likely (odds ratio 0.47) than the heterosexual women to have had a teen pregnancy (Goldberg, Reese, & Halpern, 2016). One possible reason for these pregnancy risks is the lack of targeted contraceptive messages, particularly for bisexual women (Goldberg et al., 2016). In addition, higher levels of sexual risk taking might relate to other risks that arise from marginalisation, such as earlier first sex, substance use, homelessness, mental health disparities, and greater number of sexual partners (Bowring, Vella, Degenhardt, Hellard, & Lim, 2015). Higher levels of sexual assault of lesbian and bisexual women is another well recognised issue that may contribute to unwanted pregnancy (Saewyc et al., 1999).

Sexual health and sexually transmitted infections

There has been a persistent myth that women who have sex with women (WSW) are not at risk for sexually transmitted infections (STIs) (Bauer & Welles, 2001). This myth also occurs among some healthcare professionals, as LBQ women still report being denied cervical screening due to a presumed low risk for human papilloma virus infection (Waterman & Voss, 2015). Robust research data now confirm that LBQ women are at equal or higher risk of STIs, although the types of STI can differ from those of heterosexual women depending on their sexual behaviours.

Healthcare providers should understand sexual behaviours between women in order to predict and prevent the range of STIs that are possible in any individual. This would also normalise the range of sex that occurs. An online survey study of 3,116 WSW showed that the most common sexual behaviours in the past year were genital rubbing (99.8%), vaginal fingering (99.2%), cunnilingus (98.8%), and the use of vibrators (74.1%) (Schick, Rosenberger, Herbenick, & Reece, 2012). Less than one quarter of the respondents had used a barrier. Other sexual behaviours between women that can incur some STI risk include oral-anal rimming, anal digital penetration, and fisting (hand to vagina) (J. V. Bailey, Farquhar, Owen, & Whittaker, 2003). Bisexually active women are more likely than lesbian or heterosexual women to have been diagnosed with an STI during their lifetime (Mercer et al., 2007). The STI risk factors for these women include an earlier age of first sex, childhood sexual abuse (Austin, Roberts, Corliss, & Molnar, 2008), more sexual partners, greater likelihood of sex with higher risk men, forced sex (Robin et al., 2002), intimate partner violence, and use of alcohol or drugs with sex (Coble, Silver, & Chhabra, 2017). Risky sexual behaviours have also been found to be higher amongst heterosexually identified women who have sex with women and/or men than amongst heterosexual women who have sex only with men (Nield, Magnusson, Brooks, Chapman, & Lapane, 2015).

The most common infections transmitted between women are those transmitted via skin-to-skin contact or vaginal secretions. These include bacterial vaginosis (BV), human papilloma virus (HPV), and herpes simplex virus (HSV). Other STIs are less common than among exclusively heterosexual women, but chlamydia, trichomonas, syphilis, Hepatitis B, and HIV are all possible (Gorgos & Marrazzo, 2011).

BV concordance rates between lesbian couples have been reported as high as 80% (both positive or both negative), which provides compelling evidence that BV is connected to sexual activity (Vodstrcil et al., 2015). A history of BV is common amongst all women (up to 30%) but more common amongst WSW (up to 51% lifetime rates) (Marrazzo, Koutsky, Kiviat, Kuypers, & Stine, 2001). A national US study showed that 45.2% of women with female partners had had BV compared with 28.8% of women with male partners ($p=.003$) (Koumans et al., 2007). BV can have distressing physical and emotional impacts, and this is worse with recurrent BV, which is also more common amongst WSW. Behaviours that are associated with BV include a higher number of lifetime female partners, receptive oral-anal sex, and not cleaning shared sex toys after use (Marrazzo, Thomas, Agnew, & Ringwood, 2010). It seems to be important to treat the female partner of a woman with symptomatic BV to reduce the risk of recurrence, however there are no studies to confirm the validity of this approach.

HSV is very common among WSW, particularly type 1, which traditionally has been located orally, but increasingly is diagnosed as genital herpes. A study of 393 WSW found that 46% had HSV 1 on serology, and this was more likely with a greater number of female sexual partners (Marrazzo, Stine, & Wald, 2003). HSV 2 is less likely for WSW than for heterosexual women (Xu, Sternberg, & Markowitz, 2010). HPV is also possible, even among lesbians with no history of male partners (Marrazzo et al., 1998). This underpins the need for WSW to have routine cervical screening. In the Australian Longitudinal Study of Women's Health, the rates of abnormal cervical screening over the previous three years varied: bisexual women were most likely to have had an abnormal result (42.4%), then mainly heterosexual women (33.2%), heterosexual women (24.8%), and lesbian women (16.2%, $p<.001$) (McNair, Szalacha, & Hughes, 2011).

Awareness of STI risk remains relatively low amongst WSW (McNair, Power, & Carr, 2009). This can be reinforced by healthcare providers who tend not to offer STI screening to WSW and by the lack of targeted sexual health promotion for WSW. Perceived low risk is reflected in low rates of screening. For example, in the UK National Lesbian Health Study of 6,178 lesbian (81%) and bisexual (16%) women, less than one half had had an STI test, and 75% of these women believed they were not at risk (Hunt & Fish, 2008). In a sample of 2,755 women in the UK, US, Canada, and Australia who have sex with women and men, 64.1% had not had STI screening during the past year (Mullinax, Schick, Rosenberg, Herbenick, & Reece, 2016). Gender expression rather than sexual identity was a predictor of screening, in that women with a more masculine gender expression were less likely to seek screening.

Knowledge about safer sex methods for WSW is relatively low. Women can be aware of latex methods of safer sex, including the use of dental dams to cover the genital area during oral sex, condoms on sex toys, and gloves during digital penetration. However, these methods are not commonly used and are not popular (McNair et al., 2009). For example, in an Australian community survey, only 21% of WSW had ever used condoms, 17% gloves, and 13% dams (most often only once) (Richters, Song, Prestage, Clayton, & Turner, 2005). More common activities for safer sex, and I suggest more useful activities, include changing fingers or sex toys between sites, short fingernails and no jewellery to avoid mucosal damage, and avoiding oral sex during herpes outbreaks. Discussion of safer sex practices should be part of health promotion by healthcare providers, although they often are in need of specific training (Stott, 2013).

Subgroups of transgender people are highly vulnerable to STIs due to complex inter-related factors, including lower educational attainment, lower employment, high levels of sex work, higher rates of substance abuse, and mental health concerns (McNulty & Bourne, 2017). There is a need to improve understanding about trans-specific STI risk factors amongst researchers (MacCarthy et al., 2017) and healthcare providers (Lefkowitz & Mannell, 2017) who are known to have poor knowledge in this area. A recent retrospective review of transgender people who presented at the Melbourne Sexual Health centre between 2011 and 2014 showed that 47% of the 133 people had done sex work, and relatively few people overall had used condoms with male (31%) or with female (18%) sexual partners (Bellhouse et al., 2018). This indicates a relatively high level of risk, and the researchers called for more research to contextualise sexual health promotion messages and care for transgender people. Trans women are much more likely to be studied than trans men, whose sexual health needs have been largely overlooked (Rich et al., 2017). Beyond STIs and sex work, there is a need for healthcare providers and public health officials to be more transgender "affirmative" (Reisner et al., 2016). This would result in more open conversations with transgender consumers about their bodies and positive ways to explore their sexuality. It would also involve healthcare providers asking sensitively and appropriately about body parts and sexual activities with their TGD clients to support their sexual knowledge and safety.

Health promotion

Health promotion for LBQT women needs to be targeted and evidence-based. There have been very few specific initiatives globally; assumptions may be that promotion targeted to women generally would suffice. However, we increasingly understand that some LBQT women do not respond to mainstream messages, and their physical and mental health can suffer as a result (Germanos, Deacon, & Mooney-Somers, 2015). For example, sub-groups of LBQT women are less likely to attend regular cervical or breast screenings, which then increases their risk for late diagnosis (Barefoot, Warren, & Smalley, 2017). Lesbian and bisexual women aged 65–69 in the Australian Longitudinal Study of Women's Health were much more likely never to have had cervical screening (4.7%) and never to have had a mammogram (6.9%) than heterosexual women (1.7% cervical, 3.2% mammogram) (Brown, McNair, Szalacha, Livingston, & Hughes, 2015). There have been calls for regular cervical screening for lesbian women for at least two decades based on rates of HPV transmission and cervical abnormalities (Bailey, Kavanagh, Owen, McLean, & Skinner, 2000). By contrast, breast cancer screening for LBQT women has only recently become a focus, including recommendations for breast screening services to become more LBQT affirming (Sonnenblick, Shah, Goldstein, & Reisman, 2018).

Barriers to cervical screening for LBQ women particularly relate to a lack of comfort with healthcare providers and fears of discrimination; screening is more likely if a woman is out to the provider (Reiter & McRee, 2015). TGD people with a cervix face even more barriers. Gender dysphoria can be a particular deterrent that triggers significant distress (Peitzmeier et al., 2017b), and this is coupled with more painful speculum examination for people on testosterone due to vaginal dryness (Johnson, Nemeth, Mueller, Eliason, & Stuart, 2016). TGD people are less likely to be offered screening, and experience more discrimination in healthcare generally (Johnson, Mueller, Eliason, Stuart, & Nemeth, 2016). A further issue for trans men is that they are more likely than cisgender women to have unsatisfactory screening results. For example, amongst 233 trans men and 3,625 cisgender women in a US community clinic, 10.8% of the trans men but only 1.3% of the ciswomen had inadequate sampling of cells from the cervix (Peitzmeier, Reisner, Harigopal, & Potter, 2014). This might relate to difficulty with speculum insertion, as well as the potential for testosterone to mediate atrophic cervico-vaginitis. Many TGD people with a cervix are more comfortable with self-sampling, which could improve screening rates in this group (Seay et al., 2017). This involves persons inserting a swab into their vaginas themselves to test for human papilloma virus, avoiding the need for speculum insertion.

Breast screening for LBQT women can also be difficult to access if they are fearful of discriminatory attitudes. Further, transgender people with breast tissue may be quite unaware that breast cancer screening is important for them. There is little doubt that cisgender women over the age of 50 should participate in regular breast screening, but the evidence is still scant for transgender women. There have been case reports of transgender women on oestrogen therapy developing breast cancer, and so current guidelines from both the Canadian Cancer Society (Vogel, 2014) and the US Endocrine Society (Hembree et al., 2017) recommend that they have regular breast screening over the age of 50 if they have been on oestrogen for more than five years. Trans masculine people may have other issues. A high proportion of those who practice chest binding experience breast pain and musculoskeletal and skin problems (Peitzmeier, Gardner, Weinand, Corbet, & Acevedo, 2017a), which may negatively impact their experience of breast screening. Further, if trans men have had chest reconstruction (bilateral mastectomy), there is a need to educate them about having annual chest examinations over the age of 50 to detect problems in any remaining breast tissue (Hembree et al., 2017).

Conclusion

The sexual and reproductive health of LBQ women and TGD people should involve the same successes and challenges as those for any woman. However, the context of stigma, marginalisation, and discrimination creates inequalities that require attention. Despite social enlightenment and legal reforms in many countries, LBQT people can still face family rejection, social ostracisation, and other negative attitudes that can have profound effects on their mental and physical health. They are still found to be disadvantaged in education and employment, so poverty is one of the key drivers of ill-health, particularly amongst bisexual, transgender, and gender-diverse people (Ross et al., 2016). Homelessness and loss of community connection can then be associated with substance abuse, sexual violence, risk taking, and further mental health effects, which are even more profound for indigenous and cultural minorities (Abramovich & Shelton, 2017). Responses to these health inequalities must be systemic as well as individual. Anti-discrimination laws provide some protection, but should be accompanied by social attitudes that affirm minority sexual and gender identities (Solazzo, Brown, & Gorman, 2018).

Such a systemic approach includes health care, and an LBQT-affirming health care system would have a number of characteristics. It would affirm diverse sexual and gender expressions and identities. It would enable sexual health and sexual pleasure by encouraging conversations about safer sex, autonomy, and sexual rights for LBQT people. It would include access to assisted reproductive technologies for individuals and people in a diverse range of relationships, as well as other family formation methods including surrogacy, fostering, and adoption. It would provide guidance for individuals, parents, and their children to build resilience and develop positive and healthy relationships.

Healthcare providers have a significant role to play in creating an affirming environment. This enables a more authentic relationship where LBQT people can safely discuss their identities, behaviours, and needs. The ability to disclose sexual and gender identities to a trusted healthcare provider is associated with better care for substance use and mental health, physical health screening, and health promotion (McNair, Hegarty, & Taft, 2015). We know that bisexual and pansexual women are less likely than lesbian women to disclose their identities, and therefore they receive less tailored care, such as sexual and reproductive advice (Arbeit, Fisher, Macapagal, & Mustanski, 2016). We also know that transgender people almost universally experience healthcare providers with little or no transgender knowledge and repeatedly need to educate their providers in order to receive basic care (Cruz, 2014). We can do much better than this. We should not only educate ourselves about LBQT health issues, but also make an effort to display sensitivity, facilitate disclosure, and, even better, become advocates for a more equal society. Then we will truly contribute to the health and well-being of lesbian, bisexual, queer, pansexual, transgender, and gender-diverse people.

Notes

1 Lesbian woman – a woman whose primary emotional and/or sexual attraction is toward other women.
2 Bisexual woman – a woman who may be emotionally and/or sexually attracted to women and men; or may describe herself as pansexual if she is attracted to people who are gender diverse.
3 Queer – includes a range of gender identities and sexual identities. Some use queer to mean: different; gender diverse; same-sex attracted; or, not aligned to a stereotype.
4 Transgender – a person whose gender identity or expression is different from that assigned at birth or those who sit outside the gender binary. *Trans and gender diverse* is a newer term, which is currently regarded as more inclusive. Transgender can also be shortened to trans, trans man or trans masculine, trans woman or trans feminine.
5 Gender diverse – a person whose gender expression or identity differs from the gender identity associated with the sex assigned them at birth or society's expectations, and who identifies as neither male nor female, or as both. Other terms include bigender, genderqueer, gender fluid, gender questioning, agender, and non-binary.
6 Cisgender – a person who identifies with the gender assigned at birth.
7 Gender dysphoria – a clinical psychiatric diagnosis, first listed in the 5th edition of the *Diagnostic and Statistical Manual of Mental Disorders* (American Psychiatric Association, 2013), that describes an intense distress resulting from an individual's sense of the inappropriateness of their assigned sex at birth.

References

Abramovich, I. & Shelton, J. (Eds) (2017). *Where am I going to go? Intersectional approaches to ending LGBTQ2S youth homelessness in Canada & the U.S.* Toronto, Canada: Canadian Observatory on Homelessness Press.

American Psychiatric Association (2013). *Diagnostic and statistical manual of mental disorders* (5th ed.). Washington, DC: Author.

Arbeit, M. R., Fisher, C. B., Macapagal, K., & Mustanski, B. (2016). Bisexual invisibility and the sexual health needs of adolescent girls. *LGBT Health*, *3*(5), 342–349.

Ard, K. L. & Makadon, H. J. (2011). Addressing intimate partner violence in lesbian, gay, bisexual, and transgender patients. *Journal of General Internal Medicine*, *26*(8), 930–933.

Austin, S. B., Roberts, A. L., Corliss, H. L., & Molnar, B. E. (2008). Sexual violence victimization history and sexual risk indicators in a community-based urban cohort of "mostly heterosexual" and heterosexual young women. *American Journal of Public Health*, *98*(6), 1015–1020.

Badenes-Ribera, L., Bonilla-Campos, A., Frias-Navarro, D., Pons-Salvador, G., & Monterde, I. B. H. (2016). Intimate partner violence in self-identified lesbians: A systematic review of its prevalence and correlates. *Trauma Violence & Abuse*, *17*(3), 284–297.

Bailey, J., Kavanagh, J., Owen, C., McLean, K., & Skinner, C. (2000). Lesbians and cervical screening. *British Journal of General Practice*, *50*(455), 481–482.

Bailey, J. V., Farquhar, C., Owen, C., & Whittaker, D. (2003). Sexual behaviour of lesbians and bisexual women. *Sexually Transmitted Infections*, *79*(2), 147–150.

Barefoot, K. N., Warren, J. C., & Smalley, K. B. (2017). Women's health care: The experiences and behaviors of rural and urban lesbians in the USA. *Rural and Remote Health*, *17*(1), 3875.

Barrett, C., Whyte, C., Lyons, A., Crameri, P., & Comfort, J. (2015). Social connection, relationships and older lesbian and gay people. *Sexual & Relationship Therapy*, *30*(1), 131–142.

Bauer, G. R. & Welles, S. L. (2001). Beyond assumptions of negligible risk: Sexually transmitted diseases and women who have sex with women. *American Journal of Public Health*, *91*(8), 1282–1286.

Bellhouse, C., Walker, S., Fairley, C. K., Vodstrcil, L. A., Bradshaw, C. S., Chen, M. Y., & Chow, E. P. F. (2018). Patterns of sexual behaviour and sexual healthcare needs among transgender individuals in Melbourne, Australia, 2011–2014. *Sexually Transmitted Infections*, *94*(3), 212–215.

Better, A. & Simula, B. L. (2015). How and for whom does gender matter? Rethinking the concept of sexual orientation. *Sexualities, 18*(5–6), 665–680.

Bowring, A. L., Vella, A. M., Degenhardt, L., Hellard, M., & Lim, M. S. C. (2015). Sexual identity, same-sex partners and risk behaviour among a community-based sample of young people in Australia. *International Journal of Drug Policy, 26*(2), 153–161.

Brown, R., McNair, R., Szalacha, L., Livingston, P. M., & Hughes, T. (2015). Cancer risk factors, diagnosis and sexual identity in the Australian Longitudinal Study of Women's Health. *Womens Health Issues, 25*(5), 509–516.

Callis, A. S. (2014). Bisexual, pansexual, queer: Non-binary identities and the sexual borderlands. *Sexualities, 17*(1–2), 63–80.

Campo, M. & Tayton, S. (2015). *Intimate partner violence in lesbian, gay, bisexual, trans, intersex and queer communities: Key issues.* Southbank, VIC, Australia: Australian Institute of Family Studies. Retrieved from https://aifs.gov.au/cfca/publications/intimate-partner-violence-lgbtiq-communities.

Cass, V. C. (1979). Homosexual identity formation: A theoretical model. *Journal of Homosexuality, 4*(3), 219–235.

Cass, V. C. (2006). Sexual orientation and the place of psychology: Side-lined, side-tracked, or should that be side-swiped?. *Gay and Lesbian Issues and Psychology Review, 2*(1), 27–37.

Coble, C. A., Silver, E. J., & Chhabra, R. (2017). Description of sexual orientation and sexual behaviors among high school girls in New York City. *Journal of Pediatric and Adolescent Gynecology, 30*(4), 460–465.

Crouch, S. R., Waters, E., McNair, R., Power, J., & Davis, E. (2014). Parent-reported measures of child health and wellbeing in same-sex parent families: A cross-sectional survey. *BMC Public Health, 14*, 635, doi:10.1186/1471-2458-14-635.

Cruz, T. M. (2014). Assessing access to care for transgender and gender nonconforming people: A consideration of diversity in combating discrimination. *Social Science & Medicine, 110*(0), 65–73.

Dempsey, D. (2013). *Same-sex parented families in Australia.* Southbank, VIC, Australia: Australian Institute of Family Studies. Retrieved from https://aifs.gov.au/cfca/publications/same-sex-parented-families-australia/export.

Dowshen, N., Meadows, R., Byrnes, M., Hawkins, L., Eder, J., & Noonan, K. (2016). Policy perspective: Ensuring comprehensive care and support for gender nonconforming children and adolescents. *Transgender Health, 1*(1), 75–85.

Faure, A., Bouty, A., O'Brien, M., Thorup, J., Hutson, J., & Heloury, Y. (2016). Testicular biopsy in prepubertal boys: A worthwhile minor surgical procedure? *National Review of Urology, 13*(3), 141–150.

Germanos, R., Deacon, R., & Mooney-Somers, J. (2015). The social and cultural significance of women's sexual identities should guide health promotion. *LGBT Health, 2*(2), 162–168.

Goldberg, A. E. & Gartrell, N. (2014). LGB-parent families: The current state of the research and directions for the future. Advances in Child Development and Behavior, 46, 57–88.

Goldberg, S. K., Reese, B. M., & Halpern, C. T. (2016). Teen pregnancy among sexual minority women: Results from the national longitudinal study of adolescent to adult health. *Journal of Adolescent Health, 59*, 429–437.

Gorgos, L. M. & Marrazzo, J. M. (2011). Sexually transmitted infections among women who have sex with women. *Clinical Infectious Diseases, 53*(suppl. 3), S84–S91.

Hartnett, C. S., Lindley, L. L., & Walsemann, K. M. (2017). Congruence across sexual orientation dimensions and risk for unintended pregnancy among adult U.S. women. *Women's Health Issues, 27*(2), 145–151.e142.

Hatzenbuehler, M. L., Bellatorre, A., Lee, Y., Finch, B. K., Muennig, P., & Fiscella, K. (2014). Structural stigma and all-cause mortality in sexual minority populations. *Social Science & Medicine, 103*(0), 33–41.

Hayfield, N., Clarke, V., & Halliwell, E. (2014). Bisexual women's understandings of social marginalisation: "The heterosexuals don't understand us but nor do the lesbians". *Feminism & Psychology, 24*(3), 352–372.

Hembree, W. C., Cohen-Kettenis, P. T., Gooren, L., Hannema, S. E., Meyer, W. J., Murad, M. H., Rosenthal, S. M., Safer, J. D., Tangpricha, V., & T'Sjoen, G. G. (2017). Endocrine treatment of gender-dysphoric/gender-incongruent persons: An Endocrine Society clinical practice guideline. *Journal of Clinical Endocrinology & Metabolism, 102*(11), 3869–3903.

Hunt, R. & Fish, J. (2008). *Prescription for change: Lesbian and bisexual women's health check 2008.* London, UK: Stonewall. Retrieved from www.stonewall.org.uk/campaigns/2296.asp.

Johnson, M. J., Mueller, M., Eliason, M. J., Stuart, G., & Nemeth, L. S. (2016). Quantitative and mixed analyses to identify factors that affect cervical cancer screening uptake among lesbian and bisexual women and transgender men. *Journal of Clinical Nursing, 25*, 3628–3642.

Johnson, M. J., Nemeth, L. S., Mueller, M., Eliason, M. J., & Stuart, G. W. (2016). Qualitative study of cervical cancer screening among lesbian and bisexual women and transgender men. *Cancer Nursing, 39* (6), 455–463.

Jones, T., Smith, E. M., Ward, R., Dixon, J., Hillier, L., & Mitchell, A. (2015). School experiences of transgender and gender diverse students in Australia. *Sex Education, 16*, 156–171.

Jowett, A. & Peel, E. (2010). "Seismic cultural change?": British media representations of same-sex "marriage". *Women's Studies International Forum, 33*(3), 206–214.

Koumans, E. H., Sternberg, M., Bruce, C., McQuillan, G., Kendrick, J., Sutton, M., & Markowitz, L. E. (2007). The prevalence of bacterial vaginosis in the United States, 2001–2004: Associations with symptoms, sexual behaviors, and reproductive health. *Sexually Transmitted Diseases, 34* (11), 864–869.

Langenderfer-Magruder, L., Whitfield, D. L., Walls, N. E., Kattari, S. K., & Ramos, D. (2016). Experiences of intimate partner violence and subsequent police reporting among lesbian, gay, bisexual, transgender, and queer adults in Colorado: Comparing rates of cisgender and transgender victimization. *Journal of Interpersonal Violence, 31*(5), 855–871.

Långström, N., Rahman, Q., Carlström, E., & Lichtenstein, P. (2010). Genetic and environmental effects on same-sex sexual behavior: A population study of twins in Sweden. *Archives of Sexual Behavior, 39*(1), 75–80.

Lefkowitz, A. R. F. & Mannell, J. (2017). Sexual health service providers' perceptions of transgender youth in England. *Health and Social Care in the Community, 25*, 1237–1246.

Legate, N., Ryan, R. M., & Weinstein, N. (2012). Is coming out always a "good thing"? Exploring the relations of autonomy, support, outness, and wellness for lesbian, gay, and bisexual individuals. *Social Psychological and Personality Science, 3*(2), 145–152.

LGBTIQ Domestic Violence Interagency (2014). *Calling it what it really is: A report into lesbian, gay, bisexual, transgender, gender diverse, intersex, and queer experiences of domestic and family violence.* New South Wales, Australia: . Author Retrieved from www.glhv.org.au/report/calling-it-what-it-really-report-lgbtiq-experience-domestic-and-family-violence.

Light, A. D., Obedin-Maliver, J., Sevelius, J. M., & Kerns, J. L. (2014). Transgender men who experienced pregnancy after female-to-male gender transitioning. *Obstetrics and Gynecology, 124*(6), 1120–1127.

MacCarthy, S., Poteat, T., Xia, Z., Roque, N. L., Kim, H. J., Baral, A., & Reisner, S. L. (2017). Current research gaps: A global systematic review of HIV and sexually transmissible infections among transgender populations. *Sexual Health, 14*(5), 456–468.

Marrazzo, J. M., Koutsky, L. A., Kiviat, N. B., Kuypers, J. M., & Stine, K. (2001). Papanicolaou test screening and prevalence of genital human papillomavirus among women who have sex with women. *American Journal of Public Health, 91*(6), 947–952.

Marrazzo, J. M., Koutsky, L. A., Stine, K. L., Kuypers, J. M., Grubert, T. A., Galloway, D. A., Kiviat, N. B., & Handsfield, H. H. (1998). Genital human papillomavirus infection in women who have sex with women. *Journal of Infectious Diseases, 178*(6), 1604–1609.

Marrazzo, J. M., Stine, K., & Wald, A. (2003). Prevalence and risk factors for infection with herpes simplex virus type-1 and -2 among lesbians. *Sexually Transmitted Diseases, 30*(12), 890–895.

Marrazzo, J. M., Thomas, K. K., Agnew, K., & Ringwood, K. (2010). Prevalence and risks for bacterial vaginosis in women who have sex with women. *Sexually Transmitted Diseases, 37*(5), 335–339.

McNair, R., Hegarty, K., & Taft, A. (2015). Disclosure for same-sex attracted women enhancing the quality of the patient–doctor relationship in general practice. *Australian Family Physician, 44* (8), 573–578.

McNair, R., Szalacha, L. A., & Hughes, T. L. (2011). Health status, health service use, and satisfaction according to sexual identity of young Australian women. *Women's Health Issues, 21*(1), 40–47.

McNair, R. P. & Bush, R. (2016). Mental health help seeking patterns and associations among Australian same sex attracted women, trans and gender diverse people: A survey-based study. *BMC Psychiatry, 16* (1), 1–16.

McNair, R. P., Power, J., & Carr, S. (2009). Comparing knowledge and perceived risk related to the human papilloma virus among Australian women of diverse sexual orientations. *Australia and New Zealand Journal of Public Health, 33*(1), 87–93.

McNulty, A. & Bourne, C. (2017). Transgender HIV and sexually transmissible infections. *Sexual Health*, 14(5), 451–455.

Mercer, C. H., Bailey, J. V., Johnson, A. M., Erens, B., Wellings, K., Fenton, K. A., & Copas, A. J. (2007). Women who report having sex with women: British national probability data on prevalence, sexual behaviors, and health outcomes. *American Journal of Public Health*, 97(6), 1126–1133.

Messinger, A. M. (2011). Invisible victims: Same-sex IPV in the National Violence Against Women Survey. *Journal of Interpersonal Violence*, 26(11), 2228–2243.

Monro, S., Hines, S., & Osborne, A. (2017). Is bisexuality invisible? A review of sexualities scholarship 1970–2015. *Sociological Review*, 65, 1–19.

Mullinax, M., Schick, V., Rosenberg, J., Herbenick, D., & Reece, M. (2016). Screening for sexually transmitted infections (STIs) among a heterogeneous group of WSW(M). *International Journal of Sexual Health*, 28(1), 9–15.

Nield, J., Magnusson, B., Brooks, C., Chapman, D., & Lapane, K. L. (2015). Sexual discordance and sexual partnering among heterosexual women. *Archives of Sexual Behavior*, 44(4), 885–894.

Parks, C. A. (1999). Lesbian identity development: An examination of differences across generations. *American Journal of Orthopsychiatry*, 69(3), 347–361.

Peitzmeier, S., Gardner, I., Weinand, J., Corbet, A., & Acevedo, K. (2017a). Health impact of chest binding among transgender adults: A community-engaged, cross-sectional study. *Culture, Health, & Sexuality*, 19(1), 64–75.

Peitzmeier, S. M., Agenor, M., Bernstein, I. M., McDowell, M., Alizaga, N. M., Reisner, S. L., Pardee, D. J., & Potter, J. (2017b). "It can promote an existential crisis": Factors influencing Pap test acceptability and utilization among transmasculine individuals. *Qualitative Health Research*, 27(14), 2138–2149.

Peitzmeier, S. M., Reisner, S. L., Harigopal, P., & Potter, J. (2014). Female-to-male patients have high prevalence of unsatisfactory Paps compared to non-transgender females: Implications for cervical cancer screening. *Journal of General Internal Medicine*, 29(5), 778–784.

Pennings, G. (2016). Having a child together in lesbian families: Combining gestation and genetics. *Journal of Medical Ethics*, 42(4), 253–255, doi:10.1136/medethics-2015-103007.

Pfeffer, C. A. (2012). Normative resistance and inventive pragmatism. *Gender & Society*, 26(4), 574–602.

Power, J., Perlesz, A., Brown, R., Schofield, M., Pitts, M., McNair, R., & Bickerdike, A. (2010). Diversity, tradition, and family: Australian same-sex attracted parents and their families. *Gay and Lesbian Issues and Psychology Review*, 6(2), 66–81.

Reisner, S. L., Poteat, T., Keatley, J., Cabral, M., Mothopeng, T., Dunham, E., Holland, C. E., Max, R., & Baral, S. D. (2016). Global health burden and needs of transgender populations: A review. *Lancet*, 388(10042), 412–436.

Reiter, P. L. & McRee, A. L. (2015). Cervical cancer screening (Pap testing) behaviours and acceptability of human papillomavirus self-testing among lesbian and bisexual women aged 21–26 years in the USA. *Journal of Family Planning and Reproductive Health Care*, 41(4), 259–264.

Rich, A., Scott, K., Johnston, C., Blackwell, E., Lachowsky, N., Cui, Z., Sereda, P., Moore, D., Hogg, R., & Roth, E. (2017). Sexual HIV risk among gay, bisexual and queer transgender men: Findings from interviews in Vancouver, Canada. *Culture, Health, & Sexuality*, 19(11), 1197–1209.

Richters, J., Altman, D., Badcock, P. B., Smith, A. M. A., de Visser, R. O., Grulich, A. E., Rissel, C., & Simpson, J. M. (2014). Sexual identity, sexual attraction and sexual experience: The Second Australian study of health and relationships. *Sexual Health*, 11(5), 451–460.

Richters, J., Song, A., Prestage, G., Clayton, S., & Turner, R. (2005). *Health of lesbian, bisexual and queer women in Sydney: The 2004 Sydney Women and Sexual Health survey.* (2). Sydney, Australia: Centre for Social Research in Health. Retrieved from http://nchsr.arts.unsw.edu.au.

Riggs, D. W., von Doussa, H., & Power, J. (2015). The family and romantic relationships of trans and gender diverse Australians: An exploratory study. *Sexual and Relationship Therapy*, 30(2), 243–255.

Robin, L., Brener, N. D., Donahue, S. F., Hack, T., Hale, K., & Goodenow, C. (2002). Associations between health risk behaviors and opposite-, same-, and both-sex sexual partners in representative samples of Vermont and Massachusetts high school students. *Archives of Pediatric and Adolescent Medicine*, 156(4), 349–355.

Rosario, M., Schrimshaw, E. W., & Hunter, J. (2008). Butch/femme differences in substance use and abuse among young lesbian and bisexual women: Examination and potential explanations. *Substance Use & Misuse*, 43(8–9), 1002–1015.

Ross, L. E., O'Gorman, L., MacLeod, M. A., Bauer, G. R., MacKay, J., & Robinson, M. (2016). Bisexuality, poverty and mental health: A mixed methods analysis. *Social Science & Medicine, 156*, 64–72.

Rostosky, S. S., Riggle, E. D. B., Pascale-Hague, D., & McCants, L. E. (2010). The positive aspects of a bisexual self-identification. *Psychology & Sexuality, 1*(2), 131–144.

Saewyc, E. M., Bearinger, L. H., Blum, R. W., & Resnick, M. D. (1999). Sexual intercourse, abuse, and pregnancy among adolescent women: Does sexual orientation make a difference? *Family Planning Perspectives, 31*(3), 127–131.

Schick, V., Rosenberger, J. G., Herbenick, D., & Reece, M. (2012). Sexual behaviour and risk reduction strategies among a multinational sample of women who have sex with women. *Sexually Transmitted Infections, 88*(6), 407–412.

Seay, J., Ranck, A., Weiss, R., Salgado, C., Fein, L., & Kobetz, E. (2017). Understanding transgender men's experiences with and preferences for cervical cancer screening: A rapid assessment survey. *LGBT Health, 4*(4), 304–309.

Solazzo, A., Brown, T. N., & Gorman, B. K. (2018). State-level climate, anti-discrimination law, and sexual minority health status: An ecological study. *Social Science & Medicine, 196*, 158–165.

Sonnenblick, E. B., Shah, A. D., Goldstein, Z., & Reisman, T. (2018). Breast imaging of transgender individuals: A review. *Current Radiology Reports, 6*(1), 1.

Stott, D. B. (2013). The training needs of general practitioners in the exploration of sexual health matters and providing sexual healthcare to lesbian, gay and bisexual patients. *Medical Teacher, 35*, 752–759.

Swigonski, M. E. (1995). Claiming a lesbian identity as an act of empowerment. *Affilia, 10*(4), 413–425.

Tobin, J. & McNair, R. (2009). Public international law and the regulation of private spaces: Does the convention on the rights of the child impose an obligation on states to allow gay and lesbian couples to adopt? *International Journal of Law, Policy, and the Family, 23*, 110–131.

Ussher, J. M. (2017). Unraveling the mystery of "the specificity of women's sexual response and its relationship with sexual orientations": The social construction of sex and sexual identities. *Archives of Sexual Behavior, 46*(5), 1207–1211, doi:10.1007/s10508-017-0957-x.

Ussher, J. M. & Mooney-Somers, J. (2000). Negotiating desire and sexual subjectivity: Narratives of young lesbian avengers. *Sexualities, 3*(2), 183–200.

Vodstrcil, L. A., Walker, S. M., Hocking, J. S., Law, M., Forcey, D. S., Fehler, G., Bilardi, J. E., Chen, M. Y., Fethers, K. A., Fairley, C. K., & Bradshaw, C. S. (2015). Incident bacterial vaginosis (BV) in women who have sex with women is associated with behaviors that suggest sexual transmission of BV. *Clinical Infectious Diseases, 60*(7), 1042–1053.

Vogel, L. (2014). Screening programs overlook transgender people. *Canadian Medical Association Journal, 186*(11), 823, doi:10.1503/cmaj.109-4839.

Waterman, L. & Voss, J. (2015). HPV, cervical cancer risks, and barriers to care for lesbian women. *Nurse Practitioner, 40*(1), 46–53; quiz 53–44.

Weeks, J., Heaphy, B., & Donovan, C. (2001). *Same sex intimacies: Families of choice and other life experiments*. Abingdon, UK: Routledge.

Wight, R. G., LeBlanc, A. J., & Badgett, M. V. L. (2012). Same-sex legal marriage and psychological well-being: Findings from the California Health Interview Survey. *American Journal of Public Health, 103*(2), 339–346.

Xu, F., Sternberg, M. R., & Markowitz, L. E. (2010). Women who have sex with women in the United States: Prevalence, sexual behavior and prevalence of herpes simplex virus type 2 infection-results from national health and nutrition examination survey 2001–2006. *Sexually Transmitted Diseases, 37*(7), 407–413.

Zimmerman, L., Darnell, D., Rhew, I., Lee, C., & Kaysen, D. (2015). Resilience in community: A social ecological development model for young adult sexual minority women. *American Journal of Community Psychology, 55*(1–2), 179–190.

INDEX

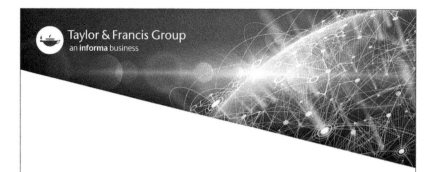

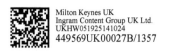

Milton Keynes UK
Ingram Content Group UK Ltd.
UKHW051925141024
449569UK00027B/1357

9 781032 475240